CLINICAL GUIDELINES
IN
CHILD HEALTH

Third Edition

Mary Virginia Graham
PhD, ARNP

Constance R. Uphold
PhD, ARNP-BC

2003

Barmarrae Books, Inc.

THIRD EDITION
Copyright © 2003 by Barmarrae Books, Inc.
Previous editions copyrighted 1994, 1999

Barmarrae Books, Inc
3017 NW 62nd Terrace
Gainesville, Florida 32606

ISBN 0-9646151-7-7

Printed in the United States of America

PREFACE

In 1994, we published the first edition of *Clinical Guidelines in Child Health.* Our original goal was to help clinicians quickly access up-to-date information regarding health maintenance and commonly occurring primary care problems. Over the decade we have been thrilled with the enthusiastic responses our book has generated. We have listened to our colleagues' comments and have added new topics and extensively updated and revised our original topics. Although the size of the book has grown to reflect the increasing complexities of patient care, the easy-to-follow format remains. We have worked to make this edition the best one to date. We have incorporated the latest advances in primary care to produce a comprehensive, yet practical and useful book for clinical practice.

A major challenge in writing this book was synthesizing the huge amount of research and literature related to primary care issues. Expert consensus or evidence-based practice guidelines developed by international, national, and professional advisory boards and organizations have grown exponentially. We have devoted extensive effort to include all the latest authoritative sources and best available evidence related to primary care in a clear and concise format.

In the third edition of *Clinical Guidelines in Child Health* we made specific changes to improve our book. Each topic has been extensively updated to reflect current advances in the field. In particular, the management approaches in certain topics such as obesity, hormonal contraception, constipation, hypertension, and HIV infection have been completely reorganized to incorporate major scientific discoveries that have led to new and improved therapies. To mirror the growing recognition that many causes of death and disability can be prevented, the chapter on health maintenance has been extensively expanded and now includes detailed information relating to nutrition as well as helpful illustrations of developmental milestones. Throughout the book, prevention and patient education are emphasized. New topics such as plantar fasciitis, chronic fatigue, penile problems, viral meningitis, skin care and sun protection in infancy and childhood have been added. This edition has more emphasis on information access. Helpful web sites are listed to help clinicians find patient education tools and to keep abreast of healthcare advances and updates in clinical guidelines. Additional tables and illustrations have been added to help the reader quickly locate information.

Mary Virginia Graham
Constance R. Uphold

DEDICATION

To my sons, Jay and Robin, and my daughter, Lori
MVG

To my family, friends, and nursing colleagues and mentors
CRU

ACKNOWLEDGEMENTS

The authors would like to thank Sharren Gibbs for her preparation of this manuscript. She worked tirelessly, typing multiple drafts of each chapter and incorporating numerous revisions as we worked diligently to include the latest information before going to press.

A special thanks to Louis Clark, our talented artist/illustrator, who managed to produce every illustration that we requested, usually by the next day! In addition, Louis designed the cover and title page, and we feel very fortunate that he was willing to join us in this endeavor.

CONTRIBUTORS

Jean E. DeMartinis, PhD, FNP-BC
Cardiology and Prevention Nurse Practitioner
Consultant in Cardiology PC
Omaha, NE

Mary Virginia Graham, PhD, ARNP
Family Nurse Practitioner
Gainesville, FL

Betsy Hernandez Warren, MSN, ARNP
Coordinator of Clinical Programs
University of Florida
Community Health and Family Medicine
Gainesville, FL

Tish Smyer, DNSc, RN
Associate Professor
Assistant Department Chair, Undergraduate Nursing
Project Director, Native American/Rural Nursing Grant
South Dakota State University College of Nursing
Brookings, SD

Constance R. Uphold, PhD, ARNP-BC
VA Research Career Development Awardee
North Florida/South Georgia Veterans Health System
Gainesville, FL

Sylvia Worden, MSN, RNCS, ARNP
Women's Health Nurse Practitioner
University of Florida Student Health Care Center
Gainesville, FL

REVIEWERS

The authors gratefully acknowledge the invaluable assistance provided by the following individuals who served as reviewers in the preparation of this edition of *Clinical Guidelines in Family Practice*.

Toni O. Barnett, PhD, FNP-C
MSN Coordinator, Family Nurse Practitioner Program
Department of Nursing, North Georgia College and State University
Dahlonega, Georgia

Madge K. Cloud, BA, MA
Consultant, Editorial Services
Elmhurst, IL

Rosemary Goodyear, EdD, RNC
Independent Consultant
Nurse Consultant Associates – www.ncassoc.org
Cardiff By The Sea, California

Lori Ann Hardcastle, MN, RNCS, FNP
Editorial Assistant
Gainesville, FL

Carol Massey Lavin, ARNP
Coordinator of Clinical Services
University of Florida Clinic at Fanning Springs
Gainesville, Florida

Anne A. Moore, MSN, RNC
Professor of Nursing
Women's Health Nurse Practitioner
Certified Nurse Colposcopist
Vanderbilt University
Nashville, TN

Grace Newsome, EdD, APRN, FNP-BC
Associate Professor
Department of Nursing, MSN/FNP Program
North Georgia College and State University
Dahlonega, Georgia   30597

Diane Stevens, MSN, APRN, FNP-BC
Clinical Coordinator
Family Nurse Practitioner Program
Husson College
Bangor, ME

Table of Contents

7 Skin Problems
MARY VIRGINIA GRAHAM

8 Problems of the Eyes
MARY VIRGINIA GRAHAM

Health Maintenance

MARY VIRGINIA GRAHAM

Child Health Supervision
Table: What is Developmental Surveillance?
Table: What is Developmental Screening?
Table: Overview of Instruments Used for Developmental Screening
Table: Snapshot of the Neonate
Table: Examination of the Neonate
Table: Snapshot of 2, 4, 6, & 9 Month Old Child
Figure: Gross Motor Developmental Milestones
Table: Snapshot of 12, 15, & 18 Month Old Child
Table: The Personal-Risk Questionnaire for Lead Exposure in Children
Table: Snapshot of 2, 3, 4, & 5 Year Old Child
Table: Snapshot of School-Age Child
Figure: Books to Recommend Related to Sexual Development
Table: Snapshot of Adolescent
Table: Recommended Childhood Immunization Schedule

Infant Nutrition

Child and Adolescent Nutrition
Table: Dietary Reference Intakes
Figure: The Food Guide Pyramid
Figure: The Food Guide Pyramid for Young Children
Table: How Many Servings Are Needed Each Day?
Table: What Counts As a Serving
Table: Ways to Increase Intake of Whole Grain Foods

Dental Health Maintenance
Figure: Primary and Permanent Dentition

Preparticipation Sports Examination
Table: Preparticipation History
Figure: Two-Minute Orthopedic Exam
Table: Conditions that Require Further Evaluation to Assess the Safety of a Given Sport for a Particular Athlete
Table: Conditions Not Necessarily Precluding Participation in Sports

CHILD HEALTH SUPERVISION

I. Definition: Periodic evaluation and implementation of measures to promote health and detect unrecognized problems in asymptomatic infants and children

   A. Health supervision visits consist of measurement of growth indices (height, weight, and head circumference [until 24 months of age]), history (initial or interval), physical examination, developmental/behavioral surveillance, procedures (such as immunizations as needed), screening (e.g., sensory and lead screening), and anticipatory guidance

   B. For every age group—newborn through adolescence—appropriate focus for all components of the health supervision visit are detailed in this section

   C. An overview of developmental surveillance and screening is presented first to provide the context for this very important component of health supervision; once children enter school, developmental assessment focuses on the child's behaviors (behavioral surveillance) related to school performance, peer and family relationships, participation in activities outside of school, and health-related behaviors

---

WHAT IS DEVELOPMENTAL SURVEILLANCE?

➡ A flexible and continuous process used by clinicians to determine the progress of infants and young children (toddlers and preschoolers) in achievement of age-appropriate milestones across the major streams of development of language, motor skills, problem solving, and psychosocial skills

➡ Components include eliciting and attending to parental concerns, obtaining a relevant developmental history, making accurate and informative observations of the child, and sharing opinions and concerns with parents and others involved in the child's care

➡ Usually accomplished vis-à-vis use of age-appropriate developmental checklists to record milestones during health supervision visits

---

WHAT IS DEVELOPMENTAL SCREENING?

➡ Developmental screening, considered one component of developmental surveillance, is a more structured and formal process using an instrument designed to identify children who should receive more intensive assessment

➡ Advantages of use of developmental screening instruments are that such tools state their norms explicitly and provide a systematic way to record observations

➡ Disadvantages of use of developmental screening instruments are that they are time consuming to administer and interpret and the time spent is usually not reimbursable by third-party payors

➡ In recent years, the science of developmental screening has greatly improved, primarily through the use of parental report instruments that have been well tested in economically and culturally diverse populations and provide accurate information about development

Adapted from American Academy of Pediatrics. (2001). Developmental surveillance and screening of infants and young children. *Pediatrics, 108*, 192-196.

Adapted from American Academy of Pediatrics. (2001). Developmental surveillance and screening of infants and young children. *Pediatrics, 108*, 192-196.

II. Neonates: Birth to One Month

A. Periodicity schedule for health supervision visits for neonates as recommended by the American Academy of Pediatrics (AAP) is as follows: At 2-4 days (for newborns discharged less than 48 hours after delivery), and by 1 month **(Note:** This schedule is designed for neonates who are receiving competent parenting, have no manifestations of important health problems, and are growing and developing satisfactorily; high risk neonates may need more frequent visits)

B. Complete a developmental surveillance of the newborn based on the milestones in the "Snapshot" below; ask appropriate history questions, and make appropriate observations during history and physical examination to assess the neonate's development

---
SNAPSHOT OF THE NEONATE

- Responds to sound by blinking, crying, quieting, changing respirations, or showing a startle response
- Fixates on human face and follows with eyes (45 - 90°)
- Lifts head momentarily when prone
- Maintains position of flexion; moves all extremities
- Sleeps for periods of 3-4 hours
- Can be comforted when crying by being held

C. Consider use of one of the developmental screening tools listed in the table above (*Overview of Instruments Used for Developmental Screening*) which use parent report to help determine if developmental milestones are being met

D. History
   1. Obtain a complete history, including prenatal, birth history, nutrition, sleep, elimination patterns, and any illnesses since birth
   2. Obtain family and social history (ask who lives in household, who provides care for infant, what the sleeping arrangements are for the infant, and if there are any smokers in the household)
   3. Inquire about parental concerns (ask "What questions or concerns about [child's name] do you have today?")

4. Observe parent-infant interaction (**Note**: To maximize the observation, have parent hold infant on lap; comment about the infant's social behavior and individuality)

E. Physical Examination
  1. Purpose of the exam is to detect abnormal findings and to model for the parent how to respond to the infant's cues and how to console the infant by quiet talking and gentle rocking movements
  2. Obtain rectal temperature, heart rate, and respiratory rate
  3. Measure and plot on growth chart the neonate's weight-for-age, length-for-age, weight-for-length, and head circumference; birth weight and length should also be charted (**Note**: National Center for Health Statistics in collaboration with the National Center for Chronic Disease Prevention and Health Promotion have developed new growth charts for infants and children which are available at http://www.cdc.gov/growthcharts)
  4. Share growth information with parent and determine if weight gain is appropriate (~1 oz/day)

EXAMINATION OF THE NEONATE	
General:	The infant should be completely undressed. Observe for position of flexion and symmetrical movement
Skin:	Observe color, hydration status, presence of lesions, evidence of trauma (always look for evidence of abuse)
Head:	Examine for symmetry, evidence of trauma, assess anterior and posterior fontanelles (expect anterior to be diamond-shaped and about 2-3 cm in diameter; posterior to be triangle-shaped and about 1 cm in diameter) **Remember:** Closure of anterior fontanelle varies (range is 7 to 19 months). Posterior fontanelle may not be palpable at birth, and is usually closed at about 3 months of age
Eyes:	Observe for position, alignment, equality, obtain red reflex, elicit pupillary reflex. Assess the newborn's ability to fixate on and follow a human face (or interesting object such as small red ball) as a gross measure of vision. (**Remember:** Infant sees best at 10-12 inch range)
ENT:	Note position of ears (low set ears are associated with renal agenesis/chromosomal abnormalities). Visualize drums. Assess ability to alert toward a human voice or interesting sound (bell) as a gross measure of hearing. Test patency of nasal canals (occlude one and then the other nostril while baby sucks on pacifier). Visualization of throat beyond uvula is usually difficult unless baby is crying
Mouth:	**Always** open baby's mouth to search for abnormalities. Insert gloved finger to feel for cleft palate. Check mouth for natal teeth, retention cysts, thrush
Chest/ Cardiovascular:	Examine for rate (average rate is 140 in newborn), rhythm, and to detect murmurs. Palpate femoral pulses (which are weak or absent with coarctation of the aorta)
Lungs:	Observe respiratory pattern. Rate in newborns ranges from 30-60 per minute. Auscultate for bronchial breath sounds bilaterally (respiration is chiefly abdominal)
Abdomen:	Listen for bowel sounds. Palpate abdomen, assess for abdominal masses (including hernias), hepato-splenomegaly (normally, liver may be palpated 2 cm below the costal margin; spleen should be nonpalpable). Inspect umbilical stump (cord should become dry one week after birth, and fall off by the time baby is 14 days old)
Genitourinary:	Males: Inspect penis for hypospadias or epispadias (in uncircumcised males, do not retract the prepuce more than is adequate for exam); palpate testicles. Females: Examine labia (labia minora usually prominent in infants); spread the labia and examine for imperforate hymen. Both genders: check for position and patency of anus
Musculoskeletal:	Palpate for clavicle fractures and check for developmental hip dysplasia (rotate the thighs with the knees flexed)
Neurological:	Elicit Moro's reflex (startle the infant by clapping your hands--infant reacts by extending, then flexing, the arms, clenching the hands, and flexing the hips and knees). Note the cry (should be lusty). Evaluate muscle tone as infant is handled throughout the exam. Assess head control and head lag by grasping both hands and gently pulling the infant from a supine to an upright position. Check for grasp, rooting, and sucking reflexes

F. Diagnostic Tests
  1. Metabolic and hemoglobinopathy screening as required by state (if not performed in hospital)
  2. Routine screening (universal screening) of newborns for hearing loss is not recommended by the US Preventive Services Task Force (USPSTF) [see http://www.ahrq.gov/clinic/uspstfix.htm for the recommendations and rationale statement relating to newborn hearing screening]
    a. Currently, universal newborn hearing screening is required by law in more than 30 states and is performed routinely in some healthcare systems in other states
    b. Selective screening of newborn infants based on risk factors for hearing loss is conducted in many settings that do not follow a policy of universal screening
    c. Clinicians should be aware of newborn screening requirements in their states (statutory requirements) and in their particular practice environments

G.   Immunizations: See RECOMMENDED CHILDHOOD IMMUNIZATION SCHEDULE on page 28

H.   Vitamin and Mineral Supplementation

> ➡ **Formula-fed term infants who are ingesting at least 500 mL per day of vitamin-D and iron fortified formula require** no vitamin and mineral supplementation during first 6 months of life (all formulas sold in the US have at least 400 IU/L of vitamin D). Once solids are introduced at 6 months, formula combined with the solid food intake is sufficient after that period as well as long as the infant is ingesting at least 500 mL/day of formula
>
> ➡ **Breastfed infants** who do not receive supplemental vitamin D or adequate sunlight exposure are at increased risk of developing vitamin D deficiency or rickets. Because it is extremely difficult to determine what is adequate sunlight exposure for an individual breastfed infant, **all breastfed infants require a supplement of 200 IU per day of vitamin D**, beginning within the first 2 months of life. A vitamin D supplement can be provided by currently available multivitamin preparations containing 400 IU of vitamin D per mL (currently available **solitary** vitamin D preparations, containing up to 800 IU/mL, are too concentrated to be safe for routine home use, and should not be recommended)
>
> ➡ **Vegetarian women who breastfeed** are at risk of providing milk that is low in Vitamin B_6 and B_{12}. These women should supplement their diets with these vitamins in order for the infant to have adequate intake

I.   Anticipatory Guidance

> **Injury and Illness Prevention**: Advise parents as follows
>
> ✓ Use rear-facing infant car seat that is properly secured in the back seat of the vehicle every time the infant rides in the car (no exceptions!) [See CAR SAFETY SEAT CHECKLIST below]
>
> ✓ Never leave infant unattended or with a young sibling or pet
>
> ✓ Put baby to sleep on side or back ("Back to Sleep") without comforters or pillows
>
> ✓ Slats in infant crib should be no more than 2 3/8 inches apart; mattress should be firm and fit snugly into crib; sides of cribs should be raised at all times when infant is in crib
>
> ✓ Keep baby's environment smoke free
>
> ✓ Install smoke alarms if not already in place; test monthly
>
> ✓ Keep infant out of direct sunlight, and ensure full shade with carriage hoods, canopies, and umbrellas; children <6 months should **never** be in direct sunlight and thus should have no need for sunscreen (which is not generally recommended for use in infants <6 months of age)
>
> ✓ Use the newborn period to begin educating parents about the importance of sun avoidance and protection from sun exposure (see section on SKIN CARE, INSECT BITE PROTECTION, AND SUN EXPOSURE PROTECTION FOR CHILDREN)
>
> ✓ If there is a gun in the household, instruct parents to keep it unloaded and locked up; ask parents if they have considered not owning a gun because of the danger to children and other family members
>
> ✓ Discuss the importance of handwashing, particularly after a diaper change and before feeding baby; always wash your own hands (preferably in the exam room) to model the importance of this behavior
>
> ✓ Emphasize to parent to never shake the baby and explain why shaking is harmful
>
> ✓ Recognize early signs of illness (see WHEN TO CALL THE HEALTHCARE CLINICIAN on page 6)

> **Car Safety Seat Checklist**
>
> **Infants from birth up to 20 pounds** should always ride in the back seat facing away from the front seat in an approved car safety seat that is attached to the read seat safety belt. The center seat in the back is the best location for placement of the safety seat
>
> ✓ Harness straps in the safety seat itself should be at or below the infant's shoulders and fit snugly with no loose areas
>
> ✓ The harness chest clip should be placed at armpit level
>
> ✓ Infants younger than 1 year who weight more than 20 pounds should ride in a safety seat equipped for a heavier child, also facing rear
>
> ✓ Refer parents to the following resources for more information
>
>   National Highway Traffic Safety Administration   National Safe Kids Campaign
>   800-424-9393 (Auto Safety Hotline)   202-662-0600
>   www.nhtsa.gov   www.safekids.org
>
> *(Continued)*

Car Safety Seat Checklist *(Continued)*

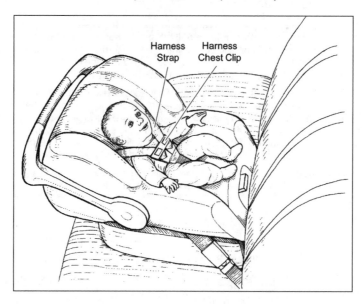

Harness Strap   Harness Chest Clip

Rear-facing Safety Seat in Center Back Seat Position of Car

Adapted from Stevens, L.M., Lynn, C., & Glass, R.M. (2002). Vehicle safety and children. *JAMA, 287*, 1212.

Nutrition

If infant is breastfed, ask: "How often and for how long do you breastfeed?" "Do you have any concerns about breastfeeding?" If infant is bottle fed, ask: "How many ounces does your baby drink per feeding, and what is the total in 24 hours?" "What kind of formula do you use and how do you mix it?"

Advise parents as follows

✓ Breastfeeding: Counsel regarding appropriate frequency and duration of feeding, breast care, and maternal nutritional requirements

✓ Bottle feeding: Counsel regarding amount and frequency of feeding, necessity of iron-fortified formula, formula preparation, and avoidance of bottle-propping; warn parent not to use microwave oven to heat formula

✓ See INFANT NUTRITION section for additional information relating to infant nutrition including **amount** and **frequency** of feedings

---

Oral health: Advise parent never to put infant to bed with bottle at any age

---

Infant care: Advise parents regarding the following aspects of care

✓ Normal sleep patterns and appropriate sleeping arrangements

✓ Bladder and bowel patterns

✓ Cord care (if cord still in place), care of circumcised and uncircumcised male; skin and nail care

✓ Importance of responding promptly to infant's crying; babies need to be held, cuddled

✓ How to comfort baby (demonstrate through role modeling if appropriate)

✓ How infant uses thumb sucking and pacifier in self-comforting

✓ Use of rectal thermometer (rectal temperature of 38.0° C/100.4° F or higher is a fever)

✓ When to call the healthcare clinician

When To Call the Healthcare Clinician: Advise parent to call if the infant/child has

➡ Fever (Rectal temp of 100.4° F or higher)   ➡ Poor feeding
➡ Vomiting, diarrhea, abdominal distention   ➡ Irritability, lethargy
➡ Inconsolable crying   ➡ Jaundice
➡ Skin rash, red eye

When to Call 911
Cyanosis (blue color)
Respiratory distress
Seizure

J. Summarize findings at the end of each visit and arrange for continuing care
1. Point out the infant's strengths and appropriately commend parents on their growing comfort with the infant
2. Praise the parent's efforts in parenting and child care
3. Encourage both parents to participate in the care of the infant
4. Remind the parents that you and your staff are available for further discussion of any areas relating to care of the infant
5. Provide suggestions, reading materials, and resources to promote health and reinforce good family health practices, and address any concerns
6. Discuss how the family should access health care (e.g., office hours, after-hours care, telephone advice lines, when to use the emergency department, how to call an ambulance)
7. Ask parent to schedule the next health supervision visit before leaving the office; prepare parent for what can be expected in next visit (e.g., immunizations, screenings)

III. Infants: **Ages 2, 4, 6, & 9 Months**

A. Periodicity schedule for health supervision visits for this age group as recommended by the AAP is as follows: At 2, 4, 6, and 9 months **(Note**: This schedule is designed for infants who are receiving competent parenting, have no manifestations of important health problems, and are growing and developing satisfactorily)

B. Complete a developmental surveillance of the infant based on the milestones in the "Snapshot" below; ask appropriate history questions, and make appropriate observations during history and physical examination to assess the infant's development

SNAPSHOT OF 2, 4, 6, & 9 MONTH OLD CHILD		
Age Group	**Activities**	
2 Months Old	Coos and vocalizes reciprocally Smiles responsively; shows interest in visual/ auditory stimuli	When prone, lifts head, neck, and upper chest with forearm support Some head control in upright position
4 Months Old	Babbles, coos, smiles, laughs, and squeals In prone position, raises body on hands Rolls from front to back; controls head well Opens hands to grasp objects, holds own hands	Reaches for objects Recognizes parent's voice and touch Has spontaneous social smile May sleep for 6 hours; able to comfort self somewhat
6 Months Old	Vocalizes single consonants ("dada") Babbles reciprocally; turns to sounds No head lag when pulled to sit; sits with support Rolls over both ways	Sits, propped on extended arm Starts to self-feed; begins to drink from cup Transfers objects from hand to hand Hands and mouth work together to explore world
9 Months Old	Responds to own name Understands a few words such as "no-no," "bye-bye" Babbles frequently, imitates vocalizations, and may say one or two words Crawls, creeps, moves forward by scooting	Sits independently; may pull to stand Pokes with index finger; uses inferior pincer grasp Plays interactive games (peek-a-boo and pat-a-cake) Feeds self with fingers May sleep through night May show stranger anxiety

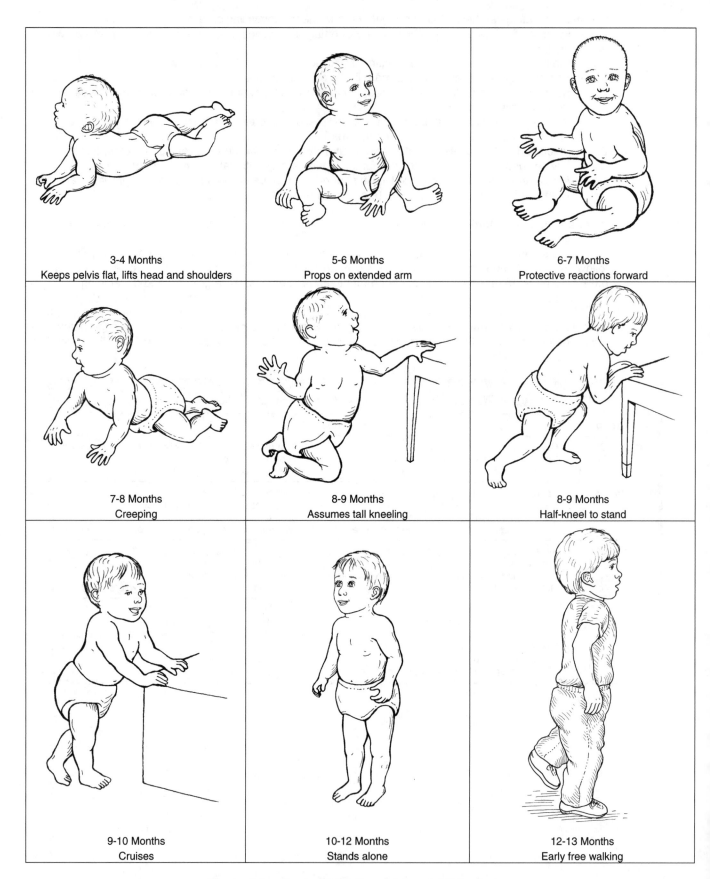

Figure 1.1. Gross Motor Developmental Milestones

C. Consider use of one of the developmental screening tools listed in the table on page 3 (*Overview of Instruments Used for Developmental Screening*) which rely on parent report to help determine if developmental milestones are being met

D. History
1. For initial visit, obtain a complete history including prenatal, birth, and family history
2. For both initial and interval visits, obtain history related to nutrition, sleep, elimination patterns, growth and development, immunization status, any illnesses since birth
3. Obtain a social history on each visit including who lives in household, who provides care for the infant, what the sleeping arrangements are for the infant, and if there are any smokers in household
4. Inquire about parental concerns; ask "What questions or concerns do you have about (child's name) today?"
5. Ask parent if infant seems to see and hear all right
6. Observe parent-infant interaction; have parent hold infant on lap; comment about infant's social behavior and individuality

E. Physical Examination
1. Measure temperature, heart rate, and respiratory rate
2. Measure and plot on growth chart the infant's weight-for-age, length-for-age, weight-for-length, and head circumference (**Note**: National Center for Health Statistics in collaboration with the National Center for Chronic Disease Prevention and Health Promotion have developed new growth charts for infants and children which are available at http://www.cdc.gov/growthcharts)
   a. Infant should double birth weight by 5-6 months
   b. Infant should triple birth weight by one year of age
3. Any infant whose weight gain is inappropriate (not following curve), whose weight is below the fifth percentile, and whose weight and length differ by more than 2 percentile lines requires further evaluation (**Note**: Infant should follow his/her own growth curve; serial [versus single measurements] allow clinician to determine if growth curve is being followed)
4. Head-to-toe examination should be completed on each visit during this age period with a **special focus** on the following

---

Focus of Infant Exam

✓ General appearance of the infant
✓ Muscle tone, symmetry of movement, responsivity
✓ Hearing and visual tracking
✓ Red reflex and alignment of eyes (eyes should be aligned by 2 months of age)
✓ Cardiac murmurs
✓ Presence of developmental hip dysplasia
✓ In males, descent of testes
✓ Examine diaper area for diaper dermatitis
✓ Evidence of abuse/neglect

F. Diagnostic Tests: Hemoglobin and/or hematocrit once between 9 and 12 months of age with 9 months being the preferred age

G. Immunizations: See RECOMMENDED CHILDHOOD IMMUNIZATION SCHEDULE on page 28

H. Fluoride, Vitamin D, and Iron Supplementation

Recommended Dietary Fluoride Supplement* Schedule			
	Fluoride Concentration in Community Drinking Water		
Age	<0.3 ppm	0.3-0.6 ppm	>0.6 ppm
Birth to 6 months	None	None	None
6 months to 3 years	0.25 mg/day	None	None
3 to 6 years	0.50 mg/day	0.25 mg/day	None
6 to 16 years	1.0 mg/day	0.50 mg/day	None

*Sodium fluoride (2.2 mg sodium fluoride contains 1 mg fluoride ion)
Adapted from Centers for Disease Control and Prevention (2001). Recommendations for using fluoride to prevent and control dental caries in the United States. *MMWR, 50* (RR14), p. 52.

Vitamin D and Iron Supplementation	
For infants less than six months of age	See Vitamin and Mineral Supplementation regarding need for vitamin D supplementation on page 5 and follow those guidelines
Breastfed infants who are ≥6 months of age	**Require iron supplementation** in the form of iron-fortified cereal, 2 servings each day, and also a supplement of 200 IU/day of vitamin D
Bottle fed infants who are ≥6 months of age	And who are receiving vitamin D and iron-fortified formula (which should be **all bottle fed infants**) do not require iron supplementation, but iron-fortified cereal is also fed to these infants beginning at six months of age

I.   Anticipatory Guidance

Injury and illness Prevention: Advise parents as follows

✓ See Injury and Illness Prevention under II.I. above and counsel parents on all those points
✓ Set hot water thermostat no higher than 120°; test water on wrist before bathing baby
✓ Keep toys with small parts, balloons, and plastic bags out of reach
✓ Keep dangerous objects/poisonous substances out of sight and reach
✓ Use safety locks on all cabinets; cover all electrical outlets with plastic covers
✓ Do not use infant walkers at any age; encourage use of expanding stair gates
✓ Never leave baby in mesh playpen/crib with drop-side down (weave on mesh sides should have small openings <1/4 inch)
✓ Keep syrup of ipecac or activated charcoal or both on hand to use as directed by Poison Control Center. The new national poison hotline is 800-222-1222; this new number can be used anywhere nationwide to call the nearest poison center
✓ Never leave infant unattended or alone with young siblings or pets
✓ Empty all buckets, tubs, or small pools immediately after use
✓ Learn infant CPR and first aid (refer parent to local classes)

Nutrition: Advise parents as follows

✓ See Nutrition under II.I. above and counsel parents as appropriate regarding breast and bottle feeding
✓ Delay introduction of solids until 6 months of age (See INFANT NUTRITION section for more detailed information)
✓ At 6 months, encourage drinking from cup
✓ At 8-9 months, add chopped table foods while child is sitting at table with family so that child is completely transitioned from pureed to chopped foods by 12 months of age
✓ Limit juice to 2-4 ounces a day (offer in cup only–not bottle); most daily calories should come from food/milk, **not** juice
✓ Avoid giving child peanuts, hot dogs, raisins, grapes, popcorn, large pieces of raw fruit/veggies to prevent aspiration/choking

Oral Health: Advise parents as follows

✓ Do not put infant to bed with a bottle containing formula or juice; (while water is acceptable, best to advise parent not to put baby to bed with a bottle at all)
✓ At 4 month visit, counsel parents regarding teething--what to expect and how to soothe painful gums
✓ As soon as teeth erupt (usually between 6 and 8 months), clean with a soft brush and plain water (no toothpaste) [see DENTAL HEALTH MAINTENANCE section for chronology of dentition in children]

Infant Care: Advise parents as follows

✓ Refer to Infant Care under II.I. above and include those items in counseling
✓ Read books to, talk and sing to, and play music for infant to comfort and to encourage vocalizations
✓ Play social games such as pat-a-cake and peek-a-boo; provide infant with age-appropriate toys
✓ Establish a bedtime routine to discourage night awakening
✓ Provide baby with the same comfort objects so that he/she can console self at bedtime or in new situations
✓ Beginning at 5-6 months, provide opportunities for exploration of the environment
✓ Beginning at 6-9 months, set limits/discipline child using distraction, structure, and routines
✓ Limit rules and enforce consistently

J.   Summarize findings at the end of each visit and arrange continuing care
1.   Emphasize strengths–point out the child's achievements and progress in development as well as the parents' increasing competence in child care
2.   Provide the parents with specific examples of ways that you observed them responding to the child's needs during the health supervision visit (if appropriate)
3.   Encourage both parents to participate in child care

4.   Remind the parents that you and your staff are available for further discussion of any areas of concern
5.   Provide suggestions, reading materials, and resources to promote health and reinforce good health practices
6.   If not done previously, discuss how the family should access healthcare (e.g., office hours, after-hours care, telephone advice lines, when to use the emergency department, how to call an ambulance)
7.   Ask parent to schedule the next health supervision visit before leaving the office; prepare parent for what can be expected in next visit (e.g., immunizations, screenings)

IV.   Toddlers: Ages 12, 15, & 18 Months

A.   Periodicity schedule for health supervision visits for this age group as recommended by the AAP is as follows: At 12, 15, and 18 months **(Note**: This schedule is designed for toddlers who are receiving competent parenting, have no manifestations of important health problems, and are growing and developing satisfactorily)

B.   Complete a developmental surveillance of the toddler based on the milestones in the "snapshot" below; ask appropriate history questions, and make appropriate observations during history and physical examination to assess the toddler's development

SNAPSHOT OF 12, 15, & 18 MONTH OLD CHILD

Age Group	Activities	
12 months	Pulls to stand, cruises	May take few steps alone
	Has vocabulary of 1-3 words, including "mama" and "dada"; imitates vocalizations	Uses precise pincer grasp; points with index finger, Plays social games (e.g., peek-a-boo and pat-a-cake)
	Waves bye-bye	Drinks from cup; feeds self finger-foods
15 months	Walks well, stoops, climbs stairs	Drinks from cup; feeds self with fingers
	Can point to one or more body parts	Has vocabulary of 3-10 words; listens to a story
	Stacks two blocks	Indicates what he/she wants by pointing, grunting
18 months	Walks quickly, runs stiffly, walks backwards	Points to some body parts; uses crayon to scribble
	Stacks 3-4 blocks; throws ball	May voice 2 or more wants; follows simple directions
	Uses vocabulary of about 15 words; imitates words	Feeds self; uses spoon and drinks from cup
	Listens to story, and names objects	Shows affection, kisses

FINE MOTOR DEVELOPMENTAL MILESTONES

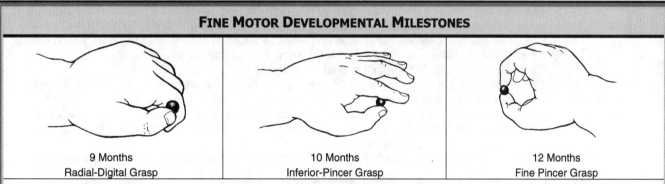

9 Months	10 Months	12 Months
Radial-Digital Grasp	Inferior-Pincer Grasp	Fine Pincer Grasp

- Refinement of voluntary grasp which begins during the second month of life (reflexive palmar grasp gradually disappears at about one month of age) follows an orderly progression, from the midline to the periphery

- Infants progress from swiping at objects held in or near midline at about 3 months of age, to using their hands as entire units to draw objects toward them at 4-5 months of age, to the development of differentiation of the parts of the hand that occurs between 5-12 months of age

- Between 5-7 months, the infant learns to adduct the thumb as the fingers squeeze against the palm in a whole hand grasp

- Shortly thereafter, the thumb moves from adduction to opposition

- At about 9 months, the infant utilizes a grasp characterized by a slight but perceptible movement of the thumb away from the palm and toward the fingertips (the radial-digital grasp as shown above)

- Beginning thumb opposition occurs at about 10 months of age (called inferior-pincer grasp as shown above), a differentiation in the use of the fingers that enables the child to explore details of an object

- The fine pincer grasp, illustrated above, represents the culmination of hand function in early infancy and is achieved at about 12 months of age. This milestone enables the infant to hold and explore tiny objects and to obtain skill in such areas as self-feeding

Adapted from Feldman, H., & Bauer, R., (1992). Developmental-behavioral pediatrics. In G.J. Zitelli & H.W. Davis (Eds.). *Atlas of pediatric physical diagnosis* (pp. 3.1-3.29). Philadelphia: Lippincott, p. 3.8.

FINE MOTOR TASKS

15 Months	24 Months	36 Months	48 Months	54 Months	60 Months
Imitates or scribbles spontaneously	Imitates vertical or circular strokes	Copies circle	Copies cross	Copies square	Copies triangle

Clinician appreciation of the above fine motor tasks and the approximate age at which they are achieved can be helpful in quickly evaluating a young child's attainment of these skills

Adapted from Feldman, H., & Bauer, R., (1992). Developmental-behavioral pediatrics. In G.J. Zitelli & H.W. Davis (Eds.). *Atlas of pediatric physical diagnosis* (pp. 3.1-3.29). Philadelphia: Lippincott, p. 3.9.

C. Consider use of one of the developmental screening tools listed in the table on page 3 (*Overview of Instruments Used for Developmental Screening)* which use parent report to help determine if developmental milestones are being met

D. History
1. For initial visit, obtain a complete history including prenatal, birth, and family history
2. For both initial and interval visits, obtain history related to nutrition, sleep, and elimination patterns, growth and development, immunization status, and illnesses since birth; ask about medications and allergies
3. Obtain a social history on each visit including who lives in household, who provides care for the infant, what the sleeping arrangements are for the infant, and if there are any smokers in household
4. Inquire about current concerns of parents
5. Observe parent-child interaction

E. Physical Examination
1. Take temperature, heart rate, and respirations
2. Measure and plot on growth chart the child's weight-for-age, length-for-age, weight-for-length, and head circumference (**Note**: National Center for Health Statistics in collaboration with the National Center for Chronic Disease Prevention and Health Promotion have developed new growth charts for infants and children which are available at http://www.cdc.gov/growthcharts)
3. By 12 months of age, birth weight should have tripled
4. During the period from 12 months to 24 months, children, on average, gain 4-6 pounds in weight and 3-5 inches in height
5. Any child whose weight gain is inappropriate (not following curve), whose weight is above the 95th percentile or below the fifth percentile, or whose weight and length (height) differ by more than 2 percentile lines requires further evaluation
6. Head-to-toe examination should be completed on each visit with special focus on the following

Focus of Exam
✓ General appearance of the child
✓ Feet and gait once walking begins
✓ Hearing and vision (subjective)
✓ Tooth eruption/baby bottle caries
✓ Red reflex and alignment of eyes
✓ Evidence of abuse/neglect

F. Diagnostic Tests: Screening for lead poisoning

CDC recommends **universal** screening for lead poisoning in all children at ages 1 and 2 and all children 36-72 months of age who have **not** been previously screened **if** their risk for lead exposure is widespread, based on responses to Personal-Risk Questionnaire screening

CDC recommends **targeted** screening for lead poisoning for children at ages 1 and 2, and children 36-72 months of age who have not previously been screened, if they meet one of the following criteria (as determined by local health department)
- ✓ Residence in a specific geographic area (e.g., a specified zip code)
- ✓ Membership in a high-risk group (e.g., Medicaid recipient)
- ✓ Responses to the personal-risk questionnaire indicating risk (see following table)

THE PERSONAL-RISK QUESTIONNAIRE FOR LEAD EXPOSURE IN CHILDREN

Interpretation: A positive response to any of the 3 items indicates risk of lead exposure
- ✓ Does your child live in or regularly visit a house that was built before 1950? This question could apply to a facility such as a home day-care center or the home of a babysitter or relative
- ✓ Does your child live in or regularly visit a house built before 1978 with recent or ongoing renovations or remodeling (within the last 6 months)?
- ✓ Does your child have a sibling or playmate who has or did have lead poisoning?

Source: Centers for Disease Control and Prevention. (1997). *Screening young children for lead poisoning: Guidance for state and local public health officials.* Atlanta: Author.

G.   Immunizations: See RECOMMENDED CHILDHOOD IMMUNIZATION SCHEDULE on page 28

H.   Supplements: Children who do not get regular sunlight exposure and who consume <500 mL/day of vitamin D-containing milk need a daily multivitamin supplement containing 200 IU of vitamin D. Also see FLUORIDE SUPPLEMENTATION RECOMMENDATIONS table on page 9

I.   Anticipatory Guidance

Promotion of Healthy and Safe Habits: Advise parents as follows
- ✓ Wash toddler's hands and own hands frequently, especially after diaper changes and toileting and before eating
- ✓ Clean toys with soap and water
- ✓ Limit television viewing to 1 hour a day; be sure the programs are appropriate and watch with child
- ✓ Expect your toddler to sleep through the night; maintain a regular bedtime routine
- ✓ Keep the environment smoke free (house and car should be nonsmoking zones)
- ✓ Protect the child from insect bites, and use the three strategies for sun protection (sun avoidance, use of protective clothing, and use of sunscreen) [see the section on SKIN CARE, INSECT BITE PROTECTION, AND SUN EXPOSURE PROTECTION FOR CHILDREN for more specific counseling]
- ✓ Participate as a family in physical activities such as taking walks, going to the park

---

Injury and Illness Prevention: Advise parents as follows

To Prevent Motor Vehicle Crashes/Other Machine-Related Injuries:
- ✓ Switch to a front-facing car safety seat and make sure it is properly secured (see CAR SAFETY SEAT CHECKLIST below)
- ✓ Keep toddler away from moving machinery, lawn mowers, backing cars

To Prevent Burn/Scalding Injuries:
- ✓ Recheck the hot water heater every 3-6 months to make certain the thermostat is <120°
- ✓ Test smoke detector frequently and change battery once a year
- ✓ Keep the toddler away from hot stoves, fireplaces, curling irons, space heaters
- ✓ Turn pot handles toward back of stove
- ✓ Ensure that electric outlets and appliances are inaccessible

To Prevent Accidental Ingestion/Poisoning:
- ✓ Keep all poisonous substances including medicines, alcohol, cleaning agents, paints, solvents out of the child's sight and reach
- ✓ Supervise the toddler constantly; do not expect young children to supervise toddler
- ✓ Keep syrup of ipecac and/or activated charcoal on hand to use as directed by Poison Control Center. The new national poison hot-line is 800-222-1222; this new number can be used anywhere nationwide to call the nearest poison center

To Prevent Drowning:
- ✓ Always supervise the toddler when around water (even if it is just a bucket of water)
- ✓ Ensure child wears a life vest if boating

To Prevent Injury from Falls:
- ✓ Continue to use gates at top and bottom of stairs, safety devices on windows
- ✓ Ensure that toddler wears a helmet when riding in a seat on an adult bike

To Prevent Other Injuries:
- ✓ Teach the child to use caution when approaching dogs
- ✓ Get down on the floor and check for new hazards now that toddler is walking
- ✓ Learn child CPR and first aid

Car Safety Seat Checklist

Children older than 1 year weighing 20 to 40 pounds may safely ride in a child seat strapped into the back seat and facing the front seat. The center seat in the back is the best location for the placement of the safety seat

✓ Harness straps in the child seat itself should be at or above the child's shoulders and fit snugly without any loose areas

✓ The harness chest clip should be at the child's armpit level

✓ Refer parents to the following resources for more information

National Highway Traffic Safety Administration
800-424-9393 (Auto Safety Hotline)
www.nhtsa.gov

National Safe Kids Campaign
202-662-0600
www.safekids.org

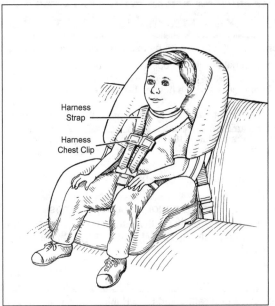

Forward-facing Safety Seat in Center Back Seat Position of Car

Adapted from Stevens, L.M., Lynn, C., & Glass, R.M. (2002). Vehicle safety and children. *JAMA, 287,* 1212.

Nutrition: Advise parents as follows

✓ Child should be eating table foods seated in highchair or booster seat with the family

✓ Give 2-3 nutritious snacks per day such as fruit, cheese, and yogurt or other dairy products; avoid sugary snacks

✓ Encourage toddler to feed self with hands at first, and then by using utensils as she/he progresses through toddlerhood

✓ Let the toddler develop clear likes and dislikes and do not allow feeding to serve as focus of power struggles

✓ Limit bottle use, avoid use of bottle in bed and never put juice or juice drinks in bottle

✓ Should be weaned from bottle/breast by about 18 months of age

✓ Decrease in appetite is normal (growth slows compared with infancy)

✓ May use whole cow's milk after 12 months of age (absolutely no low fat milk until the child is ≥ 2 years of age)

Oral Health: Advise parents as follows

✓ Continue brushing child's teeth with a soft brush and plain water (no toothpaste is recommended until age 2)

✓ Initial dental referral recommended anytime between 12 months-3 years of age (American Academy of Pediatrics [AAP])

Child Care: Advise parents as follows
✓ Praise the toddler for good behavior
✓ Encourage language development by reading books, singing songs
✓ Encourage exploration of the environment
✓ Reinforce self-care and self-expression
✓ To promote a sense of competence, invite the toddler to make choices whenever possible
✓ Encourage the toddler to play alone and with playmates, siblings, parents
✓ Set limits and discipline toddlers through distraction, gentle restraint, removal from the situation, "time out," use of routines and structure
✓ Limit the number of rules and enforce them consistently
✓ Anticipate and avoid unnecessary conflicts; do not get into power struggle with child
✓ Discipline the toddler so that he/she understands that hitting, biting are not allowed
✓ Expect the toddler to sleep through night
✓ Promote learning of self-quieting behaviors through provision of the same transitional object, such as blanket, stuffed animal so toddler can console self at bedtime and in new situations
✓ Do not begin toilet training until child is ready (dry for periods of about 2 hours, knows the difference between wet and dry and wants to be dry; can pull pants up and down, wants to learn, and can give a signal when voiding/bowel movement is imminent)
✓ Anticipate that toddler may touch genitals

J. Summarize findings at the end of each visit and arrange continuing care (see III.J. above)

V. **Toddlers and Preschoolers: Ages 2- 5 Years**

A. Periodicity schedule for health supervision visits for this age group as recommended by the AAP is as follows: At 2, 3, 4, and 5 years **(Note**: This schedule is designed for children who are receiving competent parenting, have no manifestations of important health problems, and are growing and developing satisfactorily)

B. Complete a developmental surveillance of the child based on the milestones in the "snapshot" below; ask appropriate history questions, and make appropriate observations during history and physical examination to assess the child's development

SNAPSHOT OF 2, 3, 4, & 5 YEAR OLD CHILD		
Age Group		**Activities**
2 Years Old	Goes up and down stairs one step at a time Kicks ball Can stack 5-6 blocks Imitates adults	Uses two-word phrases; follows two-step commands Makes or imitates circular strokes with crayon Has vocabulary of at least 20 words Speaks intelligibly to strangers 25% of time
3 Years Old	Goes up and down stairs using alternating feet Jumps in place, kicks a ball, balances on one foot Rides a tricycle Knows own name, age, and gender Has bladder/bowel control	Has self-care skills (feeding/dressing) Shows early imaginative behavior Follows two-step instructions; copies a circle Understands concepts of "on," "in," and "under" Speaks intelligibly to strangers 75% of time
4 Years Old	Builds a tower of 10 blocks; copies a cross Throws overhand ball; hops, jumps on one foot Can sing a song; draws a person with 3 parts Knows about things used at home (appliances)	Distinguishes fantasy from reality Talks about daily activities and experiences Is aware of gender (of self and others) Speaks intelligibly to strangers 100% of time
5 Years Old	Skips, rides bike, and uses skateboard Knows address and phone number Can count on fingers Copies square; prints some letters	Draws a person with head, body, arms, and legs Recognizes most letters of alphabet; knows colors Dresses self without help Plays make-believe and dress-up

C. Consider use of one of the developmental screening tools listed in the table on page 3 (*Overview of Instruments Used for Developmental Screening*) which use parent report to help determine if developmental milestones are being met

D. History
1. For initial visit, obtain a complete history including prenatal, birth, neonatal, and family history
2. For both initial and interval visits, obtain history related to nutrition, sleep, dental hygiene, elimination and sleep patterns, immunization status, relationship with family and playmates, play activities, discipline, child care arrangements, safety, and whether there are smokers in the household
3. Obtain past medical history; ask if child is on any medications and if child has any allergies
4. Ask about parental concerns
5. Beginning at about age 6, ask children what questions or concerns they have about their health and bodies
6. Beginning at about age 5, screen for abuse and neglect

> Ask child open-ended questions about his/her own safety such as the following (explain to the parent the purpose of the screening **prior** to asking questions)
> - ✓ Are you afraid of anyone?
> - ✓ Does anyone ever hurt you?
> - ✓ Does anyone make you keep secrets?
> - ✓ All positive responses should be followed up with more specific questions including, "What happened?" "When did it happen?" and "Who did that?"

E. Physical Examination
1. Obtain temperature, heart rate, respiratory rate; begin taking blood pressure at age 3
2. Measure and plot on growth chart the child's weight-for-age, stature-for-age, weight-for-stature, and head circumference (head circumference is routinely measured on the 2-year visit, but not on subsequent visits) [**Note**: Beginning at age 2, body mass index-for-age percentiles are calculated for both boys and girls; these new growth charts as well as the new growth charts for infants and children birth to 36 months, are available at http://www.cdc.gov/growthcharts]
3. Any child whose weight gain is inappropriate (not following curve), whose weight (BMI) is above the 95th percentile or below the 5th percentile, and whose weight and height differ by more than 2 percentile lines requires further evaluation
4. Head-to-toe examination should be completed on each visit during this age period
5. Always examine the child for evidence of abuse

F. Diagnostic Tests

> ✓ Recommendations for sensory screening—vision and hearing—are as follows
> - • Beginning at age 3, objective vision testing should be attempted (if child uncooperative, rescreen in 6 months) [see section on VISION IMPAIRMENT IN CHILDREN for vision screening guidelines]
> - • Hearing screening should be subjective in the 2 and 3 year old; beginning at age 4, objective hearing screening should be performed
> ✓ Screening for elevated blood lead levels should be done according to CDC recommendations for either **universal** or **targeted** screening (see IV.F. for guidelines)
> ✓ Urinalysis is recommended at 5 years of age (AAP)
> ✓ TB skin testing (PPD) is recommended **only** in children in whom risk factors are present

G. Immunizations: See RECOMMENDED CHILDHOOD IMMUNIZATION SCHEDULE on page 28

H. Supplements: Children who do not get regular sunlight exposure and who consume <500 mL/day of vitamin D-containing milk need a daily multivitamin supplement containing 200 IU of vitamin D. Also see FLUORIDE SUPPLEMENTATION RECOMMENDATIONS table on page 9

I. Anticipatory Guidance

Promotion of Healthy and Safe Habits: Advise parents as follows

✓ Be a role model for your child by leading a healthy life
✓ Help your child wash his hands after toileting and before eating; continue to wash your own hands
✓ Clean potty chair after each use
✓ Teach your child to cover his mouth when he coughs and to use a tissue to wipe his nose and then wash his hands
✓ Clean your child's toys with soap and water
✓ Limit "screen time" (TV, computer, and video games) to 2 hours a day; be sure the programs are appropriate and watch and talk about the program with child
✓ Expect your child to sleep through the night; maintain a regular bedtime routine; for children through 5 years of age, the suggested bedtime is 8 PM
✓ Keep the environment smoke free (house and car should be nonsmoking zones)
✓ Protect the child from insect bites, and use the three strategies for sun protection (sun avoidance, use of protective clothing, and use of sunscreen) [see the section on SKIN CARE, INSECT BITE PROTECTION, AND SUN EXPOSURE PROTECTION FOR CHILDREN for more specific counseling]
✓ Participate as a family in physical activities such as taking walks and going to the park

Illness and Injury Prevention: Advise parents as follows

To Prevent Motor Vehicle Crashes/Other Machine-Related Injuries:
✓ Continue to use an age-appropriate car safety seat or a properly secured booster in the rear seat of car until the child weighs 80 pounds or his head is higher than the back of the seat; switch to a lap/shoulder restraint after that time (see CAR SAFETY SEAT CHECKLIST below)
✓ Supervise all play near streets or driveways
✓ At age 4, teach the child pedestrian and neighborhood safety skills

To Prevent Burn/Scalding Injuries:
✓ Recheck the hot water heater every 6-12 months to make certain the thermostat is <120°
✓ Test smoke detector frequently and change battery once a year
✓ Keep the child away from hot stoves, fireplaces, curling irons, space heaters, matches, lighters, or cigarettes
✓ Turn pot handles toward back of stove
✓ Ensure that electric outlets and appliances are inaccessible
✓ Beginning at age 4, conduct fire drills at home

To Prevent Accidental Ingestion/Poisoning:
✓ Keep all poisonous substances such as medications, alcohol, cleaning agents, and solvents out of the child's sight and reach
✓ Supervise the child constantly; do not expect young children to supervise preschooler
✓ Keep syrup of ipecac and/or activated charcoal in the home to be used as directed by Poison Control Center. The new national poison hot-line is 800-222-1222; this new number can be used anywhere nationwide to call the nearest poison center. Remind parent to never use anything without first checking with Poison Control

To Prevent Drowning:
✓ Always supervise the child when in or near water
✓ Ensure child wears a life vest if boating
✓ At age 4, teach the child to swim but continue to supervise at all times

To Prevent Injury from Falls:
✓ Until the child is at least 3, continue to use gates at top and bottom of stairs, safety devices on windows
✓ Ensure that child wears a helmet when riding in a seat on an adult bike; child should also wear a helmet when riding a tricycle or a bicycle

To Prevent Other Injuries:
✓ Teach the child to use caution when approaching dogs
✓ Ensure that guns, if in the house, are locked up and that ammunition is stored separately
✓ At about age 3, teach child about body parts and good and bad touch
✓ Beginning at age 4 or 5, teach the child about safety rules for interacting with strangers

Car Safety Seat Checklist

Children weighing 40-80 pounds should ride in the back seat in a booster seat that uses the adult lap and shoulder belt
- ✓ Belt-positioning boosters should be used with the shoulder belt snugly across the child's chest and the lap belt low across the child's thighs
- ✓ Booster seats should be used until the child can sit back against the back seat with knees bent and feet touching the floor
- ✓ Refer parents to the following resources for more information

National Highway Traffic Safety Administration
800-424-9393 (Auto Safety Hotline)
www.nhtsa.gov

National Safe Kids Campaign
202-662-0600
www.safekids.org

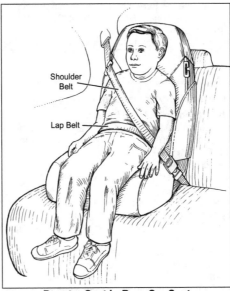

Booster Seat in Rear Car Seat

Adapted from Stevens, L.M., Lynn, C., & Glass, R.M. (2002). Vehicle safety and children. *JAMA, 287*, 1212.

Nutrition: Advise parents as follows

- ✓ Serve the child meals with the family, with 2-3 nutritious snacks per day
- ✓ Enforce reasonable mealtime behavior, but do not force the child to eat
- ✓ Avoid engaging in struggles about eating
- ✓ See section on CHILD AND ADOLESCENT NUTRITION for more counseling tips

---

Oral Health: Advise parents as follows

- ✓ At age 2, begin brushing child's teeth twice a day with a pea-size amount of fluoridated toothpaste; parent should continue to brush child's teeth until child is about 5 years of age
- ✓ Learn how to prevent dental injuries and to handle dental emergencies such as loss or fracture of tooth
- ✓ Initial dental appointment should occur between 12 months and 3 years of age, with 3 years the preferred age

---

Child Care to Promote Social Competence: Advise parents as follows

- ✓ Praise child for good behavior and accomplishments
- ✓ Model appropriate language and encourage language development by reading to child, singing with child, and communicating about what is happening
- ✓ Spend individual time with the child, playing, walking, talking together
- ✓ Beginning at about 3 years, encourage child to talk about preschool, friends, or experiences
- ✓ Appreciate the child's inquisitive nature and do not limit his explorations
- ✓ Promote physical activity in a safe environment
- ✓ In the 2 year old, encourage parallel play and do not expect shared play
- ✓ Provide opportunities for the 3 and 4 year old to socialize with other children in play groups, preschool
- ✓ By age 4, provide some type of structured learning environment for the child, whether Head Start, preschool, or Sunday school
- ✓ Reinforce self-care and self-expression; by age 2 or 3, begin to encourage the child to express his/her feelings
- ✓ To promote feelings of competence and control, give child opportunities to make choices whenever possible
- ✓ Reinforce limits and appropriate behavior
- ✓ Use time out or remove source of conflict for unacceptable behavior
- ✓ By age 3 or 4, teach the child how to manage anger and resolve conflicts without violence
- ✓ By age 3 or 4, teach the child to respect authority
- ✓ Encourage self-quieting behaviors
- ✓ Promote toilet training when the child is ready, usually at about 24 months of age
    - Is dry for periods of 2 hours
    - Wakes up from naps dry
    - Knows the difference between wet and dry and prefers being dry
    - Can pull pants up and down
    - Wants to learn
    - Can signal need to void or have bowel movement

J. Summarize findings at the end of each visit and arrange continuing care
 1. Emphasize the strengths of the child and the family
 2. Highlight both the child's developmental progress and the parents' competence in promoting the growth and development of the child
 3. Provide suggestions, reading materials, and resources to promote health, reinforce good parenting practices, and address any concerns
 4. If not done previously, discuss how the family should access health care (e.g., office hours, after-hours care, telephone advice lines, when to use the emergency department, how to call an ambulance)
 5. Provide parents with an appointment for their child's next regularly scheduled health supervision visit and briefly advise them what will be covered during the next visit

VI. School-Age Children: Ages 6 - 10

A. Periodicity schedule for health supervision visits for this age group as recommended by the AAP is as follows: At 6, 8, and 10 years (**Note**: This schedule is designed for children who are receiving competent parenting, have no manifestations of important health problems, and are growing and developing satisfactorily)

SNAPSHOT OF SCHOOL-AGE CHILD	
Six Year Old	• Eager to act independently, but unable to consistently make good decisions • Is learning about safety–crossing the street, riding a bike, interacting with strangers, but unable to adapt rules for different situations and family must set appropriate boundaries • Interested in testing the limits of his body and as he learns how his body works, he gains confidence and skills needed to enjoy physical activities and participate in individual and group sports • Spends increasing amounts of time with friends and others outside the home
Seven/Eight Year Old	• Participates in chores such as setting the table, taking out trash, and other activities which increase sense of personal competence • Able to use logic and to focus on multiple aspects of a problem; beginning to understand ways in which others' viewpoints differ from her own • Increasingly looks outside the family for new ideas and activities; identifies with children of the same gender who share her abilities and interests; may have a best friend–a milestone in interpersonal development • Increasingly responsible for health habits such as personal hygiene, nutrition, physical activity, and safety (e.g., safety belt and helmet use), but needs parental supervision
Nine/Ten Year Old	• Child has informally become a member of his peer group; has primarily same-sex friends, and friends assume greater importance; growing independence from family is now obvious • Injury prevention assumes an added dimension as children at this age may engage in risk-taking behaviors (e.g., dares, drinking, smoking, inhaling) due to peer pressure • Enhancing the child's self-esteem is especially crucial now as children who feel good about themselves are better able to handle peer pressure • With puberty approaching–and already present for some children–children at this age have many concerns about physical and emotional development and pubertal changes

B. History

1. For initial visit, obtain a complete history including prenatal, birth, neonatal, and family history
2. For both initial and interval visits, obtain history related to nutrition, sleep, dental hygiene, elimination and sleep patterns, immunization status, relationship with family and playmates, play activities, discipline, child care arrangements, safety, and whether there is a smoker in the household
3. Obtain a past medical history; ask if child is on any medications and if there are any allergies
4. Ask child what questions or concerns he/she has about own health and body **(Note:** Beginning at about age 6, the child's role as historian should be fostered so that over the next few years, the parent's role as historian [except for birth history, past medical history, and family history] is relatively diminished as the child's role emerges)
5. Ask about parental concerns
6. Screen for abuse and neglect by asking child open-ended questions about his/her own safety (refer to V.D. above for screening questions)
7. Discuss sexuality education issues with parents and with child and recommend books contained in the figure on page 21

✓ Beginning at age 9 or 10, ask if parent talks to child about sensitive subjects such as sex
✓ Ask if age-appropriate books relating to sex education are available in the home for the child to read and ask questions about
✓ At about age 10, ask parent if menstruation has been discussed (girls) or wet dreams (boys); recommend that the topics be discussed now (if not already done)
✓ At age 10, assess the child's preparation for puberty and sexual development
✓ Determine what the child already knows, and then provide additional information
✓ Begin to teach the child that delaying sexual behavior is the surest form of protection against disease and pregnancy
✓ Explore the child's understanding of sexually transmitted diseases, including AIDS

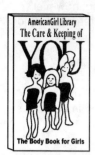
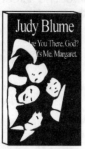
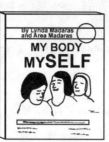
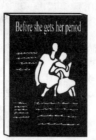
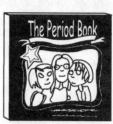
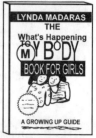

| *The Care & Keeping of You* **By Valorie Schaefer** | *Are You There God? It's Me, Margaret* **By Judy Blume** | *My Body, My Self for Girls* **By Lynda Madaras and Area Madaras** | *Before She Gets Her Period* **By Jessica B. Gillooly** | *The Period Book* **By Karen Gravelle and Jennifer Gravelle** | *What's Happening to My Body?* **By Lynda Madaras and Area Madaras** |

Figure 1-2: Books to Recommend Related to Sexual Development

C. Developmental Surveillance and School Performance

Assessment of the child should include the following areas (ask the child)

Family: "Who is in your family?" "How do you get along with your family?" "What kinds of things does your family do for fun?"

Friends: "Tell me who your friends are" "Do you have a best friend?" "What do you like to do with your friends?"

School: "What grade are you in at school?" "Who is your teacher?" "What do you like best about school?" "What don't you like about school?" (For child who is 8 or 9, "What are your grades?")

Activities: "What do you like to do for fun?" "Do you play any sports?" "What do you do after school?"

Assessment of child should include the following areas (ask the parent)

Family: "Have there been any major changes or stresses in your family since your last visit?" "How does (name) get along with his siblings?" "How are things going in the family?" "What are some of the things you do together as a family?"

Friends: "Does (name) have friends he likes to spend time with?" "What sorts of things do they do together?" "When (name) plays with other children, can he keep up with them?"

School: "How is (name) attendance at school?" "Does (name) seem to be able to follow the rules at school?" "Do you participate in school activities?" "Have you visited (name) classroom?"

Activities: "How does (name) spend her time outside of school [on weekends]?" "How much television does (name) watch each day?" "Does (name) participate in organized sports?" "Who takes (name) to practice and to games?"

D. Physical Examination
1. Measure and plot on growth chart the child's weight-for-age, stature-for-age; using the CDC growth charts, calculate the child's BMI and determine if BMI-for-age is in healthy range; the new growth charts are available at http://www.cdc.gov/growthcharts
2. Any child whose BMI is outside the healthy range requires further evaluation (see Indicators for Stature and Weight Status for Children and Adolescents in box below)
3. Head-to-toe examination should be completed on each visit during this age period
4. AAP recommended physical examination screenings during this age period in addition to measurements of height and weight are blood pressure and vision and hearing screening
5. As part of the complete physical examination, Tanner staging or Sexual Maturity Rating (SMR) should be completed to determine child's pubertal development (see section on PRECOCIOUS PUBERTY)
6. Always examine the child for evidence of abuse

Indicators for Stature and Weight Status for Children and Adolescents		
Indicator	**Anthropometric Variable**	**Cut-Off Values**
Stunting	Stature-for-age	<3rd percentile
Thinness	BMI-for-age	<5th percentile
At risk for overweight	BMI-for-age	≥85th percentile, but <95th percentile
Overweight	BMI-for-age	≥95th percentile

Source: Story, M., Holt, K., & Sofka, D. (2002). *Bright futures in practice: Nutrition.* Arlington, VA: National Center for Education in Maternal and Child Health, p. 95.

E.   Diagnostic Tests: None recommended during this age period as part of routine screening; however, consult AAP's (2000) Recommendations for Preventive Pediatric Health Care (see in reference list) for recommendations for screening of high-risk children

F.   Immunizations: See RECOMMENDED CHILDHOOD IMMUNIZATION SCHEDULE on page 28

G.   Supplements: Children who do not get regular sunlight exposure and who consume <500 mL/day of vitamin D-containing milk need a daily multivitamin supplement containing 200 IU of vitamin D. Also see FLUORIDE SUPPLEMENTATION RECOMMENDATIONS table on page 9

H.   Anticipatory Guidance

Promotion of Healthy and Safe Habits

✓ Be a role model for your child by living a healthy life
✓ Supervise your child's activities with peers; get to know the parents in the households that your child visits
✓ Be sure your child gets adequate sleep (for children 6-10 years of age, the suggested bedtime is 9 PM)
✓ Encourage regular physical activity and plan family activities that involve exercise such as biking or hiking
✓ Limit television viewing to an average of 2 hours per day; check ratings and choose appropriate programs; if computer and video games are played each day, less time should be spent in TV viewing
✓ Continue to teach your child personal care and hygiene; by age 8 or so, supervision rather than teaching should be the parent's major role in this area
✓ Remind your child to wash his/her hands after toileting and before meals (if child does not consistently perform these behaviors)
✓ Teach your child about safe use of insect repellants and how to use the three strategies for sun protection (sun avoidance, use of protective clothing, and use of sunscreen) [see the section on SKIN CARE, INSECT BITE PROTECTION, AND SUN EXPOSURE PROTECTION FOR CHILDREN for more specific counseling recommendations]
✓ Beginning at about 8 years of age, counsel your child about avoiding the use of alcohol, tobacco, drugs, and inhalants
✓ Keep the environment smoke-free

Illness and Injury Prevention: Advise parents/child as follows

To Prevent Motor Vehicle Crashes/Other Machine-Related Injuries:
✓ Continue to ensure that child wears a lap/shoulder safety belt located in the back seat of the car at all times (the back seat is the safest place for children of any age to ride) [children weighing <80 pounds or those who cannot comfortably sit back against the back seat with knees bent and feet touching the floor should use a booster seat]
✓ Do not allow the child to operate a power lawn mower or electric tools
✓ Make certain child always wears helmet when riding a bicycle and follows safety rules for biking and crossing street

To Prevent Burn/Scalding Injuries:
✓ Test the smoke detector frequently and change battery once a year
✓ Recheck the hot water heater every 6 months to make certain the thermostat is <120°
✓ Instruct child what to do in case of fire; conduct fire drills at home

To Prevent Accidental Ingestion/Poisoning:
✓ Warn child about dangers of poisonous substances
✓ Keep all medications out of sight and reach of children; make sure that safety caps are used
✓ Keep syrup of ipecac or activated charcoal in the home to be used as directed by Poison Control Center. The new national poison hot-line is 800-222-1222 and can be used anywhere nationwide to call the nearest poison center

To Prevent Drowning:
✓ Teach the child how to swim
✓ Reinforce safety rules for swimming pools and lakes (including wearing of life vest when boating)
✓ Always supervise child when in or near water

To Prevent Injury from Falls:
✓ Discuss playground safety with child
✓ Make certain that helmet is worn when biking or skating; review safety rules for biking and skating

To Prevent Other Injuries:
✓ Anticipate providing less direct supervision as child moves through age period and demonstrates more maturity
✓ Anticipate that the child may make errors in judgment due to trying to imitate (and impress) peers
✓ Ensure that guns, if in the household, are locked up and that ammunition is stored separately
✓ Reinforce with child safety rules for interacting with strangers; make sure child knows emergency numbers
✓ Make certain child is supervised before and after school in a safe environment
✓ Make sure child understands good touch and bad touch and what to do if someone tries to touch him/her in a "bad touch" way
✓ Teach child to avoid high noise levels, especially when listening to music through headphones

---

Nutrition: See section on CHILD AND ADOLESCENT NUTRITION

✓	Brush teeth after every meal (at least twice a day); parent should continue to supervise
✓	Learn to floss teeth (by age 8) [parent should do until child can do alone]
✓	Learn how to prevent dental injuries and handle dental emergencies
✓	Schedule a dental appointment every 6 months
✓	As the permanent molars erupt, ensure that child is evaluated for application of dental sealants

Child Care to Promote Social Competence: Advise parents as follows

- ✓ Praise the child for cooperation and personal successes
- ✓ As the child moves through this age period, help her choose activities in which success is likely (help child accept the reality that she will be better at some things than others)
- ✓ Encourage the child to express feelings and to talk with parent about school, friends, successes, and disappointments
- ✓ Encourage reading and hobbies such as collecting baseball cards, stamps, or making things
- ✓ Help the child learn how to get along with peers and help child learn how to follow group rules
- ✓ Promote physical activity in a safe environment
- ✓ Encourage self-discipline and impulse control; set limits and establish consequences for unacceptable behavior
- ✓ Expect the child to follow family rules such as those for bedtime, television viewing, and chores
- ✓ Teach the child to respect authority; ensure the child knows the difference between right and wrong
- ✓ As the child reaches 9 or 10 years of age, help him develop an ability to deal with peer pressure by suggesting strategies and role-playing with the child
- ✓ Teach the child how to constructively deal with conflict and anger in the family, at school, and in the neighborhood
- ✓ Provide personal space for the child at home, even if limited

I. Summarize findings at the end of each visit and arrange continuing care (see V.J. above)

VII. Adolescence: 11 - 21 Years of Age (Early Adolescence is 11-14; Middle is 15-16; Late is 18-21)

A. Periodicity schedule for health supervision visits for this age group as recommended by the AAP is as follows: Annual visits beginning at age 11 and ending at age 21 (**Note**: This schedule is designed for adolescents who are receiving competent parenting, have no manifestations of important health problems, and are growing and developing satisfactorily)

SNAPSHOT OF ADOLESCENT	
Early Adolescence 11-14 Years of Age	• Dramatic physical changes are the hallmark of early adolescence; typically, girls show signs of puberty 2 years earlier than boys • Young adolescents are egocentric and intensely preoccupied with how they look; may spend hours in front of mirror; often display erratic or moody behavior • Eating disorders may develop during this period, especially among females • Cognitive abilities and sense of morality are continuing to develop; focus is primarily on the concrete and the present—" here and now," and thinking is governed by conventional standards or rules • Parents remain important role models, serving as a consistent, stabilizing influence • School now becomes the primary setting through which peer group standards or expectations are communicated • Risk-taking behaviors during this time period are common and can have serious health consequences • More than half the injury-related deaths in this age group involve motor vehicle crashes (MVCs), with the adolescent as passenger, pedestrian, or cyclist
Middle Adolescence 15-17 Years of Age	• By the age of 15, most girls have completed the physiologic changes associated with puberty; most boys are still in the process of maturing • Extremely sensitive to the social norms of their peer group; when at home, adolescents at this age tend to seek privacy and time alone • Some 15- and 16-years-olds are beginning to make the transition from concrete to formal operational thinking, becoming more adept at abstract thought and planning for the future; often become concerned about community and societal issues during this age period • Academic success has important implications for college and career choices at this stage; economic realities lead many adolescents to seek part-time work which can negatively affect school performance (can also have many positive outcomes as well) • Risky behaviors tend to escalate among this age group; as they reach the legal age to drive, adolescents gain a mobility and independence that presents both opportunities and risks

(Continued)

Late Adolescence 18-21 Years of Age	• Are now legally responsible for themselves; key developmental tasks include focusing on achieving independence and developing a capacity for mature emotional intimacy with opposite/same sex peers while maintaining emotional ties to their families
	• Many older adolescents have developed the potential for formal operational thinking and sophisticated moral reasoning
	• While late adolescence should be a time of choice and empowerment, it can also bring intense frustration to youth with restricted options
	• Lack of family and social support systems, coupled with greater personal freedom, can increase risky behaviors which tend to peak during this time
	• MVCs, suicide, and homicide are the leading causes of death in the 18-21 year old age group

B. History

1. Determine your philosophy about seeing the adolescent (adolescent alone or with parent present for at least part of the visit) [As the adolescent transitions through this period, needs for privacy and confidentiality become increasingly important]

2. For initial visit, obtain a complete history including prenatal, birth, past medical history, and family history

3. Ask what medications are taken on a regular basis; ask about allergies

4. For both initial and interval visits, obtain history related to nutrition, sleep, dental hygiene, elimination and sleep patterns, immunization status, relationship with family and friends, activities, discipline, and safety

5. Ask about parental concerns, particularly for the younger adolescent; once the child is independent from the family (age 18 in most circumstances) role of the family will become very individualized

6. Ask adolescent what questions or concerns he has about own health and body **(Note:** By the time the child enters adolescence, he should be the primary historian with the parent supplying information about birth history, past medical history, and family history)

Ask adolescent if he/she knows what to expect as body develops

At visits during Early Adolescence (11-14 years), ask the following questions
  ✓ "Has anyone talked with you about what to expect as your body develops?"
  ✓ "Have you read about changes in your body?"
  ✓ "Do you think you are developing pretty much like the rest of your friends?"
  ✓ "How do you feel about the way you look?"

Recommend books relating to developmental changes (see under VI.B above)

At visits during Middle Adolescence (15-17 years), ask the following questions
  ✓ "How do you feel about the way you look?"
  ✓ "Do you think you have developed pretty much like the rest of your friends?"

Screen for abuse and neglect by asking adolescent open-ended questions about his/her own safety such as the following
(**Note:** These questions should be asked without the parent/caregiver present)

  ✓ Are you afraid of anyone?
  ✓ Does anyone ever hurt you?
  ✓ Does anyone make you keep secrets?
  ✓ All positive responses should be followed up with more specific questions including, "What happened?" "When did it happen?" and "Who did that?"

C. Developmental Surveillance and School Performance

Assessment of the adolescent should include the following areas: Questions that follow are intended to be used selectively to invite discussion, to gather information, and to address the needs and concerns of the adolescent; modify questions to match your own communication style

Ask the adolescent:

Family: "Are you the youngest, oldest, or middle child in your family?" "What is it like to be the oldest (youngest or middle) child?" "Who are you closest to in the family?" "How do you get along with your family?" "What kinds of chores do you have around the house?" "How are you punished?"

Friends: "Tell me who your friends are; do you have a best friend?" "What do you like to do with your friends?"

Dating/Drug Use: "Do you have a girlfriend (boyfriend)?" **Approach with a declaration such as** "Some teenagers your age have begun to be sexually active--what are most of your friends doing about sexual activity?" "How are you and your (boyfriend/girlfriend) handling this?" "I know that drugs are common on school campuses--what drugs are common at your school?" "What drugs do your friends use?" "What drugs do you use?"

School: "Tell me what happens to you on an average day at school." "What is your favorite class?" "What grade are you in at school?" "Who is your favorite teacher?" "What makes him/her so special?" "Is yours a friendly or a not so friendly school?" "Who do you have to talk with if you are having a problem at school?" "What grades do you make?" "What are some of the things that worry you?" "What makes you sad?" "What makes you angry?"

Activities: "What do you like to do for fun?" "Do you play any sports?"

Assessment of the Adolescent Using Parental Report: When is it Appropriate?

Parental report to assess the health and well-being of the adolescent **during health supervision visits** is most appropriate during the early-adolescent period (ages 11-14); by middle adolescence (15-17), many adolescents may see the healthcare clinician without the parent present (**Note:** Issues of patient confidentiality are increasingly important as the child transitions from being a minor to being independent)

Family: "Have their been any major changes or stresses in your family since your last visit?" "How does (name) get along with his siblings?" "How are things going in the family?" "What are some of the things you do together as a family?"

Friends: "Does (name) have friends she likes to spend time with?" "What sorts of things do they do together?"

Dating/Drugs: "Has (name) started dating?" "What has (name) been taught at home or in school about sex (about drugs)?" "Do you think that smoking, drinking, or using drugs is a problem for anyone in your family?"

School: "How is (name) attendance at school?" "Does (name) seem to be able to follow the rules at school?" "Do you participate in school activities?" "Have you visited (name) classroom?"

Activities: "How does (name) spend her time outside of school (on weekends)?" "How much time does (name) spend watching television, on the internet, playing video/computer games each day?" "Does (name) participate in organized sports?" "Do you go to the games?"

D. Physical Examination

1. Measure height and weight; using the new CDC growth charts based on age and gender (body mass index-for-age percentiles), calculate the BMI to determine if weight is in healthy range; growth charts are available at http://www.cdc.gov/growthcharts; measure blood pressure at each visit; any child whose BMI is outside the healthy range requires further evaluation (see *Indicators for Height and Weight Status for Children and Adolescents* under VI.D. above)

2. Head-to-toe examination should be completed on each visit during this age period

   a. Pap smear screening should begin within 3 years of onset of sexual activity or age 21, whichever comes first

   b. Screening for chlamydial infection is outlined below

Screening for Chlamydial Infection

The US Preventive Services Task Force (USPSTF) strongly recommends that clinicians routinely screen all sexually active women aged 25 and younger, and other asymptomatic women at increased risk for infection, for chlamydial infection (**Note:** Adolescents through age 20 are at **highest risk** for infection)

Optimal interval for screening is uncertain

✓ Women with a previous negative screening test should be evaluated for re-screening based on sexual activity (change in sexual partner)
✓ Women with previous positive screening test should be re-screened at 6 to 12 months because of high rates of reinfection
✓ Screening of high-risk young men is a clinical option
✓ See SEXUALLY TRANSMITTED DISEASES chapter for management of patients who test positive for chlamydial infection

---

3. Always look for evidence of abuse
4. As part of the complete physical examination, Tanner staging or Sexual Maturity Rating (SMR) should be completed to determine adolescent's pubertal development
5. In males, evaluate for gynecomastia and examine for hernias
6. Vision and hearing screening should be completed at each visit during this time period with subjective testing alternating each year with objective testing

E. Diagnostic Tests
1. Urinalysis for all males and females, once between ages 11-21 (16 years is the preferred age) [AAP]; in addition, all sexually active male and female adolescents should have an **annual** dipstick urinalysis for leukocytes
2. Hematocrit or hemoglobin for all menstruating females should be performed annually [AAP]
3. Recommended tests for screening for chlamydial infection (using endocervical specimens) include antigen-detection tests such as direct fluorescent antibody (DFA) assay and enzyme immunoassay (EIA) as well as newer technologies based on amplified DNA assays (polymerase chain reaction [PCR]), ligase chain reaction (LCR), and others
4. High risk adolescents may need additional screening; see the AAP's (2000) *Recommendations for Preventive Pediatric Health Care* (see reference list)

F. Immunizations: See RECOMMENDED CHILDHOOD IMMUNIZATION SCHEDULE on page 28

G. Supplements: See FLUORIDE SUPPLEMENTATION RECOMMENDATIONS table on page 9 for adolescents ≤16 years of age. Adolescents who do not get regular sunlight exposure or do not consume at least 500 mL of vitamin D fortified milk per day require a daily multivitamin supplement of 200 IU of vitamin D In addition, all females of childbearing age should receive a multivitamin with folic acid each day

H. Anticipatory Guidance

Promotion of Healthy and Safe Habits: Advise adolescent as follows

✓ Try to get 8 hours of sleep every night
✓ Engage in moderately strenuous physical activity for 60 minutes each day; encourage family and friends to be physically active
✓ Use the three strategies for sun protection (sun avoidance, use of protective clothing, and use of sunscreen) [see the section on SKIN CARE, INSECT BITE PROTECTION, AND SUN EXPOSURE PROTECTION FOR CHILDREN for more specific counseling]
✓ Limit TV viewing, computer and video games to 2 hours per day
✓ Learn ways to manage your activities
✓ Identify a supportive adult who can give you accurate information about sex
✓ Delay having sex until you and your partner are mature enough to assume responsibility for sexual relations
✓ Learn about contraception, use of condoms, and emergency contraception if you and your partner decide to have sex

---

Injury and Violence Prevention: Advise adolescent regarding the following

To Prevent Motor Vehicle Crashes/Other Machine-Related Injuries:
✓ Wear a lap and shoulder belt in the car (**Accident**s are the leading cause of death in this age group, with deaths from motor vehicle crashes the leading cause of accidental death). Teens should be warned against riding in the cargo bed of a pickup truck
✓ Never drink alcohol while driving and never ride with anyone who has been drinking
✓ Always wear a helmet when riding a motorcycle, ATV, or bicycle
To Prevent Burn Injuries:
✓ Test the smoke detector (or ask parent to) frequently and change battery once a year
✓ Continue to have fire drills at home
✓ Do not smoke
To Prevent Accidental Ingestion/Poisoning:
✓ Do not use drugs of any kind (most deaths from accidental poisoning occur in young adult males)
✓ Do not drink alcohol until legal age in state is reached and then only in moderation (males, no more than 2 drinks/day and females, no more than 1 drink/day)
To Prevent Drowning:
✓ Learn how to swim
✓ Do not drink alcohol or use drugs when boating or swimming
✓ Always wear a life vest when boating
To Prevent Injury from Falls:
✓ Wear appropriate safety gear at work and follow job safety procedures
✓ Make certain that helmet is worn when biking
✓ Wear protective sports gear such as mouth guard, face protector, or helmet when engaged in contact sports
To Prevent Other Injuries:
✓ Avoid high noise levels, particularly in music headsets
✓ Do not carry or use a weapon of any kind (**Note**: Homicide is the 2nd leading cause of death in the 15-24 year old age group!)
✓ Learn techniques to protect yourself from physical, emotional, sexual abuse, including rape by either strangers or acquaintances
Develop skills in conflict resolution, negotiation, and dealing with anger constructively
✓ Use care in interacting with strangers
✓ Avoid gangs and peers involved in unlawful activity

Nutrition: See CHILD AND ADOLESCENT NUTRITION

Oral Health: Advise adolescent as follows

- ✓ Brush teeth twice a day with pea-size amount of fluoridated toothpaste, and floss daily
- ✓ Schedule a dental appointment every six months
- ✓ Ask the dentist how best to handle dental emergencies such as loss or fracture of tooth
- ✓ Ensure dentist evaluates permanent molars for application of dental sealants
- ✓ Do not smoke or use smokeless tobacco

Promoting Psychosocial Development: Advise adolescent as follows

- ✓ Take on new challenges to increase self-confidence; explore new roles without hurting yourself or others
- ✓ Continue to develop your sense of identity and learning about yourself--what you think, feel, believe in
- ✓ Accept who you are and enjoy both the child and adult in you
- ✓ Talk with a trusted adult or healthcare professional if you are sad or nervous, or feel that your life is not going right (**Note:** Suicide is the 3rd leading cause of death in the 15-24 year old age group!)
- ✓ Trust your own feelings as well as listening to the ideas of good friends and adults whose opinions you value
- ✓ Understand the importance of your spiritual and religious needs and try to fulfill them
- ✓ Learn to recognize and deal with stress

Prevention of Substance Use/Abuse: Advise adolescent as follows

- ✓ Do not smoke, use smokeless tobacco, drink alcohol, or use drugs, inhalants, or diet pills
- ✓ If you engage in any of these behaviors, ask for help from a healthcare professional

---

I. Summarize findings at the end of each visit and arrange continuing care
   1. Emphasize the strengths of the adolescent and family
   2. Praise the adolescent's efforts and achievements and commend the parents (if present at the visit) on their efforts to guide and act as role models in the area of health behaviors
   3. Remind the adolescent of your availability for additional care and further confidential discussions
   4. Provide reading materials and resources to promote health and reinforce good health practices; address any concerns
   5. If not done previously, provide information about how to access care (e.g., office hours, after-hours care, telephone counseling, emergency care, and how to call an ambulance)
   6. Schedule the next health supervision visit and briefly describe the content of the next visit

Recommended Childhood and Adolescent Immunization Schedule -- United States, 2003

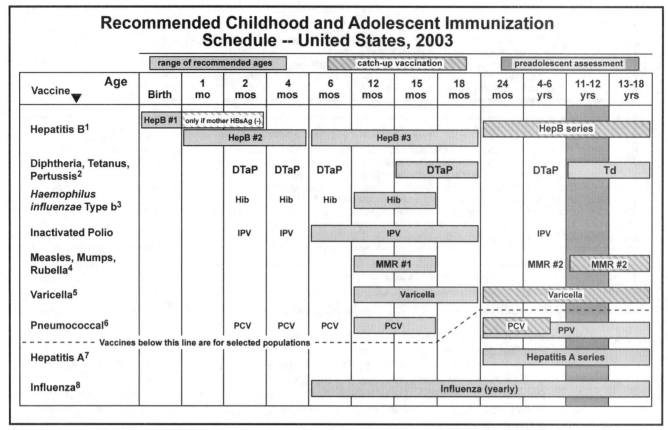

Vaccine ▼ / Age	Birth	1 mo	2 mos	4 mos	6 mos	12 mos	15 mos	18 mos	24 mos	4-6 yrs	11-12 yrs	13-18 yrs
			range of recommended ages				catch-up vaccination				preadolescent assessment	
Hepatitis B[1]	HepB #1	only if mother HBsAg (-)									HepB series	
		HepB #2				HepB #3						
Diphtheria, Tetanus, Pertussis[2]			DTaP	DTaP	DTaP		DTaP			DTaP	Td	
Haemophilus influenzae Type b[3]			Hib	Hib	Hib	Hib						
Inactivated Polio			IPV	IPV		IPV				IPV		
Measles, Mumps, Rubella[4]						MMR #1				MMR #2	MMR #2	
Varicella[5]						Varicella					Varicella	
Pneumococcal[6]			PCV	PCV	PCV	PCV				PCV / PPV		
Hepatitis A[7]										Hepatitis A series		
Influenza[8]					Influenza (yearly)							

Vaccines below this line are for selected populations

This schedule indicates the recommended ages for routine administration of currently licensed childhood vaccines, as of December 1, 2002, for children through age 18 years. Any dose not given at the recommended age should be given at any subsequent visit when indicated and feasible. ▨ Indicates age groups that warrant special effort to administer those vaccines not previously given. Additional vaccines may be licensed and recommended during the year. Licensed combination vaccines may be used whenever any components of the combination are indicated and the vaccine's other components are not contraindicated. Providers should consult the manufacturers' package inserts for detailed recommendations.

1. **Hepatitis B vaccine (Hep B).** All infants should receive the first dose of hepatitis B vaccine soon after birth and before hospital discharge; the first dose may also be given by age 2 months if the infant's mother is HBsAg-negative. Only monovalent hepatitis B vaccine can be used for the birth dose. Monovalent or combination vaccine containing Hep B may be used to complete the series. Four doses of vaccine may be administered when a birth dose is given. The second dose should be given at least 4 weeks after the first dose, except for combination vaccines which cannot be administered before age 6 weeks. The third dose should be given at least 16 weeks after the first dose and at least 8 weeks after the second dose. The last dose in the vaccination series (third or fourth dose) should not be administered before age 6 months.
   - *Infants born to HBsAg-positive mothers* should receive hepatitis B vaccine and 0.5 mL hepatitis B immune globulin (HBIG) within 12 hours of birth at separate sites. The second dose is recommended at age 1-2 month period. The last dose in the vaccination series should not be administered before age 6 months. These infants should be tested for HbsAg and anti-HBs at 9-15 months of age.
   - *Infants born to mothers whose HBsAg status is unknown* should receive the first dose of the hepatitis B vaccine series within 12 hours of birth. Maternal blood should be drawn at the time of delivery to determine the mother's HBsAg status; if the HBsAg test is positive, the infant should receive HBIG as soon as possible (no later than age 1 week). The second dose is recommended at age 1-2 months. The last dose in the vaccination series should not be administered before age 6 months.

2. **Diphtheria and tetanus toxoids and acellular pertussis vaccine (DTaP).** The fourth dose of DTaP may be administered as early as age 12 months, provided 6 months have elapsed since the third dose and the child is unlikely to return at age 15-18 months. Tetanus and diphtheria toxoids (Td) is recommended at age 11-12 years if at least 5 years have elapsed since the last dose of tetanus and diphtheria toxoid-containing vaccine. Subsequent routine Td boosters are recommended every 10 years.

3. **Haemophilus influenzae type b (Hib) conjugate vaccine.** Three Hib conjugate vaccines are licensed for infant use. If PRP-OMP (PedvaxHIB® or ComVax® [Merck]) is administered at ages 2 and 4 months, a dose at age 6 months is not required. DTaP/Hib combination products should not be used for primary immunization in infants at ages 2, 4 or 6 months, but can be used as boosters following any Hib vaccine.

4. **Measles, mumps, and rubella vaccine (MMR).** The second dose of MMR is recommended routinely at age 4-6 years but may be administered during any visit, provided at least 4 weeks have elapsed since the first dose and that both doses are administered beginning at or after age 12 months. Those who have not previously received the second dose should complete the schedule by the 11-12 year old visit.

5. **Varicella vaccine.** Varicella vaccine is recommended at any visit at or after age 12 months for susceptible children, i.e. those who lack a reliable history of chickenpox. Susceptible persons aged >13 years should receive two doses, given at least 4 weeks apart.

6. **Pneumococcal vaccine.** The heptavalent **pneumococcal conjugate vaccine (PCV)** is recommended for all children age 2-23 months. It is also recommended for certain children age 24-59 months. **Pneumococcal polysaccharide vaccine (PPV)** is recommended in addition to PCV for certain high-risk groups. See *MMWR* 2000;49(RR-9):1-35.

7. **Hepatitis A vaccine.** Hepatitis A vaccine is recommended for use in selected states and regions, and for certain high-risk groups; consult your local public health authority. See *MMWR* 1999;48(RR-12);1-37.

8. Influenza vaccine. Influenza vaccine is recommended annually for children age ≥6 months with certain risk factors (including but not limited to asthma, cardiac disease, sickle cell disease, HIV, diabetes, and household members of persons in groups at high risk; see *MMWR* 2002; 51(RR-3); 1-31), and can be administered to all others wishing to obtain immunity. In addition, healthy children age 6-23 months are encouraged to receive influenza vaccine if feasible because children in this age group are at substantially increased risk for influenza-related hospitalizations. Children aged ≤12 years should receive vaccine in a dosage appropriate for their age (0.25 mL if age 6-35 months or 0.5 mL if aged ≥3 years). Children aged ≤8 years who are receiving influenza vaccine for the first time should receive two doses separated by at least 4 weeks.

For additional information about vaccines, vaccine supply, and contraindications for immunization, please visit the National Immunization Program Website at www.cdc.gov/nip or call the National Immunization Hotline at 800-232-2522 (English) or 800-232-0233 (Spanish).

Source: American Academy of Pediatrics, Committee on Infectious Diseases. (2003). Recommended childhood immunization schedule—United States, 2003. *Pediatrics, 111*, 212-215. Also available at the National Immunization Program Website at www.cdc.gov/nip

INFANT NUTRITION

I.   The feeding experience

   A.   The process of feeding provides important opportunities for parent-child social interaction; feeding is emotional as well as physical nourishment

   B.   The feeding experience is a good barometer of overall satisfaction in the relationship between infant and parent

II.   Nutrient Requirements

   A.   In infants, the energy requirement includes the energy associated with the deposition of tissues at rates consistent with good health
      1.   Satisfactory growth is a sensitive indicator of whether energy needs are being met
      2.   The energy cost of growth as a percentage of total energy requirement decreases from 35% at one month to 3% at 12 months of age, and remains low until the pubertal growth spurt, at which time it increases to 4%

   B.   Infants double their birth weight by 4-6 months of age, and triple it by 12 months
      1.   At birth, the newborn is about 11% body fat
      2.   Progressive fat deposition in the early months results in a peak in the percentage body weight that is fat at 3-6 months (about 31%) and body fatness subsequently declines to an average 27% at 12 months
      3.   During infancy (and childhood), girls grow slightly slower than boys, and girls have slightly more body fat

   C.   In the first 4-6 months, infants gain 5-7 ounces per week (on average), and 3-5 ounces per week from 6-12 months of age

   D.   Infants increase their length by 50% in the first year; they gain about one inch a month during the first 6 months and then about one-half inch each month from 6-12 months of age

   E.   Growth rates of breastfed and formula-fed infants differ, with breastfed infants growing more rapidly in the first 2-3 months but less rapidly from 3-12 months of age

   F.   Infants who are genetically determined to be tall but who are born short may experience catch-up growth during the first 3-6 months; infants who are genetically determined to be short but who are long at birth tend to maintain the same rate of growth for several months and then experience a deceleration in growth

   G.   Full term infants require 110-120 Cal/kg and 150-180 mL of fluid per kilogram each day; by 12 months, energy requirements decrease to about 100 Cal/kg per day

   H.   Breast milk and infant formulas provide approximately 20 Cal/oz

I. Infants should be fed breast milk exclusively for the first six months of life, continuing to one year or beyond, with the addition of iron-enriched solids at about 6 months of age to complement the breast milk diet; all breastfed infants require supplementation with 200 IU of vitamin D per day supplied as part of a multivitamin preparation until they begin consuming 500 mL/day of vitamin D-fortified milk or formula

J. Nutrient requirements during first 6 months of life can also be met by a commercially prepared formula if the mother is unable or unwilling to breastfeed

III. Breastfeeding

A. Goals of the *Healthy People 2010* initiative relating to breastfeeding are contained in the box below

---

➡ To increase to at least 75% the proportion of mothers who exclusively or partially breastfeed their babies in the early postpartum period
➡ To increase to at least 50% the proportion who continue breastfeeding until their babies are 5 to 6 months old
➡ To increase to at least 25% the proportion who continue breastfeeding until their babies are 12 months of age

Status of Breastfeeding in the US
- As we enter the new millennium, US breastfeeding rates remain well below national goals and healthcare clinician expertise in the area is lacking in many respects
- In the US in 1998, 65% of mothers initiated breastfeeding in-hospital, 29% reported feeding any human milk to their infants at 6 months of age, and 16% were breastfeeding at 1 year
- These rates were less for infants born to minority women

Adapted from the US Department of Health and Human Services. (2000). *Healthy people 2010*. McLean, VA: International Medical Publishing, Inc., p. 16-46, 16-47, 16-48.

B. The benefits of breastfeeding are numerous and this must be communicated to women who are pregnant in an effort to convince them to breastfeed
  1. Experts agree that breast milk is a better source of nutrition than infant formula
  2. Breast milk contains IgA antibodies, which protect against diarrhea, middle ear infections, lower respiratory tract infections, urinary tract infections, and neonatal septicemia
  3. Breastfed infants produce more gamma-interferon, a protein that mobilizes the immune system, when infections do occur
  4. Breastfed infants produce a stronger immune response following immunization for diseases such as tetanus, diphtheria, poliovirus, and type b *Haemophilus influenzae* than do babies who receive formula
  5. In allergy-prone families, infants who are breastfed for 6 months or longer have a much lower risk of developing asthma, dermatitis, and food allergies until age 17
  6. Emphasize that breast milk contains no preservatives, is readily available, and is always the right temperature

C. Composition of human milk is summarized in the box below

Colostrum	Produced during first few days after delivery, provides enzymes that promote gut maturation and facilitate digestion. High in protein mainly due to immunoglobulins and secretory IgA
Fat	✓ Fat is the major single source of energy in the diet of infants exclusively fed human milk; the high intake of fat (55% of energy) and the energy density that it provides to the diet are important in meeting the rapid growth needs during the first 6 months of life ✓ Quality and quantity of fat in breast milk may be nutritionally superior to that in formula ✓ Breast milk contains more saturated fat–an essential nutrient for children under age 2–than does formula ✓ Breast milk also contains short- and medium-chain fatty acids, which are particularly well absorbed, and long-chain fatty acids which some research suggests may be essential to optimal neurological development and which are absent from infant formula ✓ The proportion of energy from dietary fat decreases to 40% of energy during the second 6 months of life when complementary foods, specifically infant cereals, vegetables, and fruits, are added to the diet of the infant
Carbohydrate	Lactose is present in higher concentrations in human milk than in any other mammal
Protein	Human milk has less protein than cow's milk but the protein is much more digestible
Vitamins	Breast milk is rich in vitamins A, C, and E, but low in vitamin D. Thus, breastfed infants require vitamin D supplementation (see p. 5, CHILD HEALTH SUPERVISION, Vitamin and Mineral Supplementation for more information.) Breast milk of vegetarian women may be deficient in vitamins B_6 and B_{12} unless their diet is supplemented with these vitamins
Iron	Breast milk is low in iron, but the iron is so completely utilized that breastfed babies need no iron supplementation until 6 months of age (iron-fortified cereals should be added at 6 months of age)
Fluoride	Breast milk is low in fluoride; however, fluoride supplementation is not recommended for infants under six months of age. Infants over 6 months of age may need fluoride supplements depending on water supply in household

---

D. Feeding schedule
   1. Advise the mother to allow infant to nurse every 2-3 hours during the first weeks, and to decrease the number of feedings according to the infant's signals as the milk supply increases and the infant receives more milk at each feeding
   2. Teach the mother to feed the infant when he/she is hungry; signs of hunger include hand-to-mouth activity, rooting, pre-cry facial grimaces, fussing sounds, and crying (**Note:** Crying is a late sign of hunger that often interferes with good breastfeeding)
   3. Advise the mother that each feeding may take 30 minutes or more
   4. Advise that the infant should nurse on the second side (after the first side is empty) until vigorous sucking subsides
   5. Breastfed infants should have 6-8 wet diapers per day and may produce a soft, seedy, yellow stool after each feeding

E. Supplementary feeding
   1. Advise using either expressed breast milk or formula for occasional supplementary feedings
   2. Discourage offering the infant a bottle after breastfeeding
   3. Encourage breastfeeding throughout at least the first year

F. Resources for breastfeeding information

➡ Huggins, K. (1990). *The Nursing Mother's Companion.* Harvard, MA: Harvard Common Press.

➡ Kitzinger, S. (1998) *Breastfeeding Your Baby.* Westminster, MD: Knopf.

➡ Mohrbacher, N., & Stock, J. (1997). *Breastfeeding Answer Book.* Schaumburg, IL: La Leche League International.

➡ Lawrence, R.A. (1994). *Breastfeeding: A Guide for the Medical Profession.* St. Louis: Mosby

---

IV. Formula feeding

A. Examples of commercially prepared formulas are Enfamil, Similac, and SMA. **Only iron-fortified formulas should be used!**
   1. Teach the mother to feed the infant when he/she is hungry; signs of hunger include hand-to-mouth activity, rooting, pre-cry facial grimaces, fussing sounds, and crying
   2. When using the iron-fortified versions of commercially prepared formula, no vitamin, mineral, or water supplementation are needed
   3. Formulas come in 3 forms: powder, liquid concentrate, and ready-to-feed
   4. Ready-to-feed is most expensive; powder is least expensive, but the hardest of the 3 to prepare
   5. Instruct mother about preparation and refrigeration of formula
   6. Formula taken from refrigerator does not need to be warmed before feeding
   7. Warn against warming formula in microwave which can result in esophageal burns due to overheating
   8. Bottle-fed infants should have 6-8 wet diapers per day and stools are typically tan to yellow in color, and are about the same consistency as peanut butter; may be less frequent than in breastfed infants
   9. Caution parent to use formula only—whole cow's milk should not be used in infants <1 year old

B. Feeding schedule: The following pattern is usually established:

Age (months)	Number of Feedings/Day (24 hours)	Ounces/Feeding
Birth-1	6-8	2-4
2-6	5-6	5-7
7-10	3-4	8
11-12	3-4	8

V. Introduction of complementary foods

A. Should be based on readiness of infant and **not before** 4 to 6 months of age; there is no nutritional advantage to introducing complementary foods before the infant is developmentally ready which for most infants is no earlier than 6 months of age

6 months	Cereals and fruits
7 months	Meats and vegetables
7-8 months	Egg yolks
8-9 months	Egg whites

B. Counseling relating to feeding solid foods to the infants should emphasize the following

→ Introduce one food at a time, allowing the infant time to express acceptance or rejection of that food before introducing another; gradual introduction of a variety of foods contributes to a balanced diet and helps to promote healthy eating behaviors

→ Offer iron-fortified, single-grain infant cereals (e.g., rice cereal) as the first solid food, because they are least likely to case an allergic reaction

→ Gradually introduce pureed fruits, vegetables, meats, and eggs

→ Talk to the infant during feedings; babies learn to associate feeding with pleasant social interaction

→ If the infant does not like a new food, he/she should not be forced to eat it; instead offer it again in a few weeks

→ Infants do not need salt, spices, or sugar added to their food; these are all acquired tastes that should be discouraged in the infant

→ Once the infant has mastered the art of eating solid foods (at around 7-8 months of age), finger foods can be offered (oat cereal such as Cheerios, small cubes of banana or other soft fruit)

→ With the introduction of solid foods with higher renal solute, the infant should be offered water during the day to supplement the water contained in breast milk/formula

→ Do not add cereal to bottles, and do not use "baby food nurser kits" which allow solid food to filter through the bottle nipple along with the liquid

→ No honey should be added to food, water, or infant formula because it can be a source of spores that cause botulism

C. Intake from formula or breast milk between 6-12 months or age should be no more than 28-32 oz/day

D. Once infant reaches 1 year, whole cow's milk may be given; reduced-fat milk should never be given to children <2 years of age

E. Fruit juice is unnecessary and need not be introduced before 6 months of age; intake should be limited to 1-2 ounces per day. Juice should not be used to quench thirst; encourage parent to offer infant water several times a day once solids are added at 6 months of age
   1. Remind parent to offer juice in cup only, not in bottle; prolonged exposure of the teeth to sugars is associated with dental caries
   2. Fruit juice should not replace breast milk or infant formula in the diet because it is high in carbohydrate and low in the other nutrients (compared with milk)
   3. Encourage parent to give infant mashed or pureed fruit instead of juice

F. Suggested readings relating to nutrition during childhood are contained at the end of the next section– CHILD AND ADOLESCENT NUTRITION

CHILD AND ADOLESCENT NUTRITION

I. Goals of nutrition are (1) to attain intakes of sufficient levels of essential dietary nutrients; (2) to consume a diet associated with reduced risk of chronic disease, and; (3) to maintain a balance between energy intake and physical activity

A. In children and adolescents, satisfactory growth is a sensitive indicator of whether energy needs are being met
   1. During childhood, girls grow slightly slower than boys, and girls have slightly more body fat
   2. During adolescence, gender differences in body composition are accentuated
      a. Growth in boys is characterized by the rapid attainment of fat-free mass and a modest increase in fat mass, followed by a decline; attainment of fat-free mass coincides with the rapid spurt in stature
      b. Adolescence in girls is characterized by modest increases in fat-free mass and a continual accumulation of fat mass; the pubertal increase in fat-free mass ceases at about 18 years of age, along with a decrease in the rate of gain in stature after menarche

B. During infancy and childhood, serial measurements over time of weight and stature provide an index of the child's **pattern** of growth; measurement at a single point in time provides some clinical information but growth pattern cannot be assessed

1. The 2000 CDC growth charts include a set of curves for infants (birth to 36 months), and a set for children and adolescents, 2 to 20 years of age
2. Infant growth charts consist of curves for weight-for-age, length-for-age, head circumference-for-age, and weight-for-length
3. Growth charts for children and adolescents include weight-for-age, stature-for-age, and body mass index (BMI)-for-age (growth charts available at www.cdc.gov/growthcharts)
4. In most children who are growing normally, height and weight measurements fall within two standard percentile lines of each other; children whose measurements are either above the 95th percentile or below the 5th percentile, or whose height and weight differ by more than two percentile lines require further evaluation

C. Indicators of stature and weight status for children and adolescents are contained in the box below

Indicator	Anthropometric Variable	Cut-Off Values
Stunting	Stature-for-age	<3rd percentile
Thinness	BMI-for-age	<5th percentile
At risk for overweight	BMI-for-age	≥85th percentile, but <95th percentile
Overweight	BMI-for-age	≥95th percentile

Source: Story, M., Holt, K., & Sofka, D. (2002). *Bright futures in practice: Nutrition.* Arlington, VA: National Center for Education in Maternal and Child Health, p. 95.

D. Childhood obesity has reached epidemic proportions; in 2000, 22% of preschool children were overweight and 10% were obese, making obesity the most serious and prevalent nutritional disorder in the US

II. The Food and Nutrition Board, Institute of Medicine, The National Academies, recently set forth reference values for specific nutrients with the development of Dietary Reference Intakes (DRIs), the collective term for four categories subsumed under the DRIs

A. DRIs have been established using an expanded concept that includes indicators of good health and the prevention of chronic disease, as well as possible effects of overconsumption

B. Thus, DRIs provide a more comprehensive approach to nutrition adequacy than the periodic reports called Recommended Dietary Allowances (RDAs) [now one of 4 categories encompassed by DRIs] set forth by the Food and Nutrition Board for over 50 years

C. DRI categories are defined in the table below

DIETARY REFERENCE INTAKES

➡ Recommended Dietary Allowance (RDA): The average daily dietary nutrient intake level sufficient to meet nutrient requirement of nearly all (97 to 98%) healthy individuals in a particular life stage and gender group

➡ Adequate Intake (AI): The recommended average daily intake level based on observed or experimentally determined estimates of nutrient intakes by a group of healthy people that are assumed to be adequate–used when an RDA cannot be determined

➡ Tolerable Upper Intake Level (UL): The highest average daily nutrient intake level that is likely to pose no risk of adverse effects to almost all individuals in a general population

➡ Estimated Average Requirement (EAR): The average daily nutrient intake level estimated to meet the requirements of half the healthy individuals in a particular life stage and gender group*

---

*In the case of energy, an Estimated Energy Requirement (EER) is provided; it is the average dietary energy intake that is predicted to maintain energy balance in a healthy adult of a defined age, gender, weight, height, and level of physical activity consistent with good health

Adapted from Institute of Medicine, Food and Nutrition Board, The National Academies. (2002). *Dietary reference intakes: Energy, carbohydrate, fiber, fat, fatty acids, cholesterol, protein, and amino acids, part 2.* (Prepublication copy, unedited proofs). Washington, DC: National Academies Press.

III.   Energy is required to sustain the body's various functions, including respiration, circulation, physical work, and protein synthesis; carbohydrates, proteins, and fats in the diet supply the energy

   A.   Carbohydrates (sugars and starches) provide energy to cells in the body, particularly the brain which is the only carbohydrate-dependent organ in the body
      1.   RDA for carbohydrate is set at 130 g/day for adolescents and children >1 year of age based on the average minimum amount of glucose utilized by the brain (this level is typically exceeded to meet the energy needs while consuming acceptable levels of fat and protein)
      2.   The median intake of carbohydrates is approximately 200 to 330 g/day for males and 180 to 230 g/day for females
      3.   Because of a lack of sufficient evidence on the prevention of chronic diseases in generally healthy individuals, no recommendations based on glycemic index of carbohydrate-containing foods are made (see section on DIABETES MELLITUS for more information on the glycemic index)
      4.   The current Food Pyramid–the food guide for the US–will be revised in 2004; some experts believe that the glycemic index (a quantification of the relative blood glucose response to carbohydrate containing foods) will be an important consideration in the placement of food groups within the new pyramid

   B.   Fats are a major source of fuel energy for the body and aid in the absorption of fat-soluble vitamins and other food components such as carotenoids
      1.   AI for infants 0-6 months and 6-12 months of age is set at 31 g/day and 30 g/day, respectively
      2.   For children >1 year and adolescents, neither AI nor RDA for fat has been set as there are insufficient data to determine a defined level of fat intake at which risk of inadequacy or prevention of chronic disease occurs (Acceptable Macronutrient Distribution Ranges [AMDRs], however, have been estimated for total fat and are contained in the box below)
      3.   Saturated fatty acids, monounsaturated fatty acids, and cholesterol are synthesized by the body and are not required in the diet

   C.   Proteins form the major structural components of all the cells of the body; along with amino acids (dietary components of protein), they function as enzymes, membrane carriers, and hormones; nine amino acids are indispensable and thus dietary sources must be provided. RDAs for children >6 months of age through adolescence vary by age and by gender (in adolescence)

   D.   Because carbohydrate, fat, and protein all serve as energy sources and can substitute for one another to some extent to meet caloric needs, the recommended ranges for consuming these nutrients should be useful and flexible for dietary planning; ranges for fat, carbohydrate, and protein illustrate the principle that these nutrients must be considered together

   E.   The Acceptable Macronutrient Distribution Ranges (AMDRs) for children and adolescents are estimated and represented as percent of energy intake
      1.   These ranges represent the following: Intakes that are associated with reduced risk of chronic disease; intakes at which essential dietary nutrients can be consumed at sufficient levels, and intakes based on adequate energy intake and physical activity to maintain energy balance
      2.   The AMDRs are contained in the box below

	Fat	Carbohydrate	Protein
Children 1-3 years	30-40%	45-65%	5-20%
Children 4-18 years	25-35%	45-65%	10-30%
Adults	20-35%	45-65%	10-35%

Adapted from Institute of Medicine, Food and Nutrition Board, The National Academies. (2002). *Dietary reference intakes: Energy, carbohydrate, fiber, fat, fatty acids, cholesterol, protein, and amino acids, part 2.* (Prepublication copy, unedited proofs). Washington, DC: National Academies Press.

IV.   The Food Guide Pyramid, which is the food guide for the US, translates recommendations on nutrient intake into recommendations for food intakes

   A.   Encourage patients/parents to use the Food Guide Pyramid to guide their food choices
      1.   Remind patients/parents to use plant foods as the foundation of meals
      2.   Whereas there are many ways to create a healthy eating pattern, they all start with the three food groups at the base of the pyramid–grains, fruits, and vegetables

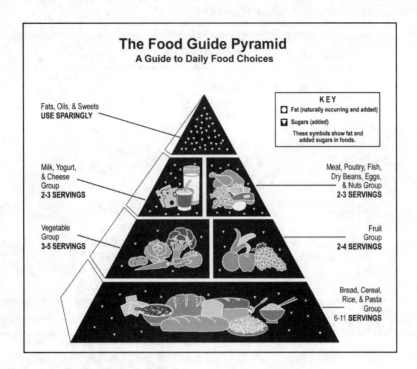

Figure 1.3. Food Guide Pyramid –Children ≥6 Years and Adolescents
Source: US Department of Agriculture/US Department of Health and Human Services. (2000). *Nutrition and your health: Dietary guidelines for Americans.* Washington, DC: Author, p. 15.

B.   The Food Guide Pyramid for Young Children was developed as a mechanism to influence the dietary intake of children ages 2-6. The basic nutritional advice is the same as the Food Guide Pyramid but it has been made more relevant for children by the use of shorter food-group names and single numbers rather than ranges to indicate the recommended daily servings. In addition, illustrations of young children playing around the pyramid are designed to send the message that physical activity is important

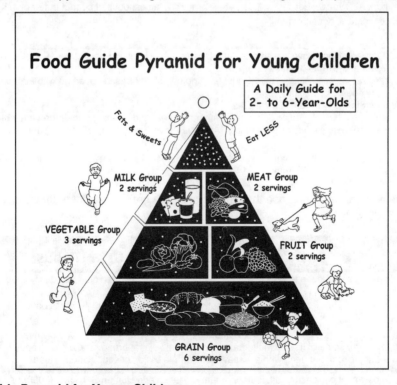

Figure 1.4. Food Guide Pyramid for Young Children
Adapted from: US Department of Agriculture/Center for Nutrition Policy and Promotion. (1999). Tips for using the Food Guide Pyramid for young children 2-6 years old. Washington, DC: Author.

C.   The recommended ranges of daily servings from each of the five major food groups for both genders and all age groups are contained in the tables below

HOW MANY SERVINGS ARE NEEDED EACH DAY?			
Food Group	Children ages 2-6 years, women, some older adults (about 1,600 calories)	Older children, teen girls, active women, most men (about 2,200 calories)	Teen boys, active men (about 2,800 calories)
Grains Group: Bread, cereal, rice and pasta group – especially whole grain	6	9	11
Vegetable Group	3	4	5
Fruit Group	2	3	4
Milk Group: Milk, yogurt, and cheese – preferably fat free or low fat	2 or 3*	2 or 3*	2 or 3*
Meat and Beans Group: Meat, poultry, fish, dry beans, eggs and nuts – preferably lean or low fat	2, for a total of 5 ounces	2, for a total of 6 ounces	3, for a total of 7 ounces

* The number of servings depends on one's age. Older children and teenagers (ages 9-18 years) and adults >50 years need 3 servings daily. Others need 2 servings daily. During pregnancy and lactation, the recommended number of milk group servings is the same as for nonpregnant women

WHAT COUNTS AS A SERVING?	

Grains Group: Bread, Cereal, Rice and Pasta – whole grain and refined:
- 1 slice of bread
- About 1 cup of ready-to-eat cereal
- 1/2 cup of cooked cereal, rice, or pasta

Vegetable Group:
- 1 cup of raw leafy vegetables
- 1/2 cup of other vegetables – cooked or raw
- 3/4 cup of vegetable juice

Fruit Group:
- 1 medium apple, banana, orange, pear
- 1/2 cup of chopped, cooked, or canned fruit
- 3/4 cup of fruit juice

Milk Group:* Milk, Yogurt and Cheese:
- 1 cup milk** or yogurt**
- 1 ½ ounces of natural cheese** (such as Cheddar)
- 2 ounces of processed cheese** (such as American)

Meat and Beans Group: Meat, Poultry, Dry Beans, Eggs, and Nuts:
- 2-3 ounces of cooked lean meat, poultry, or fish
- 1/2 cup of cooked dry beans# or 1/2 cup of tofu counts as 1 ounce of lean meat
- 2 ½-ounce soyburger or 1 egg counts as 1 ounce of lean meat
- 2 tablespoons of peanut butter or 1/3 cup of nuts counts as 1 ounce of meat

Note: Many of the serving sizes given above are smaller than those on the Nutrition Facts Label. For example, 1 serving of cooked cereal, rice, or pasta is 1 cup for the label but only ½ cup for the Pyramid
* This includes lactose-free and lactose-reduced milk products. One cup of soy-based beverage with added calcium is an option for those who prefer a non-dairy source of calcium
** Choose fat-free or reduced-fat dairy products most often
# Dry beans, peas, and lentils can be counted as servings in either the meat and beans group or the vegetable group. As a vegetable, ½ cup of cooked, dry beans counts as 1 serving. As a meat substitute, 1 cup of cooked, dry beans counts as 1 serving (2 ounces of meat)

Source: US Department of Agriculture/US Department of Health and Human Services. (2000). *Nutrition and your health: Dietary guidelines for Americans.* Washington, DC: Author, p. 14-15.

D.   Assist patients/parents to increase their intake of whole grain foods by recommending liberal use of the foods in the table below

WAYS TO INCREASE INTAKE OF WHOLE GRAIN FOODS		

Counsel patients/parents to choose foods that name one of the following ingredients first on the label's ingredient list

• Brown rice	• Oatmeal	• Whole oats
• Bulgur (cracked wheat)	• Popcorn	• Whole rye
• Graham flour	• Pearl barley	• Whole wheat

Encourage patients to try some of these whole grain foods: whole wheat bread, whole grain ready-to-eat cereal, low-fat whole wheat crackers, oatmeal, whole wheat pasta, whole barley in soup, tabouli salad

Adapted from US Department of Agriculture/US Department of Health and Human Services. (2000). *Nutrition and your health: Dietary guidelines for Americans.* Washington, DC: Author, p. 20.

E. Consuming a variety of fruits and vegetables each day provides essential vitamins, minerals, fiber, and other substances that are important to good health (most people eat fewer servings of fruits and vegetables than are recommended); assist patients/parents to select a variety of fruits and vegetables such as those featured in the box below

---

Which Fruits and Vegetables Provide the Most Nutrients?

Sources of vitamin A (carotenoids)
- Orange vegetables like carrots, sweet potatoes, pumpkin
- Dark-green leafy vegetables such as spinach, collards, turnip greens
- Orange fruits like mango, cantaloupe, apricots
- Tomatoes

Sources of vitamin C
- Citrus fruits and juices, kiwi fruit, strawberries, cantaloupe
- Broccoli, peppers, tomatoes, cabbage, potatoes
- Leafy greens such as romaine lettuce, turnip greens, spinach

Sources of folate
- Cooked dry beans and peas, peanuts
- Oranges, orange juice
- Dark-green leafy vegetables like spinach and mustard greens, romaine lettuce
- Green peas

Sources of potassium
- Baked white or sweet potato, cooked greens (such as spinach), winter (orange) squash
- Bananas, plantains, dried fruits such as apricots and prunes, orange juice
- Cooked dry beans (such as baked beans) and lentils

Adapted from US Department of Agriculture/US Department of Health and Human Services. (2000). *Nutrition and your health: Dietary guidelines for Americans.* Washington, DC: Author, p. 22.

F. Growing children and teenagers have higher needs for some minerals, specifically calcium and iron
    1. Adolescents have an especially high need for calcium (most people need to eat plenty of good sources of calcium for healthy bones throughout life); see the box below for some sources of calcium to recommend to patients and parents of young children
    2. Young children and teenage girls need enough good sources of iron; see the box below for recommendations

---

Some Sources of Calcium	Some Sources of Iron
• Yogurt	• Shellfish like shrimp, clams, mussels, and oysters
• Milk	• Lean meats (especially beef), liver, and other organ meats
• Natural cheeses such as Mozzarella, Cheddar, Swiss, and Parmesan	• Ready-to-eat cereals with added iron
• Soy-based beverage with added calcium	• Turkey dark meat (remove skin to reduce fat)
• Tofu, if made with calcium sulfate (read the ingredient list)	• Sardines
• Breakfast cereal with added calcium	• Spinach
• Canned fish with soft bones such as salmon, sardines	• Cooked dry beans (such as kidney beans and pinto beans), peas (such as black-eyed peas), and lentils
• Fruit juice with added calcium	• Enriched and whole grain breads
• Dark-green leafy vegetables such as collards, turnip greens	

Adapted from US Department of Agriculture/US Department of Health and Human Services. (2000). *Nutrition and your health: Dietary guidelines for Americans.* Washington, DC: Author, p. 17.

G. Encourage patients/parents to choose a diet that is low in saturated fat and cholesterol and within the AMDR range (see above) for children and adolescents; use recommendations based on content in boxes below to counsel patients
    1. Many experts believe that there should be a differentiation between the types of fats rather than lumping them together and placing them at the pinnacle of the Food Pyramid in the "use sparingly" category
    2. Revisions of the Food Pyramid are expected in 2004; unsaturated fats (from plant sources and some fish) may be removed from the "use sparingly" category and placed closer to the base in the new pyramid
    3. Replacing dietary fat with foods that are high in calories from sugar and other refined carbohydrates does not protect against obesity
    4. In fact, the decrease in fat intake and increase in consumption of refined carbohydrates that occurred in the US between 1977 and 1995 coincided with an 85% increase in obesity prevalence

Different Types of Fats

Saturated Fats
Foods high in saturated fats tend to raise blood cholesterol. These foods include high-fat dairy products (like cheese, whole milk, cream, butter, and regular ice cream), fatty fresh and processed meats, the skin and fat of poultry, lard, palm oil, and coconut oil. Intake of these foods should be kept low

Dietary Cholesterol
Foods that are high in cholesterol also tend to raise blood cholesterol—examples are liver and other organ meats, egg yolks, and dairy fats

Trans Fatty Acids
Foods high in *trans* fatty acids increase total and LDL cholesterol concentrations in the blood and therefore the risk of CHD; even very low intakes may increase risk. These foods include those high in partially hydrogenated vegetable oils, such as many hard margarines and shortenings. Foods with a high amount of these ingredients include many commercially fried foods and bakery goods (**Note**: The FDA recently mandated that *trans* fat [also known as *trans* fatty acids] be included on the Nutrition Facts Panel on food labels; it will be listed on a separate line from saturated fat on the nutrition label)

Unsaturated Fats
- Unsaturated fats (oils) do not raise blood cholesterol. Unsaturated fats occur in vegetable oils, most nuts, olives, avocados, and fatty fish like salmon. Unsaturated oils include both *monounsaturated fats* and *polyunsaturated fats*. Olive, canola, sunflower, and peanut oils are some of the oils high in monounsaturated fats. Vegetable oils such as soybean oil, corn oil, and cottonseed oil and many kinds of nuts are good sources of polyunsaturated fats

- Current dietary guidelines recommend consumption of fish high in omega-3 fatty acids twice weekly to prevent coronary heart disease. Good fish sources of omega-3s include salmon, bluefish, mackerel, arctic char, and sardines. For convenience, canned salmon, sardines, and herring can also be used as these products also contain high amounts of omega-3s (canned tuna contains lesser amounts)

- For an added bonus of calcium, encourage patients to eat the bones in canned sardines, salmon, and mackerel (bones are softened during cooking). For patients on salt-restricted diets, remind them that canned fish has ten times the amount of sodium as fresh fish and draining and rinsing fish in colander removes only a fair amount of salt

Food Choices Low in Saturated Fat and Cholesterol and Moderate in Total Fat
Advise patients to get most of their calories from plant foods (grains, fruits, vegetables). Counsel patients as follows:

Fats and Oils
- Choose vegetable oils rather than solid fats (meat and dairy fats, shortening)
- Decrease the amount of fat you use in cooking and at the table

Meat, Poultry, Fish, Shellfish, Eggs, Beans, and Nuts
- Choose 2-3 servings of fish, shellfish, lean poultry, other lean meats, beans or nuts daily. Trim fat from meat and take skin off poultry. Choose dry beans, peas, or lentils often
- Limit intake of high-fat processed meats such as bacon, sausages, salami, bologna, and other cold cuts. Try the lower fat varieties (check the Nutrition Facts Label)
- Limit intake of liver and other organ meats. Use egg yolks and whole eggs in moderation. Use egg whites and egg substitutes freely when cooking since they contain no cholesterol and little or no fat

Dairy Products
- Choose fat-free or low-fat milk, fat-free or low-fat yogurt, and low-fat cheese most often. Try switching from whole to fat-free or low-fat milk. This decreases the saturated fat and calories but keeps all other nutrients the same

Prepared Foods
- Check the Nutrition Facts Label to see how much saturated fat and cholesterol are in a serving of prepared food. Choose foods lower in saturated fat, cholesterol, and trans fats

Foods at Restaurants or Other Eating Establishments
- Choose fish or lean meats as suggested above. Limit ground meat and fatty processed meats, marbled steaks, and cheese
- Limit intake of foods with creamy sauces, and add little or no butter to food
- Choose fruit as dessert most often

Adapted from US Department of Agriculture/US Department of Health and Human Services. (2000). *Nutrition and your health: Dietary guidelines for Americans*. Washington, DC: Author, p. 28-29.

H. The Institute of Medicine has recently developed definitions for fiber (Dietary, Functional, and Total Fiber) and established Adequate Intakes (AI) for Total Fiber
1. Dietary Fiber is defined as nondigestible food plant carbohydrates and lignin (polymer found within "woody" plant walls) in which the plant matrix is largely intact; such sources of fiber also contain macronutrients (e.g., carbohydrate and protein such as in cereal brans) normally found in foods
2. Functional Fiber consists of isolated, nondigestible carbohydrates that have beneficial physiological effects in humans; included in this category are animal-derived carbohydrates such as connective tissue that are generally regarded as nondigestible
3. Total Fiber is the sum of Dietary and Functional Fibers
4. Benefits of fiber as well as the AI recommendations for Total Fiber are contained in the box below

---

Benefits of Fiber and Adequate Intake (AI) for Total Fiber

- Viscous fibers delay the gastric emptying of ingested foods into small intestine, which can result in a sensation of fullness (satiety)
- Delayed emptying effect also results in reduced postprandial blood glucose concentrations
- Viscous fibers can also interfere with the absorption of dietary fat and cholesterol as well as the enterohepatic recirculation of cholesterol and bile acids, which may result in reduced blood cholesterol concentrations
- Consumption of dietary and certain functional fibers, particularly those that are poorly fermented, is known to improve fecal bulk, laxation, and ameliorate constipation
- Relationship of fiber intake to colon cancer is the subject of ongoing investigation

---

Adapted from Institute of Medicine, Food and Nutrition Board, The National Academies. (2002). *Dietary reference intakes: Energy, carbohydrate, fiber, fat, fatty acids, cholesterol, protein, and amino acids, part 1.* (Prepublication copy, unedited proofs). Washington, DC: National Academies Press, p. 7-1.

Total Fiber AI Recommendations for Children, Adolescents and Adults

Group *Children*	Adequate Intake	Group *Adolescent males*	Adequate Intake
1-3 years	19 g/day		
4-8 years	25 g/day	19-21 years	38 g/day
Boys			
9-13 years	31 g/day	*Adolescent females*	
14-18 years	38 g/day		
Girls		19-21 years	25 g/day
9-18 years	26 g/day		

Adapted from Institute of Medicine, Food and Nutrition Board, The National Academies. (2002). *Dietary reference intakes: Energy, carbohydrate, fiber, fat, fatty acids, cholesterol, protein, and amino acids, part 1.* (Prepublication copy, unedited proofs). Washington, DC: National Academies Press, p. 7-36, 7-38.

I.   Help patients/parents select foods high in fiber from examples in the box below

---

Bulking Up on Fiber: Advise patients as follows:

Keep beans handy–probably the best source of fiber
- Cook a package of dried beans and freeze in usable quantities
- Canned beans are also a good source
- B & M Baked Beans Vegetarian (½ c = 7 g)
- Kidney beans, red (1 c = 13.1 g)
- Lima beans (½ c = 6.6 g)

Look for "100% whole wheat" of "whole-grain bread"
- Aim for bread with 2 or 3 g of fiber per slice

Choose high-fiber breakfast cereals
- Kellogg's Raisin Bran (1 c = 8 g) or Post 100% Bran (1/3 c = 8 g)
- For patients who don't like the high-fiber brands, suggest they mix some high-fiber brands with their preferred cereal each morning

Eat berries, a great source of fiber (1 c blueberries = 3.9 g)

Instead of drinking juice, eat the orange, grapefruit, or tomato

Eat fruits and nuts for snacks
- Medium apple with skin = 3.7 g
- Medium banana = 2.7 g
- Dates, dried (10) = 6.2 g
- Medium orange = 3 g
- Pears, canned/juice pack (1 c = 4 g)
- Prunes, dried (10) = 6 g
- Peanuts, dry roasted (1 oz) = 2.3 g

Vegetables
- Broccoli (½ c = 2.3 g)
- Campbell's Chunky Vegetable Soup (1 c = 4 g)
- Carrots, raw (1 medium = 2.2 g)
- Baked potato with skin (1 medium = 3.4 g)
- Cabbage, red (½ c = 1.5 g)

J.   Added sugars are defined as sugars and syrups added to foods in processing or preparation, not the naturally occurring sugars in foods like fruit and milk

1.   Increased consumption of added sugars can result in decreased intakes of certain micronutrients when energy dense, nutrient-poor foods are chosen

2.   In addition, increased consumption of added sugars contributes to overweight and obesity

3.   Foods containing sugars and starches can promote tooth decay; frequent consumption of sugary foods/beverages between meals is more likely to harm teeth than eating the same foods at meals and then brushing

4.   Naturally occurring sugars are primarily consumed from fruits and dairy products that also contain essential micronutrients

5.   Added sugars are listed on the "Nutrition Facts Label" of foods under "Total Carbohydrate" as "Sugars"

6.   Counsel patients/parents to limit consumption of added sugars in foods and beverages (**Note**: The number one source of added sugars in the US is nondiet soft drinks)

The Rise in Consumption of Added Sugars in US

✓ Consumption of sugar is up by 50% over that of only 50 years ago—consumption of sucrose, the refined white granules made from cane or beets is actually down

✓ What is being overeaten is fructose—not from honey or fruit—but in the form of high-fructose corn syrup (HFCS) which as added to so many foods because it is sweeter, easier to blend with other ingredients, and much cheaper than sucrose. This liquid sweetener—made from corn starch and boosted with fructose via a special manufacturing process—supplies nearly 10% of all calories consumed by Americans with the figure actually closer to 20% for many people, especially children

✓ In addition to the calories that HFCS adds to the diet, the body uses fructose differently than it does other sugars; high levels of HFCS can boost triglycerides and possibly cholesterol and may have a negative effect on the body's ability to use calcium, chromium, and other minerals

K. Counsel patients/parents to choose and prepare foods with less salt
1. Healthy children and adolescents need to consume only small amounts of salt to meet their sodium needs (no more than 2400 mg of sodium per day) [one teaspoon of salt provides about 2,000 mg of sodium]
2. Eating too little salt is not generally a concern for healthy people (lowering salt intake is safe)
3. Explain to patients that their preference for salt may decrease if they gradually add less salt or salty seasonings to food over a period of time
4. Foods that are high in convenience (frozen dinners and carry-out foods) are usually also high in sodium
5. Use information in the box below to counsel patients/parents about ways to decrease salt intake

Ways to Decrease Salt Intake

- Choose fresh, plain frozen, or canned vegetables without added salt most often
- Choose fresh or frozen fish, shellfish, poultry, and lean beef most often
- Read the Nutrition Facts label to compare the amount of sodium in processed foods – such as frozen dinners, packaged mixes, cereals, cheese, breads, soups, salad dressings, and sauces
- Leave the salt shaker in a cupboard

- Look for labels that say "low-sodium." They contain 140 mg (about 5% of the Daily Value) or less of sodium per serving
- If you salt foods in cooking or at the table, add small amounts. Learn to use spices and herbs, rather than salt, to enhance the flavor of food
- Go easy on condiments such as soy sauce, ketchup, mustard, pickles, and olives – they can add a lot of salt to your food

Adapted from US Department of Agriculture/US Department of Health and Human Services. (2000). *Nutrition and your health: Dietary guidelines for Americans*. Washington, DC: Author, p. 33.

VI. Physical inactivity is a major risk factor for development of obesity in children and adolescents

A. *Healthy People 2010* set a goal of a minimum of 30 minutes of moderate intensity physical activity most days of the week but other experts have concluded that 30 minutes per day of moderate activity is insufficient to maintain body weight in the healthy range and to achieve health benefits associated with physical activity

B. The Institute of Medicine (2002) recommends that children and adolescents engage in 60 minutes of daily moderate intensity physical activity, in addition to the activities required by a sedentary lifestyle
1. Maintaining an active lifestyle provides an important means for individuals to balance food energy intake with total energy expenditure
2. Consult the section on OBESITY for specific counseling recommendations relating to physical activity and exercise

VII. Suggested resources relating to nutrition are contained in the box below

---

General Resources

Center for Nutrition Policy and Promotion, USDA
1120 20th Street, NW, Suite 200, North Lobby
Washington, DC 20036
Internet: www.usda.gov/cnpp

Centers for Disease Control and Prevention
1600 Clifton Road
Atlanta, GA 30333
Internet: www.cdc.gov

Food and Drug Administration
200 C Street, SW
Washington, DC 20204
Internet: www.fda.gov

US Department of Agriculture
Document Delivery Services Branch
National Agricultural Library
10301 Baltimore Ave., 6th Floor
Beltsville, MD 20705-2351
301-504-5755
http://www.nal.usda.gov/fnic
circinfo@nal.usda.gov

American Cancer Society
1599 Clifton Road, NE
Atlanta, GA 30329
800-ACS-2345
http://www.cancer.org

American Diabetes Association
National Service Center
1660 Duke Street
Alexander, VA 22314
800-232-3472
http://www.diabetes.org

American Heart Association
7272 Greenville Avenue
Dallas, TX 75231
800-AHA-USA-1
http://www.amhrt.org

National Heart, Lung, and Blood Institute (NHLBI)
Information Center
PO Box 30105
Bethesda, MD 20824-0105
800-575-WELL
http://www.nhlbi.nih.gov/nhlbi/nhlbi.htm

healthfinder – Gateway to Reliable Consumer Health
Information
National Health Information Center
US Department of Health and Human Services
PO Box 1133
Washington, DC 20013-1133
Internet: www.healthfinder.gov

Food and Nutrition Information Center
National Agricultural Library, USDA
10301 Baltimore Boulevard, Room 304
Beltsville, MD 20705-2351
Internet: www.nal.usda.gov/fnic

International Food Information Council (IFIC) Foundation
1100 Connecticut Avenue, NW, Suite 430
Washington, DC 20036
http://ificinfo.health.org
E-mail: foodinfo@ific.health.org

Annotated Nutrition Links for Healthcare Professionals
Arbor Nutrition Guide
http://www.arborcom.com

National Cancer Institute
Office of Cancer Communications
31 Center Drive, MSC 2580
Building 31, Room 10A-29
Bethesda, MD 20892-2580
800-4-CANCER
http://cancernet.nci.nih.gov

OncoLink
Sponsor: University of Pennsylvania
http://www.cancer.med.upenn.edu

Vegetarian Resource Group
PO Box 1463
Baltimore, MD 21203
410-366-8343
E-mail: vrg@vrg.org
http://www.vrg.org

VIII. Suggested readings relating to nutrition during childhood and adolescence are contained in the box below

---

- Dietz, W.H. & Stern. L. (1999). *American Academy of Pediatrics Guide to Your Child's Nutrition: Making Peace at the Table and Building Healthy Eating Habits for Life.* New York, NY: Villard Books.
- Goldberg, A.C. (2000). *Feed Your Child Right from Birth Through Teens.* New York, NY: M. Evans & Company.
- Nissenberg, K.K., Bogle, M.I., & Wright, A.C. (1995). *Quick Meals for Healthy Kids and Busy Parents: Wholesome Family Meals in 30 Minutes or Less.* New York, NY: John Wiley & Sons.
- Rockwell, L. (1999). *Good Enough to Eat: A Kid's Guide to Food and Nutrition.* Scranton, PA: HarperCollins.
- Satter, E. (1987). *How to Get Your Kid to Eat . . . But Not Too Much.* Palo Alto, CA: Bull Publishing Company.
- Satter, E. (2000). *Child of Mine: Feeding with Love and Good Sense.* Boulder, CO: Bull Publishing Company.
- Shanley, E, & Thompson, C. (2001*). Fueling the Teen Machine.* Boulder, CO: Bull Publishing Company.
- Schlosser, E. (2002) *Fast Food Nation: The Dark Side of the All-American Meal.* New York: Perennial.
- US Department of Agriculture, Center for Nutrition Policy and Promotion. (1999). *Tips for Using the Food Guide Pyramid for Young Children 2 to 6 Years Old.* Washington, DC.
- Warner, P. (1999). *Healthy Snacks for Kids.* San Leandro, CA: Bristol Publishing Enterprises.
- Wood, C. (1999). *How to Get Kids to Eat Great and Love It!* Torrance, CA: Griffin Publishing Group.

DENTAL HEALTH MAINTENANCE

I.   Tooth preservation is a lifelong process

   A.   Maintaining good oral hygiene is important throughout life because poor oral hygiene can lead to gingival recession, increased tooth mobility, and eventual tooth loss

   B.   Parent may cleanse the gums of infants by wrapping a piece of gauze around her finger and gently rubbing over gums and first teeth

   C.   Generally, children are unable to clean their own teeth before the age of 7-8 years

   D.   Children are susceptible to dental caries and gum disease; factors that increase the risk of developing these oral conditions are the following
      1.   Lack of fluoridation of water supply (most effective when teeth are developing)
      2.   Diet inadequate in essential micronutrients (vitamins and minerals)
      3.   High intake of sugary foods and beverages, especially between meals
      4.   Genetics
      5.   Tobacco use; smokers are 7 times more likely to develop periodontal disease than are nonsmokers and smokeless tobacco is associated with gum recession and root damage

   E.   Healthy teeth and gums are not a given; brushing, flossing, adequate fluoride, and having regular dental checkups are all important components of maintaining oral health

II. Brushing and flossing: Counsel patients as follows regarding brushing and flossing so that they can get the most out of oral hygiene efforts

   A.   Brushing at margin of teeth and gums with a soft-textured, multi-tufted nylon bristle toothbrush is recommended after every meal or at least twice a day; use of a soft-bristled brush helps minimize wear and tear on gums (any soft bristled toothbrush will do—there is no evidence that a brush with rippled or angled bristles, tapered head, or angled handle is more effective than conventional brushes in removing plaque and keeping teeth clean)
      1.   Recommend placing brush on gumline at a 45° angle, and then brushing gums and teeth with an elliptical motion; proper brushing can disrupt or remove plaque from teeth and from the gingival sulcus groove between gums and teeth
      2.   Recommend that patient also lightly brush tongue, especially at the back, to remove additional bacteria from mouth
      3.   Stress that thoroughness, rather than vigor, is the key
      4.   Toothbrushes should be replaced every 3-4 months, or when the bristles become worn, bent, or frayed
      5.   For patients who have difficulty holding the toothbrush, toothbrush handle can be enlarged by inserting it into a sponge or tennis ball, or by wrapping the handle with foil or tape; an electric toothbrush may be easier to use for persons with dexterity problems that make brushing difficult
      6.   Use of fluoride-containing toothpaste in any age group speeds up remineralization, the process by which tooth enamel absorbs calcium and phosphorous
      7.   Tartar control or whitening toothpastes may cause gum or tooth sensitivity, and toothpastes for sensitive teeth can often lessen sensitivity

   B.   Flossing teeth after every meal can reduce plaque formation and may be even more important than brushing
      1.   Explain that waxed or unwaxed products are equally effective
      2.   For a better grip on dental floss, suggest use of a commercial dental floss holder
      3.   Tell patients to use a gentle sawing motion, and work the floss between teeth without snapping it into the gums
         a.   At the gumline, hold floss taut, bend it into a "C" shape, and then move the floss up and down on side of each tooth
         b.   The floss should go slightly below gumline until resistance is felt

   C.   For patients who cannot brush or floss after a meal, teach them to swish vigorously with a mouthful of water
      1.   Swishing with water washes away food particles and reduces mouth bacteria by 30%
      2.   In addition, swishing helps neutralize enamel-attacking acids

III.	Fluoride supplementation: Provide patients with the following information

A.	Fluoride supplements can result in reductions of 35-40% in incidence of tooth decay among children

B.	Recommended fluoride dosage schedule (mg/day) based on concentrations of fluoride in drinking water is in table under CHILD HEATLH SUPERVISION section

IV.	Dental examinations: Counsel patients regarding timing and importance of regular check-ups

A.	Regular visits to a dentist for evaluation and oral health counseling should be scheduled at least once a year

B.	Initial dental visit should be made for children between 12 months and 3 years of age, with 3 years being the preferred age in children who are experiencing no problems; thereafter, visits should be at least annually

V.	Additional counseling to promote oral health includes the following

A.	Provide dietary counseling relating to adequate intakes of essential nutrients (see section on CHILD and ADOLESCENT NUTRITION for recommendations); especially discourage intake of high sugar foods and beverages in the diet

B.	Patients who use tobacco should be counseled in accordance with the recommendations contained in the section on TOBACCO USE AND SMOKING CESSATION

C.	Encourage parents to have sealants bonded to the enamel of their child's teeth to shield the deep grooves in the chewing surfaces from bacteria

VI.	Tooth eruption of primary dentition and permanent dentition is contained in the chart below; age of exfoliation of primary dentition is also provided

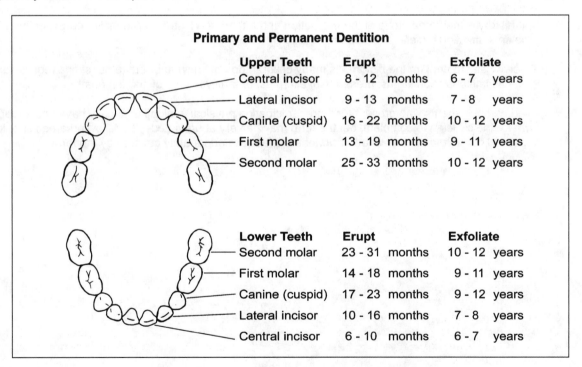

Primary and Permanent Dentition

Upper Teeth	Erupt		Exfoliate	
Central incisor	8 - 12	months	6 - 7	years
Lateral incisor	9 - 13	months	7 - 8	years
Canine (cuspid)	16 - 22	months	10 - 12	years
First molar	13 - 19	months	9 - 11	years
Second molar	25 - 33	months	10 - 12	years

Lower Teeth	Erupt		Exfoliate	
Second molar	23 - 31	months	10 - 12	years
First molar	14 - 18	months	9 - 11	years
Canine (cuspid)	17 - 23	months	9 - 12	years
Lateral incisor	10 - 16	months	7 - 8	years
Central incisor	6 - 10	months	6 - 7	years

Figure 1.5. Primary and Permanent Dentition

PREPARTICIPATION SPORTS EXAMINATION

I.   Definition: A sports-specific evaluation emphasizing recent injuries and/or any health condition affecting sports participation

II.   Overview of Evaluation

    A.   The number of preadolescent and adolescent boys and girls that are active in sports in the US increases each year and most require some type of physical evaluation before sanctioned sports participation

    B.   Objectives of evaluation
        1.   Help maintain the health and safety of athletes during both training and competition
        2.   Identify those athletes who need further conditioning, require further evaluation prior to clearance, or who require exclusion from a specific sport
        3.   Meet legal and insurance requirements

    C.   Timing of evaluation
        1.   Ideally, timing of the preparticipation examination should occur at least 6 weeks prior to preseason practice
        2.   Adequate time is needed to provide for conditioning, rehabilitation, or further evaluation, if needed

    D.   Regulations differ from state to state regarding the preparticipation exam and clearance requirements

    E.   The National Federation of State High School Associations (NFSHSA) does not require a single standardized process or forms for completion of a preparticipation sports evaluation, citing differences in local and state requirements

III.   History

    A.   The history is the cornerstone of the evaluation and a thorough history will identify approximately 75% of problems affecting athletic participation

    B.   Parents need to confirm the history, as many children do not know answers to questions regarding such areas as immunization status, presence of allergies, or family history of sudden death

    C.   Children/adolescents who present for a preparticipation physical evaluation usually have some type of form for the clinician to complete, but the form may be very abbreviated—the following areas should be assessed during the history, whether or not the areas are adequately covered by the form:

PREPARTICIPATION HISTORY

System	Questions to Ask
General	"Do you have any allergies (ask specifically, to medications, foods [such as peanuts], pollen, or insect stings)?"
	"Are your immunizations up to date?" (Proof will be required)
	"Have you ever become ill from exercising in the heat?"
	"Do you need any special protective or corrective equipment or devices that are not usually used for your sport or position (e.g., knee brace, special neck roll, hearing aid)?"
	"Do you want to weigh more or less than you do now?" "Do you lose weight regularly to meet weight requirements for your sport?"
Skin	"Do you have any current skin problems such as rashes, itching, warts, blisters, or fungal infections?"
Ears, Eyes, Nose, and Throat	"Do you have any problems with your eyes or vision?" "Have you ever had an injury to your eyes either playing sports or due to another type of accident?" "Do you have any problems hearing?"
Respiratory	"Do you cough, wheeze, or have trouble breathing during or after being physically active (e.g., running, playing tennis, racquetball)?" "Do you have asthma or seasonal asthma that requires treatment?" "Do you smoke cigarettes (or use smokeless tobacco)?" "Does anyone in your household smoke (exposure to environmental tobacco smoke)?"
Cardiovascular	During or after exercise, have you ever been dizzy, passed out, or had chest pain?" "Do you tire more easily than your friends do during exercise?" "Have you been told you have any of the following: High blood pressure? High cholesterol? Heart murmur?" "Has any immediate family member or blood relative died of heart problems or died suddenly before age 50?" "Have you had a severe viral infection within the last month?" "Have you ever been denied or restricted from participation in sports for any heart problem?"
Musculoskeletal	"Have you ever had a sprain, strain, or swelling after injury?" "Have you ever broken or fractured any bones or dislocated any joints?" "Have you ever had any other problems with pain or swelling in muscles, tendons, bones, or joints?"
Neurological	"Have you ever been knocked out, lost consciousness, or lost your memory?" "Have you ever had a seizure?" "Do you have frequent or severe headaches?" "Do you ever have numbness or tingling in your arms/hands/legs/feet?"
Psychosocial	"Do you feel stressed out?" "Is there anything that you are worried about that you would like to talk about?" "Do you ever drink alcohol or use drugs?"

Past Medical History

"Tell me about any illnesses or accidents you have had since your last check-up (or sports physical)." "Have you ever been seen in the emergency department or been hospitalized overnight?" "Do you have an on-going or chronic illness?"

Medication History

"Do you take any medications on a regular basis?" "Do you use an inhaler?" "What do you take for pain, such as a headache, or sore muscles?": "Do you take any supplements or vitamins to (1) help you lose/gain weight, or (2) improve your performance?" "Do you use any herbal remedies?"

Family History

"Has any immediate family member or blood relative died of heart problems or died suddenly before age 50?"

Females Only

Menstrual history including age at menarche, duration of, frequency of, and interval between menstrual periods, the last menstrual period (LMP, dated from the first day of the last normal menses), any intermenstrual bleeding, pain with menses, and peri-menstrual symptoms. Ask about contraceptive use

IV.   Physical Examination

    A.   The physical exam Is a screening tool emphasizing the areas of greatest concern in sports participation and areas identified in the history

    B.   Sudden death among young athletes is often the result of previously unrecognized cardiovascular disease; noncardiac causes of sudden death on the athletic field include hyperthermia, asthma-related drug reactions, and anaphylaxis

    C.   A complete physical exam including vital signs, hearing and vision screening, height/weight, calculation of BMI (Tanner staging is optional) is recommended

    D.   Orthopedic screening can be quickly completed using the two-minute orthopedic exam as illustrated in Figure 1.6 below; if a previous joint injury has occurred, stability testing of the joint should be done (see chapter on MUSCULOSKELETAL PROBLEMS for more information)

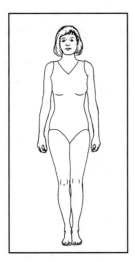

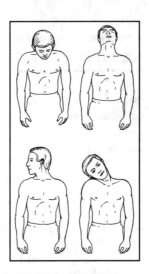

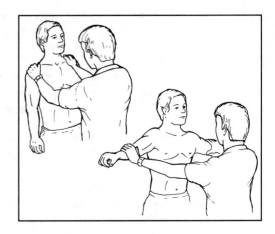

Ask patient to stand facing the examiner; observe for symmetry of trunk and upper extremities

Instruct patient to look at ceiling, floor, over both shoulders and touch ears to shoulders; observe for cervical spine range of motion

Have patient shrug shoulder with examiner resistance; check for trapezius strength Patient abducts shoulders 90° while examiner resists at 90°; check deltoid strength

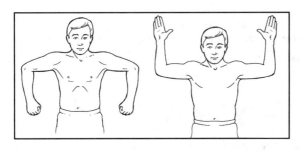

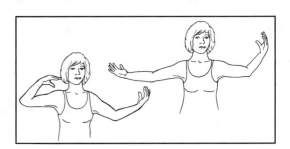

Have patient rotate shoulder—internal and external; observe for range of motion, glenohumeral joint

Ask patient to extend and flex elbow; observe for range of motion of the elbow

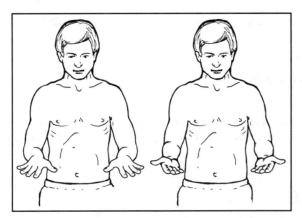

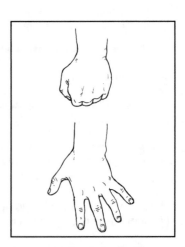

Have patient pronate and supinate hands, with arms in front and elbows flexed 90°; observe for elbow and wrist range of motion

Ask patient to spread fingers on both hands, and then make a fist with both hands; observe for range of motion of hands and fingers

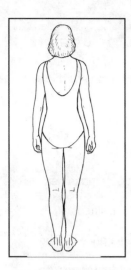 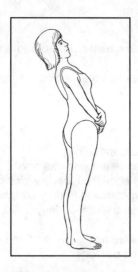 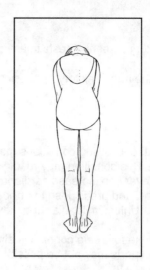 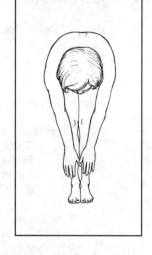

Ask patient to turn and face away from examiner; inspect for symmetry of back and upper extremities

Ask patient to stand with knees straight, back in extension, and chin tilted toward ceiling; observe for flexibility of spine

With back flexed and knees straight, patient faces toward and then away from examiner; observe for range of motion of thoracic and lumbosacral spine, for spine curvature, and for hamstring flexibility

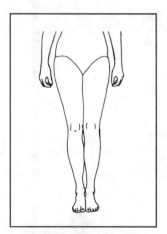 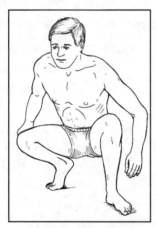 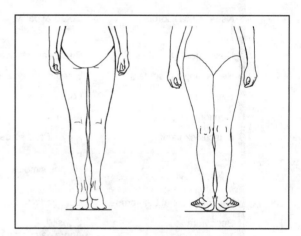

Facing examiner, ask patient to alternately contract and relax quadriceps; observe for alignment and symmetry

Ask patient to "duck walk" 4 steps toward examiner; observe for motion of hip, knee, and ankle, and also evaluate strength and balance

Tell patient to stand on toes, then on heels; observe for calf symmetry and strength, and for balance

Figure 1.6. The Two-Minute Orthopedic Exam

Adapted from American Academy of Family Physicians, American Academy of Pediatrics, American Medical Society for Sports Medicine, American Orthopaedic Society for Sports Medicine, and American Osteopathic Academy of Sports Medicine. (1997). Preparticipation physical evaluation. *The physician and sports medicine*, (p. 22). Minneapolis: McGraw-Hill

47

V. Diagnostic Tests

    A. Routine laboratory screening tests in asymptomatic athletes are not required

    B. Findings from the health history or physical examination may indicate a need to arrange specific diagnostic test

VI. Plan/Management

    A. Individuals with the following conditions may not participate in sports
       1. **Carditis**. This condition may result in sudden death with exertion
       2. **Fever**. Fever can increase cardiopulmonary effort, reduce exercise capacity, increase heat intolerance, and predispose to orthostatic hypotension during exercise
       3. **Diarrhea**. Unless mild, diarrhea may increase the risk of dehydration and heat illness

    B. Individuals with the following conditions always require further evaluation before clearance can be obtained; some sports may not be possible for some persons

CONDITIONS THAT REQUIRE FURTHER EVALUATION TO ASSESS THE SAFETY OF A GIVEN SPORT FOR A PARTICULAR ATHLETE		
Cardiovascular Disorders	Hypertension Congenital heart disease Dysrhythmia	Mitral valve prolapse Heart murmur
Neurologic Disorders	Cerebral palsy Convulsive disorder, poorly controlled	History of serious head or spine trauma, severe or repeated concussions, or craniotomy
Respiratory Disorders	Pulmonary compromise, including CF	Acute upper respiratory infection
Hematologic Disorders	Bleeding disorders	Sickle cell disease
Eyes	Loss of an eye	History of serious eye injury
Genitourinary	Absence of one kidney	
Musculoskeletal	Amy MSK disorder	Atlantoaxial instability
Skin	Boils Herpes simplex Impetigo	Scabies Molluscum contagiosum
Gastrointestinal Disorders	Enlarged spleen	Enlarged liver
Behavioral	Obesity Anorexia nervosa	Bulimia nervosa

    C. Individuals with the following conditions should not be excluded from participation in sports solely on the basis of the condition

CONDITIONS NOT NECESSARILY PRECLUDING PARTICIPATION IN SPORTS		
Endocrine	Diabetes mellitus (with proper attention to diet, hydration, and insulin therapy)	
Immunocompromised	HIV infection(all sports may be played so long as the person is able)	
Genitourinary	Absence of one ovary	Absent or undescended testicle
Respiratory	Asthma (with proper medication and education, only athletes with severe asthma will need to modify participation)	
Hematologic	Sickle cell trait	
Neurological	Convulsive disorder, well controlled (risk of convulsion during participation is minimal)	

D. Clearance is classified according to three categories
    1. **Unrestricted**—no limiting abnormality has been identified and the athlete is approved to participate in all sports
    2. **Conditional clearance**—a clearance is given, pending further evaluation
    3. **Not cleared for all sports**—includes athletes with potentially life-threatening conditions

E. A preparticipation clearance form provided by the patient/parent is used to make recommendations regarding participation
    1. Less than 2% of athletes are excluded from participation in sports based on preparticipation evaluation findings in a primary care setting
    2. However, approximately 15% require further evaluation and referral

F. Be aware of the medicolegal considerations when performing preparticipation physical evaluations
    1. Many athletes (and their parents) are unwilling to accept restrictions in sport participation
        a. A second medical opinion may be sought or an attorney may be retained by the family
        b. Under the Rehabilitation Act of 1973, and the Americans with Disabilities Act of 1990, athletes may have the legal right to participate against medical advice
    2. Healthcare providers who recommend restricted participation or exclusion from a sport should consult with experts in the medical condition in question to assist in determining the risk to the athlete of participating in the desired sport
        a. This approach limits the likelihood that the athlete will be inappropriately excluded from the sport
        b. This approach also reassures the athlete and parents if restriction or exclusion is indeed the correct course
        c. Finally, such an approach provides liability protection for the healthcare provider who is making the recommendation

REFERENCES

American Academy of Family Physicians, American Academy of Pediatrics, American Medical Society for Sports Medicine, American Orthopaedic Society for Sports Medicine, American Osteopathic Academy of Sports Medicine. (1997). *Preparticipation physical evaluation.* Minneapolis: The Physician and Sports Medicine (McGraw-Hill).

American Academy of Pediatrics, Committee on Infectious Diseases. (2003). Recommended childhood immunization schedule—United States, 2003. *Pediatrics, 111,* 212-215.

American Academy of Pediatrics, Committee on Sports Medicine and Fitness. (2001). Medical conditions affecting sports participation. *Pediatrics, 107,* 1205-1209.

American Academy of Pediatrics, Committee on Sports Medicine and Fitness. (1997). Athletic participation by children and adolescents who have systemic hypertension. *Pediatrics, 99,* 637-638.

American Academy of Pediatrics. Clinical Report. (2003). Prevention of rickets and vitamin D deficiency: New guidelines for vitamin D intake. *Pediatrics, 111,* 908-910.

American Academy of Pediatrics. Committee on Children with Disabilities. (2001). Developmental surveillance and screening of infants and young children. *Pediatrics, 108,* 192-196.

American Academy of Pediatrics. Committee on Environmental Health. (1998). Screening for elevated blood lead levels. *Pediatrics, 101,* 1072-1078.

American Academy of Pediatrics. Committee on Nutrition. (1998). Cholesterol in childhood. *Pediatrics, 101,* 141-147.

American Academy of Pediatrics. Committee on Practice and Ambulatory Medicine. (2000). Recommendations for preventive pediatric health care. *Pediatrics, 105,* 645.

American Academy of Pediatrics. Task Force on Newborn and Infant Hearing. (1999). Newborn and infant hearing loss: Detection and intervention. *Pediatrics, 103,* 527-530.

American Academy of Pediatrics. (1999). Fun in the sun: Keep your baby safe. Retrieved October 29, 2002, from http://www.aap.org/family/mnbroc.cfm

American Academy of Pediatrics. (2000). *Red book: Report of the committee on infectious diseases* (25th ed.). Elk Grove Village, IL: Author.

Barlow, S.E., & Dietz, W.H. (1998). Obesity evaluation and treatment: Expert committee recommendations. *Pediatrics, 102,* e29.

Carey, W.B. (1998). Teaching parents about infant temperament. *Pediatrics, 102,* 1311-1316.

Casamassimo, P. (1996). *Bright futures in practice: Oral health.* Arlington, VA: National Center for Education in Maternal and Child Health.

Centers for Disease Control and Prevention, National Center for Health Statistics. (2000). *CDC growth charts: United States.* Hyattsville, MD: Author.

Centers for Disease Control and Prevention. (1997). *Screening young children for lead poisoning: Guidance for state and local public health officials.* Atlanta: Author.

Colletti, T.P. (2001). Sports preparticipation evaluation. *Physician Assistant, 25,* 31-41.

DiClemente, R.J. (1999). The psychological basis of health promotion for adolescents. *Adolescent Medicine, 10,* 13-22.

Dixon, S.D., & Stein, M.T. (1992). *Encounters with children: Pediatric behavior and development.* St. Louis: Mosby.

Dworkin, P.H. (2002). Screening: General considerations. In R. A. Hoekelman, H.M. Adams, N.M. Nelson, M.L. Weitzman, & M.H. Wilson (Eds.), *Pediatric primary care* (pp. 224-227). St. Louis: Mosby.

Eiger, M.F. (2002). Nutrition: Feeding of infants and children. In R. A. Hoekelman, H.M. Adams, N.M. Nelson, M.L. Weitzman, & M.H. Wilson (Eds.), *Pediatric primary care* (pp.171-183). St. Louis: Mosby.

Feldman, H., & Bauer, R. (1992). Developmental-behavioral pediatrics. In B.J. Zitelli & H.W. Davis (Eds.). *Atlas of pediatric physical diagnosis* (pp. 3.1-3.29). Philadelphia: Lippincott.

Forbes, G.B. (2002). Nutrition: Nutritional requirements. In R. A. Hoekelman, H.M. Adams, N.M. Nelson, M.L. Weitzman, & M.H. Wilson (Eds.), *Pediatric primary care* (pp.184-198). St. Louis: Mosby.

Ford, C.A., & English, A. (2002). Limiting confidentiality of adolescent health services: What are the risks? *Journal of the American Medical Association, 288,* 752-754.

Green, M., & Palfrey, J. (2002). *Bright futures: Guidelines for health supervision of infants, children, and adults.* Arlington, VA: National Center for Education in Maternal and Child Health.

Hoekelman, R.A. (2002). Child health supervision. In R. A. Hoekelman, H.M. Adams, N.M. Nelson, M.L. Weitzman, & M.H. Wilson (Eds.), *Pediatric primary care* (pp.35-41). St. Louis: Mosby.

Institute of Medicine, Food and Nutrition Board, The National Academies. (2002). *Dietary reference intakes: Energy, carbohydrate, fiber, fat, fatty acids, cholesterol, protein, and amino acids, part 1.* (Prepublication copy, unedited proofs). Washington, DC: National Academies Press.

Institute of Medicine, Food and Nutrition Board, The National Academies. (2002). *Dietary reference intakes: Energy, carbohydrate, fiber, fat, fatty acids, cholesterol, protein, and amino acids, part 2.* (Prepublication copy, unedited proofs). Washington, DC: National Academies Press.

Luckstead, E.F. (2002). Cardiac risk factors and participation guidelines for youth sports. *Pediatric Clinics of North America, 49,* 681-707.

Patrick, K., Spear, B., Holt, K., & Sofka, D. (2001). *Bright futures in practice: Physical activity.* Arlington, VA: National Center for Education in Maternal and Child Health.

Rodriguez, J.O., Lavina, A.M., & Agarwal, A. (2003). Prevention and treatment of common eye injuries in sports. *American Family Physician, 67,* 1481-1488, 1494-1496.

Simeonsson, R.J., & Simeonsson, N.W. (2002). Developmental surveillance and intervention. In R. A. Hoekelman, H.M. Adams, N.M. Nelson, M.L. Weitzman, & M.H. Wilson (Eds.), *Pediatric primary care* (pp.274-281). St. Louis: Mosby.

Stevens, L.M., Lynn, C., & Glass, R.M. (2002). Vehicle safety and children. *JAMA, 287,* 1212-1213.

Story, M., Holt, K., & Sofka, D. (2002). *Bright futures in practice: Nutrition.* Arlington, VA: National Center for Education in Maternal and Child Health.

Sullivan, S.A., & Birch, L.A. (1994). Infant dietary experience and acceptance of solid foods. *Pediatrics, 93,* 271-277.

Tigges, B.B. (1997). Infant formulas: Practical answers for common questions. *Nurse Practitioner, 22,* 70-87.

US Department of Agriculture, Center for Nutrition Policy and Promotion. (1999). *Tips for using the Food Guide Pyramid for young children 2 to 6 years old.* Washington, DC: Author.

US Department of Agriculture/US Department of Health and Human Services. (2000). *Nutrition and your health: Dietary guidelines for Americans.* Washington, DC: Author.

US Department of Health and Human Services. (2000). *Healthy people 2010.* McLean, VA: International Medical Publishing, Inc.

US Preventive Services Task Force. (2003). Behavioral counseling in primary care to promote a healthy diet. Retrieved January 3, 2003, from http://www.preventiveservices.ahrq.gov

US Preventive Services Task Force. (2003). Screening for cervical cancer: recommendations and rationale. Retrieved February 7, 2003, from http://www.ahcpr.gov/clinic/uspstfix.htm

US Preventive Services Task Force. (2001). *Newborn hearing screening: Recommendation and rationale.* Retrieved October 29, 2002, from http://www.ahrq.gov/clinic/3rdupstf/newbornscreen/newhearr.htm

US Preventive Services Task Force. (2001). Screening for chlamydial infection: Recommendations and rationale. *American Journal of Preventive Medicine, 20,* 90-94.

US Preventive Services Task Force. (2002). Behavioral counseling in primary care to promote physical activity: Recommendation and rationale. *Annals of Internal Medicine, 137,* 205-207.

2 General

CONSTANCE R. UPHOLD

Chronic Fatigue
Table: International Consensus Definition of Chronic Fatigue Syndrome

Fever And Fever without Source
Table: Conversion of Temperature
Table: Signs of a Toxic Infant or Child
Table: Age-Specific Pulse and Respiratory Rates in Children and Infants
Table: Yale Observation Scale
Table: Criteria for Febrile Infants at Low Risk for Serious Bacterial Infection
Table: Diagnostic Tests for Sepsis, Bacteremia, and Meningitis Evaluation
Table: Acetaminophen Dosages and Available Forms for Treatment of Fevers

Lymphadenopathy
Table: Palpable Lymph Nodes, Lymphatic Drainage, and Associated Causes
Figure: Palpable Lymph Nodes of Head and Neck
Figure: Palpable Lymph Nodes of Upper and Lower Extremities

Pain
Table: Misconceptions about Pain in Children
Table: Three Step Analgesic Ladder of the World Health Organization
Table: Nonsteroidal Anti-Inflammatory Drugs (NSAIDs)
Table: Controlled Drugs
Table: Management of Opioid-Induced Adverse Events
Table: Website Resources

Weight Loss (Involuntary)
Table: Differential Diagnosis of Weight Loss by Age Group

CHRONIC FATIGUE

I.   Definition: A symptom that lasts at least six months and involves extreme, unusual tiredness, decreased physical performance, and excessive need of sleep

II.   Pathogenesis

    A.   In all age groups, fatigue is one of the prominent symptoms in the following conditions:
        1.   Infectious diseases: HIV infection, mononucleosis, hepatitis, endocarditis, Lyme disease, cytomegalovirus infection, parasitic disease
        2.   Endocrine and metabolic disorders: Addison's disease, hypothyroidism, diabetes mellitus, pituitary insufficiency, chronic renal failure, hepatocellular failure
        3.   Rheumatologic conditions: Rheumatoid arthritis, fibromyalgia, systemic lupus erythematosus
        4.   Hematologic and oncologic conditions: Cancer (especially pancreatic cancer), severe anemia
        5.   Cardiopulmonary diseases: Congestive heart disease, chronic obstructive pulmonary disease
        6.   Neurologic diseases: Parkinson's disease, multiple sclerosis, myasthenia gravis
        7.   Psychological disorders: Depression, anxiety, somatization disorder
        8.   Sleep disorders: Sleep apnea, narcolepsy, hypersomnia

    B.   Medications (antidepressants, tranquilizers, hypnotics, antihypertensives, antihistamines, illicit drugs, alcohol, excessive coffee intake) and unhealthy lifestyles (poor eating habits, lack of exercise, insufficient sleep, excessive stress) may also result in fatigue

    C.   Chronic fatigue syndrome (CFS) is a disabling systemic disease characterized by severe fatigue; unknown etiology, but many hypotheses have been proposed
        1.   Although not universal, many patients have low levels of cortisol and a blunted adrenal response to stress, suggesting a problem in the hypothalamic-pituitary-adrenal axis
        2.   Infections from Epstein-Barr virus, toxoplasmosis, and cytomegalovirus can precipitate long periods of fatigue, but it is unclear if these pathogens are causative agents or just triggers in predisposed persons
        3.   Frequently considered a psychiatric condition because of the high prevalence of somatization disorder, depression, and increased risk of suicide; however, CFS patients usually do not have low self-esteem, anhedonia, guilt, and low motivation that typify most patients with psychiatric conditions
        4.   CFS has similarities with other unexplained medical diagnoses (fibromyalgia, irritable bowel syndrome) leading some to believe that health beliefs and attributions play a major role

    D.   In childhood, fatigue is a less common complaint than in adulthood
        1.   The most common cause is recurrent or chronic infections
        2.   Hypothyroidism and diabetes mellitus are the common endocrine disorders
        3.   Rheumatoid arthritis and other rheumatoid diseases are common causes
        4.   Cyanotic heart disease and chronic advanced pulmonary disease (as seen in cystic fibrosis) are associated with severe fatigue
        5.   Leukemia or lymphoma are seen infrequently, but must be considered in the differential diagnosis

    E.   In adolescents, fatigue occurs frequently due to intense school and extracurricular activities; the following are common diseases that occur during adolescence in which fatigue is prominent:
        1.   Infectious diseases, particularly *mycoplasma* pneumonia and infectious mononucleosis
        2.   Inflammatory bowel disease
        3.   CSF is associated with depression, somatic complaints, and feeling different than others

III.   Clinical Presentation: One of the most common primary care complaints

    A.   Clinicians often attribute fatigue to psychological problems, whereas parents and patients usually fear that serious illnesses such as cancer or life-threatening infections are the causes

    B.   Fatigue is usually associated with feelings of sleepiness, irritability, boredom, and decreased efficiency

    C.   In childhood and adolescence, fatigue results in school absences and loss of contact with peers

D.   Chronic fatigue syndrome accounts for about 5-10% of all cases of chronic fatigue
1.   The 1994 case definition (see following table) is widely used for diagnosis
2.   Peak prevalence is among individuals ages 20-50 years; cases are much less common in children
3.   In adults, onset is usually acute but in children onset is insidious
4.   Approximately 20-50% of adults have some improvement after one to two years, but few fully recover; children generally have a better prognosis with recovery within 4 years

INTERNATIONAL CONSENSUS DEFINITION OF CHRONIC FATIGUE SYNDROME*†	
Criteria	**Definition**
Major	Chronic or relapsing, unexplained severe fatigue for ≥6 months that is not the result of ongoing exertion; is not substantially alleviated by rest; and results in reduction in previous levels of occupational, educational, social or personal activities
Minor	✓ Impaired memory or concentration ✓ Sore throat ✓ Tender cervical or axillary lymph nodes ✓ Muscle pain ✓ Multijoint pain ✓ New headaches ✓ Unrefreshing sleep ✓ Postexertional malaise

*The major and four or more of the minor criteria are required for case definition
†Exclusionary clinical diagnoses are the following: (1) any active medical condition that could explain the chronic fatigue (2) any previously diagnosed medical condition whose resolution has not been documented and whose continued activity may account for chronic fatigue (3) psychotic major depression, bipolar affective disorder, schizophrenia, delusional disorders, dementias, anorexia nervosa, bulimia nervosa (4) alcohol or substance abuse within 2 years prior to the onset of chronic fatigue and any time thereafter

Adapted from Fukuda, K., Straus, S.E., Hickie, I., Sharpe, M., Dobbins., J., & Komaroll, A. (1994). The chronic fatigue syndrome: A comprehensive approach to its definition and study. *Annals of Internal Medicine, 121*, 953-959.

IV.   Diagnosis/Evaluation

A.   History; patients and parents should be encouraged to share past experiences with medical personnel and frustrations they may have had with their previous care
1.   Ask to describe the development and severity of fatigue
2.   Question about associated symptoms
3.   Inquire about sleep habits and quality of sleep
4.   Ask about lifestyle behaviors such as eating habits, caffeine intake, exercising, use of alcohol, tobacco, and illicit drugs
5.   A complete medical history is often needed; always ask about symptoms of depression, fever, dyspnea, muscular weakness, blood loss, weight loss, anorexia, and pain
6.   Determine risk for HIV infection and sexually transmitted diseases
7.   Obtain a family medical history
8.   Obtain a medication history
9.   Ask about stress, significant losses, crying spells, and suicidal ideations
10. Determine how fatigue has affected occupational, educational, recreational, social, and family activities
11. Inquire about travel to areas where parasitic infections are endemic

B.   Physical Examination; a complete exam is needed to arrive at a definitive diagnosis and to assure the patient that his/her complaint of fatigue is being taken seriously
1.   Measure vital signs, including postural pulse and blood pressure, temperature, and weight
2.   Assess skin for moisture, texture, exanthems, pallor, jaundice, purpura, petechiae, and splinter hemorrhages
3.   Perform a funduscopic examination, noting diabetic retinopathy; inspect sclera for icterus
4.   Assess pharynx, noting petechiae, a sign of mononucleosis
5.   Perform a thyroid examination
6.   Examine lymph nodes
7.   Perform complete heart and lung examinations
8.   Assess the abdomen, noting organomegaly, masses, ascites, and tenderness
9.   Perform a rectal examination; check for occult blood
10. Assess the joints for signs of inflammation

11.   Perform a complete neuromuscular examination, noting focal weakness, muscle atrophy, fasciculations of muscles, deep tendon reflexes, and tremors
12.   Perform a mental status assessment

C.   Differential Diagnosis
1.   Great care must be taken to rule out underlying medical illness; most diseases have associated symptoms except for adrenal insufficiency in which fatigue is often the first and only presenting complaint
2.   Always consider unhealthy lifestyle behaviors as a possible cause

D.   Diagnostic Tests; findings from the history and physical examination should guide selection of tests; diagnostic testing should be minimized
1.   If fatigue persists, consider a basic screening evaluation including a CBC with differential, renal function tests, liver enzymes, urinalysis, an erythrocyte sedimentation rate, and thyroid function tests
2.   In patients with recent onset of persisting fatigue and adenopathy, order a heterophile test for acute mononucleosis
3.   HIV testing should be done when diffuse adenopathy is present or when there is a history of high-risk behaviors
4.   Useful tests to rule out other diseases are glucose (diabetes), chest x-ray (cardiopulmonary problems), rapid cosyntropin test (adrenal insufficiency), rheumatoid factor (rheumatoid diseases), serologies for toxoplasmosis, Epstein-Barr, or cytomegalovirus (infectious diseases), and cerebral magnetic resonance imaging (for demyelination as occurs in multiple sclerosis)
5.   Diagnosis of CFS is based on clinical findings and eliminating other diagnoses

V.   Plan/Management

A.   Treat underlying cause of fatigue; treat medical or psychiatric conditions and provide symptomatic care such as pain medications and strategies to normalize sleep patterns

B.   Treatment of chronic fatigue syndrome is variable and tailored to each patient; limited research is available on the effectiveness of treatments in children
1.   Support from family, school personnel, and health care clinics is essential to successful recovery
2.   Emphasis should be on rehabilitation rather than cure
3.   Patient education is important
   a.   Acknowledge the reality of the illness and its associated symptoms while stressing that there is no underlying organic disease
   b.   Reassure patients that CFS is not life-threatening and that most people are eventually able to return to work or school
4.   Continuous support and attention to symptomatic treatment are essential; focus on ameliorating the negative effects that fatigue is having on the patient's life; discuss the futility in continually searching for a cause and the importance of rehabilitation
5.   Cognitive-behavioral therapy helps the patient identify and reverse beliefs and coping behaviors that perpetuate disability and hinder recovery
   a.   First explore the patient's beliefs about the illness and behaviors related to the illness
   b.   Patients are encouraged to gain control of their illness and change behaviors of passivity and helplessness to active participation in their recovery
6.   Gradually increase activity; initially avoid intense exercise as this can lead to a pattern of overactivity and underactivity
7.   A targeted exercise program is effective
8.   A balanced diet and good sleep hygiene may improve symptoms
9.   Low-dose tricyclic antidepressants and/or selective serotonin reuptake inhibitors, combined with cognitive-behavioral therapy, are beneficial in adults, but no research on these therapies has been conducted with children
10. Immunologic therapy, corticosteroids, supplements, massage, and transcutaneous electrical nerve stimulation are other therapies, but evidence of their effectiveness in children is limited

C.   Follow Up
1.   Follow up is variable depending on the cause of fatigue
2.   After the first visits for evaluation and initiating treatment, patients with CFS should be scheduled for infrequent, but regular appointments

FEVER AND FEVER WITHOUT SOURCE

I.   Definition: Traditionally defined as body temperature greater than 38.0°C (100.4°F) rectally, 37.8°C (100°F) orally, or 37.2°C (98.9°F) axillary; more recently defined as early morning body temperature (measured orally) ≥37.2°C (≥98.9°F) or an afternoon temperature of ≥37.7°C (≥99.9°F) (see table that follows for conversion of temperature)

CONVERSION OF TEMPERATURE		
37°C	=	98.6°F
38°C	=	100.4°F
39°C	=	102.2°F
40°C	=	104.0°F

   A.   Fever without source (FWS): Unexplained fever (>38°C or >100.4°F, rectal temperature) of brief duration or lasting <5-7 days; source of acute febrile illness is not apparent after a careful history and physical examination. Other important definitions related to FWS in children:
   1.   Serious bacterial infection (SBI): Meningitis, sepsis, bone and joint infections, urinary tract infections, pneumonia, and enteritis
   2.   Occult bacteremia: Presence of viable bacteria in circulating blood not manifest or detectable by clinical methods alone
   3.   Sepsis: Presence of pathogenic microorganisms or their toxins in blood or other tissues
   4.   Lethargy: Level of consciousness characterized by poor or absent eye contact or the failure of the child to recognize parents or to interact with persons or objects in the environment
   5.   Toxic: Clinical presentation congruent with the sepsis syndrome (see table that follows)

SIGNS OF A TOXIC INFANT OR CHILD
➡ Altered level of consciousness
➡ Abnormal breathing
• Slow or rapid rate
• Irregular rate
• Stridor
• Prolonged expiration
• Grunting
• Nasal flaring
• Chest retractions
• Paradoxic or abdominal breathing
➡ Rapid pulse rate
➡ Elevated temperature
➡ Skin abnormalities
• Petechiae
• Central cyanosis
• Pallor
➡ Head bobbing
➡ Delayed capillary refill
➡ Poor muscle tone

   B.   Fever of unknown origin (FUO): Fever (>101°F) persisting for 3 weeks and eluding one week of intensive diagnostic testing

II.   Pathogenesis

   A.   Fever occurs when bacteria, viruses, toxins, or other agents are phagocytosed by leukocytes

   B.   Interluekin-1 and other chemical mediators (previously referred to as endogenous pyrogens) are then produced and activate the production of prostaglandins

C. Prostaglandins act on the thermoregulatory mechanism in the hypothalamus and upwardly readjust the body's thermostat

D. Raising the hypothalamic set-point initiates the process of heat production and conservation by increasing metabolism, triggering peripheral vasoconstriction, and less frequently by triggering shivering which increases heat production from the muscles

E. Infections (most common), neoplasms, and collagen-vascular diseases are the most common causes; most infections are viral in etiology

F. Other causes include the following:
1. Hypersensitivity to drugs
2. Recent immunizations with certain vaccines
3. Vascular occlusive and/or inflammatory events such as deep vein thrombophlebitis, pulmonary emboli, or myocardial infarction
4. Acute hemolytic episodes associated with acute autoimmune hemolytic anemia or sickle cell anemia
5. Central nervous system abnormalities

G. Etiology of fever without source in infants and children
1. Occult bacteremia and underlying sepsis occur in 3% of children younger than 3 years and are the primary concern in children with FWS; common pathogens are the following:
   a. *Streptococcus pneumoniae* is the most common pathogen; however, because the new conjugate pneumococcal vaccine has an efficacy rate of 90%, in the future, children will be at a much lower risk for diseases due to this pathogen
   b. *Haemophilus influenzae* vaccine has reduced the incidence of invasive disease due to this pathogen by about 90%
   c. *Neisseria meningitidis* is a potential pathogen
   d. Less common pathogens include *Salmonellae, Group A streptococcus, Staphylococcus aureus*, gram-negative enterics
2. Urinary tract infections (UTIs) are almost always occult and occur in 8-9% of female infants less than 2 years and about 3-4% of male infants less than 12 months (most UTIs in males occur in those who are uncircumcised)
3. Other less frequent causes are chronic disorders such as juvenile rheumatoid arthritis, drug reactions, allergic or hypersensitivity disorders, heat illnesses, or Kawasaki syndrome
4. In some cases, source of fever is found late in the course of the infection, such as occurs with roseola, cytomegalovirus infection, typhus, and typhoid fever; these diseases have long prodromal periods in which fever may be the only presenting symptom

H. True fever must be differentiated from hyperthermia
1. Hyperthermia occurs when there is increased body temperature but no alteration in the hypothalamic set point
2. Hyperthermia may be due to increased metabolic heat (e.g., thyrotoxicosis), excessive environmental temperature (e.g., heat stroke), defective heat loss because of environmental conditions (e.g. high humidity, overdressing, sitting in unventilated, sunny car, exercise), or dermatologic disorder (e.g., ectodermal dysplasia)

I. Occasionally, a patient may have a factitious fever or a high reading on the thermometer which was artificially produced by the patient for secondary gains

III. Clinical Presentation

A. Fever, by itself, is not a illness; rather, a sign that the body is fighting an infection or reacting to a stimulus; normal temperatures are characterized by the following:
1. Temperature is usually highest around 4 pm and lowest around 6 am
2. Normal temperature deviations occur with physical activity, stress, ovulation, and environmental heat

B. Typical symptoms include malaise, fatigue, myalgias, and tachycardia (pulse rate is often elevated by about 10-15 beats per 1°C of fever)

C. Central nervous system symptoms may occur, ranging from mild changes in alertness to delirium, particularly in young children and chronically-ill patients

D. Children's normal temperature varies from adults
1. Infants tend to have higher normal temperatures than older children; infants often have subtle signs and symptoms: Pallor, anorexia and irritability may be the only abnormalities present
2. Children will often have adaptive withdrawal or decreased activity and conversation, flushed cheeks, hot, dry skin, and an unusual glitter in their eyes
3. Febrile seizures may occur in children, particularly those children between the ages of 6 months and 5 years (see section on FEBRILE SEIZURES)

E. Although each 1°F raises the basal metabolic rate by 7%, most patients can tolerate fevers well, with a few exceptions:
1. Patients with underlying cardiac disease, chronic, debilitating disease, immunocompromised disease, history of intravenous drug abuse, implanted prosthetic devices, and those on corticosteroid or immunosuppressive therapy
2. Small infants and the elderly are at a greatest risk for dehydration and other adverse events

F. In children, the probability of having a serious bacterial infection varies
1. Toxic-appearing infants are at greatest risk, but even non-toxic appearing infants may have a SBI
2. Children who have been given oral antibiotics may have a partially treated SBI and appear less ill than other children with SBI
3. Day care attendance is a risk factor for invasive disease in children less than 2 years of age
4. The routine use of conjugate Haemophilus influenzae type b (Hib) vaccines and conjugate pneumococcal vaccines has dramatically decreased the incidence of SBIs

IV. Diagnosis/Evaluation

A. History
1. Inquire about onset, duration, and pattern of fever; ascertain that patient or parents know how to correctly measure temperature; inquire about type of thermometer used
2. Even if child is afebrile at the visit, but had a documented history of reported fever, consider the child to be febrile to the degree reported by history
3. Ask parents if child is acting differently such as more irritable, more drowsy, or not playing as usual
4. Inquire about associated symptoms such as anorexia, chills, headache, nasal congestion, earache, sore throat, cough, abdominal pain, vomiting, diarrhea, or painful urination
5. Explore hydration status by asking about amount of fluid intake and frequency and amount of fluid output
6. Ask about comfort level of patient
7. Explore possibilities of heat illness (heat stroke) or other types of environmental exposure
8. Ask whether patient started new medications, had a recent immunization, or had a recent transfusion
9. Inquire about recent travel, dental or surgical procedures, illnesses, trauma, exposure to ticks, and insect or animal bites and scratches
10. Ask about the consumption of raw or poorly cooked foods; ask about alcohol or drug use
11. Ask whether other household members are ill or have fevers
12. Obtain a complete past medical history
    a. Ask about medications, implanted prosthetic devices, discussion of previous illnesses and diseases, particularly any cardiac or chronically debilitating disorders
    b. In children, complete a thorough birth history, family history, and inquire about previous episodes of febrile seizures
13. Inquire about last dosage of an antipyretic and other self-treatment measures
14. Explore social situation and home environment (e.g., adequacy of heat and water) of the family; assess availability of transportation, telephone, thermometer, and whether family is reliable
15. A complete review of systems may be needed to uncover source of fever and to determine severity of debility due to elevated body temperature

B. Physical Examination; fevers in infants and young child necessitate a complete physical examination (remember that even a focal finding of otitis media does not rule out a more serious bacterial infection)
1. Measure temperature
    a. Always confirm initial temperature measurement
       (1) Retake temperature before ordering diagnostic tests or prescribing treatment to reduce fever
       (2) Bundled infants need temperature measurement 30 minutes after undressing
    b. Rectal temperatures are gold standard as they are accurate, reproducible, and not affected by environmental factors; rectal temperatures are approximately 1° higher than oral temperatures and 2 to 2.5° higher than axillary temperatures

    c.   Oral temperatures are reliable with cooperative patient (age >5-6) but may vary with rapid breathing and recent ingestion of hot or cold fluids

    d.   The infrared ear thermometer estimates the temperature of the tympanic membrane (TM)

        (1)   Improper placement and aiming, incomplete probe penetration into external ear canal, and obstruction/tortuosity of the external ear canal can lead to underestimating TM temperatures

        (2)   Do not measure TM temperatures in children <3 years, and possibly up to 6 years

    e.   Skin and forehead measurements are inaccurate

2.   Measure respiratory rate, pulse, and blood pressure in older children and adults; see following table for normal rates in children

AGE-SPECIFIC PULSE AND RESPIRATORY RATES IN CHILDREN AND INFANTS

Age	Range of Respiratory Rate (breaths per minute)	Heart Rate (beats per minute) Average	Heart Rate (beats per minute) Range
Term - Newborn	40-60	140	90-170
One month	30-50	135	110-180
Six months	25-35	135	110-180
One year	20-30	120	80-160
Two years	20-30	110	80-130
Three years	20-30	105	80-120

Adapted from Daaleman, T.P. (1996). Fever without source in infants and young children. *American Family Physician, 54,* 2503-2512.

3.   Pulse oximetry is a reliable predictor of respiratory problems

4.   Observation is critical; see table YALE OBSERVATION SCALE for quantifying observations in children

YALE OBSERVATION SCALE

Observation Item	Normal = 1	Moderate Impairment = 3	Severe Impairment = 5
Quality of cry	Strong or none	Whimper or sob	Weak or moaning or high-pitched
Reaction to parent stimulation	Cries briefly or appears content and not crying	Cries on and off	Persistent cry or hardly responds
State variation	If awake, stays awake or if asleep, awakens quickly	Eyes close briefly when awake or awakens with prolonged stimulation	No arousal and falls asleep
Color	Pink	Pale extremities or acrocyanosis	Pale or cyanotic or mottled or ashen
Hydration	Skin and eyes normal and moist membranes	Skin and eyes normal; mouth slightly dry	Skin doughy or tented and dry mucous membranes and/or sunken eyes
Response to social overtures	Smiles or alerts consistently (≤2 mo)	Smiles or alerts briefly (≤2 mo)	No smile, anxious, dull, expressionless; no alerting to social overtures (≤2 mo)

A total score of <11 signifies a <3% probability of serious illness
A total score of 11-15 signifies a 26% probability of serious illness
A total score of >15 signifies a >92% probability of serious illness

Adapted from McCarthy, P.L., Sharpe, M.R., Spiesel, Z., et al. (1982). Observation scales to identify serious illness in febrile children. *Pediatrics, 70,* 802-809.

5.   In infants, check for bulging fontanel, an ominous sign

6.   Observe skin for color, rashes, petechiae or purpura; absence of petechial rash below the nipples makes meningococcemia less likely

7.   Assess for signs of dehydration such as skin turgor and capillary refill

8.   Assess neck for nuchal rigidity

9.   Check for lymphadenopathy

10.   In males, note whether the child is uncircumcised, which is a predisposing factor for urinary tract infections (UTI)

11.   Assess for swollen joints

12. Perform neurologic exam, noting positive Kernig or Brudzinski signs
13. In most cases, perform a complete physical examination to find localized infection such as otitis media, pharyngitis, sinusitis, meningitis, cervical adenitis, pneumonia, urinary tract infection, arthritis, and osteomyelitis

C. Differential Diagnosis: See PATHOGENESIS section for ETIOLOGIES OF FEVER
1. Fevers almost always result in increases in pulse rates; absence of a pulse rate increase suggests factitious fever, mycoplasmal infection or typhoid fever (see table AGE-SPECIFIC PULSE RATES, IV.B.2.)
2. It is important to differentiate true fever from hyperthermia
3. Any young child with a fever without source should be evaluated for a serious bacterial infection (SBI); to help formulate a diagnosis it is important to determine if the child is at low or high risk for SBI (see following table)

CRITERIA FOR FEBRILE INFANTS AT LOW RISK FOR SERIOUS BACTERIAL INFECTION	
Clinical Criteria	**Laboratory Criteria**
History: • No previous hospitalizations • No chronic illness • No previous antibiotic therapy Physical Examination: • No toxic appearance • No focal bacterial infection (except otitis media) • Normal activity, hydration, and perfusion • No purpura • No meningeal signs Social Situation: • Parents/caregiver mature and reliable • Transportation available • Thermometer and telephone in home • Travel time to care facility <30 minutes	White Blood Cell Count: • 5,000-15,000 per mm^3 Band cell count • <1,500 per mm^3 Urinalysis • <5 WBCs per high-power field or normal gram-stained smear Stool • <5 WBCS per high-power field

Adapted from Barraff, L.J., Bass, J.W., Fleisher, G. R., et al. 1993. Practice guideline for management of infants and children 0 to 36 months of age with fever without source. *Pediatrics, 92,* 1-12.

D. Diagnostic Tests: Recommended diagnostic tests depend on patient's age, clinical presentation, and previous medical history
1. In the majority of cases, the history and physical examination will uncover likely causes of the fever and suggest selective diagnostic tests
2. Diagnostic tests for children (<3 years) with fever without source and children who have a localized infection but also one of the following: Are <3 months of age, look toxic, have an extremely elevated temperature, are immunodeficient, or have a chronic disease
   a. To partially determine whether a young child is in low risk or high risk group for serious bacterial infections order the following laboratory screening tests: CBC with differential, urinalysis, stool smear if child has diarrhea, chest-x-ray if child has tachypnea or rales
   b. Children at high risk for serious bacterial infection (see preceding table to differentiate low risk vs. high risk children in IV.C.3.), children with high fevers, immunocompromised children, and children <28 days old should have an evaluation for sepsis, bacteremia, and meningitis (see following table)

DIAGNOSTIC TESTS FOR SEPSIS, BACTEREMIA, AND MENINGITIS EVALUATION
• Cultures - cerebrospinal fluid, blood, urine* • Complete blood cell count with differential • Examination of cerebrospinal fluid for cells, glucose, and protein • Chest x-ray if child is tachypneic, has cough, or shows signs of respiratory distress • Culture of stool if child has diarrhea • (Some authorities also recommend erythrocyte sedimentation rate, Group B strep antigen detection obtained from urine and CSF, arterial blood gas, C-reactive protein, serum calcium, haptoglobin, fibrinogen)

*Urine cultures should be obtained by catheter or suprapubic aspiration

Adapted from Baraff, L.J., Bass, J.W., Fleisher, G.R., et al. 1993. Practice guideline for management of infants and children 0-36 months of age with fever without source. *Pediatrics, 92,* 1-12.

3.   Additional diagnostic tests for low risk children are dependent on age, clinical presentation, and social situation, etc.; additional tests to order are discussed in V. PLAN/MANAGEMENT

4.   Fevers of unknown origin (FUO) require an extensive diagnostic evaluation

V.   Plan/Management

A.   Hospitalize the following patients:
1.   **All infants 28 days** or less regardless of appearance or risk status
2.   All toxic-appearing infants and children
3.   All children NOT meeting low risk criteria for serious bacterial infection (see table IV.C.3.)
4.   Immunocompromised children
5.   Children and adults who are disoriented or delirious
6.   Children and adults with meningismus, petechiae or purpura

B.   Consider consultation and hospitalization for following patients:
1.   Any infant under 3 months of age needs special attention and in most cases hospitalization even if a source of the fever has been identified because of the risk of dehydration and other adverse reactions to elevated body temperatures. Also, these infants are at greater risk for sepsis, meningitis and pneumonia than other children. Remember that roseola or benign febrile seizures do not occur in infants less than 6 months of age
2.   Children between 3 months and 2 years old should not be treated on an outpatient basis without vigilant and special attention except if they have a localized, non-serious infection, are playful, drinking, voiding, and do not appear toxic. Children in this age group are more susceptible than older children to bacteremia and meningitis
3.   Patients with extremely elevated temperatures. In children bacteremia is more likely with fevers greater than 105°F. Even if a localized sign of infection is found such as otitis media, carefully consider the diagnosis of bacteremia in infants and young children with extremely high fevers
4.   Children who are lethargic and inconsolable
5.   Children with abnormal laboratory tests
6.   Patients who are immunodeficient or have a history of cardiac or another serious disease
7.   Patients who are taking corticosteroid or immunosuppressive therapy
8.   Patients who have prosthetic devices
9.   IV drug abusers
10.   Patients who are dehydrated
11.   Any patient who appears toxic (rigors, hypotension, oliguria, CNS abnormalities, petechial rash, marked leukocytosis or leukopenia, cardiorespiratory distress, new, significant cardiac murmurs)
12.   Any patient whose fever lasts longer than 7-10 days

C.   Treat cause of fever (i.e., antibiotics for bacterial infection)

D.   Treatment for **nontoxic appearing infants aged 28-90 days with fever without source**
1.   Evaluation of young children is aimed at identifying those at risk for serious bacterial infections; carefully determine if they are in low-risk group; low risk infants in this age group can be managed on an outpatient basis if close follow-up can be guaranteed. One of the following two approaches is recommended:
      a.   Approach one
            (1)   Order cultures of blood, urine, cerebrospinal fluid, and possibly stool (order if child has bloody diarrhea)
            (2)   While waiting for culture results, administer intramuscular ceftriaxone (Rocephin) 50 mg/kg/day
            (3)   Recheck in 18-24 hours, at which time a second injection of ceftriaxone can be given or admit child to hospital if condition worsens
            (4)   See **Section V.D.1.c.** for further treatment if culture results are abnormal
      b.   Approach two
            (1)   Order urine culture
            (2)   Provide careful observation
            (3)   Re-evaluate in 24 hours; if condition deteriorates patient should be admitted for sepsis evaluation and parenteral antibiotics
            (4)   See **Section V.D.1.c.(3).** for further treatment if urine culture is abnormal
      c.   Additional treatment may be needed after results of cultures are available for infants aged 28-90 days who are low-risk for SBI
            (1)   Most infants whose blood or lumbar cultures are positive should be admitted to hospital for parenteral antimicrobial therapy

        (2)   Afebrile, non-toxic-appearing infants with bacteremia caused by *Streptococcus pneumoniae* and who appear normal at recheck can be treated with second injection of ceftriaxone and 10-day course of oral amoxicillin (40 mg/kg/day in three divided doses) or penicillin (50 mg/kg/day in four divided doses) as an outpatient if careful followup can be maintained

        (3)   Afebrile, non-toxic-appearing infants with urinary tract infection without bacteremia can be treated with 10-day course of oral antibiotics (see section on URINARY TRACT INFECTION)

        (4)   Infants with otitis media without bacteremia should receive appropriate oral antimicrobial therapy (see section OTITIS MEDIA)

  2.   Fever management: see antipyretics V.F. and patient education V.H.

E.   **Treatment for non-toxic appearing children 3 months of age (>90 days) to 36 months of age with fever without source** and temperature ≥39.0 C who do not have an underlying host defense deficiency and who are in the low risk group; for children with temperature <39.0 C, no diagnostic tests or antibiotics are needed, but child should return if fever persists for >48 hours

  1.   Order following diagnostic tests:

    a.   Urine culture for the following:

        (1)   Males <6 months of age (article by Baraff [2000] also recommends uncircumcised males 6-12 months)

        (2)   Females <2 years of age (article by Baraff [2000] recommends only for females <12 months)

    b.   Stool culture if blood or mucus in stool or ≥5 WBCs/hpf in stool smear

    c.   Chest x-ray for children with dyspnea, tachypnea, rales, or decreased breath sounds (recent article by Baraff (2000) also recommends chest x-ray if SaO_2 <95% and WBC count ≥20,000)

    d.   Blood culture: Either of following approaches are acceptable

        (1)   Approach one: All children with temperature ≥39°C

        (2)   Approach two: Temperature ≥39°C and WBC ≥ 15,000

        (3)   Article by Baraff (2000) recommends that patients who have NOT received the conjugate *S. pneumoniae* vaccine and temperature ≥39.5°C should have WBC's measured; if WBC count is ≥15,000 then send blood culture and administer empiric antibiotic therapy (see V.E.2. that follows)

  2.   Empiric antibiotic therapy (prior to obtaining culture results) is usually prescribed but either of following approaches is acceptable (empiric antibiotic therapy is ceftriaxone [Rocephin] IM or some authorities suggest oral amoxicillin clavulanate [Augmentin], trimethoprim sulfamethoxazole [Septra], or erythromycin sulfisoxazole [Pediazole])

    a.   Approach one: Prescribe to all children with temperature ≥39°C

    b.   Approach two: Prescribe to only children whose temperature is ≥39°C and WBC ≥15,000

  3.   Recheck patient in 12-24 hours

  4.   Check cultures in 24-72 hours

    a.   If clinical condition deteriorates at any time or if *N. meningitidis* or *H. influenzae* are in blood cultures, hospitalize child

    b.   Children with blood culture positive for *S. pneumoniae* who are afebrile and well appearing can be treated as outpatients with second injection of ceftriaxone and 10-day course of penicillin or amoxicillin

    c.   Afebrile, non-toxic-appearing children with urinary tract infection without bacteremia can be treated with 10-day course of oral antibiotics (see section on URINARY TRACT INFECTIONS)

    d.   Children with otitis media without bacteremia should receive appropriate oral antimicrobial therapy (see section OTITIS MEDIA)

  5.   Fever management: see antipyretics V.F. and patient education V.H.

F.   Antipyretics

  1.   Reasons for NOT treating a low-grade or moderate fever in an otherwise well patient:

    a.   Antipyretics cause side effects and toxicity and do NOT alter the course or duration of disease

    b.   Antipyretics mask the signs and symptoms of a serious disease and confuse the clinical picture

  2.   However, most clinicians agree that antipyretics should be given in the following situations:

    a.   When fevers are 103°F and higher

    b.   In children with a history of febrile seizures

      c.   In patients for whom side effects of fever may be harmful (e.g. patients with compensated cardiac diseases and chronic debilitating disorders, patients who become dehydrated rapidly, patients who are alcoholics)

      d.   Patients who are uncomfortable and unable to rest

3.   In hyperthermic states such as thyrotoxicosis, heat stroke and overdressing, the set point has not been changed and antipyretic medications are not effective because they act to lower set point

4.   The drug of choice is acetaminophen (Tylenol); adolescents: 325-650 mg every 4-6 hours (maximum dose is 4 g); children: 15 mg/kg/dose every 4 hours (maximum 5 doses per day); maximum effect at 2 hours (see table that follows for doses by age and drug form)

      a.   Do not use in liver disease or transplant patients; strictly follow correct doses to prevent liver damage; typically safe in patients who drink <5 alcoholic beverages per day

      b.   Risk of toxicity is lower in children but can occur from intentional overdoses, unintended, inappropriate dosing or failure to recognize children at increased risk of toxicity (patients with diabetes, obesity, chronic undernutrition, prolonged fasting, family history of hepatoxic reaction, concomitant viral infection)

      c.   Carefully educate parents of younger children about concentration of acetaminophen in various preparations as there is potential for over dosage and under dosage (see table that follows)

ACETAMINOPHEN DOSAGES AND AVAILABLE FORMS FOR TREATMENT OF FEVERS				
Age	Drops (80 mg/0.8 mL)	Elixir (160 mg/1 tsp)	Chewable Tablets (80 mg)	Adult Tablets (325 mg)
<4 mo	0.4 mL	---	---	---
4-11 mos	0.8 mL	½ tsp	---	---
12-23 mos	1.2 mL	3/4 tsp	---	---
2-3 yrs	1.6 mL	1 tsp	2 tablets	---
4-5 yrs	2.4 mL	1 ½ tsp	3 tablets	---
6-8 yrs	---	2 tsp	4 tablets	1 tablet
9-10 yrs	---	2 ½ tsp	5 tablets	1 tablet
>10 yrs	---	---	6-8 tablets	2 tablets

5.   Although aspirin is an effective antipyretic, it should <u>never</u> be given to children and adolescents with a fever because of risk of Reye's syndrome

      a.   Adverse effects: Gastric irritation and risk of bleeding

      b.   Risk of asthma exacerbation and anaphylactic reaction, particularly in adults with history of asthma and nasal polyps

6.   Ibuprofen (Motrin) is another therapeutic option

      a.   Dosage in adolescents is 400 mg every 4-6 hours

      b.   In children with temperatures less than 102.5°F can give ibuprofen (Children's Motrin) 5 mg/kg/dose every 8 hours and 10 mg/kg/dose every 8 hours when temperatures are greater than or equal to 102.5°F. Available 50 mg/1.25 mL oral drops, 100 mg/5 mL liquid OTC, and 50 mg chewable tablets

      c.   Avoid in patients with aspirin allergies, ulcers, renal insufficiency, and bleeding disorders

      d.   Use cautiously because the long-term safety of administering ibuprofen in children has not been established

G.   Sponging may be performed but usually is unnecessary and may even be harmful because it can cause discomfort and chilling

1.   If temperature is extremely high or if aggressive fever management is necessary (such as a child with history of febrile seizures), sponge patient after giving antipyretic

2.   Sponging is an important part of the management plan in the following cases: Patients with severe liver disease who cannot take acetaminophen, neurologic problems in which temperature regulation mechanisms are abnormal, heat stroke, or in environments with excessive temperatures

3.   When sponging, water should be lukewarm and should not cause the patient to shiver (colder temperatures are used for heat illness such as heat stroke)

H. Patient Education
1. Teach parents the correct method to assess temperature
   a. If child is <3 years, use a rectal or ear thermometer (less reliable); if >3-5 years, child may be able to cooperate and use an oral thermometer
   b. Keep thermometer in place for at least 2 minutes
2. Reinforce when the parents should call a health care provider about an elevated temperature
   a. Instruct parents to immediately have their children evaluated by a clinician when there is delirium (disorientation or confusion), seizures, stiff neck, petechial or purpural rash, and signs of dehydration (can teach how to assess capillary refill)
   b. Call clinician if child of any age has associated symptoms such as swollen joints, severe cough, anorexia, lethargy (doesn't maintain eye contact or engage in environmental stimuli), inconsolability, and restlessness during sleep
   c. If child is 36 months or younger and has a fever greater than 100.4°F (38°C), call clinician
   d. For the older child, parents should call clinician for fevers above 103°F (39.4°C)
3. Teach patients and parents of children when to administer antipyretics and the correct dosage of these medications; parents often give lower than therapeutic doses
4. Teach parents to avoid over-the-counter medications which may contain aspirin (such as Pepto-Bismol) when their children have fevers
5. Remind patients and parents to read labels and find "hidden" sources of acetaminophen that are often in over-the-counter cough and cold medications and can cause toxicity
6. Teach patients to drink extra fluids; parents should be taught to offer their children fluids every 15-60 minutes depending on the child's condition
7. Daily activities should be modified to provide for additional rest, light meals, and avoidance of strenuous activities depending on patient's condition
8. Adolescents and older children should be taught to avoid overdressing when they have a fever; parents should be taught to avoid over bundling their febrile children
9. Tell patients to never use alcohol for sponging
10. Inform patients and parents of children that elevated temperatures are a normal body defense mechanism, not a disease; height of the temperature except when extremely high does not correlate well with serious diseases; assure everyone that there are almost always no adverse effects from fevers

I. Follow Up
1. Variable and depends on age, diagnosis, and clinical presentation of patient as well as the amount of friend and family support available
2. For infants, young children, and chronically-ill patients consider scheduling return visit for following morning or have telephone contact within 24 hours to assess condition
3. Instruct patients to return for further evaluation if fever persists for more than 2 or 3 days
4. For infants and children with fever without source see V. PLAN/MANAGEMENT for additional follow-up based on age and risk

LYMPHADENOPATHY

I. Definition: Lymph node enlargement (see also section on CERVICAL ADENITIS)

II. Pathogenesis

A. Following mechanisms result in lymphadenopathy
   1. Proliferation in response to an antigen
   2. Invasion of cells from cells outside the node such as malignant cells
   3. Transformation of primary nodular tissue into neoplastic cells

B. Causes of generalized lymphadenopathy (mnemonic acronym "**MIAMI**" may aid recall)
   1. **M**alignancies: Leukemia, lymphoma, immunoblastic lymphadenopathy, metastases
   2. **I**nfections (most common cause)
      a. Viral: Human immunodeficiency virus (HIV), mononucleosis, cytomegalovirus, hepatitis B, measles, rubella, rubeola
      b. Bacterial: Group A β-hemolytic *streptococcus*, cat-scratch disease, secondary syphilis
      c. Mycobacterial: atypical mycobacterial infection, miliary tuberculosis

        d.   Fungal: Histoplasmosis

        e.   Protozoal: Toxoplasmosis

    3.   **A**utoimmune disorders: Systemic lupus erythematosus, rheumatoid arthritis, Sjögren's syndrome

    4.   **M**iscellaneous: Sarcoidosis, lipid storage disease, Kawasaki disease, hyperthyroidism, hypopituitarism, hypoadrenocorticism

    5.   **I**atrogenic: Serum sickness, drug reactions (phenytoin and, less commonly, hydralazine, para-aminosalicylic acid, propylthiouracil, and allopurinol)

C.   Causes of localized lymphadenopathy: due to local infection, tumor growth, or recent immunization in area drained by involved lymph node (also see table that follows)

    1.   Although not palpable, hilar adenopathy may be found on imaging studies and associated causes are the following: Sarcoidosis, fungal infection, lymphoma, bronchogenic carcinoma, tuberculosis

    2.   Any region: Benign reactive hyperplasia, lymphomas, cat scratch disease, leukemia, sarcoidosis, malignancies

PALPABLE LYMPH NODES, LYMPHATIC DRAINAGE, AND ASSOCIATED CAUSES

Node	Drainage Area	Associated Causes
Occipital	Posterior scalp, neck	Scalp infections, insect bites, ringworm
Preauricular	Scalp, skin	Scalp infections, eye or conjunctival infections, rubella, mycobacterial infection, skin neoplasm, lymphomas, head and neck squamous cell carcinomas
Posterior auricular (mastoid)	Mastoid area	Rubella
Anterior cervical	Anterior neck, oropharynx, larynx	Mononucleosis, sarcoidosis, toxoplasmosis tuberculosis, infections of the pharynx and oral cavity, lymphomas, leukemia, squamous cell carcinoma
Posterior cervical	Scalp, neck, upper thoracic skin	Toxoplasmosis, tuberculosis, scalp infections, skin neoplasm, lymphomas, squamous cell carcinoma
Submental	Apex of tongue and lower lip	Tongue, gum, buccal mucosal, and dental infections
Submaxillary (submandibular)	Buccal cavity, tongue, cheek, and lips	Infections of the oral cavity, mononucleosis, tuberculosis, rubella, lymphomas, leukemias, squamous cell carcinoma, thyroid malignancy
Supraclavicular (Right)	Inferior neck and mediastinum	Pulmonary, mediastinal, and esophageal malignancies, mycobacterial/fungal infections, lymphomas
Supraclavicular (Left)	Inferior neck, mediastinum, and upper abdomen	Malignancies (intra-abdominal, renal, testicular, ovarian), Hodgkin's disease, lymphomas
Axillary	Breast, greater part arm, shoulder, superficial anterior and lateral thoracic and upper abdominal wall	Upper extremity infection, cat-scratch disease, tularemia, syphilis, brucellosis, leishmaniasis, breast malignancy or infection, lymphomas, leukemias
Epitrochlear	Hand, forearm, elbow	Bilateral: syphilis, tularemia, sarcoidosis, lymphomas, Unilateral: hand infection
Inguinal	Leg and genitalia	Syphilis, genital herpes, lymphogranuloma venereum, chancroid, gonococcal infection, lower extremity infection, lymphomas, skin neoplasms
Popliteal	Posterior leg and knee	Lower extremity infection

III.   Clinical presentation: The following key factors are helpful in arriving at a diagnosis:

    A.   Generalized versus localized lymphadenopathy

        1.   Generalized adenopathy is due to systemic disease

        2.   Localized adenopathy is caused by either local infection, tumor, or systemic disease

    B.   Location of node (see PATHOGENESIS, II.C.); left supraclavicular node, often called "sentinel" node, suggests Hodgkin's disease

C. Character of node
    1. Size: a large node (>1 cm) usually represents a specific pathology
    2. Metastatic cancer: Hard, painless, matted, fixed, often >3 cm
    3. Reactive: Discrete, mobile, rubbery, mildly tender
    4. Lymphadenitis: Tender, warm, red, fluctuant
    5. Infection: Firm, red, warm
    6. Lymphoma or leukemia: Firm or rubbery

D. Age of patient
    1. In children, most cases are benign or caused by infection
    2. Benign reactive hyperplasia or transient node enlargement from unknown causes occurs frequently in children and adolescents
    3. Lymph nodes in children are prominent until puberty
    4. Small palpable occipital and postauricular nodes are common in infants, but not older children; after 2 years of age, palpable cervical and inguinal nodes are common
    5. Posterior cervical node enlargement in the older child and adolescent may be mononucleosis
    6. Risk of cancer increases with age; malignant etiologies of lymphadenopathy are very low in children

E. Onset and duration
    1. Nodes of acute onset and duration are typically due to viral or pyogenic infection
    2. Chronicity suggests neoplastic disease, sarcoidosis, tuberculosis, and fungal infections although lymphadenitis may take several months to resolve

F. Rate of change: Usually nodes that are rapidly growing are more pathologic than slow-growing nodes

G. Associated symptoms
    1. Low-grade fevers with night sweats and weight loss characterize lymphoma, HIV infection, or tuberculosis
    2. Fatigue and weight loss suggest systemic infection, cancer, or connective tissue disease
    3. Hilar lymph node enlargement may cause compression of thoracic structures and result in cough, dyspnea, and wheezing

H. Associated signs
    1. Splenomegaly: Mononucleosis, lymphoma, or leukemia
    2. Thyromegaly: Hyperthyroidism
    3. Tender, warm, or enlarged joints: Collagen vascular disease, leukemia, rheumatoid arthritis
    4. Rash: Viral disease, Kawasaki disease, collagen and vascular disease

I. Epidemiologic leads
    1. Recent exposure to cats is predisposing factor in cat-scratch disease
    2. History of multiple sexual partners and IV drug use may be associated with sexually transmitted disease or HIV infection
    3. Alcohol or tobacco abuse with cervical lymphadenopathy may represent head and neck carcinoma
    4. Occupational diseases such as silicosis or asbestosis may result in hilar and mediastinal lymphadenopathy
    5. Tick bite may be associated with Lyme disease and exposure to biting insects can cause lymphadenopathy
    6. Travel-related lymphadenopathy (tuberculosis, trypanosomiasis, leishmaniasis, tularemia, plague, anthrax) is a possible diagnosis
    7. Certain medications such as phenytoin, penicillins, primidone, and trimethoprim/sulfamethoxazole can cause lymphadenopathy

IV. Diagnosis/Evaluation

A. History
    1. Ask about onset, duration, and rate of growth of all palpable nodes
    2. Question about tenderness of node(s)
    3. Ask about recent infections and trauma
    4. Inquire about systemic symptoms such as fever, weight loss, night sweats, fatigue, and diarrhea
    5. Inquire about arthralgias, muscle weakness, or rashes that suggest autoimmune diseases
    6. Question about exposure to animals, travel to foreign countries, occupational hazards, and explore other risk factors such as substance abuse, tobacco use, alcohol abuse, ultraviolet radiation, and sexual exposure

7. Ask about medications and immunization status
8. Explore past medical history and family history

B. Physical examination
   1. Assess all palpable nodes, noting size, location, consistency, tenderness, warmth, and fixation (see table in II.C. and following figures)

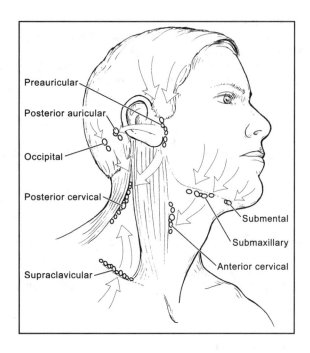

Figure 2.1. Palpable Lymph Nodes of the Head and Neck

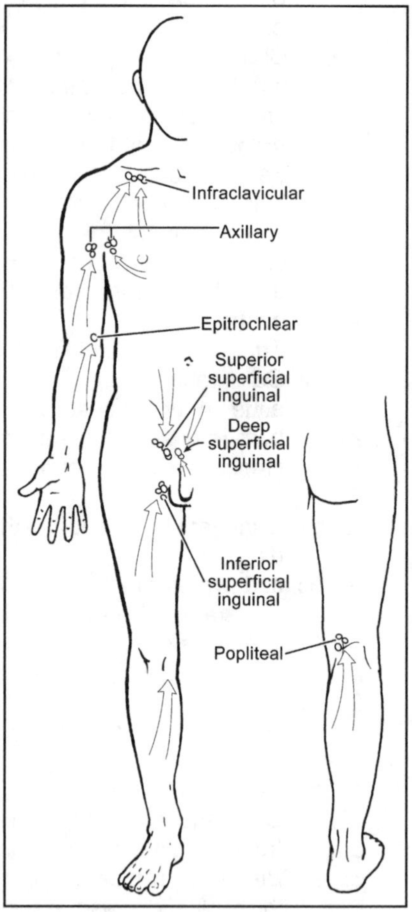

Figure 2.2. Palpable Lymph Nodes of Upper and Lower Extremities

   a. Normal, palpable nodes are discrete, freely mobile, and nontender
   b. Normal size of nodes is <1cm with two exceptions:
      (1) Inguinal nodes are normal up to 1.5 cm
      (2) Epitrochlear nodes are abnormal if >0.5 cm
   c. To assess for an enlarged supraclavicular node, ask patient to perform Valsalva maneuver during palpation of supraclavicular fossa
   2. For localized lymphadenopathy, carefully assess all body parts within the lymphatic drainage area (see preceding table in II.C.)
   3. For generalized lymphadenopathy a careful, comprehensive physical examination is needed

C. Differential Diagnosis
   1. Other structures such as enlarged parotid glands, cervical hygromas, thyroglossal and brachial cysts, hemangiomas, abscesses, lipomas, and other tumors may be confused with enlarged lymph nodes (see figure COMMON LOCATION OF MASSES OF FACE AND NECK in topic CERVICAL ADENITIS in section on PROBLEMS OF EARS, NOSE, THROAT)
   2. Potential causes range from simple and benign to complicated and serious
   3. No specific cause is found in many cases (see PATHOGENESIS, II.A.B.C. for range of etiologies)
   4. Persistent, generalized lymphadenopathy is defined as lymph node enlargement for at least three months in at least two extrainguinal sites; common causes are HIV infection, tuberculosis, syphilis, and lymphoma

D. Diagnostic Tests (if benign cause of lymphadenopathy is suspected, close observation is indicated); when the diagnosis is uncertain, stepwise testing with the following tests is needed:
1. CBC
   a. Atypical lymphocytes: Mononucleosis or other viral syndromes
   b. Increased granulocytes: Bacterial infection
   c. Increased eosinophils: Hypersensitivity states
   d. Decreased red blood cells and platelets: Malignancy
   e. Pancytopenia: HIV infection and tumor
2. Chest x-ray, which will detect pulmonary disease and hilar adenopathy, is needed for seriously ill patients and those with supraclavicular lymphadenopathy or respiratory complaints; consider ordering chest x-rays in patients who have enlarged nodes with no obvious inflammatory explanation to determine whether mediastinal or hilar nodes are also present
3. Serologic tests
   a. Monospot or Epstein-Barr virus: Mononucleosis
   b. VDRL: Syphilis
   c. HIV antibody: HIV infection
   d. Antinuclear antibody and rheumatoid factor: Collagen diseases
   e. Other serologic tests: Cytomegalovirus and toxoplasmosis infections
4. Tuberculin skin test for mycobacterial disease and hilar adenopathy
5. Cultures
   a. Throat for cervical adenopathy
   b. Urethral and cervical for inguinal adenopathy
   c. Aspirated lymph tissue for suspected fungal or mycobacterial infection
   d. Blood culture for suspected bacteremia
6. Lymph node biopsy provides a definitive diagnosis; indicated when simple testing fails to provide a diagnosis or for cases when cancer, tuberculosis, or sarcoidosis are suspected
   a. The following characteristics suggest the need for an early biopsy:
      (1) Node >2 cm
      (2) Abnormal chest x-ray
      (3) Enlarged supraclavicular node
      (4) Associated signs and symptoms of weight loss and hepatosplenomegaly
      (5) Absence of respiratory tract symptoms
   b. Nodes that remain constant in size for 4-8 weeks and those that fail to resolve in 8-12 weeks need a biopsy
7. Ultrasound and computed tomography are sometimes helpful in differentiating lymphadenopathy from nonlymphatic enlargement
8. Bone marrow examination is needed for patients with severe anemia, neutropenia, thrombocytopenia, or peripheral smear for malignant blast cells

V. Plan/Management

A. Treatment depends on diagnosis; see sections on CERVICAL ADENITIS, KAWASAKI DISEASE, PHARYNGITIS, etc.

B. Consider consultation for patients suspected of having serious disease or one of the following:
1. Undiagnosed adenopathy lasting longer than 2 months
2. Firm, matted, rapidly enlarging, nontender nodes
3. Associated signs and symptoms such as night sweats, weight loss, bone pain, hepatosplenomegaly, fever of unknown etiology, and failure to thrive in children
4. Associated CBC abnormality, positive PPD, or abnormal chest x-ray

C. Follow Up
1. Diagnosis will determine when patient should return for follow-up
2. Patients with benign clinical history, unremarkable physical examination, and no constitutional signs and symptoms can be re-evaluated in three weeks
3. For other cases in which the cause of lymphadenopathy is uncertain, watchful waiting with follow up every 3-5 days for 2 weeks is appropriate

PAIN

I. Definition: Unpleasant sensory and emotional experience related to actual or potential tissue damage

II. Pathogenesis

   A. Peripheral stimulation occurs when free nerve endings or nociceptors found in various parts of body (i.e., skin, blood vessels, viscera, muscles) are stimulated and then action potentials are transmitted along afferent nerve fibers to the spinal cord

   B. Gate control theory further develops the pathophysiology of pain
      1. The perception of pain is an interplay between the nociceptive pain fibers and the non-nociceptive or non-transmitting neurons that synapse in the spinal cord
      2. Clinically, this is important because certain treatments such as acupuncture, topical irritants, and transcutaneous electrical nerve stimulation (TENS) can stimulate the large non-nociceptive neurons and produce an analgesic effect

   C. Pain-initiated processes as well as other information are carried through the ascending spinal cord pathways (particularly the spinothalamic tract) to the brain

   D. In the brain, pain is perceived as a partial summation of two processes:
      1. Positive feedback is the nociceptive stimulus which activates pain transmission
      2. Negative feedback is the brain's modulatory network composed of the endogenous opiate system (opiate receptors, endorphins) which inhibits pain

   E. Other neurotransmitter substances such as acetylcholine, dopamine, norepinephrine, and serotonin play a role in pain transmission as well

   F. The brain controls pain sensation through an organized descending or efferent pain transmission system

III. Clinical Presentation

   A. Acute pain
      1. Arises from injury, trauma, spasm, or disease of body parts
      2. Usually is short-lived and decreases as damaged area heals
      3. Associated with hyperactivity of the sympathetic nervous system resulting in the following: tachycardia, tachypnea, elevated blood pressure, diaphoresis, and dilated pupils

   B. Persistent pain (previously called chronic pain)
      1. Pain which lasts longer than 6 months is rarely accompanied with hyperactivity of sympathetic nervous system
      2. Can be classified into 4 categories
         a. Nociceptive pain may be visceral (located in abdomen or thorax) or somatic (initiated in muscles or connective tissue)
            (1) Pain arises from tissue inflammation, mechanical deformation, ongoing injury, or destruction
            (2) Responds well to traditional pain management strategies
         b. Neuropathic pain results from a pathophysiologic process involving peripheral or central nervous system
            (1) Examples include diabetic neuropathy and post-amputation phantom limb pain
            (2) Responds to unconventional analgesics such as anticonvulsants and tricyclic antidepressants
         c. Mixed or unspecified pain such as occurs with recurrent headaches and vasculitic pain syndromes; treatment often requires experimentation with different or combined approaches
         d. Rare conditions in which psychologic disorders are cause of pain; psychiatry is needed
      3. Persistent pain is commonly a result of one of the following:
         a. Pain that persists beyond the normal healing time for an acute injury
         b. Chronic disease pain
         c. Pain without identifiable organic cause
         d. Cancer pain
      4. Depression often accompanies persistent pain; can lead to functional loss and social withdrawal

C. Pain in children is different than pain in adults
   1. Research suggests that the younger the person, the lower the pain threshold and the greater the sensitivity to pain
   2. Children are often under-treated for pain
   3. Level of cognitive development affects how the child perceives and responds to pain
      a. In infants and preverbal children, irritability, restlessness, poor feeding, excessive sweating, and sleep problems may be signs of pain
      b. Toddlers and preschool children do not understand that their pain is related to illness or injury, but instead, often believe pain is a form of punishment; children at this age become withdrawn, clingy, and quiet when in pain
      c. School-age children may respond to pain with anxiety and aggressiveness; children at this age are fearful of bodily injury and may exaggerate minor bruises and injuries
      d. By age 7, when the child is in Piaget's concept of the origin of concrete thinking, understanding that pain is a result of injury or illness is possible
      e. Children >10 years of age may be anxious and fear loss of control when in pain
      f. Adolescents need to maintain self esteem and may not display pain behaviors because of fear of embarrassment; they often feel omnipotent and may not comply with treatment regimen
      g. There are many misconceptions about pain in children (see following table)

MISCONCEPTIONS ABOUT PAIN IN CHILDREN	
Misconception	**Fact**
Infants and children do not feel pain as intensely as adults	Sensitivity to pain decreases with age; younger children exhibit a lower pain threshold than older children and adults
Infants and young children do not remember pain	By 6 months of age, children have memory of painful stimuli
Children cannot communicate where they hurt or the intensity of their pain	After infancy, children can accurately point to the location of their pain; most children by age 4 years can use simple self-report scales
The child is not experiencing pain if behavioral manifestations of pain are not present	Children can experience pain without displaying any behavioral manifestations; children use sleep and play as coping mechanisms
Children will always tell the truth about pain	Children rarely fabricate pain, but they may underreport or deny pain for fear of injections or other painful procedures
Opioids can lead to respiratory depression and addiction in children	Opioids can be safely given to neonates, infants, and children; respiratory depression is rare and there are no reports of addiction in children treated with opioids

Adapted from American Pain Society. (2002). *Guideline for the management of pain in osteoarthritis, rheumatoid arthritis, and juvenile chronic arthritis.* Glenview, IL: Author

   D. An individual's culture and belief system have a strong influence on pain perception and control

IV. Diagnosis/Evaluation

   A. History: Patient's self-report of pain is the most accurate and reliable evidence of the existence of pain
     1. Focus assessment on finding the cause of pain, determining characteristics of pain, and what factors are complicating the pain
     2. The Joint Commission on Accreditation of Healthcare Organizations recommends that pain be considered the "fifth" vital sign and that pain should be assessed each time pulse, blood pressure, temperature, and respirations are measured
     3. Mnemonic may be used to obtain patient's subjective description of pain
       a. P: palliative or precipitating factors such as stress, exertion
       b. Q: quality of pain such as sharpness, crushing, throbbing, burning
       c. R: region or radiation of pain
       d. S: subjective descriptions of severity of pain such as awakens at night or takes breath away
       e. T: temporal nature such as daytime, during meals; constant vs. intermittent
     4. Children ≥8 years can usually use a visual analog scale to quantify pain; adolescents can relate where pain falls on a line from zero (no pain) to 10 (worst pain ever experienced)
     5. In children use the "Faces" diagram/scale or for older children use Linear Analogue of "Faces" (see diagram from Beyer & Wells, 1989, in *Harriet Lane Handbook*)
     6. If the patient is a young child, ask parents to describe child's drinking pattern, activity level, amount of crying, and any unusual behaviors

7. Ask about changes in cognition and behavior such as agitation and withdrawal; inquire about sleep alterations, bowel changes, depression, and gait problems
8. Inquire about current and prior pain medication use, efficacy, and prior adverse reactions
9. Ask about previous personal or family history of chronic pain
10. Assess patient's level of functioning in all spheres of living such as family relationships, social relationships, employment, and hobbies to help determine secondary gains
11. Assess patient's attitudes, beliefs, and knowledge about pain and its management
12. Complete review of systems to determine relationship of pain to other parts of body

B. Physical Examination
1. Assess vital signs
2. Observe general appearance, gait, and posture for signs of distress
3. Observe patient's affect
4. Inspect, palpate, percuss, and auscultate, as appropriate, all areas and surrounding structures which patient perceives as painful; assess pain referral sites
5. Assess for muscle spasms, trigger points, and areas sensitive to light touch
6. Perform complete musculoskeletal, neurologic, and mental status exams
7. Observe physical function, such as ability to perform activities of daily living

C. Diagnostic tests are variable depending of patient's condition

D. Differential Diagnosis
1. Malingering for ongoing litigation or secondary gains
2. Anxiety or depression

V. Plan/Management

A. General principles of pain management
1. Resist prescribing pain medications without a diagnosis
2. The psychosocial aspects of pain are as important as the biologic aspects
3. For pediatric patients, it is important to provide a clear and realistic explanation of the problem and its treatment; allow parents to be present when a child must experience a painful procedure
4. Cultivating a sense of control by the older child and adolescent over the pain is important in both acute and chronic situations
5. Control of depression and other psychosocial factors facilitates pain management
6. In chronic situations, facilitate the patient's engagement in an active, productive life
7. Essential to involve the patient's family and friends in the management plan
8. Important to assess the patient's response to pain treatments at frequent intervals

B. Pharmacologic principles of treating pain
1. Identify source of pain and treat as appropriate
2. Use the least potent analgesic with the fewest side effects
3. Give analgesics for adequate trial time and properly titrate the dose, which means considering individual patient characteristics and needs
4. Use analgesics on a regular dosing schedule and not on a "prn" basis which promotes anxiety and contributes to future drug dependence
5. Prevent persistent pain and relieve breakthrough pain; order rescue medication equivalent to half the standing dose to start on a prn basis
6. Recognize and treat side effects; avoid excessive sedation
    a. Use neurostimulants to reduce sedative effects such as caffeine, dextroamphetamine (Dexedrine), or methylphenidate (Ritalin)
    b. Regular laxative therapy with docusate sodium and sennosides (Senokot) twice a day is often needed to prevent constipation
7. Use equianalgesic doses
8. Use appropriate route of administration
    a. Use oral medications, if possible, because of ease of administration and cost effectiveness
    b. NSAID, ketorolac (Toradol), is available in IM preparation
    c. Fentanyl (Duragesic) is available as a transdermal patch
    d. Morphine and hydromorphone are available as rectal suppositories
    e. Subcutaneous or intravenous administration of morphine and hydromorphone may be needed; patient-controlled analgesia pumps can provide individualized pain relief

9. Watch for development of tolerance; tolerance is unlikely to develop in patients with stable disease
10. For the pediatric patient, nonpharmacological approaches such as applying cold or warm compresses or hiding the injury with a Band-Aid may be helpful

C. The Three-Step Analgesic Ladder of the World Health Organization (see table that follows)
1. Designed for chronic, cancer pain but can be used as a guide for all types of pain
2. Pharmacological management of pain in children is controversial
   a. Step approach is often recommended
   b. Children **<2months of age** who receive opioids **must be monitored in intensive care unit**

Step	Oral Medications	Regimen
Step 1	Acetaminophen 650 mg Q 4-6 hrs; 10-15 mg/kg/dose q 4-6 hrs (children) Salicylates: aspirin 325-650 mg Q 4 hrs* NSAIDs (dosage in next table) Tramadol 50-100 mg Q 4-6 hrs (not recommended <16 years)	Nonopioid ± adjuvant
If pain persists, maximize nonopioid and add step 2 opioid		
Step 2	Codeine 30-60 mg Q 4 hrs; 0.5-1.2 mg/kg Q 4 hrs (children) Dihydrocodeine 16-32 mg Q 4 hrs** Hydrocodone 5-10 mg Q 4-6 hrs; 0.05-0.15 mg/kg (children) Oxycodone 5 mg Q 6 hrs; 0.05-0.10 mg/kg (children)	Opioid: mild-to-moderate pain + nonopioid ± adjuvant therapy
If pain persists at step 2, increase dose of opioid or change to step 3 opioid		
Step 3	Morphine IR 15-30 mg Q 4-6 hrs; 0.1-0.3 mg/kg Q 3-6 hrs (children) Oxycodone 7.5-10 mg Q 4-6 hrs; 0.1-0.2 mg/kg (children) Hydromorphone 4 mg Q 4 hrs; 0.04-0.08 mg/kg (children) Fentanyl 50 µg/hr Q 72 hrs**	Opioid: moderate-to-severe pain ± nonopioid ± adjuvant therapy

THREE-STEP ANALGESIC LADDER OF THE WORLD HEALTH ORGANIZATION

* Do not give to children and adolescents with fevers
** Check dosage with pediatrician

Adapted from WHO (1990). Cancer pain relief and palliative care: Report of WHO Expert Committee. *WHO Technological Report Service, 804*, 1-73.

D. Acetaminophen (Tylenol - APAP) is a nonnarcotic agent with antipyretic and analgesic effects; minimal anti-inflammatory effects
1. Onset of 0.5-1 hour; duration 3-6 hours
2. "Ceiling effect" exists; above a certain dose no further increase in analgesia is observed
3. Daily cumulative dose should not exceed 100 mg/kg/day for children and 75 mg/kg/day for infants
4. Few adverse reactions; hepatotoxicity in overdose or in chronic alcoholics following therapeutic dosage; typically safe in patients who drink <5 alcoholic beverages per day
5. Risk of toxicity is lower in children, but can occur from intentional overdoses, unintended inappropriate dosage, or failure to recognize children at increased risk of toxicity (patients with diabetes, obesity, chronic undernutrition, prolonged fasting, family history of hepatotoxic reaction, concomitant viral infection)

E. Acetylsalicylic acid (Aspirin - ASA) is a nonnarcotic agent with antipyretic, analgesic, and anti-inflammatory effects (see table on NSAIDs which follows) - Never give aspirin when the child has a viral infection
1. Typically, not used for persistent pain because of dangers of gastrointestinal toxicity
2. Onset within 0.5 hours; duration 3-6 hours
3. "Ceiling effect" exists such that single doses greater than 650 mg do not result in greater degree of pain relief
4. Stop taking drug at least one week before surgery; single therapeutic dose irreversibly inhibits platelet function for the 7-day lifetime of platelet
5. Adverse reactions include Reye's syndrome, hypersensitivity reactions (asthmatic patients particularly), dyspepsia, indigestion, gastric ulcers, irreversible inhibition of platelet aggregation, tinnitus, renal effects, anemia
6. Check hematocrit and stool guaiac periodically; order plasma salicylate level determinations when patient is prescribed high dosages
7. Avoid in patients with asthma, thrombocytopenia, GI disorders

F. Other salicylic acid derivatives have a slower onset and longer duration than ASA, but are just as potent and cause fewer gastrointestinal and central nervous system side effects (see table on NSAIDs)

G. Nonsteroidal anti-inflammatory drugs (NSAIDs) are non-narcotic agents used for mild to moderate pain and have antipyretic, analgesic, and anti-inflammatory effects (see table on NSAIDs for dosing recommendations)
   1. Useful for dental pain, rheumatoid arthritis, headaches, musculoskeletal pain, menstrual cramps, and bone pain with cancer
   2. Dosing considerations:
      a. Patients have large variability in response to individual agents; Switch to another NSAID/class if one agent is ineffective; Do not switch until an adequate trial of efficacy has been undertaken (1-2 weeks depending on half-life of drugs)
      b. Always prescribe an adequate dosage (start with low dose and gradually increase to maximum dosage for patients in moderate pain)
      c. Do not use combination of different NSAIDs
      d. It is safe to combine an NSAID and acetaminophen, but there is no net gain in pain relief by combined use
   3. Adverse effects
      a. GI distress (take with meals to lessen this effect), fluid retention, peripheral edema, hepatic problems, renal disorders, hypertension, and central nervous system effects such as dizziness and depression.
      b. For patients with gastritis and alcohol use, consider prophylaxis with misoprostol Cytotec), omeprazole (Prilosec), or sucralfate (Carafate); avoid piroxicam (Feldene)
   4. Drug interactions
      a. Be careful in prescribing if patient is on other drugs; NSAIDs may enhance oral hypoglycemic agents and coumarin
      b. May impair diuretic function and antagonize the effects of antihypertensive medications by inhibiting renal prostaglandins
   5. In adults, cyclooxygenases (COX-2 inhibitors) have a better safety profile (reduce but do not eliminate the risk of gastrointestinal bleeding and perforations) than nonselective NSAIDs, but there are few published studies on their use in children; renal toxicity, hypertension, and edema are possible adverse reactions
      a. Rofecoxib (Vioxx) is available in liquid and tablet form
         (1) Onset of action is more rapid and duration of effect longer than celecoxib (Celebrex)
         (2) Vioxx has higher risk of hypertension and myocardial infarctions than naproxen
      b. Celecoxib (Celebrex) is contraindicated for patients with allergies to sulfa; to date, when compared to nonselective NSAIDs, Celebrex had similar risk of cardiovascular adverse effects
      c. Valdecoxib (Bextra) has similar adverse effects as the older COX-2 inhibitors
   6. Baseline tests for long-term therapy include hematocrit, liver function tests, urinalysis, blood urea nitrogen (BUN), serum creatinine; often these diagnostic tests are rechecked in first month after initiation and then at 6-month intervals
   7. In children, naproxen (Naprosyn), and ibuprofen (Children's Advil, Children's Motrin), are approved for use; other nonapproved NSAIDs commonly used in children are diclofenac (Voltaren) and ketorolac (Toradol)

NONSTEROIDAL ANTI-INFLAMMATORY DRUGS (NSAIDs)

Class & Agent	Capsule/Tablet Size	Dose for persons ≥ 18 years
FENAMATES		
Mefenamic Acid (Ponstel)	250	Initial: 500 mg, then 250 mg QID; max use 1 week
INDOLES		
Indomethacin (Indocin)	25, 50	25 mg BID or TID; max 200 mg daily
Sulindac (Clinoril)	150, 200	150 mg BID; max 400 mg/day
NAPHTHYLKANONE		
Nabumetone (Relafen)	500, 750	1 g/day QD or BID; max 2 g/day
OXICAMS		
Piroxicam Feldene)	10, 20	20 mg QD or 10 mg BID
PHENYLACETIC ACID		
Diclofenac sodium (Voltaren)	25, 50, 75, 100 ext. rel.	50-75 mg BID; max 200 mg/day 100 mg ext. rel. QD
PROPIONIC ACIDS		
Ibuprofen (Motrin)[†]	200, 400, 600, 800	200-600 mg Q 4-6 hrs; max 3.2 g/day
Naproxen (Naprosyn)*	250, 375, 500	250-500 mg initially, followed by 250 mg Q 6-8 hrs
PYRANOCARBOXYLIC ACID		
Etodolac (Lodine)	200, 300, 400, 500	200-400 mg Q 6-8 hrs; max 1200 mg/day
SALICYLATES		
Acetylsalicylic acid (ASA)	Varies	325-650 mg Q 4-6 hrs; max 4 g/day
Diflunisal (Dolobid)	250, 500	500-1000 mg initially, followed by 250-500 mg q 8-12 hrs
Choline magnesium trisalicylate (Trilisate)**	500, 750, 1000	500-1500 mg BID
COX-2 INHIBITORS		
Celecoxib (Celebrex)	100, 200	100-200 mg BID
Rofecoxib (Vioxx)	12.5, 25, 50	12.5 mg QD initially; max 25-50 mg QD
Valdecoxib (Bextra)	10, 20	10 mg QD

[†]Ibuprofen (Motrin Suspension, available 100 mg/5 mL) >2yrs, 5-10 mg/kg Q 6-8 hours
*Naproxen (Naprosyn Suspension, available 125 mg/5 mL): Children >2 yrs, 2.5-5.0 mg/kg/dose BID or TID; max 15 mg/kg/day
**Choline magnesium trisalicylate (Trilisate Liquid, available 500 mg/5 mL):
    Children 12-37 kg, 50 mg/kg/day, in 2 divided doses
    Children >37 kg, 2.25 g/day, in 2 divided doses

H.   Tramadol (Ultram), a central-acting analgesic, is sometimes used for treatment of mild-to-moderate pain; well suited when pain is not relieved by acetaminophen and the patient cannot tolerate NSAIDs and wishes to defer opioid therapy; not recommended for children <16 years; use with caution in patients with seizure disorders

I.   Step 2 should be initiated when the patient continues to have mild-to-moderate pain despite taking a nonopioid analgesia; the following should occur at this step:
1.   Maximize the dose of the nonopioid analgesia - AND - add a step 2 opioid analgesia
2.   Step 2 opioids are restricted for the treatment of moderate pain because of their dose-limiting side effects or because they are prepared with fixed combinations of nonopioid analgesics (see table CONTROLLED DRUGS for classification)
    a.   Value of codeine (CIII) is limited because of increasing risk of side effects at doses above 1.5 mg per kg; available in elixir containing 120 mg acetaminophen and 12 mg codeine per 5 mL
    b.   Hydrocodone (Lortab) (CIII) and oxycodone (Percocet) (CII) are limited because of their combinations with acetaminophen; both drugs are available in elixirs combined with acetaminophen

CONTROLLED DRUGS

CII:	High potential for abuse which may lead to severe psychological or physical dependence. Prescriptions must be written in ink or typewritten and signed by practitioner. Verbal prescriptions cannot be made
CIII:	Use of these products may lead to moderate or low physical dependence or high psychological dependence. Prescriptions can be oral or written and may be redispensed
CIV:	These drugs have a low abuse potential, use may lead to limited physical or psychological dependence. Prescriptions may be oral or written and may be redispensed up to 5 times within 6 months
CV:	These drugs have a low abuse potential, may or may not require a prescription, and are subject to state and local regulation

J.　Step 3: If pain persists even when taking highest, safe dose of step 2 opioid, add a step 3 opioid to treat moderate to severe pain
　　1.　Morphine is first line agent and the most widely used opioid for management of acute pain in children; available in immediate release tablets (MSIR) (CII), sustained release tablets (MS Contin) (CII), extended release tablets (Avinza) (CII), rectal suppository, liquid, injection, and intravenous
　　2.　Other choices
　　　　a.　Oxycodone (OxyContin) (CII)
　　　　b.　Hydromorphone (Dilaudid) (CII); 5 times as potent as morphine in children
　　　　c.　Fentanyl (Duragesic) (CII) transdermal patches can control pain for 72 hours; to avoid over-medication, remember that the drug continues to be delivered approximately 18 hours after removal of the patch; patch is not currently approved for children, but a 12.5 µg/hour patch is under investigation
　　　　d.　Methadone (Dolophine) (CII) and levorphanol (Levo-Dromoran) are useful for severe pain, but because of long half-lives are not recommended for initial therapy; carefully assess and titrate to prevent delayed sedation
　　3.　Adverse effects of opioids are respiratory depression, nausea, ileus, itching, and urinary retention in children (see following table on management of adverse effects)

MANAGEMENT OF OPIOID-INDUCED ADVERSE EFFECTS*

Respiratory Depression
- Naloxone, 0.01-0.02 mg/kg up to a full reversal dose of 0.1 mg/kg

Excessive Sedation Without Evidence of Respiratory Depression
- Methylphenidate: 0.3 mg/kg/dose PO (typically, 10-20 mg to a teenager) before breakfast and lunch. Do not administer to patients taking clonidine, because dysrhythmias may develop.
- Change opioid or decrease the dose

Nausea and Vomiting
- Trimethobenzamide: PO or PR; <15 kg, 100 mg q6h; >15 kg, 100-200 mg q6h.
- Ondansetron: 0.15 mg/kg, up to 8 mg, IV q6-8h, not to exceed 32 mg/day (also available as a sublingual tablet)
- Change opioid

Pruritus
- Diphenhydramine: 0.5 mg/kg PO q6h
- Hydroxyzine: 0.5 mg/kg PO q6h
- Cyproheptadine: 0.1-0.2 mg/kg PO q8-12h; maximum dose, approximately 12 mg
- Change opioid

Constipation
- Encourage consumption of water, a high-fiber diet, and vegetable roughage
- Bulk laxatives: Metamucil, Maltsupex
- Surfactants: Docusate sodium (Colace)

* PO = per os (orally); PR = per rectum

K.　The following opioids are not recommended
　　1.　Meperidine (Demerol) has a short half-life and its metabolite, normeperidine, is toxic
　　2.　Propoxyphene (Darvon) has a long half-life and there is risk of accumulation of norpropoxyphene, a toxic metabolite

3. Mixed narcotic agonist-antagonists such as pentazocine (Talwin) (CIV), butorphanol (Stadol) (CIV), and buprenorphine (Buprenex) (CIV) cause less constipation and biliary spasmodic activity but have the tendency to cause psychotomimetic responses

L. Adjuvant analgesics; limited data are available on the efficacies of these analgesics in children, but they are commonly used in this population
   1. Tricyclic antidepressants (TCAs) such as amitriptyline (Elavil) (most frequently used, but has most side effects), imipramine (Tofranil), and desipramine (Norpramin) may be beneficial
      a. Have direct analgesic effects and may potentiate opiate analgesia
      b. Useful in treatment of pain due to nerve injury such as diabetic neuropathy
   2. Selective serotonin reuptake inhibitors (SSRIs) such as fluoxetine (Prozac) or sertraline (Zoloft) have fewer adverse effects than TCAs and may be beneficial
   3. Caffeine may increase analgesic effect when given with other pain medications
   4. Phenothiazines such as prochlorperazine (Compazine) 5-10 mg TID or QID (children >2yrs: 0.4 mg/kg/day in three or four divided doses, available 5 mg/5 mL syrup) or promethazine (Phenergan) 25 mg BID (children >2yrs: 0.1 mg/kg/dose Q 6 hours, available 6.25 mg/5 mL syrup) are useful as antiemetics when used in combination with other pain medications
   5. Anticonvulsants are useful for management of brief lancinating pain in chronic neuralgia such as trigeminal neuralgia and postherpetic neuralgia; use one of following:
      a. Carbamazepine (Tegretol)
      b. Gabapentin (Neurontin)
   6. Mexiletine (Mexitil) is beneficial for neuropathic pain
   7. Corticosteroids are beneficial in patients with acute nerve compression, visceral distention, increased intracranial pressure, and soft-tissue infiltration

M. Treatment of metastatic bone pain includes radionuclides (strontium-89 and samarium-153 lexidronam) and bisphosphonates

N. A recent concept in acute pain therapy is preemptive analgesia that involves introducing an analgesic regimen prior to onset of noxious stimuli to prevent sensitization of the nervous system to subsequent stimuli that could amplify pain

O. Nonpharmacologic modalities to treat pain include meditation, relaxation, distraction, exercise, massage, imagery, aromatherapy, biofeedback, hypnosis, acupuncture, surgery (cordotomy), neuroablative blocks (chemical destruction of nerves), and nervous system stimulators such as dorsal column stimulators (DCS) and transcutaneous electrical nerve simulators (TENS)

P. Interdisciplinary pain management can reduce the patient's reliance on opiates through nonpharmacological methods such as biofeedback, visual imagery, and stress management

Q. Patient education
   1. Research has shown that patient education alone can significantly improve pain management
   2. Provide information about nature of pain, medications, and nonpharmacologic approaches
   3. Explain the difference between addiction that rarely occurs with chronic opioid use and dependence or tolerance that may occasionally occur
   4. Explain that patients typically develop tolerance to most adverse effects such as nausea, vomiting, and sedation
   5. When using opioid analgesics, instruct adolescent not to drive; patient and parents should be warned about potential for falls and accidents (precautions should be undertaken)
   6. Remind patients and parents to carefully read labels of over-the-counter medications (especially cold, cough, fever, and headache drugs) because these drugs often have analgesic components (e.g., acetaminophen) that may cause over-medication, adverse reactions, and toxicity
   7. Warn patients that chewing or crushing continuous-release tablets destroys their controlled-release properties and may result in overdosage
   8. Explain to patient and family that chronic pain is a chronic disease and goals of treatment are to improve functioning and quality of life rather than eliminate pain; cognitive coping strategies that help patients gain control of pain management also are effective
   9. Behavioral strategies such as controlling pain by relaxation methods, increasing pleasurable activities, and pacing activities are beneficial
   10. Meditation, which helps the patients accept pain, and distraction strategies (imagery, focal point, counting method) are effective
   11. Website resources are available (see table WEBSITE RESOURCES)

R.   Follow up evaluation is important if patient is on long-term pain management regimen
    1.   Regularly evaluate for drug efficacy
    2.   Carefully evaluate for side effects
        a.   For patients on NSAIDs, monitor for gastrointestinal blood loss, renal insufficiency, edema, hypertension
        b.   For patients on opioids, monitor for sedation, fatigue, confusion, and constipation
        c.   Monitor for drug-drug and drug-disease interactions
    3.   Periodically evaluate for inappropriate or dangerous drug-use patterns

WEIGHT LOSS (INVOLUNTARY)

I.   Definition: Process that occurs when the number of calories available for utilization is below the patient's daily needs (also see topic UNDERNUTRITION AND FAILURE TO THRIVE)

II.   Pathogenesis

A.   Reduced food intake and/or anorexia can result in a calorie deficit from the following causes:
    1.   Psychological problems such as anorexia nervosa, depression, and anxiety
    2.   Physical and financial factors that limit purchasing, preparing, or eating food
        a.   Poor dentition
        b.   Immobility problems
        c.   Dysphagia
    3.   Drug-related problems such as digitalis excess or amphetamine abuse
    4.   Esophageal disease
    5.   Infections such as human immunodeficiency virus (HIV) infection, tuberculosis, and fungal disease
    6.   Malignancy
    7.   Uremia
    8.   Hepatitis
    9.   Vitamin B deficiencies
    10.   Neurologic disorders, including trauma
    11.   Substance abuse and tobacco use
    12.   Competitive athletics (especially wrestling)

B.   Calorie loss can occur because of malabsorption from the following conditions:
    1.   Crohn's disease
    2.   Pancreatic insufficiency
    3.   Cholestasis
    4.   Parasitic disease such as giardiasis
    5.   Blind loop syndrome
    6.   Food sensitivity in celiac disease, lactose intolerance, and milk allergy

C.   Calories can be lost in the urine or stool from the following illnesses:
    1.   Uncontrolled diabetes mellitus
    2.   Diabetes insipidus
    3.   Diarrhea and vomiting

D.   Accelerated metabolism can contribute to weight loss in the following conditions:
1.   Hyperthyroidism
2.   Pheochromocytoma
3.   Fever
4.   Malignancy
5.   Spastic states

E.   Causes of weight loss vary by age group (see following table):

DIFFERENTIAL DIAGNOSIS OF WEIGHT LOSS BY AGE GROUP		
Newborns and Infants	Older Infants, Preschoolers, and Schoolchildren	Adolescents
✓ Inadequate intake of milk from breast or formula feeding ✓ Inappropriate dilution or choice of formula ✓ Infection ✓ Metabolic disorders ✓ Craniofacial abnormalities ✓ Central nervous system disorders ✓ Congenital heart disease ✓ Somnolence from maternal medications or substance abuse ✓ Vomiting due to congenital gastrointestinal malformations (duodenal atresia, volvulus) ✓ Polyuria from diabetes insipidus or renal disease	✓ Pyloric stenosis ✓ Gastroesophageal reflux ✓ Malabsorption syndromes ✓ Inflammatory bowel disease ✓ Cystic fibrosis ✓ Hirschsprung's disease ✓ Vomiting ✓ Diarrhea ✓ Infection ✓ Diabetes mellitus ✓ Hyperthyroidism ✓ Tuberculosis ✓ Congenital heart disease ✓ Malignancy or tumors ✓ HIV infection ✓ Psychological problems such as parental or childhood depression or eating disorder	✓ Inflammatory bowel disease ✓ Diabetes mellitus ✓ Hyperthyroidism ✓ Tuberculosis ✓ Malignancy ✓ HIV infection ✓ Psychological problems such as depression or eating disorder

III.   Clinical presentation of common causes of weight loss

A.   In children and adolescents, unintentional weight loss is an uncommon, but highly significant finding that signals a serious problem; although uncommon, organic causes should always be carefully ruled-out (see table II.E.)
1.   Newborns and young infants: A loss of more than 10% to 12% of birth weight in the few days after birth is uncommon and needs to be investigated
a.   Breast-fed infants should regain lost birth weight by 2 weeks of age; loss of weight is typically due to infrequent, small feedings, failure of the let-down reflex, or improper positioning of infant for feeding
b.   Bottle-fed infants rarely lose more than 5% of birth weight in first few days and should be above birth weight at 2 weeks; loss of weight is typically a result of errors in feeding due to parental inexperience
2.   Older infants, preschoolers, and schoolchildren
a.   Loss of 3% to 5% of baseline body weight occurring in less than 30 days is significant
b.   Consider pyloric stenosis or gastroesophageal reflux in young infants with weight loss and vomiting
c.   Loss of fluids due to vomiting and diarrhea is the most common cause of acute weight loss in older infants and toddlers
d.   Fever due to infections is another common cause
e.   Although uncommon, eating disorders have been found in children as young as 7 years
3.   Adolescents
a.   Anorexia nervosa and bulimia nervosa occur mainly in adolescents and young adult females who have body image disturbances and intense fear of becoming obese (see EATING DISORDERS section)
b.   Depression and other affective disorders may also contribute to weight loss

B.   Patients with HIV infection often have chronic anorexia, nausea, vomiting, and diarrhea due to drugs or to infections of the hepatobiliary system

C. Malignancies are less common in children than adults
1. May be present without major signs and symptoms
2. Dramatic, rapid weight loss accompanied by aversion to food and later jaundice and abdominal pain characterizes pancreatic cancer

D. Uremia often presents initially with anorexia and subsequent weight loss

E. Patients with uncontrolled diabetes mellitus often have weight loss and increased food intake

F. Hyperthyroidism or thyrotoxicosis is a common endocrine disease; patients often have increased appetite, food intake, and motor activity.

G. In malabsorption syndrome, foul-smelling, bulky, greasy stools are typical

H. Signs and symptoms of malnutrition may occur with any illness if there is a loss of 10 to 20% of normal body weight
1. Typical complaints include fatigue, depressed immune function, increased susceptibility to infection, skin breakdown, and changes in emotional stability such as irritability and apathy
2. Laboratory tests: Serum albumin <3.4 g/dL and lymphocyte count <1,500 are indicative of malnutrition

IV. Diagnosis/Evaluation (also see topic UNDERNUTRITION AND FAILURE TO THRIVE)

A. History
1. Carefully ascertain amount of weight loss; ask about change in clothing size if unable to elicit number of pounds lost
2. Validate amount of weight loss from a family member or significant other
3. In infants, carefully determine the number of ounces of formula ingested or, in breast-fed infants ask about number of times infant nursed
4. Obtain a 24 hour daily food intake
5. Determine whether patient has loss of appetite, normal appetite, or increased appetite; in patients with malignancies, depression, and adverse drug reactions, food often has an unappealing appearance, taste, and odor
6. Ask about abnormal or bad taste in mouth (occurs in hepatitis, drugs, sinusitis, vitamin B deficiencies, zinc deficiency, psychological disorders)
7. If decreased food intake is suspected, explore symptoms of depression, poor dentition, dysphagia, alcohol and drug use, pain, nausea, vomiting, fatigue, and symptoms of heart failure
8. Question about chewing or swallowing difficulties (occurs in neurologic, dental, oral, esophageal or pulmonary diseases)
9. If anorexia nervosa is suspected ask about eating habits, self-image and attitudes about weight control
10. Assess patient's emotional well-being
11. If malabsorption is suspected determine character of stools, signs of jaundice, easy bruising, sore tongue, and paresthesias
12. If loss of calories in stool or urine is suspected, inquire about polyuria, polydipsia, nausea, and character of the stools
13. If accelerated metabolism is suspected inquire about fever, fatigue, melena, cough that has changed in character, and symptoms of hyperthyroidism such as tachycardia, nervousness, heat intolerance, menstrual disturbances, and palpitations
14. Obtain history of tobacco dependence, alcohol consumption, and drug use
15. Inquire about participation in competitive athletics
16. Inquire about previous history of hepatitis exposure, renal disease, and endocrine problems
17. Determine family history, particularly noting any history of cancer in first-degree relatives
18. In children, it is particularly important to assess family functioning

B. Physical Examination; assessment should focus on nutritional status as well as identification of the underlying cause of weight loss
1. Measure height and weight, comparing with previous measurements (see OBESITY section for determining optimal weights)
   a. Body weight measurement is not always a good indicator of weight loss
   b. Occasionally loss of body tissue is accompanied by equal gain in extracellular fluid such as ascites or edema; thus, it is important to observe face and limbs for loss of soft-tissue mass
2. Assess for orthostatic hypotension which accompanies dehydration and malnutrition
3. Observe general appearance for wasting such as sunken eyes, sallow complexion, and hair loss

4. Assess for signs of depression such as inappropriate dress and dull affect
5. Assess skin for pallor, ecchymosis, jaundice, and turgor
6. In infants, palpate fontanelle
7. Examine mouth for poor dentition, glossitis, lesions, and excessive dryness
8. Palpate neck for thyromegaly and lymphadenopathy
9. Perform a complete cardiovascular examination
10. Auscultate the lungs; obtain oxygen saturation level
11. Inspect abdomen for shape, scars, and masses
12. Auscultate abdomen for bowel sounds
13. Palpate and percuss abdomen for tenderness, ascites, masses, and organomegaly
14. Perform a rectal examination
15. Assess extremities for edema, muscle wasting, and skin turgor
16. Assess position and vibratory senses
17. Assess deep tendon reflexes; check for prolonged relaxation phase of reflexes that often occurs with thyroid disorders

C. Differential Diagnosis (also see table in II.E.)
1. Feeding problems are most common causes in infants
2. Vomiting, diarrhea, and infections are common causes in children
3. Depression and psychological problems are the most common causes in older children
4. When weight loss occurs with increased food intake, consider diabetes, thyrotoxicosis, malabsorption, or possibly leukemia and lymphoma as the likely diagnosis
5. When food intake is normal or decreased, consider psychological problems, malignancy, infection, renal disease, or endocrine problems as the likely diagnosis

D. Diagnostic tests should be ordered based on history and physical examination
1. The following are recommended as the initial battery of tests to order:
   a. CBC to provide an overview of nutritional status and to screen for cancer
   b. Erythrocyte sedimentation rate (ESR) may be elevated in chronic infections, collagen vascular diseases, certain cancers, and inflammatory bowel disease; may be abnormally low in anorexia nervosa
   c. Serum electrolyte, blood urea nitrogen, and creatinine to assess dehydration, to rule-out renal or adrenal disease, and to determine pernicious or self-induced vomiting
   d. Serum protein and albumin to assess liver function, to diagnose malnutrition, and to rule-out protein malabsorption
   e. Three stool specimens for occult blood and tests of malabsorption to determine gastroenteritis, inflammatory bowel disease, and various causes of malabsorption
   f. Urinalysis and urine culture to diagnose diabetes mellitus, diabetes insipidus, dehydration, urinary tract infection, and renal disease; the urine pH may be elevated (> 8) in adolescents who have eating disorders, particularly if they are vomiting
   g. Serum glucose to diagnose diabetes mellitus
2. Consider ordering the following tests:
   a. Chest x-ray to detect infection and malignancies
   b. Thyroid stimulating hormone and T_4 to diagnose thyroid problems; also order thyroid tests in patients who have not had reduced food intake with weight loss
   c. Serum iron, transferrin, total iron-binding capacity, RBCs, folate, B_{12}, and zinc levels if malnutrition is suspected
   d. For patients with impaired absorption, a quantitative stool fat examination by means of a 72-hour stool collection or a breath test (definitive test); but screening for malabsorption can also be performed with Sudan stain of stool for fat and serum tests for carotenoids and folic acid
   e. Consider colonoscopy or flexible sigmoidoscopy, barium enema, upper endoscopy, or upper gastrointestinal series with small bowel follow-through, abdominal ultrasonography, computerized tomography of the abdomen, or magnetic resonance imaging if concerns of abdominal malignancy exist
   f. Consider serum amylase and lipase if a pancreatic disorder is suspected
   g. Stool for ova and parasites is ordered when giardiasis is suspected
   h. To assess nutritional status consider the following: serum albumin concentration, grip strength, triceps skin-fold thickness, arm muscle circumference, total lymphocyte count, bioimpedance analysis, serum transferrin, and transthyretin (prealbumin) concentrations

V.   Plan/Management (also see topic UNDERNUTRITION AND FAILURE TO THRIVE

A.   Treat underlying cause of weight loss (i.e., treat depression with antidepressant medications or pancreatic insufficiency with oral pancreatic enzyme preparations)

B.   Consider hospitalization for children with the following:
1.   Any child with significant weight loss
2.   Newborns with weight loss more than 12% to 15% of birth weight
3.   Older infants, children, and adolescents with excessive weight loss (more than 5% to 10% of previous weight)
4.   Children of any age who have the following:
   a.   Excessive fluid loss (vomiting, diarrhea, polyuria)
   b.   Evidence of dehydration
   c.   New onset diabetes mellitus
   d.   Severe febrile illness such as septicemia, osteomyelitis, meningitis
   e.   Electrolyte abnormalities
   f.   Congenital abnormalities
   g.   Severe malnutrition
   h.   Significant psychosocial dysfunction
5.   Infants who have extreme passivity when feeding; older children and adolescents who have acute food refusal, uncontrollable binge eating or purging, or severe anorexia nervosa

C.   Consultation with a dietitian/nutritionist is beneficial

D.   Symptomatic therapy includes the following:
1.   Suggest patient eat small, frequent feedings (6 times per day) of foods with high-calorie density
2.   Suggest dietary supplements such as Ensure (see section on HIV INFECTION)
3.   Consider ordering vitamin supplementation
4.   For nausea, suggest salty foods, cool clear beverages, gelatin, popsicles; avoid sweet, greasy, or high fat foods
5.   Appetite stimulants such as dronabinol (Marinol) and megestrol acetate (Megace) are recommended for AIDS patients, but are not FDA approved for unknown causes of weight loss

E.   Follow Up
1.   Scheduling of subsequent visits will depend on underlying cause of weight loss and age of patient: follow-up evaluations should be more frequent in infants and young children
2.   Encourage patient or parents to keep daily record of food intake, activity level, and symptoms

REFERENCES

Agency for Healthcare Research and Quality. (2001). *Defining and managing chronic fatigue syndrome.* (AHRQ Pub. No. 01-E061). Rockville MD: US Government Printing Office.

Agency for Healthcare Research and Quality. (2002). *Systematic Review of the Current Literature Related to Disability and Chronic Fatigue Syndrome.* Summary, Evidence Report/Technology Assessment: Number 66. AHRQ Publication No. 03-E006. Rockville MD. http://www.ahrq.gov/clinic/epcsums/cfsdissum.htm

American Academy of Pediatrics, Committee on Drugs. (2001). Acetaminophen toxicity in children. *Pediatrics, 108,* 1020-1024.

American Academy of Pediatrics, Committee on Psychosocial Aspects of Child and Family Health, & American Pain Society, Task Force on Pain in Infants, Children, and Adolescents. (2001). The assessment and management of acute pain in infants, children, and adolescents. *Pediatrics, 108,* 793-797.

American Pain Society. (2002). *Guideline for the management of pain in osteoarthritis, rheumatoid arthritis, and juvenile chronic arthritis.* Glenview, IL: Author.

Bazemore, A.W., & Smucker, D.R. (2002). Lymphadenopathy and malignancy. *American Family Physician, 66,* 2103-2110.

Bandyopadhyay, S., Bergholte, J., Blackwell, C.D., Friedlander, J.R., & Hennes, H. (2002). Risk of serious bacterial infection in children with fever without a source in the post-*Haemophilus influenzae* era when antibiotics are reserved for culture-proven bacteremia. *Archives of Pediatric and Adolescent Medicine, 156,* 512-517.

Baraff, L.J. (2000). Management of fever without source in infants and children. *Annals of Emergency Medicine, 36,* 602-614.

Baraff, L.J., Bass, J.W., Fleisher, G.R,. Klein, J.O., McCracken, G.H., Powell, K.R., et al. (1993). Practice guidelines for the management of infants and children 0 to 36 months of age with fever without source. *Pediatrics, 92,* 1-12.

Berde, C.B., & Sethna, N.F. (2002). Analgesics for treatment of pain children. *New England Journal of Medicine, 347,* 1094-1103.

Beyer, J.E., & Well, N. (1989). Multidimensional pain assessment of children. *Pediatric Clinics of North America, 36,* 387.

Craig, T., & Kakumanu, J. (2002). Chronic fatigue syndrome: Evaluation and treatment. *American Family Physician, 65,* 1083-1090, 1095.

Daaleman, T.P. (1996). Fever without source in infants and young children. *American Family Physician, 54,* 2503-2512.

Fitzgerald, G.A., & Patrono, C. (2001). The coxibs, selective inhibitors of cyclooxygenase-2. *New England Journal of Medicine, 345,* 433-442.

Fainsinger, R.L. (2002). Symptomatic care pending diagnosis: Pain. In R.E. Rakel, & E.T. Bope (Eds.), *Conn's current therapy 2002.* Philadelphia: Saunders.

Finkelstein, J.A., Christiansen, C.L., & Platt, R. (2000). Fever in pediatric primary care: Occurrence, management, and outcomes. *Pediatrics, 105,* 260-2666.

Fletcher, R. H. (1997). Lymphadenopathy. In L. Dornbrand, A.J. Hoole, & R.H. Fletcher (Eds.), *Manual of clinical problems in adult ambulatory care* (3rd ed.). Philadelphia: Lippincott-Raven.

Franck, L.S., Greenberg, C.S., & Stevens, B. (2000). Pain assessment in infants and children. *Pediatric Clinics of North America, 47,* 487-512.

Fukuda, K., Straus, S.E., Hickie, I., Sharpe, M., Dobbins., J., & Komaroll, A. (1994). The chronic fatigue syndrome: A comprehensive approach to its definition and study. *Annals of Internal Medicine, 121,* 953-959.

Garralda, M.E., & Rangel, L. (2002). Annotation: Chronic fatigue syndrome in children and adolescents. *Journal of Child Psychology and Psychiatry, 43,* 169-176.

Golianu, B., Krane, E.G., Galloway, K.S., & Yaster, M. (2000). Pediatric acute pain management. *Pediatric Clinics of North America, 47,* 559-587.

Gorman, T.E. (2000). Approach to the patient with chronic nonmalignant pain. In A.H. Goroll, & A.G. Mulley, Jr. (Eds.), *Primary care medicine.* Philadelphia: Lippincott.

Goroll, A.H., & Mulley, A.G. (2000). Evaluation of chronic fatigue. In A.H. Goroll & A.G. Mulley, Jr., (Eds.). *Primary care medicine: Office evaluation and management of the adult patient* (4th ed). Philadelphia: Lippincott.

Goroll, A.H., & Mulley, A.G. Jr. (2000). Evaluation of weight loss. In A.H Goroll, & A.G. Mulley, Jr. (Eds.). *Primary care medicine: Office evaluation and management of the adult patient* (4th ed). Philadelphia: Lippincott.

Gottschalk, A., & Smith, D.S. (2001). New concepts in acute pain therapy: Preemptive analgesia. *American Family Physician, 63,* 1979-1984.

Graham, D.B. (2002). Weight loss. In R.B. Taylor (Ed.). *Manual of family practice* (2nd edition). Philadelphia: Lippincott.

Greene, M.G. (1991). *The Harriet Lane Handbook.* St. Louis: Mosby.

Koch, W.C. (2002). Fever. In: F.D. Burg, J.R. Ingelfinger, R.A. Polin, & A.A. Gershon (Eds.), *Gellis & Kagan's' current pediatric therapy,* Philadelphia: Saunders.

Levine, P.H. (1998). What we know about chronic fatigue syndrome and its relevance to the practicing physician. *American Journal of Medicine, 105,* 100S-109S.

Luszczak, M. (2001). Evaluation and management of infants and young children with fever. *American Family Physician, 64,* 1219-1226.

Marcus, D.A. (2000). Treatment of nonmalignant chronic pain. *American Family Physician, 61,* 1331-1338.

McCarthy, P.L., Sharpe, M.R., Spiesel, Z., et al. (1982). Observation scales to identify serious illness in febrile children. *Pediatrics, 70,* 802-809.

Ozuah, P.A.O., & Sigler, A.T. (2001). Fatigue and weakness. In R.A. Hoekelman (Ed.). *Primary pediatric care.* St. Louis: Mosby.

Plaisance, K.I., & Mackowiak, P.A. (2000). Antipyretic therapy: Physiologic rationale, diagnostic implications, and clinical consequences. *Archives of Internal Medicine, 160,* 449-456.

Reid, S., & Wessely, S. (2002). Chronic fatigue syndrome. In R.E. Rakel & E.T. Bope (Eds.). *Conn's current therapy 2002.* Philadelphia: Saunders.

Rodriguez, R. (2002). The challenge of evaluating fatigue. *Journal of American Academy of Nurse Practitioners, 12,* 329-338.

Schechter, W.S. (2002). Pediatric pain management. In: F.D. Burg, J.R. Ingelfinger, R.A. Polin, & A.A. Gershon, (Eds.), *Gellis & Kagan's' current pediatric therapy,* Philadelphia: Saunders.

Segel, G.B., & Hall, C.B. (2001). Lymphadenopathy. In R.A. Hoekelman (Ed.), *Primary pediatric care.* St. Louis: Mosby.

Simon, H.B. (2000). Evaluation of fever. In A.H. Goroll, & A.G. Mulley, Jr. (Eds.), *Primary care medicine: Office evaluation and management of the adult patient* (4th ed). Philadelphia: Lippincott.

Simon, H.B. (2000). Evaluation of lymphadenopathy. In A.H. Goroll, & A.G. Mulley, Jr. (Eds.), *Primary care medicine: Office evaluation and management of the adult patient* (4th ed). Philadelphia: Lippincott.

Stashwick, C.A. (2001). Weight loss. In R.A. Hoekelman (Ed.), *Primary pediatric care.* St. Louis: Mosby.

Straus, S.E., & Gartner, J.C., Jr. (2002). Chronic fatigue syndrome (CFS). In: F.D. Burg, J.R. Ingelfinger, R.A. Polin, & A.A. Gershon, (Eds.), *Gellis & Kagan's' current pediatric therapy,* Philadelphia: Saunders.

Tan, E.M., Sugiura, K., & Gupta, S. (2002). The case definition of chronic fatigue syndrome. *Journal of Clinical Immunology, 22,* 8-12.

Welker, M.J. (2002). Symptomatic care pending diagnosis: Fever. In R.E. Rakel, & E.T. Bope (Eds.), *Conn's current therapy 2002.* Philadelphia: Saunders.

Wessely, S. (2001). Chronic fatigue: Symptom and syndrome. *Annals of Internal Medicine, 134,* 838-843.

WHO (1990). Cancer pain relief and palliative care: Report of WHO expert committee. *WHO Technological Report Service, 804,* 1-73.

Wright, J.B., & Beverley, D.W. (1998). Chronic fatigue syndrome. *Archives of Diseases in Children, 79,* 308-374.

Yaster, M., Kost-Byerly, S., Khandwala, R.S., & Maxwell, L.G. (2001). Management of acute pain in children. In R.A. Hoekelman (Ed.), *Primary pediatric care.* St. Louis: Mosby.

Behavioral Problems

MARY VIRGINIA GRAHAM

Alcohol Problems

Attention Deficit Hyperactivity Disorder

Eating Disorders

Encopresis

Obesity

Primary Nocturnal Enuresis

Sleep Patterns and Problems in Infants and Young Children

Tobacco Use and Smoking Cessation

Undernutrition and Failure to Thrive

ALCOHOL PROBLEMS

I. Definition: Problems caused by alcohol that may be acute or chronic, may range from mild to severe and vary in their response to treatment; problems exist on a continuum of increasing severity ranging from at-risk use to alcohol abuse to alcohol dependence

II. Pathogenesis

   A. Causes of alcohol problems are incompletely understood, but factors that contribute to teenage alcohol use are in the table below

   B. Alcohol affects several brain neurotransmitters, including dopamine, γ-aminobutyric acid, glutamate, serotonin, adenosine, norepinephrine, and opioid peptides and their receptors

   C. A dopaminergic pathway projecting from the ventral tegmental area to the nucleus accumbens mediates the pleasurable effects of alcohol; humans tend to repeat any action that provides pleasure

---

FACTORS CONTRIBUTING TO ALCOHOL USE AND ABUSE IN CHILDHOOD AND ADOLESCENCE

Genetic and Family Factors

Family history of alcoholism
✓ Predisposes children to problem drinking; in the US, 7 million children younger than 18 years have alcoholic parents
✓ Sons of alcoholic men have a 1 in 4 risk of becoming alcoholics and daughters of alcoholics are more likely to marry alcoholic men that are daughters of nonalcoholics

Parental attitudes and behavior related to alcohol use
✓ Often shapes how children view its use and whether they will drink
✓ Home is the primary source of alcohol for adolescents
✓ Some families not only accept but may encourage excessive drinking, especially among males of any age

Adolescent Development

✓ Teen drinking is often accepted as normal behavior in US society
✓ Because of their smaller body size, and limited experience with the effects of alcohol, teens may become intoxicated with less alcohol intake than adults
✓ Further, teens are less able to recognize and compensate for the neuropsychiatric effects of alcohol use due to biologic, cognitive, and psychological immaturity

Peer Influence

✓ Alcohol use is often reinforced by peers, and being part of the peer group has special meaning and importance during childhood and adolescence
✓ Adolescents who use alcohol spend most of their time with others who use in order to keep the code of secrecy

Media Influence

✓ An analysis of alcohol ads demonstrates that the ads often link drinking with such valued attributes as physical attractiveness, sociability, elegance, romance, relaxation, and adventure
✓ Most middle-school students reported in a recent survey that alcohol advertising encourages them to drink and these children also hold positive beliefs about the social benefits of beer consumption
✓ In order to capitalize on the Internet's strong appeal to children and adolescents, many of the major alcoholic beverage companies use the Internet to advertise and promote their products through a variety of marketing techniques

Community Attitudes

✓ Alcohol use is often the centerpiece of many community celebrations whether for sports victories or for national holidays such as July 4th
✓ Children and teens are often confused by the conflicting messages conveyed by the drive-through convenience stores that sell alcohol to the customer who is operating a motor vehicle and purchasing alcohol at the same time

---

III. Clinical Presentation

   A. Underage drinking continues to be one of the most serious public health problems in the US, exacting a tremendous toll on productivity and negatively impacting individuals who drink, as well as their families and communities
      1. Seventy-eight percent of high school students have tried alcohol (defined as at least 1 drink of alcohol other than sips of wine for religious purposes) and more than 5 million (30%) admit to binge drinking (consuming ≥5 alcoholic drinks on 1 occasion) at least once a month
      2. The incidence of lifetime alcohol abuse and dependence is greatest for those who begin drinking between the ages of 11 and 14 years of age

B. Although the minimum legal drinking age is 21 in all 50 states, alcohol is the leading drug of abuse by children and adolescents
    1. The 2000 National Household Survey on Drug Abuse (NHSDA) found that the average age of initiation of use among 12- to 20-year olds is now 14 years
    2. The proportion of children who begin drinking in eighth grade or earlier increased by 33% from 1975 to 2001

C. Underage drinkers (aged 12-20 years) account for 19.7% of total alcohol consumption in the US; underage drinkers accounted for an estimated $22.5 billion of total consumer expenditures in 1999

D. Underage alcohol use may range from occasional consumption of small amounts of alcohol, to "problem drinking," to alcohol abuse, and finally to alcohol dependence

---

What is Problem Drinking?

From a law enforcement/legal perspective, *any* consumption of alcohol by underage individuals (even occasional use of small amounts of alcohol) represents "problem drinking" in that it is an illegal activity

From a health perspective, underage drinking can cause physical damage to the brain, interfere with mental and social development, undermine academic progress, increase chances of risky sexual behavior, and result in unintentional injury and death

Despite the fact that underage drinking is often perceived as "normal behavior," when alcohol use leads to problems with friends and family, poor school attendance and performance, trouble with teachers, trouble with police, and driving after drinking, there is no dispute that this constitutes "problem drinking"

E. **Alcohol abuse** is the continued use of alcohol in spite of adverse consequences (UCR mnemonic--*U*se, followed by adverse *C*onsequences, followed by *R*epetition). Consequences may be physical, social, or psychological (see CRITERIA FOR ALCOHOL ABUSE table)

CRITERIA FOR ALCOHOL ABUSE	
Pattern of alcohol use in which 1 (or more) of the following 4 criteria are present within a 12-month period	
Recurrent alcohol use resulting in	✓ Failure to fulfill major role obligations (home, work, school) ✓ Placing self and others in potentially hazardous situations (DUI) ✓ Legal problems (e.g., arrest for DUI)
Continued alcohol use despite	✓ Persistent or recurrent social/interpersonal problems due to effects of alcohol

Adapted from the American Psychiatric Association. (2000). *Diagnostic and statistical manual of mental disorders*, (4th ed.), Text Revision. Washington, DC: Author.

F. Alcohol dependence is a chronic disease characterized by impaired control over drinking, preoccupation with the drug alcohol, use of alcohol in spite of adverse consequences, and distortions in thinking, primarily denial (see CRITERIA FOR ALCOHOL DEPENDENCE table)

CRITERIA FOR ALCOHOL DEPENDENCE
Pattern of alcohol use in which 3 (or more) of the following 7 criteria are present within a 12 month period
✓ Physical tolerance (increased amounts are required for desired effect)   ✓ Withdrawal symptoms when substance is discontinued   ✓ Larger amounts of alcohol are used than intended   ✓ Unsuccessful efforts to control use   ✓ Much time and energy are spent in obtaining, using, and recovering from effects of alcohol   ✓ Many social, work-related, and recreational activities are reduced because of alcohol use   ✓ Continued use in spite of knowledge that alcohol causes physical and/or psychological problems

Adapted from the American Psychiatric Association. (2000). *Diagnostic and statistical manual of mental disorders*, (4th ed.), Text Revision. Washington, DC: Author.

G. Binge drinking—consumption of 5 or more alcoholic beverages on a single occasion—is most prevalent among males aged 18-25
    1. Episodes of binge drinking result in acute impairment and cause a substantial fraction of all alcohol-related deaths in the US each year

2.   Adverse health consequences specifically associated with binge drinking include unintentional injuries (e.g., motor vehicle crashes, falls, drownings, and burns), suicide, alcohol poisoning, acute myocardial infarction, gastritis, and poor control of diabetes

H.   Motor vehicle crashes resulting from driving under the influence of alcohol are the leading cause of death in the 15-24 year old age group

---

Facts about Alcohol-Related Traffic Deaths

- Alcohol-related traffic death rate in the US has dropped substantially in the last 20 years
- In 1982, 60% of traffic deaths were related to alcohol compared with 41% in 2001 (most dramatic decreases have been among the youngest drivers)
- State with highest alcohol-related death rate: South Carolina, followed by Montana, Louisiana, and the District of Columbia
- State with the lowest rate: Utah, followed by Vermont, New York, Minnesota, New Jersey, and Massachusetts
- Men killed in traffic crashes are nearly 2 times as likely to be legally intoxicated as women
- Beer consumption is the cause of up to 80% of all alcohol-related crashes and fatalities
- In spite of the success of tougher drunk-driving laws, more than 17,000 persons still die each year in the US in alcohol-related crashes

---

I.   Children of alcoholics are from 2 to 4 times more likely to develop the disease
1.   The genetic underpinnings of alcoholism are not well understood; one likely contributor is the body's inherited ability to make a liver enzyme that is efficient at metabolizing alcohol—a high enzyme level gives even young persons the ability to drink their peers under the table
2.   Growing up in an alcoholic family seems to play a role apart from the genes—children in alcoholic families must realize that they are at an increased risk for the disease and need to figure out how to say "no" to drinking until adulthood

J.   Parents of an adolescent with alcohol problems may report presence of warning signs such as the following: A new set of friends the teen never brings home, being unusually argumentative, testy, sad, or losing motivation in school, even if grades remain good

IV.   Diagnosis/Evaluation

A.   History
1.   Keep in mind that the history (including interview and use of standardized questionnaires) is by far more sensitive and specific than are physical exam and laboratory findings
2.   All patients should be screened for alcohol problems, beginning in early adolescence (11-14 years). Approach with a declaration – "I know that alcohol and drug use are common among kids your age." **First ask 'Do your friends use alcohol?' Then ask 'Do you ever drink alcohol?'**
3.   If patient **ever** drinks, ask **quantity-frequency** questions which deal with level of consumption, and can help distinguish infrequent from at-risk drinking and identify binge drinking (see LEVEL OF CONSUMPTION and GENERAL EQUIVALENCIES OF ALCOHOLIC BEVERAGES tables)

LEVEL OF CONSUMPTION	
Frequency	How many days in a week do you usually have something to drink?
Quantity	On days that you drink, how many drinks do you have?
Maximum	What is the most you had to drink on any one day during the past month?
Last drink	When was your last drink? (Persons with a problem know exactly)

Adapted from Bower, K.T., & Severin, J.D. (1997). Alcohol and other drug-related problems. In D.J. Knesper, M.B. Riba, & T.L. Schwenk (Eds.), *Primary care psychiatry*. Philadelphia: Saunders.

GENERAL EQUIVALENCIES OF ALCOHOLIC BEVERAGES*

Hard liquor (80 proof spirits)		Beer (4% to 5% alcohol)	
1 shot or highball (1.5 ounces)	= 1 drink	1 12-ounce bottle or can	= 1 drink
1/2 pint of liquor	= ~5 drinks	1 40-ounce container	= ~3 drinks
1 pint of liquor	= ~10 drinks	1 6-pack of beer	= 6 drinks
Wine (11% to 12% alcohol)		**Wine Coolers (5% alcohol)**	
1 glass of wine (5 ounces)	= 1 drink	1 wine cooler (12 ounces)	= 1 drink
1 bottle of wine (750 mL)	= 5 drinks		

* One drink contains approximately 12 g of alcohol

4.   Follow quantity-frequency questions with the CAGE Questionnaire or with the CRAFFT Questionnaire, a screening instrument specifically designed for use with adolescents

CAGE QUESTIONNAIRE

C	Have you ever felt you ought to **C**ut down on your drinking?
A	Have people **A**nnoyed you by criticizing your drinking?
G	Have you ever felt bad or **G**uilty about your drinking?
E	Have you ever had a drink the first thing in the morning (**E**ye opener) to steady your nerves or get rid of a hangover?
Scoring and Interpretation	Person receives one point for each positive answer. One "yes" answer indicates hazardous drinking and two or more "yes" answers indicate alcohol abuse or dependence

Source: Bush, B., Shaw, S., Cleary, P., Delbanco, T.L., & Aronson, M.D. (1987). Screening for alcohol abuse using the CAGE questionnaire. *American Journal of Medicine, 82*, 231-235.

CRAFFT QUESTIONNAIRE

C	Have you ever ridden in a CAR driven by someone (including yourself) who was "high" or had been using alcohol or drugs?
R	Do you ever use alcohol or drugs to RELAX, feel better about yourself, or fit in?
A	Do you ever use alcohol or drugs while you are by yourself or ALONE?
F	Do you ever FORGET things you did while using alcohol or drugs?
F	Do your family or FRIENDS ever tell you that you should cut down on your drinking or drug use?
T	Have you ever gotten into TROUBLE while you were using alcohol or drugs?

Source: Knight, J.R., Shrier, L.A., Bravender, T.D., Farrell, M., Vanderbilt, J., & Shaffer, J.J. (1999). A new brief screen for adolescent substance abuse. *Archives of Pediatric & Adolescent Medicine, 153*, 591-596

5.   If patient answers "yes" to a CAGE or CRAFFT question, prompt for more details
6.   If screening using quantity-frequency questions and CAGE or CRAFFT questions indicates problems with alcohol, ask more specific questions based on criteria for alcohol abuse and dependence
7.   Finally, carefully screen for use of other substances (high concomitant use of tobacco and other drugs by persons with alcohol problems)

B.   Physical Examination
1.   Note that an absence of findings on physical exam does not indicate that the patient is free of alcohol problems (most early manifestations of alcohol abuse/dependence are psychosocial, not physical)
2.   Assess general appearance (should be normal); evaluate heart and lungs
3.   Perform abdominal exam for hepatomegaly and right upper quadrant tenderness (rare in teens)
4.   Perform neurologic exam; much of the exam in a healthy young patient can be done simply by watching the person walk into the examining room, sit on exam table (or a chair) and engage in conversation with you during the history. Further testing of mental status, cranial nerves, motor, cerebellar, and sensory status can be done only if indicated

5. During exam, note if patient smells of alcohol as alcohol on breath during primary care visit indicates that there is impaired control over drinking

C. Differential Diagnosis: Other mental disorders such as mood and anxiety disorders, psychosis, delirium, dementia; abuse of other psychoactive substances such as opioids, marijuana, hallucinogens, PCP, inhalants, and sedatives

D. Diagnostic Tests
1. CBC (elevated mean corpuscular volume is a marker of excessive alcohol consumption; may be elevated due to other causes such as liver disease or smoking)
2. Liver enzyme tests
   a. A γ-glutamyltransferase level that is 2 times the normal level in patients with an aspartate aminotransferase:alanine aminotransferase ratio of at least 2:1 strongly suggests a diagnosis of alcohol abuse
   b. Use of γ-glutamyltransferase level as a single test to diagnose alcohol abuse is not recommended because of its lack of specificity
3. Carbohydrate-deficient transferrin can detect heavy drinking; may be useful for monitoring alcohol-dependent patients; this test is not yet readily available to most clinicians

V. Plan/Management

A. When clinicians assess the a patient's use of alcohol as a routine part of risk behavior assessment and discuss alcohol refusal skills with him/her, they may reinforce nonuse behaviors, especially when risk factors for problem drinking, such as family history of alcoholism are present

B. Management is determined by the **identification** and **confirmation** that the patient has problems with alcohol and by his/her **willingness to change** behavior

C. **Identification** of problem-drinking is determined primarily from screening using the CAGE or CRAFFT and the Level of Consumption questions; the physical examination and the laboratory testing may provide additional evidence that a problem exists

D. **Confirmation** of the problem is based on the extent to which the patient meets the criteria for alcohol abuse or dependence and involves two important diagnostic issues
1. What happens when the patient uses alcohol? (adverse consequences)
2. What happens when the patient tries to stop? (impaired control, tolerance and withdrawal)

E. Diagnostic Issues
1. **First diagnostic issue**. Assess problem areas first (adverse consequences) then link them to substance use. (Example: How are things going at home? At school? In your social life? and so on. As the patient introduces problems, be empathetic, but ask patient "How do you think your use of alcohol fits in with this?")
2. **Second diagnostic issue**
   a. Determine degree of **impaired control** by asking questions such as "Do you drink more than you intend to?" "Why do you think that happens?" "Do you ever make rules for your drinking?" "Are you able to follow those rules?"
   b. Assess **tolerance**. "Do you need more to get the same effect?"
   c. Ask about **withdrawal**. "Do you ever feel bad or sick when you try to stop drinking?"

F. **Motivation** for change on the patient's part is crucial to the success of any treatment plan. Appropriate questions to assess motivation are the following: "Are you concerned about your use of alcohol?" "Are you interested in changing?"; success of any intervention is dependent on the patient's willingness to participate in treatment goals

G. **Brief interventions have been demonstrated through research to be highly effective**
1. Can be conducted in the office for the following groups of patients: Underage drinkers who occasionally use alcohol or who have early signs of problem drinking
2. Brief, nonspecific interventions by primary care clinicians often result in outcomes equal to more intensive interventions by highly trained specialists

BRIEF INTERVENTIONS FOR UNDERAGE DRINKERS IN TWO GROUPS: THOSE WHO OCCASIONALLY USE SMALL AMOUNTS OF ALCOHOL AND THOSE WHO HAVE EARLY SIGNS OF PROBLEM DRINKING

Underage drinking should be discouraged in all patients by a number of approaches

Implement approaches in a matter-of-fact, nonjudgmental manner

- First, teens should be reminded that underage drinking is illegal and that there can be consequences if caught in this behavior
- Second, facts and figures related to the health consequences of drinking (including risk of injury or death from a motor vehicle crash) should be pointed out (see above under III)
- Finally, the special risks encountered by children of alcoholic parents should be emphasized (if appropriate) because of the child's increased risk of developing an addiction

Alcohol refusal skills should be discussed with all children and teens; parents should be encouraged to develop alcohol-free activities in the community

Specific management techniques such as the use of contracts and designated driver programs are also options, although the efficacy for such recommendations are not yet conclusive

H.   Refer all adolescents with drinking problems resulting in problems with law-enforcement, with school officials, with family, and all patients determined to be abusers of alcohol or alcohol dependent to experts for further assessment and management

I.   Recommend self-help books for both patients and family members (see table below)

SELF-HELP BOOKS FOR ALCOHOL PROBLEMS

For the patient (author of book is a woman, so particularly useful for females)	Knapp, C. (1991). *Drinking: A love story*. New York: Doubleday Delacorte Press
For the patient (emphasis is on lifestyle as well as behavioral change)	Washington, A., & Boundy, D. (1990). *Willpower is not enough: Understanding and recovering from addictions of every kind*. New York: Harper-Perennial
For parents of a teen with alcohol problems (written by former US Senator George McGovern)	McGovern, G. (1996). *Terry: My daughter's life and death struggle with alcoholism*. New York: Villard
For children of alcoholics and their risk issues	Black, C. (1981). *It will never happen to me: Children of alcoholics as youngsters-adolescents-adults*. New York: Ballantine

J.   Provide teen and family with appropriate resources from the box below and strongly encourage participation in a self-help group

Teen Health Issues	Web site: http://health4teens.org
Alcoholics Anonymous *A self-help group founded to help alcoholics stay sober by sharing their experience, strength, and hope. This 12-step recovery program is based on spiritual principles*	Web site: http://alcholics-anonymous.org (or check your local phone book)
Alateen *A fellowship of young Al-Anon members whose lives have been affected by someone else's drinking. A 12-step program*	Telephone: 1-800-356-9996 Website: http://www.al-anon.alateen.org
Al-Anon *A 12-step group designed for the support and recovery of significant others who are affected by the person with alcoholism*	Telephone: 1-800-356-9996 Website: http://www.al-anon.org
National Council on Alcoholism and Drug Dependence	Telephone: 1-800-475-HOPE
Mothers Against Drunk Driving	Telephone: 1-800-GET-MADD
Students Against Drunk Driving	Check your local phone book

K. Be familiar with at least one specialized treatment facility for adolescents in your area
   1. Clinicians **must be ready with a plan** when the drinker is ready to quit
   2. For a list of programs as well as a discussion of approaches, visit the American Society of Addiction Medicine at www.asam.org
   3. Feedback from patients will help you learn which programs in your area are most effective
   4. Referral for family therapy may be indicated when complex problems are present

L. Pharmacologic treatment: The FDA has approved two drugs for use in those >18 years of age to treat alcohol dependence; however, alcohol treatment centers are reluctant to prescribe drugs
   1. Naltrexone (ReVia) is an opioid antagonist that blocks the alcohol-induced release of dopamine in the nucleus accumbens
      a. Reduces the craving for alcohol
      b. May deter patients who sample alcohol from progressing to relapse
      c. Dosing is 50 mg once daily for 12 weeks
      d. Consult PDR for prescribing information, contraindications, precautions, and adverse effects
   2. Disulfiram (Antabuse) is an aversive drug which has been available for many years, but is little used today
      a. Controlled clinical trials in recent years cast serious doubt on its efficacy
      b. Nonetheless, a small minority of clinicians continue to prescribe it
      c. Usual dose is 250 mg once daily (available in 250 and 500 mg tabs)
      d. Consult PDR regarding dosing, contraindications, precautions, and adverse effects

M. Another opiate antagonist that is currently in clinical trials in the US is acamprosate; based on clinical trials in Europe, this medication appears to be highly efficacious and should be available in 2003

N. Teens who are alcohol dependent and who also have a psychiatric disorder must be referred for treatment for the underlying disorder as these patients are complex and require expert management

O. Follow up is variable depending on type of treatment
   1. Patients for whom brief intervention is conducted: Follow up in first few weeks with two or more visits/telephone contacts to monitor patient's progress and assess need for additional approaches (aim for 4 contacts in 6 weeks)
   2. Patients who have been referred to alcohol treatment (either residential or outpatient) should be followed for ongoing support; the natural course of alcohol problems includes remission as well as relapse; these patients should be attending AA meetings on regular basis
   3. For both groups of patients (brief intervention and intensive treatment), supportive relapse visits should include the following

QUESTIONS/DISCUSSION FOR THE SUPPORTIVE RELAPSE VISIT	
Ask	"When was the date of the last drink?" "Have you used other drugs?" "Are you continuing with Alcoholics Anonymous/Narcotics Anonymous meetings?" "Do you have a sponsor?"
Discuss	Nutrition, exercise, sleep, school attendance, and spiritual activities which are important to relapse prevention Problematic areas in early recovery—peer and family relationships; spend time talking about this with the patient
Look for	Overconfidence Recurrence of negativity Declining interest in AA

ATTENTION DEFICIT/HYPERACTIVITY DISORDER

I.   Definition: Descriptive category for cluster of symptoms that include inattention, impulsivity, and motor hyperactivity that are more frequent and severe than seen in persons of the same developmental level

II.   Pathogenesis

A.   Probably encompasses several distinct disorders involving multiple genetic, neurological, temperamental, and environmental factors

B.   Current research has found that certain brain regions might malfunction in persons with ADHD and that defective genes may also play a role in the expression of the disorder
1.   Several studies support involvement of the prefrontal cortex, part of the cerebellum, and two basal ganglia--the caudate nucleus and the globus pallidus
2.   Genes that dictate the way in which the brain uses dopamine have also been implicated (imaging studies have implicated frontostriatal circuitry [which is rich in dopaminergic innervation] in ADHD)

III. Clinical Presentation

A.   The most common neurobehavioral disorder of childhood with an estimated prevalence of about 8% to 10% and a male to female ratio of almost 10:1

B.   Once believed to largely resolve in childhood/adolescence, evidence now exists indicating that it can persist into adulthood. **Important**: Not an acquired disorder of adulthood

C.   Presentation during preschool years
1.   Most common time of onset
2.   Child often described as "driven by motor"
3.   Constant supervision required
4.   Child-proofing house required beyond what is normally needed

D.   Presentation during school-age years
1.   Usually presents soon after entry to school when cognitive/behavioral abilities are challenged by teacher/situation expectations (classroom is a powerful screening tool as sedentary activities are difficult for affected children to endure)
2.   Frequent teacher attention required to keep child "on task"
3.   Child frequently disrupts classroom with motor activity (leaving desk without permission) and/or impulsivity (talking out of turn)

E.   Presentation during adolescence (represents persistence from childhood)
1.   Almost without exception, adolescents with ADHD have **continuing** symptoms from childhood
2.   Adolescent-onset ADHD is not a primary diagnosis but may occur secondary to a neurologic insult or to a psychiatric disorder
3.   Regarding activity level, adolescents with ADHD are usually more active than other adolescents, but less active than they were as preadolescents
4.   Low self-esteem from academic failure/social rejection becomes more of an issue during this age period

F.   **Hyperactivity is no longer a required diagnostic criterion for ADHD at any age**

G. Diagnostic criteria for ADHD are contained in the following table
1. Note there are **two** dimensions, inattention and hyperactivity/impulsivity, with behaviors specific to each dimension
2. From these two dimensions, three subtypes are derived
a. Predominantly inattentive type (criteria are met on inattention dimension, but **not** on the hyperactivity/impulsivity dimension)
b. Predominantly hyperactive/impulsive type (criteria are met on hyperactive/impulsive dimension but **not** on the inattention dimension)
c. Combined type (criteria are met for both dimensions)
3. The diagnostic criteria are meant to be age neutral but are **most** applicable to the school-age child

---

ADHD DIAGNOSTIC CRITERIA

Either 1 or 2

1. Six or more symptoms of inattention have persisted for at least a 6 month period to the degree that is maladaptive and inconsistent with developmental level:

Inattention-- The person **often**	➡ Fails to pay close attention to details resulting in careless mistakes
	➡ Has difficulty sustaining attention in activities (whether play or other tasks)
	➡ Does not seem to listen when being spoken to
	➡ Does not follow through on instructions and fails to complete schoolwork, chores, or duties in the workplace (not due to oppositional behavior or inability to understand directions)
	➡ Has difficulty with organization
	➡ Avoids, dislikes, or is reluctant to undertake activities that require sustained mental effort (such as schoolwork or homework)
	➡ Loses items necessary for tasks or activities
	➡ Becomes easily distracted by extraneous stimuli
	➡ Is forgetful in daily activities

2. Six or more symptoms of hyperactivity-impulsivity have persisted for at least a 6 month period to a degree that is maladaptive and inconsistent with developmental level:

Hyperactivity-- The person **often**	➡ Fidgets with hands or feet or squirms in seat
	➡ Leaves seat in situations where remaining in seat is expected
	➡ Runs or climbs excessively in situations in which it is inappropriate to do so (in adolescents or adults, this may be limited to subjective feelings of restlessness)
	➡ Has difficulty engaging in quiet play or leisure activities
	➡ Is "on the go" or seems driven by a motor
	➡ Talks excessively
Impulsivity-- The person **often**	➡ Blurts out answers before question has been asked
	➡ Has difficulty waiting turn
	➡ Interrupts or intrudes on others (butts into conversations or games)
In addition, the following must be true	➡ Some hyperactive-impulsive or inattentive behaviors were present **before** age 7 years
	➡ Some impairment from the symptoms is present in two or more settings (home, school or work)
	➡ Clear evidence of clinically significant impairment in social, academic, or work-related functioning must exist
	➡ Symptoms may not better be accounted for by another mental disorder (e.g., mood, anxiety, personality, psychotic)

Adapted from American Psychiatric Association. (2000). *Diagnostic and statistical manual of mental disorders* (4th ed.), Text Revision, Washington, DC: Author

IV.   Diagnosis/Evaluation

A.   History

OBTAIN HISTORY

Overview of History Taking

✓   Focus of history taking is to determine whether patient meets the diagnostic criteria for *DSM-IV* criteria for ADHD as outlined in the table above

✓   Use both open-ended questions (e.g., "What are your concerns about [child's name] behavior in school?" and focused questions such as "Explain what you mean by [child's name] is hyper all the time; what specifically does he do?")

✓   History **must** come from multiple sources with the two primary sources being parents and teachers

✓   Use of selected ADHD-specific rating scales/questionnaires by parents and teachers is extremely important; the Conners' Rating Scales (two versions, one for parents and one for teachers) are rated highly by experts (Agency for Health Care Policy and Research [see reference under Green, M. et al., in reference list]); use of global questionnaires (scales that assess a variety of behavioral conditions [also called broadband]) are not recommended

Specific Information to Obtain

✓   Ask about age of onset. "When did the symptoms begin?" Gather specific examples of child's behaviors according to the two dimensions--inattention and hyperactivity/impulsivity

✓   Ask about duration of symptoms. "Have the symptoms been present at least 6 months?"

✓   Establish that symptoms are present in 2 or more settings

✓   If child is school age, obtain evidence from classroom teacher regarding the core symptoms of ADHD, the duration of symptoms, and the degree of functional impairment; ask about presence of coexisting conditions

✓   In preschoolers, obtain evidence from caregivers in other settings (e.g., grandparent, daycare provider)

✓   Obtain social history, development history, past and present medical history, and **current medications**

✓   Consider the presence of coexisting conditions: most common are oppositional defiant and conduct disorders, anxiety, depression, and learning disabilities (description of these disorders/conditions is beyond the scope of this book)

✓   Interview the child, particularly the child who is ≥5, as the child can provide insight into his/her feelings (may not provide accurate reports of behaviors, however); ask adolescent about substance use

---

ADHD RATING SCALES

Children ages 6-17
    Conners' Rating Scales – Revised (CRS-R) (versions for parent and for teacher)
    Conners' Parents Rating Scale – Revised (CPRS-R) and Conners' Teachers Rating Scale – Revised (CTRS-R)

      Source: Psychological Corporation, 800-211-8378, www.psychcorp.com

---

B.   Physical Examination
    1.   Perform complete neurologic exam including gait, muscular strength and tone, deep tendon reflexes, sensory responses
    2.   Results of the PE are usually negative

C.   Differential Diagnosis
    1.   Anxiety (suspect if symptoms present in only one setting, e.g., home, but not at school)
    2.   Substance abuse (suspect if child/adolescent exhibits symptoms uncharacteristic of previous behavior)
    3.   Mood disorders/depression
    4.   Conduct disorder and oppositional defiant disorder
    5.   Learning disability (children with comprehension difficulties often appear restless, inattentive)

D.   Diagnostic Tests
    1.   Keep in mind that ADHD is a clinical diagnosis based primarily on history and secondarily on in-office observation and neuropsychological testing
    2.   Other diagnostic tests are not routinely indicated to establish the diagnosis of ADHD; screening children for high lead levels and for abnormal thyroid hormone levels are not recommended unless there is some clinical reason to do so

V.   Plan/Management

   A.   The evaluation of a child who presents with inattention, hyperactivity, impulsivity, academic underachievement, or behavior problems requires several visits as well as consultation with other adults (teachers) and completion of rating scales by parents and teachers in order to have an accurate picture of the child

   B.   Once the diagnosis of ADHD has been made based on *DSM-IV* criteria, a treatment plan can be developed and implemented

   C.   Information, counseling, and support to the child, parents, and teachers in combination with **behavior therapy** and use of **psychostimulant medications** are core features of the treatment plan
      1.   Before treatment options are discussed, the parents must have some understanding of ADHD
      2.   Child also must be provided with age-appropriate education about the condition
      3.   In addition to providing information in a counseling setting, recommend resources and books for parents, teachers, and children from the tables that follow

---

RESOURCES FOR PATIENTS WITH ADHD AND THEIR FAMILIES

Children and Adults with Attention Deficit Disorders (CHADD), National Headquarters, Suite 185, 1859 North Pine Island Road, Plantation, FL 33322, 800-233-4050 and www.chadd.org

Attention Deficit Disorder Association, 4300 West Park Blvd., Plano, TX 75093 and www.add.org

National Institute of Mental Health/IRIB, 5600 Fishers Lane, Room 7C-02, Rockville, MD 20857 and www.nimh.nih.gov

---

READINGS FOR PARENTS, ADOLESCENT PATIENTS, AND TEACHERS

Taking Charge of ADHD: The Complete, Authoritative Guide for Parents by R.A. Barkley. Published by Guilford Press, New York, 1995	Basic book with comprehensive information for parents
The Time-Out Solution: A Parent's Guide for Handling Everyday Behavior Problems by L. Clark. Published by Contemporary Books, Chicago, 1989	Provides practical details on use of time-out as well as other ways to increase appropriate behavior
Driven to Distraction: Recognizing and Coping with Attention Deficit Disorder from Childhood Through Adulthood by E. Hallowell & J. Ratey. Published by Pantheon Books, New York, 1994	Especially good reference for understanding ADHD
ADHD: A Guide to Understanding and Helping Children with Attention Deficit Hyperactivity Disorder in School Settings by L. Braswell, M. Bloomquist, & S. Pederson. Published by the University of Minnesota, Department of Professional Development and Conference Services, Continuing Education and Extension, 315 Pillsbury Drive, SE, Minneapolis, MN 55455; 612-625-3502	An outstanding resource for teachers

---

BOOKS FOR CHILDREN WITH ADHD

Primary School-Age Children
Eukee the Jumpy Elephant by C.L. Corman & E. Trevino. Plantation, FL: Specialty Press, 1995
Otto Learns About His Medications by M. Galvin. New York: Magination Press, 1988

Middle School-Age Children
Sometimes I Drive My Mom Crazy, But I Know She's Crazy About Me by L.E. Sharpiro. King of Prussia, PA: Center for Applied Psychology, 1993

Adolescents
Distant Drums, Different Drummers: A Guide for Young People with ADHD by B.D. Ingersoll. Bethesda, MD. Cape Publications, 1999

   D.   Behavior therapy represents a broad set of specific interventions that include behavior modification and environmental manipulation aimed at increasing appropriate and decreasing inappropriate behaviors
      1.   Successful programs require a mental health counselor who is skilled in this area
      2.   Usually requires parents to work with counselor to learn techniques
      3.   Teachers often need additional support to implement these techniques

E. General guidelines for parents whose child is awaiting referral to a mental health counselor
   1. A substantial commitment of time and energy by parent is required
   2. A structured environment in which expectations are clear is the appropriate milieu for the child
   3. Regular and frequent exercise, a well-balanced diet, and good sleep hygiene are important; martial arts training for the child may be very helpful
   4. Limit rules to those that impact health and safety
   5. Find tolerant baby-sitters for respite

F. The goal of psychostimulant medications is to decrease motor activity, control impulsivity, and increase attention span
   1. Indicated when there is clear evidence that a child's attentional difficulties affect school performance, present problems with social adjustment, or are associated with a behavioral disorder
   2. An estimated 70% of children respond to stimulant drugs; attentiveness improves, and interpersonal interactions with peers and adults are less confrontational (academic performance usually does not improve as dramatically as behavior)
   3. Benefits of stimulants persist over time and tolerance does not develop, but the effects of drugs on behavior wear off quickly
   4. If referral of children to an expert in the evaluation and treatment of children with ADHD is not possible, consultation with an expert is necessary prior to initiation of therapy to insure that the child is being appropriately treated

G. The table below contains stimulant medications used to treat children with ADHD

SELECTED STIMULANTS USED IN THE TREATMENT OF CHILDREN WITH ADHD

Overview of Dosing Guidelines for Methylphenidate and Dextroamphetamine

- ✓ Ranges of doses of methylphenidate and dextroamphetamine are narrow and cannot be predicted based upon the child's age, body mass, level of hyperactivity, or measurement of plasma drug concentrations—these are class II (controlled) drugs
- ✓ Begin with a low dose and titrate upward; there is marked individual variability in the dose-response relationship
- ✓ The **initial** dose of standard methylphenidate or dextroamphetamine is 2.5 to 5 mg once daily; dose may be increased every 3-5 days while adverse effects, behavior, and academic function are assessed through reports from parents and teachers
- ✓ Once the lowest effective dose is determined, a decision regarding the need and timing of additional doses can be made in order to improve the duration of desired behaviors in the child
- ✓ The dose must be adjusted in each patient to obtain the maximal benefit in terms of both behavior and academic function with the minimal adverse effects
- ✓ Whereas some authorities recommend a drug holiday (on weekends and vacations) others believe drug holidays can destabilize control (ADHD often creates problems and stress at home, e.g., inability to do chores, get along with siblings and playmates). Decisions to use a 5-day versus 7-day schedule should be individualized
- ✓ Consult PDR for prescribing information, contraindications, precautions, and adverse reactions

(Continued)

SELECTED STIMULANTS USED IN THE TREATMENT OF CHILDREN WITH ADHD *(CONTINUED)*

Medication	Usual Daily Dosing Schedule	Effect Duration	Comments
Methylphenidate Short-Acting Ritalin (standard)	≥6 years of age: 2.5-5 mg PO BID (Before breakfast & lunch)	1-4 hrs	If an additional dose is needed, the 3rd dose should be given at 4 PM May gradually increase dose by 5-10 mg/day at weekly intervals Maximum total dose per day is 60 mg
Intermediate-Acting Ritalin SR	≥6 years of age: 20 mg QD in AM	3-9 hrs	May use in place of standard Ritalin once dosing with standard Ritalin has been titrated to a therapeutic level
Long-Acting Concerta	≥6 years of age: 18 mg QD in AM	8-12 hrs	Typical pediatric dose is 36 mg in AM When switching from standard or sustained release Ritalin to Concerta, consult PDR for equivalencies
Dextroamphetamine Short-Acting Dexedrine (standard)	3-5 years of age 2.5 mg QD ≥6 years of age 2.5-5 mg BID (in AM and early afternoon [4-6 hours apart])	1-8 hrs	Gradual increases if needed; maximum total dose per day is 40 mg
Long-Acting Adderall XR	≥6 years of age 10 mg QD in AM	8-12 hrs	May increase by 10 mg weekly; maximum total dose per day is 30 mg

Overview of Adverse Effects

Adverse effects of standard and sustained-release preparations of methylphenidate and dextroamphetamine are dose dependent and similar in terms of frequency, duration, and severity

Common
- ✓ Decreased appetite occurs in about 80% of children (often mild and limited to daytime eating)
- ✓ Weight loss (substantial) occurs in about 10% to 15% of children
- ✓ Insomnia reported in up to 85% of children with sleep delays of about an hour

Less Common
- ✓ Abdominal pain, irritability, headaches, dry mouth, dizziness, and depression
- ✓ Cardiovascular effects involve variable increases in heart rate and blood pressure (most evident at rest and diminish with activity)
- ✓ Consult PDR for a complete list of adverse effects

Comparing Dextroamphetamine and Methylphenidate

- For both standard and sustained-release preparations, the peak plasma concentration and plasma half-life are higher and longer for dextroamphetamine than for methylphenidate

- For standard preparations of both drugs, the duration of maximal behavioral benefit parallels the absorption phase—1-2 hours for methylphenidate and 3-4 hours for dextroamphetamine

- Sustained-release preparations do not always provide more prolonged action than do the standard preparations, because the slower rates of absorption of the sustained-release preparations may delay their onset of action

---

H.   Approximately 30% of children, adolescents, and adults with the disorder to do not respond to, or cannot tolerate, treatment with a stimulant medication making the need for non-stimulant pharmacological treatment options evident

   1.   Atomoxetine (Strattera) is the first non-stimulant drug to be approved by the FDA for the treatment of ADHD, and is also the first FDA-approved treatment that is not a controlled (class II) drug

   2.   A selective norepinephrine reuptake inhibitor, atomoxetine is presumed to work by blocking a neurotransmitter that plays an important role in modulating the brain systems that control attention and activity

   3.   Not associated with stimulant or euphoric effects, thus it avoids the abuse-potential of other FDA-approved drugs for ADHD (which makes it an attractive option for adolescents)

   4.   Available in 10-, 18-, 25-, 40-, and 60-mg caps

   5.   Dosing of atomoxetine for children and adolescents is contained in the box below

Children (≥6 years)/adolescents ≤70 kg: Starting does is 0.5 mg/kg/day; after a minimum of 3 days, the dose can be increased to the target dose of about 1.2 mg/kg/day. Maximum dose is 1.4 mg/kg/day or 100 mg, whichever is lower

Children (≥6 years)/adolescents >70 kg: Starting dose is 40 mg/day and increased after a minimum of 3 days to a target dose of about 80 mg/day. Maximum dose is 100 mg/day

The total daily dose may be taken in a single dose in the AM, or in 2 evenly divided doses in the AM and late afternoon or early evening

Patients with moderate hepatic dysfunction should take half the usual dose

Consult PDR for indications, precautions, contraindications, interactions, and side effects. Long-term safety, especially the effect on growth, remains undetermined

I. When selected management of child with ADHD has not met target outcomes:
   1. Re-evaluate the original diagnosis
   2. Assess compliance with treatment plan
   3. Consider the presence of a coexisting condition
   4. Consult with an expert for recommendations

J. Follow Up
   1. Evaluation of children suspected of having ADHD is a very time-consuming process; therefore, these patients are best managed in a specialized treatment center if one is available
   2. Initial diagnosis and evaluation requires 2-3 visits (1-2 weeks apart); thereafter, follow-up schedule is variable depending on whether patient is being managed in a specialty treatment center or in a primary care setting
   3. For all patients on medications, titration of dose to therapeutic levels must be done at least weekly for first month or so, then monthly thereafter; very frequent monitoring for efficacy and for adverse events is essential (see table above for assessing response to medication and for overview of adverse effects)

EATING DISORDERS

I. Definition: Symptomatic disturbances of eating behavior unique to the developed world, with anorexia nervosa (AN) and bulimia nervosa (BN) being the two major types

II. Pathogenesis

   A. Eating disorders are best understood using a multidimensional model that encompasses biologic vulnerability, family issues, and societal pressure

   B. Eating behavior is a complex integration of a person's attitude toward food and internal physiology resulting in individual concepts of hunger and satiety

III. Clinical Presentation

   A. Disordered eating represents a spectrum of behavior that is unique to the developed world and is overwhelmingly a disease of young women (about 5% to 10% of all cases of eating disorders occur in males and the incidence of the disorder in males has increased in recent years)

   B. Participation in activities that promote thinness, such as gymnastics, dance, modeling, as well as being a type 1 diabetic are associated with a higher prevalence of AN
      1. Other proposed risk factors include perfectionism and sensitivity to negative comments about body appearance from others
      2. New evidence suggests there is also a genetic basis for increased risk

C. Using strict diagnostic criteria for AN, the prevalence in the young female population—the group most often affected—is approximately 1 to 2%
1. AN is further divided into 2 subtypes: restricting and purging (see table below for diagnostic criteria)
2. The more common of the two is the restricting subtype in which patients severely limit their food intakes

D. Adequate caloric intake, weight gain, and body fat are necessary for the progression of normal growth and pubertal development
1. Over time, severely limited caloric restriction causes linear growth retardation in the adolescent
2. Several hormonal changes may contribute to growth retardation in AN—low thyroxine (T_4) and triiodothyronine (T_3), elevated cortisol, and low sex hormone levels
3. Female adolescents with AN, despite being extremely hypoestrogenic, have low levels of follicle-stimulating hormone and luteinizing hormone (there is a blunted response to the pulsatile release of hypothalamic gonadotropin-releasing hormone)
4. In males with AN, hypothalamic hypogonadism can present as decreased levels of serum testosterone

E. Menstrual disorders are among the most common reasons that female anorectic teens seek medical attention—hypothalamic-induced amenorrhea is a universal feature of anorexia nervosa
1. Whereas such patients are concerned about amenorrhea, they seem unconcerned about their weight loss, in contrast to medically ill patients
2. Patients with mild cases of AN may or may not experience amenorrhea, but instead may seek care for nonspecific symptoms, such as asthenia, dizziness, and lack of energy

F. AN has the highest premature mortality rate of any psychiatric disorder; most deaths are caused by cardiac arrest secondary to arrhythmias (a prolonged QT interval, common in patients with this disorder, may be a marker for risk of sudden death)

G. Bulimia is much more common than AN, with a prevalence of up to 5% in adolescent females—bulimic patients often have an unremarkable appearance thus their disease may initially go unrecognized (in contrast, the cachectic appearance of patients with severe anorexia is readily apparent)
1. Bulimic patients may purge through self-induced vomiting, abuse of laxatives or diuretics, or excessive exercise
2. About half of patients with anorexia eventually develop bulimia

H. Both bulimic and anorectic patients commonly engage in excessive amounts of exercise—weight obsession and compulsive exercise training often precede the development of disordered eating
1. Runners experience "withdrawal" symptoms if they cannot run and insist on running even when sick or injured
2. Of the two disorders, males are much more likely to have bulimia and overexercise is quite common

I. Diagnostic criteria for AN according to *DSM-IV* (2000) are contained in the following table

DIAGNOSTIC CRITERIA FOR ANOREXIA NERVOSA
➡ Refusal to maintain weight at or above a minimally normal weight for age and height (body weight is less than 85% of expected)
➡ Intense fear of weight gain even though underweight
➡ Amenorrhea (in postmenarcheal females)
➡ Severe body-image disturbance in which weight has undue influence on feelings of self-worth; denial that current low body weight is problematic
➡ Types of anorexia nervosa:
• Restricting Type: During current episode of AN, person has not regularly engaged in binge eating or purging behavior
• Binge-Eating/Purging Type: During current episode of AN, person has regularly engaged in binge eating or purging behavior

Adapted from American Psychiatric Association. (2000). *Diagnostic and statistical manual of mental disorders* (4th ed.) Text Revision, Washington, DC: Author

J. Diagnostic criteria for BN according to *DSM-IV* (2000) are contained in the following table

---

DIAGNOSTIC CRITERIA FOR BULIMIA NERVOSA

➡ Recurrent episodes of binge eating which include **both** of the following
- Eating, in a discrete time period, an amount of food substantially larger than most people would consume in the same time period
- A sense of lack of control over eating during episode

➡ Recurrent inappropriate compensatory behavior to prevent weight gain such as laxative, diuretic, enema use, induced vomiting, fasting, excessive exercise

➡ The above two behaviors occur, on average, at least 2 times/week for 3 months

➡ Feelings of self-worth unduly influenced by weight

➡ Disturbance does not occur exclusively during episodes of AN

➡ Types of bulimia nervosa:
- Purging Type: During the current episode of BN, person has engaged in self-induced vomiting, laxative, diuretic, or enema use on a regularly basis
- Nonpurging Type: During the current episode of BN, person has used compensatory behaviors such as fasting or excessive exercise, but has not regularly engaged in self-induced vomiting, laxative, diuretic, or enema use

---

Adapted from American Psychiatric Association. (2000). *Diagnostic and statistical manual of mental disorders* (4th ed.) Text Revision. Washington, DC: Author

K. Using less strict diagnostic criteria, a much higher percentage of young women regularly engage in disordered eating including rigid dieting, binging and purging, all behaviors that place them at risk for a number of sequelae

IV. Diagnosis/Evaluation

A. History
1. Obtain weight history including highest and lowest weights over the past 12 months, methods of losing weight, and how patient defines "ideal" weight; ask patient if she thinks she is too fat
2. Through appropriate questioning, establish the presence or absence of criteria for eating disorders (see DIAGNOSTIC CRITERIA FOR ANOREXIA AND BULIMIA NERVOSA in the preceding tables)
3. If possible, obtain additional information from family/friends as patient may lack the capacity to accurately describe own behavior
4. Inquire about other behaviors that can support the presence of an eating disorder such as preference for eating alone, severely limited food preferences, unusual eating habits (ritualistic patterns); ask how often vomiting is induced because of feeling uncomfortably full; ask patient if food dominates life
5. Obtain a careful diet history, with a focus on overall caloric intake and intake of specific nutrients such as calcium
6. Obtain a complete menstrual history; if patient has amenorrhea, determine how long it has been present
7. Question about exercise patterns (overexercise believed to be especially prevalent in males with eating disorders)
8. Ask what medications have been used or are currently being used to induce weight loss; ask specifically about use of appetite suppressants as well as diuretics and laxatives

B. Physical Examination
1. Measure weight with the patient undressed and gowned; measure height and calculate BMI (see OBESITY section for calculation of BMI and definition of "healthy weight")
2. Take vital signs including lying and standing blood pressure and pulse at initial evaluation and at all follow-up visits; pulse in patients with AN is often bradycardic (<60) and majority of ANs have hypotension with pressures <90/60
3. Perform complete physical examination, observing for the stigmata of vomiting which include parotid enlargement, soft palate lesions, dental erosions, and calluses on the dorsal surface of the hand (most frequently seen at the metacarpal-phalangeal joints)
4. Neurologic exam should include mental status, cranial nerves, motor and sensory systems, and cerebellar system

C.	Differential Diagnosis
1.	Numerous **medical conditions** can mimic presentation of eating disorders; however, persons with medical conditions that cause loss of appetite, weight loss, unexplained vomiting **lack the attitudinal features** of a primary eating disorder (obsession with thinness and body image distortion); in addition, the young age of the patient further simplifies the evaluation
    a.	Inflammatory bowel diseases (stool is often positive for blood; erythrocyte sedimentation rate is increased in IBD, and usually subnormal in eating disorders)
    b.	Thyroid disease (physical findings of hyperthyroidism are usually present and laboratory findings confirm the diagnosis)
    c.	Diabetes mellitus (laboratory findings confirm the diagnosis) [eating disorders are almost twice as common in adolescent females with type 1 diabetes as in their non-diabetic peers]
    d.	Central nervous system lesions and occult malignancies anywhere in the body (appropriate imaging studies)
    e.	Chronic infections such as tuberculosis and acquired immunodeficiency
2.	Psychiatric disorders can also present with decreased appetite and weight loss

D.	Diagnostic Tests
1.	Initial laboratory evaluation should include CBC with differential, serum electrolytes, calcium, magnesium, and phosphorous levels, liver function tests, blood urea nitrogen (BUN) level, creatinine level, urinalysis, TSH, and electrocardiogram
    a.	In bulimics, metabolic alkalosis and hypokalemia are the most common abnormalities encountered
    b.	Anorectic patients who lose weight exclusively through caloric intake restriction usually have normal electrolyte levels
2.	Patients who have been underweight >6 months: consider evaluating for osteopenia and osteoporosis (DEXA, estradiol level, and testosterone level [in males])
3.	Patients with atypical presentations should have laboratory evaluation based on history and physical examination in order to rule out other diagnoses
4.	Serum amylase levels are elevated during active vomiting and return to normal within 72 hours after vomiting ceases (may be helpful in documenting presence of bulimia or to follow treatment response [in patients with bulimia, serum amylase elevations are **almost always** caused by a salivary source and not by pancreatitis; can be confirmed by lipase measurement which is elevated in pancreatitis but normal in patients with amylase elevations due to a salivary source as occurs in purging])

V.	Plan/Management

A.	Goals of treatment include restoring and maintaining normal weight, and management of physiologic and psychologic abnormalities; treatment at a specialty center is ideal
1.	Weight gain is crucial for recovery; aim is a 2-3 pound per week gain in a structured treatment setting once patient has begun to cooperate with treatment (most outpatient programs find weight gain goals of 0.5-1 pound/week to be realistic)
2.	The goal is to obtain ideal body weight (IBW) [defined as a BMI in the healthy weight range]; in general, the target goal weight should be within 90% of the IBW; most experts believe that a healthy weight for adolescents is one in which menstruation and ovulation are restored; in premenarcheal girls, a healthy goal weight is one at which normal physical and sexual development resumes

Calculating the Target Goal Weight
✓ Based on the assumption that the ideal body weight for a person who is 5 feet tall is 100 pounds, 5 pounds should be added for each additional inch of height
✓ The target goal weight should be within 90% of this ideal body weight

B.	In-patient versus outpatient management depends on the severity of the condition as well as availability of local resources and insurance status of the patient
1.	Patients who are emaciated or who have hemodynamic instability, significant hypovolemia, arrhythmias, heart failure, or cardiomyopathy must be hospitalized
2.	Failure of appropriate outpatient treatment is also a criterion for hospitalization

C.	Most outpatient treatment for patients with serious but less severe weight loss is managed by a decentralized team, with patients seeing a variety of providers (including a psychotherapist and nutritionist) who communicate with each other about the progress of the patient

D. Cognitive behavioral treatment is the treatment of choice for eating disorders
  1. Objectives of cognitive techniques are to change faulty thought processes such as all-or-none thinking, judgmental thinking, and catastrophizing
  2. Objectives of behavioral techniques are to break patterns of disordered eating through the use of food monitoring, thought monitoring, meal regularity, and nutritional monitoring
  3. Until the acute physiological effects of malnutrition are reversed, behavior change with counseling therapies is difficult; therefore, this treatment approach should be delayed until patient is stabilized
  4. Family therapy is often an important component of treatment as well

E. Role of the primary care clinician
  1. Identify patients with eating disorder and facilitate appropriate treatment
  2. Refer for treatment (AN patients are much less likely to agree to treatment than are patients with BN)
  3. Monitor the medical aspects of the condition (weekly weigh-ins, vital sign measurement, and periodic laboratory testing [CBC, serum electrolytes, and serum amylase levels])
  4. Most patients with AN will recover menses within 6 months of attaining 90% of IBW
  5. Coordinate the efforts of the other professionals involved in care

F. Role of Medications
  1. In patients with AN, need for antidepressants is best assessed following weight gain when the effects of malnutrition are resolving
  2. In patients with BN, antidepressants are effective as one component of an initial treatment program for most patients
  3. For both groups of patients, selective serotonin reuptake inhibitors (SSRIs) are currently considered to be the safest antidepressants and may be especially helpful for patients with significant symptoms of depression, anxiety, and obsessive-compulsive tendencies

G. Risk for osteoporosis
  1. Peak bone mass achieved as a young adult is an important determinant of bone density and fracture risk later in the postmenopausal years
  2. Osteopenia and osteoporosis are among the most serious sequelae of amenorrhea and weight loss in young women with anorexia; AN is associated with markedly reduced bone density, particularly at the lumbar spine but also at the proximal femur and distal radius, increasing the long-term risk for any fracture almost 3-fold
  3. Osteopenia in AN is believed to be a low-turnover condition, associated with increased bone resorption and high serum cortisol levels, and thus is different from the osteopenia of postmenopausal women
  4. Because normalized weight is the best predictor of bone density, the restoration of weight and the avoidance of bone loss are important treatment goals; calcium and vitamin D supplementation are necessary, however
  5. Adolescent patients with moderate to severe anorexia, especially after amenorrhea has occurred, require evaluation and management by a pediatric endocrinologist for close monitoring of bone mineral density; an increase in body weight may be insufficient to completely restore bone mineral density as AN becomes more chronic and more aggressive therapies are indicated

H. Refer patients to the following resources

  ✓ The National Eating Disorders Organization, 6655 South Yale Avenue, Tulsa, OK 74136; 918-481-4044; http://www.laureate.com
  ✓ The American Anorexia/Bulimia Association, 293 Central Park West, Suite 1R, New York, NY 10024; 212-501-8351; http://members.aol.com/amanbu
  ✓ National Association of Anorexia Nervosa and Associated Disorders, Box 7, Highland Park, IL 60035; 847-831-3438

I. Follow Up: See V.E. above for role of the primary care clinician

ENCOPRESIS

I. Definition: A chronic disorder in which young children have bowel movements in unacceptable sites (usually underwear) after age 4

II. Pathogenesis

    A. There are two types of encopresis: retentive in which there is involuntary leakage of fecal material from an impaction and nonretentive in which normal movements are passed into underwear

    B. In retentive encopresis, an impaction occurs when constipation has been present for about a week; pressure of the impaction dilates internal anal sphincter rendering it incompetent so that leakage of stool occurs due to gravity, exercise, or relaxation
        1. A small minority of children become impacted due to organic factors
        2. Most children in this category voluntarily withhold stool because of fear of pain or because of control issues with parent

    C. In nonretentive encopresis, child has normal stool in underwear rather than in toilet
        1. Child is not constipated
        2. In preschoolers, a deliberate resistance to bowel training is likely cause
        3. In school-age child, reluctance to use public toilets or to leave enjoyable activity is likely cause

III. Clinical Presentation

    A. Varying degrees of disorder exist in all cultures, though exact prevalence rates are unknown

    B. Encopresis has a prevalence of about 1% in first- and second-graders; about 80% of those with encopresis are boys

    C. Children with retentive encopresis (most common type) have a history of stool-withholding, with resultant constipation, fecal impaction, and fecal soiling from liquid stool that seeps around the impaction
        1. Such children respond to urge to defecate by contracting the anal sphincter and gluteal muscles in an attempt to withhold stool
        2. They may wriggle, fidget, or assume unusual postures such as rising on toes and rocking back and forth while stiffening their buttocks and legs—all in an attempt to withhold stool
        3. After a while, the rectum habituates to the stimulus of the enlarging fecal mass and the urge to defecate subsides
        4. Over time, the retentive behavior becomes an automatic reaction, and as the rectal wall stretches, fecal soiling may occur

    D. Children with nonretentive encopresis (affecting about 10-20% of children with encopresis) present with no history of constipation and have 1-2 normal stools per day in underwear

IV. Diagnosis/Evaluation

    A. History
        1. Distinguish between retentive and nonretentive encopresis by asking appropriate questions (see KEY QUESTIONS TO DISTINGUISH TYPES OF ENCOPRESIS table below)
        2. Determine if there is a history of stool withholding and, if so, how long this behavior has been present
        3. Take a complete dietary history including intake of dairy products, fruit juice, and fiber
        4. Inquire about pattern of toilet sitting—when and how often it occurs during day and whether toilet sitting is voluntary or coerced by parent/teacher/daycare provider
        5. Take a psychosocial history including family structure, number of persons living in child's home and their relationship to child, interactions child has with peers, and the possibility of abuse
        6. Remember to talk to the child! Child should be a primary historian after about age 7 (except of course, in the areas of past medical history). What are child's perceptions of problem and parental responses to the problem?

KEY QUESTIONS TO DISTINGUISH TYPES OF ENCOPRESIS		
Question	**Retentive**	**Nonretentive**
Are there symptoms of constipation?	Yes	No
What is the frequency of soiling?	Weekly to 1-2 x day	1-2 x day
What is the stool size?	Small	Normal
What is the stool consistency?	Liquid	Normal
Is there a history of need for laxatives?	Yes	No
Does child experience pain with stooling?	Yes	No
Is there passage of huge stools that clog toilet?	Yes	No

B. Physical Examination
1. Perform abdominal exam; in retentive soiling an abdominal mass most commonly involving the rectosigmoid area is usually palpable; mass is midline, suprapubic, irregular, and mobile
2. Inspect the perineal and perianal areas; at least one digital exam of the anorectum is recommended in order to assess perianal sensation, anal tone, size of the rectum, and presence of an anal wink
3. Digital exam also allows for the determination of amount and consistency of stool and its location within the rectum (in impacted children, rectum is dilated and packed with wet-clay consistency stool)
4. In nonretentive stooling, rectal exam should reveal either normal stool or nothing
5. Perform a neurologic exam to rule out any sensory or motor deficits

C. Differential Diagnosis
1. Constipating medications or diet
2. Hirschsprung disease

D. Diagnostic Tests
1. Urinalysis for nitrites and leukocytes (impaction can cause partial bladder emptying and retention)
2. An abdominal radiograph is not indicated to establish the presence of a fecal impaction if the rectal exam shows the presence of a large amount of stool
3. When there is doubt about whether an impaction is present (for example, when child is very obese or when child refuses a rectal exam), a plain abdominal radiograph is reliable in establishing presence of impaction, and may be useful in some children

V. Plan/Management

A. Management of retentive encopresis is described in the following table

MANAGEMENT OF RETENTIVE ENCOPRESIS

➡ Initial Counseling/Education
- ✓ Counsel parent and child that withholding stool is the primary cause of soiling
- ✓ "Demystify" the problem; include a diagram and review of colonic function
- ✓ Remove blame from both parents and child; explain to parents that soiling from overflow incontinence is not a willful and defiant maneuver on the child's part
- ✓ Outline treatment plan in a positive, supportive manner

➡ Disimpaction
- ✓ Removal of impaction is absolutely necessary if child is to maintain bowel control
- ✓ Can be carried out with either oral or rectal medications, or a combination of the two, based on parent/child preferences after the options have been discussed
- ✓ Oral approach is not invasive and gives a sense of control to the child but adherence may be a problem
- ✓ Rectal approach is quicker but is invasive (more than one enema is often needed)
- ✓ Example of oral medication—polyethylene glycol with electrolytes (GoLYTELY), 10-20 mL/kg/dose x 1-2 doses, depending on extent of impaction (not very palatable and children may resist drinking this drug)
- ✓ Example of rectal medication—hypertonic sodium phosphate enema (Fleet enema), [for children ≤11 years, use Fleet enema for children; for children 12 years and older, use Fleet enema for adults] x 1-3 days, depending on extent of impaction

➡ Maintenance Regimen
- ✓ Once the impaction has been removed, maintenance therapy should be initiated—cornerstone of maintenance therapy is behavior modification, dietary interventions, and use of medications to overcome the child's stool-withholding behavior
- ✓ Behavior modification includes the following counseling to parents
  - • Retrain the child in proper bowel habits
    Encourage child not to ignore urge to defecate, even though it may be inconvenient
    Child should sit on toilet, with proper foot support to allow hip flexion and to help leverage for 5-10 minutes after breakfast and the evening meals to take advantage of the gastrocolic reflex
    Child should be rewarded with stickers and given positive reinforcement such as having parent play a game or read a story as a reward for proper toileting
- ✓ Dietary interventions include the following counseling to parents
  - • Provide the child with a balanced diet that includes whole grains, fruits and vegetables (see section on CHILD AND ADOLESCENT NUTRITION for more detailed dietary recommendations to guide counseling to parents, including recommended dietary intake of fiber)
  - • Encourage the child to drink 4-6 ounces of a sorbitol-containing juice such as prune, pear, or apple each day
  - • Encourage the child to drink water frequently throughout the day
- ✓ Medications that will overcome stool-withholding behavior and prevent reimpaction should be given on a long-term basis (maintenance therapy is usually necessary for many months)
  - • Mineral oil, magnesium hydroxide, lactulose, or sorbitol are equally efficacious and the choice among these should be based on cost, the child's preference, ease of administration, and the clinician's experience; all 4 drugs are considered safe for long-term use, although none have FDA approval for long-term use
    Lactulose, 10 g/15 mL; 1-3 mL/kg/day in divided doses (well tolerated long-term), OR
    Mineral oil, 1-3 mL/kg/day, OR
    Magnesium hydroxide, 1-3 mL/kg/day of 400 mg/5 mL (inexpensive), OR
    Sorbitol, 1-3 mL/kg/day in divided doses (less expensive than lactulose)
  - • Instruct parent as follows
    Adjust dose to induce a daily bowel movement for at least 3 months before attempting to wean child from drug
    Drug should be promptly reinstated if relapse occurs
    See V.B. below for management of relapses

B. Advise parents to expect relapses
  1. A stimulant laxative may be necessary intermittently for short periods of time (the use of stimulant laxatives is termed "rescue therapy")
  2. If more than 48 hours pass without a BM, instruct parent to administer a stimulant laxative such as Senokot (>5 years, 10 mL syrup; adolescents, 15 mL syrup) or Dulcolax (>5 years, one 5 mg tab; adolescents, two 5 mg tabs)
  3. If soiling begins to recur, advise child/parent that rectum is full and impaction is returning; vigorous intervention is indicated (increasing dose of maintenance laxative and disimpaction with either an oral or rectal medication) in order to restore normal stool patterns

C. Follow up pattern for retentive encopresis
1. Visits every 4-10 weeks, depending on severity, need for support; duration could be as short as 6 months or as long as 2-3 years
2. Telephone availability is important to provide support and to adjust dosing when needed
3. The successful treatment of encopresis, especially when overflow incontinence is frequent, requires a family that is well organized, can complete time-consuming interventions, and is sufficiently patient to tolerate gradual improvements and relapses
4. Some families may need counseling support to help them effectively deal with the problem

D. Referral to a pediatric gastroenterologist is necessary when management is complex or when the child fails therapy

E. Management of nonretentive encopresis
1. Decreasing involvement of the parent in this problem (except for providing incentives to child) and increasing the responsibility of the child are keys to success
2. Advise parents to discontinue any pressure on child regarding stooling (there should be no lectures, no reminders, no questions relating to toilet use, and absolutely NO PUNISHMENT for stooling in underwear)
3. Advise parents to provide incentives for stooling in toilet (praise, hug, playing favorite game with child)
4. Advise parents not to ignore soiling; parent should instruct child (if old enough) to immediately clean self up when soiling occurs; this should be a quick, impersonal interaction in which child is not made to feel shame
5. Medications are not indicated because stool withholding is not the issue
6. For non-retentive encopresis, continue to follow-up every 2 months for 6 months to evaluate progress; refer to a psychologist who specializes in behavioral problems in children if there is no improvement in 3-6 months

OBESITY

I. Definition: Excessive accumulation of body fat

II. Pathogenesis

A. In all persons, obesity is caused by ingesting more energy than is expended over a long period of time

B. Multiple factors interact and contribute to development of overweight and obesity: a genetic predisposition combines with environmental factors to produce the disorder

C. The role of individual hormones and neurotransmitters in the etiology of obesity remains unknown; however, the recent discovery of the hormone leptin may revolutionize the field of obesity in the next few years

III. Clinical Presentation

A. *Classifying Weight Status*: The Centers for Disease Control and Prevention (CDC) recommends the use of body mass index (BMI) to determine overweight and obesity in children, by comparison of individuals to age- and sex-specific percentiles from a reference population
1. Children older than 2 and adolescents with BMIs at or above the 95th percentile for age and sex are considered overweight
2. Children older than 2 and adolescents with BMIs for age ≥85th percentile but <95th percentile are considered at risk for becoming overweight (the new growth charts using BMI are available at http://www.cdc.gov/growthcharts)
3. Infants less than 2: Overweight is defined as weight-for-length above the 95th percentile or weight greater than 120% of the median weight for a given height (new growth charts for this age group are also available at http://www.cdc.gov/growthcharts)

B. *Prevalence*: Childhood obesity has reached epidemic proportions in the US with the number of overweight children more than doubling over the past three decades making overweight the most common nutritional disorder among today's children

    1. Most of the increase in body weight has occurred since 1980. In 1983, 18.6% of preschool children in the US were defined as overweight, and 8.5% were defined as obese; by 2000, 22% of preschool children were overweight and 10% were obese.

    2. Similar increases in the prevalence of obesity have been observed worldwide

    3. The prevalence of overweight has increased by 21.5% among non-Hispanic black children, 21.8% among Hispanic children, and 12.3% among non-Hispanic white children

    4. The tracking of obesity from childhood to adulthood increases as children age, especially through adolescence

    5. To illustrate, the odds ratios for childhood obesity to result in adult obesity increases from 1.3 for obesity at 1 or 2 years of age to 17.5 for obesity at 15 to 17 years of age

C. *Genetics and Overweight*: The adiposity of a child's parents influences the child's likelihood of becoming obese in adulthood. This correlation applies especially to younger children with overweight parents

    1. A toddler with no obese parent is far more likely to avoid adult obesity than is a child with one or two obese parents

    2. After 10 years of age, the adiposity of the parent is less important than is the adiposity of the child in predicting adulthood obesity

    3. Nonetheless, parental obesity increases the risk for obesity by two- to threefold in children at all ages

D. *Developmental Changes and Overweight*: Data suggest that humans are especially prone to the development of obesity during certain critical periods in their development

---

PATTERNS OF WEIGHT GAIN BASED ON DEVELOPMENTAL STAGES

- BMI increases in the first year of life and then decreases until the child is approximately 6 years of age
- After age 6, BMI again increases, a period known as adiposity rebound
- Research suggests that those children whose BMI increases before age 5.5 years are significantly more likely to show persistent obesity compared with those children who begin to fatten later; thus, children with a rapidly increasingly BMI prior to age 5.5 years should be considered at risk for obesity regardless of whether they are overweight at that point
- During childhood (as in infancy), girls grow slightly slower than boys, and girls have slightly more body fat
- During adolescence, the gender differences in body composition are accentuated, with girls experiencing a continual accumulation of fat mass (FM) and a modest increase in fat-free mass (FFM). Adolescence in boys, on the other hand, is characterized by rapid acquisition of FFM and a modest increase in FM in early puberty, followed by a decline
- Thus, girls are especially disposed to developing persistent obesity during puberty—a period during which the amount of body fat in females tends to increase by about 40%; adolescent boys, on the other hand, experience an increase in lean body mass and a decrease of about 40% in body fat during this time period
- Body weight subsequently normalizes in about 70% of obese male adolescents, but normalization of body weight occurs in only about 20% of obese adolescent females

---

E. *Fitness and Overweight*: Both an increase in energy intake and a decline in physical activity are responsible for this recent epidemic of obesity

    1. Walking and bike riding by children ages 5 to 15 years decreased 40% between 1977 and 1995

    2. Daily participation in high school physical education decreased from 42% to 29% between 1991 and 1999

    3. Data from numerous surveys indicate that low physical activity is particularly common among minority children

F. *Sedentary Activities and Overweight*: Excess TV watching (more than 30% of children now watch more than 5 hours per day of TV), playing video games, and computer activities contribute to the sedentary lifestyle of many children

    1. TV watching not only decreases time available for physical activity, it also encourages snacking and consumption of energy-dense foods with little nutritional value

    2. More than 90% of foods advertised on TV are high in fat, sugar, or salt and most such marketing is specifically designed to appeal to children

G. *Dietary Factors and Overweight*: Children who are overweight take in more calories than they expend, and many of the calories come from high-fat, high-sugar foods

    1.   Recent surveys indicate that American children obtain 50% of their calories from added fat and sugar and only one percent of children regularly ate diets conforming to the recommendations of the Food Guide Pyramid; 45% failed to achieve *any* of the Pyramid recommendations

    2.   Parental guidance remains a critical determinant of children's dietary intake; however, once children reach school-age, factors outside parental control also influence what children eat

    3.   Current trends that have a substantial impact on the dietary intake of US children are summarized in the box below

---

Influence of Current Trends on Dietary Intake of Children

- About 60% of US middle and high schools sell soft drinks in vending machines; in 2002, approximately 240 US school districts participated in exclusive "pouring rights" contracts with soft drink companies in which the school district is rewarded for selling soda to students (in some cases, the school's revenues are directly linked to the amount of soda sold)

- Soft drink companies aim advertising campaigns at children in an effort to develop lifetime brand loyalties with entire conferences devoted to strategies for marketing to kids

- Commonly available food portions exceed the USDA's standard portion sizes. This trend is part of the "supersizing" phenomenon first seen at fast food establishments

- Unfortunately, there has also been a shift to larger portion sizes in the foods consumed at home—a shift that indicates marked changes in eating behavior in general

- Over the past two decades, food portion sizes have increased both inside and outside the home for the following categories: Salty snacks—increased from 1.0 to 1.6 oz; soft drinks—from 12.1 to 19.9 fl oz; hamburgers—from 5.7 to 7.0 oz; french fries—from 3.1 to 3.6 oz; and Mexican food—from 6.3 to 8.0 oz

- The decrease in fat intake and increase in consumption of refined carbohydrates that occurred in the US between 1977 and 1995 coincided with an 85% increase in obesity prevalence

- Consumption of sugar is up by 50% over that of only 50 years ago—consumption of sucrose, the refined white granules made from cane or beets is actually down

- What is being overeaten is fructose—not from honey or fruit—but in the form of high-fructose corn syrup (HFCS) which is added to so many foods because it is sweeter, easier to blend with other ingredients, and much cheaper than sucrose. This liquid sweetener—made from corn starch and boosted with fructose via a special manufacturing process—supplies nearly 10% of all calories consumed by Americans with the figure actually closer to 20% for many people, especially children

- In addition to the calories that HFCS adds to the diet, the body uses fructose differently than it does other sugars; high levels of HFCS can boost triglycerides and possibly cholesterol and may have a negative effect on the body's ability to use calcium, chromium, and other minerals

---

H. *Medical Complications and Overweight*: Obesity related diseases that typically are seen in adults, such as insulin resistance, type 2 diabetes mellitus, hyperlipidemia, hypertension, orthopedic complications, sleep apnea, gallbladder disease, and nonalcoholic steatohepatitis (NASH) are now being seen with increasing frequency in children

I. *Psychosocial Outcomes and Overweight*: Whereas in most cases the health-related consequences of obesity in children do not occur for decades, the social and emotional components of obesity in children are of immediate consequence

    1.   Overweight and obesity are known to affect self-esteem, body image, and social mobility in children, just as it does in adults

    2.   The effects of chronic obesity on the development of psychopathology such as depressive disorders are less clear

J. *Early Timing of Puberty Among Girls and Overweight*: Higher percent body fat and greater abdominal adiposity at 5 and 7 years and greater increases in these variables across middle childhood have been associated with earlier timing of puberty at 9 years

    1.   Overweight and obesity and early timing of puberty among girls have been linked to negative health and psychological outcomes

    2.   Increase in the risks of cardiovascular disease, diabetes, and cancer is a direct consequence of chronic obesity

    3.   Negative outcomes associated with early puberty include higher rates of delinquent behaviors, greater risk of reproductive cancers, and a greater likelihood of elevated weight status during adulthood

IV.   Diagnosis/Evaluation:

    A.   History
        1.   Obtain prenatal history, weight milestones, growth pattern
        2.   Obtain diet history to identify if patterns of excessive eating or drinking exist

---

FOCUS OF DIET HISTORY IN OVERWEIGHT CHILD

Note: Questions about food consumption should be framed in a matter-of-fact, non-judgmental manner

- Ask parent (or child/adolescent) to describe the meals and snacks in a typical day (Note: Purpose is to determine pattern of eating and snacking habits and quality of diet—should not be used to determine caloric intake)

- Ask to estimate daily consumption of high-calorie and high-fat foods, such as chips, cookies, candy, granola bars; ask about intake of high-calorie liquids such as soda, juice, whole milk

- Determine if meals prepared outside the home are important sources of high-calorie eating (from "take-out," fast-foods, school, daycare, or with grandparents, etc.)

---

        3.   Complete a psychosocial history to detect emotional stresses at home or school which may be aggravating problem
        4.   Determine amount and type of physical activity engaged in each week and time spent in sedentary activities, such as TV viewing, video game playing, computer activity, and talking on the telephone
        5.   Ask about motivation for weight loss and types and results of past attempts to lose weight
        6.   Obtain past medical history for orthopedic problems (most often hip or knee pain or limited range of motion), current medications
        7.   Inquire about family history of overweight, dyslipidemia, diabetes, hypertension, premature CHD, or sudden death experienced by father or other male first-degree relative at or before 55, or experienced by the mother or other female first-degree relative at or before 65 years of age

    B.   Physical Examination
        1.   Measure blood pressure, taking care to use the correct size cuff. A common source of false measurement is the use of an incorrectly sized cuff. Correctly sized cuffs have a bladder width of 40% of the child's arm circumference when measured at a point midway between the olecranon and the acromion—the bladder should cover 80% to 100% of the child's arm circumference
        2.   Assess for overweight and at risk for becoming overweight

---

Note:
- ✓ Measure height and weight and determine BMI for children older than 2 and adolescents (based on gender and age) and plot on CDC's new growth chart (see III.A. above for availability); see III.A. above for criteria for overweight and at risk for being overweight in children
- ✓ For infants <2, measure length and weight, and plot on CDC's new growth chart (see III.A. above for availability of charts and for criteria for overweight

---

        3.   Examination of the severely obese patient may be difficult (auscultation of the lungs and heart is compromised as is exam of the abdomen)
        4.   Skin over the neck may be hyperpigmented, thicker, and have a velvet appearance (acanthosis nigricans, associated with insulin resistance in obese adults, also occurs in children with NIDDM and in insulin-resistant children)
        5.   In adolescent females, observe for intertriginous dermatitis under breasts and abdominal panniculus
        6.   In adolescent males, examination of the genitalia may require that the prepubic fat tissue be lifted upward in order to visualize the penis which may be hidden by surrounding fat
        7.   Perform musculoskeletal exam for range of motion
        8.   Determine stage of sexual maturation for both males and females

C. Differential Diagnosis
1. Most obesity is the result of overeating; identifiable exogenous causes of obesity are rare
2. Major endocrine disorders that may manifest with obesity are the following:
   a. Pituitary and adrenal dysfunction (hirsutism and truncal obesity occur in Cushing's syndrome and prominent violaceous striae should prompt an evaluation with a urine free cortisol or dexamethasone suppression test)
   b. Thyroid disease
   c. Polycystic ovarian disease
   d. Hypothalamic disease
3. Psychologic disorders (eating disorders, depression)

V. Plan/Management

A. Plan of care for children who are overweight or at risk of becoming overweight should be based on several underlying principles
   1. Overweight and obesity are important chronic medical problems that are treatable; this fact should be communicated to the child and parents
   2. Sensitive and compassionate care is critical to any successful program
   3. Time spent in understanding each family's particular circumstances is time well spent if the clinician is to support the efforts of the child and family
   4. Changing eating and activity habits is an active process involving the entire family

B. For a weight-management program to be successful, the parent (in the case of children) or adolescent must be ready to make changes; unsuccessful programs can diminish the child/adolescent's self-esteem, thereby jeopardizing future attempts to attain a healthy weight

---

A Practical Approach to Assess Readiness to Make Changes in Diet and Activity

✓ Ask the child and parents how concerned they are about the child's weight
✓ Ask if they believe weight loss is possible
✓ Ask what practices they believe need to be changed
✓ (**Note:** Families who are not ready to change may express a lack of concern about the child's obesity, may believe that obesity is inevitable, and are not interested in modification of eating or activity)

C. For patients/families who are ready to make changes, a program aimed at correcting obesity through healthy eating and activity patterns should be implemented
   1. For young children whose eating and activity are largely under parental control, motivation to participate in an intervention aimed at changing eating and activity behaviors is not necessarily important
   2. On the other hand, for older children who make many of their decisions about eating and physical activity, motivation to change behaviors is crucially important

D. Experts recommend that children younger than 2 years of age be referred to a pediatric obesity center for management
   1. If such referral is not possible, focus should be on slowing excessive weight gain; weight reduction is inappropriate during this period (if referral is not possible, clinician should at the least seek expert consultation)
   2. Discourage feeding infant high calorie foods, such as puddings/desserts and limit juice to 2-4 ounces/day
      a. Advise parent to offer infant pacifier between feedings
      b. Children younger than 2 years of age should never be placed on reduced fat milk
      c. Refer to nutritionist for counseling (WIC if family is eligible)
   3. Refer to section on INFANT NUTRITION for more information
   4. Monitor child's weight gain monthly to make certain child is gaining weight, but at an appropriate level

E. The initial step in management for all overweight children who are between 2 years and 7 years of age is to maintain baseline weight; prolonged weight maintenance allows for a gradual reduction in weight for height
   1. Beginning at age 2, it is acceptable to gradually reduce the amount of fat in the diet (**Remember**: Some fatty acids--linoleic and linolenic acid--are essential for growth and must be supplied by food)
   2. As children move through this age period, they can consume fewer calories from fat; nutrient-rich foods such as grain products, fruits, vegetables, and reduced fat dairy products should supply more of their caloric needs

3. Recommend that parents reward children with affection and attention, not food, money, or gifts
4. Remind parents to provide many opportunities for active play and limit television viewing to 1 hour/day
5. Refer to nutritionist for counseling (refer eligible children to WIC)
6. Expert consultation should be sought as limiting the energy intake of growing children is risky

F. For children older than 7 years of age, with a BMI >95th percentile, weight maintenance is the initial goal, and once that goal is achieved, additional changes in eating and activity to achieve actual weight loss of about 1 pound per month is appropriate
   1. By age 7, a child's pattern of eating should conform to the same dietary guidelines as older children and adults (see section on NUTRITION)
      a. The focus should be on consuming well-balanced meals not just for the overweight child but for the entire family
      b. Encourage families to use the Dietary Guidelines for Americans which provide general nutritional principles, and the Food Guide Pyramid which shows how to select different types of foods for optimal nutrition (see NUTRITION sections)
   2. Discuss with parents approaches that promote the successful treatment of overweight and obesity

---

PARENTING APPROACHES THAT PROMOTE SUCCESSFUL TREATMENT OF OVERWEIGHT AND OBESITY

- Emphasize healthy eating and activities for the entire family, not just for the overweight child—all family members should eat a healthy diet and participate in energy expending activities
- Find reasons to praise the child; many children eat when what they really need is nurturing
- Avoid the use of food as a reward; instead, use time and activities involving the parents or friends as a reward for desired behavior
- Establish daily family meals and snack time; parents determine what food is offered and child can decide whether to eat
- Sit-down meals involving the entire family are ideal; with this approach, dinner time is not just about eating, but also involves building relationships and developing social skills
- Offer only healthy options at meals and snacks—child can choose between apple and popcorn, not between cookie and apple
- Offer daily activities that involve a substantial expenditure of energy—child can choose between riding bike in park or going roller skating, not between doing a craft project or riding bike in park
- Limit eating at fast-food restaurants to 1 or 2 times a month (see Eric Schlosser's *Fast-Food Nation: The Dark Side of the All-American Meal*, New York: Harper Collins, 2002)

G. Exercise programs for children should be age-appropriate; the best type of exercise is any form that is sustainable
   1. Parents need to provide opportunities for child to increase his/her activity
   2. Ideally, exercise programs should increase the interaction between parents and children (family walks, basketball games, tennis, biking)
   3. Activities with other children are also ideal (e.g., participating in karate with a friend)
   4. Sedentary behaviors, such as watching TV and playing video games should be limited to 1 hour or less per day
   5. Exercise also helps to promote self-esteem; research has shown that adolescents who exercise regularly are more likely to perceive themselves as attractive
   6. Current recommendations are for children to engage in 60 minutes or more of daily moderate intensity physical activity

H. Follow Up
   1. Successful weight loss and maintaining weight loss are long-term endeavors and frequent follow-up is important to monitor weight loss and provide support; face-to-face contact is not always necessary. Alternate office visits with telephone calls or e-mails to keep in contact with patients and follow their progress
   2. Distinguishing between lapse and relapses may be a useful concept in assisting the child to lose weight and then maintain that weight loss
      a. Lapses are defined as slips and temporary setbacks, considered a normal part of any behavioral change; it is important to explain to the child and family that lapses are inevitable and should be considered learning experiences rather than a sign of failure
      b. Relapses, on the other hand, are defined as the permanent abandonment of a weight-control program. When relapses occur, causes for the failure need to be identified and a new approach should be implemented as soon as possible, if the child is willing
   3. Referral to a behavioral psychologist is often necessary to facilitate change

PRIMARY NOCTURNAL ENURESIS

I.   Definition: Involuntary discharge of urine that occurs only at night beyond the age of 5 years in girls and 6 years in boys

II.   Pathogenesis

    A.   Enuresis is considered to be multifactorial in etiology

    B.   Various theories have been proposed to explain this disorder

> - Developmental delay explanations have focused on a delay in adequate neuromuscular control
> - Organic theories suggest disorders of the genitourinary and nervous systems; however, only about 3-4% of children with enuresis have organic pathology
> - Psychological factors may have an impact on the expression of enuresis although the incidence of behavioral problems in enuretic children is difficult to determine
> - Early sleep studies suggested that "disorder of arousal" may have role in enuresis but, more recently, it has been concluded that sleep stage is unrelated to episodes of enuresis
> - A lack of circadian rhythm in the secretion of arginine vasopressin, the antidiuretic hormone appears to play a major role in nocturnal enuresis
>   - ✓ A rise in the hormone decreases the amount of urine produced at night
>   - ✓ Without this rise in hormone secretion, an amount of urine is produced that overwhelms the bladder's ability to retain urine until morning
> - Genetic predisposition or family history has an important role in development of enuresis with a 45% chance that a parent who was enuretic will have one or more children who is enuretic

III.   Clinical Presentation

    A.   Approximately 15% of all 5 year olds, 7% of 8 year olds, and 3% of 12 year olds have nocturnal enuresis, with males predominating in all age groups

    B.   Prevalence rates are highest among lower socioeconomic status (SES) groups, less educated groups, and those children who are institutionalized

    C.   Fewer than 10% of all enuretics also wet in the daytime (diurnal enuresis)

    D.   Primary enuresis exists when a child has never achieved consistent dryness

    E.   Secondary enuresis exists when child has had a period of dryness for 3-5 months and then relapses; most children fall into this category

    F.   In general, for the diagnosis of nocturnal enuresis to be established, a child 5-6 years of age must have ≥2 bedwetting episodes per month, and a child >6 years of age must have ≥1 episodes per month

    G.   Children who have chronic constipation or encopresis may present with bed-wetting

IV.   Diagnosis/Evaluation

    A.   History
        1.   Determine if enuresis is primary or secondary, nocturnal or diurnal
        2.   Ask about onset, duration, severity (number of wet nights per week, for example 4/7)
        3.   Ask if either parent was enuretic as a child
        4.   Obtain prenatal, birth history including gestational age, birth weight; inquire about developmental milestones
        5.   Inquire about toilet training and how parent has managed the enuresis thus far
        6.   Review of systems should focus on genitourinary and nervous systems
        7.   Inquire about presence of encopresis

8. Determine attitudes of the parent toward the child and toward the problem by observing interactions with child and by listening to the content of their statements about the child and the problem

9. Remember to talk to the child! Child should be the primary historian after about age 7 (except, of course, in the area of past medical history). What are child's perceptions of problem and parental responses to the problem?

B. Physical Examination
1. Measure blood pressure, height, weight, and plot on growth chart (poor growth and/or elevated blood pressure suggest renal disease)
2. Examine genitals, looking for major and minor anomalies
3. Perform neurological exam including gait, muscular strength and tone, deep tendon reflexes, sensory responses, and rectal sphincter tone
4. If possible, observe child voiding and note stream, ability to initiate and interrupt in midstream (usually not possible)

C. Differential Diagnosis
1. Urinary tract infection
2. Genitourinary or neurologic anomalies

D. Diagnostic Tests
1. Urinalysis and urine culture
2. Complicated enuresis (severe voiding dysfunction, associated encopresis, urinary tract infection, and an abnormal neurologic exam) requires further study
    a. Renal or bladder sonogram
    b. Voiding cystourethrogram (VCUG)
    c. Urodynamic measurement

V. Plan/Management

A. Supportive counseling should be provided to all families with an emphasis on the following:
1. Enuresis is a common problem with a spontaneous cure rate of approximately 15% a year after the child reaches 5 years of age
2. It is an involuntary process and the child has no control of the behavior; thus child should not be made to feel guilty, nor should parents punish the child
3. Acceptance of the behavior as an individual difference by parent and child is important and may hasten spontaneous resolution

B. In general, initiation of treatment for nocturnal enuresis is deferred until the child reaches 6 years of age because of the high spontaneous cure rates that occur with maturation (enuresis is very common among 5 year olds)

C. Reassurance is the therapy of choice for younger children (<6 years) or for children who develop transient enuresis in response to environmental stress

D. For children ≥6 years of age, pharmacologic treatment is the most common approach to management of nocturnal enuresis
1. Parents and child must understand that this is not a cure for the disorder but rather controls the symptoms
2. Discontinuation of the medication usually results in the recurrence of enuresis, unless the child has reached the age at which he/she would have outgrown the problem without any therapy

E. The most commonly used pharmacologic treatment is desmopressin (DDAVP), an effective and safe medication when used as directed; acts on the renal tubule to increase the absorption of filtered water, increasing urinary concentration and decreasing urinary volume; success rate reported to be 60 to 70%
1. Available as a nasal spray and in tablet form (**Note:** Dosage is not titrated by patient weight; there are conflicting reports regarding optimal dose which appears to vary according to the individual child)

Nasal spray	✓ Children <6 years of age, not recommended
	✓ Children ≥6 years, 20 micrograms (half of dose per nostril) at bedtime and may be increased gradually to 40 micrograms in order to achieve dryness (**Note:** Some children respond to as little as 10 micrograms)
Tablet form	✓ Children <6 years of age, not recommended
	✓ Children ≥6 years, 0.2 mg at bedtime; may be increased gradually to 0.6 mg in order to achieve dryness

2. If there is good response to the drug, the program is maintained for several months and then the child is weaned off the DDAVP (using only every other night for several weeks and then stopping altogether)

3. Caution parents that this medication, like others, must be used only as directed; daytime use can result in retention of water and subsequent dilutional hyponatremia

F. The tricyclic antidepressant imipramine (Tofranil) has been used extensively in the past to treat enuresis but is **not commonly used today**. Consult PDR for details regarding dosing, adverse reactions, contraindications, and drug interactions

G. Use of a bed wetting alarm is probably the most effective therapy (success rate of 75%) in treating enuresis in children ≥7 years, but most parents are not receptive to this therapy
   1. Alarm works by negative reinforcement or avoidance
   2. Uses a moisture activated sensor which attaches to child's underwear
   3. A small pin-on battery powered alarm awakens child (can be equipped with a buzzer)
   4. Average of 60 days of treatment is needed to achieve success; relapses frequently occur (about 40%) but retreatment is usually successful
   5. Alarms are inexpensive ($40-$60) but can be noisy, frequently awakening the entire household
   6. Improved technology makes the alarms a more attractive option than in the past
   7. Devices commonly used include

> ✓ **WetStop** by Palco Laboratories, 1595 Soquel Drive, Santa Cruz, CA 95065; 800-346-4488 (www.palcolabs.com)
> ✓ **Potty Pager** (silent alarm), Ideas for Living, 1285 N. Cedarbrook, Boulder, CO 80304 (www.pottypager.com)
> ✓ **Nytone Alarm** by Nytone Medical Products, 2424 S. 900 West, Salt Lake City, UT 84119 (www.nytone.com)

H. Bladder training therapy is designed to increase child's bladder capacity through stretching; efficacy is unproven, but some parents may want to try this nonpharmacologic approach
   1. Based on the observation that many enuretic children have decreased bladder capacity
   2. Children are instructed to try to avoid urinating for as long as possible during the day
   3. Parents should measure voiding volumes on a daily basis to monitor progress
   4. Normal bladder volume can be estimated as one ounce per age in years plus 2 (**Example:** 6 year old = 6 ounces plus 2 = 8 ounces of bladder capacity, on average)
   5. Limitations of the approach is that increased bladder capacity does not necessarily translate to nighttime dryness

I. Treatment failures and relapses are common, but a trial of 4-6 weeks should be given for an approach to have a fair chance of working

J. The presence of coexistent emotional problems and poor family interaction patterns suggests need for referral for counseling

K. Follow Up
   1. In 2 weeks for patients on pharmacologic therapy to titrate dose, then monthly x 3 months
   2. Important to follow up at regular intervals to provide encouragement
   3. The efficacy of all of the treatment modalities is enhanced by active clinician involvement

SLEEP PATTERNS AND PROBLEMS IN INFANTS AND YOUNG CHILDREN

I.   Definition:

    A.   Sleep patterns are age and developmentally determined sleep behaviors

    B.   Sleep problems are difficulty falling asleep or staying asleep as perceived by the parent; excessive daytime sleepiness (hypersomnolence) and abnormal behaviors associated with sleep (parasomnias) such as night terrors, sleepwalking, bruxism, and enuresis are not considered here

II.   Pathogenesis

    A.   Sleep patterns are carefully controlled by underlying circadian pacemakers

- The task of the newborn is twofold: To organize behavior into specific states—waking, non-rapid eye movement (NREM) sleep and rapid eye movement (REM) sleep—and to organize these states into a 24-hour rhythmic pattern
- Over a period of 24 hours, newborns sleep 16-17 hours; by 16 weeks of age, total sleep time has slowly decreased to 14-15 hours, and by 6-8 months of age, has decreased even further to about 13-14 hours per day
- By 3 weeks of age, sleep is spread out over the 24-hour day in approximately equal segments between feedings
- By about 6 weeks of age, a clear diurnal/nocturnal distribution of wake and sleep emerges in most infants
- By 3 months of age, day/night differentiation is defined in most infants; sleep is largely distributed in the night hours and daytime sleep becomes consolidated into better defined daytime naps; thus waking periods also become longer
- By 4 months of age, the infant lengthens his/her longest sleeping period; between birth and 4 months, the sleeping stretch usually doubles to about 8 hours
- By 6 to 9 months of age, most infants have developed pattern of well-consolidated nighttime sleep, a significant milestone in the infant's development of a mature sleeping pattern
- Between 2 and 5 years of age, REM sleep decreases from between 30-35% of total sleep time to the adult level of 20-25%; the total sleep time decreases for most children during the preschool years from about 14 hours to 12 hours per day
- From entry to first grade (at age 6 years) to the beginning of adolescence, the total amount of sleep steadily decreases from about 10 hours to 8-9 hours

    B.   Daytime sleep or napping changes substantially during infancy and early childhood

- Infants at 4 months of age take two to three naps each day and about half of 15 month old toddlers take 2 naps per day, for a total of about 2.5 hours
- Most preschoolers continue to nap, with 90% of 3 years olds, over half of 4 year olds, and about one-fourth of 5 year olds taking one nap in the early afternoon on most days of the week
- Little is known about napping patterns in school-age children, but napping behavior is believed to be uncommon among this age group

    C.   Night wakings are an important aspect of infant and toddler development and follow a predictable pattern

- Brief awakening from sleep is more frequent during the early months than at older ages in infancy
- Most infants awaken for brief periods throughout the night and return to sleep without their parents being aware that wakings have occurred
- Infants who put themselves back to sleep without their parents' knowledge are called *self-soothers*; infants who cry to awaken their parents are called *signalers*
- *Settling* is defined as sleeping throughout most of the night, with self-soothing behaviors used to return to sleep on one's own
- In general, as infants mature, they become increasingly more able to settle into sleep without signaling the parent
- Development of the ability to settle by infants is believed to be affected by parenting practices, feeding and soothing styles, as well as by individual characteristics of the infant
- Good sleepers are able to soothe themselves to sleep after waking up, whereas night wakers require the parent's presence to return to sleep

D.   Problems with sleep have many causes, but there are five major areas that must be considered

- Parental misperceptions regarding age-appropriate sleep patterns in infants and children
- Parental behaviors that are well-intended but that promote disrupted sleep in the infant or child
- Transient physical discomfort associated with colic, teething, or a minor illness
- Serious medical problems causing disturbed sleep via the mechanism of partial or complete airway obstruction during sleep
- Family problems such as marital discord or maternal guilt that create or maintain a sleep disturbance for the child

III.   Clinical Presentation

A.   Sleep occupies a major portion of young children's lives with newborn infants spending almost 70% of the first few weeks in the sleep state

B.   Sleep comprises such a significant part of the infant and young child's life that it is assumed to play a critical role in the child's development

C.   The complaint of sleep disturbance almost always comes from the parent and not from the child, even when the child is an adolescent

D.   Night wakings, prolonged bedtime routines, and other sleep/wake behaviors often concern parents, either because the behaviors themselves are inconvenient and disturb the parents' sleep, or because they may be considered symptomatic of more serious difficulties

E.   On occasion, infants' and young children's sleep is disrupted because of physical problems such as colic, discomfort from teething, or respiratory tract infections; more often, however, there is no physical cause for disrupted sleep

F.   The most common cause of disturbed sleep in infants, toddlers, and preschoolers is parental mismanagement

IV.   Diagnosis/Evaluation

A.   History
        1.   Ask parent to give an overview of the problem as a beginning point (the focus should be on exactly what happens most nights and days and under what circumstances)

- Parents tend to say the child "never sleeps," so they must be assisted in focusing their account on specifics rather than on generalizations
- Keep in mind that parents often like to describe worst-case scenarios, and may have difficulty relating what patterns the infant or child typically follows, saying "There is **not** one"
- Focus on the current pattern of sleep; past patterns are important, but the current problem is most relevant

        2.   If the child is at least 4 years of age, include him/her as appropriate in the history taking process (for example, determine how he/she views the problem [if it is viewed as a problem])
        3.   Ask about evening routines in the family such as what time the evening meal is consumed (in infants, what time the last feeding is provided), what time the child is placed in (or goes to) bed, what sorts of bedtime rituals there are prior to, and after child is placed in (or goes to) bed, how long the child takes to fall asleep, what problems occur with sleep onset and how these are handled by the parent
        4.   Ask about the sleep environment, specifically determine **where** the child sleeps and who else sleeps in the room or in the bed with the child; ask about the lighting in the room at night; ask about nighttime noises (are there lullaby tapes, radios, televisions on in the room?)[Note: Unsupervised watching of TV in bed is a common cause for sleep disturbances in school-age children]
        5.   In infants and toddlers, ask about the use of pacifiers, the use and significance of transitional objects such as blankets and stuffed toys; ask if infant/toddler is placed in bed with a bottle and what liquid is in the bottle (water, milk, juice)

6. Obtain daytime schedule for weekdays and weekends (which are different for children in daycare or school), with a focus on amount of daytime sleep (how many naps, what time the naps occur, and how long the naps last)

7. Ask about bedwetting (in children over 3 in whom nighttime dryness has usually been established), walking or talking while asleep, nightmares, teeth grinding, snoring, complaints of nighttime leg discomfort, head banging while in bed

8. Obtain developmental history and psychosocial history

> - Ascertain that the child's development is age appropriate; perform a screening test using parental report (e.g., Ages and Stages Questionnaire or Parents' Evaluation of Developmental Status [see section on CHILD HEALTH SUPERVISION])
> - Interaction between social problems and sleep problems are well documented
> - A parent with problems with alcohol, drugs, depression or anxiety creates tension within the family that may be expressed as disordered sleep in the child
> - Sleep problems in the child may be an early symptom of an emerging psychiatric disturbance, but this is very uncommon

9. Obtain past medical history, and ask what medications, if any, are presently being taken by the child; ask if child has any allergies

B. Physical Examination
   1. The focus of the exam should be to establish normality and to rule out any underlying medical problems (**Note**: Physical findings to explain sleeplessness in an infant and child are rare)
   2. Obtain weight-for-age, stature-for-age, weight-for-stature, head circumference (for children ≤24 months of age); beginning at age 2 body mass index-for-age percentiles are calculated; plot on the child's growth chart, and compare with previous recordings to determine if child is following his/her growth curve
   3. Observe the child for any facial abnormalities
   4. Assess the nose and throat to evaluate nasal airflow, tonsillar size
   5. Perform a cardiopulmonary assessment including blood pressure measurement
   6. Perform a neurologic assessment

C. Differential Diagnosis
   1. Underlying behavioral or emotional problem in which disturbed sleep is an associated feature
   2. Medical problem including allergies, large adenoids or tonsils, or birth defects–all of these conditions can cause partial or complete airway obstruction during sleep
   3. Problems between the parents or within the family

D. Diagnostic Testing
   1. None indicated unless underlying medical problem is suspected
   2. If there are suspected respiratory deficits, referral to a pediatric sleep specialist for sleep studies to evaluate the quality of breathing during sleep or referral to an otolaryngologist (if allergies or enlarged adenoids or tonsils are believed to be the problem) is indicated

V. Plan/Management

A. The exact management strategy should be geared to the developmental level of the child and to the particular circumstances of the individual child and family

B. The following tables contain age-specific sleep patterns and parental behaviors that can promote good sleep habits in infants and children

BIRTH TO 4 MONTHS

➡ Parents should understand the usual cycles of sleep/waking in the newborn and early infant period; babies should always be fed when they are hungry and consoled when they cry; parents should anticipate when the baby will become drowsy and prepare for these periods of sleep

➡ When the infant is ready for sleep, some parents prefer to soothe the baby for several minutes, and then put the baby on her back in the crib whether or not she is asleep; other parents prefer to always hold the baby until she is in a deep sleep, and then put the baby in the crib asleep

➡ Either of the methods described above is acceptable but it is probably best for parents to allow infant to learn to get to sleep in bed rather than in parent's arms so that the infant learns to fall asleep without parent present

➡ Establishment of bedtime routines should be started during this time period—bedtime song or music box, use of a pacifier or blanket for comfort

➡ The goal in this age group is not to impose a rigid sleep schedule but instead to synchronize care giving with the infant's circadian sleep-wake rhythms and to develop an orderly routine that is predictable and helps the infant achieve the developmental task of trust

➡ Parents should expect newborns and infants to awaken every 3-4 hours during the night for feedings (breastfed infants may awaken every 2-3 hours during the neonatal period)

➡ Parents of colicky infants should expect to spend more time holding and soothing the infant than parents of noncolicky infants

INFANTS 4 TO 9 MONTHS OF AGE

➡ Circadian rhythms continue to mature during this age period, and parents can begin to look more to clock time as an aid to predict nap time, bed time, and morning awakening time

➡ By 9 months of age, most infants take lengthy naps at 9 AM and 1 PM and then fall asleep at around 7 or 8 PM; babies often wake up for a feeding once or twice each night until 9 months of age (especially infants who are breastfed)

➡ If there is a night-waking problem during this age period, parents should be advised to stop attending to all but one or two night wakings

- If infant is overtired, parent can try an earlier bedtime and put their infant in bed either awake or asleep after the established soothing period and bedtime rituals (story, song, pacifier, blanket)

- If this schedule is maintained, protest crying at bedtime or at night-waking should rapidly (over 3-4 nights) disappear

- Remind the parent that consistency is the key; intermittent reinforcement by the parent has the effect of increasing crying in the infant

INFANTS 9 TO 15 MONTHS OF AGE

➡ Children in this age group should have consolidated night sleep with no night waking and one or two naps during the day, at 9 AM and 1 PM; 90% of 9 month olds, 80% of 12 month olds, and 45% of 15 month olds take two naps a day (total duration of naps during the day is 2-3 hours)

➡ Bed time does not have to be on a rigid schedule; it can be variable, but always early, and based on the child's apparent degree of tiredness, whether naps occurred, and nap duration

➡ Soothing to sleep rituals should always be regular and predictable in terms of what the parent does to soothe the child to sleep; by this time, bedtime rituals should be firmly in place, with changes in the rituals based on developmental level (for example, reading a story is not as appropriate for a 3 month old as it is for a 15 month old)

➡ Children in this age group have more persistence, autonomy, and willfulness; sleep problems are likely to be more common and more easily mismanaged by the parent

➡ Desire for the parent's company may prompt child to cry or call out for the parent; it is important that parents not respond once they have assured themselves that the child is not ill

TODDLERS 15 TO 24 MONTHS OF AGE

➡ Toddlers in this age group should be taking one nap per day in the early afternoon

➡ Toddlers who have difficulty transitioning from two to one nap per day should have an earlier bedtime; parents should be told that an earlier bedtime does not mean an earlier wake-up time

➡ Consistency in bedtime rituals at sleep times and reasonable regularity when the child is tired help to establish structured sleep habits

➡ Toddlers who get out of crib or bed should be firmly and silently placed back in the bed to teach the child that this behavior is not acceptable

➡ Limited interaction and an unemotional attitude reduce the social rewards that reinforce night waking

➡ Parents should understand that they cannot force the child to sleep but that they can insist that the child remain in his/her crib or bed

CHILDREN 2 TO 3 YEARS OF AGE

➡ Between ages two and three years of age, children sleep an average of 14 hours a day

➡ Virtually all children are napping at 2 (most often around lunch time for 2-3 hours) but about 10% have discontinued napping by age 3

➡ Children in this age group resist going to sleep even when going-to-sleep rituals have been firmly established

➡ To provide the toddler with feelings of control (and thereby promote his feelings of autonomy), encourage parents to let him make as many choices as possible at bedtime—let him select which book to read, which stuffed toy to take to bed, etc.; make certain the night light is on as this promotes feelings of security

  • If the child cries when the parent leaves the room, the parent should wait 10 minutes, then return to settle him down again

  • Parent should be advised not to reinforce this behavior by giving child food or their company. If the child cries again, wait 10 minutes to give him the opportunity to settle down, then repeat the process

  • The child should not be scolded or punished, but firmly settled down and left alone to get to sleep

➡ By age 3, sleep rules can be instituted to help motivate the child in good sleep hygiene; a poster can be made with the sleep rules and placed in the child's room

  • The sleep rules are simple ones that a 3 year old can understand and can consist of the following: "At sleep time, we stay in bed, we close our eyes, and we rest"

  • Parents can recite these rules with child at nap time and at bed time

  • The child is rewarded for following the rules (the reward needs to be highly motivational and should not involve food)

  • Children younger than 3 who do not understand sleep rules should be quietly and unemotionally returned to bed

➡ Children in this age group are often very demanding and parents find themselves spending more and more time in bedtime routines and soothing behaviors; to limit this, parents can place a timer (with a very soft bell or pleasing musical sound) on the night stand set to go off after a reasonable period

➡ **A word about nightmares**: When nightmares awaken the toddler, it is important that the parent comfort the child by holding him, asking him to talk about the dream (a 3 year old may be able to do this), and stay with him until he is calm enough to fall asleep

BOOKS ABOUT BEDTIME, SLEEP, AND DREAMS

Goodnight Moon by Margaret Wise Brown
In the Night Kitchen by Maurice Sendak
Bedtime for Frances by Russell Hoban
Goodnight Gorilla by Peggy Rathmann
There's a Nightmare in My Closet by Mercer Mayer
Ben's Dreams by Chris van Allsberg

C. Consider referral to a pediatric sleep specialist if the problem is chronic and severe, or if the problem has seriously disrupted the family and there is lack of agreement between the parents regarding how to deal with the problem

D. Follow Up: Telephone follow up once a week or so for a month can be very helpful to parents who are dealing with sleep problems in their child; visits should be scheduled on an as-needed basis

TOBACCO USE AND SMOKING CESSATION

I. Definition: Destructive health behavior involving use of tobacco (cigarettes, chewing tobacco, and snuff)

II. Pathogenesis

A. Tobacco smoke contains numerous substances which are toxic, mutagenic, or carcinogenic

B. In addition to harmful volatile substances such as carbon monoxide, the particulate phase of cigarette smoke contains nicotine and tars

C. The consequences of a product of combustion (smoke) being drawn into close contact with delicate pulmonary tissues are devastating

D. The etiology of tobacco dependence is multidimensional with physiological, psychological, and social/behavioral factors
   1. Physiological factors include activation of the mesolimbic dopaminergic system ("reward circuit") and locus ceruleus (vigilance and arousal)
   2. Psychological factors evolve from positive feedback provided by pleasurable sensations
   3. Social/behavioral factors include the following: smoking becomes a habit or an automatic and intrinsic part of daily activities, and smoking can be used as self-medication to reduce unpleasant sensations that occur with tobacco withdrawal or stress

III. Clinical Presentation

A. Tobacco addiction, a pervasive disease in the US, usually begins in childhood and adolescence; unfortunately, children who begin tobacco use at an early age are more likely to continue to smoke into adult life

B. Every day in the US, approximately 6000 young people start smoking, and half of these youth will become daily smokers
   1. Prevalence rates for some adolescent groups (e.g., high school seniors) is 31% which actually exceeds the adult smoking rate in the US, which is about 25%
   2. This rate does not include those youth who drop out of school and are more likely to use tobacco than those who are in school
   3. Ethnic and cultural variations in tobacco use reflect interactions among multiple factors including income, tobacco price, availability, culture, stress, genetics, age, gender, and targeted advertising
   4. Cigarette smoking is more prevalent among low-income, low socioeconomic populations

C. Tobacco use is the leading preventable cause of death in the US, responsible for more than 400,000 deaths annually, or 1 of every 5 deaths
   1. Almost all smokers acknowledge that tobacco use is harmful to health, but tend to underestimate the risk to their **own** health
   2. Many smokers believe the benefits of smoking in the present outweigh the risk of disease in the future
   3. Half of regular smokers die prematurely of a tobacco-related disease

D. As with cigarette smoking, the use of smokeless tobacco, such as chewing tobacco and snuff, produces addiction to nicotine and has serious health consequences
   1. Use of these products has increased in recent years, especially among white youth who live in the South and Midwest regions
   2. Health risks from use of these products include gingival recession, periodontal bone loss, leukoplakia, oral cancer, and cardiovascular disease

E. Cigar smoking, which increased dramatically over the past decade, also poses serious health risks: smokers are at higher risk for coronary heart disease, COPD, lung and other cancers, with evidence of dose-dependent effects

F. In the US, 43% of children aged 2 to 11 are exposed to environmental tobacco smoke (ETS)
   1. Consequences of ETS increase based on exposure; the more cigarettes smoked in the child's environment, the more particulate matter is discharged into the air
   2. Children exposed to ETS have increased risk of growth disorders, sudden infant death syndrome, asthma, middle ear disease, pneumonia, cough, and upper respiratory infection

G. The addictive nature of nicotine (it causes tolerance and physical dependence) is the primary physiological barrier to quitting tobacco use
   1. Withdrawal syndrome is characterized by symptoms of anxiety, irritability, anger, impatience, restlessness, difficulty concentrating, sleep disturbances, increased appetite and depressed mood
   2. Symptoms begin a few hours after the last cigarette, peak 2-3 days later, and then decline over a period of weeks or months

H. Psychological barriers to quitting include the fact that tobacco use is an integral part of the individual's daily routine
   1. Smokers develop certain patterns of tobacco-use behavior such as smoking after meals, and to relax at the end of the day
   2. Smokers also frequently use tobacco to handle stress and negative emotions such as anxiety and anger

I. Primary care clinicians have an unprecedented opportunity to reduce tobacco use rates in the US
   1. More than 70% of smokers visit a health care setting each year where they could consistently receive effective tobacco interventions
   2. Effective treatments now exist

J. Thirty-three states have established telephone quitlines to deliver cessation-counseling services to smokers who want to quit smoking

IV. Diagnosis/Evaluation

    A. History
        1. Ask how long the child/adolescent has been smoking
        2. Determine the degree of nicotine dependence by using the assessment tool in the box below

---

Brief Fagerstrom Test for Nicotine Dependence

How soon on waking do you smoke your first cigarette?

If answer is	Within 5 minutes,	Score = 3
	Within 30 minutes, excluding the first 5 minutes	Score = 2
	Within 60 minutes, excluding the first 30 minutes	Score = 1
	After 60 minutes	Score = 0

How many cigarettes do you smoke a day?

If answer is	31 or more	Score = 3
	21 to 30	Score = 2
	11 to 20	Score = 1
	10 or fewer	Score = 0

Scoring and Interpretation: Calculate score from 2 questions and determine level of dependence based on total score
        5-6 = High nicotine dependence
        3-4 = Moderate nicotine dependence
        0-2 = Light nicotine dependence

Adapted from Heatherton, T.F., Kozlowski, L.T., Frecker, R.C., & Fagerstrom, K.O. (1991). The Fagerstrom test for nicotine dependence: A revision of the Fagerstrom tolerance questionnaire. *British Journal of Addiction, 86*, 1119-1127.

        3. Ask about past attempts at quitting, including length of smoking cessation, problems encountered, and reasons for relapse
        4. Explore smoke-related symptoms such as cough, sputum production, shortness of breath, recurrent respiratory infections
        5. Review family history and personal medical history of tobacco-related diseases such as coronary heart disease, chronic obstructive pulmonary disease, and cancer

    B. Physical Examination: Use the examination as an intervention, highlighting the damage that smoking can do to each body system which is assessed
        1. Monitor vital signs, particularly blood pressure which adds an additional risk of heart disease if elevated
        2. Examine ears, nose, sinuses, mouth, and pharynx, noting signs of inflammation due to irritation from tobacco
        3. Perform complete exam of lungs
        4. Perform complete exam of heart and peripheral vascular system

    C. Diagnostic Tests
        1. Consider spirometry
            a. If normal, stress the benefits of smoking cessation before damage occurs
            b. If abnormal, stress the importance of cessation before further damage occurs
        2. Other diagnostic testing not indicated

    D. Differential Diagnosis: Not applicable

V. Plan/Management

    A. Major intervention categories for treating tobacco use and dependence are as follows
        1. *Brief clinical interventions*--can be provided by any clinician but are most relevant to primary care clinicians who treat a wide variety of patients and who have severe time constraints; can be effectively implemented in 3 minutes and can increase cessation rates significantly
        2. *Intensive clinical interventions*--can be provided by any trained clinician who has the time and resources available; produce higher success rates and are most cost-effective in the long term than less-intensive interventions
        3. *Systems interventions*--involve healthcare delivery systems that institutionalize the consistent identification, documentation, and treatment of every tobacco user seen in the setting

B. **Ask**–the first step in implementing an effective smoking cessation program for all patients in your practice is to implement an office-wide system to identify all tobacco users at every visit
    1. Expand vital sign section to include "tobacco use," with categories of "current," "former," or "never"
    2. As an alternative, put "tobacco use status" stickers on every chart
    3. If electronic charts used, incorporate into clinical reminder system
    4. **Note:** The rate at which clinicians provide advice on smoking cessation is now a standard measure for assessing quality of care delivered by health plans in US
    5. Evidence-based guidelines relating to tobacco use interventions at the systems (versus individual) level of healthcare delivery are available at http://www.thecommunityguide.org

C. **Advise** all smokers to stop
    1. *Be clear.* In a straightforward manner tell the patient that you believe it is important for him/her to quit smoking now, and that you can help; cutting down is not enough
    2. *Speak strongly.* Emphasize that quitting smoking is the single most important thing that patient can do for future health
    3. *Personalize advice.* Point out reasons that smoking cessation will improve the personal health as well as the health of loved ones exposed to ETS. See GOOD REASONS FOR YOUR PATIENT TO QUIT SMOKING in the table that follows

GOOD REASONS FOR YOUR PATIENTS TO QUIT SMOKING	
Teenagers	Bad breath, stained teeth, cost, potential decrease in athletic performance, frequent respiratory infections
Pregnant Teens	Increased rate of spontaneous abortion, fetal death, low birth weight
Parents	Increased respiratory infections among children of smokers, poor role model for children
New Smokers	Easier to stop now

Adapted from Glynn T, & Manley M. (1991). *How to help your patients stop smoking: A National Cancer Institute manual for physicians.* Bethesda, MD: National Institutes of Health.

D. **Assess** willingness to make a quit attempt
    1. Ask every patient if he/she is willing to make a quit attempt at this time (e.g., within the next 30 days)
    2. Based on patient response, select an appropriate intervention

SELECT AN INTERVENTION BASED ON PATIENT RESPONSE TO "ARE YOU WILLING TO QUIT AT THIS TIME"?
If the answer is "*Yes, in the next 30 days,*" go to V.E. through F. below
If the answer is "*Yes, but not now,*" go to V.G. below
If the answer is "*No,*" go to V.H. below

E. **Assist** patient who is willing to quit now through a combination of *counseling* and *pharmacotherapy*; each approach is effective by itself, but the two in combination achieve the highest success rates
    1. *Counseling*–Three types of counseling and behavioral therapies have been found to be especially effective and should be used with all patients who are attempting tobacco cessation
        a. Provision of practical counseling
        b. Provision of intratreatment social support (from clinician and staff)
        c. Help in securing extratreatment social support (from family/friends, community resources)

COUNSELING TO ASSIST PATIENT WITH A QUIT PLAN

Advise the smoker to
- ➡ Set a quit date, ideally within 2 weeks
- ➡ Inform friends and family of plans to quit, and ask for support
- ➡ Remove cigarettes from home and car
- ➡ Anticipate challenges, particularly during critical first few weeks, including nicotine withdrawal symptoms

Provide practical counseling (problem solving/skills training)
- ➡ Total abstinence is essential--not even a single puff
- ➡ Review previous quit attempts--what helped, what led to relapse
- ➡ Drinking alcohol is strongly associated with relapse and is also an illegal activity for persons <21 years of age
- ➡ Withdrawal typically peaks within 1-3 weeks after quitting
- ➡ Having other smokers in the household hinders successful quitting; patient should encourage family members to quit or at least not smoke in his/her presence

Provide intratreatment social support
- ➡ Provide a supportive clinical environment while encouraging patient in his/her quit plan
- ➡ "My office staff and I are available to assist you"
- ➡ Use the telephone to deliver cessation-counseling services, thereby establishing an office "quitline"

Help patient obtain extratreatment social support
- ➡ Assist patient in development of social support for his/her quit attempt in environment outside of treatment
- ➡ "Ask your family and friends to support you in your quit attempt"
- ➡ If there is a telephone quitline for smokers in the state, provide patient with contact information
- ➡ Refer adolescent to resources in the box below

Make culturally and age appropriate materials on cessation techniques readily available in your office
Such materials have little efficacy when used alone but may augment other interventions

Adapted from Fiore, M.C., Bailey, W.C., Cohen, S.J., Dorfman, S.F., Goldstein, M.G., Gritz, E.R., et al. (2000). Treating tobacco use and dependence. *Clinical practice guideline.* Rockville, MD: USDHHS, Public Health Service.

Community Resources for Smoking Cessation Programs

American Cancer Society (ACS) offers FRESHSTART, a straightforward, no-nonsense program that consists of four, 1-hour sessions held during a 2-week period
- • Works best for teens who prefer the structure and support of a group
- • Emphasizes quitting as a two-part process: stopping and staying stopped
- • Meetings focus on the following:
  - ✓ Individual needs of smokers
  - ✓ Information and strategy
  - ✓ Understanding smoking as a chemical addiction, habit, and psychological dependency
  - ✓ Stress management
  - ✓ Weight control
- • Also available on video and audiocassette for those unable to attend the sessions
- • Refer patients to ACS at 800-ACS-2345

American Lung Association (ALA) offers Freedom From Smoking
- • Within the Freedom From Smoking program, smokers can seek help in a group setting, individually with self-help materials (both written and audiotapes), and with materials that involve the entire family
- • Tobacco-Free Teens is available within the Freedom From Smoking program
- • Refer patients to ALA at 800-LUNG-USA

2. *Pharmacotherapy*–There are six products to assist patient with smoking cessation
    a. The FDA has approved six products for smoking cessation for persons ≥18 years: five nicotine-replacement products (transdermal patch, gum, lozenge, nasal spray, and vapor inhaler) and sustained-released bupropion
    b. Recent research suggests that pharmacotherapy can be useful and safe in adolescent tobacco users. However, pediatric and adolescent patients should be considered candidates for nicotine replacement therapy and for non-nicotine therapy **only** when there is clear evidence of nicotine dependence and a clear desire to quit, as use of these products in children under 18 years does not have FDA approval
    c. Suggestions for the clinical use of these products are contained in the tables that follow

SUGGESTIONS FOR THE CLINICAL USE OF NON-NICOTINE THERAPY

Patient Selection	Appropriate as a first-line pharmacotherapy for smoking cessation: FDA-approved for this indication in patients ≥18 years of age Behavioral/educational support is recommended with this therapy; should be especially considered in patients with a history of depression
Precautions	***Pregnancy:*** Pregnant smokers should first be encouraged to attempt cessation without pharmacologic treatment. Bupropion SR should be used during pregnancy only if the benefits outweigh the risks. Similar factors should be considered in lactating women ***Cardiovascular Diseases:*** Generally well tolerated; infrequent reports of hypertension ***Contraindications:*** Contraindicated in individuals with a history of seizure disorder, a history of an eating disorder, who are using another form of bupropion (Wellbutrin or Wellbutrin SR), or who have used an MAO inhibitor in the past 14 days

Product	Daily Dose	Duration	Comments	Advantages	Disadvantages	Common Side Effects
Sustained-release bupropion (Zyban or Wellbutrin SR)	150 mg every morning for 3 days then 150 mg twice daily (begin treatment 1-2 weeks prequit)	7-12 weeks maintenance up to 6 months	May be used with nicotine replacement. Do not crush, chew, or divide tablets. Stop smoking within 1-2 weeks of starting drug. Avoid bedtime dosing. Do not use with other forms of bupropion	Easy to use (pill), no exposure to nicotine	Increases risk of seizure (≤0.1%)	Insomnia, dry mouth, agitation

SUGGESTIONS FOR THE CLINICAL USE OF NICOTINE-REPLACEMENT THERAPY

Patient Selection	Appropriate as first-line pharmacotherapy for smoking cessation; FDA-approved for this indication in persons ≥18 years of age. Behavioral/educational support is recommended with this therapy
Precautions	***Pregnancy:*** Pregnant smokers should first be encouraged to attempt cessation without pharmacologic treatment. Nicotine-replacement therapy (NRT) should be used during pregnancy only if the benefits outweigh the risks. Similar factors should be considered in lactating women ***Cardiovascular Diseases:*** NRT is not an independent risk factor for acute myocardial events. NRT should be used with caution among particular cardiovascular patient groups: those within the immediate (within 2 weeks) postmyocardial infarction period, those with serious arrhythmias, and those with serious or worsening angina pectoris

Product	Daily Dose	Duration	Comments	Advantages	Disadvantages	Common Side Effects
Transdermal patch 24 hr (e.g., Nicoderm CQ)	21 mg/24 hrs* 14 mg/24 hrs 7 mg/24 hrs	4 weeks 2 weeks 2 weeks	Apply to clean, dry, nonhairy site on trunk or upper outer arm. Rotate sites. Remove after 16-24 hours	Provides steady level of nicotine; easy to use; unobtrusive; available without prescription	User cannot adjust dose if craving occurs; nicotine released more slowly than in other products	Local skin irritation, insomnia
16 hr (e.g., Nicotrol)	15-mg patch worn for 16 hrs	8 weeks	Apply to clean, dry, nonhairy site on hip or upper outer arm. Remove at bedtime. Rotate sites. Not for use in light smokers.			
Nicotine polacrilex gum (Nicorette)** 2 mg (<25 cig/day) 4 mg (≥25 cig/day)	1 piece/hr (<24 pieces/day)	Up to 12 weeks	• Proper chewing technique needed to avoid side effects and achieve efficacy** • Instruct to chew gum on a fixed schedule (at least 1 piece/1-2 hrs) for 1-3 months may be more beneficial than *ad lib* use • Use 4 mg strength for highly nicotine-dependent patients, or if failed with 2 mg	User controls dose; oral substitute for cigarettes; available without prescription	User cannot eat or drink while chewing the gum; can damage dental work; difficult for denture wearers to use	Mouth irritation, sore jaw, dyspepsia, hiccups

(Continued)

Product	Daily Dose	Duration	Comments	Advantages	Disadvantages	Common Side Effects
Nicotine polacrilex lozenge (Commit) 2 mg (if first cigarette smoked ≥30 min after waking) 4 mg (if first cigarette smoked ≤30 min after waking)	One lozenge every 1-2 hours (at least 9/day) for 6 weeks, then every 2-4 hours for 3 weeks, then stop (maximum dose is 20 lozenges/day)	12 weeks	Dissolve over 20-30 min; minimize swallowing	User controls dose; oral substitute for cigarettes; available without prescription Avoids sore jaw and dental work damage associated with gum	Cannot eat or drink for 15 minutes before and during use	Mouth and throat irritation
Vapor inhaler (Nicotrol Inhaler)	6-16 cartridges/ day (delivered dose, 4 mg/ cartridge)	3-6 months	20 minutes of active puffing releases 4 mg of nicotine (about 2 mg absorbed, equivalent to about 2 cigarettes)	User controls dose; hand-to-mouth substitute for cigarettes	Frequent puffing needed; device visible when used	Mouth and throat irritation; cough
Nasal spray (Nicotrol NS)	1-2 doses/hr (1 mg total; 0.5 mg in each nostril) (maximum 40 mg/day)	3-6 months	Do not sniff, swallow, or inhale spray. Nasal vasoconstrictors may delay absorption	Most irritating nicotine-replacement product to use; device visible when used	User controls dose; offers most rapid delivery and highest nicotine levels of all NRTs	Nasal irritation; sneezing, cough, teary eyes

* The starting dose is 21 mg/day unless the smoker weighs less than 45.5 kg (100 lb) or smokes fewer than 10 cigarettes per day, in which case the starting dose is 14 mg/day. The starting dose should be maintained for 4 weeks, after which the dose should be decreased every week until it is stopped

** Gum should be slowly chewed until a "peppery" taste emerges, then "parked" between cheek and gum to facilitate nicotine absorption. Gum should be intermittently "chewed and parked" for about 30 minutes. Acidic beverages (e.g., coffee, juices, soft drinks) interfere with the buccal absorption of nicotine, so eating and drinking anything except water should be avoided for 30 minutes before and during chewing

Adapted from Fiore, M.C., Bailey, W.C., Cohen, S.J., Dorfman, S.F., Goldstein, M.G., Gritz, E.R., et al. (2000). Treating tobacco use and dependence. *Clinical practice guideline.* Rockville, MD: USDHHS, Public Health Service.

F. Follow up for patients who are attempting to quit at this time is outlined in the box below

---

Schedule follow-up contact either in person or by telephone (be proactive in your approach)
➡ Timing
   ✓ First follow-up contact within 2 weeks of quit date, preferably during first week
   ✓ Second contact within the first month
   ✓ Schedule further follow-up contacts as needed
➡ Actions during follow-up visits
   ✓ Congratulate success
   ✓ If a relapse occurred, obtain recommitment to abstinence
   ✓ Remind patient that relapse can be used as learning experience
   ✓ Identify problems encountered and anticipate challenges in the immediate future
   ✓ Assess pharmacotherapy use and problems

Preventing relapse
➡ Congratulate, encourage, and stress importance of abstinence at every opportunity
➡ Review benefits derived from cessation
➡ Inquire about problems encountered and offer possible solutions
➡ Anticipate problems or threats to maintaining abstinence
➡ Help patient identify sources of support
➡ Emphasize that beginning to smoke (even a puff) will increase urges and make quitting more difficult
➡ Assess pharmacotherapy use and problems
➡ Referral for intensive tobacco dependence interventions (such as FRESHSTART or Freedom From Smoking [described under V.E. above]) should be considered for all tobacco users willing to participate in them
   ✓ Should not be limited to any subpopulation of tobacco users (e.g., heavily dependent smokers)
   ✓ May be used in addition to the brief strategies to help patients that are clinician provided
   ✓ Effective when provided by trained counselors and includes repeated contacts over a period of at least 4 weeks
   ✓ Either individual or group counseling may be used; telephone counseling is also effective

G.   Brief clinical intervention for smokers who are willing to quit but at a later date (smokers who answer, "Yes, but not now," when asked "Are you willing to quit at this time?") are contained in the following table

BRIEF CLINICAL INTERVENTIONS FOR PATIENTS WHO ARE WILLING TO QUIT SMOKING, BUT NOT AT THIS TIME

• **Identify and address barriers to quitting in a nonjudgmental, supportive way**
   ✓ Nicotine dependence
   ✓ Fear of failure
   ✓ Lack of social support
   ✓ Lack of confidence
   ✓ Concern about weight gain
   ✓ Concurrent depression
▪ **Identify reasons to quit smoking**
   ✓ Health-related
   ✓ Economic
   ✓ Health of household members
▪ **Follow up with patient at the next visit**

Adapted from Rigotti, N.A. (2002). Treatment of tobacco use and dependence. *New England Journal of Medicine, 346*, 508

H.   Brief clinical intervention for smokers who are not willing to quit smoking (Smokers who answer, "No," when asked "Are you willing to quit at this time?")
   1.   Motivation is enhanced via use of the "5 Rs"-- *R*elevance, *R*isks, *R*ewards, *R*oadblocks, and *R*epetition
   2.   See the table that follows for strategies to use with this intervention

BRIEF CLINICAL INTERVENTIONS FOR PATIENTS WHO ARE NOT WILLING TO QUIT	
Why patient may be unwilling to quit: Misinformation, concern about the effects of quitting and demoralization from previous unsuccessful quit attempts	
Use of a motivational intervention: Use the "5R's," *Relevance, Risk, Rewards, Roadblocks*, and *Repetition*	
Relevance: Encourage patient to tell you why quitting would be personally relevant to him/her	▪ Relevant to disease status or risk, family, social situation, school, etc. ▪ Ask to be as specific as possible
Risks: Ask the patient to identify potential negative consequences of tobacco use	▪ Acute risks: SOB, worsening of asthma, harm to pregnancy, impotence ▪ Long-term risks: Heart attacks and strokes, lung and other cancers, COPD ▪ Environmental risks: Exposure of family members and friends to environmental tobacco smoke (ETS)
Rewards: Ask the patient to identify potential benefits of stopping tobacco use (clinician may suggest and highlight those that seem most relevant to patient)	▪ Improved health ▪ Food will taste better ▪ Improved sense of smell ▪ Save money ▪ Feel better about self/feel better physically ▪ Can stop worrying about quitting ▪ Set a good example for others in the family ▪ Perform better in physical activities ▪ Reduced wrinkling/aging of skin
Roadblocks: Ask the patient to identify barriers to quitting and note elements of treatment (problem-solving, pharmacotherapy) that could address barriers. Typical barriers might include:	▪ Withdrawal symptoms ▪ Fear of failure ▪ Weight gain ▪ Lack of support ▪ Depression ▪ Enjoyment of tobacco
Repetition: Motivational intervention should be repeated every time an unmotivated patient visits the clinical setting; teens who have failed in previous attempts to quit should be reminded that most people make repeated attempts before they successfully quit	• Clinicians are most likely to use repetition when there is an office-wide system in place to identify all tobacco users at every visit • Without such a system, repeating the message to stop smoking is not likely to consistently occur

Adapted from Fiore, M.C., Bailer, W.C., Cohen, S.J., et al. (2000). Treating tobacco use and dependence. *Clinical practice guideline.* Rockville, MD: USDHHS. Public Health Service.

➡ Recommend starting or increasing physical activity

➡ Discourage "dieting"; instead, emphasize the importance of a healthy diet

➡ Reassure patient that some weight gain after quitting is common; usually limited to 10 pounds

➡ Encourage patient to tackle one problem at a time; quitting smoking should be the focus now

➡ Don't minimize patient's concern about weight gain; be empathetic, but help patient to re-focus

➡ Maintain the patient on pharmacotherapy known to delay weight gain (e.g., bupropion SR, NRTs, particularly nicotine gum)

➡ Refer patient to a specialist or program such as FRESHSTART or Freedom From Smoking

I. Follow-Up
    1. For patients willing to quit at this time: See V.F. above
    2. For patients willing to quit, but not at this time: See V.G. above
    3. For patients who are not willing to quit: See V.H. above

UNDERNUTRITION AND FAILURE TO THRIVE

I. Definition: Inadequate physical growth, or the inability to maintain the expected rate of growth over time in a young child

II. Pathogenesis

    A. Immediate cause of failure to thrive is inadequate nutrition; ultimate cause is often difficult to determine

    B. Organic causes include the following:
        1. Inadequate caloric intake due to such conditions as cleft palate, inability to suck and swallow or masticate
        2. Food assimilation defect due to conditions such as cystic fibrosis, celiac disease
        3. Loss of ingested calories such as occurs in chronic diarrhea, vomiting, or gastroesophageal reflux
        4. Increased energy requirements due to conditions such as chronic infection, heart disease, or renal disease
        5. Prenatal causes including intrauterine infection, maternal malnutrition, exposure to alcohol, drugs, or cigarettes during prenatal period

    C. Nonorganic causes include the following:
        1. Underfeeding the child due to improper mixing of formula (overdilution) or parental misconceptions about nutritional needs of the child; parent unintentionally fails to feed child enough to support growth
        2. Economic and psychosocial factors, as well as child neglect and abuse, also result in failure to thrive

    D. Approximately 50% of cases of FTT admitted to tertiary care centers and almost all cases managed in primary care settings have nonorganic etiologies

III. Clinical Presentation

    A. There is a wide range of variation in the growth rate of infants and children
        1. Growth occurs in spurts, even in healthy children
        2. Problems with measurement precision and high variability in individual growth rates over short periods complicate the interpretation of growth velocity data

    B. Diagnostic criteria for failure to thrive are based on weight and stature for age using National Center for Health Statistics (NCHS) growth charts from the Centers for Disease Control and Prevention (2000) (available online at http://www.cdc.gov.growthcharts); children with weight less than 80% of ideal (median) for age are considered to meet the criteria

C. Failure to thrive is a common problem usually identified during the first three years of life with approximately **80% of cases in children less than 18 months of age**

D. Children whose slowed velocity of weight gain results in "crossing percentiles" (for example, dropping from 50th to 15th percentile for weight) may also be considered in the failure to thrive category. This is especially true after the child reaches 18-24 months of age, when changes in growth velocity are rarely physiologic

E. Whereas weight is the major criterion, in more severe cases, linear growth and head circumference may be affected over time

F. In early infancy, feeding difficulties are the predominant cause, including lactation failure, inadequate feeding frequency or volume, and formula-mixing errors

G. Condition is seen in all socioeconomic levels, but incidence is particularly high among families living in poverty as growth failure and malnutrition are inextricably linked

H. Children with failure to thrive are at increased risk for developmental and behavioral problems in addition to growth problems

IV. Diagnosis/Evaluation

A. History
1. Obtain a detailed perinatal history including prenatal exposures to tobacco, alcohol and other drugs, gestational age, weight, length, and head circumference at birth
2. Obtain detailed weight history including somatic measurements at every age since birth (obtain records from other agencies as needed)
3. Inquire about illnesses since birth, including vomiting, diarrhea, and the child's energy level
4. In order to determine if the child is receiving adequate calories, take a comprehensive feeding history, including type of formula/food, amount fed in 24 hour period, frequency of feeding, exactly how the formula is mixed (have patient bring in a can of the formula she uses), who feeds the child at each feeding, if the bottle is propped, and if there are any problems with sucking, swallowing, or regurgitation. **Important**: Caution should be used when interpreting a dietary history as parental guilt may lead to inaccuracies in reporting
5. In breast-fed infants, determine if there are any problems with milk supply, sore nipples, inadequate let-down reflex; ask mother about any ingestion of substances (alcohol, medications) that might affect the milk supply
6. Assess the development of the child to determine if age-appropriate
7. Determine if there is a family history of short stature or growth-retarding illnesses such as cystic fibrosis or malabsorption syndromes
8. Obtain a psychosocial history to determine family composition and functioning; look for strengths as well as risk factors

B. Physical Examination
1. Measure blood pressure to screen for acute or chronic renal disease
2. Carefully measure and plot weight (unclothed and using a balance-beam scale), length (recumbent under 2 years, standing height over age 2), and head circumference (even in children >2 years). Plot weight-for-length. (Children with genetic short stature will have concordant weight and length)
3. Relate measurements to previous measurements to see pattern of growth; note if pattern of growth has been steady or if growth slowed at a specific point in time
4. Examine child for dysmorphic features, hypotonia, murmur, protuberant abdomen (associated with celiac disease, malabsorption, or cystic fibrosis), defects in soft and hard palate
5. Perform a neurologic examination, including an oral motor evaluation (suck, gag, and swallow reflexes), test cranial nerves, deep tendon reflexes, muscle strength, and passive and active muscle tone
6. Look for signs of abuse and neglect during the exam; infants experiencing environmental deprivation manifest behaviors such as minimal smiling, decreased vocalization, resistance to being held, self-stimulating rhythmic behaviors, and "frozen watchfulness"
7. Perform a developmental screening using one of the parent report instruments recommended in section on CHILD HEALTH SUPERVISION
8. If child still on breast/bottle feeding, observe mother feeding child (**Note: This is very important!**); observe for gagging, choking, refusal to feed, or unusual parent-infant interactions

C. Differential Diagnosis
1. Failure to thrive may be the result of a number of both organic and inorganic causes listed under Pathogenesis, above
2. Because birth weight and length are influenced to a greater degree by maternal size and intrauterine influences than by genetic factors, there are increases or decreases in growth velocity during the first 2 years of life to adjust for maternal factors and for genetic potential to be achieved. Therefore, some children experience a decrease in growth rate (a shift in height or weight of more than 25 percentile points) during the first 2 years of life. This may represent a physiologic adjustment, rather than true failure to thrive; in most of these cases, the growth rate does stabilize and follows a predictable pattern

D. Diagnostic Tests
1. Basic laboratory tests include a complete blood count, urinalysis, serum electrolytes, and perhaps an erythrocyte sedimentation rate; if even mild GI symptoms are present, a stool culture, pH, reducing substances test, and stool for occult blood are also indicated
2. History, physical examination, and observation are the most important aspects of the diagnostic evaluation

V. Plan/Management

A. Important to keep in mind that advocacy of the child must be maintained without becoming an adversary of the parents

B. Development and maintenance of an alliance with the family is of paramount importance

C. If no underlying organic disease is uncovered in H&P and diagnostic tests, and the cause appears to be inadequate caloric intake, the treatment plan outlined below is reasonable
1. Refer immediately to nutritionist (WIC if eligible) for counseling on feeding techniques and high calorie diet; refer all breastfeeding mothers to a certified lactation consultant
2. Caloric intake higher than normal is required for child to experience growth recovery (**Example:** Infants under one year have nutritional requirements, on average, of 100 kcal/kg of body weight per day; a caloric intake of 150 kcal/kg/day may be needed in order to "catch up")
3. Have parent keep a detailed diary of feedings, and the frequency, volume, and consistency of stools and vomitus
4. Most children with calorie-deprivation failure to thrive respond to intensive feeding efforts by the caregiver by gaining weight in just a few days (expect infants less than 6 months of age, a period of rapid growth, to respond by gaining weight in just 2-3 days)
5. If child fails to exhibit catch up growth within 7-10 days, (in infants <6 months, within 5 days) hospitalization is necessary as nutrition is crucial for brain development during the first two years of life

D. Follow Up
1. In 1-2 weeks for growth check and response to plan
2. Then every 2-4 weeks until growth recovery is steadily progressing

REFERENCES

American Academy of Pediatrics, Committee on Substance Abuse. (2001). Tobacco's toll: Implications for the pediatrician. *Pediatrics, 107,* 794-798.

American Academy of Pediatrics, Committee on Substance Abuse. (2001). Alcohol use and abuse: A pediatric concern. *Pediatrics, 108,* 185-189.

American Academy of Pediatrics. (2000). Clinical practice guideline: Diagnosis and evaluation of the school-aged child with attention-deficit/hyperactivity disorder. *Pediatrics, 105,* 1158-1170.

American Academy of Pediatrics. (2001). Clinical practice guideline: Treatment of the school-aged child with attention-deficit/hyperactivity disorder. *Pediatrics, 108,* 1033-1044.

American Academy of Pediatrics. (2001). Tobacco's toll: Implications for the pediatrician. *Pediatrics, 107,* 794-798.

American Academy of Pediatrics. (2001). Alcohol use and abuse: A pediatric concern. *Pediatrics, 108,* 185-189.

American Gastroenterological Association, Clinical Practice Committee. (2002). AGA technical review on obesity. *Gastroenterology, 123,* 882-932.

American Psychiatric Association. (2000*). Diagnostic and statistical manual of mental disorders,* (4th ed.), Text Revision. Washington, DC. Author.

American Psychiatric Association. (2000). Practice guideline for the treatment of patients with eating disorders (revision). *American Journal of Psychiatry, 157*(Suppl. 1), 1-39.

Anderson, S.E., Dallal, G.E., & Must, A. (2003). Relative weight and race influence average age at menarche: Results from two nationally representative surveys of US girls studied 25 years apart. *Pediatrics, 111,* 844-850.

Barlow, S.E., & Dietz. (1998). Obesity evaluation and treatment: Expert committee recommendations. Retrieved May 1, 2002, from http://www.pediatrics.org/cgi/content/full/102/3/e29

Barlow, S.E., Dietz, W.H., Klish, W.J., & Trowbridge, F.L. (2002). Medical evaluation of overweight children and adolescents: Reports from pediatricians, pediatric nurse practitioners, and registered dietitians. *Pediatrics, 110,* 222-228.

Barnes, H.N., & Samet, J.H. (1997). Brief interventions with substance abusing patients. *Medical Clinics of North America, 81,* 867-880.

Bobo, J.K. (2002). Tobacco use, problem drinking, and alcoholism. *Clinical Obstetrics and Gynecology, 45,* 1169-1180.

Brower, K.J., & Steverin, J.D. (1997). Alcohol and other drug-related problems. In D.J. Knesper, N.B. Riba, & T.L. Schwenk (Eds.), *Primary care psychiatry.* Philadelphia: Saunders.

Bush, B., Shaw, S., Cleary, P., Delbanco, T.L., & Aronson, M.D. (1987). Screening for alcohol abuse using the CAGE questionnaire. *American Journal of Medicine, 82,* 231-235.

Centers for Disease Control and Prevention. (2002). Trends in cigarette smoking among high school students—United States, 1991-2001. *Morbidity and Mortality Weekly Report, 51,* 409-412.

Centers for Disease Control and Prevention. (2002). Childhood growth charts. *Pediatrics, 110,* 141-142.

Cohen, M.W. (2001). Enuresis. In R.A. Hoekelman (Ed.), *Primary pediatric care* (pp. 833-837). Philadelphia: Mosby.

Davison, K.K., Susman, E.J., & Birch, LL. (2003). Percent body fat at age 5 predicts earlier pubertal development among girls at age 9. *Pediatrics, 111,* 815-821.

Devlin, M.J. (2001). Binge-eating disorder and obesity. *Psychiatric Clinics of North America, 24,* 325-335.

Elia, J., Ambrosini, P.J., & Rapoport, J.H. (1999). Treatment of attention-deficit/hyperactivity disorder. *New England Journal of Medicine, 340,* 780-789.

Enoch, M., & Goldman, D. (2002). Problem drinking and alcoholism: Diagnosis and treatment. *American Family Physician, 65,* 441-449.

Fiore, M.C., Bailey, W.C., Cohen, S.J., Dorfman, S.F., Goldstein, M.G., Gritz, E.R., et al. (2000*). Treating tobacco use and dependence.* Clinical Practice Guideline. Rockville, MD: US Department of Health and Human Services.

Fontaine, K.R., Redden, D.T., Wang, C., Westfall, A.O., & Allison, D.B. (2003). Years of life lost due to obesity. *JAMA, 289,* 187-193.

Fried, E., & Nestle, M. (2002). The growing political movement against soft drinks in schools. *JAMA, 288,* 2181-2182.

Gahagain, S., & Holmes, R. (1998). A stepwise approach to evaluation of undernutrition and failure to thrive. *Pediatric Clinics of North America, 45,* 169-188.

Gimpel, G.A., Warzak, W.J., Kurh, B.R., & Walburn, J.N. (1998). Clinical perspectives in primary nocturnal enuresis. *Clinical Pediatrics, 37,* 23-30.

Green, M., Wong, M., Atkins, D., Taylor, J., & Feinleib, M. (1999). *Diagnosis of attention-deficit/hyperactivity disorder.* Technical Review No. 3. AHCPR Publication No. 99-0050. Rockville, MD: Agency for Health Care Policy and Research.

Iglowstein, I., Jenni, O.G., Molinari, L., & Largo, R.H. (2003). Sleep duration from infancy to adolescence: Reference values and generational trends. *Pediatrics, 111,* 302-307.

Ikeda, J.P., & Mitchell, R.A. (2001). Dietary approaches to the treatment of the overweight pediatric patient. *Pediatric Clinics of North America, 48,* 955-968.

Jadad, A.R., Boyle, M., Cunningham, C., Kim, M., & Schachar, R. (1999). Treatment of attention-deficit/hyperactivity disorder. Evidence Report/Technology Assessment No. 11. AHRQ Publication No. 00-E005. Rockville, MD: Agency for Healthcare Research and Quality.

Manson, J.F., & Bassuk, S.S. (2003). Obesity in the United States: A fresh look at its high toll. *JAMA, 289,* 229-230.

Maynard, L.M., Wisemandle, W., Roche, A.F., Chumlea, W.C., Guo, S.S., & Siervogel, R.M. (2001). Childhood body composition in relation to body mass index. *Pediatrics, 107*, 344-350.

Miller, K.J., & Wender, E.H. (2001). Attention-deficit/hyperactivity disorder. In R.A. Hoekelman (Ed.), *Primary pediatric care* (pp. 756-766). Philadelphia: Mosby.

Modan-Moses, D., Yaroslavsky, A., Novikov, I., Segev, S., Tolendano, A., Materany, E., & Stein, D. (2003). Stunting of growth as a major feature of anorexia nervosa in male adolescents. *Pediatrics, 111*, 270-276.

Mokdad, A.H., Ford, E.S., Bowman, B.A., Dietz, W.H., Vinicor, F., Bales, V.S., & Marks, J.S. (2003). Prevalence of obesity, diabetes, and obesity-related health risk factors, 2001. *JAMA, 289*, 76-79.

Mustillo, S., Worthman, C., Erkanli, A., Keeler, G., Angold, A., & Costello, E.J. (2003). Obesity and psychiatric disorder: Developmental trajectories. *Pediatrics, 111*, 851-859.

National Institutes of Health; National Heart, Lung, and Blood Institute; & North American Association for the Study of Obesity. (2000). *The practical guide: Identification, evaluation, and treatment of overweight and obesity in adults.* Bethesda, MD: Author.

O'Connor, P.G. & Schottenfeld, R.S. (1998). Patients with alcohol problems. *New England of Medicine, 338,* 592-602.

Pereira, M.A., & Ludwig, D.S. (2001). Dietary fiber and body-weight regulation. *Pediatric Clinics of North America, 48*(4), 969-981.

Powers, P.S., & Santana, C.A. (2002). Eating disorders: a guide for the primary care physician. *Primary Care Clinics in Office Practice, 29,* 81-99.

Racine, A.D. (2001). Failure to thrive. In R.A. Hoekelman (Ed.), *Primary pediatric care* (pp. 1072-1079). Philadelphia: Mosby

Rigorn, N.A. (2002). Treatment of tobacco use and dependence. *New England Journal of Medicine, 346,* 506-513.

Rocchini, A.P. (2002). Childhood obesity and a diabetes epidemic. *New England Journal of Medicine, 346*, 854-855.

Rosen, D.S., & Demitrack, M.A. (1997). Eating disorders and disordered eating. In D.J. Knesper, N.B. Riba, & T.L. Schwenk (Eds.), *Primary care psychiatry.* Philadelphia: Saunders.

Schmitt, B.D. (2001). Encopresis. In R.A. Hoekelman (Ed.), *Primary pediatric care* (pp. 828-833). Philadelphia: Mosby

Southern, M.S. (2001). Exercise as a modality in the treatment of childhood obesity. *Pediatric Clinics of North America, 48,* 995-1014.

Stettler, N., Zemel, B.S., Kumanyika, S., & Stallings, V.A. (2002). Infant weight gain and childhood overweight status in a multicenter cohort study. *Pediatrics, 109,* 194-131.

Story, M.H., & Sofka, D. (Eds.) (2002*). Bright futures in practice: Nutrition* (2nd ed.). Arlington, VA: National Center in Maternal and Child Health.

Strauss, R.S. (2002). Childhood obesity. *Pediatric Clinics of North America, 49,* 175-195.

Strauss, R.S., & Pollock, H.A. (2001). Epidemic increase in childhood overweight, 1986-1998. *JAMA, 286*, 2845-2848.

Styne, D.M. (2001). Childhood and adolescent obesity: Prevalence and significance. *Pediatric Clinics of North America, 48*(4), 823-849.

Szymanski, M.L., & Zolotor, A. (2001). Attention-deficit/hyperactivity disorder: Management. *American Family Physician, 64,* 1355-1362.

Tobacco Use and Dependence Clinical Practice Guideline Panel. (2000). A clinical practice guideline for treating tobacco use and dependence. *Journal of the American Medical Association, 283,* 3244-3255.

Treasure, J., & Serpell, L. (2001). Osteoporosis in young people: Research and treatment in eating disorders. *Psychiatric Clinics of North America, 24,* 359-367.

Weissbluth, M. (1999). Sleep disturbances in young children. In R.A. Dershewitz (Ed.), *Ambulatory pediatric care* (pp. 813-819). Philadelphia: Lippincott-Raven.

Whitaker, R.C. (2002). Understanding the complex journey to obesity in early adulthood. *Annals of Internal Medicine, 136,* 923-925.

Yanovski, S.Z., & Yanovski, J.A. (2002). Obesity. *New England Journal of Medicine, 346,* 591-602.

Zhu, S., Anderson, C.M., Tedeschi, G.J., Rosbrook, B., Johnson, C.D., Byrd, M., et al. (2002). Evidence of real-world effectiveness of a telephone quitline for smokers. *New England Journal of Medicine, 347,* 1087-1093.

4 Mental Health

TISH SMYER & MARY VIRGINIA GRAHAM

Depression

Domestic Violence: Child Abuse and Neglect

Grief

DEPRESSION

I. Definition: Unipolar mood disorders characterized by physical and psychological symptoms that cause significant distress and impairment in functioning and occur in the absence of elevated mood (mania or hypomania)

II. Pathogenesis

  A. Theories related to a biologic etiology of depression include the following:
    1. Biogenic amine hypothesis: Occurs as result of depletion of levels of serotonin
    2. Receptor suprasensitivity hypothesis: Results from suprasensitive catecholamine receptors in response to decreased levels of catecholamine in brain
    3. Genetic predisposition plays a role in etiology as well as treatment. There is some evidence that patients will respond to an antidepressant medication that has been successful in a first-degree relative.

  B. Theories related to a psychosocial etiology of depression include the following:
    1. Psychoanalytic: Mourning of symbolic object loss with rigid superego that leads one to experience feelings of worthlessness
    2. Cognitive: Cognitive triad of (a) automatic negative thoughts and negative self-view, (b) negative interpretation of experience and pessimistic view of the world, and (c) negative view of future

III. Clinical Presentation

  A. Unipolar depressive disorders are psychiatric disorders with specific diagnostic categories and criteria as set forth by the American Psychiatric Association in the *Diagnostic and statistical manual of mental disorders (4th edition), Text Revision (DSM-IV)* (2000)
    1. Using *DSM-IV* nomenclature, the three unipolar depressive disorders are major depression, dysthymic disorder, and minor depression (**Note:** Minor depression is the most common form of a diagnostic category called "depressive disorder, not otherwise specified," a category that includes several disorders)
      a. Major depression is the most severe form of unipolar depression and consists of history of one or more major depressive episodes
      b. Dysthymic disorder is a milder and chronic form of depression
      c. Minor depression is characterized by fewer than five symptoms of major depression
    2. Diagnostic criteria for each of the three disorders are summarized in the following tables

---

DIAGNOSTIC CRITERIA FOR MAJOR DEPRESSION

At least five of the following symptoms (one of which **must** be either [1] depressed mood or [2] loss of interest or pleasure) are present nearly every day during the same 2-week period

  ✓ Depressed mood (can be irritable mood in children/adolescents)
  ✓ Loss of interest or pleasure in most activities
  ✓ Significant weight loss/gain or decreased/increased appetite
  ✓ Insomnia or hypersomnia
  ✓ Psychomotor agitation or retardation
  ✓ Loss of energy or fatigue
  ✓ Feelings of worthlessness or excessive/inappropriate guilt
  ✓ Diminished ability to think/concentrate or indecisiveness
  ✓ Recurrent thoughts of suicide or death
  ✓ Symptoms cause clinically significant distress or impairment in social, occupational or other important areas of functioning

DIAGNOSTIC CRITERIA FOR DYSTHYMIC DISORDER

Depressed mood (can be irritable mood in children/adolescents present for at least **one year**) for most of the day, for more days than not, for at least 2 years

During periods of depressed mood, at least two of the following additional symptoms are present:

- Appetite disturbance
- Insomnia or hyposomnia
- Low energy or fatigue
- Low self-esteem
- Poor concentration or difficulty making decisions
- Feelings of hopelessness

DIAGNOSTIC CRITERIA FOR MINOR DEPRESSION

- Presence of fewer than five symptoms of major depression
- Duration of symptoms (must include either depressed mood or loss of interest or pleasure in most activities) at least 2 weeks
- Disturbance does not occur exclusively during course of psychotic disorders

Previous three tables adapted from American Psychiatric Association. (2000). *Diagnostic and statistical manual of mental disorders* (4th ed.) Text revision. Washington, DC: Author.

B. According to the World Health Organization (WHO), by the year 2020, childhood neuropsychiatric disorders will rise proportionally by 50%, internationally, to become one of the five most common causes of morbidity, mortality, and disability among children and adolescents
1. A number of epidemiological studies have reported that up to 2.5% of children and up to 8.3% of adolescents in the US suffer from depression
2. In childhood, boys and girls appear to be at equal risk for depressive disorders, but during adolescence, girls are twice as likely to develop depression
3. Research indicates that depression onset is occurring earlier in life today than in past decades; early-onset depression often persists, recurs, and continues into adulthood

C. Depressive disorders adversely affect mood, energy, interest, sleep, appetite and overall functioning
1. In contrast to the normal emotional experiences of sadness, feelings of loss, or passing mood states, symptoms of depression are extreme and persistent and can have a significant impact on a child's ability to function at home, in school, and with peers
2. Depressive disorders are associated with an increased risk of suicidal behavior

D. **Major depression** affects approximately 2% of children and between 4% and 8% of adolescents in adolescents, peak age of onset is 14-15 years and 16-17 years
1. Children who develop major depression are more likely to have a family history of the disorder; although adolescents with depression are also likely to have a family history of depression, the correlation is not as high as it is for children
2. Syndrome is often under-recognized and under-treated; thus, many children and adolescents continue to suffer the negative psychological consequences of persistent depression for many years
3. See DIAGNOSTIC CRITERIA table above for clinical presentation description

E. **Dysthymic disorder** frequently begins in childhood or early adolescence
1. Symptomatically is less severe than major depression, but much more persistent with a duration criterion of one year
2. See DIAGNOSTIC CRITERIA table above for clinical presentation description

F. **Minor depression** is a diagnostic category for children and adolescents who have too few depressive symptoms to qualify for a diagnosis of major depression, as well as duration too brief to fit into the dysthymic disorder category
1. Associated with high use of health services; should be considered in the differential diagnosis in patients presenting with chronic unexplained headaches, stomachaches, and other vague complaints featuring symptom complexes that fail to fit into any pattern, and with an unpredictable and disappointing response to all therapeutic interventions
2. See DIAGNOSTIC CRITERIA table above for clinical presentation description

G. Children and adolescents who present with depressive symptoms in primary care settings may not meet the rigid diagnostic criteria for the above disorders
   1. Whereas the core symptoms for the disorders are the same for children and adults, the prominence of the symptoms may change depending on the developmental stage of the child, and the expression of symptoms may also differ based on age—a major influence on cognitive and emotional maturity
   2. The following list of behaviors may more accurately reflect depression in children and adolescents

> ✓ Withdrawal from friends and from participation in activities
> ✓ Outbursts of shouting, complaining, unexplained irritability, or crying
> ✓ Alcohol or substance use
> ✓ Social isolation, poor communication, difficulty with relationships
> ✓ Persistent boredom, difficulty concentrating
> ✓ Extreme sensitivity to rejection or failure
> ✓ Persistent boredom, difficulty concentrating, or decline in the quality of schoolwork
> ✓ Frequent vague, nonspecific physical complaints, such as stomachaches, headaches, or fatigue
> ✓ Intolerance of praise and reward
> ✓ Frequent absences from school or poor performance in school
> ✓ Talk of or efforts to run away from home

H. Depression in children and adolescents is associated with an increased risk of suicidal behaviors; facts about suicide in children and adolescents are contained in the table below

FACTS ABOUT SUICIDE IN CHILDREN AND ADOLESCENTS

- Suicide is the third leading cause of death among adolescents ages 15-24, and accounts for 13% of the mortality in this age group; it is the fourth leading cause of death among 10-14 year olds
- Since 1950, the suicide rate in 15- to 19-year-olds has more than tripled; in recent years an increase has been recorded for 10- to 14-year-olds
- The suicide rate among black males, once much lower than that among white males, has increased dramatically in recent years and is now about 80% of that of whites; young native Americans have a very high suicide rate, especially those who live in tribes characterized by family disorganization and alcoholism
- The completed suicide rate is much higher among males, whereas the attempt rate is much higher among females; this may be related to males having higher rates of aggressive and antisocial behavior
- Among children and adolescents, the rate of attempted and completed suicide increases greatly with age—although prepubertal children consider suicide, their cognitive immaturity often limites their ability to successfully plan and carry out the act
- In general, suicide in adolescents younger than 16 years of age is more difficult to predict because it arises less often within the context of chronic and severe psychopathology, tends to be more impulsive than suicide in older adolescents, and appears to be greatly influenced by the presence of firearms in the home
- Adolescent suicide risk is especially high after the suicide of a friend, classmate, or acquaintance; after a suicide has been reported in the media; and after a popular television show or film glamorizes suicide (called "contagion effect")
- In the US, the most common methods of suicide in order by decreasing frequency are firearms, hanging, jumping, asphyxiation by carbon monoxide, and self-poisoning; in contrast, self-poisoning is the most common method of suicide attempt, followed by wrist cutting
- About 30% of suicide victims show a very strong wish to die, as evidenced by a great deal of planning such as use of an irreversible method, timing the suicide so as not to be discovered, leaving a note, and verbalizing intent prior to the act. On the other hand, approximately 60% of adolescents who attempt suicide actually **do not** wish to die; instead, they act impulsively with the motivation of gaining attention, communicating their love or anger, or to escape a difficult or painful situation

I. There are several tools that are useful for screening children and adolescents for possible depression

IV. Diagnosis/Evaluation

A. History: (Child/adolescent should be seen initially with the parent(s) present and then interviewed alone, with the parent's permission; some clinicians suggest that patient be asked to complete a preliminary depression screening questionnaire prior to the interview in order to guide the process)

1. Determine the presenting symptoms from both the child and parent, and ask about onset, duration, and description of symptoms. Ask about symptoms that characteristically occur by referring to tables above that contain diagnostic criteria for major depression, dysthymic disorder, and minor depression (or if a brief screening instrument for depression has been completed by the patient prior to being seen, use the responses to guide the history taking)

2. Determine if these symptoms are new or if they have been present for some time (or have occurred before but remitted)

3. Ask if anything makes the symptoms go away. If yes, ask what, and ask how long the remissions usually last (i.e., how long do the symptoms *stay* away?)

4. Ask about the impact of these symptoms on the major areas of functioning for the child—family, school, peer relationships, and community

---

Family: Tell me how are things going with your family. Tell me how you get along with your family. Do you talk to your mom or dad about how you are feeling? How much time each week do you spend doing things with your family (e.g., eating meals, watching TV, going to movies, playing board or computer games)? How often do you get in shouting matches, name-calling with family members (siblings or parents)? Do you ever think about running away from home?

School: How are things going at school? How is school attendance? Are you able to turn in your assignments on time? What were your grades during the last grading period? Tell me how you get along with your teachers. Have you been suspended from school during the past 6 months for any reason?

Peer Relationships: How are things going with your friends? How often do you do things with your friends? How do you and your friends spend your time together? (Adolescents) Do you have a girlfriend/boyfriend? How are things going with the relationship?

Community: What kinds of things do you do for fun? Do you have any hobbies? Do you play competitive sports? Do you go to the Y or other places in the community to participate in activities? Have you ever been in trouble with the law? Do you belong to any clubs or youth groups? Do you belong to a gang?

---

5. Ask about presence of identifiable stressors using these categories:

Major discrete stressors: Ask about losses (e.g., death in family, death of family pet, break-up with girlfriend/boyfriend, divorce of parents) over the past months

Chronic stressors: Ask about presence of marital discord between parents, on-going chronic illness of family member, or any other situation that is a source of long-term stress in the family

Minor daily stressors: Ask if demands in school, in organized sports are worrisome to the child (does child feel pushed beyond his/her capabilities?)

---

6. Always consider the possibility of abuse and ask appropriate questions (see section on DOMESTIC VIOLENCE: CHILD ABUSE AND NEGLECT for more information)

7. Ask if there are problems sleeping. If yes, inquire about bedtime, nighttime awakening, waking of parents, having bad dreams, nap taking, and so on

8. Ask child if he/she is tired a lot, if takes naps after school, if puts head on desk and falls asleep during school

9. Ask about alcohol and substance use
10. Obtain past medical history and medication history
11. Ask about suicidal thinking, impulses, and personal history of suicide attempts; a suggested format is contained in the table below

---

SUICIDE RISK ASSESSMENT

Initial and follow-up screening evaluations must include very specific questions
- Approach with a declaration such as: "It sounds as if you are having a really hard time."
- Then ask, "Do you ever think of hurting yourself or taking your own life?"
- If the answer is "Yes," ask, "When you have such thoughts, are you able to put them out of your mind, or do you find yourself dwelling on them?"
- Regardless of the answer, ask, "Do you feel that you might act on these thoughts?" or "Do you have a plan?"

Patients who have suicidal thoughts must be referred for emergency psychiatric evaluation

---

B. Physical Examination: Should be directed toward ruling out an infectious, neoplastic, metabolic, or neurologic disorder that might account for symptoms

C. Differential Diagnosis
1. Bipolar disorder
2. Psychotic disorders, particularly schizophrenia
3. Bereavement
4. Substance abuse
5. Conduct disorder
6. Anxiety disorder
7. Medical conditions such as thyroid dysfunction, other endocrine disorders, neurological problems, as well as medications that treat those disorders

D. Diagnostic Tests
1. Use of a screening test for depression in children/adolescents can be very helpful (see III.I. above)
2. All positive screening tests should trigger full diagnostic interviews with a pediatric mental health specialist
3. Consider the following screening tests based on history/physical examination findings to rule out an organic cause or substance use: CBC, sedimentation rate, VDRL, chemistry profile, thyroid profile, and drug screen

V. Plan/Management

A. Suicidal ideation warrants *emergent* psychiatric evaluation and close supervision of the child until that evaluation can be accessed

B. Children who are clearly in distress (but are not suicidal) or who, based on history (including responses to depression screening instrument, if used) have difficulty functioning in the main spheres of home, school, peer relationships, or community, require *urgent* referral for a more thorough diagnostic psychiatric evaluation

C. Given the challenging nature of depression in children and adolescents, referral to a child psychiatrist or psychologist for further evaluation, diagnosis, and treatment is necessary when depression is suspected based on initial findings in the primary care setting
1. Depressive disorders in children are often overlooked and undertreated; thus it is crucial that appropriate referral is made when these patients present in primary care settings
2. Primary care clinicians should not feel obligated to treat any psychiatric disorder or target psychiatric symptom beyond their level of comfort
3. The scientific literature on treatment of children and adolescents with depression is far less extensive than that relating to adults; in the last 4 or 5 years, however, a number of studies have confirmed the short-term efficacy and safety of treatments for depression in youth, but longer trials are needed to determine which treatments work best

D. Depression in children and adolescents is often the product of multiple forces that have shaped expression of the disorder, and because comorbidity is not unusual, the treatment plan is rarely one dimensional; instead, the treatment plan usually recommends multiple modalities for intervention in efforts to address biologic issues, psychological issues, and social, family, and educational concerns (obviously, what may be realistic in terms of family and community resources must also be considered)

E.   The stigma of mental illness and the fears of parents that they are responsible for their child's problems either through biologic inheritance or their failure as parents may be a barrier to accepting a referral for psychiatric evaluation of their child

F.   Based on the efficacy of psychotherapy, and also because of the potential adverse effects of psychotropic medications, a form of psychotherapy is often the first line of treatment for children and adolescents with mild to moderate depression

G.   The major types of psychotherapy are briefly described in the tables below

COGNITIVE-BEHAVIORAL THERAPY (CBT)	
Central Concept	**Therapeutic Techniques**
Based on the premise that persons with depression have cognitive distortions in their views of themselves, the world, and the future	✓ Therapist provides specific "homework" assignments to be completed by patient ✓ Purpose of the assignments is to enable patient to accumulate information and experience that challenge his/her often erroneous negative cognitive sets ✓ Rather than simply attempting to develop new thought patterns, patients also learn to respond to familiar triggers with different actions (e.g., the patient who usually isolates himself in his room when he feels sad, responds to sad feelings by getting out of the house and going for a walk instead) ✓ Over time, and with practice, patient gains new skills, enhanced confidence, and broadens his/her social circle ✓ Other techniques are the teaching of relaxation techniques and slow-breathing so that these become conditioned responses to cues
Comments: CBT is the most studied type of talk therapy; rates of remission with the use of CBT tend to be highest in patients with the mildest forms of depression	
Usually administered in 20 weekly sessions and requires a high degree of collaboration between the patient and therapist (children may be too young to benefit from this type of therapy)	

INTERPERSONAL PSYCHOTHERAPY FOR ADOLESCENTS (IPT-A)		
Central Concept	**Therapeutic Techniques**	**Comments**
Depression can be considered within the context of a patient's interpersonal relationships based on the assumption that depression can both result from and contribute to difficulties in these relationships Initially developed for use in adults, IPT has been modified for the treatment of adolescents	✓ Four main problems areas—grief, interpersonal disputes, role transitions, and interpersonal deficits—are considered in therapy (if appropriate, an additional problem area, living in a single-parent family may also be considered) ✓ The adolescent and therapist select one or two areas to be the major focus for the main portion of therapy	Use of IPT-A warrants further study; however research to date indicates that this therapy results in decreases in depression and improvement in social functioning in depressed adolescents Attrition rates from IPT-A therapy appear to be low, making it an attractive treatment option since adherence is a recurrent problem in the treatment of mental disorders A standard treatment course is 12 weekly sessions and often involves the adolescent's family in therapy

SYSTEMIC BEHAVIORAL FAMILY THERAPY (SBFT)		
Central Concept	**Therapeutic Techniques**	**Comments**
Underlying assumption is that difficulties in family relationships and poor communication among family members contributes to the depression of one family member	✓ Family works with therapist to identify areas for improvements in relationships and to develop strategies for bringing about positive changes in family dynamics	A standard treatment course is 12 weekly sessions and the entire family stands to benefit using this therapeutic approach

H. Medication as a first-line treatment should be considered for children and adolescents with severe symptoms that would prevent effective psychotherapy, those who are unable to undergo psychotherapy, those with psychosis, and those with chronic or recurrent episodes
1. The selective serotonin reuptake inhibitors (SRRIs) appear to be the safest of the antidepressants for children and adolescents. The FDA recommends that paroxetine (Paxil) not be used to treat depression in adolescents or children, but warns against discontinuing the drug too quickly if the medication has been prescribed prior to this recommendation
2. Baseline laboratory tests are not routinely required before beginning SSRI therapy in medically healthy children
3. The long-term safety of SSRIs, especially their effects on personality development and behavior in children, is unknown
4. Wide use of SSRIs (in adults) has been associated with declines in suicide rates, not increases

I. Currently, the National Institutes of Mental Health has a large-scale, controlled clinical trial at 10 sites across the US to compare the long-term effectiveness of fluoxetine, CBT, and the combination of these interventions for treatment of depression in adolescents. More information about this trial, called the Treatment of Adolescent with Depression Study (TADS) can be found through the following web site: http://www.nimh.nih.gov/studies/index.cfm

---

INFORMATION RESOURCES FOR CLINICIANS

National Institute of Mental Health
Office of Communications
Information Resources Inquiries Branch
6001 Executive Blvd., Room 8184, MSC 9663
301-443-4513
Mental Health FAX 4U: 301-443-5158
E-mail: Nimhinfo@nih.gov
NIMH home page: www.nimh.nih.gov

American Psychological Association
750 First Street, NE
Washington, DC 20002
202-336-5500
www.apa.org

Child & Adolescent Bipolar Foundation
1187 Willmette Avenue, PMG #331
Willmette, IL 60091
847-256-8525
www.pgkids.org

Depression & Bipolar Support Alliance (DBSA)
730 N. Franklin Street, #501
Chicago, IL 60610-7224
312-988-1150
FAX: 312-642-7243
www.DBSAlliance.org

National Alliance for the Mentally Ill (NAMI)
Colonial Place Three
2107 Wilson Blvd., Suite 300
Arlington, VA 22201
800-950-NAMI (6264) or 703-524-7600
www.nami.org

National Mental Health Association (NMHA)
2001 N. Beauregard Street, 12th Floor
Alexandria, VA 22311
800-969-6942 or 703-684-7722
www.nmha.org

National Institutes of Health
National Library of Medicine's clinical trials database
www.clinicaltrials.gov

American Academy of Child and Adolescent Psychiatry
3625 Wisconsin Avenue, NW
Washington, DC 20016
202-966-7300
www.aacap.org

American Psychiatric Association
1400 K Street, NW
Washington, DC 20005
202-682-6000
www.psych.org

J. Follow-up: Should be by the pediatric mental health specialist to whom the patient and family were referred

DOMESTIC VIOLENCE: CHILD ABUSE AND NEGLECT

I. Definition: Any physical or mental nonaccidental injury to a child; any failure to provide a child with adequate food, clothing, shelter, supervision, and care

II. Pathogenesis

    A. There is no single set of factors that produce neglectful and abusive parents

    B. There appear to be some common themes in parental behavior that is abusive and neglectful; these are listed here:
        1. Often, parent was victim of abuse him/herself
        2. Increased family stress is correlated with abuse in many cases
        3. Low income is associated with increased rates of neglect and abuse
        4. Some psychiatric conditions in parents are related to abuse and neglect
        5. **Alcohol and drug abuse are associated with high rates of neglect and abuse** (almost half of cases involve substance abuse)
        6. Characteristics of the child such as male gender, being fussy as an infant, being slow to develop, and being handicapped increase rates of abuse and neglect

III. Clinical Presentation

    A. There were 903,000 victims of maltreatment that were substantiated by child protective services agencies in 1998 and there were 1100 deaths due to neglect and abuse in the US

    B. Surveys of adults indicate that approximately 30% of girls and 20% of boys are sexually assaulted by the age of 18 years. The majority do not have diagnostic physical findings on exam, thus history becomes very important

    C. An estimated 1.3 to 1.5 million cases of child neglect are reported each year

    D. Physical indicators of abuse:
        1. Retinal hemorrhages (shaken baby syndrome), unexplained fractures, burns, bruises, welts, bald spots, human bite marks
        2. Bruises or bleeding in external genitalia
        3. Vague complaints such as abdominal pain and sleep disturbances

    E. Behavioral indicators of abuse:
        1. Withdrawn, clothing worn is inappropriate to season and may be worn to cover injuries; history of being a runaway
        2. Role reversal (overly concerned for siblings); sudden school difficulties, habit disorders (sucking, rocking), peer problems, isolation
        3. Sexual display/acting out, excessive or public masturbation, promiscuity

    F. Physical indicators of neglect:
        1. Abandonment, inappropriate dress, poor hygiene, unattended medical needs
        2. Undernutrition or failure to thrive

    G. Behavioral indicators of neglect:
        1. Often tardy or absent from school; school dropout (adolescent)
        2. Listless, withdrawn, substance abuse

IV. Diagnosis/Evaluation

    A. History
        1. Obtain social history including information about parents, care takers, family functioning
        2. Screening for abuse and neglect should be part of every health supervision visit

> → Parents should be asked routine questions about current family stressors, discipline, child behavior, and home safety
> → Children should be asked open-ended questions about their own safety such as the following:
>   • "Are you afraid of anyone?"
>   • "Does anyone ever hurt you?"
>   • "Does anyone make you keep secrets?"
> → Children older than 10 should be interviewed in private, without the parent present
> → All positive responses are followed up with more specific questions including:
>   • "What happened?"
>   • "When did it happen?"
>   • "Who did that?"

3. If physical injury is present, ask detailed questions including "When did it happen?", "How did it happen?", and "Who did it?"
    a. Long interval between injury and seeking help is red flag
    b. Story that is inconsistent, contradictory, or fails to adequately explain injury is a red flag
    c. Important to keep in mind that many injuries are accidental
4. Important to get history in child's own words, using child's vocabulary, and if appropriate, using an anatomically correct doll to help clarify what the child is describing
5. If behavioral problems are evident, ask appropriate questions to determine etiology
6. Question about child's past or present medical or behavioral problems in the following areas:
    a. Difficulties with pregnancy, labor, delivery, or neonatal period
    b. Feeding difficulties or problems with toilet training
    c. Behavioral problems, especially of recent onset
    d. Previous trauma, ingestions, or frequent visits for vague complaints
    e. Enuresis or encopresis
7. History should be carefully recorded as it may be part of court case; stories that change over time are suggestive of abuse -- thus statements made as part of the initial disclosure take on added significance

B. Physical Examination
    1. Measure height and weight; record on growth chart, comparing it to norms and the child's own growth curve (undernutrition may be a sign of neglect)
    2. Observe child's behavior during exam for fearfulness, listlessness, and withdrawn behavior
    3. Inspect skin for hygiene, burns, bruises, bites, and lacerations
        a. Use measuring tape and record on anatomic diagrams on chart
        b. Injuries from accidental trauma generally occur on extensor surfaces; trauma to other areas deserves more evaluation
    4. Examine head, focusing on any patchy hair loss, Battle's sign (bruising over mastoid process behind ears) raccoon eyes, and blood behind the tympanic membranes
    5. Observe eyes for retinal hemorrhages
    6. Examine abdomen for signs of injury. **Note:** Cutaneous signs of abdominal injury are rare. Blunt trauma to abdomen can cause serious injury difficult to detect with physical exam alone
    7. Examine genitalia for injury. **Note:** The majority of children who have been sexually abused have no detectable genital injury
    8. If child <6 years of age, consider developmental screening (see Child Health Supervision section)

C. Differential Diagnosis
    1. Unintended injury
    2. Poverty resulting in poor clothing/hygiene

D. Diagnostic Tests
    1. History and physical exam dictate tests
    2. Sexual abuse requires meticulous collection of laboratory and forensic evidence, and its description is beyond the scope of this book. (Consult your state health department or social service agency for requirements in your state)

V. Plan/Management

A. Goal of management in cases of suspected abuse and neglect is protection of the child from further harm, identification of risks and how these might be dealt with, and compliance with legal reporting requirements

B. In cases where severe injury or serious threat of further abuse is present, child must be removed from the situation and immediate legal intervention must be sought

C. In most cases of suspected abuse or neglect, child can be left in the care of the parent/guardian while an investigation takes place
  1. All states require that healthcare providers (as well as teachers and child care providers) report suspected cases of abuse and neglect
  2. Suspicion, not certainty, of child abuse and neglect is what mandates reporting
  3. Immunity from liability is provided for all reports made in good faith, even if the abuse is not confirmed through investigation
  4. The National Child Abuse Hot-Line number is 800-422-4453 or go online to http://www.childhelpusa.org/child/hotline.htm. This hotline can be used by anyone needing more information about reporting mechanisms and requirements
  5. State reporting requirements can be accessed at http://endabuse.org/statereport/list.php3
  6. Additional family violence resources are listed in the following table:

NATIONAL FAMILY VIOLENCE RESOURCES
➤ National Domestic Violence Hot Line: 800-799-SAFE (TDD hearing impaired: 800-787-3224) or online at http://www.ndvh.org
➤ National Resource Center on Domestic Violence: 800-537-2238 or online at: http://www.pcadv.org
➤ Department of Justice Response Center: 800-421-6770 or online at: http://www.ojp.usdoj.gov/ovc/publications/infores/firstrep/welcome.html
➤ Centers for Disease Control and Prevention (domestic violence information) http://www.cdc.gov/ncipc/dvp/fivpt/spotlite/home.htm
➤ Family Violence and Sexual Assault Institute: 858-623-2777 or online at: http://www.fvsai.org
➤ National Center for Assault Prevention: 908-369-8972 or online at: http://www.ncap.org/aboutncap.htm
➤ National Coalition Against Domestic Violence: 303-839-1852 or online at: http://www.ncadv.org/
➤ National Council on Child Abuse and Family Violence: 202-429-6695 or online at: http://www.americancampaign.org/programs.htm
➤ Family Violence Prevention Fund (http://www.fvpf.org); national agency that focuses on prevention at all levels - primary, secondary, and tertiary
➤ Domestic Violence: A Practical Approach for Clinicians: http://www.sfms.org/domestic.html
➤ Stop Abuse for Everyone (SAFE): http://www.safe4all.org/

D. Explain to parent that you are required by law to report your concerns to the state's child protection agency; many states also require that healthcare providers file a written report within a specified time period (see C.5. above for state reporting requirements' website)

E. Once the report has been made, the child protection agency is responsible for investigating the case
  1. The goals of child protective services are to keep the child safe and to identify solutions to problems that jeopardize child safety
  2. If possible, the family unit is preserved and the child is removed from the family as a last resort

F. Documentation is critical in all cases of suspected abuse and neglect; when possible, consult with an expert in child abuse and neglect

G. Follow Up: Primary care clinicians have a responsibility to follow up closely on all cases of abuse and neglect involving children

GRIEF

I. Definition: A variable but normal response to loss, deprivation, injury, illness, or disenfranchisement

II. Pathogenesis

A. A full depressive syndrome that is a normal reaction to loss

B. Persons with uncomplicated bereavement regard the feeling of depressed mood as normal and transitory

III. Clinical Presentation

A. Feelings of depression and associated symptoms of poor appetite, weight loss, and insomnia following loss are usually present

B. Feelings of guilt, if present, are usually related to things done or not done at time of death by the survivor (if the loss is via death)

C. Approximately 80% of persons are markedly improved in 10 weeks after the loss

D. Morbid preoccupation with feelings of worthlessness and prolonged functional impairment indicate abnormal grieving and the development of major depression

E. By age 18, approximately 4% of US children will experience death of a parent, one of the most stressful life events

F. Children usually show affective, cognitive, and behavioral symptoms during the first year of bereavement

G. Children under age 6 who have lost a parent are likely to have difficulty with separation from the surviving parent, to be very fearful and to demonstrate increased dependency needs; those older than 6 experience symptoms of anger, aggression, depression, and problems with discipline

IV. Diagnosis/Evaluation

A. History
1. Determine when loss occurred, how child is accepting and coping with loss
2. Prior experience with child/family is crucial in making an assessment of adjustment
3. Ask about functional status (if able to carry out usual activities)
4. Ask about presence of support system
5. Determine if child is able to mourn
6. Determine if child is experiencing despair to the level of self-harm

B. Physical Examination: Not indicated

C. Differential Diagnosis: Major depression

D. Diagnostic Tests: None indicated

V. Plan/Management

A. Differentiating between children/families who are experiencing a normal grief process and those who exhibit significant pathology requiring referral to a mental health provider is an important first step in management
1. Continued preoccupation with feelings of worthlessness, marked functional impairment that is prolonged, and significant psychomotor retardation suggest a major depressive episode
2. Bereavement that is unduly severe or prolonged indicates the need for management by a mental health provider

B. Interventions for acute grief
1. Encourage child to mourn, and to express grief in ways that are consistent with his/her age and particular personality (children, like adults, mourn differently). Message to child should be "You have the right to mourn"
2. Children typically need frequent, brief discussions of the loss rather than a few long discussions (advise parents regarding this); brief, episodic discussion over a period of months may be important to the child
3. Spontaneously occurring discussions, when the child seems to want to talk, are much more helpful than "planned talks" by the parent
4. Encourage family and small group of people who knew deceased to talk about him/her in presence of the grieving child
5. Parents should not lie to child, but should use the term "death" when appropriate
   a. By age 4-5, child can understand a brief explanation about how the deceased person died (child should not be told the deceased is "asleep")
   b. Child's questions should be answered at that time and later as they arise
   c. Children should attend and be involved in funeral activities

6. Emphasize that grief is normal, and the goal is not to get rid of it as quickly as possible
7. Recognize that your presence is the most important comfort you have to offer. Avoid the pressure to provide your own philosophy of death and loss or to talk about your own losses). Don't worry about what to say; being present and listening are what the patient needs, not your advice. Message should be "I care"
8. Accept child's grief for loss that conventional society may not acknowledge as very important (such as loss of pet)
9. Recognize that providers are not equally capable of intervening effectively in situations of acute loss

C. Return to routines: Children do much better if their normal routine is re-established quickly; thus, they should return to normal routines as soon as is practical (no more than 2 weeks between death and return to school and other activities)

D. Physical exercise: Recommend daily exercise which can be very beneficial in dealing with depression

E. Support groups: Some children and families benefit from sharing with a group; others do not; prior knowledge about family functioning should guide referral

F. Child or family with significant preexistent psychopathology cannot be expected to adjust in the same way as healthy persons and should be referred for counseling

G. Children's books relating to death and grieving which may be helpful to children are in the table below:

CHILDREN'S BOOKS RELATING TO DEATH AND GRIEVING	
Author	Book
Blackburn, Lynn	Timothy Duck
Buchanan-Smith, Doris	A Taste of Blackberries
Carrick, Carol	The Accident
Conley, B.H.	Butterflies, Grandpa and Me
Fassler, Joan	My Grandpa Died Today
Viorst, Judith	The Tenth Good Thing About Barney
Walker, Alice	To Hell With Dying*

* In this very special book, the Pulitzer Prize-winning author relates the experiences of a young girl and her brother with the death of a cherished neighbor, Mr. Sweet. The book is beautifully written and illustrated, but the title may be offensive to some parents

H. Follow-up: Frequently by telephone/mail over the period of acute grief during the first few weeks' can offer checkup during the first 9 months, depending on mourner's wishes or needs. Beware of delayed grief reaction. These reactions may occur close to anniversary of a death (anniversary reaction)

REFERENCES

Abramowicz, M. (2003). Are SSRIs safe for children? *The Medical Letter, 45*, 53-54.

American Psychiatric Association. (2000). *Diagnostic and statistical manual of mental disorders* (4th ed.). Text Revision. Author.

Asarnow, J.R., Jaycox, L.H., & Anderson, M. (2002). Depression among youth in primary care: Models for delivering mental health services. *Child and Adolescent Psychiatric Clinics of North American, 11*, 477-497.

Ascherman, L.I., Dowben, J., & Velosa, J.F. (2002). Psychiatric disorders in children and adolescents. In F.D. Burg, J.R. Ingelfinger R.A. Polin, & A.A. Gershon (Eds.) *Kagan's current pediatric therapy* (pp. 366-370). Philadelphia: Saunders.

Birmaher, B., Brent, D.A., & Benson, R.S. for the American Academy of Child and Adolescent Psychiatry (1998). Summary of the practice parameters for the assessment and treatment of children and adolescents with depressive disorders. *Journal of the American Academy of Child and Adolescent Psychiatry, 37*, 1234-1238.

Brent, D.A. (2001). Mood disorders in children and adolescents. In R.A. Hoekelman (Ed.), *Pediatric primary care* (pp. 922-926). St. Louis: Mosby.

Brown, J., Cohen, P., & Johnson, J.G. (1999). Childhood abuse and neglect: Specificity of effects on adolescent and young adult depression and suicidality. *Journal of the American Academy of Child and Adolescent Psychiatry, 38,* 1490-1496.

Casarett, D., Kutner, J.S., & Abrahms, J. (2001). Life after death: A practical approach to grief and bereavement. *Annals of Internal Medicine, 124,* 208-215.

Chaney, S.E. (2000). Child abuse: Clinical findings and management. *Journal of the American Academy of Nurse Practitioners, 12,* 467-471.

Eyler, A.E., Cohen, M., & Kershaw, M.O. (1997). Domestic violence and abuse. In D.J. Knesper, M.B. Riba, & T.L. Schwenk, (Eds.). *Primary care psychiatry.* Philadelphia: Saunders.

Fawcett, J. (2000). Predictors of early suicide: Identification and appropriate interventions. *Journal of Clinical Psychiatry, 49,* 7-8.

Houry, D., Sachs, C.J., Feldhaus, K.M., & Linden, J. (2002). Violence inflicted injuries: Reporting laws in 50 states. *Annals of Emergency Medicine, 39,* 56-60.

Jayson, D., Wood, A., & Kroll, L. (1998). Which depressed patients respond to cognitive-behavioral treatment? *Journal of the American Academy of Child and Adolescent Psychiatry, 37,* 35-39.

Kaplan, H.I., & Sadock, B.J. (2000). *Synopsis of psychiatry* (8th Ed.). Philadelphia: Williams & Wilkins.

Klein, D.N., Schwartz, & Rose, S. (2000). Five-year course and outcome of dysthymic disorder: A prospective, naturalistic follow-up study. *American Journal of Psychiatry, 157,* 931-939.

Krug, E.G., Kresnow, M., & Peddicord, J.P. (1998). Suicide after natural disasters. *New England Journal of Medicine, 228,* 273-378.

Lahoti, S.L., McClain, R.N, Girardet, R., McNeese, M., & Cheung, K. (2001). Evaluating the child for sexual abuse. *American Family Physician, 63,* 883-895.

Lewisohn, P.M., Rohde, P., & Seeley, J.F. (1999). Life events and depression in adolescence: Relationship loss as a prospective risk factor for first onset of major depressive disorder. *Journal of Abnormal Psychology, 108,* 606-614.

Margolis, S., & Swartz, K. (2001). Depression and anxiety. *The Johns Hopkins White Papers.* New York: Medletter Associates.

McCormack, S., Pine, D., & Mufson, L. (2002). Depression in children and adolescents. In F.D. Burg, J.R. Ingelfinger R.A. Polin, & A.A. Gershon (Eds.) *Kagan's current pediatric therapy* (pp. 362-366). Philadelphia: Saunders.

Neufeld, B. (1996). SAFE questions: Overcoming barriers to the detection of domestic violence. *American Family Physician, 53,* 2575-2580.

Reinecke, M.A., Ryan, N.E., & DuBois, D.L. (1998). Cognitive-behavioral therapy of depression and depressive symptoms during adolescence: A review and meta-analysis. *Journal of the American Academy of Child and Adolescent Psychiatry, 37,* 26-34.

Rosenbaum, J.F., & Fava, M. (1998). Approach to the patient with depression. In T.A. Stern, J.B. Herman, & P.L. Slavin (Eds.). *The MGH guide to psychiatry in primary care.* New York: McGraw-Hill.

Sahler, OJ. (2000). The child and death. *Pediatric Review, 21,* 350-353.

Schaffer, D., & Craft, L. (1999). Methods of adolescent suicide prevention. *Journal of Clinical Psychiatry, 60*(Suppl 2), 70-76.

Schneider, R.K., & Levenson, J.L. (2002). Update in psychiatry. *Annals of Internal Medicine, 136,* 293-301.

Trimm, R.F. (2002). The child and the death of a loved one. In F.D. Burg, J.R. Ingelfinger R.A. Polin, & A.A. Gershon (Eds.) *Kagan's current pediatric therapy* (pp. 362-366). Philadelphia: Saunders.

US Preventive Services Task Force. (2001). Screening for depression. Recommendations and rationale. *Annals of Internal Medicine, 136,* 760-764

Weisman, A. (1998). The patient with acute grief. In T.A. Stern, J.B. Herman, & P.L. Slavin (Eds.). *The MGH guide to psychiatry in primary care.* New York: McGraw-Hill.

Weissman, M. M., Wolk, S., & Goldstein, R.B. (1999). Depressed adolescents grown up. *Journal of the American Medical Association, 281,* 1701-1713.

Whooley, M.A., & Simon, G.E. (2000). Managing depression in medical outpatients. *New England Journal of Medicine, 343,* 1942-1950.

Metabolic and Endocrine Problems

CONSTANCE R. UPHOLD

DIABETES MELLITUS

I.   Definition: Group of metabolic diseases characterized by hyperglycemia from defects in insulin secretion, insulin action, or both

II.   Pathogenesis and etiologic classification of diabetes mellitus (DM)

    A.   Type 1 (formerly known as insulin-dependent [IDDM or juvenile-onset diabetes]: Due to β-cell destruction which usually results in absolute insulin deficiency

    B.   Type 2 (formerly known as non-insulin dependent type [NIDDM or adult-onset diabetes]): A complex metabolic disorder characterized by resistance to the action of insulin and a relative or predominant impairment of insulin secretion

    C.   Other specific types of diabetes
        1.   Genetic defects in β-cell function and insulin action
        2.   Genetic defects in insulin action (type A insulin resistance, leprechaunism, lipoatrophic diabetes)
        3.   Diseases of the exocrine pancreas (pancreatitis, trauma, infection, cancer)
        4.   Endocrinopathies such as acromegaly, Cushing's syndrome, pheochromocytoma
        5.   Drug or chemical-induced diabetes (steroids, thiazide diuretics, phenytoin, nicotinic acid, thyroid hormones, α-interferon)
        6.   Infections such as congenital rubella or cytomegalovirus
        7.   Immune-mediated diabetes ("stiff man" syndrome and anti-insulin receptor antibodies)
        8.   Other genetic disorders such as Down's, Klinefelter's, and Turner's syndromes

    D.   Gestational diabetes mellitus (GDM): Glucose intolerance with onset during pregnancy (will not be discussed further in this section)

    E.   Impaired glucose tolerance (IGT) or impaired fasting glucose (IFG)
        1.   Plasma glucose levels are higher than normal but are not diagnostic of diabetes mellitus
        2.   Intermediate stage between glucose homeostasis and diabetes
        3.   Insulin resistance syndrome or metabolic syndrome is associated with IGT and is a state in which insulin-sensitive tissues have a reduced sensitivity to effects of insulin on glucose uptake

III. Clinical Presentation

    A.   Criteria for diagnosing diabetes mellitus in children and adolescents (see following table)

DIAGNOSTIC CRITERIA FOR DIABETES MELLITUS*

- Symptoms of diabetes (polydipsia, polyuria, and weight loss) plus casual plasma glucose concentration ≥200 mg/dl (11.1 mmol/L); "casual" is any time of day without regard to time since last meal

        OR

- Fasting plasma glucose (FPG) ≥126 mg/dl (7.0 mmol/L); "fasting" is no caloric intake for at least 8 hours

        OR

- 2 hour plasma glucose ≥200 mg/dl during an oral glucose tolerance test (OGTT); OGTT should be performed using a glucose load containing the equivalent of 75-g anhydrous glucose (in children, use 1.75 g/kg to maximum of 75 g glucose load)

---

*These criteria should be confirmed by repeat testing on a different day, except in the case of unequivocal hyperglycemia with acute metabolic decompensation

Adapted from American Diabetes Association. (2003). Report of the Expert Committee on the diagnosis and classification of diabetes mellitus. *Diabetes Care, 26(*Suppl. 1), S5-S20

    B.   Criteria for diagnosing impaired fasting glucose (IFG) or IGT: FBG ≥110 mg/dl (6.1 mmol/L) and <126 mg/dl (7.0 mmol/L) or 2-hour glucose ≥140 mg/dl (7.8 mmol/L) and <200 mg/dl (11.1 mmol/L)

    C.   Type 1 diabetes in children and adolescents
        1.   Second most common chronic disease in children, following asthma
        2.   Most common type that occurs in childhood
        3.   About three-quarters of all newly diagnosed cases occur in persons <18 years of age

4. Most children have the classic symptoms that appear within a short time period: Polydipsia, polyphagia, polyuria, weight loss, blurred vision, and frequent infections, such as dermatologic fungal infections

5. Children may also have fatigue, weakness, and listlessness; however, in some, failure to grow may be the only sign

6. After the initial presentation of symptoms, the newly diagnosed patient often undergoes a "honeymoon" period or remission phase that may last from several months to 2 years

7. Children have more infections and sick days than adults which complicates their care

8. Certain clinical manifestations vary by age of child
   a. Morbidity and mortality are greatest in infants; infants who have persistent vomiting and lethargy are at high risk of rapid progression to dehydration
   b. Nocturnal enuresis may occur in a previously toilet-trained child; an infant may need his/her diaper changed constantly
   c. Prior to age 6 or 7, children lack the cognitive capacity to recognize hypoglycemic symptoms

9. Unlike adults, ketoacidosis may be the first manifestation of diabetes in children and adolescents

10. Type 1 diabetic children are at risk for retinopathy and microalbuminuria

D. Type 2 diabetes in children and adolescents
   1. Epidemiology
      a. Occurs mainly in adults >30 years, but the incidence is increasing in children and adolescents
      b. Children from high risk ethnic groups are more frequently affected (Native American, African American, Latino, Asian American, Pacific Islander)
      c. Almost always found in children after the onset of puberty
         (1) Normal physiology of puberty helps explain this increased occurrence during puberty
         (2) At onset of puberty there is an increase in insulin resistance that returns to normal insulin sensitivity at the end of puberty
   2. Risk factors
      a. Obesity is the hallmark in children as it is in adults
      b. Most children have a family history
      c. Diabetic gestation; increased prevalence in children whose mothers had diabetes during pregnancy
      d. Children who were underweight or overweight for gestational age are at increased risk
   3. Symptoms
      a. Most children do not have classic symptoms of hyperglycemia
      b. Many children are asymptomatic, however, fatigue may be a problem
      c. Acanthosis nigricans is present in 90% of children; characterized by velvety, hyperpigmented patches that are most prominent in intertriginous areas
      d. In females, polycystic ovarian syndrome (PCOS), a reproductive disorder, is common; characterized by hyperandrogenism and chronic anovulation
      e. In females, recurrent vaginal candidiasis is often present
   4. It is difficult to classify the type of diabetes in pubertal children and thus diagnosis of diabetes type may be inaccurate
      a. Post pubertal children who are obese usually have type 2 diabetes, but this is not always the case
      b. Type 2 diabetics do not usually have autoantibodies
      c. Insulin and C-peptide levels are usually higher at diagnosis in patients with type 2 diabetes
   5. Hypertension and dyslipidemia may occur
   6. Hyperosmolar hyperglycemic nonketotic coma (see III.E.2.) and ketoacidosis (see III.E.1.) may occur
   7. Although the long-term complications are relatively unknown, children are probably at risk in adulthood for coronary heart disease, stroke, and peripheral vascular disease

E. Diabetic ketoacidosis (DKA) and hyperosmolar hyperglycemic state (HHS) (See table that follows for diagnostic criteria)
   1. Ketoacidosis can occur in children who have both type 1 and type 2 diabetes
      a. Because some insulin is present in children with type 2 diabetes, the condition is less prevalent in type 2 diabetics
      b. Symptoms include nausea, vomiting, abdominal pain, dehydration, Kussmaul respirations, fruity or acetone odor to breath, and impaired consciousness
   2. Hyperosmolar hyperglycemic state (HHS) is predominant in type 2 diabetes
      a. Characterized by blood glucose >600 mg/dL, minimal ketosis, serum osmolality >320 mosmol/L, and profound dehydration
      b. Often precipitated by hyperglycemic-inducing drugs (steroids, diuretics), therapeutic procedures (surgery, dialysis, hyperalimentation), chronic disease, and acute stress

DIAGNOSTIC CRITERIA FOR DKA AND HHS

	DKA			HHS
	Mild	Moderate	Severe	
Plasma glucose (mg/dL)	>250	>250	>250	>600
Arterial pH	7.25-7.30	7.00-7.24	<7.00	>7.30
Serum bicarbonate (mEq/L)	15-18	10 to <15	<10	>15
Urine ketones*	Positive	Positive	Positive	Small
Serum ketones*	Positive	Positive	Positive	Small
Effective serum osmolality (mOsm/kg)**	Variable	Variable	Variable	>320
Anion gap†	>10	>12	>12	Variable
Alteration in sensorial or mental obtundation	Alert	Alert/drowsy	Stupor/coma	Stupor/coma

* Nitroprusside reaction method
** Calculation: 2[measured Na (mEq/L)] + glucose (mg/dL)/18
† Calculation: $(Na^+) - (Cl^- + HCO_3^-)$ (mEq/L).

Source: American Diabetes Association. (2003). Hyperglycemia crisis in patients with diabetes mellitus. *Diabetes Care, 26*(Suppl), S109-S117.

F. Impaired glucose tolerance (IGT) or insulin resistance syndrome
1. IGT is associated with insulin resistance syndrome, which is also known as the metabolic syndrome (syndrome X)
2. Syndrome with its related components—hyperinsulinemia, obesity, hypertension, and hyperlipidemia—is a major precursor to cardiovascular disease
3. Prevalence in children is unknown; recent study found that 9%of children with obesity seeking medical attention had IGT
4. Puberty increases the extent of insulin resistance; the pubertal transition from Tanner stage 1 to Tanner stage III was associated with a 32% reduction in insulin sensitivity and an increase in fasting glucose in a recent study
5. Patients are asymptomatic but are at risk for developing coronary heart disease and diabetes

G. Macrovascular and microvascular complications occur in type 1 and type 2 diabetes of sufficient duration; retinopathy and microalbuminuria are two complications that can occur in adolescents
1. Retinopathy is the leading cause of new adult blindness in US
   a. Background retinopathy or nonproliferative retinopathy involves microaneurysms and dot hemorrhages but does not impair vision unless it involves the macula
   b. Prevalence is related to the duration and type of diabetes; occurs in almost every patient with type 1 diabetes for 20 years or more and in >60% of patients with type 2 diabetes
   c. Proliferative retinopathy can lead to blindness and involves neovascularization (new vessels develop) with retinal detachment and vitreous hemorrhages
2. Nephropathy
   a. Develops in 35-45% of adult patients with type 1 and 20% with type 2 diabetes
   b. Progresses from the development of microalbuminuria to overt proteinuria and finally to end-stage renal disease (ESRD); this process may take as long as 23 years but once clinical albuminuria appears, the risk of ESRD is high in type 1 diabetes and significant in type 2 diabetes
   c. Diabetes is the most common single cause of ESRD in US
3. Neuropathy occurs primarily in adults
   a. Most common manifestation is a peripheral, symmetric sensorimotor neuropathy which is usually only minimally uncomfortable
   b. A minority of patients have lancinating or burning pain
   c. Autonomic neuropathy may affect gastric or intestinal motility, erectile function, bladder function, cardiac function, and vascular tone
4. Cardiovascular disease: diabetes is a major risk factor
5. Other complications include an increased prevalence of infections, cognitive impairment, and contractures of digits (hammer toes, stiff fingers)

IV. Diagnosis/Evaluation

A. History
1. To establish the diagnosis, explore the following:
   a. Symptoms such as polyuria, polydipsia, polyphagia, weight loss, and fatigue
   b. Frequency of skin infections and other infections
   c. Eating and exercise patterns

        d.   Family history of diabetes and other endocrine problems

        e.   Neonatal history including maternal smoking, the weight and condition of the child at birth, and whether complications occurred during the mother's pregnancy or at the time of labor and delivery

        f.   To uncover polyuria in children, inquire about bedwetting, nocturia, number of diapers used, or whether the child frequently leaves the classroom to urinate

        g.   In peripubertal females, ask about menses to detect PCOS

    2.   In patients who are already diagnosed, inquire about the following:

        a.   Frequency, severity, and cause of hypoglycemia or ketoacidosis

        b.   Symptoms and treatments of chronic eye, kidney, nerve, genitourinary (including sexual), bladder, gastrointestinal function, heart, peripheral vascular, foot, and cerebrovascular complications

        c.   Prior or current infections

        d.   Previous and current pharmacological, nutritional, and self-management treatment plans

        e.   Patterns and results of glucose monitoring, laboratory tests, and special examinations such as ophthalmoscopic exams

        f.   Dietary habits (especially amount of carbohydrates such as juices and soft drinks), nutritional status, and weight history; in children ask about growth and development

        g.   Amount, intensity, and frequency of exercise

        h.   Risk factors for atherosclerosis such as smoking, hypertension, obesity

        i.   Contraceptive, reproductive, and sexual history

        j.   Psychological, sociological and economic factors that may impact on management plan

B.   Physical Examination; perform at diagnosis and then at least annually

    1.   Measure height and weight (and compare to norms)

    2.   During peripubertal period, determine sexual maturation stages

    3.   Measure vital signs including orthostatic blood pressure to detect autonomic neuropathy

    4.   Examine skin

        a.   In children, inspect for hyperpigmented patches of acanthosis nigricans

        b.   Inspect sites of previous insulin administration if applicable

    5.   Complete a thorough ophthalmoscopic examination (best done with dilation)

    6.   Perform a thorough mouth and dental examination

    7.   Palpate thyroid

    8.   Perform complete cardiac examination

    9.   Palpate and auscultate pulses

    10.   Perform abdominal examination; check for liver enlargement

    11.   Assess hand, finger, and wrist, including mobility and presence of contractures

    12.   Carefully examine feet; exam should include use of Semmes-Weinstein monofilament, tuning fork, palpation, and inspection

    13.   Perform complete neurological exam

    14.   May need to do a complete physical exam to exclude any sources of occult infection

C.   Differential Diagnosis

    1.   Glucosuria without hyperglycemia occurs in benign renal glucosuria or in renal tubular disease

    2.   Diabetes insipidus presents with polyuria and polydipsia but not hyperglycemia

    3.   Transient hyperglycemia is present when patients have severe stress from trauma, burns or infection or are on glucocorticoids; this occurs much more commonly in children than adults

    4.   Salicylate intoxication mimics ketoacidosis

    5.   Children with inborn errors of metabolism may present with modest hyperglycemia and acidosis

D.   Diagnostic Tests

    1.   Screening for type 1 diabetes in children and adolescents

        a.   Generally, patients with type 1 diabetes present with acute symptoms of diabetes and markedly elevated blood glucose levels

        b.   For asymptomatic patients screening for type 1 diabetes is usually reserved for individuals ≥45 years, however, as noted in the table that follows, consider testing for certain patients at a younger age

➡ Testing should be considered at a younger age or be performed more frequently in individuals who
- are overweight (≥120% desirable body weight or a BMI ≥25 kg/m^2)
- have a first-degree relative with diabetes
- are members of a high-risk ethnic population (e.g., African-American, Hispanic-American, Native American, Asian-American, Pacific Islander)
- have delivered a baby weighing >9 lb or have been diagnosed with GDM
- are hypertensive (≥140/90 mm Hg)
- have an HDL cholesterol level ≤35 mg/dl (0.90 mmol/L) and/or a triglyceride level ≥250 mg/dl (2.82 mmol/L)
- on previous testing, had IGT or IFG
- have habitual inactivity and polycystic ovarian syndrome
- have history of vascular disease

➡ Fasting Plasma Glucose (FPG) is test of choice (fast for 8 hours prior to test)

➡ If FPG is ≥126 mg/dl, repeat test on different day to confirm diagnosis

➡ If FPG is <126 mg/dl and there is high suspicion for diabetes, an OGTT should be performed. A 2-hour postload in OGTT ≥200 mg/dl is a positive test and should be confirmed on an alternate day

➡ Random plasma glucose measurements can be made when food or drink has been ingested within 3 hours preceding test; ≥200 mg/dL is considered a positive screening test and the diagnosis of diabetes should be confirmed with an additional test, preferably a fasting plasma glucose (FPG) test

Adapted from American Diabetes Association. (2003). Report of the Expert Committee on the diagnosis and classification of diabetes mellitus. *Diabetes Care, 26(*Suppl. 1), S5-S20

2. Screening for type 2 diabetes in children; order every 2 years for high-risk children
   a. Initiate at age 10 or onset of puberty
   b. FPG is preferred test
   c. Criteria for "at risk" status: overweight (BMI >85th percentile for age and sex, weight for height >85th percentile, or weight >120% of ideal [50th percentile] for height) and has any two of the following risk factors:
      (1) Family history of type 2 diabetes in first- and second-degree relatives
      (2) Belongs to a high risk ethnic group (Native American, African American, Latino, Asian American, Pacific Islander)
      (3) Signs of insulin resistance or conditions associated with insulin resistance (acanthosis nigricans, hypertension, dyslipidemia, polycystic ovarian syndrome)

3. Screening for autoantibodies related to type 1 diabetes is not recommended outside the context of research studies

4. Consider screening lean new-onset diabetic patients for type 1 diabetes by measuring postprandial serum C peptide

5. Tests to determine the degree of glycemic control
   a. Glycated hemoglobin (GHb) also referred to as glycohemoglobin, glycosylated hemoglobin, A1C, HbA1, or HbA1C
      (1) Reflects mean glucose levels for the preceding 2-3 months
      (2) Order at baseline and then at least every 6 months for well-controlled patients
      (3) Order more often (every 3 months) in diabetics with poor control or when beginning new therapies
      (4) Levels <7% are the goal of treatment for adults; it is controversial if this same goal should be applied to children and adolescents (see V.A.)
      (5) Falsely low levels may occur in the presence of anemia and falsely elevated levels may occur in presence of uremia, alcoholism, and aspirin use
   b. Glycemic control is best evaluated by a combination of results of patient's self-monitoring of blood glucose (SMBG) and the current A1C
      (1) AIC is also used to check accuracies of the patient's self-reported results and the patient's glucose meter
      (2) Following table shows correlation between A1C levels and mean plasma glucose levels

CORRELATION BETWEEN A1C LEVEL AND MEAN PLASMA GLUCOSE LEVELS		
	Mean plasma glucose	
A1C (%)	mg/dl	mmol/L
6	135	7.5
7	170	9.5
8	205	11.5
9	240	13.5
10	275	15.5
11	310	17.5
12	345	19.5

From: American Diabetes Association. (2003). Standards of medical care for patients with diabetes mellitus. *Diabetes Care, 26*(Suppl. 1), S33-S50.

    c.   Glycated serum protein indicates glycemic control in a short period of time and needs to be performed monthly; currently this test is not recommended

6.   Tests helpful in defining associated complications and risk factors:

    a.   Testing for diabetic retinopathy

        (1)   Comprehensive eye examination by an ophthalmologist or optometrist should be completed within 3-5 years after onset of type 1 diabetes and shortly after diagnosis in type 2 diabetes

        (2)   Assess annually or more often if retinopathy is progressing

    b.   Order fasting lipid profile: total cholesterol, high-density lipoprotein (HDL) cholesterol, low density lipoprotein (LDL) cholesterol, and triglycerides

        (1)   Order when diabetes is first diagnosed in children >2 years

        (2)   In children whose values fall within acceptable levels and with low risk and no family history, repeat tests every 5 years; see section on DYSLIPIDEMIA for monitoring in children with abnormal levels

    c.   Order annual serum creatinine if proteinuria is present in children

    d.   Order a urinalysis: ketones, glucose, protein, sediment

        (1)   If protein is positive, a quantitative measure should be performed

        (2)   If protein is negative, a test for the presence of microalbuminuria is necessary (see IV.D.6.e.), which immediately follows

    e.   Testing for microalbuminuria

        (1)   In adolescents with type 2 diabetes, test at the time of diagnosis and then yearly

        (2)   Because microalbuminuria rarely occurs with short duration of type 1 diabetes or before puberty, individuals with type 1 diabetes should begin testing with puberty and after 5 years duration

        (3)   Because of marked day-to-day variability in albumin excretion, at least two of three collections measured in a 3- to 6-month period should show elevated levels before arriving at a diagnosis

        (4)   Testing for microalbuminuria can be performed by 3 methods

            (a)   Measurement of the albumin-to-creatinine ratio in a random, spot collection (usually assessed first)

            (b)   24 hour collection with serum creatinine which allows for simultaneous measurement of creatinine clearance

            (c)   Timed collection such as 4 hours or overnight

        (5)   Microalbuminuria is defined in following table:

DEFINITIONS OF ABNORMALITIES IN ALBUMIN EXCRETION			
Category	24-h Collection	Timed Collection	Spot Collection
Normal	<30 mg/24 h	<20 µg/min	<30 µg/mg creatinine
Microalbuminuria	30-299 mg/24 h	20-199 µg/min	30-299 µg/mg creatinine
Clinical albuminuria	≥300 mg/24 h	≥200 µg/min	≥300 µg/mg creatinine

Two of three specimens collected within a 3- to 6-month period should be abnormal before considering a patient to have crossed one of these diagnostic thresholds. Exercise within 24 hours, infection, fever, congestive heart failure, marked hyperglycemia, and marked hypertension may elevate urinary albumin excretion over baseline values

Adapted from American Diabetes Association. (2003). Diabetic nephropathy. *Diabetes Care, 26*(Suppl. 1), S94-S98.

      f.   In type 1 patients, order T_4 and thyroid stimulating hormone; order in type 2 patients if clinical presentation indicates a need

      g.   Some, but not all authorities, also suggest regular serum BUN and CBC tests

      h.   Consider screening for celiac disease

7. Testing for diabetic ketoacidosis and hyperosmolar hyperglycemic state

      a.   Order plasma glucose, blood urea nitrogen/creatinine, serum ketones, electrolytes (with calculated anion gap), osmolality, urinalysis, urine ketones by dipstick, initial arterial blood gases, complete blood count with differential, and electrocardiogram

      b.   If infection is suspected, order bacterial cultures of urine, blood, and throat

      c.   If indicated, order chest x-ray

      d.   Patients with hyperglycemic emergencies typically have leukocytosis, decreased serum sodium, and elevated serum potassium (also see table DIAGNOSTIC CRITERIA FOR DKA AND HHS, III.E.)

8. Testing for insulin resistance

      a.   Best tested with complicated method: the euglycemic insulin clamp; at present this test is reserved for research purposes

      b.   A reasonable alternative to euglycemic clamp is measurement of fasting insulin levels (normal <15 mU/L, borderline high 15-20 mU/L, high >20 mU/L

V. Plan/Management

A. Glycemic control: goals should be discussed with patient and/or family; degree of glycemic control must be individualized and balanced with the risk of developing hypoglycemia

    1. Tight glycemic control is recommended in adults, but is controversial in children

    2. Children younger than 5 years of age do not have the cognitive capacity to recognize symptoms of hypoglycemia and are also at most risk for central nervous system damage because myelin lipid development is still occurring; thus, some experts recommend less stringent treatment goals for very young children

    3. Other experts state that intensive treatment regiments that are flexible with sufficient education and support prevent the risk of hypoglycemia in children and that strict treatment goals should be maintained

    4. Typical goals are the following:

      a.   Infants and toddlers: 100-200 mg/dL range

      b.   Older children and adolescents: 70-180 mg/dL range

      c.   HbA1C level near 7% is recommended, but this is difficult to attain in children; infants and toddlers usually need higher goals to avoid hypoglycemia

B. Hospitalization should be considered for individuals with ketoacidosis or hyperosmolar nonketotic coma, infection, or dehydration

C. Children who are newly diagnosed should be referred to a pediatric endocrinologist or hospitalized

D. All diabetic patients benefit from medical nutritional therapy (MNT), exercise, and extensive patient education

E. Patient and family education is essential; education must be integrated with all aspects of the plan (also, see patient education in each of the following sections)

    1. Discuss basic pathophysiology

    2. Explain long-term complications, emphasizing that these complications can be prevented or delayed when blood glucose is well controlled

    3. Encourage patient to wear Medic-Alert tags

    4. Discuss contraception and emphasize the importance of glucose control before conception and during pregnancy in females of childbearing age

    5. Recommend annual influenza immunization

    6. See following table for good resources. The Small Steps•Big Rewards•Prevent type 2 Diabetes Campaign is first national diabetes prevention program. (See National Diabetes Education Program website for clinicians tool kit as well as tools for patients to determine if they are at risk for type 2 diabetes and a "game plan food and activity tracker" to help lose weight)

RESOURCES FOR PATIENTS	
Organization	**Website**
American Diabetes Association (ADA)	http:// www.diabetes.org
American Association for Clinical Endocrinologists	http://www.aace.com
ADA Diabetes Care & Educational Practice Group	http://www.eatright.org
National Diabetes Education Program	http://www.ndep.nih.gov

F. Nutritional recommendations or medical nutrition therapy (MNT)
1. Collaboration or referral to a dietitian is beneficial; MNT should be individualized with respect to age, personal and cultural preferences, individual's wishes, and willingness to change
2. For youth with type 1 diabetes, goal is to promote adequate energy for normal growth and development, and integrate insulin regimens into usual eating and activity habits
3. For youth with type 2 diabetes, goal is to facilitate changes in eating and physical activity that reduce insulin resistance and improve metabolic status
4. Type 1 diabetes cannot be treated with diet alone
   a. Monitor blood glucose levels and adjust insulin based on the amount of food usually consumed
     (1) Individuals on intensified insulin programs can make adjustments in rapid or lispro insulin to cover carbohydrate content of meals and/or snacks and for deviations from typical eating and exercising habits
     (2) For individuals on fixed insulin doses, day to day consistency in the amount of carbohydrate is needed
       (a) Plan meals to provide the amount of calories and nutrients that are expected to be metabolized when insulin is administered
       (b) Keep timing and amount of calories and nutrients in meals the same each day
     (3) Have a consistent, daily pattern of exercise and physical activity (may need supplemental snacks before and after exercise; may need to alter insulin dosage before activity)
   b. Carbohydrate counting in which the patient takes insulin based on the amount of insulin consumed for a meal may be effective; approximately 1 unit of insulin will cover 10-15 grams of carbohydrate consumed
5. For adolescents with type 2 diabetes the following are helpful:
   a. Moderate weight loss alone may control diabetes
   b. Spacing of meals throughout day and regular exercise improve control
   c. Portion control is important
   d. For long-term weight loss, structured weight loss programs are often needed
6. Dietary recommendations for both types of diabetics are similar to recommendations of nondiabetic children
   a. Carbohydrates and fats
     (1) Unrefined carbohydrates (whole grains, vegetables [excluding potatoes], fruits, legumes, lowfat milk) and fiber should be eaten whenever possible; avoid refined starchy foods and concentrated sugar
     (2) Select foods with a low glycemic index and low glycemic load (see following table)
       (a) Glycemic index and glycemic load are systems for classifying carbohydrate-containing foods according to glycemic response
       (b) High-glycemic foods produce an initial period of high blood glucose and insulin levels, followed in many persons by reactive hypoglycemia, counterregulatory hormone secretion, and increased serum free fatty acid concentration
       (c) Regular consumption of high-glycemic meals results in higher average 24-hour blood glucose and insulin levels

GLYCEMIC INDEX AND GLYCEMIC LOAD VALUES FOR MAJOR CARBOHYDRATE SOURCES (RELATIVE TO WHITE BREAD)

Foods	Serving Size	Glycemic Index (%)	Carbohydrate (Grams)	Glycemic Load*
Potatoes, mashed	1 cup	104	37	38
Bread, white	1 slice	100	12	12
Orange juice	6 ounces	75	20	15
Banana	1 medium	88	27	23
Rice, white	1 cup	102	45	45
Pizza	2 slices	86	78	67
Pasta	1 cup	71	40	28
Coke	12 ounces	90	39	35
Apple	1 medium	55	21	12
Milk, skim	1 cup	46	12	5.4
Pancake	2 six-inch	119	56	66
Sugar, table	1 tsp.	84	4	3.4
Jam	1 tbsp.	91	14	13
Candy	1 ounce	99	27	27
Ice cream	½ cup	42	16	7
Carrots, raw	½ cup	131	4	5
Baked beans	1 cup	60	27	16
Cornflakes	1 cup	114	24	27
Cheerios	1 cup	106	22	23
Total	1 cup	109	32	35
Bran Flakes	1 cup	74	31	23
Oatmeal	1 cup	82	25	21

* Glycemic load calculated by multiplying grams of carbohydrate by glycemic index of bread (100%=1.0)

Glycemic index taken from: Jenkins, D.J.A., et al. (1981). Overview of implications in health and disease. *American Journal of Clinical Nutrition, 76*(Suppl.), 266S-273S.

Adapted from Willett, W.C. (2001). *Eat, drink, and be healthy: The Harvard Medical School guide to healthy eating.* New York: Simon & Schuster.

b. Protein intake
  (1) Reduce intake if renal function is abnormal
  (2) In children, protein intake should be sufficient for optimal growth
  (3) Choose healthy sources of protein (beans, nuts, fish, poultry, eggs)
c. Saturated fats (whole milk, ice cream, red meat, butter, coconut oil) should be restricted to <10% of total calories and cholesterol to <300 mg/day; unsaturated fats (olive, canola, corn, safflower oils, fish, peanuts) should replace saturated fats
d. Patients can use nutritive and nonnutritive sweeteners
e. Excessive alcohol increases risks of hypertriglycemia and pancreatitis and contributes to hypoglycemia in persons with type 1 diabetes

G. Physical activity is an integral component of diabetes management
  1. Positive effects: increases metabolism and, over an extended period, reduces insulin resistance, reduces cardiovascular risk factors, improves weight loss, and promotes well being
  2. Encourage at least 30 minutes of moderate physical activity most days of week and preferably every day
  3. For patients on insulin therapy, the following guidelines are helpful:
    a. Avoid exercising at times when insulin is at its peak action
    b. Monitor blood glucose before and after exercise to identify when changes in insulin or food intake are necessary and to learn glycemic response to different exercise conditions
    c. Avoid exercise if FPG levels are <80 mg/dl or >250 mg/dl and ketosis is present or if glucose levels are >300 mg/dl, regardless of whether ketosis is present
    d. Ingest added carbohydrates if glucose levels are <100 mg/dl
    e. Eat added carbohydrates as needed to avoid hypoglycemia; keep carbohydrate-based food available during and after exercise; in general, one serving of carbohydrates increases plasma glucose about 40 points
    f. Avoid exercising extremities in which insulin has recently been injected
  4. For patients with type 2 diabetes, exercise should be a high priority; benefit is probably greatest when it is begun early in course of disease

H. Insulin therapy: Goals of normalized glycohemoglobin must be balanced with risks of hypoglycemia; insulin is required for management of type 1 diabetes and in some patients with type 2 diabetes

1. Newly diagnosed children and adolescents should be referred to a pediatric endocrinologist; frequent consultation with a specialist is often needed, particularly during times of illness, stress, and growth spurts, when changing insulin regimens, or when initiating Lispro insulin

2. Consider type of insulin to use

a. If patients are on pork insulin, do not switch if they are well-controlled

b. Newly diagnosed diabetics should be on human insulin because of its lower incidence of insulin allergy, resistance, and lipoatrophy (see table VARIOUS HUMAN INSULIN PREPARATIONS for brand names of human insulin)

VARIOUS HUMAN INSULIN PREPARATIONS			
Type	Onset (hours)	Peak (hours)	Duration (hours)
Rapid acting analog			
Humalog (Lispro)	<0.25	1	3.5-4.5
NovoLog (Aspart)	<0.25	0.75	3-5
Short acting			
Humulin R	0.5	2-4	6-8
Novolin R	0.5	2.5-5	8
Velosulin BR	0.5	1-3	8
Intermediate acting			
Humulin N (NPH)	1-2	6-12	18-24
Novolin N (NPH)	1.5	4-12	24
Humulin L (Lente)	1-3	6-12	18-24
Novolin L (Lente)	2.5	7-15	22
Long acting			
Humulin U (Ultralente)	4-6	8-20	24-48
Lantus (Glargine)	1.1	none	≥24
Premixed: Insulin isophane suspension (NPH)/regular insulin (R)*			
Humulin 70/30	0.5	2-12	24
Humulin 50/50	0.5	3-5	24
Novolin 70/30	0.5	2-12	24
Premixed: Lispro Protamine/Lispro*			
Humalog Mix 75/25	≤0.25	0.5-1.5	24
Premixed: Aspart Protamine/Aspart*			
NovoLog 70-30	<0.25	1-4	24

*Do Not use premixed with Type 1 diabetics as it severely limits flexibility

3. Persons without diabetes produce insulin continuously (basal insulin) in order to suppress hepatic glucose production, with increases or boluses of insulin at meal times to utilize prandial glucose; these same basal and postprandial patterns should be followed in persons with diabetes for insulin therapy to be effective

4. Insulin is commercially available in concentrations of 100 or 500 units/ml (designated U-100 and U-500, respectively); use U-100 insulin, as U-500 is used only in rare cases when patient requires extremely large doses

5. Children with established diabetes usually require 0.5-1.2 units/kg/day
    6. The adolescent may need 1.25-1.50 units/kg/day during the pubertal growth spurt
    7. Adjust insulin levels to meet target blood glucose ranges
        a. Preschool child should be in the range of 90-140 mg/dL preprandially and 90-200 mg/dL postprandially
        b. School-aged children should be in the range of 80-120 mg/dL preprandially and 80-180 mg/dL postprandially
    8. Most children and adolescents seem to benefit from multiple daily injection regimens and are typically started on 2-4 daily injections of intermediate or long-acting and rapid or short-acting insulin (see table COMMON INSULIN REGIMENS that follows)
    9. Because of the danger of hypoglycemia to the developing brain, cautiously lower blood glucose in young children
    10. About 1/3 of children under 3 years of age develop hypoglycemia at nighttime on split/BID dosing regimen which can lead to cognitive and neurological deficits; instruct parents to occasionally check blood glucose at 3 AM and if low, reduce evening dose of insulin by 10% every few days until control is reached
    11. Some experts recommend lispro (Humalog) insulin for toddlers and adolescents who have difficulty adhering to a strict mealtime routine; for example, Humalog can be injected immediately after a meal for toddlers who may refuse to eat
    12. Premixed insulins may not be practical for young children
    13. In adolescent, consider an eating disorder if glycosylated hemoglobin levels are >12%; adolescents may intentionally miss doses to lose weight
    14. Honeymoon phase: after initial therapy is instituted this phase occurs and may last 12-18 months; insulin dosages may be reduced to 0.2-0.5 units/kg/day (important to tell patients and families about this phase to prevent false beliefs that the diabetes is partially cured)
    15. Long-term insulin therapy
        a. Dosage: 0.6-0.8 units/kg/day; children may need 1.0-1.2 units/kg/day; adolescents may need 1.0-1.5 units/kg/day
        b. Determine the pattern or regimen of insulin therapy (see table COMMON INSULIN REGIMENS)
    16. Persons with type 2 diabetes vary considerably and may require small (5-10 units) to several hundred units per day

COMMON INSULIN REGIMENS

Regimen	Dosing	Comments
Single daily injection	Intermediate or long lasting at bedtime (usually start ~10 units)	• Only for type 2 • Use when daily doses are <30 units/day; for larger daily insulin doses, 2 or more injections are needed unless using Lantus (Glargine) • Suppresses hepatic glucose production • Often used in combination with daytime oral agent
2-injection -or- split/mix	2/3 of total daily dosing in AM* 1/3 of total daily dosing in PM* **THEN** AM 2/3 NPH + 1/3 rapid or short acting** PM 1/2 NPH + 1/2 rapid or short acting**	• Best in type 2 and early type 1 • Disadvantages: poor peaking of noon insulin & excess insulin at night (to resolve this problem, limit noon meal and eat a bedtime snack)
3-injection	Of total daily dose (approximate): AM* 20-30% NPH & ~ 25% rapid or short acting** PM* ~ 25% rapid or short acting** Bedtime 20-30% NPH **OR** AM* ~ 20-30% rapid or short acting** PM* ~ 20-30% rapid or short acting** Bedtime insulin glargine (~50%)	• Best in type 1 • Advantages: less risk of nighttime hypoglycemia & better control of dawn phenomenon or persistent AM hyperglycemia • Disadvantage: poor peaking of insulin at noon (to resolve this problem, limit noon meal)
4-Injection or prandial/basal	Of total daily dose (approximate): Prandial insulin (before each meal) ~15-20% rapid or short acting** (best to vary dose depending on food intake, i.e., higher dose at dinner) Basal insulin ~ 50% glargine at bedtime or ~25% NPH or ~ 25% lente in AM and bedtime	• Best in type 1 • Requires committed patient and care-provider, with frequent self-blood-glucose monitoring • Advantage: clear relationship between insulin dose and glucose level • Insulin glargine and lispro combination can lessen risk of hypoglycemia and result in a pattern that resembles endogenous insulin release
Continuous subcutaneous insulin infusion -or- insulin pump therapy	-Continually delivers rapid or short acting -Provides both basal insulin release and adjustable pre-meal bolus release	• Indications: inability to control glucose with 2 or more injections; recurrent, major hypoglycemia due to hypoglycemic unawareness, loss of counter-regulatory mechanisms or variable absorption of modified insulins • Prerequisites: Family must be motivated and capable of working to achieve control • Advantages: closely resembles endogenous insulin release; results in more predictable insulin absorption and fewer dosage errors • Disadvantages: expensive; blood glucose must be monitored 4 times/day

* AM is before breakfast: regular or short acting insulins should be taken 30-45 minutes before meal and rapid acting insulins should be taken within 15 minutes of meal; PM is before evening meal or supper

**Rapid acting insulins are often more convenient for patients because they can be injected immediately before (or after) meals and can lessen the likelihood of late post-prandial hypoglycemia and nocturnal hypoglycemia but they are more expensive and need more intensive monitoring than regular insulins

17. Adjusting insulin is based on daily blood glucose levels and on peak effect of a given insulin dose (patients should record their blood glucose and insulin doses with comments on a flow sheet)
    a. Self-monitoring of blood glucose is essential
        (1) Patients with type 1 diabetes should monitor 3-4 times a day
        (2) Patients with type 2 diabetes should monitor at various times such as some mornings, at bedtimes, and 1-2 hour after meals
    b. Adjustments are made to individual components of insulin regimen in 5-10% increments or decrements
    c. Downward adjustments should be made the day following a "below range blood glucose" to avoid repeat hypoglycemia
    d. Upward adjustments should be delayed for 2 days to establish a pattern

e. When increasing a long lasting or evening intermediate insulin, instruct patient to monitor blood glucose at 2-3 AM for hypoglycemia

f. Consider timing and type of insulin when making adjustments (see following table):

ADJUSTING INSULIN THERAPY

Insulin	Affected Blood Glucose Value
AM* Intermediate	Post-lunch Pre-supper
AM* Short or rapid acting	Post-breakfast Pre-lunch
PM** Intermediate	Early morning
PM** Short or rapid acting	Bedtime
Bedtime Intermediate or long acting	Early morning

*AM is before breakfast
**PM is before evening meal or supper

18. Tips on administering insulin therapy (see following table)

TIPS ON INSULIN THERAPY

- Insulin should approximate the natural release of insulin by the beta cell
- Administer Insulin to provide a basal amount in 40-60% of total daily dose as well as peaks after each meal
- One time a day insulin therapy is **not** sufficient for patients with type 1 diabetes
- Be careful in adjusting insulin with type 1 diabetics; they are very sensitive to adjustments because they have no endogenous insulin secretion
- Consider giving PM NPH at bedtime to reduce early morning hyperglycemia
- Combination insulin therapy of glargine and lispro insulins can lessen risk of hypoglycemia (however, do not mix insulin glargine in same syringe with other forms of insulin)
- Use NPH when there is a need to mix with another type of insulin
- Consider the following when blood glucose is not controlled with insulin: malignant insulin resistance, occult infection, noncompliance, poor coping skills

19. Patient education concerning the administering, storage, and disposal of insulin is essential (see following table)

PATIENT EDUCATION - INSULIN THERAPY

- Insulin in use can be kept at room temperature, for one month only, to limit local irritation at injection site; unopened insulin should be refrigerated
- Opened cartridges and prefilled pens can be kept for varying amounts of time (10-28 days) depending on the type
- When mixing insulin, the clear, rapid-acting and short-acting insulins should be drawn into syringe first
- Lantus (Glargine) and lente should not be mixed with other insulin
- Syringes can be prefilled and stored in a vertical position in the refrigerator for 3 weeks (do not allow if using rapid)
- Usually, regular or short-acting insulin should be given 30 minutes before eating; rapid should be given within 15 minutes of eating
- Subcutaneously inject insulin into upper arm, anterior and lateral aspects of thigh, the buttocks and abdomen (with exception of a circle with a 2-inch radius around the navel); do not frequently rotate to different anatomical sites, but do make injections in different areas of one anatomical site; absorption is most rapid and consistent from the abdomen
- Do not use clear insulin that is cloudy or discolored or any insulin that has sediment or other visible changes
- Dispose syringes in resistant disposal container and contact local public health unit or local trash-disposal authority for appropriate disposal provisions
- Proper procedure of syringe reuse involves cleaning needle after use and putting in refrigerator (only teach patients who have good cognitive and psychomotor functioning)
- Syringe alternatives such as jet injectors, pen-like devices, and insulin-containing cartridges are usually expensive but may be more convenient and improve technique of insulin injection

I. Treatment of children and adolescents with type 2 diabetes
1. Normalization of blood glucose, A1C, and associated comorbidities (hypertension, hyperlipidemia, obesity) is goal
2. If child presents with high blood glucose or significant symptoms (dehydration, ketosis) start on insulin; insulin may be tapered and oral agents, diet (MNT), and exercise added as glycemic control improves
3. Less ill children may be treated with MNT and exercise
   a. Low glycemic index foods are associated with greater weight loss than a standard reduced fat diet
   b. Lifestyle changes that incorporate the entire family increase the success rate
4. Drug therapy; most children eventually require drug therapy; however, with exception of metformin there are limited efficacy and safety data available (see table ORAL HYPOGLYCEMIC AGENTS for drugs approved by the Food and Drug Administration [FDA] for adults)
   a. Metformin is the oral agent of choice
      (1) Do not use if child has impaired renal function, hepatic disease, or alcohol abuse
      (2) Reduces fasting blood glucose, insulin concentrations, and moderates weight gain
      (3) May normalize ovulatory function in adolescents with polycystic ovarian syndrome; preconception and pregnancy counseling is imperative
      (4) Administer before meals to reduce side effects
      (5) Usual starting dose is 500 mg BID; may titrate in increments of 1 table (500 mg) every week up to a maximum of 2550 mg/day
      (6) Temporarily discontinue metformin during acute illness associated with dehydration or hypoxemia, before administration of radiocontrast material, and before surgery
   b. If monotherapy is not successful after 3-6 months, some experts recommend the following:
      (1) Adding a sulfonylurea or insulin
      (2) Non-sulfonylurea secretagogues and α-glucosidase inhibitors are acceptable, but used less frequently
      (3) Repaglinide may be useful in adolescents who have irregular eating schedules
      (4) Thiazolidinediones: Safety information is limited for children; use very cautiously
   c. Treatment of complications:
      (1) Control of hypertension is critical
         (a) Angiotensin-converting enzyme (ACE) inhibitors may be helpful in treating microalbuminuria
         (b) α-blockers, calcium channel blockers (long-acting), low-dose diuretics, and β-blockers are also acceptable in selected patients
      (2) Dyslipidemia should be treated; if weight loss, diet, glycemic control, and exercise do not lower lipid levels, medications should be used

J. Management of insulin resistance
1. Periodically measure blood pressure, fasting plasma glucose, and lipids
2. Assessment, prevention, and treatment of overweight/obesity should be a priority
3. Weight control, lifestyle modification, and early detection of type 2 diabetes is recommended to improve risk profiles for cardiovascular disease and type 2 diabetes

ORAL HYPOGLYCEMIC AGENTS*

Drug	Mechanism of Action	Advantages	Major Adverse Reactions and Disadvantages	Food and Drug Administration Approval Status
Sulfonylureas (SUs) Glyburide (Micronase/DiaBeta) Glyburide, micronized (Glynase Pres Tabs) Glipizide (Glucotrol XL) Glipizide (Glucotrol) Glimepiride (Amaryl)	↑ Pancreatic insulin secretion	• Well established • Decreases microvascular risk • Daily dosing	• Weight gain • Hypoglycemia	• Monotherapy • Combine with insulin, metformin, thiazolidinediones, α-glucosidase inhibitors
Non-Sulfonylurea Secretagogues Repaglinide (Prandin) Nateglinide (Starlix)	↑ Pancreatic insulin secretion	• Possibly less hypoglycemia and weight gain than SUs • Targets postprandial glycemia	• Hypoglycemia (skip dose if miss meal) • Weight gain • Complex dosing • No long-term data	• Monotherapy • Combine with metformin • Combine with thiazolidinediones
Biguanides Metformin (Glucophage) Metformin (Glucophage XR)	↓ Hepatic glucose production ↑ Insulin action on muscle glucose uptake	• Well established • Weight loss • No hypoglycemia • Decreases microvascular and macrovascular risks • Decreases lipid levels • Increases fibrinolysis • Decreases hyperinsulinemia • Daily dosing	• Diarrhea and other GI effects • Lactic acidosis with incorrect dosing or renal disease • Many contraindications	• Monotherapy • Combine with insulin, SU, non-SU secretagogue, thiazolidinedione
α-Glucosidase Inhibitors Acarbose (Precose) Miglitol (Glyset)	↓ Delays carbohydrate digestion	• Targets postprandial glucose • No hypoglycemia • Nonsystemic	• Complex dosing • GI effects • No long-term data	• Monotherapy • Combine with SU
Thiazolidinediones Pioglitazone (Actos) Rosiglitazone (Avandia)	↑ Insulin action on muscle and fat glucose uptake	• Reverses prime defect of type 2 diabetes • Possible beta cell preservation • No hypoglycemia • Decreases lipid levels • Increases fibrinolysis • Decreases hyperinsulinemia • Improves endothelial function • Daily dosing	• Weight gain • Edema • Liver function test monitoring (especially with insulin, monitor every 2 months for first year) • Slow onset of action • Resumption of pre-menopausal ovulation in anovulating women (may result in pregnancy)	• Monotherapy • Combine with insulin, SU, metformin
Combination Sulfonylurea & Biguanide Glyburide & metformin (Glucovance) Glipizide & metformin (Metaglip)	See SU and biguanides above	See SU and biguanides above	See SU and biguanides above	See SU and biguanides above
Combination Thiazolidinedione & Biguanide Rosiglitazone & metformin (Avandamet)	See thiaz. and biguanides above	See thiaz. and biguanides above	See thiaz. and biguanides above	See thiaz. and biguanides above

* Begin at a low dose and gradually titrate upwards according to clinical effect (especially in elderly, malnourished, debilitated, or those with renal and/or hepatic dysfunction.)
Adapted from Inzucchi, S.E. (2002). Oral antihyperglycemic therapy for type 2 diabetes: Scientific review. *JAMA, 287,* 360-372.

K. Self-monitoring of blood glucose has replaced urine testing as a method to assess glucose control; however, type 1 patients need to check urine for ketones whenever their blood glucose levels are >300 mg/dL, during illness, stress, pregnancy, or when symptoms of ketoacidosis such as nausea, vomiting, or abdominal pain are present
1. Frequent monitoring is essential when patients are on intensive insulin therapy or insulin pump therapy; monitor blood glucose three or more times, typically before meals, at bedtime and occasionally in the middle of night
2. Less frequent monitoring may be appropriate for some patients, but even these patients should adhere to the following recommendations:
a. When medications are altered should do the following:
(1) Check blood glucose before each meal, at bedtime, and at 2-4 AM for 3 days
(2) Next 7 days, check blood glucose before breakfast and dinner
b. After glucose is initially controlled, check once a day at different times
c. When glucose is stabilized, check 2-4 times per week at different times
3. In children, blood glucose testing should be performed at the school or day care setting before lunch and when signs/symptoms of abnormal glucose levels occur
4. FDA has approved the GlucoWatch Biographer, a device that monitors patterns of glucose levels in adults without puncturing the skin; used as a supplement rather than a replacement for standard home glucose monitoring systems

L. Contingency plan for managing hypoglycemia (BG <70 mg/dL with or without symptoms)
1. Teach patient and family the signs and symptoms of hypoglycemia such as shakiness, sweating, restlessness, hunger, headache, confusion, or seizures
2. Instruct patient to carry source of oral glucose (glucose tablets, Lifesavers, raisins) with them at all times
a. For BG 50-70 mg/dl, ~15 grams of carbohydrate (3-4 glucose tablets, 8 Lifesavers, 2 tablespoons of raisins, 4 oz. of fruit juice or soft drink, 8 oz milk) should raise BG 30-45 mg/dl
b. For BG <50 mg/dl, ~30 grams should be taken
3. Family or friends should be instructed in administering a subcutaneous or intramuscular injection of glucagon if patient is unresponsive or unable to swallow; if patient does not respond in 15 minutes, may give 1-2 more doses
a. Adolescent dose: 1 mg
b. Children <5 years: 0.25-0.5 mg; Children 5-10 years: 0.5-1 mg
c. After consciousness is regained, patient should ingest oral carbohydrates to prevent further hypoglycemia
4. Encourage patient to carry medical identification

M. Managing diabetes when the patient is ill; teach the following:
1. Especially in children who have more frequent and severe episodes, illnesses can be life-threatening and require careful monitoring
2. Although difficult to predict, blood glucose usually increases; perform self-blood-glucose monitoring several times a day and check urine for ketones (twice a day)
3. Imperative to call clinician in following circumstances:
a. Vomiting with ketosis (may indicate diabetic ketoacidosis that requires immediate medical care to prevent complications and even death)
b. Inability to drink fluids
c. Blood glucose >240 mg/dL and urine positive for ketones
4. Continue to take usual dose of insulin or oral agent; patients with oral agents may temporarily require insulin
5. If patients are able to drink, increase intake of non-caloric fluids
6. Drink small, continuous amounts of sugar-containing liquids such as juice, Gatorade or Coke in conjunction with the readings from their self-monitoring and if they are vomiting or nauseated

N. Management of associated problems and complications. Growing recognition that tight glycemic control prevents or delays many of the following problems
1. Treatment of hyperglycemic crisis
a. Correct dehydration; typically IV isotonic saline is infused
b. Unless the episode is mild, regular insulin by continuous intravenous infusion is usually recommended
c. To prevent hypokalemia, potassium replacement in the IV infusion is started after serum potassium levels fall below 5.5 mEq/L, assuming urine output is adequate
d. Assess need for bicarbonate therapy; bicarbonate may be beneficial in patients with a pH <6.9

e. To avoid cardiac and skeletal muscle weakness and respiratory depression due to hypophosphatemia, careful phosphate replacement may be indicated in patients with cardiac dysfunction, anemia, or respiratory depression and in those with serum phosphate concentration <1.0 mg/dL

f. Cerebral edema is a rare but frequently fatal complication of DKA and HHS; prevention involves gradual correction of glucose and osmolality as well as judicious use of isotonic or hypotonic saline depending on the sodium and the hemodynamic status of the patient

2. Diabetic retinopathy: refer to ophthalmologist; laser therapy and vitrectomy have been effective

3. Nephropathy: Achieving normoglycemia and lowering blood pressure have proven to delay progression

O. Follow Up: Scheduling of return visits will depend on type of diabetes, degree of glucose control, changes in therapeutic regimen, and presence of illnesses or complications of diabetes

1. Patients beginning insulin or who are making a major change in their insulin program need frequent contact with the health team, possibly daily, until control is achieved and risk of hypoglycemia is low

2. Patients beginning treatment with medical nutrition therapy or oral glucose-lowering agents may need weekly visits until control is achieved

3. Most patients should be seen at least quarterly until their treatment goals have been achieved; thereafter, the frequency of visits can be decreased to every 6 months

4. Increase visits if patients are involved in intensive insulin therapy, not meeting glycemic or blood pressure goals, or there is progression in microvascular/macrovascular complications

DYSLIPIDEMIA

I. Definition: Elevation of one or more of the following: cholesterol, cholesterol esters, phospholipids, or triglycerides

II. Pathogenesis

A. Pathophysiology
1. An elevated cholesterol level is an independent and significant risk factor for coronary heart disease (CHD); evidence linking higher cholesterol levels in children and adolescents with atherosclerotic lesions in coronary and other arteries is increasing

2. Blood lipid levels are regulated by lipoproteins or "carriers" which are a combination of lipids (fats) and proteins

3. High-density lipoproteins (HDL), major carriers, are thought to prevent or delay atherogenesis because of their low fat content and their probable role in carrying lipids away from blood vessels to the liver for degradation

4. The other major carriers, low density lipoproteins (LDL), are considered harmful lipoproteins because they keep cholesterol in the blood vessels, forming fatty deposits

5. Chylomicrons transport triglycerides from the gut and are largest lipoproteins with the lowest density

6. Very low density lipoproteins (VLDL) are triglyceride-rich lipoproteins produced by the liver and are associated with increased cardiovascular disease risk

B. Etiology
1. Primary hyperlipidemia results in defects in lipid metabolism and transport; occurs in individuals with specific inherited traits

2. Several secondary factors can contribute to hyperlipidemia
   a. Obesity
   b. Low activity levels
   c. High dietary saturated fat, cholesterol, carbohydrate, and calorie intake
   d. Endocrine disorders such as diabetes mellitus, Cushing's syndrome, polycystic ovarian syndrome, hypothyroidism, lipodystrophies, anorexia nervosa, and acute intermittent porphyria
   e. Renal disorders such as uremia and nephrotic syndrome,
   f. Hepatic disorders such as obstructive liver disease, primary biliary cirrhosis, acute hepatitis, and hepatoma
   g. Immunologic disorders such as systemic lupus erythematosus

	h.	Stress
	i.	Medications such as thiazide diuretics, loop diuretics, beta-blockers without intrinsic sympathomimetic activity, progestins, anabolic steroids, corticosteroids, and HIV protease inhibitors
	j.	Alcohol

III. Clinical Presentation

A. Empirical evidence is accumulating that atherosclerosis begins in childhood and that there is a relationship between childhood and adult cholesterol levels

B. High levels of total cholesterol and LDL and low levels of HDL are major risk factors for CHD

C. Vascular problems are the most frequent adverse clinical sequela
   1. In the most severe forms of hyperlipidemia, which are due to specific inherited traits, cholesterol levels can reach as high as 1200 mg/dL and these patients develop coronary heart disease (CHD) in childhood and usually die before age 30
   2. In contrast, many patients with other types of hyperlipidemia do not develop symptoms of CHD until they are in their 60s or 70s
   3. There is limited evidence at present that expensive, lengthy interventions to lower cholesterol levels in children are more efficacious in lowering coronary artery disease than shorter, less-costly interventions which are begun during adulthood

D. Except for children and adolescents with the inherited forms of dyslipidemia, other manifestations do not usually occur; older patients with severe dyslipidemia may present with the following:
   1. Dermatological manifestations can occur: Xanthomas which are cutaneous or subcutaneous papules, plaques, or nodules may develop in the tendons, extensor surfaces of the extremities, buttocks, knees, skin folds, scars, and eyelids
   2. Gastrointestinal problems may develop, particularly with hypertriglyceridemia
      a. Severe abdominal pain which is often associated with pancreatitis can occur
      b. Hepatomegaly or splenomegaly may be present
      c. Less severe symptoms include mild pain, nausea, vomiting, and diarrhea
   3. Other clinical manifestations include premature arcus cornea, aortic stenosis, Achilles tendinitis, hyperinsulinemia, hyperuricemia, arthritis, and possibly cholelithiasis
   4. History of thyroid disease, liver disease, renal disease, or diabetes is a warning sign

E. Insulin resistance is associated with hyperlipidemia as well as hyperinsulinemia, obesity and hypertension in children and adolescents
   1. The body becomes resistant to the actions of insulin, resulting in overproduction of this hormone by the pancreas and the subsequent development of hyperinsulinemia
   2. This syndrome is a precursor of atherosclerotic cardiovascular disease and type 2 diabetes
   3. Puberty increases the extent of insulin resistance

IV. Diagnosis/Evaluation

A. History
   1. Ask about previous or present cardiovascular disease
   2. Inquire about presence or absence of CHD risk factors (see table CORONARY HEART DISEASE RISK FACTORS)

CORONARY HEART DISEASE RISK FACTORS OTHER THAN LOW-DENSITY LIPOPROTEIN CHOLESTEROL

Positive
- Family history of premature CHD
- Smoking
- Hypertension
- HDL cholesterol <35 mg/dL (0.9 mmol/L)
- Diabetes

Negative
- HDL cholesterol ≥60 mg/dL (1.6 mmol/L)

---

3. Explore past medical history including pancreatitis, renal disease, liver disease, vascular disease, diabetes mellitus, hypothyroidism, Cushing's syndrome, and immunologic disorders
4. Complete a medication history, focusing on drugs that elevate cholesterol levels (II.B.2.i.)
5. Explore amount of alcohol consumption
6. Determine amount and intensity of physical activity
7. Ask about occurrence of xanthomas and abdominal pain
8. If female, ask about menstrual history and type of hormone replacement therapy if applicable
9. Inquire about typical diet over a 24-hour period; to assess intake of LDL-raising nutrients, see table BRIEF DIETARY CAGE QUESTIONS

BRIEF DIETARY CAGE QUESTIONS

- **C** - Cheese (and other sources of dairy fats such as whole milk, ice cream, cream, whole fat yogurt)
- **A** - Animal fats (hamburger, hotdogs, sausage, fried foods, bologna, fatty cuts of meat)
- **G** - Got it away from home (high-fat meals purchased from or eaten in restaurants)
- **E** - Eat (extra) high-fat commercial products (candy, pastries, pies, doughnuts, cookies)

Adapted from National Institutes of Health. (2001). *Third report of the National Cholesterol Education Program (NCEP) Expert Panel on Detection, Evaluation, and Treatment of High Blood Cholesterol in Adults (Adult Treatment Panel III).* (NIH Publication 01-3670). Bethesda, MD: National Institutes of Health.

B. Physical Examination
   1. Measure blood pressure
   2. Measure height and weight
   3. Observe skin for cutaneous xanthomas
   4. Palpate thyroid
   5. Perform a complete heart and vascular exam
   6. Perform a complete abdominal exam; assess for hepatomegaly and splenomegaly

C. Differential Diagnosis: rule out all secondary causes listed under pathogenesis

D. Diagnostic Tests
   1. Selectively screen children >2 years of age in the following groups:
      a. Children whose parents, grandparents or first degree aunts or uncles have a history of coronary or peripheral vascular disease before the age of 55 years; fasting lipoprotein analysis is recommended
      b. Children whose parents have blood cholesterol levels ≥240 mg/dL; screen for total blood cholesterol level (may be nonfasting, but fasting provides better information)
         (1) If child's total blood cholesterol level is ≥200 mg/dL, obtain lipoprotein analysis
         (2) If child's total cholesterol level is borderline (170-199 mg/dL), repeat and average results; if the average of these two total cholesterol levels is >170 mg/dL perform lipoprotein analysis
      c. For children and adolescents with several risk factors for future CHD (smoking, obesity, diabetes mellitus, nephrotic syndrome, hypertension, sedentary lifestyle, excessive alcohol intake, use of certain medications such as retinoic acid, oral contraceptives, or anticonvulsants) or whose family history cannot be accurately determined, screening is at the discretion of the clinician and involves total blood cholesterol level and then lipoprotein if needed
   2. Lipoprotein analysis includes the following:
      a. Measurement of fasting levels of total cholesterol, total triglyceride, and HDP cholesterol
      b. From the values above, LDL cholesterol is calculated: LDL cholesterol + (Total cholesterol – HDL cholesterol) – (Triglycerides/5)
   3. Results from lipoprotein analysis will determine when patient needs further diagnostic testing (see section on Plan/Management, V.B.) and table that follows for classification of levels

ATP III Classification of LDL, Total, and HDL Cholesterol (mg/dL)

LDL cholesterol

<110	Acceptable
110-129	Borderline
≥130	High

Total cholesterol

<170	Acceptable
170-199	Borderline
≥200	High

HDL cholesterol

<35	Considered a risk factor

Triglycerides

>200	Significance of elevated triglycerides unknown; >200 is related to obesity

Adapted from National Cholesterol Education Program Report of the Expert Panel on Blood Cholesterol Levels in Children and Adolescents (1991). Bethesda, MD: National Heart, Lung, and Blood Institute Information Center

V. Plan/Management

   A. Recommendations for primary prevention of hyperlipidemia in children
      1. No restriction of fat or cholesterol for infants <2 years of age; skim or low-fat milk is not recommended in the first 2 years of life
      2. After age 2, children and adolescents should gradually assume a healthy diet by eating a wide variety of foods and caloric intake should be adequate for growth and development to reach or maintain desirable body weights
         a. Children should consume 5 or more daily servings of fruits and vegetables
         b. Children should consume 6-11 daily servings of whole-grain and other grain foods
         c. Children should consume adequate amounts of dietary fiber (Age +5 g/day)
      3. Children and adolescents (2-18 years) should have the following pattern of nutrient intake:
         a. Saturated fatty acids <10% of total calories
         b. Total fat over several days of ≥30% of total calories and no less than 20% of total calories
         c. Dietary cholesterol <300 mg per day
      4. Selectively screen "at risk" children >2 years of age (see Section IV. Diagnostic Tests for recommended screening procedures)
      5. Efforts should be made to identify and eliminate risk factors for coronary heart disease
      6. Encourage children at any age to have an active life-style with strenuous exercise and the avoidance of tobacco
      7. Recommend that family access government-sponsored websites (see following table)

Government-Sponsored Websites

Diet	www.nhlbi.nih.gov/chd
	www.nhlbi.nih.gov/subsites/index.htm -- then click Healthy Weight
	www.nhlbi.nih.gov/hbp
	www.nutrition.gov
Physical activity	www.fitness.gov
Body weight	www.nhlbi.nih.gov/subsites/index.htm -- then click Healthy Weight
Cholesterol	www.nhlbi.nih.gov/chd
Blood pressure	www.nhlbi.nih.gov/hbp
Smoking cessation	www.cdc.gov/tobacco/sgr_tobacco_use.htm

B. Management plan for children >2 years of age who were selectively screened because of parental history of hyperlipidemia, family history of coronary artery disease (CAD), and several risk factors for CAD (see section IV.D. Diagnostic Tests); refer children <2 years of age to a specialist
   1. Children who have acceptable LDL cholesterol level (LDL-C <110 mg/dL) need routine care (counseling about prudent diet, elimination of risk factors and maintaining a healthy life style) and repeat lipoprotein analysis every 5 years
   2. For children who have borderline LDL cholesterol (LDL-C 110-129 mg/dL) offer advice about risk factors for cardiovascular disease, begin Step-One diet and other risk factor interventions; re-evaluate lipid profile in one year (see V.D. for dietary therapy and table on following page)
   3. For children who have high LDL cholesterol (LDL-C ≥130 mg/dL) examine for secondary causes (thyroid, liver, and renal disorders) and familial disorders, screen all family members, begin Step-One diet, and then, Step-Two diet if necessary
   4. Consider drug therapy only after consulting lipid specialist
      a. Consider drug therapy in children >10 years of age after an adequate trial of diet therapy (6-12 months) whose LDL cholesterol level remains >190 mg/dL or whose LDL cholesterol remains ≥160 mg/dL and there is a family history of premature cardiovascular disease or two or more risk factors
      b. Limited data are available in children regarding the long-term efficacy of drug therapy
         (1) Statins (HMG-CoA reductase inhibitors) are used most frequently today
         (2) In the past, bile acid sequestrants were the most commonly used first-line drugs but they have gastrointestinal adverse affects and their efficacy may be lower than other classes
         (3) See tables (SUMMARY OF STATINS, BILE ACID SEQUESTRANTS, NICOTINIC ACID, FIBRIC ACID DERIVATIVES, EZETIMIBE) for lipid-lowering drugs available for use in adults

C. Treatment of triglyceridemia in children
   1. Refer any child with triglyceride levels >300 mg/L to a lipid specialist
   2. Nonpharmacologic therapy as weight reduction in overweight patients and increased physical activity is recommended
   3. Children are often prescribed a fibric acid drug, or a combination of a fibric acid drug and a preparation of fish oil containing at least 35% eicosapentaenoic acid and docohexapentanoic acid

D. Dietary therapy occurs in 2 steps, Step I and Step II diets, and is aimed at reducing intake of saturated fatty acids, cholesterol and at promoting weight loss in overweight patients by eliminating excess total calories and increasing physical activity (see following table on foods to eat and avoid in diet therapy)
   1. Step I Diet should be prescribed and explained; involves intake of the following:
      a. Saturated fat: 8-10% of total calories
      b. Total fat: 30% or less of total calories
      c. <300 mg of cholesterol per day
   2. Step II Diet or intensive dietary therapy (often dietician is consulted or implements the diet therapy); involves intake of the following:
      a. Saturated fat intake: <7% of calories
      b. Cholesterol: <200 mg per day
      c. Weight reduction of overweight patients and increased physical activity should be encouraged

NUTRITION RECOMMENDATIONS

Food Items to Choose More Often	Food Items to Choose Less Often	Recommendation for Weight Reduction	Recommendations for Increased Physical Activity
Breads and Cereals ≥6 servings per day, adjusted to caloric needs Refined whole-grain breads and cereals, brown rice, dry beans, and peas **Vegetables** 3-5 servings per day fresh, frozen, or canned, without added fat, sauce, or salt **Fruits** 2-4 servings per day fresh, frozen, canned, dried **Dairy Products** 2-3 servings per day Fat-free, ½%, 1% milk, buttermilk, yogurt, cottage cheese; fat-free & low-fat cheese **Eggs** ≤2 egg yolks per week Egg whites or egg substitute **Fish, Meat, Poultry** ≤5 oz per day Fish, lean cuts loin; extra lean hamburger; cold cuts made with lean meat or soy protein; skinless poultry **Fats and Oils** Amount adjusted to caloric level Unsaturated fats: Olive oil, canola oil, peanut oil, vegetable oils, nuts, fish **TLC Diet Options** Stanol/sterol-containing margarines (Benacol); viscous fiber food sources; barley, oats, psyllium, apples, bananas, berries, citrus fruits, nectarines, peaches, pears, plums, prunes, broccoli, Brussels sprouts, carrots, dry beans, peas, soy products (tofu, miso)	**Breads and Cereals** Many bakery products, including doughnuts, biscuits, butter rolls, muffins, croissants, sweet rolls, Danish, cakes, pies, coffee cakes, cookies Many grain-based snacks, including chips, cheese puffs, snack mix, regular crackers, buttered popcorn **Vegetables** Vegetables fried or prepared with butter, cheese, or cream sauce **Fruits** Fruits fried or served with butter or cream **Dairy Products** Whole milk, 2% milk, whole-milk yogurt, ice cream, cream, cheese **Eggs** Egg yolks, whole eggs **Meat, Poultry, Fish** Higher fat meat cuts: ribs, t-bone steak, regular hamburger, bacon, sausage; cold cuts: salami, bologna, hot dogs; organ meats: liver, brains, sweetbreads; poultry with skin; fried meat; fried poultry; fried fish. **Saturated Fats** Coconut oil, butter, stick margarine	**Weigh Regularly** Record weight, BMI & waist circumference **Lose Weight Gradually** Goal: lose 10% of body weight in 6 months. Lose ½ to 1 lb per week **Develop Healthy Eating Patterns** ✓ Choose healthy foods (see Column 1) ✓ Reduce intake of foods in Column 2 ✓ Limit number of eating occasions ✓ Select sensible portion sizes ✓ Avoid second helpings ✓ Identify and reduce hidden fat by reading food labels to choose products lower in saturated fat and calories, and ask about ingredients in ready-to-eat foods prepared away from home ✓ Identify and reduce sources of excess carbohydrates such as fat-free and regular crackers; cookies and other desserts; snacks; and sugar-containing beverages	**Make Physical Activity Part of Daily Routines** ✓ Reduce sedentary time ✓ Walk, wheel, or bike-ride more, drive less; take the stairs instead of an elevator; get off the bus a few stops early and walk the remaining distance; mow the lawn with a push mower, rake leaves; garden; push a stroller; clean the house; do exercises or pedal a stationary bike while watching television; play actively with children; take a brisk 10-minutes walk before work, during your work break and after dinner **Make Physical Activity Part of Exercise or Recreational Activities** ✓ Walk, wheel, or jog; bicycle or use an arm pedal bicycle; swim or do water aerobics; play basketball; join a sports team; play wheelchair sports; golf (pull cart or carry clubs); canoe; cross-country ski; dance; take part in an exercise program at work, home, school or gym

SUMMARY OF STATINS (HMG-CoA REDUCTASE INHIBITORS)

Available drugs	Atorvastatin (Lipitor) Lovastatin (Mevacor) Simvastatin (Zocor) Pravastatin (Pravachol) Fluvastatin (Lescol)
Lipid/lipoprotein effects	LDL decrease 18-55% HDL increase 5-15% TG decrease 7-30%
Contraindications	Active or chronic liver disease
Use with caution	Concomitant use of cyclosporine, gemfibrozil, niacin, antifungal agents
Major adverse effects	Elevated hepatic transaminase, myopathy, upper and lower gastrointestinal complaints; use with anticoagulant may increase prothrombin time
Comments	Dosages should be adjusted at 6-week intervals Order liver function tests at baseline, 12 weeks after starting, and periodically thereafter Advise patient to stop therapy and order creatine kinase if patient reports muscle discomfort, weakness, or brown urine Pravastatin metabolism is least affected by other drugs Atorvastatin has the greatest LDL lowering effect Do not take at same time as grapefruit juice Generally, take at evening meal or at bedtime In general, every doubling of dose lowers LDL by approximately 6% Statins reduce the level of C-reactive protein (an inflammatory marker & emerging risk factor for CHD)

SUMMARY OF BILE ACID SEQUESTRANTS

Available drugs	Cholestyramine (Questran Light) Colestipol (Colestid tablets) Colesevelam (Welchol)
Lipid/lipoprotein effects	LDL decrease 15-30% HDL increase 3-5% TG no change or increase
Contraindications	Familial dysbetalipoproteinemia Triglycerides >400 mg/dL
Use with caution	Triglycerides >200 mg/dL
Major adverse effects	Gastrointestinal distress, constipation Decreased absorption of other drugs (take other meds at least one hour before or four to six hours after the sequestrants) Pancreatitis in patients with hypertriglyceridemia
Comments	To reduce GI complaints suggest the following: • Take medicine slowly, reducing amount of swallowed air • Increase fluid and fiber intake and drink with pulpier liquids such as orange juice • May combine with psyllium hydrophilic mucilloid such as Metamucil

SUMMARY OF NICOTINIC ACID

Available drugs	Nicotinic acid derivative* (Niaspan) Crystalline (immediate release) Sustained (timed-release)
Lipid/lipoprotein effects	LDL decrease 5-25% HDL increase 15-35% TG decrease 20-50%
Contraindications	Chronic liver disease, severe gout
Use with caution	High doses (>3 g/day) in type 2 diabetes mellitus; gout, or hyperuricemia
Major adverse effects	Flushing (less with Niaspan) and itching of skin, gastrointestinal distress, hepatotoxicity (especially sustained-release form); hyperglycemia, hyperuricemia or gout limit its use
Comments	Take enteric-coated aspirin before dose to lessen adverse effects Liver function should be evaluated before beginning niacin and 6-8 weeks after reaching a daily dose of 1,500 mg, 6-8 weeks after reaching the maximum daily dose, then at least annually Blood glucose and uric acid should be monitored initially, then 6-8 weeks after starting therapy, then annually or more frequently if indicated Lowers Lp(a), an emerging risk factor for CHD

*Swallow whole; take at bedtime with low-fat meal or snack. Avoid concomitant alcohol and hot beverage.

SUMMARY OF FIBRIC ACID DERIVATIVES

Available drugs	Gemfibrozil (Lopid) Fenofibrate (Tricor) Clofibrate (Atromid-S)
Lipid/lipoprotein effects	LDL decrease 5-20% (may be increased in patients with high TG) HDL increase 10-20% TG decrease 20-50%
Contraindications	Severe renal disease Severe hepatic disease
Use with caution	Patients with history of gallstones; increased risk of rhabdomyolysis with statins; potentiates effects of anticoagulants
Major adverse effects	Gastrointestinal distress, cholesterol gallstones, myopathy
Comments	Fenofibrate appears to reduce LDL by a greater amount than other fibrates

SUMMARY OF EZETIMIBE

Lipid/lipoprotein effects	LDL decrease HDL increase TG decrease
Contraindications	Hepatic insufficiency
Use with caution	Data unavailable
Major adverse effects	Upper and lower gastrointestinal complaints; myopathy
Comments	Research is limited Patients may take drug with or without food

E. Management of insulin resistance
    1. Periodically measure blood pressure, fasting plasma glucose, and lipids
    2. Assessment, prevention, and treatment of overweight/obesity should be a priority
    3. Weight control, lifestyle modification, and early detection of type 2 diabetes is recommended to improve risk profiles for cardiovascular disease and type 2 diabetes

F. Follow-up is based on results of screening cholesterol levels and, if needed, subsequent lipoprotein analysis; patients on drug therapy should be reevaluated at 6-8 weeks with frequent follow-up appointments

HYPERTHYROIDISM

I. Definition: Condition that results when tissues are exposed to an excess of thyroid hormone; clinical manifestation is termed thyrotoxicosis

II. Pathogenesis:

A. Typically results from the uncontrolled secretion or release of thyroid hormones, thyroxine (T_4) and triiodothyronine (T_3), into the blood stream

B. Congenital hyperthyroidism or neonatal thyrotoxicosis occurs almost exclusively in infants of mothers with Graves' disease; due to transplacental passage of maternal-stimulating immunoglobulins

C. Acquired hyperthyroidism in childhood and adolescence is typically due to the following:
    1. Graves' disease is by far the most common cause, accounting for over 95% of pediatric cases; Graves' disease is an autoimmune condition that is also referred to as diffuse toxic goiter and is related to abnormalities associated with TSH receptor antibodies
    2. Next more common cause is lymphocytic thyroiditis or Hashimoto's thyroiditis
    3. Uncommon causes are subacute thyroiditis, thyroid nodule, and postpartum thyroiditis

III. Clinical Presentation (see table DIFFERENTIATING FEATURES OF CONDITIONS)

A. Congenital hyperthyroidism; disease can be life-threatening
    1. Self-limited disease that lasts several weeks to over 6 months
    2. Signs include low birth weight, failure to gain weight despite hyperphagia, microcephaly, hyperactivity, tachycardia, tachypnea, prominent eyes, and thyromegaly
    3. Clinical manifestations include irritability, vomiting, diarrhea, hepatosplenomegaly, jaundice, thrombocytopenia, and cardiac failure

B. Graves' Disease
    1. Often has an insidious onset; patients may be asymptomatic for months
    2. Patients typically have one or more of the following complaints:
        a. Nervousness which manifests as irritability, inability to concentrate, emotional lability, or insomnia
        b. Weight loss may be present even though appetite is often increased
        c. Increase in bowel movements or diarrhea
        d. Heat intolerance is a common symptom
        e. Palpitations may be a troublesome, intermittent complaint
    3. Children often have acceleration of growth and advanced skeletal maturity
    4. The following are signs:
        a. Hair may be fine and silky; thinning of hair may occur
        b. Nails may develop onycholysis (irregular separation of the nail plate from the nail bed near its distal end), psoriasis (ridges in nail), or onychomycosis (thickening and yellowing of nail)
        c. Skin may have diffuse hyperpigmentation, particularly over the extensor surfaces of the elbows, knees, and small joints
        d. Pretibial myxedema that is characterized by erythematous, mildly scaly, indurated, nontender plaques on the skin of the ankles and pretibial areas may occur

      e.   Eye changes are usually milder in children than adults and are often transitory; symptoms disappear when euthyroidism is restored
- (1)   Conjunctivitis
- (2)   Lid lag
- (3)   Lid retraction with increased scleral visibility above and below the iris often gives the patient the appearance of "staring"

      f.   Thyroid may be visibly or palpably enlarged; thrill can sometimes be palpated or bruit can sometimes be auscultated

      g.   Postural tremor, particularly of the hands, is commonly found

      h.   Skeletal muscle wasting with proximal myopathy develops as the disease progresses

      i.   Long-standing conditions may lead to osteoporosis and back pain

      j.   In severe cases, signs of heart failure may be present

      k.   Other autoimmune diseases such as type 1 diabetes mellitus, rheumatoid arthritis, nephritis, and vitiligo may coexist with Graves' disease

C.   Thyroid storm, a life-threatening syndrome, occurs with decompensated hyperthyroidism
1.   Stressful events such as trauma and infection often precipitate an episode
2.   Symptoms such as nausea, vomiting, and abdominal pain may precede the storm
3.   Agitation, confusion, delirium, psychosis, or coma with high fever and diaphoresis may occur
4.   Tachycardia is always present; tachyarrhythmias may occur

D.   Lymphocytic thyroiditis or Hashimoto's thyroiditis
1.   Presentation is similar to Graves' disease
2.   Hashimoto's thyroiditis tends to subside whereas Graves' disease is more persistent
3.   Thyroid gland feels rubbery, enlarged, and sometimes asymmetrical

E.   Subacute thyroiditis (also called painful thyroiditis or de Quervain's thyroiditis)
1.   Symptoms frequently develop after a respiratory or viral prodrome
2.   Severe pain in the thyroid area which often extends to ear on same side may occur
3.   Low grade fever and symptoms of hypermetabolism are often present
4.   With exception of exophthalmus and pretibial myxedema, presentation is similar to Graves' disease
5.   Typically the erythrocyte sedimentation rate (ESR) is markedly elevated
6.   As the disease progresses, patients may become mildly hypothyroid and eventually return to a euthyroid state with complete recovery within approximately 2-6 months

F.   Hyperfunctioning nodules: Extent of patient's condition is positively related to mass of the nodule; nodules >4 cm in diameter often produce signs and symptoms of thyrotoxicosis

G.   Postpartum thyroiditis
1.   Develops in 5-10% of females within the first year after delivery
2.   Typically has an initial hyperthyroid phase, followed by hypothyroidism, and eventually returns to euthyroid state; symptoms may persist for months

DIFFERENTIATING FEATURES OF CONDITIONS CAUSING THYROTOXICOSIS

Cause	Thyroid Gland	FT$_4$I	TSH	RAIU
Graves' disease	Diffusely enlarged	↑	Suppressed	↑
Subacute thyroiditis	Tender, firm, nodular	↑	Suppressed	↓
Hashimoto's thyroiditis	Nontender, enlarged	↑	Suppressed	↓
Postpartum thyroiditis	Small, painless	↑	Suppressed	↓
Hyperfunctioning nodule	Firm, enlarged	↑	Suppressed	↑
TSH-secreting pituitary tumor	Enlarged	↑	Normal or high	↑

FT$_4$I: free thyroxine index; TSH: thyroid stimulating hormone; RAIU: radioactive iodine uptake

IV.   Diagnosis/Evaluation

    A.   History
1.   A complete review of systems is needed because symptoms may be subtle and involve every system of the body
2.   Inquire about changes in weight; ask about growth and development
3.   Obtain a complete medication history

4. Inquire about personal and family medical history; risk factors include previous thyroid dysfunction, goiter, surgery affecting thyroid gland, diabetes, vitiligo, pernicious anemia, leukotrichia (prematurely gray hair), and autoimmune diseases
5. Inquire about abnormal laboratory tests that suggest hyperthyroidism: hypercalcemia, elevated alkaline phosphatase, and elevated hepatocellular enzymes

B. Physical Examination
1. Observe general appearance, paying particular attention to signs of nervousness or hyperactivity
2. Measure blood pressure, resting pulse, temperature, and weight
3. Inspect and palpate skin, noting pigmentation pattern, moistness, and turgor
4. Inspect hair for texture and thickness, nails for ridges, discoloration or splitting
5. Examine fingers and toes for thickening
6. Examine eyes, noting exophthalmos, lid lag, and/or extraocular movements
7. Test visual acuity
8. Palpate for lymphadenopathy
9. Observe the neck and palpate the thyroid, noting thrills, nodules, diffuse enlargement, firmness, and tenderness; measure size (see section on HYPOTHYROIDISM)
10. Auscultate thyroid for bruits
11. Auscultate the heart, noting murmurs and rate and rhythm
12. Assess the abdomen for hepatomegaly and splenomegaly
13. Do a complete neuromuscular exam, noting fast relaxation of tendon reflexes
14. Evaluate for tremor (can place piece of paper on outstretched hand to observe for movement of paper with slight tremors)
15. Test muscular strength; focusing on signs of proximal muscle weakness
16. Assess lower extremities, noting pretibial myxedema

C. Differential Diagnosis
1. Neoplasm is often suspected due to weight loss and weakness that typically accompany hyperthyroidism
2. Congestive heart failure and atrial fibrillation
3. Psychological problems such as panic disorder and depression
4. Tremors such as essential, physiological, and cerebellar
5. Suppressed TSH and elevated T_4 levels occur in conditions not associated with hyperthyroidism
   a. Estrogen administration or pregnancy raises thyroid binding globulin, resulting in high T_4 levels but normal free T_4 and sensitive TSH
   b. Glucocorticoids, amiodarone therapy, dopamine therapy, severe illness, and pituitary dysfunction may result in suppressed TSH in the absence of hyperthyroidism

D. Diagnostic Tests (see table DIFFERENTIATING FEATURES OF CONDITIONS in III.G. for typical test results with various types of hyperthyroidism)
1. Consider ordering a free T_4 to confirm the diagnosis (expected values should be higher than normal); always order both T_4 and T_3 if pituitary problems are suspected
   a. Free T_4 measures unbound thyroxine in serum
   b. The alternative, second-line test, a total T_4, can be altered with estrogen and pregnancy
2. If free T_4 levels are normal, order T_3 level because approximately 5% of hyperthyroid patients have normal T_4 levels
3. Consider ordering 24-hour radioiodine uptake (RAIU) test in two situations
   a. To determine the correct dosage of radioactive iodine to treat Graves' disease or toxic multinodular goiter
   b. To differentiate Graves' disease and multinodular goiter from subacute thyroiditis and silent thyroiditis (in both types of thyroiditis the RAIU test will be low; whereas in Graves' disease and multinodular goiter it is elevated); test probably not needed to confirm diagnosis of Graves' disease if patient has ophthalmopathy, clinical hyperthyroidism, and diffusely enlarged thyroid
4. Thyroid autoantibodies including TSH receptor antibody (TSI, TSHRab or TRab): not ordered routinely except in selected cases such as pregnancy
5. Thyroid scan (either ^{123}I or technetium-99m) particularly useful in assessing the functional status of palpable thyroid irregularities or nodules related to a toxic goiter
6. In females, consider performing a urine pregnancy test
7. Computed axial tomography (CAT scan) or magnetic resonance imaging (MRI) of the orbit is often recommended for patients with eye problems, particularly those patients with unilateral eye signs
8. Consider dual energy radiographic absorptiometry to determine osteoporosis

V. Plan/Management

A. Treatment of congenital hyperthyroidism (refer to pediatric endocrinologist); needs immediate treatment to prevent dangerous sequelae to nervous system

B. Three treatments (radioactive iodine, antithyroid drugs, and surgery) are available for acquired hyperthyroidism; patients and/or parents should be advised of risks and benefits of each treatment and collaborate in making decisions about their plans of care

C. Radioactive iodine (sodium iodide, I^{131}, Iodotope) is treatment of choice for most adults and adolescents who have Graves' disease and severe symptoms of thyrotoxicosis with multinodular goiter and single hyperfunctioning adenoma; recommended by some specialists for children as well
   1. Many experts recommend an ablative dose of radioactive iodine whereas some prefer to render the patient euthyroid with smaller doses
   2. Radioactive iodine works slowly; most patients become euthyroid in 8-26 weeks
   3. Monitor free T_4 and T_3 every 6-8 weeks (see section on HYPOTHYROIDISM)
      a. Many patients become hypothyroid and require lifelong thyroid replacement therapy
      b. Therapy with levothyroxine is started when patient become either euthyroid or hypothyroid (see section in HYPOTHYROIDISM)
   4. Radioactive iodine is not associated with increased risk of malignancy or genetic damage; however, many clinicians are reluctant to use in children, particularly <5 years of age
   5. Other considerations include the following:
      a. Eye symptoms usually improve
      b. Therapy contraindicated in pregnant females; always order pregnancy testing in patients who are scheduled for this therapy
      c. Females should use birth control 6 months after therapy, even though studies have not found teratogenic effects from therapy
      d. Breast-feeding is contraindicated

D. Antithyroid drugs, propylthiouracil (PTU) and methimazole (Tapazole)
   1. Often preferred initial treatment for children, pregnant females, and patients scheduled for surgery
   2. Antithyroid drugs should **not** be continued long-term
   3. Drugs will control excessive production of thyroid hormone, but about half of patients will have a remission if no other treatment is instituted
   4. One of the following drugs is usually prescribed:
      a. Methimazole (Tapazole) is often first choice because it is long-acting; initial dose: 0.4 to 1.0 mg/kg/day divided in 3 doses; as soon as euthyroidism is achieved, reduce dose to 5-10 mg/day
      b. Propylthiouracil (PTU) has the most rapid onset with initial dose of 5-10 mg/kg/day in three divided doses
   5. May need to give both these drugs at higher dosages if patient is severely ill
   6. It takes 4-6 weeks for patients taking methimazole and 6-12 weeks for patients taking PTU to reach euthyroid state; monitor with thyroid tests every 6 weeks
   7. Patients usually remain on drugs for 1-2 years, then drug is gradually withdrawn with the hope of permanent remission
   8. Instruct patient to call provider if severe sore mouth, sore throat, or fever develop (signs of agranulocytosis, a rare side effect of both drugs)
   9. Order WBC count before initiating therapy and then periodically during the first 3 months of treatment; however, agranulocytosis occurs so rapidly that periodic monitoring is not considered cost-effective by some experts
   10. A transient rash may occur; symptomatically treat with an antihistamine

E. β-blockers may be initiated to control cardiovascular hypersensitivity during the 4-8 week period before maximal clinical response to drug therapy is reached

F. Surgical therapy is a less frequently considered option due to potential complications such as hypoparathyroidism and vocal cord paralysis

G. Thyroid storm, a medical emergency, requires prompt therapy
   1. Antithyroid drugs are often recommended and coadministered with corticosteroids, beta-adrenergic blockers and iopanoic acid (Telepaque)
   2. Other supportive measures include fluids, nutritional support, and electrolyte corrections

H. Ophthalmopathy
    1. For mild cases prescribe eye lubricants such as artificial tears, petrolatum, or mineral oil ocular ointment (Lacri-Lube), apply 1/4" as needed
    2. Local mechanical therapies such as sunglasses, elevation of head of bed, and eye protectors during sleep are helpful

I. Hashimoto's thyroiditis does not require pharmacological treatment, however thyroid hormone levels must be monitored periodically as approximately 50% of these patients develop hypothyroidism
    1. Advise patient that condition will usually disappear in 4-10 weeks
    2. If symptoms are bothersome, β-blockers may be given

J. Subacute thyroiditis is a self-limiting condition and does not require permanent therapy
    1. Nonsteroidal anti-inflammatory agents may be prescribed to relieve the pain; occasionally oral prednisone 20-40 mg per day in divided doses and tapered over two to four weeks is needed to control pain
    2. May prescribe β-blockers or anti-thyroid drugs when patient has thyrotoxic symptoms

K. Treatment of single, hyperfunctioning adenoma is radioactive iodine

L. Postpartum thyroiditis
    1. Acute symptoms are treated with β-blockers
    2. Antithyroid drugs are not indicated because the symptoms are caused by release of preformed T_3 and T_4 from the damaged gland
    3. When patient's symptoms are severe or longstanding in the hypothyroid phase, replacement of the thyroid hormone is indicated

M. Immediately refer patients with pituitary tumors to an endocrinologist

N. Patient education
    1. Consider a supplemental multivitamin; additional calcium and vitamin D may rebuild bone density lost during period of hyperthyroidism; remind patients that increased thyroid hormone is a risk factor for osteoporosis
    2. Successful treatment of hyperthyroidism may be followed by serious depression; warn patient and family of this potential risk and frequently monitor mental health

O. Follow Up
    1. Patients treated with radioactive iodine
        a. Order free T_4 levels every 4-8 weeks until patient becomes euthyroid or hypothyroid and thyroid hormone replacement is needed
        b. Once patients are stable, schedule visits at 3 months, then 6 months, and then annually
    2. Patients on antithyroid drugs
        a. Free T_4 level should be measured after a month of treatment and every 2-3 months thereafter
        b. Order WBC after several weeks of therapy and after any changes in drug doses
        c. Order liver enzymes every 3-6 months when patient is stable
    3. Patients on β-blockers should be initially followed every 1-3 months, and then periodically depending on symptoms
    4. Patients who are not treated with medications should be followed periodically based on their diagnosis and clinical presentation (i.e., every 3-12 months)

HYPOTHYROIDISM

I.   Definition: Condition in which serum thyroid hormone levels are not sufficient to maintain normal intracellular hormone levels

II.   Pathogenesis

A.   Congenital hypothyroidism
1.   Permanent primary hypothyroidism is due to one of the following:
a.   Most common cause is irreversible failure of thyroid gland to produce sufficient thyroid hormone due to an ectopic thyroid gland which failed to migrate properly during fetal development
b.   Second most common cause is hypoplasia or aplasia of the thyroid gland
c.   Third most common cause is an enzymatic deficiency resulting in an inborn error of thyroid hormone synthesis, secretion, or utilization
2.   Another type is transient primary hypothyroidism related to maternal iodine deficiency, fetal or neonatal exposure to iodine, maternal antithyroid drugs, or maternal antibodies
3.   Permanent secondary hypothyroidism can occur and is usually associated with congenital hypopituitarism

B.   Acquired hypothyroidism
1.   Primary hypothyroidism, the most common form, is the result of a defect in the thyroid gland causing it to produce insufficient thyroid hormone
a.   Frequent cause is Hashimoto's thyroiditis (also called chronic thyroiditis)
b.   Idiopathic hypothyroidism is most likely an autoimmune disease
c.   Post-therapeutic hypothyroidism occurs after treatment (usually for Graves' disease) with radioactive iodine, surgery, or thioamide drugs
d.   Transient hypothyroidism is often associated with acute or subacute thyroiditis which may have a viral etiology
e.   Hypothyroidism can occur after hyperthyroidism in females following pregnancy (postpartum thyroiditis)
f.   Less common causes include iodine ingestion, neck irradiation, and certain medications such as lithium or para-aminosalicylic acid
2.   Secondary hypothyroidism is due to the failure of the pituitary gland to stimulate the thyroid to produce sufficient T_4 levels; often occurs from postpartum pituitary infarction, granulomatous disease, or cranial mass lesion
3.   Tertiary hypothyroidism is due to the malfunctioning of the hypothalamic-pituitary axis as a result of deficient secretion of thyroid releasing hormone (TRH) from the hypothalamus or lack of thyroid stimulating hormone (TSH) from the pituitary

III. Clinical Presentation

A.   Newborns with congenital hypothyroidism often have the following:
1.   Since the advent of screening programs for newborns, affected children are usually diagnosed and treated early before development of symptoms
2.   Symptoms may appear in the first 2 weeks, but some infants are asymptomatic for the first month
3.   Subtle abnormalities (persistent jaundice [bilirubin >10 mg/dl after 3 days of age], temperature instability, hypoactivity, poor feeding, delayed first stooling) appear first
4.   Later, classic signs and symptoms appear: Thickened tongue, coarse facies, facial edema, hirsute forehead, umbilical hernia, lethargy, irritability, delayed growth, short extremities, persistently open posterior fontanelle, and large anterior fontanelle
5.   Irreversible mental changes may occur before any symptoms are present
6.   If treated from early months, infants usually have normal intellectual function and linear growth; if therapy is delayed for three months, there is risk of mental retardation

B.   Severity of acquired hypothyroidism depends on the duration and extent of hormone deficiency; symptoms range from subtle symptoms to severe, multisystem problems with myxedema
1.   Onset is often insidious and children with this disorder may not be identified for a long time after onset
2.   In children, initial complaint may be shortness of stature or poor growth

3. Early symptoms have an insidious onset and consist of fatigue, dry skin, nail changes, slight weight gain, cold intolerance, constipation, and, in female adolescents, heavy menses
4. As disease progresses, following symptoms present: dry skin, yellow skin, coarse hair, hair loss of lateral eyebrows, eyelid edema, decreased sweating, slight alopecia, hoarseness, weight gain, cognitive changes, slow speech, forgetfulness, depression, and hypersomnia
5. Myxedematous changes occur in the later stage with thickened, scaly and "doughy" skin, enlarged tongue, muscle weakness, joint complaints, hearing impairment, bradycardia, possibly cardiac enlargement, pleural effusion, and ascites
6. Children have the following additional manifestations: poor growth and development, decreased activity level, skeletal maturation delay and limb length reduction which leads to increased upper to lower segment ratio, delayed puberty; mental retardation does not occur
7. Myxedema coma is an infrequent sequelae of long-standing disease
   a. Is often precipitated by intercurrent illness
   b. Symptoms, in addition to obtundation or coma, include hypothermia, bradycardia, respiratory failure, and possibly cardiovascular collapse
8. Patients with acquired hypothyroidism due to Hashimoto's thyroiditis have variable symptoms and typically experience transient hyperthyroidism that progresses to hypothyroidism whereas others remain euthyroid; in rare cases, the patient may change from hypothyroid to euthyroid or hyperthyroid

C. With malfunctioning of the hypothalamic-pituitary axis, there may be loss of axillary and pubic hair, amenorrhea, and postural hypotension; low levels of TSH and T_4 will be present

D. Nodules
   1. Goiter or thyroid nodules can occur; almost always benign and treatment is symptomatic, common in iodine-deficient areas
   2. Solitary nodules are uncommon in children

E. The following groups of individuals are at high risk for developing hypothyroidism
   1. Newborns
   2. Patients with a strong family history of thyroid disease
   3. New mothers in the postpartal period
   4. Individuals with autoimmune diseases (e.g., type 1 diabetes, Addison's disease)
   5. Patients exposed to certain medications (lithium carbonate, iodide, amiodarone)

IV. Diagnosis/Evaluation

A. History
   1. A complete review of systems is needed because symptoms are subtle and may involve every system of the body
   2. Ask about pain and swelling or enlargement in the neck
   3. Ask about history of radiation to the neck
   4. Inquire about previous endocrine problems in past or family medical history
   5. Obtain a complete medication history
   6. In adolescent females, determine date, characteristics, and duration of last menstrual period
   7. If patient was previously diagnosed with thyroid disease, ascertain past symptoms, treatments, and responses; in past, patients were frequently treated with medications for reasons that are unacceptable by today's standards

B. Physical Examination
   1. Observe overall appearance, noting slow movements and dull facies
   2. Measure height and weight; in children plot on growth chart, comparing with past measurements
   3. Measure blood pressure, resting pulse, temperature, and weight
      a. Diastolic pressure may be increased
      b. Heart rate may be low or normal
   4. Perform a complete dermatologic examination
   5. Inspect head for coarseness and thinning of hair, thinning of eyebrows, thickened tongue
   6. Perform a complete eye examination
   7. Assess for lymphadenopathy
   8. Inspect the neck; fully extend neck and observe from front and side; observe for prominences and scars (evidence of previous surgery)

9.	Palpate neck and thyroid for the following:
	a.	Tenderness
	b.	Consistency (i.e., firmness, fluctuance)
	c.	Measure size of gland
	d.	Note whether there is a focal nodule or diffuse growth
	e.	The easiest method to palpate infant's thyroid is to place the infant supine with the neck hyperextended
10.	Auscultate thyroid for bruits
11.	Determine point of maximal impulse (PMI) as an indirect method for uncovering dilation and hypertrophy of the heart
12.	Auscultate heart, noting rate, rhythm, and murmurs
13.	Do a complete lung exam
14.	Palpate for splenomegaly
15.	Auscultate the abdomen, noting bowel sounds which may be diminished in hypothyroidism
16.	Perform a musculoskeletal examination
17.	Perform a complete neurological exam; tendon reflexes may have a brisk contraction and a prolonged relaxation period in hypothyroidism
18.	Perform a mental status examination

C.	Differential Diagnosis: The following conditions mimic certain characteristics of hypothyroidism
	1.	Ischemic heart disease
	2.	Nephrotic syndrome
	3.	Cirrhosis
	4.	Depression

D.	Diagnostic Tests
	1.	Screening for congenital hypothyroidism
		a.	Newborn screening is performed in all US states, but approaches vary
		b.	In most states newborns are tested for thyroxine (T_4) and/or thyroid stimulating hormone (TSH); generally a T_4 value <10% or a TSH >20 mU/L serves as cutoff for further testing
		c.	Timing of screening also varies
			(1)	TSH surges immediately after birth, thus most facilities perform screening close to discharge to avoid false-positive results; the most desirable time is 2-6 days of age
			(2)	In some states, two screening samples are routinely collected—one at birth and a second sample at 2-6 weeks of age
		d.	Neonates with normal thyroid tests can develop hypothyroidism during the first weeks of life; retest all infants who present with symptoms of hypothyroidism
		e.	Infants with abnormal screening results need confirmatory diagnosis with an additional sample to measure serum free T_4 and TSH
			(1)	If diagnosis is confirmed, technetium scans or thyroid sonography are usually ordered to determine exact cause of thyroid underactivity
			(2)	Treatment should never be delayed for testing
	2.	Screen for thyroid disease in the following individuals:
		a.	All symptomatic individuals
		b.	Children with Down syndrome should be retested at age 3 months
		c.	Past history of medically or surgically treated thyroid disease (screen annually)
		d.	Past history of receiving supervoltage x-ray therapy to neck for nonthyroid cancer
		e.	Patients with other autoimmune diseases and those with cognitive dysfunction, unexplained depression, and hyperlipidemia
		f.	Patients on lithium therapy
		g.	Patients with type 1 diabetes; 10% of these patients develop hypothyroidism in their lifetimes; obtain sensitive TSH levels at regular intervals, particularly if a goiter develops
		h.	Consider screening for patients with infertility problems, repeated pregnancy losses, menstrual irregularities, and a family history of thyroid disease
	3.	Diagnostic testing for acquired hypothyroidism includes the following: (all tests may be normal in patients with chronic thyroiditis and certain medications [corticosteroids, dopamine] as well as illnesses and starvation may interfere with results of thyroid function tests)
		a.	A sensitive thyroid-stimulating hormone (TSH) assay (normal TSH concentration is	0.02 mIU/L or less)
			(1)	TSH is elevated in hypothyroidism
			(2)	If serum TSH is normal, there is no need for additional thyroid tests as 98% of the time T_4 is normal when TSH is normal

b. Free T$_4$ assay in following circumstances:
    (1) When TSH is elevated, a low free T$_4$ level will confirm the diagnosis of acquired hypothyroidism
    (2) When hypothyroidism associated with pituitary or hypothalamic failure is suspected
        (a) TSH may be normal, low, or mildly elevated (TSH does not rise proportionally to low T$_4$)
        (b) Further evaluation is needed with results suggesting secondary or tertiary hypothyroidism: neuroradiologic studies, measurement of serum prolactin, and assessment of pituitary-adrenal and pituitary-gonadal function are indicated

c. If autoimmune thyroiditis is suspected, order either antimicrosomal antibody (anti-TPO antibody) which is test of choice or antithyroglobulin antibody; positive in 95% of patients with Hashimoto's thyroiditis

d. Thyroid scan or sonogram may be needed to evaluate suspicious structural thyroid abnormalities

e. The free thyroxine index provides an indirect estimate of free T$_4$ and is rarely ordered today

4. Consider ordering the following:
    a. Serum electrolytes, blood urea nitrogen, creatinine, glucose, calcium, PO$_4$, and albumin
    b. Urine pregnancy test
    c. Urinalysis to detect proteinuria
    d. Lipid studies for hyperlipidemia which often occurs with hypothyroidism

V. Plan/Management

A. Treatment of congenital hypothyroidism
1. Consult pediatric endocrinologist immediately to prevent or minimize the adverse effects that can occur to the developing nervous system
2. Treatment should be started immediately
3. Although controversial, some experts recommend treating newborns with borderline hypothyroidism
4. Treatment is daily oral thyroxine 10-15 μg/kg/day for severe forms of hypothyroidism; in newborns the usual daily dose is 37.5 μg
5. Optimum dose of thyroxine is the minimum level needed to maintain TSH values within normal range
6. Educate parents concerning the etiology of the disease, impact of early diagnosis and treatment in preventing mental retardation, importance of follow-up care, and the manner of administering drug

B. Consult specialist when patient is myxedemic, has significant cardiac disease, has secondary hypothyroidism, or is chronically ill or hospitalized with abnormal thyroid function tests

C. Pharmacological treatment with levothyroxine is the recommended first-line therapy for acquired hypothyroidism; prescribe a high-quality brand preparation (Synthroid, Levothroid, Levoxyl) and always prescribe the same brand throughout treatment
1. In children, give once daily on empty stomach; initial doses are the following:
    a. 0-3 months: 10-15 micrograms/kg/day
    b. 3-6 months: 8-10 micrograms/kg/day
    c. 6-12 months: 6-8 micrograms/kg/day
    d. 1-5 years: 5-6 micrograms/kg/day
    e. 6-12 years: 4-5 micrograms/kg/day
    f. >12 years: 2-3 micrograms/kg/day
2. Continually monitor response to medication
    a. TSH assay should be ordered every 4-8 weeks until concentration is normalized (keep in mind that TSH levels may remain elevated for several months despite effective treatment; rapid increase in medication based on TSH levels should be avoided because of the risk of thyrotoxicosis or excessive thyroid hormones)
    b. Ask patient about symptoms of thyrotoxicity such as tachycardia, nervousness, tremor and evaluate with diagnostic tests
        (1) If hyperthyroidism is confirmed the current dose of levothyroxine should be withheld for one week and restarted at a lower dose
        (2) Some patients remain asymptomatic even with elevated free T$_4$ and/or TSH abnormalities; these patients should have their doses reduced until TSH concentration is normalized to prevent development of osteoporosis which may occur with levothyroxine over-replacement
    c. Signs and symptoms of hypothyroidism should improve within 2 weeks and resolve within 3-6 months

       d.   Need careful monitoring of growth and development and diagnostic tests (TSH and T_4) in children who begin drugs; these children may have school and behavioral problems due to decreased attention spans and increased activity; parents and teachers need to be warned about this possibility

    3.   Maintenance treatment is lowest dosage required to maintain euthyroidism with a nonelevated serum TSH and a normal or slightly elevated T_4

    4.   Drug interactions

       a.   Drugs such as cholestyramine, ferrous sulfate, calcium, sucralfate, and aluminum hydroxide antacids may interfere with levothyroxine absorption from the stomach; space levothyroxine at least 4 hours from these medications

       b.   May need to increase dose of levothyroxine when used with phenytoin, carbamazepine, and rifampin as they increase the metabolism of thyroxine

       c.   Females on estrogen may need a higher dose as estrogen increases serum thyroxine binding globulin

D.   Triiodothyronine (T_3) is the active form of thyroid hormone

    1. T_3 or liothyronine sodium (Cytomel) is rarely used as an alternative medication

    2.   Low doses have been used in combination with levothyroxine (T_4) as T_3 may improve mood and neuropsychological function

E.   Follow Up

    1.   Congenital hypothyroidism:

       a.   Important to monitor serum T_4, free T_4, and TSH levels frequently and adjust dosage of thyroxine accordingly

       b.   Assess at 2 and 4 weeks after diagnosis and then every 1-2 months in first year, and every 4 months thereafter

       c.   Every 6 months is usually adequate in older children if the thyroxine dose is stabilized

    2.   Acquired hypothyroidism

       a.   When beginning medication therapy, patient's therapeutic response should be monitored every 4-8 weeks until TSH is normalized

       b.   After medication dosage is stabilized, schedule visits every 6-12 months and order serum TSH assays

       c.   If drug dosage is changed, patient should have repeat TSH in 2-3 months

       d.   Values within normal limits imply adequate treatment

       e.   Undetectable TSH levels suggest over-treatment and medications should be decreased; over-treatment increases the risk of osteoporosis

       f.   Elevated TSH indicates under-treatment or noncompliance; after ascertaining that patient is taking medication, increase dose

GYNECOMASTIA

I.   Definition: Proliferation of glandular component of male breast

II.   Pathogenesis: Due to an imbalance between serum estrogen and androgen levels with an excess of estrogens resulting in breast duct proliferation

A.   Physiologic causes

    1.   Neonatal period: Palpable breast tissue is due to transplacental passage of estrogens

    2.   Puberty: Breast enlargement is associated with lower free testosterone levels and excessive levels of estrogen created by peripheral conversion of adrenal androgens

B.   Pathological causes

    1.   Carcinomas: testicular, adrenal, pituitary, breast, lung, pancreas, colon

    2.   Chronic diseases: liver disease, renal disease and dialysis, pulmonary disease, congestive heart failure, nervous system damage

    3.   Malnutrition

    4.   Hyperthyroidism or hypothyroidism

    5.   Adrenal disorders

    6.   Primary gonadal failure

    7.   Secondary hypogonadism

8. Drugs such as hormones (i.e., androstenedione), anti-infectives (e.g., isoniazid, ketoconazole, metronidazole), antiulcer drugs, cardiovascular drugs (e.g., digoxin, verapamil, captopril, spironolactone), psychoactive agents (e.g., diazepam, tricyclic antidepressants, phenothiazines), drugs of abuse (e.g., alcohol, amphetamines, heroin, marijuana), protease inhibitors for HIV infection, finasteride, phenytoin, and penicillamine
9. Enzymatic defects of testosterone production
10. Androgen-insensitivity syndromes
11. Idiopathic gynecomastia
12. Familial gynecomastia

C. The most common causes are idiopathic gynecomastia and gynecomastia due to puberty; drugs and alcohol, cirrhosis, malnutrition, and primary hypogonadism are other common causes

D. The following are risk factors for developing gynecomastia: Klinefelter's syndrome, obesity, testicular failure, recovery from prolonged severe illness associated with malnutrition and weight loss, positive family history, Peutz-Jeghers syndrome, male pseudohermaphroditism, and alcoholism

III. Clinical Presentation

A. Physiological
1. Occurs in most newborn males during the first 3 weeks of life with resolution by time infant is 4 months old
2. In puberty, gynecomastia is characterized by the following:
    a. High prevalence; occurs in approximately 38-65% of pubertal boys
    b. Average age at onset is between 12-14 years
    c. Usually occurs during Tanner stages II, III, or IV
    d. More common in obese boys due to excessive conversion of androgens to estrogens in the adipose tissue
    e. Transitory tenderness often occurs
    f. Breasts may be of a firm, rubbery consistency or consistency may be similar to female breasts
    g. There is an absence of ulceration or nipple retraction
    h. Often unilateral but may progress to bilateral disease
    i. Enlargement resolves spontaneously in several months to 2 years; in the following cases enlargement never fully regresses: breast development which has progressed beyond Tanner stage II, breasts in which there is greater than 2 cm of palpable tissue in the first year, or palpable tissue that enlarges to >4 cm
    j. Patients' testes are normal in size and volume for Tanner stage and no other physical abnormalities are present

B. Pathological
1. Tumors
    a. Suspect a neoplasm in children <10 years who have gynecomastia
    b. Risk of breast cancer in males is proportional to the amount of breast tissue present; increased risk in patients with substantial gynecomastia
2. Familial gynecomastia may be an X-linked recessive or sex-linked autosomal dominant trait
3. Patients with other pathological causes present with variable signs and symptoms

IV. Diagnosis/Evaluation

A. History
1. Carefully determine the age of onset of gynecomastia, and its course and duration
2. Ask about pain and discharge from breast
3. Ask whether the breast(s) is(are) growing or shrinking
4. Explore the relationship of breast enlargement to other pubertal events
5. Ascertain the pattern and timing of pubertal events
6. Inquire about medication history; inquire about use of androstenedione
7. Inquire about alcohol use and illegal drug use
8. Obtain a complete nutrition history
9. Determine whether patient is active in athletics and/or lifts weights to identify breast enlargement due to pectoral muscle hypertrophy
10. Inquire about family history of breast enlargement
11. Inquire about previous medical history including liver, renal, pulmonary, nervous, adrenal, pituitary, and endocrine disorders

12. In adolescent males, ask about changes in libido
13. Inquire about any recent weight loss or gain
14. Explore the impact of the gynecomastia on the patient's lifestyle and self-image

B. Physical Examination
   1. Obtain measurements of height, weight, and arm span to detect Klinefelter's syndrome
   2. Assess general health and observe for evidence of feminization, such as lack of male hair distribution and a eunuchoid body habitus
   3. Assess skin for signs of hepatocellular failure (jaundice, spider angiomata, palmar erythema) and hyperthyroidism (warm, sweaty)
   4. With patient lying supine, grasp breast between thumb and forefinger and gently bring the 2 fingers toward the nipple; a disk-like mound of tissue is often felt with gynecomastia
     a. Measure dimensions of glandular tissue and areolae
     b. Note consistency, tenderness, and mobility of any lesion or mass; squeeze nipple and note any discharge
     c. Asymmetry and nodules deserve special attention
   5. Palpate for axillary lymphadenopathy
   6. Check for signs of thyroid hormone excess such as thyromegaly, tachycardia, diaphoresis, and exophthalmus
   7. Perform a cardiopulmonary examination for signs of congestive heart failure
   8. Check for signs of liver dysfunction such as hepatomegaly
   9. Deeply palpate upper abdomen for tumor of the adrenal glands or kidney
   10. Determine Tanner staging of sexual development
   11. Perform complete testicular examination
     a. Measure size of testes (small, firm testes are characteristic of Klinefelter's syndrome)
     b. Palpate for masses or tumor

C. Differential Diagnosis: gynecomastia may be a normal physiologic phenomenon or a result of a pathologic condition
   1. Pseudogynecomastia presents with smooth, fatty enlargement of breasts without glandular proliferation; more common in obese males
   2. In patients with Klinefelter's syndrome, gynecomastia occurs around puberty and patients have long limbs and small, firm testes
   3. Patients with cirrhosis and gynecomastia have loss of libido, loss of body hair, and testicular atrophy
   4. Breast cancer, uncommon in males, is characterized by a unilateral, hard or firm mass which is fixed to the underlying tissues and may be associated with dimpling of the skin, ulceration, retraction or crusting of the nipple, nipple discharge or bleeding, or axillary lymphadenopathy
   5. Neurofibromas, lipomas, and dermoid cysts are other breast masses that may present like gynecomastia

D. Diagnostic Tests: ordered on the basis of patient's clinical presentation
   1. Order mammogram or fine-needle aspiration biopsy if breast enlargement is not characteristic of typical physiologic gynecomastia
   2. Laboratory tests are usually not needed if patient has signs and symptoms of pubertal gynecomastia (see preceding clinical presentation)
   3. When the following characteristics exist, there is a need for further evaluation:
     a. Breast development that occurred in prepubertal boy without genital changes
     b. Males with genital abnormalities such as small testes with penile enlargement, hypospadias, or incomplete testicular descent
     c. Gynecomastia that persists beyond 2 years or is unusually prominent
     d. Males >18 years with recent onset of enlarging and tender breasts
     e. Males who have physical abnormalities of unknown etiology
     f. Breast masses which are large (>4 cm in diameter)
   4. Consider the following workup for the above mentioned group of males who need further evaluation (consultation with a specialist is recommended)
     a. Begin with measurement of luteinizing and follicle-stimulating hormone
       (1) High concentrations are associated with testicular failure, Klinefelter's syndrome, and hCG-secreting tumors
       (2) Low concentrations may result from use of exogenous steroid such as androstenedione or may be more worrisome and due to autonomous androgen or estrogen production

b. Next, consider ordering the following tests:
   (1) Free testosterone to detect testicular failure and carcinomas
   (2) Serum estradiol; elevated in interstitial-cell tumors and feminizing adrenal tumors
   (3) Serum β-hCG level (may be elevated in carcinomas)
c. Consider the following additional tests in special cases:
   (1) Dehydroepiandrosterone (may be abnormal in adrenal diseases)
   (2) Prolactin (may be elevated in pituitary tumors)
   (3) Thermography and testicular ultrasound should be considered when patient has a suspected testicular tumor
   (4) Chest film to screen for pulmonary tumors and metastatic lesions
   (5) Thyroid, liver function tests, BUN, and creatinine, if indicated
   (6) Chromosomal karyotype (if both testes are small)

V. Plan/Management

A. Consultation with an endocrinologist is recommended in the following situations: any male with physical abnormalities, prepubertal and pubertal males whose breast development has occurred without genital changes, breast enlargement which persists (>2 years) or is >4 cm, males older than 18 years of age

B. If the patient has pubertal gynecomastia reassurance should be given that the condition is physiological and transient in nature

C. Postpubertal males who have had a thorough negative evaluation will also need assurance that the breast enlargement is not pathological

D. Males that have residual fibrous tissue may benefit from referral to a surgeon if they are embarrassed or emotionally distressed by the breast enlargement

E. Medical approaches to treating gynecomastia have included use of antiestrogens (i.e., clomiphene, tamoxifen), testosterone, nonaromatizable androgens, and danazol in pubertal boys, and diethylstilbestrol (DES) in elderly men

F. Follow Up
   1. Follow up will vary depending on patient's clinical diagnosis
   2. Males with pubertal gynecomastia should be re-evaluated every 3-6 months

PRECOCIOUS PUBERTY

I. Definition: Onset of puberty before the age of 9 years in males and before the age of 8 in females; a new cut-off of 6 to 7 years for girls was proposed by the Lawson Wilkins Pediatric Endocrine Society (Kaplowitz, et al, 1999), but recently Midyette, Moore, and Jacobson (2003) concluded that these new cut-off values will result in failure to detect important conditions

A. Isosexual precocity is advanced sexual development appropriate to the phenotype of the child

B. Heterosexual precocity is advanced sexual development at a variance with the phenotype of the child

II. Pathogenesis

A. Central or true isosexual precocious puberty results from stimulation of the hypothalamic-pituitary axis with gonadotropin secretion and resultant sex steroid secretion
   1. May be classified as constitutional in some early-school-age children who are actually in the lower range of normal on the distribution curve; usually these children have a family history of early puberty
   2. Often there is no abnormal organic cause (idiopathic); 90% of female cases and 50% of male cases are idiopathic

3. Other causes are central nervous system (CNS) abnormalities such as the following:
    a. Congenital anomalies (hydrocephalus)
    b. Benign or malignant tumors in the hypothalamus region
    c. Head trauma
    d. Infections such as encephalitis, meningitis, or brain abscess
    e. Syndromes such as neurofibromatosis or tuberous sclerosis
4. Severe hypothyroidism may also cause abnormal development

B. Pseudo-precocious isosexual puberty occurs independent of the stimulation of the hypothalamic-pituitary axis with elevated sex hormones but low gonadotropins
    1. In females, possible causes are ingestion of oral contraceptives or other estrogen-containing agents, estrogen-producing tumors of the ovary and adrenal glands, gonadotropin-producing tumors, and McCune-Albright syndrome
    2. In males, possible causes are abuse of androgenic agents, untreated congenital adrenal hyperplasia, adrenal tumors, testicular tumors, and familial Leydig cell hyperplasia

C. Heterosexual precocious puberty has the following etiologies
    1. In females, ovarian abnormalities, adrenal problems such as tumors or congenital adrenal hyperplasia, adrenal enzyme deficiencies, and exogenous androgens are likely causes
    2. In males, adrenal tumors, estrogen-producing teratomas, neurofibromatosis, and iatrogenic factors are possible factors

D. Variations of pubertal development occur frequently and are related to the following factors
    1. Premature thelarche or premature breast development often has no known causative factor but may be a result of ovarian cysts or ingestion of exogenous estrogens such as birth control pills
    2. Premature adrenarche or premature development of sexual hair is often due to organic abnormalities such as adrenal hyperplasia, adrenal tumors, gonadal tumors, or possible central nervous system abnormalities

III. Clinical Presentation

A. Most girls have idiopathic central precocious puberty whereas boys have an identifiable cause of precocity such as tumor, congenital adrenal hyperplasia, or familial gonadotropin-independent precocity

B. Children with central isosexual precocious puberty have the following characteristics:
    1. Complete sexual development (pubic hair, axillary hair, breasts, and phallus)
    2. Pattern of progression of pubertal events is normal
    3. Potential to be fertile due to production of mature sperm or ova
    4. Accelerated linear growth and advanced bone age is typical; at first child is tall for age, but owing to premature closure of epiphyses, smallness of stature is usually the end result
    5. Pubertal levels of luteinizing hormone (LH), follicle stimulating hormone (FSH), and sex steroids
    6. Common symptoms are emotional lability, high energy levels, and increased appetite
    7. Girls may have white vaginal secretion (leukorrhea) and/or vaginal bleeding due to menarche
    8. Patients with precocity due to central nervous system abnormalities have neurological symptoms and signs such as headache, visual impairments, and seizures

C. In pseudo-precocious isosexual puberty, children have the following characteristics:
    1. Elevated sexual hormones but low gonadotropins
    2. Infertility due to immature sperm or ova
    3. Clinical presentation is variable and will depend on the causative factor
        a. In males, enlargement of one testis may indicate a testicular tumor
        b. In females, a palpable mass on bimanual examination may indicate an ovarian tumor

D. Heterosexual precocious puberty is uncommon, occurs mainly in newborns, and results in virilization in females and feminization in males

E. Variations of puberty have the following characteristics:
    1. Girls with thelarche have enlarged breasts usually without nipple and alveolar development
        a. Commonly occurs in girls between 2 months and 4 years of age
        b. Enlarged breasts often regress within several months to a year
        c. There are no others signs of premature pubertal development and no linear growth acceleration

2. Children with adrenarche have development of sexual hair which gradually increases
    a. Usually occurs between 5-8 years of age
    b. Most common in African-American or Hispanic girls
    c. Typically, children have no or slightly accelerated growth and slightly advanced bone age
    d. Some children have mild neurologic problems

IV. Diagnosis/Evaluation

    A. History
      1. Carefully explore the pattern and times of pubertal changes (compare with following table)

PATTERN OF PUBERTAL DEVELOPMENT		
	Mean Age (years)	
Sign	Females	Males
Breast buds	11	
Enlargement of testes		11
Pubic hair	11	13
Maximum linear growth rate	12	14
Menses	12	
Axillary hair	13	15
Facial hair		16+

      2. Ask about associated symptoms such as headaches, changes in vision, changes in appetite, thirst, vaginal discharge, vaginal spotting, menses, hot flashes, seizures, mood lability
      3. Ask about past medical history, particularly past central nervous system infections and abnormalities, thyroid problems, adrenal disorders, and gonadal disorders
      4. Ask at what age grandparents, parents, and other siblings experienced first pubertal changes
      5. Inquire about family history of accelerated height
      6. Inquire about ingestion of steroids (oral contraceptives, estrogen creams, phytoestrogens, and supplements such as DHEA-S and androstenedione)
      7. Inquire about quality of family and peer relationships
      8. Ask about school performance; inquire about aggressive behaviors

    B. Physical Examination
      1. Measure for height (standing and sitting) and weight; plot on growth chart and compare with previous measurements
      2. Observe skin for facial sebaceous glands, café au lait markings, neurofibromatosis lesions, or lesions of McCune-Albright syndrome (one or more large brown macules with irregular borders)
      3. Palpate thyroid for enlargement or tenderness
      4. Check for axillary hair and odor
      5. Check for amount of breast tissue and whether the nipples and areolas are enlarging and thinning
      6. Perform a complete abdominal and rectal exam
      7. In females, consider performing pelvic and speculum examinations
        a. Depending on the age of and clinical condition of the child, external examination of the genitalia may be all that is necessary
        b. If speculum and bimanual exams are done, note uterine and ovarian size and look for evidence of maturation such as pink and dull vagina following estrogenization or developing fullness of the labia minora (normal uterus measures 1-2 cm and the ovaries measure 0.5-1.0 cm until puberty)
      8. In males, measure length and width of stretched penis
      9. In males, perform testicular exam, noting size and evidence of masses
        a. If both testes are pubertal in size, suspect gonadotropin-stimulated precocious puberty
        b. If one testis is enlarged, suspect a testicular tumor
        c. If both testes are small, suspect exogenous androgens or adrenal disorders
      10. Perform a complete neurological exam
      11. Assess for sexual maturity stages or Tanner stages (see tables which follow)

SEXUAL MATURITY STAGES IN GIRLS

Stage	Breasts
1	Preadolescent - only papilla is elevated above level of chest wall
2	Breast budding - Breast and papilla elevated as small mound, increased diameter of areola
3	Continued breast and areola enlargement, no contour separation
4	Areola and papilla form secondary mound
5	Mature - Nipple projects, areola is part of general breast contour
	Pubic Hair
1	Preadolescent - None or vellus hair in pubic area
2	Sparse, straight, lightly pigmented along medial border of labia
3	Darker, coarser, curlier and in increased amount
4	Abundant but has not spread to medial surface of thighs
5	Adult feminine, inverse triangle, spread to medial surface of thighs

SEXUAL MATURITY STAGES IN BOYS

Stage	Penis, Testes, and Scrotum
1	Preadolescent - all are size and proportion seen in early childhood (testes 1 cm)
2	Slight enlargement, with alteration in color (more reddened) and texture of scrotum (testes 2.0-3.2 cm)
3	Further growth and enlargement (testes 3.3-4.0 cm)
4	Penis significantly enlarged in length and circumference; further development of glans; enlargement of testes and scrotum with darkening of scrotal skin (testes 4.1-4.9 cm)
5	Genitalia of adult size (testes 5.0 cm)
	Pubic Hair
1	Preadolescent - None or vellus hair in pubic area
2	Sparse, straight, lightly pigmented at base of penis
3	Darker, coarser, curlier and in increased amount
4	Abundant but less quantity than adult type
5	Adult distribution, spread to medial surface of thighs

Adapted from Tanner, J.M. (1962). *Growth at adolescence*. Oxford: Blackwell Scientific Publications.

C. Differential Diagnosis
   1. Aimed at distinguishing idiopathic precocity from those conditions which have correctable and possibly life-threatening causes
   2. Typically, earlier onset and faster progression of puberty are suggestive of pathology

D. Diagnostic Tests: Order tests based on what is uncovered in history and physical exam
   1. Consider measurement of luteinizing hormone (LH), follicle-stimulating hormone (FSH), human chorionic gonadotropin levels, testosterone, and estradiol levels to determine whether precocity is central or pseudo-precocious
   2. An easy way to determine whether a girl is in active puberty is a vaginal smear obtained by cotton swab and fixed immediately to assess estrogen effect (vaginal cells change from immature parabasal cells toward intermediate and finally superficial squamous cells under the influence of estrogen)
   3. A GnRH stimulation test is helpful in determining central or peripheral precocious puberty
   4. If congenital adrenal hyperplasia is suspected order 17-OH progesterone, 17-pergnenolone, DHEA (unsulfonated), androstenedione, and total testosterone
   5. Consider tests to determine bone age (radiographs of the nondominant hand and wrist)
   6. Consider computed tomography (CT) or magnetic resonance imaging (MRI) of the head if CNS abnormality is suspected; studies have found that small CNS tumors were present in children believed to have idiopathic precocity
   7. Abdominal CT, MRI, or ultrasound should be considered if ovarian cysts/tumors, testicular tumors, or adrenal gland tumors or abnormalities are suspected
   8. Consider ordering urinary 17-ketosteroids and plasma dehydroepiandrosterone and its sulfate in boys with premature adrenarche

9. For premature thelarche:
    a. Consider ordering a βhCG to rule out a possible hCG-producing tumor
    b. Consider ordering plasma FSH, LH, and estradiol and an ultrasound to rule out ovarian cyst
10. For premature adrenarche, consider 17-hydroxyprogesterone, androstenedione, and testosterone
11. Consider ordering thyroid stimulating hormone (TSH) levels

V. Plan/Management

A. Cases which involve organic abnormalities are usually referred to an endocrinologist

B. True isosexual precocity which is idiopathic centers on removal of the underlying cause and may be treated in the following manner with consultation of an endocrinologist:
    1. Observe child for 3-12 months to determine whether status is changing
    2. If condition remains unchanged, continue to observe
    3. When sexual maturation is progressing:
        a. Typical treatments involve the following medications to suppress the hypothalamic-pituitary-gonadal axis: GnRH agonist therapy is usually the treatment of choice and is available in intramuscular (depot), subcutaneous, and nasal formulations; medroxyprogesterone acetate (progestational steroid), danazol (androgen), or cyproterone acetate (antiandrogen) are other pharmacological therapies that may be beneficial
        b. Investigational agent, testolactone, has been used in girls
        c. Antifungal drug, ketoconazole, has been used in males

C. Medical treatment of peripheral precocious puberty depends on the etiology and includes medroxyprogesterone acetate, testolactone, ketoconazole, cyproterone acetate, and spironolactone

D. Treatment of premature thelarche and adrenarche
    1. If all organic causes have been eliminated, no treatments are necessary
    2. Close follow up is essential as both conditions are clinically indistinguishable from the early stages of precocious puberty

E. Patient education and counseling are extremely important

F. Follow Up
    1. Confer with endocrinologist about frequency of follow-up visits for children with precocity due to organic causes
    2. Children with idiopathic isosexual precocious puberty or premature thelarche or adrenarche should be re-evaluated at least every 3-6 months

DELAYED PUBERTY

I. Definition: Absence of breast budding by age 13 in females or lack of testicular enlargement by age 14 in males as well as arrest in pubertal maturation

II. Pathogenesis is due to failure at any point along the hypothalamic-pituitary-gonadal axis and is associated with one of the following factors:

A. Constitutional delayed puberty
    1. Involves slow maturation but with secretion of appropriate amounts of hormones
    2. Heredity probably plays an important role

B. Gonadotropin-releasing hormone (GnRH) secretion can be inhibited by functional causes:
    1. Inadequate nutrition or poor eating habits; anorexia nervosa
    2. Congenital heart disease
    3. Chronic diseases such as Crohn's disease, celiac disease, chronic pulmonary disease, chronic renal failure, sickle cell anemia, collagen vascular disease
    4. Environmental stress
    5. Intensive athletic training or exercise
    6. Hypothyroidism and diabetes mellitus
    7. Drugs such as opiates

C. The ability of the hypothalamus to secrete GnRH:
1. Brain tumors
2. Central nervous system infections
3. Trauma
4. Genetic and molecular causes such as Prader-Willi syndrome, Kallmann's syndrome, Laurence-Moon-Bardet-Biedi syndrome

D. The pituitary may not be able to respond to the GnRH with gonadotropin production:
1. Tumor
2. Infection
3. Excess prolactin secretion
4. Trauma
5. Pituitary adenoma

E. The gonads may be unable to respond to the luteinizing hormone (LH) and follicle-stimulating hormone (FSH) for the following reasons:
1. Gonadal dysgenesis in association with abnormalities of sex chromosomes (Turner syndrome, Klinefelter's syndrome)
2. Infections (orchitis, oophoritis, gonorrhea, tuberculosis)
3. Mechanical causes such as torsion, surgery, or congenital anorchia
4. Radiation or chemotherapy

III. Clinical Presentation

A. Criteria used to determine pubertal delay in females
1. Breast stage 1 (see SEXUAL MATURITY STAGES IN GIRLS in Precocious Puberty section) persisting beyond age 13 or pubic hair stage 1 beyond age 14
2. Greater than 4 to 5 years elapsing between initiation of breast growth and menarche
3. Failure to menstruate beyond age 16

B. Criteria used to determine a pubertal delay in males
1. Genital stage 1 (see SEXUAL MATURITY STAGES IN BOYS in Precocious Puberty section) persisting beyond age 14 or pubic hair stage persisting beyond age 15
2. More than 4 to 5 years elapsing from initiation to completion of genital growth

C. Delayed puberty is more common in males

D. Constitutional delay
1. Most common type; 90-95% of delayed puberty is constitutional
2. Frequently, children with this delay have been slow growers throughout their childhood with growth curves below the third percentile
3. Final, adult height is often shorter than average
4. Patient has negative review of systems, normal diagnostic tests, normal physical exam, but bone age is slightly delayed

E. Other types of delayed puberty will have abnormal physical findings (e.g., gynecomastia in a male with a gonadal disorder or abnormal cranial nerve function in a child with gonadotropin deficiency) and abnormal diagnostic tests (e.g., low testosterone response to hCG in gonadotropin deficiency)

IV. Diagnosis/Evaluation

A. History
1. Ask about onset and pattern of pubertal changes
2. Obtain a neonatal history which includes previous maternal miscarriages and congenital lymphedema (Turner's syndrome)
3. Gather a thorough medical history including history of chronic disease, congenital anomalies, previous surgery, radiation exposure, chemotherapy, or drug use
4. Pay particular attention in the review of systems to weight changes, dieting, stress, exercise, athletics, gastrointestinal symptoms, neurologic complaints, and symptoms of thyroid disorders
5. Ask about family history of infertility and endocrine disorders
6. Inquire about heights of parents, siblings, grandparents
7. Inquire about age of menarche in mother and adolescent sisters
8. Explore quality of family and peer relationships
9. Ask about school performance

B. Physical Examination
1. Observe for general body habitus to determine nutritional status
2. Measure height, weight, and plot on growth chart, noting pattern in relationship to previous measurements
3. Check thyroid for nodules and enlargement
4. Measure dimensions of areolae and any glandular breast tissue
5. Perform a complete chest exam to eliminate any chronic lung problems
6. Perform a complete heart exam, noting evidence of congenital heart disease
7. Palpate for liver and spleen enlargement
8. In males, measure testicular length, width, midshaft diameter, and stretched length of penis
9. In females, assess estrogen effect on external genitalia (pale, pink vaginal mucosa with white discharge indicates estrogen exposure)
10. Speculum and bimanual pelvic exams are not always necessary in the initial evaluation of girls with delayed sexual development but should be done in the girl who has normal pubertal development but delayed menarche
11. Note any evidence of heterosexual development such as clitoromegaly or hirsutism in females or gynecomastia in males
12. Perform a complete neurological exam to eliminate intracranial abnormalities
13. Determine sexual maturity rating

C. Differential Diagnosis
1. Constitutional delayed puberty is common but is a diagnosis of exclusion; all correctable and organic causes must be ruled out
2. A child whose delayed puberty is associated with nutritional deficiency due to an eating disorder or a chronic disease will show a greater decline in weight gain than height, whereas in children with pubertal delay due to endocrine factors, there is a greater slowing of linear growth than weight

D. Diagnostic Tests
1. Order complete blood count and erythrocyte sedimentation rate (screen for chronic disease)
2. Order LH, FSH, dehydroepiandrosterone sulfate, and testosterone or estradiol levels (elevated levels are suggestive of primary gonadal failure)
3. Consider test for bone age (delayed bone age will be seen in adolescents with hypopituitarism, hypothyroidism, chronic illness, and constitutional delay in puberty; normal bone age is seen in patients with Turner's syndrome)
4. Consider thyroid function tests
5. Consider lateral skull x-ray to rule out CNS disorders
6. Other tests are necessary in some workups:
   a. Karyotype to rule out Turner's syndrome
   b. Growth hormone measurements to determine whether a growth hormone deficiency exists
   c. To rule out hypogonadotropic hypogonadism, order hCG test
   d. Prolactin level, computerized tomography (CT), and magnetic resonance imaging (MRI) to rule out central nervous system abnormality

V. Plan/Management

A. Children with pubertal delay who have abnormal physical findings or diagnostic tests are referred to an endocrinologist

B. Treatment of constitutional pubertal delay
1. Usually no treatment is necessary, but close follow up and monitoring is essential
2. In boys with constitutional delay and severe psychological problems, injections of human chorionic gonadotropin or testosterone can be prescribed to initiate secondary sexual development after conferring with an endocrinologist

C. Counseling and education are integral parts of the plan

D. Follow up of constitutional pubertal delay is at least every 6 months

REFERENCES

American Association of Clinical Endocrinologists and American College of Endocrinology. (1995). AACE clinical practice guidelines for the evaluation and treatment of hyperthyroidism and hypothyroidism. *Endocrine Practice, 1,* 56-62.

American Association of Clinical Endocrinologists. (2001). AACE Consensus Conference guidelines for glycemic control. *Endocrine Practice.*

American Association of Clinical Endocrinologists. (2002). Medical guidelines for the management of diabetes mellitus: The AACE system of intensive diabetes self-management – 2002 update. *Endocrine Practice, 8*(Suppl. 1), 41-82.

American Diabetes Association. (2000). Type 2 diabetes in children and adolescents (Consensus Statement). *Diabetes Care, 23,* 381-389.

American Diabetes Association. (2002). Care of children with diabetes in the school and day care setting. *Diabetes Care, 25*(Suppl. 1), S122-S125.

American Diabetes Association. (2003). Evidence-based nutrition principles and recommendations for the treatment and prevention of diabetes and related complications. *Diabetes Care, 26*(Suppl. 1), S51-S61.

American Diabetes Association. (2003). Hospital admission guidelines for diabetes mellitus. *Diabetes Care 26*(Suppl. 1), S118.

American Diabetes Association. (2003). Hyperglycemic crisis in patients with diabetes mellitus. *Diabetes Care, 26*(Suppl. 1), S109-S117.

American Diabetes Association. (2003). Immunization and the prevention of influenza and pneumococcal disease in people with diabetes. *Diabetes Care, 26*(Suppl. 1), S126-S128.

American Diabetes Association. (2003). Implications of the United Kingdom prospective diabetes study. *Diabetes Care, 26*(Suppl. 1), S28-S32.

American Diabetes Association. (2003). Insulin administration. *Diabetes Care, 26*(Suppl. 1), S121-S124.

American Diabetes Association. (2003). Report of the Expert Committee on the diagnosis and classification of diabetes mellitus. *Diabetes Care, 26*(Suppl. 1), S5-S20.

American Diabetes Association. (2003). Screening for diabetes. *Diabetes Care, 26*(Suppl. 1), S21-S24.

American Diabetes Association. (2003). Standards of medical care for people with diabetes mellitus. *Diabetes Care, 26*(Suppl. 1), S33-S50.

American Diabetes Association. (2003). Tests of glycemia in diabetes. *Diabetes Care, 26*(Suppl. 1), S106-S108.

American Heart Association. (2001). Summary of the scientific conference on dietary fatty acids and cardiovascular health. *Circulation, 103,* 1034-1039.

Bhatnagar, D. (2002). Should pediatric patients with hyperlipidemia receive drug therapy? *Pediatric Drugs, 4,* 223-230.

Biondi, B., Palmeri, E.A., & Fazio, S. (2000). Endogenous subclinical hyperthyroidism is not a benign process. *Journal of Clinical Endocrinology and Metabolism, 85,* 4701-4705.

Brown, A.B. (2001). Individualizing insulin therapy for optimum glycemic control. *Patient Care, 35,* 35-47.

Chumlea, W.C., Schubert, C.M., Roche, A.F., Kulin, H.E., Lee, P.A., Himes, J.H., & Sun, S.S. (2003). Age at menarche and racial comparisons in US girls. *Pediatrics, 111,* 110-113.

Cooke, D.W., & Plotnick, L. (2002). Diabetes mellitus in children and adolescents. In R.E. Rakel & E.T. Bope. *2002 Conn's current therapy.* Philadelphia: Saunders.

Deblinger, L, Colwell, J.A., & Feinglos, M.N. (2001). Using insulin in type 2 diabetes. *Patient Care, 35,* 36-48.

Decsi, T., & Molnar, D. (2003). Insulin resistance syndrome in children: Pathophysiology and potential management strategies. *Pediatric Drugs, 5,* 291-299.

DeFronzo, R.A. (1999). Pharmacologic therapy for type 2 diabetes mellitus. *Annals of Internal Medicine, 131,* 281-303.

DeWitt, D.E., & Hirsch, I.B. (2003). Outpatient insulin therapy in type 1 and type 2 diabetes mellitus. *JAMA, 289,* 2254-2264.

Donaghue, K.C., Fairchild, J.M., Craig, M.E., Chan, A.K., Hing, S., Cutler, L.R., et al. (2003). Do all prepubertal years of diabetes duration contribute equally to diabetes complications. *Diabetes Care, 26,* 1224-1229.

Dötsch, J., Rascher, W., & Dörr, H.G. (2003). Graves' disease in childhood: A review of the options for diagnosis and treatment. *Pediatric Drugs, 5,* 95-102.

Freemark, M., & Bursey, D. (2001). The effects of metformin on body mass index and glucose tolerance in obese adolescents with fasting hyperinsulinemia and a family history of type 2 diabetes. *Pediatrics, 107,* E55.

Goroll, A.H., & Mulley, A.G. (2000). Approach to the patient with hyperthyroidism. In A.H. Goroll & A.G. Mulley. *Primary care medicine: Evaluation of the adult patient* (4th ed.). Philadelphia: Lippincott.

Goroll, A.H., & Mulley, A.G. (2000). Approach to the patient with hypothyroidism. In A.H. Goroll & A.G. Mulley. *Primary care medicine: Evaluation of the adult patient* (4th ed.). Philadelphia: Lippincott.

Goroll, A.H., & Mulley, A.G. (2000). Evaluation of gynecomastia. In A.H. Goroll & A.G. Mulley. *Primary care medicine: Evaluation of the adult patient.* (4th ed.). Philadelphia: Lippincott.

Holmboe, E.S. (2002). Oral antihyperglycemic therapy for type 2 diabetes: Clinical applications. *JAMA, 287,* 373-376.

Hueston, W.J. (2001). Treatment of hypothyroidism. *American Family Physician, 64,* 1717-1724.

Hung, W. (2001). Thyroid disorders of infancy and childhood. In K.L. Becker (Ed.), *Principles and practice of endocrinology and metabolism* (3rd ed.). Philadelphia: Lippincott.

Inzucchi, S.E. (2002). Oral antihyperglycemic therapy for type 2 diabetes. *JAMA, 287,* 360-372.

Jackson, I.M., & Hennessey, J.V. (2001). Thyroiditis. In K.L. Becker (Ed.), *Principles and practice of endocrinology and metabolism* (3rd ed.). Philadelphia: Lippincott.

Jenkins, D.J.A., Kendall, C.W.C., Augustin, L.S.A., Franceschi, S., Hamidi, M., Marchie, A., et al. (2002). Glycemic index: Overview of implications in health and disease. *American Journal of Clinical Nutrition, 76*(Suppl.), 266S-273S.

Jones, K.L., Arslanian, S., Peterokova, V.A., Park, J.S., & Tomlinson, M.J. (2002). Effect of metformin in pediatric patients with type 2 diabetes. *Diabetes Care, 25,* 89-94.

Kaplowitz, P.H., Oberfield, S.E., & the Drug and Therapeutics and Executive Committees of the Lawson Wilkins Pediatric Endocrine Society. (1999). Reexamination of the age limit for defining when puberty is precocious in girls in the United States: Implications for evaluation and treatment. *Pediatrics, 104,* Part 1 of 2, 936-941.

Knopp, R.H. (1999). Drug treatment of lipid disorders. *New England Journal of Medicine, 341,* 498-511.

Kulmala, P. (2003). Prediabetes in children: Natural history, diagnosis, and preventive strategies. *Pediatric Drugs, 5,* 211-221.

Ladenson, P.W., Singer, P.A., Ain, D.B., Bagchi, N., Bigos, S.T., Levy, E.G., Smith, S.A., & Daniels, G.H. (2000). American Thyroid Association guidelines for detection of thyroid dysfunction. *Archives of Internal Medicine, 160,* 1573-1575.

Litton, J., Rice, A., Friedman, N., Oden, J., Lee, M.M., & Freemark, M. (2002). Insulin pump therapy in toddlers and preschool children with type 1 diabetes mellitus. *Journal of Pediatrics, 141,* 490-495.

Ludvigsson, J., & Bolli, G.B. (2001). Intensive insulin treatment in diabetic children. *Diabetes Nutrition Metabolism, 14,* 292-304.

Ludwig, D.S. (2002) The glycemic index: Physiological mechanisms relating to obesity, diabetes, and cardiovascular disease. *JAMA, 287,* 2414-2423.

Ludwig, D.S., & Ebbeling, C.B. (2001). Type 2 diabetes mellitus in children: Primary care and public health considerations. *JAMA, 286,* 1427-1430.

Luna, B., & Feinglos, M.N. (2001). Oral agents in the management of type 2 diabetes mellitus. *American Family Physician, 63,* 1747-1756.

Mansfield, M.J. (1999). Precocious puberty. In R.A. Dershewitz (Ed.), *Ambulatory pediatric care* (2nd ed.). Philadelphia: Lippincott

Mansfield, M.J., & Landay, H. (1999). Delayed puberty. In R.A. Dershewitz (Ed.), *Ambulatory pediatric care* (2nd ed.). Philadelphia: Lippincott.

Mansfield, M.J., & Landay, H. (1999). Gynecomastia. In R.A. Dershewitz (Ed.), *Ambulatory pediatric care* (2nd ed.). Philadelphia: Lippincott.

Midyette, L.K., Moore, W.V., & Jacobson, J.D. (2003). Are pubertal changes in girls before age 8 benign? *Pediatrics, 111,* 47-51.

Mohn, A., Dunger, D.B., & Chiarelli, F. (2001). The potential role of insulin analogues in the treatment of children and adolescents with Type 1 diabetes Mellitus. *Diabetes Nutrition Metabolism, 14,* 349-357.

Nathan, D.M. (2002). Initial management of glycemia in type 2 diabetes mellitus. *New England Journal of Medicine, 347,* 1342-1349.

National Cholesterol Education Program Report of the Expert Panel on Blood Cholesterol Levels in Children and Adolescents. (1991). Bethesda, MD: National Heart, Lung, and Blood Institute Information Center.

National Cholesterol Education Program. (1997). *Cholesterol lowering in the patient with coronary heart disease.* (NIH Publication No. 97-3794). Bethesda, MD: National Institutes of Health, National Heart, Lung, and Blood Institute.

National Institutes of Health. (2001). *Third Report of the National Cholesterol Education Program Expert Panel on Detection, Evaluation, and Treatment of High Blood Cholesterol in Adults (Adult Treatment Panel III).* (NIH Publication 01-3670). Bethesda, MD: National Institutes of Health.

Neuman, J.F. (1997). Evaluation and treatment of gynecomastia. *American Family Physician, 55,* 1835-1844.

Plotnick, L., & Henderson, R. (1998). *Clinical management of the child and teenager with diabetes.* Baltimore: Johns Hopkins University Press.

Plotnick, L.P., & Kritzler, R.K. (2001). Puberty: Normal and abnormal. In R.A. Hoekelman (Ed.), *Primary pediatric care.* St. Louis: Mosby.

Rosenbloom, A.L. (2002). Increasing incidence of type 2 diabetes in children and adolescents: Treatment considerations. *Pediatric Drugs, 4,* 209-221.

Rovet, J., & Daneman, D. (2003). Congenital hypothyroidism: A review of current diagnostic and treatment practices in relation to neuropsychologic outcome. *Pediatric Drugs, 5,* 141-149.

Sadeghi-Nejad, A. (2002). Thyroid disorders. In F.D. Burg, J.R. Ingelfinger, R.A. Polin, & A.A. Gershon. *Gellis & Kagan's current pediatric therapy 17.* Philadelphia: Saunders.

Schwetz, B.A. (2001). New diabetes glucose test. *JAMA, 285,* 56.

Shamir, R., & Fisher, E.A. (2000). Dietary therapy for children with hypercholesterolemia. *American Family Physician, 61,* 675-682, 685-686.

Shapiro, L.E., & Surks, M.I. (2001). Hypothyroidism. In K.L. Becker (Ed.), *Principles and practice of endocrinology and metabolism* (3rd ed.). Philadelphia: Lippincott.

Slatosky, J., Shipton, B., & Haney, W. (2000). Thyroiditis: Differential diagnosis and management. *American Family Physician, 61,* 1047-1054.

Smallridge, R.C. (2000). Postpartum thyroid disease: A model of immunologic dysfunction. *Clinical and Applied Immunology Reviews, 1,* 89-103.

Spieth, L.E., Harnish, J.D., Landers, C.M., Raezer, L.B., Piera, M.A., Hangen, J., & Ludwig, D.S. (2001). A low-glycemic diet in the treatment of pediatric obesity. *Archives of Pediatrics and Adolescent Medicine, 154,* 947-951.

Stein, E.A. (2001). Statins in children. Why and when. *Nutrition, Metabolism, Cardiovascular Disease, 1*(Suppl 5), 24-29.

Styne, D.M. (1997). New aspects in the diagnosis and treatment of pubertal disorders. *Pediatric Clinics of North America, 44,* 505-529.

Taha, D. (2002). Hyperlipidemia in children with type 2 diabetes mellitus. *Journal of Pediatric Endocrinology Metabolism, 15*(Suppl 1), 505-507.

Tamborlane, W.V., Bonfig, W., & Boland, E. (2001). Recent advances in treatment of youth with Type 1 diabetes: Better care through technology. *Diabetic Medicine, 18,* 864-870.

Tanner, J.M. (1962). *Growth at adolescence.* Oxford: Blackwell Scientific Publications.

White, J.R., Campbell, R.K., & Yarborough, P.C. (2001). Diabetes management therapies. In M.E. Franz (Ed.). *A core curriculum for diabetes educators* (4th ed.). Chicago: American Association of Diabetes Educators.

Willett, W.C. (2001). *Eat, drink, and be healthy.* New York: Simon & Shuster.

Williams, C.L., Hayman, L.L., Daniels, S.R., Robinson, T.N., Steinberger, J., Paridon, S., et al. (2002). Cardiovascular health in childhood: A statement for health professionals from the Committee on Atherosclerosis, Hypertension, and Obesity in Young (AHOY) of the Council on Cardiovascular Disease in the Young, American Heart Association. *Circulation, 106,* 143-160.

Wolfsdorf, J.I., & Weinstein, D.A. (2002). Diabetes mellitus in children and adolescents. In F.D. Burg, J.R. Ingelfinger, R.A. Polin, & A.A. Gershon. *Gellis & Kagan's current pediatric therapy 17.* Philadelphia: Saunders.

Cat Scratch Disease

Fifth Disease (Erythema Infectiosum)

Influenza
Table: Websites for Information on Influenza
Table: Selection of an Antiviral Drug for Treatment
Table: Properties of Antiviral Drugs
Table: Target Groups for Influenza Vaccine
Table: Dose and Schedule for Influenza Vaccine
Table: Persons for Whom Chemoprophylaxis Is Indicated

Kawasaki Disease
Table: Diagnostic Criteria (Principal Clinical Findings) of Kawasaki Disease

Lyme Disease
Table: Recommended Treatment

Meningitis and Encephalitis, Viral

Mononucleosis, Infectious

Rocky Mountain Spotted Fever

Roseola (Exanthem Subitum)

Rubella (German Measles)

Rubeola (Measles)

Varicella (Chickenpox)
Table: Clinical Features that Distinguish Chickenpox from Smallpox

CAT SCRATCH DISEASE

I. Definition: Infection causing unilateral regional adenitis, usually due to scratch of a cat

II. Pathogenesis

    A. *Bartonella henselae* (previously *Rochalimaea)* is the causative pathogen in most cases

    B. Pathogen enters the body through a break in the skin, primarily caused by the scratch of a cat (usually cats are immature and not ill); dogs, monkeys, and fleas are other possible transmitters; no evidence of person-to-person transmission

    C. Period of communicability is unknown

III. Clinical Presentation

    A. Diagnosis of cat scratch disease (CSD) is based on the presence of 3 out of 4 of the following criteria:
        1. History of animal (usually cat) contact, with presence of a scratch or inoculation lesion of the eye, skin, or mucous membrane
        2. Positive cat scratch disease skin test
        3. Regional lymphadenopathy (predominant sign) with normal laboratory results for other causes of lymphadenopathy
        4. Biopsied lymph node that has characteristic histopathologic features

    B. Natural history:
        1. Cat scratch occurs and produces a primary cutaneous lesion 7-12 days later; lesion typically begins as a macule, progresses to a papule, then to a vesicle
        2. Nodes that drain the site of inoculation enlarge in 1-2 weeks after lesion appears
            a. Node is usually singular, but may present in a cluster; typically node measures between 1.5-5.0 cm
            b. Area around affected node is usually tender, warm, erythematous, and indurated

    C. In most cases, the illness is self-limited with minimal malaise, headaches, and generalized aching; approximately 30% of cases have fever and mild systemic symptoms

    D. Lymphadenopathy usually regresses within 2-4 months, but may persist for more than a year

    E. Occasionally, Parinaud oculoglandular syndrome develops
        1. Soft granuloma or polyp develops on palpebral conjunctiva
        2. Preauricular lymphadenopathy is usually present
        3. Patient typically does not recall cat scratch; hypothesized that pathogen is transmitted in saliva left on cat's fur; patient pets cat, rubs eye, and transmits organism to conjunctiva

    F. Rare complications include encephalitis, splenomegaly, and hepatic granulomata

IV. Diagnosis/Evaluation

    A. History
        1. Ask about onset and duration of all symptoms
        2. Determine whether patient lives in household with a cat (particularly kitten) or other animals
        3. Carefully determine whether patient saw scratch or bite of any animal
        4. Specifically ask whether any skin lesion was noticed within the last 2-3 months
        5. Ask about symptoms which typically accompany CSD such as low-grade fever and myalgia
        6. Ask about symptoms which are related to other illnesses that present with lymphadenopathy such as pharyngitis (mononucleosis), weight loss and fatigue (malignancy), exanthem (Kawasaki disease), cough (tuberculosis), ear pain (otitis media), facial tenderness (sinusitis), mouth pain (dental abscess)
        7. Inquire about symptoms which would denote complications of CSD such as abdominal pain, neurological complaints, conjunctivitis

B. Physical Examination
1. Obtain vital signs, noting temperature
2. Carefully examine skin for inoculation lesion, which may be hidden in the interdigital webs of fingers, eyelids, or scalp
3. Observe skin for exanthem
4. Palpate all areas where lymph nodes are present, noting any node enlargement, erythema, or tenderness (see section on LYMPHADENOPATHY)
5. If a node is enlarged, assess the area that the node drains for signs of infection
6. Inspect eyes for signs of conjunctivitis
7. Perform complete examinations of ears, eyes, nose, and throat to rule out infection
8. Auscultate heart and lungs
9. Palpate abdomen for organomegaly, masses, and tenderness
10. Perform a neurological examination to rule out complications

C. Diagnostic Tests: usually no tests are needed
1. Indirect fluorescent antibody test for detection of serum antibody to antigens of *Bartonella* species is useful for diagnosis (available through the Centers for Disease Control and Prevention)
2. Polymerase chain reaction assays are available in some commercial laboratories
3. A stain (Warthin-Starry silver impregnation stain) can identify the pathogen if lymph node, skin, or conjunctival tissue is available; test is not specific for *Bartonella henselae*
4. Pathologic and microbiologic examinations are useful to exclude other diseases

D. Differential Diagnosis: Involved lymph node in CSD is usually tender, whereas nodes are nontender in noninfectious diseases (see sections on LYMPHADENOPATHY and CERVICAL ADENITIS)

V. Plan/Management

A. Management is usually symptomatic (e.g., pain management); complete resolution occurs without medications in 2-4 months

B. Antibiotic therapy may be beneficial in immunosuppressed patients and other patients who are severely ill but is <u>NOT</u> recommended for healthy patients
1. Oral antibiotics (rifampin [Rifadin], trimethoprim-sulfamethoxazole [Bactrim], ciprofloxacin [Cipro], azithromycin [Zithromax], or intramuscular gentamicin [Garamycin]) are possible choices
2. Therapy is discontinued when enlarged node has decreased in size (about 10 mm), the patient has no systemic symptoms, and has been afebrile for at least one week

C. Node aspiration is done when nodes are tender and fluctuant to relieve symptoms; node excision is generally unnecessary

D. Patient Education
1. Animals do not need to be destroyed or removed from the house
2. No person-to-person transmission so patients do not need to be isolated
3. Instruct patients to always thoroughly cleanse animal scratches and bites to prevent CSD
4. Persons with immune deficiencies should avoid contact with cats that scratch or bite
5. Recommend that care of cats should include flea control

E. Follow-up: None needed if patient's condition is stable

FIFTH DISEASE (ERYTHEMA INFECTIOSUM)

I. Definition: Mild viral disease with an erythematous eruption

II. Pathogenesis

A. Causal agent is human parvovirus B19

B. Mode of transmission probably is through contact with infected respiratory secretions or blood and from vertical transmission between mother and her fetus

C. Incubation period is 4-14 days from acquisition of infection to onset of initial symptoms

D.   Period of communicability: Greatest before onset of rash; probably not communicable after onset of rash; patients with aplastic crises are contagious from before the onset of symptoms and at least through the week after onset

III.   Clinical Presentation

A.   Parvovirus B19 infections are ubiquitous and cases can occur as a community outbreak or sporadically in the late winter and early spring

B.   >50% of individuals have serologic evidence of past infection by age 15 years and are immune; young children are usually susceptible to infection

C.   First manifestation is typically a rash which usually appears without fever or other symptoms; in some cases there may be a mild prodrome with fever, headache, conjunctivitis, coryza, and pharyngitis; about 20% of infected individuals are asymptomatic

D.   Rash is characteristic and may be pruritic
   1.   First erupts as a bright, erythematous rash on cheeks and forehead with circumoral pallor; adults often do not have rash on face
   2.   A maculopapular rash on the trunk occurs next
   3.   Rash gradually spreads, leaving a lacelike appearance as it clears; this stage lasts 2-4 days
   4.   In third stage, rash appears transiently when skin is traumatized by pressure, sunlight, or extremes of hot and cold

E.   Complications
   1.   Although uncommon in children, arthritis and arthralgia occur frequently in adults, especially in women; usually resolve in one or two weeks, but may last for several months
   2.   Thrombocytopenia and neutropenia may occur
   3.   Chronic bone marrow failure may occur in immunocompromised patients, and aplastic crisis may occur in patients with hemolytic anemia

F.   Infection during pregnancy can result in fetal hydrops and death (risk of fetal death is <10% after proven maternal infection in first half of pregnancy and even less in second half of pregnancy)

IV.   Diagnosis/Evaluation

A.   History
   1.   Question about degree, onset, and duration of fever or prodromal symptoms
   2.   Ask patient to describe progression of rash
   3.   Ask whether rash becomes more visible when patient is in sunlight or becomes overheated
   4.   Determine whether there are other accompanying symptoms
   5.   Determine whether other family or household members have similar symptoms
   6.   Inquire about symptoms which would denote complications such as joint pain and stiffness
   7.   Determine medication use
   8.   Inquire about present and past health history of patient and other household members; specifically question about immunosuppression and pregnancy in women

B.   Physical Examination
   1.   Measure vital signs
   2.   Assess general appearance
   3.   Carefully inspect skin; apply pressure to skin noting whether rash becomes more visible
   4.   To rule out other viral exanthems, may need to perform examinations of the head, eyes, ears, nose, throat and mouth
   5.   Assess neck for nuchal rigidity and adenopathy
   6.   Auscultate heart and lungs
   7.   Assess joints for tenderness, swelling, and range of motion

C.   Differential Diagnosis: "Slapped cheek" appearance, lacy rash, and transient nature of rash with heat, cold, and pressure are characteristic of fifth disease and lead to diagnosis; consider other conditions such as rubella, enteroviral diseases, and drug rashes, but these typically have different rash patterns

D. Diagnostic Tests
1. No tests are needed unless diagnosis is uncertain or when treating immunosuppressed patients or pregnant women
2. Assay for serum B19-specific IgM antibody is available for confirming recent infection; serum IgG antibody indicates previous infection and immunity
3. If exposure is highly suspicious in pregnant woman, additional testing is needed; consult specialist who will typically order IgG and IgM titers and then alpha-fetoprotein (MSAFT) levels if titers are positive; serial ultrasonography is needed if MSAFT is elevated
4. Tests such as nucleic acid hybridization assay or polymerase chain reaction assay are available; typically ordered to determine chronic infection in immunocompromised patients

V. Plan/Management

A. Treatment is symptomatic for healthy persons; usually the condition is benign and self-limited

B. Patients with aplastic crisis may need blood transfusions

C. For immunosuppressed patients with chronic infection, intravenous immunoglobulin therapy is effective

D. Control procedures
1. Precautions for pregnant women:
   a. Routine exclusion from the workplace where disease is occurring is not recommended due to the high prevalence of B19, the low incidence of ill effects on fetus, and the fact that avoidance of child care or teaching classrooms can only reduce but not eliminate the risk of exposure
   b. Explanation of the relatively low potential risk and option of serologic testing should be given to pregnant women who have been in contact with patients in the incubation period of disease or who were in aplastic crisis; fetal ultrasound can be offered to assess damage to the fetus
2. Children with fifth disease may attend child care or school as they are not contagious
3. Good hand washing and disposal of facial tissues containing respiratory secretions lessen transmission of infection

E. Follow Up: None needed unless complications develop

INFLUENZA

I. Definition: Acute viral disease of the respiratory tract

II. Pathogenesis

A. Causal agents: Influenza A (accounts for 99.5% of cases) and influenza B cause epidemic human disease

B. Mode of transmission: Spread from person to person by inhalation of small particle aerosols, by direct contact, by large droplet infection, or by articles recently contaminated with nasopharyngeal secretions

C. Incubation period: Ranges from 1- 4 days with an average of 2 days: in young children the incubation period is 1-6 days

D. Period of communicability: Patients are most infectious in the first 24 hours before onset of symptoms and during the period of peak symptoms; viral shedding in nasal secretions usually stops within 7 days of onset of infection, but in children shedding may last for >10 days

III. Clinical Presentation

A. Influenza virus infection occurs in epidemics that last approximately 5-6 weeks and may be associated with attack rates as high as 10-20% of population

B. Reason for continuing problems with epidemic influenza is the phenomenon of antigenic variation in which there are alterations in the structure of antigens, leading to variants against which the general population has little or no resistance

C.	Antigenic shift is primarily due to changes in the viral hemagglutinin and results in widespread and lethal pandemics; occurs at irregular intervals of 10 or more years

D.	Characterized by abrupt onset of fever, malaise, diffuse myalgia, headache, anorexia, rhinitis, and nonproductive cough
1.	Less common symptoms are sore throat, nasal congestion, and sneezing
2.	Cough is usually the most frequent and troublesome symptom and may be associated with substernal discomfort
3.	Symptoms usually last about 3-4 days, but cough and malaise may persist for 1-2 weeks

E.	Otitis media, nausea, vomiting, and diarrhea occur in children, but are less common in adults

F.	Influenza can affect metabolism of certain medications such as theophylline; toxicity from high serum concentrations may occur

G.	Complications include primary influenza pneumonia, secondary bacterial pneumonia, myositis (calf tenderness, refusal to walk in children), myocarditis, pericarditis, Reye's syndrome, and central nervous system problems; influenza can exacerbate underlying medical conditions such as cardiopulmonary disease

H.	Healthy children <24 months are at greater risk of influenza-associated hospitalization than adults >50-64 years

IV.	Diagnosis/Evaluation

A.	History
1.	Inquire about onset, duration, and character of symptoms
2.	To assess for complications, ask about chest pain, hemoptysis, severe muscle pain, and central nervous system manifestations such as confusion
3.	Determine whether household members or close contacts of patient are ill
4.	Determine history of previous influenza vaccinations
5.	Obtain a medication history; especially ask about use of theophylline

B.	Physical Examination
1.	Measure vital signs
2.	Observe general appearance for lassitude and distress
3.	Assess hydration status
4.	Perform complete eyes, ears, nose, and throat examinations
5.	Palpate sinuses for tenderness
6.	Examine neck for nuchal rigidity and cervical adenopathy
7.	Auscultate heart
8.	Perform complete lung exam
9.	Always perform abdominal and neurological exams in patients with severe cases

C.	Differential Diagnosis: Difficult to differentiate influenza from other respiratory infectious diseases
1.	Onset of symptoms is more abrupt in influenza than the common cold
2.	Sore throat, nasal congestion, and sneezing are less common in influenza than the common cold
3.	Myalgia and malaise are predominant symptoms in influenza, but may not be present in other respiratory infectious diseases; fever, anorexia, headache, fatigue, and chest discomfort are more common in patients with influenza than patients with common colds
4.	Always consider illnesses associated with biological warfare: Inhalational anthrax, smallpox, inhalational tularemia, pneumonic plague, and hemorrhagic fever (such as would be caused by Ebola or Marburg viruses)

D.	Diagnostic Tests
1.	Epidemiologic data are usually sufficient to make diagnosis in uncomplicated cases (when it is known that a certain influenza type is prevalent in a community, most persons with acute, febrile, respiratory symptoms and myalgia can safely be assumed to have influenza); epidemiologic information can be obtained from the health department, as well as websites (see table that follows)

CDC = Centers for Disease Control and Prevention
*-From October through May, the CDC collects and reports influenza surveillance data (voice information telephone system: 888-232-3228; fax 888-232-3299 [request document number 361100]

2. Consider cultures of nasopharyngeal secretions; must collect within the first 72 hours of illness
3. Rapid diagnostic kits are available commercially to detect antigens from nasopharyngeal secretions; sensitivity and specificity varies
   a. Order rapid tests for all patients hospitalized with acute respiratory infection during an epidemic period
   b. Not necessary for initiating treatment in outpatient settings but provides reassurance that therapy is appropriate and permits clinician to withhold antibiotics with confidence
   c. Be aware that CDC estimates that up to 30% of samples may produce false-negative results
4. Change in antibody titer between acute and convalescent sera using complement fixation, hemagglutination inhibition, neutralization, or enzyme immunoassay tests can help confirm diagnosis retrospectively
5. Consider CBC and urinalysis

V. Plan/Management

A. Antiviral drugs for treatment
   1. Consider treatment for the following persons:
      a. All high-risk individuals regardless of vaccination status
      b. Persons with severe influenza
      c. Consider for others to shorten duration of illness
      d. Potential benefit of treatment is the reduction in transmission to household members
   2. Start therapy as soon as possible; treatment is effective only when begun within first 2 days of symptom onset; however, zanamivir and oseltamivir may reduce risk of complications in high-risk persons on the third or fourth day of their illnesses
   3. Selection of an antiviral drug (see table that follows): In adults, zanamivir and oseltamivir are preferred because they have lower complication rates, lower risks of drug resistance, and are effective against influenza B; zanamivir also preferred for children >7 years

SELECTION OF AN ANTIVIRAL DRUG FOR TREATMENT					
	FDA Approved	**Cost**	**Complication Rate**	**Risk of Drug Resistance**	**Effective against Influenza B**
Amantadine (Symmetrel)	Adults & children ≥1 year	Low	High*[†]	High	No
Rimantadine (Flumadine)	Adults[‡]	Low	Moderate[†]	High	No
Zanamivir (Relenza)	Adults & children ≥7 years	High	Low	Low	Yes
Oseltamivir (Tamiflu)	Adults & children ≥1 year	High	Low[†]	Low	Yes

* Incidence of CNS-related (anxiety, depression, insomnia, etc.) adverse effects highest when amantadine is used; adverse effects are more common in patients with seizure disorders, psychiatric disorders, and renal insufficiency.
[†] Amantadine, rimantadine and oseltamivir occasionally cause nausea, vomiting, and dyspepsia
[‡] Rimantadine can be safely given to children ≥1 year, although not FDA approved for children

   4. Duration of therapy: 2-5 days or for 24-48 hours after patient becomes asymptomatic; immunocompromised patients may require longer course (do not exceed 10 to 14 days, regardless of patient's status)
   5. See table PROPERTIES OF ANTIVIRAL DRUGS for prescribing medications

6. Adverse effects of antiviral drugs
    a. Amantadine: Insomnia, lightheadedness, nervousness, difficulty concentrating, delirium, hallucinations, and seizures
    b. Rimantadine has CNS effects but they are less prevalent than with amantadine
    c. Zanamivir: Cough, nasal and throat discomfort, headache, and in patients with asthma, bronchospasm
    d. Oseltamivir: Nausea, vomiting, headache

PROPERTIES OF ANTIVIRAL DRUGS				
		Daily Dose		
Drug	**Route**	Children	Adults	**Available Form**
Amantadine	Oral	1-9 yrs: 5 mg/kg/day in 1-2 doses[†]	100 mg BID[‡]	Tablets and syrup
Rimantadine	Oral	Not recommended	100 mg BID[‡]	Tablets and syrup
Zanamivir	Oral inhalation	≥7 yrs: 10 mg (2 inh) BID	10 mg (2 inh) BID*	Powder for an inhaler
Oseltamivir	Oral	1-13 yrs: ≤15 kg: 30 mg BID 15-23 kg: 45 mg BID 23-40 kg: 60 mg BID	75 mg BID[‡]	Capsules

[†] The daily dose in children must not exceed 150 mg
[‡] The dose should be reduced in persons with renal insufficiency
* Is not generally recommended in patients with COPD, asthma, or other underlying airway disease
Adapted from Couch, R.B. (2000). Prevention and treatment of influenza. *New England Journal of Medicine, 343*, 1778-1787.

B. Patient Education
    1. Symptomatic treatment of fever, myalgia, and cough may be needed; especially important in young children who are at risk for febrile seizures (**do not give salicylates to children and adolescents because of risk of Reye's syndrome**)
    2. Recommend rest and increased fluids
    3. Encourage cessation of smoking in household
    4. Instruct patient to return to clinic if chest pain, dyspnea, hemoptysis, wheezing, increased temperature, agitation, behavioral changes, or confusion occur
    5. Instruct patient who is taking amantadine to be cautious of concurrent medications that affect the central nervous system, such as antihistamines and anticholinergic drugs

C. Control Measures
    1. Consider annual influenza vaccine for certain groups of individuals (see following table, TARGET GROUPS FOR INFLUENZA VACCINE)
    2. Administer influenza vaccine in the fall (optimal time is October to November), before the start of the influenza season (see following table DOSE AND SCHEDULE OF INFLUENZA VACCINE)
        a. Persons with certain chronic diseases may develop lower postvaccination antibody titers than healthy, young adults but vaccine is still effective in preventing secondary complications and reducing risk of death in this age group
        b. Do **not** administer vaccination to persons known to have anaphylactic hypersensitivity to eggs or other components of the vaccine without consulting an expert in infectious disease
        c. Minor illnesses with or without fever should not contraindicate use of vaccine
        d. Inactivated vaccine can also reduce incidence of otitis media in young children during influenza season
        e. Adverse reactions include soreness at site of vaccination and fever in young children; severe reactions are rare (concern about Guillain-Barré syndrome should not deter persons from receiving vaccine)
        f. American Academy of Pediatrics encourages immunizations of the following persons:
            1. Healthy children between 6-24 months
            2. Household contacts and out-of-town caregivers of children <24 months
            3. Immunization of close contacts of children <6 months is particularly important, as these children are not to be immunized
        g. Do not immunize children <6 months

TARGET GROUPS FOR INFLUENZA VACCINE

Groups at Increased Risk for Influenza-Related Complications
- ✓ Persons ≥50 years of age
- ✓ Residents of nursing homes or chronic-care facilities
- ✓ Adults and children with chronic disorders of the pulmonary or cardiovascular system, including children with asthma and cystic fibrosis
- ✓ Adults and children who have chronic metabolic diseases (e.g. diabetes mellitus), renal dysfunction, hemoglobinopathies or immunosuppression (including immunosuppression caused by medications or by HIV)
- ✓ Children (6 months-18 years) receiving long-term aspirin therapy who might be at risk for developing Reye's syndrome
- ✓ Women who will be in the second or third trimester of pregnancy during the influenza season

Groups That Can Transmit Influenza to Persons at High Risk
- ✓ Health care providers in both hospitals and outpatient settings, including emergency response workers
- ✓ Employees of nursing homes and chronic-care facilities who have contact with residents
- ✓ Providers of home care to persons at high risk
- ✓ Household members (including children) of persons in high risk groups including high risk infants
- ✓ Home caregivers for children and adolescents in high-risk groups

Special Groups
- ✓ Persons with HIV infection: vaccine is effective in persons with mild AIDS-related symptoms and high CD4+ T-lymphocyte counts; may not produce protective antibody titers in patients with advanced HIV disease and low CD4+ T-lymphocytes
- ✓ Breast-feeding is not contraindicated for vaccination
- ✓ Persons traveling to foreign countries: risk of exposure to influenza varies depending on season and destination; if persons traveling were not vaccinated the previous fall or winter, encourage vaccine
- ✓ General population: administer to any person who wishes to receive; especially encourage persons who provide community services and students or other persons living in institutional settings
- ✓ Children aged 6-23 months are at increased risk for hospitalizations related to influenza; vaccination for this age group is encouraged when feasible

Adapted from Advisory Committee on Immunization Practices. (2002). Prevention and control of influenza: Recommendations of Advisory Committee on Immunization Practices (ACIP). *MMWR, 51*(RR-3), 1-31.

DOSE AND SCHEDULE FOR INFLUENZA VACCINE *[†]

Age Group	Product	Dosage	# Doses
6-35 months	Split virus only	0.25 mL	1-2[§]
3-8 years	Split virus only	0.50 mL	1-2[§]
9-12 years	Split virus only	0.50 mL	1
>12 years	Whole or split virus	0.50 mL	1

* The recommended site of vaccination is the deltoid muscle for older children. The preferred site for infants and young children is the anterolateral aspect of the thigh
[†] Dosages are those recommended in recent years; refer to product circular each year for correct dosage
[§]Two doses given at least 1 month apart are recommended for children <9 years who are receiving vaccine for the first time

Adapted from Advisory Committee on Immunization Practices. (2002). Prevention and control of influenza: Recommendations of Advisory Committee on Immunization Practices (ACIP). *MMWR, 51*(RR-3), 1-31.

D. Chemoprophylaxis with antiviral drugs is an adjunct for influenza vaccine for control and prevention of influenza; antiviral drugs are **not** a substitute for vaccination
   1. Chemoprophylaxis in vaccinated persons may provide additional protection and does not interfere with the immune response, particularly useful for high-risk persons if influenza outbreak occurs before or <2 weeks after vaccination (see following table)
   2. For maximal effectiveness of prophylaxis, drug must be taken each day for duration of influenza activity in community; to be cost effective, prophylaxis should only be prescribed during period of peak influenza activity; typically prophylaxis is continued up to 6-8 weeks

Adapted from Advisory Committee on Immunization Practices. (2001). Prevention and control of influenza: Recommendations of Advisory Committee on Immunization Practices (ACIP). *MMWR, 50*(RR04), 1-46.

3. Prophylactic doses
    a. Amantadine (Symmetrel)
        (1) Children 1-9 years and children <40 kg: Amantadine 5 mg/kg/day in 1-2 doses (not to exceed 150 mg/day)
        (2) Persons ≥10 years and children who weigh ≥40 kg: Amantadine 100 mg BID
    b. Rimantadine (Flumadine)
        (1) Children 1-9 years and children <40 kg: Rimantadine 5 mg/kg/day in 1-2 doses (not to exceed 150 mg/day)
        (2) Persons ≥10 years and children who weigh ≥40 kg: Rimantadine 100 mg BID
        (3) In persons with renal insufficiency and hepatic dysfunction, the dose should be reduced to 100 mg/day or below 100 mg/day
    c. Oseltamivir (Tamiflu) 75 mg QD is approved for chemoprophylaxis of influenza among persons ≥13 years; zanamivir (Relenza) is waiting for approval for prophylaxis

E. Influenza surveillance information is available at http://www.cdc.gov/ncidod/diseases/flu/weekly.htm

F. Follow Up: None needed unless symptoms persist >7-10 days

KAWASAKI DISEASE

I. Definition: Febrile, erythematous, multi-system disease often referred to as mucocutaneous lymph node syndrome

II. Pathogenesis: Unknown etiology, but the following causative factors have been hypothesized:

A. Infection caused by rickettsiae, viruses (Epstein-Barr virus and retrovirus) and bacteria (*Group A Streptococcus*, other streptococci, and *propionibacteria*)

B. Disease may be related to living near bodies of water or exposure to house dust mites or recently shampooed carpets

III. Clinical Presentation

A. Leading cause of acquired heart disease in children in the US

B. Approximately 80% of cases occur in children <5 years of age; peak occurrence is 18-24 months of age

C. Highest incidence is in children of Asian ancestry

D.   The following clinical criteria are available to assist in formulating the diagnosis (see following table)

DIAGNOSTIC CRITERIA (PRINCIPAL CLINICAL FINDINGS) OF KAWASAKI DISEASE*

Fever of at least 5 days duration[†] **AND**

Presence of 4 of the following principal features:
- ✓ Changes in extremities (acute: erythema and edema of hands and feet; convalescent: membranous desquamation of fingertips)
- ✓ Polymorphous exanthema
- ✓ Bilateral painless conjunctival injection without exudate
- ✓ Changes in the lips and oral cavity (erythema and cracking of lips, strawberry tongue, diffuse injection of oral and pharyngeal mucosae)
- ✓ Cervical lymphadenopathy (usually unilateral and involving at least one node ≥1.5 cm in diameter)

Exclusion of other diseases with similar findings (see DIFFERENTIAL DIAGNOSIS)

---

*Patients (usually infants) with fever and <4 principal features can be diagnosed as having Kawasaki disease when coronary artery disease is detected by 2-dimensional echocardiogram or coronary angiography. The clinician should be aware that some children with illness not fulfilling these criteria have developed coronary artery aneurysm
[†]Many experts believe that, in the presence of classic features, the diagnosis of Kawasaki disease can be made by experienced observers before the fifth day of fever

Adapted from Council on Cardiovascular Disease in Young, Committee on Rheumatic Fever, Endocarditis, and Kawasaki Disease, American Heart Association. (2001). Diagnostic guidelines for Kawasaki disease. *Circulation, 87,* 335-336.

E.   Fever is one of the prominent symptoms, lasting 1-2 weeks or longer despite the use of antibiotics and the standard dose of antipyretics

F.   Within 3 days of fever other characteristic signs appear:
  1.   Swollen, indurated erythematous, and tender palms of both hands and soles of the feet
  2.   Polymorphous, erythematous rash involving the entire body and accentuated in the perineal region
  3.   Cervical lymphadenopathy which is usually unilateral and involves at least one node that is greater than 1.5 cm in diameter
  4.   Other signs include bilateral conjunctival injection, cracking of lips, strawberry tongue, erythema of the oropharyngeal mucosa and mouth ulcerations

G.   Approximately by the sixth day of illness, patient has drying, cracking, and fissuring of lips, followed by periungual desquamation and peeling of palms and soles during second to third week; in the last phase of disease, the patient may have deep transverse grooves across the nails or Beau's lines

H.   Cardiac problems are the primary cause of morbidity and mortality
  1.   Coronary aneurysms occur in approximately 20-25% of untreated patients
  2.   Carditis can involve the pericardium, myocardium, and endocardium
  3.   Mitral and aortic regurgitation may develop
  4.   Myocardial infarction is the major cause of death; in the US, the mortality rate is <0.5%

I.   Noncardiac problems are also associated with Kawasaki disease:
  1.   Joints: Arthritis and arthralgias
  2.   Gastrointestinal: Diarrhea, vomiting, and abdominal pain are frequent manifestations; mild obstructive jaundice, liver problems, hydrops of gallbladder and paralytic ileus are less common
  3.   Respiratory: Cough, rhinorrhea, otitis media, or pulmonary infiltrates
  4.   Neurological: Striking irritability and, rarely, facial palsy and aseptic meningitis

J.   Course of disease:
  1.   Without treatment, mean duration of fever is 12 days
  2.   Other symptoms and complications resolve by 6-8 weeks of onset illness, although myocardial infarction and sudden death can occur months to years later: In US, mortality rate is <0.5%

K.   Atypical Kawasaki is often misdiagnosed; criteria for diagnosis are two of the principal features and a coronary artery aneurysm
  1.   Most common in infants <1 year who have a greater chance of coronary artery aneurysm and other complications
  2.   Severe, life-threatening thrombocytopenia has been reported

IV. Diagnosis/Evaluation

    A.   History
        1.   Inquire about onset and duration of symptoms
        2.   Ask about occurrence, pattern, and degree of fever and effectiveness of self-care measures to reduce fever
        3.   Explore associated symptoms such as rash, swollen and tender hands/feet, mouth lesions, conjunctivitis, upper respiratory complaints, gastrointestinal disturbances, arthralgias, and chest pain
        4.   Inquire about previous streptococcal infection
        5.   Inquire about exposure to infectious agents
        6.   Complete a thorough medication history
        7.   Carefully determine whether patient is up-to-date with all immunizations

    B.   Physical Examination
        1.   Quickly assess whether patient is in distress or has signs of dehydration such as decreased capillary refill, poor skin turgor, and dry mucous membranes
        2.   Measure vital signs, carefully determine temperature
        3.   Inspect skin for erythema, edema, induration, rashes, drying, cracking, and desquamation
        4.   Perform a complete eye examination
        5.   Assess ears, nose, and throat for signs of infection
        6.   Carefully assess neck for lymphadenopathy and nuchal rigidity
        7.   Perform complete heart and cardiovascular exams (gallop rhythm or distant heart sounds are characteristic of Kawasaki disease)
        8.   Auscultate the lungs
        9.   Palpate abdomen for organomegaly and tenderness
        10.   Assess the joints for swelling, erythema, and tenderness
        11.   Perform a neurological exam, noting irritability, change in mental status, and facial palsy
        12.   In males, check for testicular swelling

    C.   Diagnostic Tests: Diagnosis is based primarily on clinical presentation and exclusion of other illnesses
        1.   No specific tests are available but consider ordering the following:
            a.   CBC (typically in acute stage has leukocytosis with left shift and mild anemia; in subacute phase has thrombocytopenia)
            b.   Erythrocyte sedimentation rate (ESR) (almost universally elevated)
            c.   C-reactive protein (almost universally elevated)
            d.   Urinalysis (sterile pyuria and occasional proteinuria are typical)
            e.   Serum transaminases (usually elevated)
            f.   Albumin (decreased in acute phase)
            g.   Lumbar puncture (mononuclear pleocytosis in cerebrospinal fluid)
        2.   Order a baseline echocardiogram, followed by subsequent echocardiograms at 3 and 8 weeks after onset of illness; additional echocardiograms will depend on degree of coronary artery involvement
        3.   Coronary angiography is considered by some experts as the "gold standard" to detect vascular artery disease, but has risks

    D.   Differential Diagnosis
        1.   Infectious diseases such as rubeola, scarlet fever, Lyme disease, Rocky Mountain spotted fever, infectious mononucleosis, and roseola
        2.   Drug reactions; Stevens-Johnson syndrome
        3.   Scalded skin syndrome
        4.   Toxic shock syndrome
        5.   Juvenile rheumatoid arthritis
        6.   Mercury poisoning
        7.   Illnesses caused by intentional release of biologic agents: anthrax, smallpox, and hemorrhagic fever caused by Ebola or Marburg viruses

V.   Plan/Management: Treatment consists of supportive care, detection of coronary artery disease, and anti-inflammatory therapy

    A.   Consult specialist and arrange hospitalization for patients with suspected Kawasaki disease; patients should be managed by a cardiologist

B.	Therapy should begin when diagnosis is established or strongly suspected; treat with the following 2 agents in the first 10 days of illness: intravenous gamma globulin and aspirin; treatment on or before 5 days of fever may prevent coronary inflammation and damage to arteries

C.	Subsequent immunizations
1.	Do not administer varicella and measles vaccines for at least 11 months after gamma globulin therapy; other immunizations should be given at routine times
2.	To reduce risks of Reye's syndrome in children on long-term aspirin therapy, administer influenza vaccine yearly to patients 6 months to 18 years of age

D.	Patient Education
1.	Due to risk of Reye's syndrome in patients with influenza or varicella receiving salicylates, instruct parents whose children are receiving aspirin to contact health care provider immediately if child develops symptoms or is exposed to either disease
2.	Teach parents about the signs and symptoms of possible complications such as arthralgias, chest pain, and palpitations
3.	Explain that Kawasaki disease is not spread from person-to-person contact so there is no need to preventively treat family members

E.	Follow Up
1.	Patients should be examined frequently during the first 2 months of onset of illness to detect arrhythmias, heart failure, valvular problems, and myocarditis
2.	Echocardiogram should be ordered in acute phase and then 6-8 weeks after onset of illness
3.	Follow-up care of patients with cardiac problems should be managed by a cardiologist

LYME DISEASE

I.	Definition: Infection caused by *Borrelia burgdorferi*, a member of the family of spirochetes or corkscrew-shaped bacteria

II.	Pathogenesis

A.	Ticks of the *Ixodes ricinus* complex transmit the disease

B.	Small mammals, particularly rodents, are important hosts of ticks and critical for maintenance of *B. burgdorferi* in nature; deer are hosts for the adult tick

C.	Adult ticks are less likely to transmit disease because they are readily noticed and removed; transmission of the disease is unlikely if tick attachment is less than 48-72 hours

D.	Incubation period is 3-31days (typically 7-14 days); late manifestations occur months to years later

III.	Clinical Presentation

A.	Epidemiology
1.	Leading vector-borne disease in US
2.	Incidence is increasing and there has been an expansion of the affected geographic area
3.	Occurs in the Northeast from Maine to Maryland, in the Midwest, especially Wisconsin and Minnesota, and in the West, particularly northern California and Oregon
4.	Most human infections occur during late spring and early summer months
5.	Less than 50% of all patients with Lyme disease remember receiving a tick bite

B.	Case definition for the national surveillance of Lyme disease (Centers for Disease Control and Prevention, 1990)
1.	Erythema migrans observed by clinician; to be counted for surveillance purposes, a solitary lesion must reach a size of at least 5 cm; however, recent studies have found that some patients with Lyme disease do not present with erythema migrans but rather have only systemic symptoms such as fever, chills, malaise, and occipital headaches

2. At least one manifestation and laboratory confirmation of infection
   a. Nervous system: lymphocytic meningitis, cranial neuritis, radiculoneuropathy, or rarely, encephalomyelitis
   b. Cardiovascular system: acute-onset, high-grade (2nd or 3rd degree) atrioventricular conduction defects that resolve in days or weeks
   c. Musculoskeletal system: recurrent, brief attacks (lasting weeks to months) of objectively confirmed joint swelling in one or a few joints
   d. Laboratory evidence: isolation of *B. burgdorferi* from tissue or body fluid, or detection of diagnostic levels of antibody against the spirochete by the two-test approach of enzyme-linked immunosorbent assay and Western blotting

C. First stage is called early localized and is characterized by the following:
   1. Erythema migrans (EM) is a lesion that starts as a red macule or papule at the site of a recent tick bite and enlarges over days or weeks to form a large, round lesion, often with central clearing; occurs in about 80% of patients with Lyme disease in the US
   2. Patient may not have erythema migrans or may have a rash that mimics cellulitis (erythematous plaque); rash may have a vesicular center
   3. Fever, malaise, headache, neck stiffness, and arthralgia may occur with rash; these symptoms may be intermittent over several weeks

D. Second stage is called early disseminated disease and presents as the following:
   1. Multiple erythema migrans lesions typically develop 3 to 5 weeks after tick bite and appears as annular erythematous lesions which are smaller but similar to primary lesion
   2. Other common manifestations are palsies of cranial nerves, meningitis, conjunctivitis, and systemic symptoms such as arthralgia, myalgia, headache, and fatigue; carditis, which presents as various degrees of heart block, is a rare occurrence

E. Third stage is called late disease and signs and symptoms in this stage may not present until months or years after tick bite; characterized by following:
   1. Recurrent arthritis which is pauciarticular and affects large joints, particularly the knees
   2. Central nervous system manifestations include subacute encephalopathy and polyradiculoneuropathy
   3. Third stage occurs infrequently in children treated with antibiotics in early stages of disease

F. After an episode of appropriately treated Lyme disease, some persons have subjective complaints (such as myalgia, arthralgia, fatigue) and have been classified as having "chronic Lyme disease" or "post-Lyme disease syndrome"; there is insufficient data to regard this syndrome as a separate diagnostic entity and repeated or prolonged courses of antibiotics have been ineffective

IV. Diagnosis/Evaluation

A. History
   1. Ask about possible exposure to tick bites such as recent camping trip, frequent yard work, and pets who are outside in vegetation
   2. Ask patient to describe the duration, characteristics, and course of any skin lesion
   3. Question about fatigue, headache, fever, myalgias
   4. Inquire about late manifestations such as arthritis and neurologic and cardiac problems

B. Physical Examination
   1. Carefully inspect the skin
   2. Palpate for lymphadenopathy
   3. Perform a thorough cardiac exam
   4. Inspect joints for swelling, tenderness, or erythema
   5. Perform a neurological examination

C. Differential Diagnosis
   1. Infectious diseases such as Reiter's syndrome, Rocky Mountain spotted fever, acute rheumatic fever, tularemia, viral syndrome, or meningitis/encephalitis
   2. Rheumatoid arthritis
   3. Systemic lupus erythematosus
   4. Bell's palsy

D. Diagnostic Tests; accurate identification of the tick is useful and is often available free of charge from the health department

    1. Serologic testing at time of tick bite is usually **not** recommended; antibodies to *B. burgdorferi* do not have sufficient time to develop at time of tick bite

    2. Patients who meet case definition for Lyme disease (III.B.), who have rash resembling erythema migrans, or who have a history of characteristic rash and a previous tick bite should have empiric antibiotic therapy; no diagnostic tests are needed

    3. Closely monitor persons who remove attached ticks for signs and symptoms of Lyme disease for up to 30 days, specifically assessing for skin lesion at site of bite or temperature >38°C

    4. Carefully assess and consider testing and therapy for any person who develops skin lesion or clinical symptoms within one month of removing tick; **Patients with singular symptoms of arthralgias, myalgia, headache, fatigue, or palpitations** have a low chance of having Lyme disease and **should not be tested**

    5. Although the Infectious Disease Society of America does not recommend testing for tick-borne infectious organisms, some clinicians obtain serologic tests for antibodies, especially for those persons who live in communities with high incidence of Lyme disease; tests should be performed in a reference rather than a commercial laboratory

        a. First, order an enzyme-linked immunosorbent assay (ELISA) or an immunofluorescence assay (IFA); these tests often have false positive results

        b. For specimens that give positive or equivocal ELISA or IFA results, order a Western immunoblot to test for antibodies

    6. Other diagnostic tests are not usually ordered but may be beneficial:

        a. In persons with suspected early disease and a negative serologic test, changes in antibody levels in paired acute-phase (close to time of tick bite) and convalescent-phase (6-8 weeks later) serum samples may help diagnose disease, but published data are not yet available to determine the clinical utility of this approach

        b. Seek consultation with a specialist on testing of patients with suspected central nervous system involvement; antibody testing of cerebrospinal fluid may be recommended

        c. Investigational tests such as polymerase chain reaction (PCR) are more sensitive and specific, but their clinical usefulness is unproven

    7. To establish or exclude diagnosis in patients who have received the recombinant outer surface protein A (rOspA) vaccine, order the Western immunoblot test

V. Plan/Management

    A. Treat the following patients with antibiotics (see following table on RECOMMENDED TREATMENT)

        1. Patients with erythema migrans

        2. Consider treatment for any person who develops skin lesion or clinical symptoms (i.e., temperature >38°C) within one month of removing tick; Patients with singular symptoms of arthralgias, myalgia, headache, fatigue, or palpitations have a low chance of having Lyme disease and should not be treated

        3. Consider treatment for patients who live in high incidence area and who have positive results from the two-test protocol (ELISA or IFA and Western blot)

    B. Do not treat patients whose only evidence of Lyme disease is a positive immunologic test; the risks of empiric antibiotic treatment outweigh the benefits

RECOMMENDED TREATMENT

Disease Category	Drug/Duration	Adult Dosage	Pediatric Dosage
Early Localized Disease*	Doxycycline (Vibramycin) 14-21 days	100 mg BID	Not recommended <8 years of age
	Amoxicillin (Amoxil) 14-21 days	500 mg TID	25-50 mg/kg/day divided into 2 doses; max. 2 g/day
Early Disseminated and Late Disease			
• Multiple erythema migrans	Same as early disease except duration is 21 days		
• Isolated facial palsy	Same as early disease, except duration is 21-28 days[‡]		
• Arthritis	Same as early disease except duration is 28 days		
• Persistent or recurrent arthritis[§] • Carditis • Meningitis or encephalitis	Ceftriaxone (Rocephin) IV or IM for 14-21 days OR Penicillin G IV for 14-21 days	2 g QD or 1 g BID OR 20 million units in 4 divided doses	75-100 mg/kg QD (maximum, 2 g/day) OR 300,000 U/kg/day given in divided doses every 4 hours (maximum 20 million U/day)

*Cefuroxime axetil (500 mg BID or 30 mg/kg/day in 2 doses for children) is alternative drug for patients allergic to penicillin; other alternatives are erythromycin or penicillin

[†]Do not give corticosteroids

[‡]Antibiotics do not affect resolution of nerve palsy; purpose is to prevent late disease

[§]Considered persistent when there is objective evidence of synovitis for at least 2 months after treatment is initiated. Some experts use a second course of an oral agent before using an IV antibiotic

Adapted from American Academy of Pediatrics. (2000). In L.K. Pickering (Ed.). *2000 Red Book: Report of the Committee on Infectious Diseases* (25th ed.). Elk Grove Village, IL: American Academy of Pediatrics.

C. Prevention
  1. Patient education
     a. Avoidance of tick-infested areas is the most important preventive measure
     b. Keep grass mowed and remove leaves, brush, tall grass, and woodpiles from around houses and at the edges of gardens
     c. Always inspect body carefully after being outdoors; pay special attention to exposed hairy regions of the body
     d. Daily inspect pets and remove ticks
     e. Wear lightly colored clothing so that ticks can be seen more easily
     f. Prevent ticks from getting under clothing; tuck pant legs into socks or tape area where pants and socks meet, and tuck shirt into pants
     g. Wear a hat and long-sleeved shirt
     h. Avoid overhanging grass and brush by walking in the center of trails
     i. Spray permethrin on clothing or treat clothes with permethrin which kills ticks on contact and prevents tick attachment
     j. Spray insect repellent containing n,n-diethyl-m-toluamide (DEET) on all exposed skin other than face, hands, and abraded skin (must reapply every 1-2 hours); use DEET sparingly because of rare reports of serious neurologic complications after use (wash treated skin with soap and water after being outdoors)
     k. Remove clothing and wash and dry it in high temperature after outdoor exposure
  2. Remove attached ticks with fine tweezers or blunt, medium-tipped angled forceps as close to skin as possible; pull tick straight back with a slow steady force; remove tick completely, including the mouth part; disinfect skin before and after tick is removed; do not use nail polish, alcohol, or matches to remove tick
  3. Routine use of antimicrobial agents to prevent disease is not recommended because therapy is associated with potential risks and costs and is not efficacious; however, a recent study found that a single, 200 mg dose of doxycycline prevented infection after a nymphal tick bite, particularly when duration of attachment was prolonged
  4. Lyme disease vaccine was removed from the market in 2002 due to poor sales

D.   Follow Up
      1.   Patients treated with oral antibiotics should be reevaluated at the end of treatment
      2.   Patients with severe symptoms should be seen more frequently based on their clinical condition

MENINGITIS AND ENCEPHALITIS (VIRAL)

I.   Definition: Viral infection of the central nervous system

      A.   Aseptic meningitis: Inflammatory process of the meninges in which the cerebrospinal fluid (CSF) is sterile
            for bacteria

      B.   Encephalitis: Acute inflammatory process involving brain tissue

      C.   Meningoencephalitis: Inflammation of the brain tissue and the adjacent meninges

II.   Pathogenesis

      A.   Pathogens are identified in only about 20% of cases

      B.   Enteroviruses cause about 80-85% of cases in which an agent is identified

      C.   The remaining cases with an identified agent are primarily due to the following:
            1.   Arboviruses: St. Louis encephalitis virus (most common), West Nile virus, eastern equine
                  encephalomyelitis virus, western equine encephalomyelitis virus; all of which are transmitted by
                  mosquitos
            2.   Herpes simplex virus
            3.   Human immunodeficiency virus
            4.   Less common viruses are adenovirus, varicella zoster virus, cytomegalovirus, Epstein-Barr virus,
                  influenza virus, and mumps virus
            5.   Rare viruses are parvovirus B19, rotavirus, measles, rubella, and rabies

III. Clinical Presentation

      A.   Onset is usually acute, but signs and symptoms are usually preceded by a nonspecific febrile illness and
            sometimes, an upper respiratory tract infection

      B.   Signs and symptoms vary by age
            1.   Infants
                  a.   Nonspecific symptoms of fever, irritability, and lethargy occur first
                  b.   Poor feeding and a bulging fontanelle are later manifestations
            2.   Older children:
                  a.   Initially, children have headache, fever, altered consciousness, disorientation, and
                        behavioral and speech alterations
                  b.   Other manifestations include vomiting, stiff neck, back and leg pain, photophobia

      C.   Children who have enteroviral meningitis usually recover completely; however, some studies have
            reported that very young infants have lower intelligence and delayed speech development following this
            infection

      D.   When encephalitis accompanies meningitis the patient's condition is much more severe; patients with
            severe encephalitis may have stupor, coma, bizarre movements, and seizures

IV. Diagnosis/Evaluation

    A. History; discussion with local public health authorities is important to determine which viruses are circulating in the area
1. Question about onset of symptoms
2. In infants, ask about feeding patterns, irritability, and lethargy
3. Inquire about fever, rash, vomiting, headache, eye complaints, speech abnormalities, and mental status changes
4. To determine the possibility of malignancies, ask about weight loss, anorexia, bleeding, and fatigue
5. Ask about recent infections and exposure to others with infectious diseases
6. Ask about history of immunosuppression
7. Inquire about history of travel, exposure to an epidemic, exposure to toxins, and animal exposure
8. Ask about medications and recent immunizations
9. Inquire about alcohol abuse

    B. Physical Examination; because of the possible severity of this condition, a complete physical examination of all systems is usually required
1. Assess general appearance
2. Measure vial signs
3. Examine head; in infants observe for a bulging fontanelle that may occur with viral meningitis
4. Examine skin; rashes may occur, but are more common in bacterial meningitis and in other conditions (Rocky Mountain spotted fever, Kawasaki disease, toxic shock syndrome)
5. Perform funduscopic examination; papilledema is uncommon in both viral and bacterial meningitis
6. Examine ears, eyes, nose and throat to detect other conditions that mimic meningitis (pharyngitis, peritonsillar abscess)
7. Palpate for lymphadenopathy to detect other infectious diseases (cat-scratch disease, cervical adenitis, Kawasaki disease)
8. Perform cardiovascular, respiratory, gastrointestinal, and genitourinary examinations to rule-out other conditions that mimic meningitis
9. Perform musculoskeletal examination; arthralgia and myalgias may occur (more common in bacterial meningitis than viral meningitis)
10. Perform complete neurologic examination
11. Perform tests to check for meningeal inflammation
    a. Kernig's sign
      (1) Place patient supine and extend the leg at the knee while the hip is flexed at 90 degrees
      (2) Positive for inflammation when the maneuver causes extensor spasm of the knee and pain in the hamstrings when the leg is extended to about 135 degrees
    b. Brudzinski's sign
      (1) Place patient in supine position and flex neck
      (2) Positive for inflammation when the maneuver causes involuntary flexing of hips and knees
12. Assess mental status

    C. Differential Diagnosis
1. Bacterial meningitis (important to quickly detect and treat to prevent complications and death)
    a. Highest incidence is in infants within the first month of life
    b. Typically children with this condition have a more acute condition and are more critically ill than those with viral meningitis, but this is not always the case
    c. Children with bacterial meningitis usually have more meningeal signs than children with viral infections
    d. Untreated bacterial meningitis is quickly fatal
    e. Mortality rate is 5-10% of all cases
    f. About 15-25% of survivors have long-term morbidity (developmental delays, seizure disorders, spasticity, and hearing loss)
2. Nonviral, nonbacterial causes of CNS infection: Rickettsiae, mycoplasmas, parasites, fungi
3. Postimmunization encephalitides
4. Kawasaki disease
5. Rocky Mountain spotted fever
6. Cat-scratch disease
7. Toxic shock syndrome
8. Neurosyphilis
9. Subdural empyema

10. Noninfectious disorders may cause CNS disturbances
   a. Metabolic: Hypoglycemia, electrolyte imbalance, uremia, hepatic encephalopathy
   b. Malignancies: Leukemia, tumors
   c. Collagen vascular diseases (systemic lupus erythematosus)
   d. Intracranial hemorrhage
   e. Medications (oral trimethoprim/sulfamethoxazole, intravenous immunoglobulin, some nonsteroidal antiinflammatory agents)
   f. Toxins (lead)
11. Other disorders may mimic clinical manifestations of meningitis, but have normal CNS findings
   a. Pharyngitis
   b. Retropharyngeal abscess
   c. Cervical adenitis
   d. Cervical spine arthritis
   e. Osteomyelitis
   f. Pyelonephritis
   g. Sepsis
   h. Pneumonia
   i. Torticollis
   j. Tetanus

D. Diagnostic Tests; it is important to search for an etiologic agent to identify a treatable pathogen, to detect a possible impending epidemic for which preventive measures can be implemented, and to determine the patient's long-term prognosis
   1. Perform lumbar puncture unless patient has papilledema or there is concern about a space-occupying lesion or increased intracranial pressure; typical findings include the following:
      a. 30-500 white blood cells (WBCs) per cubic millimeter; early in course of disease, polymorphonuclear neutrophils predominate, but after 8-12 hours, lymphocytes predominate
      b. Protein may be slightly elevated
      c. Glucose is normal
      d. Gram's stain is negative
      e. Cerebrospinal fluid (CSF) culture is negative for bacteria
      f. Immunofluorescence antibody assays or polymerase chain reaction (PCR) assays are available to identify the virus
      g. Serologic tests of the (CSF) by IgM antibodies can confirm eastern equine encephalitis, western equine encephalitis, LaGrosse encephalitis, and St. Louis encephalitis
   2. Obtain culture of nasopharynx or throat fluids and a rectal swab
   3. Obtain blood cultures if bacterial meningitis is a possible diagnosis
   4. The following tests are also routinely recommended: complete blood count with differential and platelets, electrolytes, glucose, calcium, magnesium, blood urea nitrogen/creatinine, liver function tests, erythrocyte sedimentation rate, toxicology screen, thyroid function tests, antinuclear antibodies, HIV test, rapid plasma reagin, Epstein-Barr virus panel, urinalysis, chest x-ray
   5. For patients with fever and CNS manifestations consider ordering electroencephalography, computed tomography, technetium brain scans, and magnetic resonance imaging

V. Plan/Management

A. All children with altered states of consciousness, severe symptoms, and suspected bacterial meningitis should be hospitalized (usually in an intensive care unit) and observed closely

B. Any child less than 1 year of age should be hospitalized because at this age viral meningitis is difficult to distinguish from bacterial meningitis; thus, parenteral antibiotics are usually given for 48-72 hours until a bacterial cause is excluded

C. Treatment of older children with viral meningitis who have mild symptoms:
   1. These children can be treated as outpatients if they can tolerate fluids orally, have responsible caregivers, and can return to health care centers quickly in case their conditions worsen
   2. Provide symptomatic therapy with antipyretics, oral fluids, and vigilant observation

D. Treatment of children with viral encephalitis
   1. Hospitalization is recommended
   2. Pharmacological treatment
      a. If patient has herpes simplex virus encephalitis, prescribe intravenous acyclovir (Zovirax)
      b. No specific antiviral therapy is available for the other forms of meningitis and encephalitis

3. Care is supportive
   a. Hydration; but avoid overhydration as this can exacerbate cerebral edema
   b. Treat fever
   c. Carefully provide pain medication as overmedication may mask symptoms or confuse the clinical picture
   d. Provide rest in a quiet, dark environment
   e. Provide for seizure precautions
   f. Prevent complications such as deep venous thrombosis, decubiti, urinary tract infections
   g. Carefully monitor for increased intracranial pressure

E. Followup
   1. Followup is variable depending on severity of condition
   2. Patients with mild symptoms who are treated as outpatients should be evaluated within 8-24 hours and then daily or every 3-4 days depending on their condition

MONONUCLEOSIS, INFECTIOUS

I. Definition: Acute viral syndrome with classic triad of fever, pharyngitis, and adenopathy

II. Pathogenesis

   A. Causal agent is the Epstein-Barr virus (EBV)

   B. Spread person-to-person by the oropharyngeal route (via saliva); rarely via blood transfusion

   C. Incubation period is from 30 to 50 days

   D. Period of communicability is indeterminate but may be prolonged
      1. Respiratory tract viral excretion may persist for many months or more after illness
      2. Asymptomatic carriage is common

III. Clinical Presentation

   A. Common infection in college-age individuals and adolescents living in group settings such as educational institutions; in infants and young children, the disease is frequently unrecognized and generally mild

   B. Spectrum of disease is variable; patients may be asymptomatic or suffer from fatal infection

   C. Common signs and symptoms include the classic triad of fever, exudative pharyngitis, adenopathy (particularly posterior cervical), as well as fatigue, eyelid edema, headache, pain behind eyes, and a palatal petechial rash

   D. Atypical lymphocytosis and abnormal liver function tests often accompany the disease

   E. Splenic enlargement may occur; usually resolves within the first month of the illness

   F. Duration of the illness is variable with the average, uncomplicated illness lasting 3-4 weeks; some patients have a low level of fatigue for 6-12 months

   G. Complications occur more often in patients <10 years, >50 years, and those who are immunocompromised; complications include central nervous system (CNS) disorders such as aseptic meningitis, encephalitis, and the Guillain-Barré syndrome; rare complications include splenic rupture, thrombocytopenia, agranulocytosis, myocarditis, hemolytic anemia

IV. Diagnosis/Evaluation

   A. History
      1. Ask about onset, pattern, and character of symptoms
      2. Ascertain that patient does not have trouble breathing or severe swallowing difficulty

3. Question about severe headaches, weakness, and confusion (CNS complications of mononucleosis)
4. Question about recent history of exposure to others with mononucleosis

B. Physical Examination
1. Observe general appearance
2. Measure vital signs
3. Observe skin for exanthems
4. Perform complete ears, nose, and throat examinations
5. Auscultate the heart
6. Auscultate the lungs, making certain that the patient does not have upper airway obstruction from enlarged tonsils and lymphoid tissue
7. Palpate abdomen for organomegaly
8. Perform a neurological examination to rule out CNS complications

C. Differential Diagnosis
1. Streptococcal or viral pharyngitis (posterior cervical adenopathy and splenomegaly help distinguish pharyngitis of infectious mononucleosis from other types of pharyngitis)
2. Viral syndromes
3. Hepatitis
4. HIV infection
5. Cytomegalovirus infection
6. Toxoplasma infection
7. Secondary syphilis

D. Diagnostic Tests
1. Order complete blood count with differential; absolute lymphocytosis in which more than 10% of cells are atypical is characteristic
2. Order nonspecific serologic tests for heterophil antibody (Paul-Bunnell test and slide agglutination reaction are most widely available)
   a. Often negative in children younger than 4 years but will identify 90% of cases in older children and adults
   b. Early in the course of this illness, some infected persons will have a negative test because the level of antibodies in the blood has not reached sufficient levels; if patient continues to have symptoms repeat test in 7-10 days
   c. A positive result may remain positive for up to a year after the initial illness
3. Multiple specific serologic antibody tests for EBV are available
   a. Most commonly used test is for IgG and IgM antibodies against viral capsid antigen (VCA); particularly useful for evaluating patients who have heterophil-negative infectious mononucleosis (testing for other viral agents such as cytomegalovirus is needed for these patients)
   b. Testing positive for IgM antibodies indicates recent infection
   c. Positive IgG antibodies with findings of negative IgM antibodies, indicates past infection
4. Consider obtaining throat swab and perform rapid strep test. If the rapid strep test is negative (3-30% of patients with mononucleosis also have streptococcal infection) send a throat culture
5. Consider ordering liver function tests

V. Plan/Management

A. Patients with uncomplicated acute mononucleosis require only symptomatic therapy

B. For patients with more severe symptoms, consult specialist and consider the following:
1. Corticosteroid therapy is considered only for patients with complications such as obstructive tonsillar enlargement, hemolytic anemia, aplastic anemia, encephalitis, myocarditis, and massive splenomegaly; prescribe prednisone 1mg/kg/day orally for 7 days and then taper
2. Acyclovir is not currently recommended

C. If patient has concomitant streptococcal pharyngitis treat with erythromycin (see section on PHARYNGITIS); Do not prescribe ampicillin or amoxicillin-containing agents because they cause a rash; infrequently, penicillin can also cause a rash

D. Patient Education
1. Help patient plan a realistic schedule of rest with modification of work and/or school responsibilities depending on patient's condition
2. Increased fluid intake may be beneficial
3. Instruct patient to immediately report pain in left upper area of abdomen or in shoulder as this could be a sign of splenic rupture
4. Isolation is not needed, but good hand washing technique, avoidance of sharing eating or drinking utensils with others, and avoidance of kissing or sharing oral secretions are important
5. Avoid contact sports, heavy lifting, and strenuous activity for at least one month or until resolution of splenomegaly because an enlarged spleen is susceptible to rupture
6. Avoid alcohol consumption for at least a month to decrease the work of the liver
7. Instruct patient with a recent history of mononucleosis to avoid donating blood
8. Avoid ampicillin or amoxicillin during course of disease as a drug-related rash may develop
9. Inform patient that recovery is typically in 2 to 4 weeks, but that some patients have a slow recovery of 2 to 3 months

E. Follow Up: every 1-2 weeks until symptoms resolve for uncomplicated cases

ROCKY MOUNTAIN SPOTTED FEVER

I. Definition: Systemic, small vessel vasculitis with characteristic rash that results from bite of infected tick

II. Pathogenesis

A. Infectious agent is *Rickettsia rickettsii*

B. Mode of transmission
1. Tick must attach and feed on blood for approximately 4-6 hours to become infectious in humans
2. No person-to-person transmission

C. Incubation period ranges from 2-14 days

III. Clinical Presentation

A. Primarily occurs in children <15 years of age during the months of April through October

B. Most cases are in south Atlantic, southeastern, and south central states; other areas include the upper Rocky Mountain states, Canada, Mexico, and South and Central America

C. Patient typically presents with sudden onset of moderate to high fever (which persists if untreated for 2-3 weeks), severe headache, myalgia, conjunctival injection, nausea, and vomiting; other symptoms include photophobia and myalgia (bilateral calf pain is classic)

D. Characteristic maculopapular rash that usually blanches with pressure often appears before the sixth day of illness
1. Rash spreads from wrists and ankles to trunk, neck, and face
2. In untreated patients, the lesions become petechial in about 4 days, then purpuric and coalesced
3. In severe cases, rash can involve entire body and mucous membranes and result in gangrene or necrosis

E. Thrombocytopenia develops in most patients; anemia is present in about 30% of cases

F. Disease can persist for 3 weeks and can be severe with CNS, cardiac, pulmonary, gastrointestinal, and renal involvement as well as disseminated intravascular coagulation which can lead to shock and ultimately to death; death is uncommon when diagnosis and treatment are prompt

IV. Diagnosis/Evaluation

    A.   History
        1.   Inquire about onset, duration, and characteristics of all symptoms
        2.   Ask patient to describe characteristics and progression of any rashes or skin lesions
        3.   Inquire about possible exposure to tick bites such as a recent camping trip or frequent yard work
        4.   May need to do a complete review of systems to detect complications from the infection

    B.   Physical Examination
        1.   Measure vital signs, noting fever
        2.   Observe general appearance for signs of distress and lethargy
        3.   Carefully inspect skin for rashes and lesions
        4.   Inspect eyes for conjunctival injection
        5.   Palpate for lymphadenopathy
        6.   Perform complete heart, lung, gastrointestinal, genitourinary, and neurological examinations to rule out complications

    C.   Differential Diagnosis
        1.   Most often confused with viral syndrome
        2.   In advanced disease, bacterial sepsis, meningitis, and meningococcemia are part of differential diagnosis
        3.   Cutaneous anthrax as a result of bioterrorism
            a.   Rash occurs primarily on exposed areas of hands, arms, or face
            b.   An area of local edema develops into a painless, pruritic macule or papule that enlarges and ulcerates after 1-2 days
            c.   Subsequently, a painless, depressed black eschar develops
            d.   Lymphangitis and painful lymphadenopathy are often present
            e.   Without antibiotic treatment (ciprofloxacin, doxycycline), mortality can reach 20%
        4.   Other illnesses caused by intentional release of biologic agents such as smallpox and hemorrhagic fever due to Ebola or Marburg viruses

    D.   Diagnostic Tests
        1.   Consider ordering acute and convalescent sera, group-specific serologic tests (a fourfold rise in antibody titer is diagnostic of the disease)
            a.   Titers can be determined by indirect fluorescent antibody, enzyme immunoassay, complement fixation, latex agglutination, indirect hemagglutination, or microagglutination
            b.   Never delay initiation of antimicrobial treatment to confirm diagnosis
        2.   Consider ordering a CBC with differential, BUN, serum albumin, serum electrolytes, and liver function studies

V. Plan/Management (consult specialist)

    A.   Important to treat patients with antimicrobial therapy early in the course of disease; mortality sharply increases when therapy is delayed until the fifth day of illness

    B.   Doxycycline (Vibramycin) is the drug of choice in all patients
        1.   Previously, chloramphenicol was recommended for children <8 years and those with severe disease; today doxycycline is considered to be most efficacious agent and the risk of teeth staining is less than previously believed
        2.   In children, prescribe oral doxycycline (Vibramycin) 2-4 mg/kg/day in two divided doses; available in 50 mg/5 ml syrup
        3.   Adult dose is doxycycline 100 mg BID after a loading dose of 200 mg
        4.   Therapy is continued until patient is afebrile for at least 2-3 days; usual course is 7-10 days

    C.   Patients who have any signs of complications should have a specialist consult and probably be admitted to the hospital because of the dangers of vascular collapse

    D.   Prevention: Teach patient about measures to avoid tick bites (see section on LYME DISEASE)

E.	Follow Up
1.	Because of the possible dangerous complications, close monitoring is needed
2.	Teach patients to return to clinic if any danger signs such as alterations in mental status, stiff neck, severe headache, prolonged nausea and vomiting, shortness of breath, decreased urine output, high fever, severe weakness, and dizziness occur
3.	Patients should return to clinic within 24-48 hours of initial visit; and patient should be re-evaluated at the end of the antimicrobial therapy

ROSEOLA (EXANTHEM SUBITUM)

I.	Definition: Acute viral infection occurring primarily in children under 3 years of age

II.	Pathogenesis

A.	Causal agent is human herpesvirus-6 (HHV-6) or a virus closely related to HHV-6

B.	Mode of transmission is unclear; infants may become infected by asymptomatic shedding of persistent virus in secretions of close contacts

C.	Incubation period ranges from 5-15 days

D.	Period of communicability is unknown, but is most likely greatest during the febrile phase, before the appearance of the exanthem

III.	Clinical Presentation

A.	Children between the ages of 6 to 24 months have the highest rates; uncommon in infants <3 months and children >3 years

B.	Most common exanthem of children <3 years; most children are infected with the virus early in life but have no symptoms and the condition usually goes unrecognized

C.	Usually child is asymptomatic; child with symptoms presents with acute onset of prodromal fever, lasting 3-7 days, which can be as high as 106°F (41°C), mild adenopathy, and inflamed tympanic membranes

D.	Abrupt resolution of fever and eruption of a rash often occur together
1.	Rash begins on trunk and spreads to face and extremities
2.	Discrete, pinkish maculopapular rash which lasts only one or two days

E.	Complication is the onset of febrile seizures due to high fever

IV.	Diagnosis/Evaluation

A.	History
1.	Question about degree, onset, and duration of fever
2.	Question about self-treatment of fever
3.	Ask parents to describe progression of rash
4.	Determine whether there are other symptoms such as coryza, cough, sore throat, watery eyes (accompanying symptoms suggests a diagnosis other than roseola)
5.	Determine whether other family or household members have similar symptoms (infection of close contacts suggests a diagnosis other than roseola)
6.	Determine medication use (side effects of several medications present with rash)
7.	Ask about history of febrile seizures

B. Physical Examination
   1. Measure vital signs, carefully assessing temperature
   2. Assess general appearance, noting lethargy and respiratory distress
   3. Carefully inspect skin
   4. To rule out other viral exanthems assess head, eyes, ears, nose, throat, and mouth
   5. Assess neck for nuchal rigidity and adenopathy (adenopathy may be present with roseola)
   6. Auscultate heart and lungs (normal findings are present with roseola)

C. Differential Diagnosis: The rash accompanying roseola may be confused with other viral exanthematous diseases; the following characteristics differentiate roseola from other conditions
   1. Roseola occurs in children 3 months to 3 years (children younger than 3 months who have exanthem do not have roseola)
   2. Children with roseola are often playful without change in appetite even with the high fever (typically, with other viral exanthems, children are uncomfortable or lethargic)
   3. Abrupt onset of fever followed by rash with rapid resolution of both is characteristic of roseola

D. Diagnostic Tests: No tests are needed unless diagnosis is uncertain

V. Plan/Management

A. Treatment is symptomatic
   1. Administer acetaminophen to control temperature (see section on FEVER for dosage)
   2. Encourage fluids to prevent dehydration from high fever

B. Patient Education
   1. Parents need reassurance that the high fever does not mean a serious disease
   2. Teach parents to be alert for symptoms such as lethargy, decreased fluid intake, cough, and irritability that suggest a diagnosis other than roseola and the need for further evaluation

C. Follow Up: No follow up is needed if there are no further problems

RUBELLA (GERMAN MEASLES)

I. Definition: Febrile viral disease with diffuse maculopapular rash; postnatal rubella is usually mild and congenital rubella is associated with high incidence of congenital anomalies

II. Pathogenesis

A. Causal agent is rubella virus which is a RNA virus

B. Postnatal rubella is spread by direct or droplet contact with secretions of nose and throat

C. Incubation period ranges from 14-21 days

D. Period of communicability
   1. One week before and 5-7 days after onset of rash
   2. Infants with congenital rubella may shed virus for months after birth

III. Clinical Presentation

A. Epidemiology
   1. Importance of this viral illness is not the morbidity of the disease itself, but rather the consequences that can occur to a fetus during a maternal infection
   2. Before the use of vaccines, rubella was a wide-spread disease; today the incidence of disease has declined by more than 99% from the prevaccine era
   3. Most cases today occur in young, unvaccinated adults and outbreaks in colleges and occupational settings; approximately 10% of young adults are susceptible to rubella

B. Postnatal rubella
   1. Prodrome may or may not be present; typically lasts 1-5 days; younger children present with mild coryza and diarrhea; older children and adolescents have headaches and sore throats
   2. Mild disease with rash, impressive lymphadenopathy (suboccipital, postauricular, cervical), and slight fever; rarely involves complications
   3. Exanthem is typically a pink, maculopapular eruption which begins on the face and spreads downward to the trunk and extremities
      a. Rash is usually completely cleared by third or fifth day after initial presentation
      b. Lesions remain discrete and pink which contrasts with the rash of rubeola which is deep red and becomes confluent
   4. Transient polyarthralgia and polyarthritis are common in adolescents and adults; rare in children
   5. Disease is usually self-limited and patient does not have complications

C. Congenital rubella
   1. Most common anomalies: eye (cataracts, congenital glaucoma, retinopathy), heart (patent ductus arteriosus, pulmonary artery stenosis), sensorineural deafness, and neurologic disorders (meningoencephalitis, mental retardation)
   2. Growth retardation, hepatosplenomegaly, thrombocytopenia, and purpuric skin lesions also frequently occur in infants
   3. Occurrence of congenital defects is at least 50% if infection occurs during first month of gestation, 20-30% if during the second month, and falls to 5% during the 3rd or 4th month

IV. Diagnosis/Evaluation

A. History
   1. Inquire about duration and occurrence of rash, fever, and enlarged lymph nodes which indicate rubella as well as other symptoms such as cough, coryza, conjunctivitis, and pharyngitis which are associated with other exanthematous diseases
   2. Ask about recent exposure to persons with a rash
   3. Ask about medication and drug use
   4. Inquire about history of rubella illness and/or illnesses with exanthems (history of rubella illness is not a reliable indicator of immunity; identification of immune status is based on the presence of demonstrable antibody)

B. Physical Examination
   1. Measure vital signs
   2. Inspect skin, noting characteristics of exanthem
   3. To eliminate other exanthematous diseases as the diagnosis, examine the following:
      a. Eyes, noting signs of conjunctivitis
      b. Head, ears, nose, and throat
      c. Mouth for signs of Koplik's spots which indicate measles, not rubella
      d. Neck, noting nuchal rigidity and adenopathy
      e. Heart, noting murmurs associated with Kawasaki syndrome

C. Differential Diagnosis
   1. Infectious diseases such as rubeola, roseola, Rocky Mountain spotted fever, scarlet fever, Kawasaki syndrome, infectious mononucleosis
   2. Enteroviral infections are a common cause of exanthems
      a. Enteroviruses consist of different strains of echoviruses, coxsackieviruses, and polioviruses that typically cause infection in summer and fall
      b. Patients typically have a nonspecific febrile illness with rhinitis, pharyngitis, pneumonia, vomiting, diarrhea, abdominal pain, or conjunctivitis
      c. Patients infected with coxsackievirus A16 or enterovirus 71 may have hand, foot, and mouth syndrome; papulovesicular lesions occur in mouth, palms, fingers, soles, and occasionally on buttocks
      d. Severe cases may have aseptic meningitis, encephalitis, paralysis, hepatitis, acute hemorrhagic conjunctivitis, myopericarditis
      e. Treatment is symptomatic for most cases; consult specialist for serious cases
   3. Drug reaction

D. Diagnostic Tests
1. The virus can be isolated from nasal specimens by inoculation of appropriate cell culture; notify laboratory personnel that rubella is suspected, because additional testing is required
2. Throat swabs, blood, urine, and cerebrospinal fluid can also be used to detect the virus, particularly in congenitally infected infants
3. A fourfold or greater rise in antibody titer or seroconversion between acute and convalescent sera is indicative of infection
4. Detection of specific rubella IgM antibodies indicates a recent postnatal or congenital infection
5. Congenital infection can also be confirmed by stable or increasing levels of rubella-specific IgG over several months
6. Serologic screening tests include latex agglutination, fluorescence immunoassay, passive hemagglutination, hemolysis-in-gel, or enzyme immunoassay

V. Plan/Management

A. Treatment: Only symptomatic treatment (such as rest and increased fluid intake) is needed

B. Primary prevention of rubella (see immunization schedule in HEALTH MAINTENANCE section)

C. Treatment of exposed persons
1. Pregnant women need blood specimens tested for rubella antibody; consult specialist for further treatment of exposed pregnant women; routine use of immune globulin is not recommended and only considered if termination of pregnancy is not an option
2. Live rubella vaccine given within 3 days after exposure to nonpregnant persons does not theoretically prevent the disease, but may be indicated, and will provide protection against developing rubella in the future

D. Control procedures
1. All cases of rubella and congenital rubella should be reported to the local public health unit
2. In institutions such as hospitals, patients suspected of having rubella should be isolated
3. Patients should not go to work or school for 5-7 days after onset of rash; patients with congenital rubella should be considered contagious until they are one year old, unless nasopharyngeal and urine cultures after 3 months of age are repeatedly negative
4. Efforts should be made to identify and counsel all pregnant females who had contact with patient with infection

E. Follow up is not needed except for cases in which convalescent titers after 2-3 weeks of initial illness are required

RUBEOLA (MEASLES)

I. Definition: Acute, highly communicable viral disease consisting of fever, rash, and presence of cough, coryza, or conjunctivitis

II. Pathogenesis

A. Causal agent is the measles virus which is an RNA virus

B. Transmitted by direct contact with infectious droplets, or less frequently, by airborne spread

C. Incubation period is 8-12 days from exposure to onset of symptoms

D. Period of communicability: Patient is infectious 1-2 days before onset of symptoms and 3-5 days prior to rash to approximately 4 days after rash

III.   Clinical Presentation

A.   Epidemiology
1.   One of most serious exanthematous diseases
2.   Prior to widespread immunization, measles were common in childhood; effective immunization programs have reduced rate by 99%
3.   Most recent cases result from importations rather than indigenous spread

B.   Center for Disease Control's clinical case definition is as follows:
1.   Generalized rash lasting 3 or more days
a.   Deep, macular rash on face and neck that spreads down trunk and extremities
b.   Begins as discrete lesions, but later becomes confluent and salmon-colored
2.   Fever greater than 38.3°C (100.9°F)
3.   At least one of the following symptoms: Cough, coryza, and conjunctivitis (sometimes referred to as the 3 "C"s); symptoms typically last 1-4 days and patient is usually very ill

C.   Typically, patients have a prodrome with fever and the 3 "C"s which lasts between 1-4 days; patients are usually very ill during this time

D.   As prodromal symptoms reach a peak, the exanthem appears and is characterized by the following:
1.   Deep, red macular rash which begins on face and neck and spreads down trunk and extremities
2.   Rash begins as discrete lesions but then becomes confluent and salmon-colored (referred to as a morbilliform rash)
3.   When fever subsides, around the sixth day, a faint brown stain on the skin remains and desquamation of the skin often begins

E.   Koplik's spots are pathognomonic for measles; this enanthem presents as tiny, bluish white spots on an erythematous base which cluster adjacent to the molars on the buccal mucosa

F.   Most patients recover rapidly after the first 3-4 days

G.   Complications are common and include otitis media, pneumonia, croup, and encephalitis

IV.   Diagnosis/Evaluation

A.   History
1.   Ask about occurrence and duration of rash, cough, conjunctivitis, coryza, and Koplik's spots
2.   Inquire about other symptoms that denote complications such as chest pain, ear pain, and confusion
3.   Ask about immunization status
4.   Ask about recent exposure to persons with a rash
5.   Inquire about medical history (immunosuppressed patients may need different treatment regimens; patients who are chronically ill often develop life-threatening symptoms)
6.   Ask about medication use

B.   Physical Examination
1.   Measure vital signs
2.   Inspect skin, noting characteristics of exanthem
3.   Examine eyes, noting signs of conjunctivitis
4.   Examine head, ears, nose, and throat because complications often involve these areas
5.   Examine mouth for signs of Koplik's spots
6.   Examine neck for adenopathy and nuchal rigidity
7.   Carefully perform heart, lung, neurological, and mental status examinations

C.   Differential Diagnosis
1.   Infectious diseases such as rubella, roseola, Rocky Mountain spotted fever, scarlet fever, infectious mononucleosis, secondary syphilis, enterovirus, or Kawasaki syndrome
2.   Drug reaction
3.   Illnesses caused by release of intentional biologic agents: Anthrax, smallpox, and hemorrhagic fever caused by Ebola or Marburg viruses

D. Diagnostic Tests:
    1. Usually none are needed
    2. Detection of measles specific IgM antibodies (present 3-4 weeks after rash) or a significant rise in IgG antibody concentrations between acute and convalescent sera confirms the diagnosis

V. Plan/Management

A. The following patients in US should be considered for Vitamin A supplementation:
    1. Children 6 months to 2 years of age who are hospitalized with measles and its complications
    2. Patients >6 months with measles who have one of the following risk factors: Immunodeficiency, evidence of vitamin A deficiency (night blindness, Bitot's spots, or xerophthalmia), impaired intestinal absorption, moderate to severe malnutrition, and recent immigration from areas where high mortality rates from measles have occurred
    3. Recommended dose: Available in 50,000 IU/mL solution
        a. Single dose of 100,000 IU orally for children 6 months to 1 year of age
        b. Single dose of 200,000 IU orally for children 1 year of age and older
        c. Dose needs to be repeated the next day and at 4 weeks for children who have ophthalmologic evidence of vitamin A deficiency

B. Symptomatic treatment: Rest, fluids, and avoidance of bright lights to lessen photosensitivity

C. Treatment of exposed persons
    1. Give live measles vaccine if exposure was within 72 hours; recommended dose is 0.5 mL, given subcutaneously
    2. In addition to vaccine, give immune globulin (IG) within 6 days of exposure to susceptible household contacts, particularly immunocompromised contacts, contacts <1 year of age, and pregnant women
        a. Induces passive immunity and prevents or modifies symptoms
        b. Recommended dose is 0.25 mL/kg/dose IM (immunocompromised patients should receive 0.5 mL/kg). Maximum dose is 15 mL

D. Primary prevention of measles (see immunization schedules in HEALTH MAINTENANCE section)

E. Control Procedures
    1. Infected patients should be isolated for at least 4 days after appearance of rash
    2. Persons exposed to measles who are susceptible to developing the infection should be isolated from 5th day post-exposure up to and including the 21st day
    3. All reports of measles cases should be reported to the local health unit and investigated promptly
    4. All patients who cannot provide documentation of measles immunity should be vaccinated or excluded from school, work, or other public places
    5. Investigate immune status of family members and other immediate contacts; prescribe vaccine if appropriate

F. Patient Education
    1. Teach patient to take daily temperature readings; fever lasting more than 4 days suggests presence of complications
    2. Teach patient and/or parents to monitor for signs of complications of measles such as how to count respirations and how to assess for changes in respiratory status and changes in level of consciousness

G. Follow Up
    1. Clinical assessment (can be performed by nurse) is needed daily during acute phase to rule out complications
    2. Patient should then be seen in the clinic about 3-4 days after onset of rash for full-examination

VARICELLA (CHICKENPOX)

I. Definition: Viral disease with a pruritic, vesicular exanthem that appears in crops

II. Pathogenesis

    A. Causal agent is varicella-zoster virus (VZV), a member of the herpesvirus family

    B. Transmission (highly contagious disease):
        1. Direct contact with patients with varicella or zoster (shingles)
        2. Airborne spread from respiratory tract secretions
        3. Contact with fluid from vesicles

    C. Incubation period is 10-21 days with an average of 14-16 days

    D. Patient is communicable one to two days before the rash is apparent until all the vesicles have crusted, typically 5 days after onset of rash

III. Clinical Presentation

    A. Number of cases has significantly declined due to increased vaccination coverage rates

    B. Most cases in US occur in children <10 years

    C. In children, there is usually no prodrome or a mild prodrome with slight malaise and a low-grade fever; adolescents have more severe prodrome

    D. A few hours to days after the prodrome, a rash on the scalp, neck, or upper trunk emerges:
        1. Exanthem occurs in stages: begins as macules, but then turns to papules, and then to vesicles, all within 12-24 hours
        2. When vesicles begin to resolve, crusts develop
        3. Rash spreads centrifugally (away from center) and lesions may occur on mucous membranes of mouth, conjunctivae, esophagus, trachea, rectum, and vagina
        4. Usually patient has little scarring unless infection of skin occurs

    E. Certain groups of patients have more severe cases
        1. Neonates and patients with leukemia may suffer severe, prolonged, or fatal chickenpox
        2. Older children and adults often have prolonged and severe illness
        3. Immunocompromised children often have eruption of lesions and high fever for 2 weeks
        4. HIV-infected patients may develop chronic chickenpox
        5. Severe and **fatal varicella has occurred in healthy individuals receiving intermittent courses of corticosteroids**

    F. Complications are uncommon but may include the following:
        1. Secondary bacterial skin infection, cerebellar ataxia, meningoencephalitis, thrombocytopenia, glomerulonephritis, and pneumonia (rare in normal children, but the most common complication in older patients)
        2. Reye's syndrome was more common in the past due to salicylate therapy

    G. Varicella reinfections may occur and are more common than previously thought

    H. The virus remains in a latent form after the primary infection; zoster or shingles occurs with reactivation

IV. Diagnosis/Evaluation

    A. History
        1. Inquire about recent exposure to chickenpox
        2. Ask patient to specifically describe when and where the first lesion occurred
        3. Ask about the spread, characteristics, and changes in the lesions
        4. Ask about prodromal symptoms

5. Question about associated symptoms or potential complications such as pulmonary and neurological problems
6. Obtain a medication history; especially noting use of corticosteroids
7. Ask about any self-treatments
8. Determine whether patient is immunocompromised or has any other risk factors
9. Ask whether any household contacts lack immunity to varicella and if there are immunocompromised individuals who were exposed to infected patient

B. Physical Examination
1. Observe skin and describe types of lesions, location of lesions, arrangement of lesions
2. Palpate for adenopathy
3. Auscultate heart and lungs
4. Perform a focused neurological examination

C. Differential Diagnosis
1. Scabies or insect bites
2. Skin disorders such as herpes simplex, folliculitis, impetigo, contact dermatitis
3. Viral exanthems such as coxsackievirus and echovirus have vesicles, but these vesicles do not usually crust as occurs in chickenpox
4. Drug eruptions
5. Secondary syphilis
6. Smallpox, a bioterrorism agent (see table below that distinguishes smallpox from varicella)

CLINICAL FEATURES THAT DISTINGUISH CHICKENPOX FROM SMALLPOX

	Chickenpox	Smallpox
Pruritus	Yes	No
Lesion location	More central and involve the scalp; palms and soles are not involved	More on face and extremities; affects palms and soles
Development of lesions	Appears in crops or groups over several days	Synchronous in their stages of development
Depth of lesions	More superficial, thin-walled, and easily ruptured	Deeply embedded in dermis

Adapted from Relman, D.A., & Olson, J.E. (2002). Smallpox: A brief overview. *Consultant, 177-178.*

D. Diagnostic Tests: Usually none needed
1. Virus can be isolated from scrapings of the vesicle base and vesicle scrapings during the first 3 days of eruption; can use tissue cultures, DFA, or Tzanck smears
2. Acute and convalescent titers by standard serologic assays can retrospectively confirm diagnosis (significant increase in serum varicella IgG antibodies confirms diagnosis)

V. Plan/Management

A. Consider oral acyclovir (Zovirax) therapy
1. Results in only moderate decrease in symptoms and is not recommended routinely for treatment of uncomplicated varicella in otherwise healthy children, but is used in healthy adolescents and adults
2. Oral acyclovir is recommended, if it can be initiated **within the first 24 hours (or possibly 48 hours) after the onset of rash**, in the following groups:
   a. Otherwise healthy, nonpregnant individuals 13 years of age or older
   b. Persons with chronic cutaneous or pulmonary disorders
   c. Persons receiving long-term salicylate therapy
   d. Persons receiving short, intermittent or aerosolized course of corticosteroids (if possible, corticosteroids should be discontinued)
   e. Some experts also suggest oral acyclovir for secondary household cases who typically have most severe infection
3. Prescribe oral acyclovir 80 mg/kg/day in 4 divided doses for 5 days; maximum dose is 3200 mg/day; patient should be well-hydrated
4. Intravenous acyclovir is recommended treatment of immunocompromised patients
5. In the pregnant woman with uncomplicated varicella, oral acyclovir therapy is not recommended

B. Measures to control pruritus:
   1. Calamine or Cetaphil lotion to lesions
   2. Prescribe hydroxyzine (Atarax). Adolescent dosage is 25 mg TID/QID; in children prescribe 2 mg/kg/day in 3-4 divided doses (available in syrup 10 mg/5 mL)
   3. Alternatively, prescribe diphenhydramine HCl (Benadryl). Adolescent dosage is 25-50 mg TID/QID; in children, prescribe 5 mg/kg/day in 3-4 divided doses (available in 12.5 mg/5 mL liquid)
   4. Bathe with baking soda or Aveeno and cut nails to prevent bacterial superinfection

C. Symptomatic treatment to reduce fever and discomfort: Use acetaminophen (Tylenol); **never use aspirin in children and adolescents**; NSAIDs may also increase risk of more severe varicella

D. Control measures: Patients may return to school/work after all the lesions are crusted which may be several days in mild cases to several weeks in severe cases

E. Care of exposed persons: Potential therapies for susceptible persons exposed to varicella include varicella vaccine **or** varicella-zoster immune globulin (VZIG)
   1. Administer varicella vaccine (one dose) to susceptible persons within 72 hours and possibly up to 120 hours after exposure
   2. Administer varicella-zoster immune globulin (VZIG) within 96 hours after exposure to varicella to susceptible persons at high risk for severe varicella
      a. Obtain VZIG from American Red Cross Blood Services or FFF Enterprises (telephone number is 1-800-843-7477)
      b. VZIG should be given to the following persons if they have had significant exposure such as residing in same household, indoor face-to-face contact, hospital contact:
         (1) Immunocompromised children without history of varicella
         (2) Immunocompromised adolescents
         (3) Susceptible, pregnant women
         (4) Newborns whose mothers had onset of varicella within 5 days before or within 2 days after delivery
         (5) Hospitalized premature infants
            (a) ≥28 weeks gestation whose mother has no history of varicella or seronegativity
            (b) <28 weeks of gestation or ≤1000 g regardless of maternal history or serostatus
      c. Dosage: One vial VZIG containing 125 units is given intramuscularly (IM) for each 10 kg of body weight; maximum dose is 625 units or 5 vials
   3. Consider a 7-day course of acyclovir to susceptible adults beginning 7-9 days after varicella exposure if vaccine is contraindicated or to adults with late presentations

F. Active or primary immunization (see immunization schedule in HEALTH MAINTENANCE section)

G. Follow Up
   1. Teach patients to identify potential complications such as secondary skin infections, central nervous system problems, and pneumonia
   2. In uncomplicated cases, no follow up is needed

REFERENCES

American Academy of Pediatrics. (2000). In L.K. Pickering (Ed.). *2000 red book: Report of the Committee on Infectious Diseases* (25th ed.). Elk Grove Village, IL: Author.

American Academy of Pediatrics, Committee on Infectious Diseases. (2000). Prevention of Lyme disease. *Pediatrics, 105,* 142-146.

American Academy of Pediatrics, Committee on Infectious Diseases. (2002). Reduction of the influenza burden in children: Policy statement: Organizational principles to guide and define the child health safety system and/or improve the health of children. *Pediatrics, 110,* 1246-1252.

Breman, J.G., & Henderson, D.A. (2002). Diagnosis and management of smallpox. *New England Journal of Medicine, 346,* 1301-1304.

Buckinham, S.C. (2002). Rocky Mountain spotted fever: A review for pediatrics. *Pediatric Annals,* 31, 163-168.

Centers for Disease Control and Prevention. (1990). Case definition for public health surveillance. *MMWR, 39(RR-13),* 1-43.

Centers for Disease Control and Prevention, Advisory Committee on Immunization Practices. (1999). Recommendations for the use of Lyme disease vaccine. *MMWR, 48(RR07)*, 1-17.

Centers for Disease Control and Prevention. (2001). Control and prevention of rubella: Evaluation and management of suspected outbreaks, rubella in pregnant women, and surveillance for congenital rubella syndrome. *MMWR, 50(RR12)*, 1-23.

Centers for Disease Control and Prevention. 2002. Measles – United States 2000. *MMWR, 51*(06), 120-123.

Centers for Disease Control and Prevention, Advisory Committee on Immunization Practices. (2003). Prevention and control of influenza: Recommendations of Advisory Committee on Immunization Practices (ACIP). *MMWR, 52(RR08)*, 1-36.

Chin, J. (Ed.). (2000). *Control of communicable diseases manual* (17th ed.). Washington DC: American Public Health Association.

Colgan, R., Michocki, R., Greisman, L. , & Moore, T.A.W. (2003). Antiviral drugs in the immune competent host. Part II. Treatment of influenza and respiratory syncytial virus infections. *American Family Physician, 67*, 763-766.

Couch, R.B. (2000). Prevention and treatment of influenza. *New England Journal of Medicine, 343*, 1778-1787.

Council on Cardiovascular Disease in Young, Committee on Rheumatic Fever, Endocarditis, and Kawasaki Disease, American Heart Association. (2001). Diagnostic guidelines for Kawasaki disease. *Circulation, 87*, 335-336.

Dennehy, P.H. (2002). Viral meningitis and encephalitis. In F.D. Burg, J.R., Ingelfinger, R.A. Polin, & A.A. Gershon (Eds.). *Gellis & Kagan's current pediatric therapy 17.* Philadelphia: Saunders.

Gammons, M., & Salam, G. (2002). Tick removal. *American Family Physician, 66*, 63-64.

Hall, S., Maupin, T., Peterson, C., Goldman, G., Mascola, L, Sewart, J., et al. (2002). The second varicella infections: Are they more common than previously thought? *Pediatrics, 109*, 1068-1073.

Hanson, C.M. (2001). Fifth disease. *American Journal for Nurse Practitioners, 5*, 35-40.

Iglesias, E.A., & Fisher, M. (2002). Infectious mononucleosis. In R.E. Rakel, & E.T. Bope (Eds.), *Conn's current therapy 2002.* Philadelphia: Saunders.

Ingelsby, T.V., O'Toole, T., Henderson, D.A., et al. (2002). Anthrax as a biological weapon, 2002: Updated recommendations for management. *JAMA, 287*, 2236-2252.

Montalto, N.J. (2003). An office-based approach to influenza: Clinical diagnosis and laboratory testing. *American Family Physician*, 67, 111-118

Montalto, N.J., Gum, K.D., & Ashley, J.V. (2000). Updated treatment of influenza A and B. *American Family Physician, 62*, 2467-2476.

McCrindle, B., Shulman, S., Burns, J., Kato, H., Gersony, W., & Newburger, J. (2000). Meeting report: Summary and abstracts of the Sixth International Kawasaki Disease Symposium. *Pediatric Research, 47*, 544-548.

Relman, D.A., & Olson, J.E. (2002). Smallpox: A brief overview. *Consultant,* 177-178.

Reef, S.E., Frey, T.K., Theall, K., Abernathy, E., Burnett, C.L., Icenogle, J., et al. (2002). The changing epidemiology of rubella in the 1990s: On the verge of elimination and new challenges for control and prevention. *JAMA, 287*, 464-472.

Seward, JF., Watson, B.M., Peterson, C.L., Mascola, L., Pelosi, J.W., & Zhang, J.X. (2002). Varicella disease after introduction of varicella vaccine in the United States, 1995-2000. *JAMA, 287*, 606-611.

Shapiro, E.D. (2001). Doxycycline for tick bites – Not for everyone. *New England Journal of Medicine, 345*, 113-114.

Sood, S.K. (2003). Lyme borreliosis. *Advanced Studies in Medicine, 3*, 22-26.

Steere, A.C. (2001). Lyme disease. *New England Journal of Medicine, 345*, 115-125.

Tselis, A. (2002). Viral meningitis and encephalitis. In R.E. Rakel, & E.T. Bope (Eds.). *Conn's current therapy 2002.* Philadelphia: Saunders.

Thanassi, W. D., & Schoen, R.T. (2000). The Lyme disease vaccine: Conception, development, and implementation. *Annals of Internal Medicine, 132,* 661-668.

Weinberg, G.A. (2001). Meningitis. In R.A. Hoekelman (Ed.). *Pediatric primary care.* St. Louis: Mosby.

Wormser, G.P., Nadelman, R.B., Dattwyler, R.J., Dennis, D.T., Shapiro, E.D., Rush, T.J., et al. (2000). Practice guidelines for the treatment of Lyme disease: Guidelines from the Infectious Disease Society of America. *Clinical Infectious Diseases, 31*(Suppl 1), S1-S14.

Skin Problems

MARY VIRGINIA GRAHAM

Fungal and Yeast Infections

Candidiasis

Dermatophyte Infections

Tinea Versicolor

Infestations and Bites

Scabies

Pediculosis (Lice Infestation)

Cutaneous Larva Migrans (Creeping Eruption)

Papulosquamous Disorders

Psoriasis
Pityriasis Rosea

Disorders of Pigmentation

Pityriasis Alba
Café au Lait Spots

Viral Infections

Herpes Simplex

Molluscum Contagiosum
Warts

CARE OF DRY AND OILY SKIN

I. Definition: Care aimed at preserving or restoring the normal physiologic state of the skin

II. Pathogenesis

    A. Dry skin results from reduced water content of the stratum corneum and may occur because of genetic influences and/or environmental factors such as exposure to irritating substances (household/industrial chemicals), decreased humidity (optimal humidity for skin is ≥70%; during winter, indoor humidity can get as low as 10%), and frequent or prolonged exposure to water

    B. Oily skin is a result of excess sebum production by sebaceous glands which are largest and most numerous on face, chest, and upper back

III. Clinical Presentation

    A. Dry skin presents as scaly, dry appearing skin which feels dry to touch, and is most often located on the hands and extensor surfaces of legs and arms

    B. Dry skin is sensitive (that is, easily irritated) and usually pruritic

    C. Oily skin presents as moist appearing, shiny skin which feels oily to touch and is most often located on face, chest, and upper back

    D. Oily skin may occur at any age, but is most common among adolescents

IV. Diagnosis/Evaluation

    A. History
        1. Inquire about distribution, onset, duration
        2. Ask about skin cleansing practices, occupational, and household exposures
        3. Ask about treatments tried and results

    B. Physical Examination
        1. Examine entire skin surface
        2. For patients complaining of dry skin, focus on legs, extensor surfaces, and hands, where drying is likely to be worse
        3. For oily skin, focus on face, upper back, and chest

    C. Differential Diagnosis
        1. Atopic dermatitis
        2. Contact dermatitis
        3. Ichthyosis
        4. Dyshidrotic eczema

    D. Diagnostic Tests: None indicated

V. Plan/Management

A. For dry skin, provide the following recommendations:

ADVICE FOR PATIENTS WITH DRY SKIN

→ Keep skin well hydrated by daily baths or showers in water no warmer than 90°

→ Use mild, super-fatted soaps such as Dove, Keri, Basis, Caress, or Eucerin; use soap in the axilla and groin area and avoid rubbing over entire body; avoid over-aggressive use of wash cloth that can exfoliate and remove the stratum corneum (avoid Ivory Soap which tends to be drying)

→ A waterless liquid cleanser such as Cetaphil or Aquanil may also be used, especially for washing face

→ Omit use of bubble baths and bath oils which pose hazard (falls)

→ After bath, brush away excess water with hands, then pat or blot skin with towel

→ Apply moisturizers from the list below immediately after bathing, while skin is somewhat moist to seal in moisture

→ **Note:** Lotions are the least moisturizing but the most acceptable to patients; ointments are the most moisturizing and should always be recommended to patients with very dry skin

Moisturizing Lotions	**Moisturizing Creams**	**Moisturizing Ointments**
Petrolatum-based	Petrolatum-based	Petrolatum-based
Dermasil	Purpose Dry Skin Cream	Vaseline Pure Petroleum Jelly
DML Lotion	Cetaphil Cream	(Fragrance, preservative, and
Moisturel Lotion	Keri Cream	lanolin free)
Replenaderm		
Mixtures of lanolin and petrolatum	Mixtures of lanolin and petrolatum	Mixtures of lanolin and petrolatum
Eucerin Lotion	Eucerin Creme	Aquaphor Natural Healing Ointment
Lubriderm Lotion		(Fragrance and preservative free)
Nivea Moisturizing		
Without lanolin or petrolatum	Without lanolin or petrolatum	
Corn Huskers Lotion	Neutrogena Norwegian Formula	
Cetaphil Lotion	Hand Cream	

B. Consult the box below for a listing of relatively inexpensive moisturizers that were given high ratings for moisturizing effectiveness by *Consumer Reports* (**Note:** Efficacy in skin care products does not necessarily correlate with cost; cheaper products are often as good as, if not better than, more expensive ones)

MOISTURIZERS RATED BEST BY *CONSUMER REPORTS*

Face
L'Oreal Plenitude Active Daily Moisture SPF15
Pond's Nourishing Moisturizer SPF15

Body
Vaseline Intensive Care Advanced Healing with Skin Protection Complex
Curel Therapeutic Moisturizing Original Formula

Hands
Curel Soothing Hands Moisturizing with Chamomile
Neutrogena New Hands Restorative SPF15

Adapted from Editors (2000). The skin game. *Consumer Reports*, January 2000, 38-41

C. Agents containing lactic acid or urea should be used judiciously as these products draw water from the environment and thus don't work well unless the surrounding humidity is relatively high; they are also very irritating to dry skin and **make the skin more sensitive to the sun**; burning and stinging limit the usefulness of these products in young children
1. Strictly speaking, such agents are not moisturizers
2. They enhance shedding of superficial cells and this exfoliation results immediately in a smoother, more uniform surface

---

Urea Creams and Lotions
- Cream 10% (Aquacare, Nutraplus)
- Cream 20% (Carmol 20)
- Lotion 10% (Aquacare, Carmol 10)

Lactic Acid-Containing Lotions
- 5% (LactiCare)
- 12% (Lac-Hydrin) [Rx product for children>2 years]

D. For oily skin, provide the following recommendations:

ADVICE FOR PATIENTS WITH OILY SKIN

➡ Use a deodorant soap such as Dial or Safeguard containing an antibacterial or a mildly drying soap (Ivory)
➡ Avoid using preparations containing oils
➡ Use an astringent or toner on face
➡ For adolescent girls, use cosmetics such as those listed below

---

COSMETICS FOR ADOLESCENT GIRLS WITH OILY SKIN

Allercreme
Matte-Finish Makeup (waterbase, oil free)
Charles of the Ritz
T-Zone Controller
Clinique
Pore Minimizer Makeup (fragrance and oil free)
Stay True Oil-Free (for sensitive skin, SPF 15)
Covergirl
Fresh Complexion, 100% oil-free
Esteé Lauder
Tender Matte Makeup (fragrance and oil free)
Simply Sheer
Lucidity Makeup

Lancome
Maquicontrol, Oil-Free Liquid Makeup
L'Oreal
Mattique Illuminating Makeup
Monteil
Habitat Natural Light Makeup
Max Factor
Shine-Free Makeup
Revlon
Spring Water Matte Makeup
Shisheido
Pureness Oil-Control Makeup
Ultima II
The Nakeds: The Foundation Oil-Free Formula

E. Use every opportunity to discuss the role of sun exposure in photoaging (see section on SKIN CARE, INSECT BITE PROTECTION, and SUN EXPOSURE PROTECTION for recommendations relating to sun avoidance counseling)

F. Follow-up: None indicated

BENIGN SKIN LESIONS OF INFANTS AND CHILDREN

I. Definition: Cutaneous disorders commonly present in infants and children that are of no consequence in terms of the child's physical health

II. Pathogenesis

A. Milia: Superficial epithelial cysts in the papillary dermis; the cyst cavity is filled with keratin

B. Mongolian spots: Spindle-shaped pigment cells located deep in dermis

C. Erythema toxicum: Associated with obstruction of the pilosebaceous orifice; unknown etiology

D. Sebaceous gland hyperplasia: Increase in volume, size, and number of sebaceous cells caused by maternal androgenic stimulation

E. Sucking blisters: Vigorous sucking in utero is believed to be cause

F. Vascular birthmarks (nevus flammeus): Caused by developmental errors in vessel formation

G. Freckles: Areas with increased pigment secondary to sun exposure

H. Lentigines: Increased numbers of melanocytes along the basal layer of the epidermis

III.   Clinical Presentation

BENIGN SKIN LESIONS IN INFANTS AND CHILDREN: CLINICAL PRESENTATION	

Milia	Multiple, white, 1-2 mm papules occurring on forehead, cheeks, and nose of infant
	Called Epstein's pearls when in oral cavity
	  ✓ Up to 40% of newborns have on skin and 60% on palate
	  ✓ Rupture and exfoliate and disappear a few weeks after birth

Mongolian spots	Blue-black macule found in lumbosacral area in up to 90% of African-American, Asian, Hispanic, and Native American infants ✓ Tend to fade with time and usually disappear by age 3 years

Erythema toxicum	Blotchy, erythematous macules 2-3 cm in diameter, with a tiny central vesicle or pustule; usually begin at 24 to 48 hours of age and occur in about 50% of term infants (in the past called "flea-bite" dermatitis)
	  ✓ Occur on face, back, chest, and extremities of infants, sparing the palms and soles
	  ✓ Usually clear in 4 to 5 days; smear of central vesicle or pustule contents reveals numerous eosinophils on Wright-stained preparations

Sebaceous gland hyperplasia	Yellow macules or papules, about 1 mm in diameter that occur at opening of pilosebaceous follicles over the nose and cheeks of newborns
	  ✓ Occur in about 50% of infants
	  ✓ Recede completely by 4 to 6 months of age

Sucking blisters	Usually solitary intact oval blisters on noninflamed skin in newborn ✓ Occur on forearms, wrists, fingers, or upper lip

Vascular birthmarks	Salmon patch appears as a pale red macule over the nape of neck, upper eyelids, and glabella; usually more apparent with episodes of crying
	  ✓ Present over back of neck in over 40% of infants
	  ✓ Fade with time, but remnants may remain well into adulthood

Freckles	Small, 1-5 mm light brown pigmented macules that occur in UVL exposed skin
	  ✓ Most frequent in light-haired, blue-eyed children; become less common with age
	  ✓ Autosomal dominant and first appear at ages 3-5 years on face and extensor surfaces of extremities

Lentigines	Small 1-2 mm brown to brown-black macules found sparsely scattered over body including mucous membranes
	  ✓ Do not change with sun exposure
	  ✓ First appear during school age and number 15-20 in any one individual

IV.   Diagnosis/Evaluation

    A.   History
        1.   Ask about onset, location, and a description of the lesion
        2.   Ask if there are any associated symptoms
        3.   Inquire about treatments tried and results

    B.   Physical Examination
        1.   Examine the entire skin surface
        2.   Use good lighting and magnification if needed
        3.   Determine patient skin type and sun sensitivity and use this information to teach parents about importance of sun exposure avoidance

SKIN TYPES AND SUN SENSITIVITY	
Skin Type	*Description*
I	Fair skin, always burns, never tans
II	Fair skin, usually burns, sometimes tans
III	Lightly pigmented, usually tans, sometimes burns
IV	Pigmented, always tans, never burns
V	Moderately pigmented, never burns
VI	Heavily pigmented (black) skin

    C.   Differential Diagnosis
        1.   Milia: Molluscum contagiosum (does not appear in immediate neonatal period) and sebaceous gland hyperplasia (yellow rather than whitish in appearance)
        2.   Mongolian spots: Bruising secondary to trauma
        3.   Erythema toxicum: Central vesicle may mimic herpes simplex or bacterial folliculitis (Wright-stained slide from pustule of erythema toxicum will show a predominance of eosinophils)
        4.   Sebaceous gland hyperplasia: May resemble milia, but milia are white rather than yellow

5. Sucking blisters: Herpesvirus infection and bullous impetigo are in the differential, but both lesions from these infections have an erythematous base and are not usually solitary lesions as is found with sucking blisters

D. Diagnostic Tests: None indicated unless there is a need to rule out a viral or bacterial infection

V. Plan/Management

A. Milia: No treatment needed; reassure parents that it's a normal variation which disappears in weeks

B. Mongolian spots: No treatment needed; reassure parents that it's a normal variation which disappears over months

C. Erythema toxicum: No treatment necessary as eruption fades spontaneously within 5-7 days

D. Sebaceous gland hyperplasia
1. No treatment necessary
2. Recedes completely by 4 to 6 months of age

E. Sucking blisters: No treatment necessary as they resolve in a few days

F. Vascular birthmarks: Salmon patch
1. No treatment necessary
2. Generally, eyelid lesions fade by 6 to 12 months; glabellar lesions by 5 to 6 years, and the lesions on the neck are more likely to persist for many years

G. Freckles and lentigines: No treatment necessary

H. Parent education
1. Use all clinical encounters with parents of infants and children to discuss skin care, use of insect repellents, and especially sun protection
2. Provide parents with a list of cleansers and moisturizers appropriate for use in infants and children
3. Advise parents that protection against insect bites is best achieved by avoiding infested habitats, dressing child in protective clothing, and applying insect repellent (see table in section on SKIN CARE, INSECT BITE PROTECTION, AND SUN EXPOSURE PROTECTION for recommendation regarding use of insect repellents)
4. Counsel parents regarding the dangers of sun exposure (see table in section on SKIN CARE, INSECT BITE PROTECTION, AND SUN EXPOSURE PROTECTION)

I. Follow Up: None indicated for these benign conditions

SKIN CARE, INSECT BITE PROTECTION, AND SUN EXPOSURE PROTECTION

I.   Definition: Care aimed at preserving or restoring the normal physiologic state of the skin and hair, protecting against arthropod bites, and protecting against ultraviolet radiation (UVR)

II. Pathogenesis:

A.   The epidermal barrier of the skin is only 0.05 to 0.1 mm thick but is very effective in preventing penetration from outside and retaining substances inside
1.   Disruption of the water and lipid content of the epidermis through the use of chemical or mechanical means alters the integrity of the barrier, compromising its function
2.   Maintenance (or restoration) of the normal epidermal barrier is accomplished through the avoidance of harsh chemicals, gentle cleansing, and the use moisturizers

B.   Arboviruses transmitted by mosquitoes continue to cause sporadic outbreaks of encephalitis
1.   Since the identification of West Nile virus in New York City in 1999, enzootic activity has been documented in 27 states and continued geographic expansion is likely
2.   West Nile virus encephalitis has recently been added to the list of designated nationally notifiable arboviral encephalitides

C.   Bites from non-disease carrying mosquitoes can cause extreme pruritus and dermatitis in children

D.   Tanning/burning rays from the sun represent ultraviolet radiation
1.   Exact cause of ultraviolet radiation damage is unknown, but is believed to be a combination of direct effects, generation of toxic oxygen species, and production of inflammatory mediators
2.   Accumulated exposure to ultraviolet radiation produces damage to the skin including hyperkeratosis of the stratum corneum, flattened rete ridges, keratinocyte atypia and dyskeratosis, dermal elastosis, and dilated cutaneous vessels
3.   Long term effects are expressed as photoaging (dry, mottled skin with fine and deep wrinkling) and UV light-induced precancerous lesions—actinic keratosis

III. Clinical Presentation

A.   Many parents have questions and concerns about which bath products, shampoos, lotions, and powders are appropriate for use on infants and children

B.   Parents may be unaware of the importance of protecting children from arthropod bites and how best to achieve that protection

C.   Many parents fail to appreciate the degree of sun sensitivity in children and underestimate the dangers of sun exposure
1.   Nearly two-thirds of an individual's lifetime ultraviolet (UV) radiation dose is received by 18 years of age
2.   By the time children reach adolescence, they are usually fairly resistant to use of sun protection, unless that behavior has been learned at an early age
3.   The myths that tans are "healthy," and that tanning devices are safe are pervasive in the US, particularly among adolescents

IV. Diagnosis/Evaluation

A.   History
1.   Ask parent/child if there are any skin problems as part of the review of systems in every health supervision visit; if yes, ask appropriate questions regarding onset, location, appearance, associated signs and symptoms, treatments tried and results
2.   Ask parent/child about which bath products, shampoos, lotions, or other hygiene products are used on the child
3.   During summer months, ask parent about what specific practices are implemented to keep child from being bitten by mosquitoes

4. During every season of the year (but especially during spring and summer), ask parent what specific practices are implemented to protect child from sun exposure

B. Physical Examination
1. Examine child's skin, noting condition of skin and scalp
2. Look for evidence of dry or damaged skin (tanning and/or sunburn)
3. Inspect the skin for bites
4. Determine skin type and sun sensitivity (see table in BENIGN SKIN LESIONS OF INFANTS AND CHILDREN)

C. Differential Diagnosis: N/A

D. Diagnostic Tests: N/A

V. Plan/Management

A. The table below contains recommendation for bath and skin care products for use on infants and children

RECOMMENDATIONS FOR BATH AND SKIN CARE PRODUCTS	
Soaps	✓ Function of soaps is to emulsify oils and suspend small solid particles on skin surface which can then be removed by rinsing with water ✓ All soaps are at least mild irritants and parents should be advised of this ✓ Products such as Johnson's Baby Wash and Dove are mild neutral pH cleansers and are acceptable for washing infants and older children; examples of other neutral soaps are Neutragena, Lowila, and Basis ✓ Soaping the skin is best restricted to short contact time (less than 5 minutes) ✓ When bath time is used for play in toddlers and preschoolers, the tub should be filled with plain water for play, and then bathing with soap should be left for the last few minutes in the tub ✓ Bubble bath products often contain additives that can cause skin problems for some children; parents should be aware of this possibility and use judiciously
Shampoos	✓ Shampoos are synthetic detergents especially formulated for cleansing the hair ✓ Shampoos contain both cleansing agents and lather enhancers as well as a number of other additives such as preservatives (required by law), buffers, fragrances, and dyes ✓ Baby shampoos contain fewer additives than regular shampoo and are pH adjusted with a pH of 6.0 to 6.5 which approaches the pH of water (7.0); this adjusted pH is responsible for the "no tears" quality that make washing the infant/child's hair more pleasant for both child and parent ✓ Product examples are Johnson's Baby Shampoo and L'Oreal for Kids
Skin Care Products	✓ Moisturizers are important especially in the colder months ✓ Product examples are Lubriderm Lotion, Fragrance-Free, and Keri Lotion for Sensitive Skin, which are general purpose moisturizers that can be used on skin of infants and children; encourage parent to apply sparingly and to be alert for any adverse reaction ✓ There are hundreds of products on the market, many of which are safe for infants and children; in general, parents should avoid products with more than three active ingredients and those with many additives ✓ For the diaper area, Desitin ointment combines zinc oxide (40%) with cod liver oil in a petrolatum-lanolin base and is a good product for preventing (and treating) irritant diaper rash; provides a physical barrier by forming a protective coating over skin which serves to reduce effects of irritants such as urine and stool (also available as Desitin Creamy, which contains 10% zinc oxide) ✓ Use of powder of any type on infants should be discouraged because of the tendency of some parents to use incorrectly

B. Protection from mosquito bites is best achieved using a three-pronged program
1. Limit exposure to infested habitats, particularly at dusk and after dark
2. Dress the child in protective clothing, thereby limiting the access of skin to the insect
3. Apply repellents which may be the only feasible approach in certain circumstances (the American Academy of Pediatrics recommends that repellents containing no more than 10% DEET be used on children [when DEET-containing products are used])

SELECTED TOPICALLY-APPLIED INSECT REPELLENTS AND THEIR INGREDIENTS

Overview
✓ Insect repellents currently available are either synthetic chemicals or are derived from plants
✓ Most widely marketed chemical-based repellents contain DEET, a broad-spectrum agent that is effective against many species of mosquitoes, biting flies, chiggers, fleas, and ticks
✓ Most plant-based repellents contain essential oils from one or more of the following plants–citronella, cedar, eucalyptus, peppermint, lemongrass, geranium, and soybeans

	Active Ingredient and Concentration	Average Protection Time (In minutes)
Plant-Based Repellents		
Bite Blocker for Kids (HOMS)	Soybean Oil, 2%	94
Skin-So-Soft Bug Guard Plus (Avon)	IR3535, 7.5%	22.9
Buzz Away (Quantum) oil, 2%	Citronella, 10%, peppermint	13.5
DEET-Containing Repellents		
Off! Skintastic for Kids (SC Johnson)	DEET, 6.65%	112.4
Off! Skintastic MagiColor	DEET, 7.12%	N/T*
Cutter All Family	DEET, 6.65%	N/T*
Cutter Skinsations Gel	DEET, 6.65%	N/T*

Advice to parents
✓ Remind parents to read directions on label carefully; some products are designed to be used on clothing only, not on the child's skin

✓ Avoid use of wristbands impregnated with either DEET or citronella because these provide little or no protection from bites (repellents are not able to protect beyond 4 cm around site of application)

✓ DEET-based repellents are safe to use when applied with common sense; there is no need to completely avoid these products despite the substantial attention paid by the lay press every year to DEET's safety

*Not tested in the above referenced study; however, since the DEET concentration is as high or higher than the product that **was** tested, one would anticipate that the average complete protection time (elapsed time of exposure to the first bite) would be similar

Adapted from Fradin, M.S., & Day. J.F. (2002). Comparative efficacy of insect repellents against mosquito bites. *New England Journal of Medicine, 347,* 1-18.

C.   The three main strategies for sun protection in order of effectiveness are sun avoidance, use of protective clothing, and sunscreen use
   1.   Explain to parent the child's skin type (see section on Benign Skin Lesions of Infants and Children); sunburn occurs quickly in fair-skinned children who have less melanin protection than darker-skinned children; nonetheless, intense sun exposure can produce sunburn in children with dark skin as well
   2.   Provide counseling related to the three strategies for sun protection based on recommendations in the table that follows

RECOMMENDATIONS FOR COUNSELING PARENTS REGARDING SUN PROTECTION IN INFANTS AND CHILDREN

- The message that must be repeated to parents and children is that tanning is **always** a sign of ultraviolet injury to the skin
- Sun protection habits must be formed in early childhood; such habits are unlikely to be adopted during the teen years (this attitude is likely to persist until there is a change in current social norms that find tanned skin desirable)
- Incorporate these talking points into your counseling:

Strategy One
✓ **Sun avoidance** is the **most** effective way to protect children from sun damage
✓ Infants <6 months should **never** be subjected to direct sun exposure during the spring and summer months (or during winter in sunny climates)
✓ Infants and children >6 months of age should have time spent in sun **severely limited**; no mid-day exposure (10 AM to 4 PM) and indirect sunlight exposure during the other hours of the day
✓ Outdoor activities should not be planned during this time of day during the spring and summer
✓ If children must be out, advise parent to use an umbrella for shade or seek shade from trees

Strategy Two
✓ **Protective clothing** is better at sun protection than sunscreens and is the **second** most effective way to provide sun protection
✓ Advise use of a broad-brimmed hat to shade ears, nose, and lips (can prevent 70% of UV rays from reaching the face)
✓ Have child wear shirt and special sun-protective clothing with an SPF such as Solumbra and Frogskin (available from LL Bean and others) SunSafe (toll-free 1-877-Sun-Safe), and Radicool (www.radicoolaustralia.com)

(Continued)

Strategy Three	✓	**Sunscreen use** is the **weakest** strategy to protect children from ultraviolet radiation
	✓	Sunscreen should **not** be used for the purpose of increasing the amount of time the child is exposed to mid-day sun and this point should be made to parents and to older children
	✓	Sunscreens are classified as chemical sunscreens or physical blocks. A common example of a chemical sunscreen is para-aminobenzoic acid. A new product recently approved by the FDA, (Parsol 1789) provides added protection against UVA rays as well as UVB protection found in older ingredients. Examples of physical blocks include zinc oxide and titanium dioxide—although these products previously appeared white on the skin (which reduced their acceptably, particularly among teens), new technology has produced smaller particles that allow for invisible application. These ingredients also block both UVA and UVB rays
	✓	Advise parents/patients to use sunscreen products with a SPF of 30 or greater; the SPF numbers refer mostly to protection against the ultraviolet B (UVB) rays, which are the most damaging to skin
	✓	Most products currently on the market provide good sun protection against a broad spectrum of the sun's rays
	✓	Apply to skin 30 minutes before sun exposure; reapply every hour while exposed because it is washed off with sweating and swimming
	✓	To be effective, the product must be applied generously and uniformly over the skin; water-resistant products should hold up for up to 40 minutes of immersion in water and a **very** water resistant (formerly designated waterproof) product should retain its SPF for up to 80 minutes of immersion
	✓	Interestingly, in a recent survey of youth in the US regarding sunburn and sun exposure, more than one third of youths reporting having applied sunscreen with SPF 15+ prior to receiving their most serious summer sunburn. Obviously, it is not enough to remind children to **use** sunscreen; more emphasis needs to be placed on correct use and also on sun avoidance
	✓	Suggest the use of gel-based formulations to adolescents; gels do not feel greasy and rub in more easily than creams and lotions; sprays are wasteful; much of the active ingredient is lost in the air
	✓	Reflection of sun off snow, water, or sand can be very damaging to skin

D. Follow up: None required; however, use all clinical encounters with patients to reinforce importance of good skin care (if needed), need for use of insect repellents, and especially the crucial importance of sun protection

ACNE

I. Definition: A disease of the pilosebaceous unit that is most intense in areas where sebaceous glands are numerous

II. Pathogenesis

    A. A number of factors and events work in concert to make the pathogenesis of acne multifactorial in nature

    B. Excessive sebum produced by the androgen-dependent sebaceous glands, combined with excessive numbers of desquamated cells from the walls of the sebaceous follicles cause obstruction of the follicles (which are located primarily on the face and trunk)

    C. As a consequence of this obstruction, microcomedones are formed that may eventually evolve into either comedones or inflammatory lesions

    D. A resident anaerobic organism, *Propionibacterium acnes* (found in very low numbers on normal skin) finds the environment created by the excessive sebum and desquamated follicular cells very conducive to growth and produces chemotactic factors and proinflammatory mediators that may lead to inflammation

III. Clinical Presentation

    A. Acne is the most common skin disorder, affecting almost 80% of persons at some point in their lives, most often between the ages of 11 and 30
        1. Acne begins in the pre-pubertal period when the adrenal glands begin secreting increased amounts of adrenal androgens which leads to increased production of sebum
        2. Androgen production and sebaceous gland activity are further stimulated with gonad development during puberty

B. Most patients with acne are probably hyper-responsive to androgens rather than overproducers of androgens; androgen excess, however, has been implicated in the development of acne

C. **Comedonal acne** represents the **earliest** clinical expression of acne, occurring in the pre-teen and early teenage years
   1. Characteristic lesions are noninflammatory comedones located on central forehead, chin, nose, paranasal area
   2. Comedones are open (blackheads) or closed (whiteheads)
   3. Colonization with *P. acnes* has not yet occurred; thus, no inflammatory lesions are present

D. **Mild inflammatory acne** usually develops in teenagers **after the first phase** of non-inflammatory comedonal acne; also occurs in adult women in their 20s
   1. Characterized by scattered small papules or pustules with a minimum of comedones and rarely results in scarring
   2. Arises from microcomedones in which two factors are present
      a. Abnormal desquamation of epithelial cells in the follicles
      b. Proliferation of *P. acnes*

E. **Inflammatory acne** represents the **final** phase in the evolution of acne from noninflammatory comedonal acne, to small numbers of inflammatory lesions on the face, to a more generalized eruption, first on the face, and then on the trunk
   1. Most patients with acne have inflammatory acne, with comedones, papules, and pustules on the face and trunk
   2. In a minority of patients, large, deep inflammatory nodules (called cysts) develop reflecting the presence of a very destructive type of inflammation
   3. Cystic acne requires prompt attention since ruptured cysts may result in scar formation

IV. Evaluation/Diagnosis

   A. History
      1. Question regarding onset, type of lesions, distribution
      2. In females, question about history of cyclic menstrual flares, use of oral contraceptives
      3. Inquire about types of cleansers and lubricants used on face
      4. Document previous treatments and results

   B. Physical Examination
      1. Examine skin to determine form of acne:
         a. Comedonal acne—noninflammatory comedones
         b. Mild inflammatory acne—scattered small papules or pustules with a minimum of comedones
         c. Inflammatory acne—comedones, papules, and pustules on the face and trunk
         d. Inflammatory acne with large, deep inflammatory nodules
      2. Determine areas of involvement and document in patient record

   C. Differential Diagnosis
      1. Rosacea
      2. Steroid rosacea
      3. Molluscum contagiosum
      4. Folliculitis

   D. Diagnostic Tests: None indicated

V. Plan/Management

   A. Explain the mechanism of acne and treatment plan to the patient
      1. Emphasize that little improvement may be evident for 2-3 months
      2. Use written patient education materials to reinforce teaching

   B. Counsel patient regarding the following general measures:
      1. Cleanse affected areas gently with mild soap (Purpose, Basis) or cleansers such as Cetaphil lotion no more than 2-3 x day (emphasize that use of topical agents such as soaps and astringents have no effect on sebum production but only remove sebum from the surface of the skin which has little therapeutic value)
      2. Avoid picking at lesions as it may cause scarring

242

3. Avoid oil-based cosmetics, hair styling mousse, and face creams which have no effect on sebum production but do increase the amount of oil on the face

4. Use nonacnegenic moisturizers such as Moisturel, and cosmetics from the table that follows

---

NONACNEGENIC COSMETICS FOR TEENS

Allercreme
- ✓ Matte-Finish Makeup (Waterbase, oil free)

Charles of the Ritz
- ✓ T-Zone Controller

Clinique
- ✓ Pore Minimizer Makeup (Fragrance and oil free)
- ✓ Stay True Oil-Free (For sensitive skin, SPF 15)

Covergirl
- ✓ Fresh Complexion, 100% Oil-Free

Esteé Lauder
- ✓ Tender Matte Makeup (Fragrance and oil free)
- ✓ Simply Sheer Fresh Air Makeup Base, Oil-free

Lancome
- ✓ Maquicontrol, Oil-Free Liquid Makeup

Mary Kay Cosmetics
- ✓ Oil-Free Foundation (Fragrance and oil-free)

Max Factor
- ✓ Shine-Free Makeup

Revlon
- ✓ Spring Water Matte Makeup

Shisheido
- ✓ Pureness Oil-Control Makeup

---

5. Dietary factors have no effect on sebum production, and patient should be counseled to eat a well-balanced diet

C. Consider whether patient is a candidate for oral contraceptive use (see section on Contraception in GYNECOLOGY chapter); the FDA has approved several OCs (e.g., Ortho Tri-Cyclen and Estrostep Fe) for acne therapy in female teenagers without contraindications who desire contraception (not considered a first-line drug for acne)

D. Treatment of acne in adolescents using both topical and oral agents is outlined in the following table

TREATMENT OF ACNE IN ADOLESCENTS

Treatment Aims	Treatment	Comments

Comedonal Acne
 	
• Reduce or counteract abnormal desquamation of follicular epithelium
	Topical comedolytic agents are the treatment of choice
	Select a comedolytic agent from the following list of topical agents
	
	Tretinoin
	(Retin-A) available as cream, gel, or liquid
	  Cream: 0.025%, 0.05%, and 0.1%, supplied as 20 g, 45 g
	  Gel: 0.01%, 0.025%, supplied as 15 g, 45 g (contains alcohol 90%)
	  Liquid: 0.05%, supplied as 28 mL (contains alcohol 55%)
	(Retin-A Micro) sustained release delivery system, available as 0.04%, 0.1% aqueous gel, supplied as 20 g, 45 g
	(Avita) available as cream, gel (0.025%), supplied as 20 g, 45 g
	Apply QD at bedtime, beginning with a lower concentration of the cream, gel, or liquid and increasing if mild local irritation does not occur (adjust dose/frequency if irritation is more than "mild")
	(**Note:** Considered the standard against which all other comedolytics are judged)
	
	Adapalene *(Differin)*, a naphthoic derivative with retinoid activity, available as cream, gel, solution, and pledgets
	  Cream and Gel: 0.1%, supplied as 15 g, 45 g (alcohol-free)
	  Solution: 0.1%. supplied as 30 mL (contains alcohol 30%)
	  Pledgets: 0.1%, supplied as 60 pledgets (contains alcohol 30%)
	Apply QD at bedtime, beginning with a lower concentration of the solution or gel, and increasing if mild local irritation does not occur
	(**Note:** Causes less irritation than topical tretinoin and is often effective in patients who cannot tolerate topical tretinoin)
	
	Azelaic acid *20% (Azelex)* has both comedolytic and antibacterial effects, available as cream (one concentration only); supplied as 30 g
	Apply BID, in the morning and evening to clean dry skin; if persistent irritation occurs, decrease to once daily
	(**Note:** May cause less irritation than tretinoin and often causes hypopigmentation which may be desirable for some patients)
		↑ Advise patient to apply thin layer of the topical agent to the entire face, not just the individual lesions
		
		↑ Warn about increased photosensitivity – patient must apply sunscreen daily for any sun exposure
		
		↑ Patient should reduce frequency or discontinue if prolonged or more than mild irritation occurs
		
		↑ Gels are usually preferred in hot/humid climates and creams in cold/dry climates
		
		↑ Several months may be necessary to achieve good results
		
		↑ Treatment should be continued until no new lesions are developing

Mild Inflammatory Acne • Reduce or counteract abnormal desquamation of follicular epithelium • Prevent proliferation of *P. acnes*	*Topical therapy with a combination of a comedolytic **and** an antibiotic is the treatment of choice* **Select a comedolytic agent from the list above** **Select a topical antibiotic agent from the list below** (**Note:** When used in combination, **once** daily dosing for the comedolytic and the topical antibiotic is acceptable; each product should be used at separate times of day. Use comedolytic in AM and antibiotic in PM. **The BID dosing schedule for both comedolytic and antibiotic agents in the lists given here are the dosing recommendations when the agents are used alone!**) **Topical Antibiotics** *Benzoyl peroxide, (Benzac)* available as a gel with alcohol-base in 5%, 10% concentrations (contains alcohol 12%); also available as aqueous-base gel (Benzac-W) in 2.5%, 5%, 10% concentrations (alcohol-free) Both products supplied as 60 g Apply QD to clean, dry skin (**Note:** Very effective anti-*P. acnes* agent; major disadvantage is irritation which can be minimized by using lower concentrations and water-base form)	↑ Most patients respond to treatment after 2-4 weeks ↑ Treatment should be continued until no new lesions develop, then slowly discontinued ↑ Many products available, some of which are generic and less expensive *(Continued)*

244

TREATMENT OF ACNE IN ADOLESCENTS (CONTINUED)

Treatment Aims	Treatment	Comments
Mild Inflammatory Acne (Continued)		
	Erythromycin, 2% solution and alcohol-base gel (A/T/S) Supplied as solution—60 mL, and gel—30 g Apply BID to clean, dry skin	↑ Many products available, some of which are generic and much less expensive ↑ Advise patient to discontinue if excessive irritation occurs
	Clindamycin, 1% (Cleocin-T) available as solution, pledgets, lotion, and alcohol-base (50%) gel Supplied as solution—30 mL, 60 mL; pledgets—boxes of 60; lotion—60 mL; gel—30 g, 60 g Apply BID to clean, dry skin	
	Benzoyl peroxide plus erythromycin (Benzamycin), contains 3% erythromycin and 5% benzoyl peroxide in gel form (alcohol base) Supplied as gel—23.3 g, 46.6 g Apply BID to clean, dry skin (**Note:** Considered by many to be the **most effective** topical antibiotic therapy against *P. acnes*)	
Inflammatory Acne		
• Reduce or counteract abnormal desquamation of follicular epithelium • Prevent proliferation of *P. acnes* and the resultant inflammation produced by the organism	*Topical therapy with comedolytic and systemic antibiotic therapy (all acne begins with follicular impaction)* **Select a comedolytic agent from the list above** **Select an antibiotic from the following list** **Oral antibiotics** *Doxycycline (Vibramycin)*, available as 50 mg, 100 mg caps 100 mg BID x 1 day, then 50 mg BID; dose can be reduced to 50 mg QD after improvement *Minocycline (Minocin)*, available as 50 mg, 100 mg caps 50 mg BID; dose can be reduced to 50 mg QD after improvement (**Note:** Above two agents are more lipid-soluble than tetracycline and erythromycin and are generally considered to be more effective than tetracycline and erythromycin) *Tetracycline (Achromycin V)*, available as 250 mg, 500 mg caps 1 g/day in 2 divided doses, then 125-500 mg/day with further reduction after improvement *Erythromycin (E-Mycin)*, available as 250 mg, 333 mg tabs 500 mg BID or 333 mg BID, with reduction after improvement	↑ Deciding between topical and systemic antibiotics should be guided by two factors: Extent of skin involvement and severity of inflammation ↑ **Do not use tetracycline derivatives** in pregnant women, nursing mothers, or children under the age of 12 ↑ Patients treated with oral antibiotics may also be given topical antibiotics once the oral dose is reduced to a maintenance level

E. Refer patients with widespread, nodular cystic lesions to a dermatologist for treatment aimed at therapy to suppress sebum production

F. Follow Up: Three follow up visits (over 8-10 weeks) are generally needed to establish a successful treatment program
   1. For patients with comedonal and mild inflammatory acne on topical agents:
      a. Use chart to document location, type, and number of lesions to determine treatment response on each visit
      b. Adjust strength and frequency of topical agents depending on irritation and effectiveness
      c. If skin dryness is a problem that interferes with compliance, suggest use of a nonacnegenic moisturizer such as Moisturel, Purpose lotion, or Neutrogena Moisture after application of gel, or switch to a cream preparation
   2. For patients with inflammatory acne using **topical** comedolytics as well as **oral** antibiotics:
      a. Do a., b., and c. in F.1. above.
      b. Begin tapering oral antibiotic dose after 4-6 weeks of treatment (depending upon when development of new inflammatory lesions ceases); once the oral dose is reduced to a maintenance level, can add topical antibiotics to provide control
      c. Most patients require prolonged courses (months) or frequent, intermittent courses before complete and final remission occurs. **Consult PDR regarding need to monitor blood, renal, and hepatic function in patients on long-term antibiotic use!**
   3. For patients who are not on a successful treatment program after a total of 10-12 weeks of therapy, referral to a pediatric dermatologist is indicated

ATOPIC DERMATITIS

I. Definition: Extremely pruritic skin disorder involving cutaneous hypersensitivity

II. Pathogenesis

   A. A hereditary disorder whose exact pathogenesis is unknown

   B. Recently, factors involved in both epidermal barrier function and immunity (such as the serine protease inhibitor SPINK-5 and interleukin-4 mutations) have been implicated in the pathogenesis

III. Clinical Presentation

   A. Generally, begins in infancy/childhood, has periods of remission, exacerbation, and resolves by age 30. Highest incidence is among children

   B. Abnormally dry skin and lowered threshold for itching are significant factors

   C. Itching occurs in paroxysms and may be severe, especially in evenings

   D. Once itch-scratch cycle is established, characteristic lesions are created secondary to trauma cause by scratching

   E. Patterns of inflammation begin with severe pruritus and erythema. As skin changes are produced by trauma from scratching, skin becomes dry and scaly (xerosis)

   F. Several patterns of lesions may be produced: erythematous papular lesions that become confluent; diffuse erythema and scaling; lichenification (thickening of dermis with accentuation of skin lines)

   G. Involvement of the eyelids is common in all phases of atopic dermatitis

   H. Atopic dermatitis is divided into 3 phases which are outlined in the following table

ATOPIC DERMATITIS	

Infant phase (birth to 2 years)	Usually appears at about 3 months of age especially during cold, dry weather
	    Erythema and scaling of cheeks, chin with sparing of perioral and paranasal areas is frequently seen and there is sparing of the diaper area as well. May have generalized eruption of papules that are erythematous and scaly
	    Exudative lesions (oozing, weeping) are typical in infancy

Childhood phase (2-12 years)	Characteristic appearance at this age is flexural area involvement; perspiration produced by act of flexing and extending stimulates itching and itch-scratch cycle
	    Erythematous papules coalesce into plaques and scratching produces lichenification
	    Foot dermatitis is common in school-age children as well as in adolescents
	    Exudative lesions are seen less frequently

Adult phase (12 years to adult)	New onset as adult is rare
	    Onset of puberty may be associated with exacerbation
	    Localized inflammation of flexural areas with lichenification is most common pattern
	    Hand dermatitis occurs much more frequently in the adult phase

IV.   Diagnosis/Evaluation

    A.   History
        1.   Inquire about personal or family history of atopy—allergic rhinitis, asthma, atopic dermatitis--and age of onset
        2.   Question about itching, appearance and distribution of lesions, if dermatitis is chronic or chronically relapsing
        3.   Question regarding hand dermatitis
        4.   Ask about routine skin care at home including frequency of bathing and products used

    B.   Physical Examination
        1.   Have patient disrobe completely
        2.   Examine the skin methodically and determine the extent of the eruption and its distribution
        3.   Determine the primary lesion and the nature of the secondary lesions
        4.   Examine flexural areas for erythema and scaling but also look for lichenification in these areas
            a.   Examine the hands. Look for erythema and scaling on dorsal aspects of hands
            b.   Look for dry, fissured fingertip pads

    C.   Differential Diagnosis
        1.   Contact dermatitis, irritant or allergic
        2.   Seborrheic dermatitis
        3.   Nummular dermatitis
        4.   Scabies
        5.   Tinea

    D.   Diagnostic Tests: Not routinely indicated

V.   Plan/Management

    A.   Patients with acute, severe dermatitis (as well as all infants <6 months old) should be referred to an expert for management

    B.   For patients with less acute and less severe forms of the disorder, emphasize that this is a chronic condition and exacerbating factors must be controlled for successful management

    C.   Dry skin is a constant feature of atopic dermatitis; counsel patient/family how to control exacerbating factors using guidelines in the following table

KEYS TO REDUCING OR ELIMINATING FACTORS THAT PROMOTE DRYNESS AND INCREASE DESIRE TO SCRATCH

➡ Keep environment slightly cool and well humidified (home humidifiers)

➡ Avoid frequent hand washing; wear plastic gloves for wet work

➡ Keep skin well hydrated by daily baths in water no warmer than 90 degrees and soak for 10 minutes; always use a mild cleansing bar such as Dove, Basis, Eucerin to wash in axilla and groin areas; use plain water on other parts of body

➡ Avoid over-aggressive use of wash cloth which can exfoliate and remove the stratum corneum

➡ Skin should be patted dry after bath and moisturizers applied immediately to still-moist skin (see table below)

➡ Wear loose-fitting 100% cotton clothing; avoid wool

➡ Use fragrance-free laundry products such as Ivory Snow Flakes, Cheer-Free

➡ Recognize that emotional stress can worsen (by possibly increasing desire to scratch) but not cause the disorder

D. Lubrication of the skin done daily on a consistent basis is the key to control
1. Bathing should always be followed by immediate use of emollients applied after patting the skin dry
2. Remind patient to moisturize skin throughout the day if the skin feels dry; more frequent lubrication is necessary during winter months
3. Recommend moisturizers from the table below
4. In terms of moisturizing, ointments are the most moisturizing but leave a greasy feel to the skin; creams are thicker and more lubricating than lotions; very dry skin benefits the most from ointments and patients should always be encouraged to use ointments at least at night

RECOMMENDED MOISTURIZERS		
Moisturizing Lotions	**Moisturizing Creams**	**Moisturizing Ointments**
Petrolatum-based ✓ Dermasil ✓ Moisturel Lotion ✓ Replenaderm Lotion	Petrolatum-based ✓ Purpose Dry Skin Cream ✓ Cetaphil Cream ✓ Keri Cream	Petrolatum-based ✓ Vaseline Pure Petroleum Jelly (Fragrance, preservative, and lanolin free)
Mixtures of lanolin and petrolatum ✓ Eucerin Lotion ✓ Lubriderm Lotion ✓ Nivea Moisturizing Lotion	Mixtures of lanolin and petrolatum ✓ Eucerin Creme Without lanolin or petrolatum ✓ Neutrogena Norwegian Formula Hand Cream	Mixtures of lanolin and petrolatum ✓ Aquaphor Natural Healing Ointment (Fragrance and preservative free)
Without lanolin or petrolatum ✓ Corn Huskers Lotion ✓ Cetaphil Lotion		

E. Pharmacologic therapy: Mainstays of therapy are topical steroid ointments and oral antihistamines
1. To reduce inflammation, it is often necessary to use topical steroid preparations applied thinly 2x/day until controlled (up to 7 days in children, up to 14 days in adolescents)
   a. Infants and children: Hydrocortisone ointment 2.5% (use 1% on face and intertriginous areas) (**Note**: Systemic absorption of topical corticosteroids in infants and children can cause growth retardation and hypothalamic-pituitary-adrenal axis suppression!)
   b. Adolescents: Triamcinolone acetonide ointment 0.1% (Aristocort ointment 0.1%, supplied as 15, 60 g)
   c. In milder cases, may use steroid cream instead of ointment; ointments leave a greasy feel to the skin which many patients dislike
   d. Lubricants can also be applied to the skin not being treated with the steroid ointment; (lubricant creams/ointments should **not** be applied over the steroid ointment)
   e. Once inflammation is controlled, substitute lubricants for the steroid ointments to improve skin barrier function
   f. Use the topical corticosteroid of the lowest potency that will control the condition
2. Pruritus control with the use of antihistamines and topical antipruritics is the other mainstay of pharmacologic therapy (see following table); focus is on relief of itching so that patient is not constantly fighting the urge to scratch

PRURITUS CONTROL USING PHARMACOLOGIC INTERVENTIONS

Oral Antihistamines (Second-Generation H₁-Receptor Blockers)

Fexofenadine (Allegra), supplied as 30, 60, 180 mg tabs
Children 6-11 years: 30 mg BID
Children ≥12 years: 60 mg BID or 180 mg once/day

Loratadine (Claritin), supplied as 5 mg/5 mL syrup, 10 mg tabs, and 10 mg disintegrating (Reditabs)
Children, 2-5 years: 5 mg once/day
Children ≥6 years: 10 mg once/day
All formulations of Claritin have been approve for OTC sale

Desloratadine (Clarinex), supplied as 5 mg tabs
Children ≥12 years: 5 mg once/day

Cetirizine (Zyrtec), supplied as 1 mg/mL syrup, and 5, 10 mg tabs
Children, 6-23 months: 2.5 mg once/day
Children, 2-5 years: initially 2.5 mg once daily, max 5 mg once daily or 2.5 mg Q 12 hrs
Children ≥6 years: 5-10 mg once/day

➡ Of the second-generation H₁-receptor blockers above, Allegra seems to offer the best combination of effectiveness and safety (see Abramowicz, M., (2001). Newer antihistamines. *Medical Letter, 43*, 35-36.)
➡ Any of the H₁-receptor blockers listed above is preferred over first-generation H₁-receptor blockers which can impair psychomotor performance even in the absence of sedation

Oral Antihistamines (First-Generation H₁-Receptor Blockers)

Hydroxyzine (Atarax), supplied as 10 mg/5 mL syrup and 10, 25, 50, 100 mg tablets
Infants and children ≤6 years, 0.5 mg/kg/dose TID PRN
Children >6 years, 25 mg/dose TID PRN
A single dose at bedtime is frequently all that is necessary

➡ A good choice for use at bedtime; cost is much less than the second-generation antihistamines (loratadine will be generic and thus will also be somewhat more affordable by the end of 2002)

Topical Antipruritic Agents

Sarna lotion, Prax lotion, Eucerin Itch-Relief Moisturizing Spray, and *Itch-X gel* are all OTC products

➡ Instruct patients to use products only as directed on the label, making sure to avoid the eyes and not use on broken skin

Topical agents may be used in addition to or instead of oral antihistamines

F.   Counsel patient to avoid exposure to chemicals, and to use gloves when engaging in "wet work"

G.   Patients who do not respond to conventional therapies after a 2-4 weeks trial should be referred to a specialist for management

H.   Tacrolimus (Protopic) and pimecrolimus (Elidel) are new prescription products—first in a new class of topical immunomodulators
    1.   Tacrolimus, an ointment, has been approved by the FDA for short-term and intermittent long-term therapy in children ≥2 years of age with **moderate to severe** atopic dermatitis in whom the use of conventional therapies is inadvisable, ineffective, or not tolerated
        a.   Use either 0.03% or 0.1% formulation depending on age of child; continue for one week after resolution
        b.   Apply BID in thin layer to affected areas; do not occlude or apply to wet skin
    2.   Pimecrolimus, a cream, has been approved by the FDA for short-term or intermittent long-term treatment of **mild to moderate** atopic dermatitis in children ≥2 years of age when conventional therapies are inadvisable, ineffective, or not tolerated
        a.   Available in 1% cream formulation
        b.   Apply BID to affected areas; do not occlude
    3.   Consult PDR for prescribing information, precautions, contraindications, and adverse reactions before prescribing this or any other medication

I. Follow up
1. The first follow-up visit should be within 2-4 weeks to determine the effectiveness of therapy
2. Monthly visits are appropriate until patient is using lubricants only; then every 3-6 months
3. Patient should understand that this is a chronic, recurrent disorder and should be offered practical counseling on each visit regarding ways to deal with the disorder
4. Reliable parents and adolescents should be given ample refills of topical corticosteroids so that they can control the condition themselves (if there is not a concern about overuse/inappropriate use)
5. Patients who do not respond to conventional therapies after a 2-4 week trial should be referred to a specialist for management

CONTACT DERMATITIS

I. Definition: Skin inflammation due to irritants (irritant contact dermatitis) or allergens (allergic contact dermatitis)

II. Pathogenesis

A. Irritant contact dermatitis
1. Damage to one of the components of the water-protein-lipid matrix of the outer layer of the epidermis of the skin caused by irritants including chemicals, dry, cold air, and friction
2. An eczematous response in the skin is produced that is nonallergic in origin

B. Allergic contact dermatitis
1. A form of cell mediated immunity that occurs in 2 phases
2. The sensitization phase which occurs when allergens penetrate the epidermis and produce proliferation of T lymphocytes (sensitization phase; can take days or months)
3. In the elicitation phase, the antigen-specific T lymphocytes present in the skin combine with the subsequent exposures to the allergen to produce inflammation

III. Clinical Presentation

A. Irritant contact dermatitis
1. About 80% of cases of contact dermatitis involve irritants rather than allergens
2. Hands are commonly affected in adolescents
3. Intensity of inflammation is related to the concentration of the irritant, the exposure time, and the state of the epidermal barrier
4. Acute irritant contact dermatitis is characterized by papules and/or vesicles on an erythematous patchy background with weeping and edema; burning usually predominates over itching
5. Persistent, chronic dermatitis is characterized by lichenification, patches of erythema, and fissures in the skin
6. Frequent hand washing is a very common cause in adolescents; jobs involving repeated wet work such as food service, child care, health care, and hair styling predispose workers to irritant contact dermatitis
7. Irritant diaper dermatitis is the form most commonly seen in infants

---

CLINICAL FEATURES OF IRRITANT DIAPER DERMATITIS

- Results from prolonged contact of urine and/or feces; feces are implicated in perianal distribution and urine in thigh and waistband lesions; affected skin is very erythematous
- Two most common presentation are the chafing type and the perianal involvement type

Chafing type:
  ✓ Most common of the two types
  ✓ Involves convex skin surfaces that are in contact with diaper (thighs, buttocks, waist area)
  ✓ Usually absent in skin folds
  ✓ Observed most often at 7-12 months when urine capacity exceeds absorbent capacity of diaper (even superabsorbents)

Perianal type:
  ✓ Limited to the perianal area
  ✓ Observed most often in newborns or in infants who have diarrhea
  ✓ Sharply circumscribed area of erythema in perianal area

B. Allergic contact dermatitis
1. Much less common than irritant contact dermatitis
2. A genetically predisposed hypersensitivity reaction
3. May correspond exactly to contactant (e.g., fabric treatments, clothing, nickel in jewelry, latex in gloves, ingredients in cosmetics or topical medications)
4. Hands, forearms, and face are common sites
5. Skin findings include vesicles, edema, erythema, and pruritus
6. Poison ivy, oak, and sumac are by far the most common causes in the US
   a. In classic presentation, vesicular lesions on erythematous base are in a linear distribution on exposed skin caused from leaves brushing skin or from streaking oleoresin when scratching
   b. Extreme pruritus is usually present
   c. Diffuse patterns may occur when oleoresin is contacted from contaminated pets or smoke from burning plants

C. Distribution often provides clues to diagnosis
1. Scalp and ears: Hair care products, jewelry
2. Eyelids: Cosmetics, contact lens solution
3. Face/neck: Cosmetics, cleansers, medications, jewelry
4. Trunk/axilla: Clothing, deodorants
5. Arms/hands: Poison oak, ivy, sumac, soaps, detergents, frequent hand washing, jewelry, rubber gloves
6. Legs/feet: Clothing, shoes
7. Preservatives in OTC and prescriptive topical products may produce dermatitis at area of application

IV. Diagnosis/Evaluation

A. History
1. Question regarding location of eruption, time and rate of onset (abrupt or insidious), and associated symptoms such as pruritus; ask if others in household have similar symptoms
2. Ask about job exposures and recreational pursuits
3. Question regarding exposures to such substances as chemicals, detergents, medications, poison plants, lubricants, cleansers, and rubber gloves, both at home and at work or in recreational pursuits
4. Obtain family history, personal history of allergies, treatments tried and results

B. Physical Examination
1. Examine skin to determine the location of the inflammation
2. Determine the primary lesion
3. Determine the distribution of the eruption as a clue to diagnosis

C. Differential Diagnosis
1. Atopic dermatitis (usually more chronic, occurs in flexural distribution, onset in childhood)
2. Scabies (usually begins in fingerwebs, wrists, spreading to groin, axilla and itching is prominent; other household contacts are symptomatic)
3. Nummular dermatitis (discrete, coin-shaped, erythematous, scaling plaques)
4. Dermatitis herpetiformis (usually localized to elbows, knees, buttocks, posterior scalp)

D. Diagnostic Tests: None indicated

V. Plan/Management: Irritant contact dermatitis

A. In adolescents, a common type of irritant contact dermatitis involves the hands

B. The first step in management is to identify the offending agent and eliminate or at least limit further exposure (preventive measures)

C. Hands: For adolescents with hand involvement who must engage in wet work
1. Suggest the wearing of cotton gloves under vinyl gloves which may reduce need to wash hands as frequently
2. Use mild soap when washing hands
3. Appropriate protective gloves should be worn for specific solvent or chemical exposures
4. Frequent application of occlusive ointments such as Vaseline or Aquaphor should be used (remind patient that ointments should not be applied over steroid ointments or creams if also using as this creates too much occlusion)
5. Topical steroid ointment applied BID can help in reducing erythema
   a. Triamcinolone acetonide 0.1% (Aristocort A) ointment
   b. Supplied as 15, 60g
   c. Use for 10-14 days then use lubricant only

D. Diaper Dermatitis: For both variations of irritant contract diaper dermatitis—chafing and perianal involvement—the basis of treatment is to eliminate the irritants and to protect the skin. Advise parents as follows:
1. Change diaper frequently (at least every two hours); recommend use of Pampers Rash Guard diapers which deliver petrolatum to diaper area
2. Expose diaper area to air when practical (place infant on disposable waterproof pad)
3. Never use hair dryer to dry diaper area (even at air setting)
4. Caution against over scrubbing of diaper area (a minimum of mild cleansers such as Dove or Basis may be used in this area with gentle rinsing once or twice a day) (Ivory Soap or detergent soaps such as Dial should not be used)
5. Explain to parents that nothing is absolutely necessary for cleansing the diaper area besides warm water and a soft cloth; use of baby wipes is ubiquitous in US and is acceptable
6. Apply barrier ointments such as zinc oxide (Desitin) to diaper area/perianal area
7. Caution against use of other creams and powders in the diaper area (powders can be accidentally inhaled by infant)

E. Irritant diaper dermatitis predisposes infant to secondary *C. albicans* infection (see section on CANDIDIASIS for diagnosis and treatment of this condition)

VI. Plan/Management: Allergic contact dermatitis

A. Avoidance of allergens is necessary for recovery and to prevent recurrences

B. If poison ivy, oak, sumac are identified as the source, advise patient as follows:
1. Wash skin immediately with soap and water to remove oleoresin (must be done within 15 minutes of exposure, so this is information most useful in preventing future episodes rather than dealing with the present episode)
2. Apply cold, wet compresses to affected areas (can use Burrow's solution or tap water) 3-4 times daily for 20 minutes during acute phase (vesicles present) to suppress inflammation and reduce itching
3. Bathing with Aveeno may be helpful
4. Use of calamine lotion may be helpful and is drying which makes it beneficial for exudative inflammation; avoid use of topical products containing diphenhydramine
5. Other topical antipruritic agents include Prax (pramoxine), PrameGel (pramoxine and menthol), and Sarna (menthol, camphor, and phenol)

C. Prescribe topical steroids to clear the dermatitis and decrease discomfort
1. Adolescents: Refer to V.C.5. above for use on hands, arms, legs, and trunk; use lower potency for face and groin area (hydrocortisone 2.5% cream)
2. Children: Hydrocortisone 2.5% cream (Hytone); apply thin layer BID for 7 to 10 days; use lower potency for face and groin area (hydrocortisone 1% cream)

D. Also prescribe oral antihistamines for pruritus control (see table *Pruritus Control* in section on ATOPIC DERMATITIS) for products and dosing information or prescribe topical antipruritic agents such as Sarna lotion, or Prax lotion (OTC products)

E. When skin involvement is extensive, the face and/or groin areas are involved, or pruritus is poorly controlled with oral and topical therapies, refer child to an expert for management

F. Follow Up
1. None indicated if dermatitis is mild
2. In 3-4 days for moderate dermatitis requiring topical corticosteroid use

KERATOSIS PILARIS

I. Definition: An eruption consisting of follicle-based, scaling papules most commonly on the posterolateral aspects of the upper arms, anterior thighs, and the buttocks that is common in person with atopic dermatitis

II. Pathogenesis

A. Results from mild follicular plugging and peri-follicular inflammation

B. Exact mechanism of pathogenesis is unknown, but may be caused by a disorder in keratinization so that follicular plugging with keratin debris occurs

C. May also represent a response to drying of the skin surface; the scaling produced is trapped in follicular opening

III. Clinical Presentation

A. Commonly occurs in individuals with atopic dermatitis with children, adolescents, and young adults most often affected; occurrence peaks in adolescence

B. Appears as small, pinpoint, follicular papules and pustules on the extensor aspects of the extremities, and the buttocks—a "gooseflesh" appearance

C. The affected skin surface feels rough and dry; hair in the center of the papule/pustule confirms a follicular location

D. Condition is aggravated by cold, dry climates, and is usually associated with extremely dry skin

IV. Diagnosis/Evaluation

A. History
1. Ask about location of eruption, onset, duration, and appearance of lesions
2. Determine if there is a history of atopic dermatitis
3. Ask if condition gets better or worse at any time of the year
4. Question about associated symptoms (there should be none)

B. Physical Examination
1. Examine skin, focusing on areas typically affected—extensor aspects of arms, legs, and the buttocks
2. Touch affected areas for rough skin texture; examine all skin surfaces for signs of dryness

C. Differential Diagnosis
1. Microcomedones of acne (distribution of acne is face, chest, upper back)
2. Molluscum contagiosum (lesions are waxy-appearing with central umbilication)
3. Drug eruption (drug eruption usually has acute onset and keratosis pilaris is chronic)

D. Diagnostic Tests: None indicated

V. Plan/Management

A. Mild forms: Recommend application of lubricants applied to moist skin immediately after bathing (see CARE OF DRY AND OILY SKIN for table of moisturizers)

B.   Moderate to severe forms

> - Recommend/prescribe products containing alpha hydroxy acids (glycolic, lactic, and citric acids)
> - A property of all alpha hydroxy acids is that they enhance shedding of surface corneocytes and the exfoliation of the dried out corneocytes results in a smoother, more uniform surface
> - Lactic acid 12% cream (Lac-Hydrin) applied BID usually controls the condition (children >2 years)
> - Advise patient to continue to use lubricants (recommended under V.A. above)
> - Patient should be advised to use cautiously on face and to **avoid sun exposure** to treated skin

C.   Advise patient to soak 3-4 x per week for 10 minutes in tepid water, to use cleansers such as Dove, Purpose, or Basis, and to apply moisturizers after bathing while skin is still damp after having been patted dry (**Note:** Persons who shower typically use hotter water than those who take tub baths–brief soaking in tepid water (bathing) may be a good alternative to help keep skin hydrated)

D.   Follow up: None indicated

POMPHOLYX

I.   Definition: A disease of unknown etiology that disrupts the skin of the palms and soles

II.   Pathogenesis: Recurrent eczematous dermatitis of unknown etiology; also referred to as dyshidrosis or dyshidrotic eczema

III.   Clinical Presentation

A.   Condition is characterized by sudden eruptions of itchy vesicles on the palms, or on lateral fingers, or on the plantar feet (acute phase)

B.   Waves of vesiculation may occur; vesicles are 1-5 mm in size, are symmetrical in distribution, and are filled with clear fluid making the eruption look like tapioca

C.   Moderate to severe itching usually precedes the emergence of the vesicles

D.   Over 1-3 weeks vesicles slowly resolve, and are replaced by scaling, redness, and lichenification (chronic phase)

IV.   Diagnosis/Evaluation

A.   History
    1.   Question about location of lesions, onset, duration, and changes in lesions over time
    2.   Ask about associated symptoms
    3.   Inquire about skin allergies
    4.   Ask about treatments tried and results

B.   Physical Examination
    1.   Examine lesions looking for vesicles, or if the acute process has ended, exfoliation of skin revealing a red, cracked base
    2.   Examine all skin surfaces to determine if vesicles are located in areas other than palms and soles

C.   Differential Diagnosis
    1.   Contact dermatitis
    2.   Tinea
    3.   Atopic dermatitis
    4.   Pustular psoriasis of palms and soles (with this disease, vesicles are cloudy with purulent fluid; pain rather than itching is the chief complaint); referral is needed

D.   Diagnostic Tests: None indicated

V.   Plan/Management

    A.   Initial treatment consists of use of cold, wet compresses and application of topical corticosteroids
        1.   Cold wet compresses: Apply cold, sopping wet compresses (using either cold tap water or Burrow's solution) twice a day to affected area; leave in place at least 30 minutes
        2.   Follow wet dressings with application of triamcinolone acetonide cream, 0.025% (Aristocort A cream, 0.025%) to affected areas BID x 7-10 days

    B.   Oral antihistamines can be prescribed to relieve pruritus (see section on ATOPIC DERMATITIS for table of medications and dosing recommendations)

    C.   Follow up: None indicated

SEBORRHEIC DERMATITIS

I.   Definition: A common, chronic, inflammatory skin disorder with a characteristic pattern for different age groups

II.   Pathogenesis

    A.   The yeast *Pityrosporum ovale* is believed to play a role in the etiology

    B.   Both genetic and environmental factors seem to influence onset and course of disease

III.   Clinical Presentation

    A.   In children, two age groups are affected: infants and adolescents

    B.   Mild seborrheic dermatitis presents as fine, dry, white or yellow greasy scale, on an inflamed base

    C.   More severe eruptions appear as dull, red plaques with thick, white or yellow scale in a diffuse distribution

    D.   Occurs in seborrheic areas
        1.   Infants: Scalp ("cradle cap"), scalp margins, and forehead
        2.   Adolescents: Scalp, scalp margins, eyebrows, base of lashes, paranasal, nasolabial folds, external ear canals, posterior auricular fold, presternal areas, and upper back

    E.   Seborrheic dermatitis is one of the most common early cutaneous manifestations of HIV infection

    F.   White scaling that adheres to the eyelashes and lid margins is characteristic of seborrheic blepharitis (see section on BLEPHARITIS)

IV.   Diagnosis/Evaluation

    A.   History
        1.   Question regarding onset, duration, and location of lesions
        2.   Inquire about personal or family history of seborrheic dermatitis
        3.   Determine if immunosuppressed
        4.   Ask about treatments tried and results

    B.   Physical Examination
        1.   Examine skin for characteristic lesions: fine, dry, white or yellow scale on inflamed base or dull, red plaques with thick white or yellow greasy appearing scale
        2.   Determine distribution

    C.   Differential Diagnosis
        1.   Tinea capitis/faciale (fungal culture/KOH prep can help differentiate; tinea faciale is usually unilateral)
        2.   Acne rosacea (central facial erythema and a significant flushing component are present with this condition; also telangiectasia and inflammatory papules may be present)

D. Diagnostic Tests: None indicated if typical lesions, distribution

V. Plan/Management

A. Infants with seborrheic dermatitis should be treated as follows

TREATMENT OF INFANTS & SMALL CHILDREN

Cradle cap: Use bland shampoo such as Johnson's Baby Shampoo left on 2-3 minutes while gently scrubbing scalp with soft brush to remove scale and crust; rinse thoroughly
   ✓ Repeat 2-3x/week
   ✓ Apply topical steroid lotion of low potency such as hydrocortisone lotion 1% BID for 2 weeks
On the face: Use low potency topical steroid cream such as Hytone cream 1% once a day or every other day
   ✓ Use no longer than 2 weeks

B. Adolescents ≥16 years of age with seborrheic dermatitis should be treated as follows

TREATMENT OF ADOLESCENTS

For scalp involvement that is mild, use of a medicated shampoo to remove and control mild scale is usually effective
   ✓ Selenium sulfide: Exsel, Selsun Blue, and Reme-T (OTC)
   ✓ Sulfur and salicylic acid combination: Sebulex (OTC)
   ✓ Coal tar: Denorex, T/Gel, Tegrin (OTC)
   ✓ Above shampoos must be left on a minimum of 5-10 minutes before rinsing
   ✓ Ketoconazole 2%: Nizoral shampoo (Rx): Use 2-3 x/week x 1 month; may need to use once a week for maintenance (also available OTC as Ketoconazole 1% (Nizoral A-D shampoo)
 	
For scalp involvement that is more extensive, (or for milder cases in which initial treatment [above] was not successful), treatment involves the removal of some of the scale prior to use of the medicated shampoo
   ✓ Instruct patient to apply warm peanut oil or olive oil to the scalp at bedtime to loosen scale; in AM, shampoo hair with one of the medicated shampoos listed above
 	
For facial involvement, dermatitis usually responds to ketoconazole (Nizoral Topical 2% cream) [apply BID up to 4 weeks]; alternative is antidandruff shampoo diluted with water and used daily as a facial wash
   ✓ For more severe facial involvement, prescribe ciclopirox (Loprox Gel) applied once daily for up to 2 weeks (not for use in adolescents <16 years of age)
 	
For intertriginous involvement, hydrocortisone 2.5% cream (Hytone cream 2.5%) should be used for 7 days; ointments should not be used on intertriginous areas (opposition of two skin surfaces greatly enhances absorption)
 	
For chest involvement, medicated shampoos may be used on chest skin; may also use triamcinolone 0.1% lotion BID OR topical ketoconazole 2% (Nizoral cream) BID until clear; then use once or twice weekly

C. Recalcitrant cases should be referred to a specialist for management

D. Follow up: Not indicated except in treatment failures

IMPETIGO AND ECTHYMA

I.   Definition: Bacterial skin infection caused by invasion of the epidermis by pathogenic *Staphylococcus aureus* or *Streptococcus pyogenes,* or a combination of these organisms

II.   Pathogenesis

    A.   Most skin microorganisms in healthy persons are nonpathogenic

    B.   Microscopic breaks in the epidermal barrier allows penetration by the two major pathogens found on the skin—*S. aureus* and/or *S. pyogenes*

    C.   The depth of invasion in impetigo is superficial; the entire epidermis is involved in ecthyma

    D.   Poststreptococcal glomerulonephritis may follow skin infections involving strains of nephritogenic streptococci; rheumatic heart disease is not a sequelae of this infection

III.   Clinical Presentation

    A.   Impetigo begins as small (1-2 mm) superficial vesicles with fragile roofs that are quickly lost; vesicles rupture leaving erosions covered by moist, honey-colored crusts

    B.   Multiple lesions are usually present, and face and extremities are the **most common** sites of involvement

    C.   The terms bullous and nonbullous impetigo have been used to describe two patterns of infection with bullous impetigo suggesting staphylococcal origin and nonbullous, streptococcal origin. The preferred term presently is simply, "impetigo," since differentiation is difficult based on appearance, and many infections are caused by both organisms

    D.   In ecthyma, ulcers form with a dry, dark crust, and surrounding erythema; lesions are usually found on legs

    E.   Both ecthyma and impetigo may occur simultaneously

    F.   Both infections occur most frequently in children but also occur in adults

    G.   Enhanced by poor hygiene and warm, moist climates; disease is self-limiting

IV.   Diagnosis/Evaluation

    A.   History
        1.   Question about location of lesions, onset, duration, and any associated symptoms
        2.   Ask if other family members are affected; treatments tried and results

    B.   Physical Examination
        1.   Determine if febrile
        2.   Examine skin (focus on areas of typical involvement—face, arms, legs) looking for erosions covered by moist, honey-colored crusts that characterize impetigo, and firm, dry, dark crusts with surrounding erythema that characterize ecthyma
        3.   Check for regional lymphadenopathy

    C.   Differential Diagnosis
        1.   Tinea (with tinea, there is central clearing, and KOH test is positive)
        2.   Herpes simplex infections (HSV is characterized by clusters of lesions, and can be confirmed via fluorescent antibody testing of smears from intact vesicles)
        3.   Second-degree burn may be confused with ecthyma (careful history is important; Gram stain for bacteria should be negative unless burn site contaminated with bacteria)
        4.   Allergic contact dermatitis (itching is prominent symptom in allergic contact dermatitis)
        5.   Cutaneous anthrax may be confused with ecthyma; bacterial culture would be needed

D. Diagnostic Tests: None required as clinical features are so characteristic; if uncertain about diagnosis, perform Gram stain on fluid from intact vesicle/pustule looking for gram-positive cocci in clusters (*S. aureus*) or chains (*S. pyogenes*); see IV.C. above for other diagnostic tests

V. Plan/Management

A. For multiple lesions, systemic antibiotics are the preferred therapy and there are several options

B. Dicloxacillin, supplied as suspension, 62.5 mg/5 mL, and caps, 250, 500 mg
   1. Children: 15 to 50 mg/kg/day divided into 4 doses x 10 days
   2. Adolescents (≥16 years): 250 mg QID x 10 days, OR

C. Cephalexin (Keflex), supplied as suspension (250 mg/5 mL), caps (250, 500 mg) and tabs (250, 500 mg)
   1. Children: 25 mg/kg/day divided into 2 doses (Q 12 hrs) x 10 days
   2. Adolescents (≥16 years): 500 mg BID x 10 days
   3. Better compliance with this drug than with dicloxacillin

D. If only a few lesions are present, consider use of topical mupirocin ointment (Bactroban) which has been shown to be as efficacious as oral cephalexin for mild infections
   1. Apply to affected areas TID x 7-10 days or until all lesions have cleared
   2. Re-evaluate if no response in 3-5 days

E. Gentle washing of lesions to remove loose crusts may be helpful and must be done if mupirocin is used; scrubbing of lesions with antibacterial soaps has not been shown to be effective and is not recommended

F. Good hand washing (for both the caregiver [if patient is a young child] and the patient) and personal hygiene are recommended to reduce likelihood of spread; use of a mild antibacterial soap such as Lever 2000 for hand washing and bathing may be helpful

G. Highly contagious nature of the infection should be emphasized; child can return to school 24 hours after beginning antibiotic therapy

H. Follow up: In one week to determine response to treatment

CELLULITIS

I. Definition: An acute, diffuse inflammation of the skin and subcutaneous structures characterized by hyperemia, edema, and leukocytic infiltration

II. Pathogenesis

A. Invasion of bacteria (usually pathogenic streptococci) into the dermis and subcutaneous fat with subsequent spread through the lymphatics

B. Many other bacteria are causative agents including *Staphylococcus aureus and Haemophilus influenzae* (less common in US since introduction of the *Haemophilus influenzae*, Type B [Hib] vaccine)

C. May develop in apparently normal skin, but more often trauma to the skin provides a portal of entry for invading organisms

III. Clinical Presentation

A. Erythema, warmth, edema, and pain are usual clinical features; the erythematous plaque is usually tender-to-painful to touch without a sharply demarcated border and may cover a small to large area of the skin

B. Fever, chills, malaise, and lymphadenopathy are frequently present

C. Typically, there is a preceding wound or trauma to the skin which compromises lymphatic drainage

D. Findings that signal an emergent condition are listed in the following table

<table>
<tr><td colspan="2">INDICES OF AN EMERGENT CONDITION</td></tr>
<tr><td>✓</td><td>Extensive, rather than limited, localized cellulitis</td></tr>
<tr><td>✓</td><td>Fever, or other signs and symptoms of septicemia (toxic presentation)</td></tr>
<tr><td>✓</td><td>Diminished arterial pulse in a cool, swollen, infected extremity</td></tr>
<tr><td>✓</td><td>Presence of cutaneous necrosis</td></tr>
<tr><td>✓</td><td>Closed space infections of the hand</td></tr>
<tr><td>✓</td><td>Periorbital cellulitis because of proximity to brain</td></tr>
<tr><td>✓</td><td>Immunosuppressed or diabetic host</td></tr>
<tr><td>✓</td><td>Infants and children <2 years of age</td></tr>
</table>

E. Erysipelas, a distinctive type of superficial cellulitis is virtually always caused by group A streptococci

F. In erysipelas, infection is more superficial, with margins that are more clearly demarcated from normal skin than in cellulitis

G. Lower legs, face, and ears are most frequently involved in erysipelas

H. Lymphatic involvement ("streaking") is prominent in erysipelas which also differentiates it from other types of cellulitis

IV. Diagnosis/Evaluation

A. History
1. Question about location, onset, duration, degree of spread, and presence of pain
2. Ask if there was a pre-existing wound or trauma to involved area
3. Determine if systemic symptoms are present (fever, chills, malaise)

B. Physical Examination
1. Vital signs and BP to determine if febrile, and to evaluate cardiovascular status
2. Examine involved area of skin to determine how extensive infection is, degree of erythema, presence of purulent discharge, presence of necrotic tissue
3. Examine adjacent skin/lymph nodes to determine presence of "streaking," degree of lymphadenopathy

C. Differential Diagnosis
1. Pressure erythema
2. Contact dermatitis
3. Swelling over septic joint

D. Diagnostic Tests
1. Obtain Gram stain and culture and sensitivity of wound before treatment is instituted
2. Obtain CBC and blood cultures if cellulitis is extensive or associated with systemic toxicity and refer for emergent care

V. Plan/Management

A. Treatment of erysipelas and cellulitis depends on the patient's condition and underlying risk factors

B. Refer all patients who meet criteria for emergent conditions (see table above) for expert care

C. Adolescents and children >2 years of age with nontoxic presentation and localized and limited skin involvement can be treated empirically with oral antibiotics aimed at staphylococcal and streptococcal organisms

D. For uncomplicated cases, choose ONE of the following antibiotics, and **treat for 10-14 days** (except for Zithromax which has a treatment course of 5 days):

1. Dicloxacillin
   a. Children: 50 mg/kg/day divided into 4 doses (Q 6 hours)
   b. Adolescents (≥16 years): 500 mg QID, **OR**
2. Cephalexin (Keflex) supplied as suspension, 250 mg/5 mL; caps, 250, 500 mg; tabs, 250, 500 mg
   a. Children: 50-75 mg/kg/day in 2 divided doses (Q 12 hours)
   b. Adolescents (≥16 years): 500 mg BID, **OR**
3. Amoxicillin/clavulanic acid (Augmentin) supplied as suspension, 125 mg/5 mL, 250 mg/5 mL, 400 mg/5 mL; tabs, 250, 500, 875 mg; chewable tabs, 125, 200, 250, 400 mg
   a. Children: 45 mg/kg/day in 2 divided doses (Q 12 hours)
   b. Children >40 kg: 500 mg TID **OR**
4. Azithromycin (Zithromax) supplied as suspension, 100 mg/5 mL, 200 mg/5 mL; Z-Pak (6 tabs)
   a. Children: 10 mg/kg (maximum 500 mg/day) once daily x 1 day, then 5 mg/kg (maximum 250 mg/day) once daily for next 4 days (days 2-5)
   b. Adolescents: 500 mg on day 1, then 250 mg/day on days 2-5

E. In all cases, antibiotic therapy may require changing based on culture results and clinical response

F. Local measures such as immobilization, elevation, application of moist heat (3-4 x day for 15-20 minutes) should be used with all patients to provide symptomatic relief and speed resolution of the infection

G. Follow up in 24-48 hours to determine response to therapy

FOLLICULITIS, FURUNCLES, AND CARBUNCLES

I. Definition: Bacterial invasion of the follicular wall

II. Pathogenesis

   A. Most commonly due to *Staphylococcus aureus*

   B. Other organisms may be involved, and, in general, the microbiology of cutaneous infection reflects the microflora of the part of body involved

III. Clinical Presentation

   A. Folliculitis is inflammation of the hair follicle caused by infection, chemical irritation, or injury

   B. Furuncle (abscess or boil) is a deep folliculitis, consisting of a walled-off, pus filled mass that is painful, firm, or fluctuant; fever is uncommon
      1. Furuncle may appear at any site
      2. Most often occurs in areas of friction (waistline, groin, buttocks, axilla)

   C. Carbuncles are aggregates of infected, abscessed follicles located deep in dermis; it points and drains through multiple openings
      1. Very painful and systemic signs such as chills, fever may be present
      2. Occur in areas with thick dermis (back of neck, lateral aspect of thigh)

   D. Furuncles and carbuncles are uncommon in children

IV. Diagnosis/Evaluation

   A. History
      1. Ask about location, appearance of lesion, onset, duration, and if purulent drainage is exuding from surface
      2. Inquire about associated symptoms of pain and systemic symptoms of fever and chills
      3. Inquire about frequency of occurrence

B. Physical Examination
1. Take temperature to determine if systemic involvement
2. Inspect lesion(s) for signs of local inflammation (erythema, swelling, and pustular surface)
3. Palpate surface of lesion for fluctuance, which indicates accumulation of purulent matter; palpate adjacent lymph nodes

C. Differential Diagnosis
1. Acne pustules
2. Epidermal cyst
3. Hidradenitis suppurativa

D. Diagnostic Tests: Wound culture should be done to verify antibiotic choice

V. Plan/Management

A. For folliculitis in which skin involvement is limited, treatment with topical antibiotics is usually sufficient; use **one** of the following
1. Mupirocin (Bactroban) cream may be used: Apply small amount TID to affected area x 7-10 days
2. Erythromycin 2% solution (A/T/S) BID x 7-10 days
3. Clindamycin solution (Cleocin T) BID x 7-10 days

B. For folliculitis in which skin involvement is more extensive, oral antistaphylococcal antibiotics are indicated (see V.E. below for antibiotic choices and dosing information)

C. For carbuncles and furuncles, frequent warm, moist compresses provide relief and promote localization and spontaneous draining

D. Incision and drainage is commonly required for carbuncles and furuncles

E. Systemic antistaphylococcal antibiotics should be used to treat furuncles and carbuncles
1. Treatment of choice is dicloxacillin supplied as suspension, 62.5 mg/5 mL, and caps, 250, 500 mg
   a. Children: 15-50 mg/kg/day divided into 4 doses x 10 days
   b. Adolescents (≥16 years): 250 mg QID x 10 days
2. Alternative treatment is cephalexin (Keflex) supplied as suspension, 250 mg/5 mL; caps, 250, 500 mg; tabs
   a. Children: 25-50 mg/kg/day divided into 2 doses (Q 12 hours) x 10 days
   b. Adolescents (≥16 years): 500 mg BID x 10 days

F. Refer children with cutaneous abscesses located on face, scalp, and neck

G. Culture recurrent abscesses and refer patients for evaluation for diseases that may underlie recurrent furunculosis: Immunodeficiency, diabetes mellitus, alcoholism, malnutrition, and severe anemia

H. Patients with recurrent abscess formation who are otherwise healthy may benefit from mupirocin 2% ointment (Bactroban Nasal); apply 0.25 g to inside of each nostril BID for 5 days in order to eradicate nasal carriage of *S. aureus*

I. To prevent recurrence, stress role of good hygiene to patient and family. Most useful: frequent hand washing and daily skin cleansing with an antibacterial soap such as Dial or Hibiclens antimicrobial skin cleanser

J. Follow Up: None indicated if patient is responding to treatment

CANDIDIASIS

I. Definition: Skin and mucous membrane infections caused by the yeast-like fungus, *Candida albicans*

II. Pathogenesis: *C. albicans* is part of the normal flora of skin and mucous membranes; invasion of the epidermis occurs when moisture, warmth, and breaks in epidermal barrier allow overgrowth

III. Clinical Presentation

   A. **Oral** cavity: In infants, appears as white plaque on erythematous base (thrush). In immunocompromised patients, acute process is similar to the infection in infants. Tongue is almost always involved; may spread into trachea, esophagus, and angles of mouth, and become a chronic process

   B. **Diaper** area: Beefy red, well-demarcated lesions with elevated margins and satellite lesions; may also present as erosions, pustules, and erythematous papules

   C. **Intertriginous** areas: Occurs most often in obese individuals (inframammary, axillary, neck, and inguinal body folds). Presents as red, moist, glistening plaque or moist red papules and pustules

   D. **Vagina**: Appears as a cheesy discharge with white plaques on erythematous base. External genitalia become red, swollen, with some skin erosions (see GYNECOLOGY section for discussion of vulvovaginal candidiasis)

   E. **Male genitalia**: Occurs mainly in uncircumcised but also occurs in circumcised. Multiple, round red erosions on glans and shaft (candida balanitis); usually painful. Often involves scrotum whereas tinea spares scrotum

   F. **Nails**: A common result of thumb/finger sucking in children; tender erythema and swelling at cuticle area (paronychia)

   G. Pain, discomfort usually symptoms regardless of site. Itching usually occurs with vulvovaginitis

IV. Diagnosis/Evaluation

   A. History
      1. For infants/young children, inquire about location of lesions (remember that with thrush, there is frequently co-existing diaper dermatitis and vice versa). If nail involvement, ask if child sucks involved thumb/finger
      2. In adolescents, inquire about location of lesions, medications used (e.g., inhaled steroids or oral corticosteroids) and underlying chronic conditions (diabetes, HIV+)
      3. If genitalia involved, ask about associated symptoms of discharge, itching, and burning

   B. Physical Examination
      1. Examine skin, mucous membranes, and nails for characteristic lesions
         a. White plaques on erythematous base (oral); red moist plaques with satellite lesions (diaper/intertriginous)
         b. Red erosions on glans, shaft (penis); non-tender erythema of nail margins (nail)
         c. For vulvovaginal candidiasis, see under GYNECOLOGY
      2. Palpate adjacent lymph nodes

   C. Differential Diagnosis is outlined in the box below

Oral:	Diaper:	Intertriginous areas:	Vaginal:	Male genitalia:	Nails:
Geographic tongue	Bacterial infection	Miliaria	See GYNECOLOGY	Bacterial	Bacterial
Aphthous stomatitis	Linea IgA dermatosis	Bacterial	section	Psoriasis	Tinea
Leukoplakia	Irritant contact dermatitis			Tinea	

   D. Diagnostic Tests
      1. None indicated when typical lesions present
      2. Potassium hydroxide (KOH) wet mount that is positive for pseudohyphae and budding spores confirms the diagnosis

V.   Plan/Management

A.   Oral candidiasis: For the majority of patients, topical treatments are effective

---

TREATMENT FOR ORAL CANDIDIASIS

Topical treatment is preferred for limited disease in normal hosts
  ➡ Nystatin (Mycostatin) oral suspension (100,000 U/mL) QID x 10 days
   • Infants: 2 mL (1/2 dose in each side of mouth)
   • Older children: 4-6 mL (1/2 dose in each side of mouth)
   • Medication should be retained in mouth as long as possible before swallowing
  ➡ Alternative for adolescents with thrush or angular cheilitis: 10 mg clotrimazole (Lotrimin) buccal troches, dissolve 1 PO 5x day for 2 weeks
Systemic therapy is necessary for moderate to severe disease that occurs in immunocompromised persons (see HIV/AIDS section for treatment recommendations)

B.   Treatment of diaper candidiasis is outlined below

TREATMENT FOR DIAPER CANDIDIASIS

  ➡ Wash skin with plain water with each diaper change
  ➡ Dry completely; allow to air dry 15 minutes, 4 x day
  ➡ Discontinue all powder, creams; once infection is resolved, may judiciously use zinc oxide (Diaparene), a barrier cream
  ➡ Nystatin cream, applied with each diaper change for 3 days
  ➡ Suggest use of Pampers Rash Guard diapers which deliver petrolatum to diaper area

---

C.   For candidal vaginitis, see GYNECOLOGY section

D.   Candidal balanitis: For limited disease, select one of the topical agents from the table

---

TREATMENT FOR CANDIDAL BALANITIS

  ➡ Nystatin cream, 2-3 x day for 10 days
  ➡ Miconazole (Monistat-Derm) or clotrimazole (Lotrimin) cream 2 x day for 10 days
  ➡ Econazole (Spectazole) cream, BID x 10 days
  ➡ Relief occurs quickly once treatment begins; remind patient to use for 10 days even though discomfort is gone

---

E.   Candidal intertrigo: Select one of the topical agents from the table

---

TREATMENT FOR CANDIDAL INTERTRIGO

  ➡ Miconazole (Monistat Derm) cream applied BID x 10-14 days
  ➡ Econazole (Spectazole) cream; apply QD x 14 days
  ➡ Clotrimazole (Lotrimin) cream, solution, lotion; apply BID x 10 days
  ➡ Oxiconazole (Oxistat) cream; apply QD or BID x 14 days
  ➡ Counsel regarding weight reduction and elimination of conditions leading to maceration of skin
  ➡ If there is maceration, use wet Burrow's compress 3-4 x day for 15-20 minutes to promote drying
  ➡ Advise patient to expose areas to light and air several times a day to promote drying
  ➡ Once infection has resolved, recommend use of absorbent powder such as Zeasorb which acts as a dry lubricant in intertriginous areas

---

F.   Candida paronychia (chronic): The following treatment is recommended

```
┌──────────────────────────────────────────────────────────────┐
│            TREATMENT FOR CANDIDAL PARONYCHIA                  │
├──────────────────────────────────────────────────────────────┤
│  ➡ 3% thymol in 95% ethanol (must be compounded by           │
│     pharmacist) TID                                          │
│  ➡ In addition, select one of the following to be used       │
│     BID 2-4 weeks                                            │
│     •  Clotrimazole  (Lotrimin) solution                     │
│     •  Ciclopirox  (Loprox)  lotion (children ≥10 years)     │
│     •  Mycostatin (Nystatin) cream                           │
│  ➡ Advise patient to avoid excess exposure to water          │
│  ➡ For refractory cases, refer to specialist                 │
└──────────────────────────────────────────────────────────────┘
```

G.   Treat predisposing factors. Rule out HIV+ and diabetes mellitus in patients with recurring infection

H.   Follow up is not indicated; patient should return if no improvement after 2 weeks and cause for the treatment failure should be determined

DERMATOPHYTE INFECTIONS

I.   Definition: Infections by a group of fungi that have the ability to infect and survive only on keratin

II.   Pathogenesis

A.   Causative organisms belong to 3 genera: *Microsporum, Trichophyton*, and *Epidermophyton*

B.   Predisposing factors include debilitating diseases, poor nutrition, poor hygiene, tropical climates, and contact with infected persons or animals

III. Clinical Presentation

A.   **Tinea capitis**, fungal infection of the scalp
1.   *Trichophyton tonsurans* infection accounts for 95% of all tinea capitis in US
2.   Occurs mainly in prepubertal children (ages 2-10)
3.   Erythema and scaling of the scalp with patchy hair loss are characteristic
4.   Usually asymptomatic unless kerion, a tender, boggy, lesion representing a hypersensitivity reaction to the fungal infection is present

B.   **Tinea corporis**, fungal infection of the body and face (excluding beard area in men)
1.   Occurs in all age groups; more common in warm climates
2.   Lesion is generally circular, erythematous, well demarcated with a raised, scaly, vesicular border
3.   The central area becomes hypopigmented, and less scaly as the active border progresses outward
4.   Pruritus is common

C.   **Tinea cruris**, fungal infection of the groin and upper thighs
1.   Frequent in males, usually obese ones; rare in females
2.   Eruption is sharply demarcated, scaling patches; usually extremely pruritic
3.   Involvement of the scrotum is uncommon (unlike candidal infections in which scrotal involvement is common)

D.   **Tinea pedis**, fungal infection of the foot
1.   Common infection in adolescents (uncommon in prepubertal children)
2.   Lesions are fine, vesiculopustular or scaly and usually itch
3.   Any area of the foot may be involved, but likely to occur on the instep or between the toes

E.   **Tinea unguium**, fungal infection of the nails (onychomycosis)
1.   Occurs in adolescents; rare in young children
2.   May occur simultaneously with hand or foot tinea or present independently
3.   Usually involves only 1 or 2 nails; toenails more often than fingernails
4.   Distal thickening and yellowing of the nail plate are characteristic features

IV. Diagnosis/Evaluation

    A.   History
        1.   Question regarding onset, duration, distribution, appearance of lesions, and presence of symptoms
        2.   Question regarding contact with others (or infected dogs, cats) with similar lesions, symptoms
        3.   Ask about predisposing conditions—sweaty feet, occlusive footwear
        4.   Inquire about treatments used and outcomes

    B.   Physical Examination
        1.   Examine skin to determine type, distribution of lesions
        2.   Use of Wood's light may aid in exam as some species cause tinea to fluoresce (pale or brilliant green). The most common fungus infecting the scalp, *T. tonsurans* **does not** fluoresce. Lint, scales, serum exudate, and hair preparations containing petrolatum fluoresce a bluish or purplish color which may be confusing

    C.   Differential Diagnosis
        1.   Seborrheic dermatitis
        2.   Psoriasis
        3.   Alopecia areata
        4.   Atopic dermatitis
        5.   Contact dermatitis

    D.   Diagnostic Tests

DIAGNOSTIC TESTS FOR DERMATOPHYTE INFECTIONS

Microscopic examination for fungus
- ➡ Scrape the border of lesion with a sterile scalpel blade (No. 15) moistened with tap water to contain scales; can also "pluck" 2 or 3 hairs using a hemostat. Transfer specimen to slide with a small droplet of plain water
- ➡ Add 1 or 2 drops of KOH solution, put on coverslip and warm the slide carefully for 15-30 seconds with a flame
- ➡ Examine the specimen under low power with minimal illumination
- ➡ Identify hyphae—thin, often branching strands of uniform diameter; switch to high dry (43X) objective to confirm finding
- ➡ While a positive exam establishes the diagnosis, a negative test does not rule out the disease

Dermatophyte test medium (DTM) for diagnosis of tinea capitis
- ➡ Using a hemostat, remove 5-10 hairs from a scaling area or rub a moistened 2 x 2 gauze (or previously sterilized toothbrush) [a painless technique for the patient] vigorously over an area of scaling and alopecia
- ➡ Inoculate the plucked hair/scrapings from the gauze directly onto the culture medium, breaking the agar surface, and incubate at room temperature (with cap on loosely)
- ➡ After 1-2 weeks, phenol red indicator in agar will turn from yellow to red in area surrounding dermatophyte colony

---

V. Plan/Management

    A.   Treatment for tinea capitis is contained in the table below

---

TREATMENT FOR TINEA CAPITIS

Tinea capitis requires systemic antifungal therapy

Griseofulvin microsize (Grifulvin V), supplied as 250, 500 mg tabs; 125 mg/5 mL suspension
- ➡ Dosing: 30-50 lbs, give 125-250 mg daily. >50 lbs, give 250-500 mg daily x 6-8 weeks. Give as a single daily dose
- ➡ Take with high fat food such as whole milk, peanut butter, or ice cream to enhance absorption
- ➡ Treat for up to 12 weeks
- ➡ Continue medication for 2 weeks after clinical resolution

Selenium sulfide, 2.5% shampoo used 2 x week for 2 weeks may reduce fungal shedding
- ➡ If kerion present, a short course of oral steroid therapy to reduce inflammation and prevent scarring of scalp may be needed
- ➡ Prednisone, 1-2 mg/kg/day (adolescents >16 years 25-50 mg/day) for 10-14 days is recommended
- ➡ **Taper dose over last half of therapy**
- ➡ Children receiving treatment may attend school
- ➡ Cutting hair, shaving head, or wearing cap unnecessary
- ➡ Advise parent/child that hair regrowth is slow

Laboratory monitoring for 12 week course of this medication is not necessary
Repeat fungal culture after treatment ends to document clearance

---

B.   Selected topical treatments for tinea corporis, pedis, and cruris are contained in the table below; all of these products are by prescription only

SELECTED TOPICAL TREATMENTS FOR TINEA CORPORIS, PEDIS, AND CRURIS

Topical Antifungal Agents	Supplied As	Dosing	Duration of Treatment	Use in Children
Miconazole (Monistat-Derm)	Cream, 15 g, 1 oz, 3 oz	BID	Tinea corporis, cruris - 2 wks Tinea pedis - 4 wks	Yes
Terbinafine (Lamisil) Solution	Solution, 30 mL Pump-spray	QD for tinea corporis, cruris; BID for tinea pedis	1 week	<18 - not recommended
Econazole (Spectazole)	Cream, 15, 30 g	QD	Tinea corporis, cruris - 2 wks Tinea pedis - 4 wks	Yes
Ciclopirox (Loprox)	Cream, 15, 30, 90 g Lotion, 30, 60 mL	BID	Up to 4 weeks	<10 - not recommended
Ketoconazole (Nizoral)	Cream, 15, 30, 60 g	QD	Tinea corporis, cruris - 2 wks Tinea pedis - 6 wks	<18 - not recommended
Oxiconazole (Oxistat)	Cream, 15, 30 g Lotion, 30 mL	QD or BID	Tinea corporis, cruris - 2 wks Tinea pedis - 4 wks	Yes
Sulconazole (Exelderm)	Cream, 15, 30, 60 g Solution, 30 mL	BID for tinea pedis (use cream only) QD or BID for tinea corporis, cruris	Tinea pedis - 4 wks Tinea corporis, cruris - 3 wks	<18 - not recommended
Butenafine 1% (Mentax)	Cream, 15, 30 g	BID or QD for tinea pedis QD for corporis, cruris	Tinea pedis - 1 wk (BID) **OR** 4 wks (QD) Tinea pedis, cruris - 2 wks	<18 - not recommended

C.   General measures: Advise patient as follows:
1.   **T. pedis**: If moist lesions, soak affected foot/feet in Burrow's solution BID until skin has dried. Expose feet to air as much as possible by going barefoot—wearing sandals is next best. Wear synthetic socks which wick away moisture; change socks during the day in hot weather. Air out shoes between use and do not wear the same pair day in, day out. Use strand of lamb's wool (Dr. Scholl's Lamb's Wool) between toes, if there is interdigital/toe web involvement. May apply powder such as Zeasorb to dry feet after infection has resolved. Avoid the use of powders containing cornstarch that may actually promote fungal growth
2.   **T. cruris and corporis**: If moist lesions, apply wet compresses using Burrow's solution BID until skin has dried; apply Zeasorb powder after infection has resolved

D.   For resistant infections, refer to expert for management

E.   Treatment for onychomycosis in adolescents ≥18 years is outlined in the table below; select **one** of the following (see F.3. below for monitoring requirements)

ORAL AND TOPICAL AGENTS FOR TREATMENT FOR ONYCHOMYCOSIS IN ADOLESCENTS ≥18 YEARS OF AGE

Medication	Fingernail	Toenail
Oral		
Terbinafine	250 mg/d for 6 weeks	250 mg/d for 12 weeks
Itraconazole (continuous)	200 mg/d for 6 weeks	200 mg/d for 12 weeks
Itraconazole (pulse)	200 mg twice daily for 1 week on and 3 weeks off, repeated for 2 pulses	200 mg twice daily for 1 week on and 3 weeks off, repeated for 3 pulses*
Topical		
Ciclopirox nail lacquer 8%	Daily application for up to 48 weeks	Daily application for up to 48 weeks

* Not FDA approved for this indication

F.   Follow Up
1.   For mild cases of T. corporis, cruris, no follow up is required unless there is a treatment failure
2.   For T. capitis, a visit in 2-4 weeks to evaluate the effectiveness of the griseofulvin therapy; repeat KOH examination, and culture to determine need for increasing length of therapy; if lesions are KOH and culture negative, a total of 6 weeks of therapy may be all that is required
3.   For onychomycosis, need to monitor CBC, ALT, and AST levels before initiating oral treatment, at 4 weeks into treatment, and then monthly for duration of treatment

TINEA VERSICOLOR

I.   Definition: Common non-inflammatory fungal infection of the skin caused by lipophilic yeast

II.   Pathogenesis

    A.   Fungal infection of skin caused by *Pityrosporum orbiculare*

    B.   *P. orbiculare* is part of normal flora; overgrowth occurs for unknown reasons

III.   Clinical Presentation

    A.   Occurs at any age, but most likely to occur in adolescence and young adulthood

    B.   Presents as multiple small, circular macules of various colors—white, pink, or brown—(color is uniform in each patient)—thus the name "versicolor"; fine scale is present on surface of macules which can be appreciated by scraping lightly with a #15 surgical blade

    C.   Infection is limited to the outermost layers of the skin

    D.   Upper trunk most commonly affected, rarely located on face (except in young children); may itch, but usually asymptomatic; may be contagious

    E.   Proliferation exacerbated by heat, humidity, pregnancy, corticosteroid therapy, oral contraceptives, and immunosuppression

    F.   Infection is most evident in summer because the organism produces azelaic acid, a substance that inhibits pigment transfer to keratinocytes

IV.   Diagnosis/Evaluation

    A.   History
        1.   Ask about location, onset, duration, and appearance of lesions
        2.   Inquire if associated symptoms present
        3.   Ask if any medications, including oral contraceptives are being taken
        4.   Determine if patient is immunocompromised

    B.   Physical Examination
        1.   Examine skin for characteristic lesions
        2.   Use Wood's light to look at skin. While not useful as a diagnostic aid (because fluorescence is not predictably present) can demonstrate extent of the infection better than ordinary light

    C.   Differential Diagnosis
        1.   Vitiligo
        2.   Tinea corporis
        3.   Seborrheic dermatitis
        4.   Pityriasis alba

    D.   Diagnostic Tests
        1.   Microscopy of KOH-cleared scrapings
        2.   Short, curved hyphae and clusters of round yeast cells ("spaghetti and meatballs") pattern are diagnostic

V.   Plan/Management

    A.   For limited disease, **topical** therapies are usually effective. Select **one** from the following table

---

TREATMENT FOR TINEA VERSICOLOR USING TOPICAL THERAPIES

Selenium sulfide 2.5% lotion (Selsun), supplied as 4 oz
➡ Apply daily x 7 consecutive days; rinse off after 10 minutes
➡ Advise patient to apply Selsun from neck down
➡ Allow skin to repigment for one month; if not cleared in one month, have patient repeat above treatment
➡ Repeat the treatment monthly until satisfactory result obtained; treatment is cheap and usually effective

Ketoconazole (Nizoral A-D) 1% [OTC] shampoo (children ≥12 years)
➡ Apply to damp skin in affected area with wide margins
➡ Lather, and leave in place for 5 minutes before rinsing
➡ May be used as a single application or used daily for 3 days

---

B. Use **oral therapies** for extensive or recalcitrant infection (poor response to topical therapy) in adolescents ≥18 years of age

1. Ketoconazole (Nizoral) 400 mg PO x 1 dose (adolescents ≥18 years of age only). Small risk of liver toxicity with this drug **OR**
2. Fluconazole (Diflucan) 300 mg PO as an initial dose; repeat this dose (300 mg) after 2 weeks (adolescents ≥18 years of age only)
3. Sweating may improve transfer of these drugs to skin surface
4. Advise patient not to bathe for 12 hours after treatment with oral medication to allow accumulation of drug on skin
5. Not FDA approved for this indication (off-label use

C. Tell patients that clearing may be temporary; since infection is caused by an inhabitant of normal skin, it often recurs

D. Recommend prophylactic monthly use of selenium sulfide lotion (especially during summer) to prevent recurrences

E. Advise that treatment does not repigment the skin; once the infection is cleared up, the skin will normally repigment itself, but it will take 2 months or longer

F. Follow Up: In one month to evaluate therapy

SCABIES

I. Definition: Skin infestation of the mite, *Sarcoptes scabiei*

II. Pathogenesis

A. A fertilized female mite excavates a burrow in the stratum corneum and deposits eggs and fecal pellets

B. The larvae hatch and reach maturity in about 14 days, mate, and repeat the cycle

C. Humans are the source of infestation with transmission occurring most often by prolonged, close personal contact (a mild self-limited infestation can be acquired from dogs)

D. A hypersensitivity reaction rather than a foreign-body response is responsible for the intense pruritus

E. Incubation period in persons without previous exposure is 4-6 weeks

III.   Clinical Presentation

A.   Occurs mainly in children and adolescents; also among institutionalized persons of all ages

B.   Primary lesions are serpiginous burrows, vesicles, and papules
1.   Burrows appear as gray or skin-colored ridges up to a few centimeters in length; scratching destroys burrows, so they may be difficult to find
2.   Vesicles are isolated, pinpoint, and filled with serous fluid; may contain mites
3.   Papules are small, isolated, represent a hypersensitivity reaction, and rarely contain mites

C.   Secondary lesions with erythema and scaling caused by scratching are present in more chronic cases

D.   In infants <2 years of age, lesions are often vesicular and are likely to occur on the head, neck, palms, and soles, areas that are largely spared in older children; this is caused by a hypersensitivity reaction to the proteins of the parasite

E.   In older children and adolescents, common sites are hands (90%), especially fingerwebs, flexor aspects of the wrists, belt line, thighs, navel, intergluteal cleft, penis, areola, and axillae

F.   Main symptom is intense itching which is usually worse at night and the diagnosis should be considered with widespread pruritus presenting primarily with skin excoriation

G.   Although uncommon, a generalized urticarial rash may occur in debilitated, immunodeficient, or malnourished persons; called Norwegian scabies, this condition is the result of penetration of the underlying epidermis by hundreds of mites and results in widespread, crusted, hyperkeratotic lesions

IV.   Diagnosis/Evaluation

A.   History
1.   Question regarding onset, duration, morphology, and location of lesions
2.   Ask if itching is present, and if it is worse at night
3.   Ask about exposures to friends or family members with similar symptoms
4.   Inquire what treatments have been tried and their effectiveness

B.   Physical Examination
1.   Examine the skin for typical burrows
2.   Pay particular attention to the hands, especially the fingerwebs and wrists (flexor aspect), axillary folds, belt line, navel, penis, areas surrounding the areolae
3.   A magnifying glass and good lighting are essential

C.   Differential Diagnosis
1.   Atopic dermatitis
2.   Allergic and irritant contact dermatitis
3.   Papular urticaria
4.   Pediculosis

D.   Diagnostic Tests
1.   Microscopic identification of mite, ova, or feces proves the diagnosis. Two ways to do this:
a.   Locate tiny black dot at end of burrow; insert a 25 gauge hypodermic needle at dot. Mite, ova, or feces (dot) will stick to it and can be transferred to immersion oil on slide; cover with slip and examine under low power
b.   Slice off whole burrow with sterile scalpel blade (# 15) held parallel to skin; put slice on slide, add immersion oil, cover with slip, and examine under low power
2.   If no burrows are found, no diagnostic test indicated

V.   Plan/Management

A.   Use a scabicide from the following table

TREATMENT OF SCABIES

Recommended regimen is 5% permethrin (Elimite) cream
- ➡ Children: Apply cream over the entire body from the neck down
- ➡ Infants >2 months and toddlers: Apply cream over the head, neck, and body (avoid the eyes)
- ➡ Remove by bathing in 8-14 hours
- ➡ Of drugs available to treat scabies, this drug is safest for use in infants, young children, and pregnant and lactating women

Alternative regimens:
- ➡ Lindane (Kwell, Scabine) lotion (1 oz) or cream (30 g)
  - • Apply as for permethrin cream above except remove in 8 hours
  - • *Caution: Lindane should not be used in infants, toddlers, and pregnant and lactating women;* should not be used immediately after a bath or shower, and should not be used by persons who have extensive dermatitis

- ➡ Ivermectin 200 µg/kg orally, repeated in 2 weeks
  - • Not recommended for pregnant and lactating women
  - • Safety of ivermectin in children who weigh <15 kg has not been determined

Adapted from Centers for Disease Control and Prevention. (2002). Sexually transmitted diseases treatment guidelines. *MMWR, 51* (RR-6), 68-69.

B. Appropriate treatment of crusted scabies (Norwegian scabies) remains unclear; substantial treatment failure might occur with single topical scabicide or oral ivermectin treatment
   1. Some experts recommend combined treatment with a topical scabicide and oral ivermectin or repeated treatments with ivermectin
   2. Lindane should be avoided because of risks of neurotoxicity with heavy applications and denuded skin
   3. Consult infectious disease specialist for treatment of patients with this variant of scabies

C. To control itching which can be intense, prescribe hydroxyzine (Atarax) which also provides sedation at night [the time of day when itching is most intense] and recommend topical agents to control pruritus
   1. Hydroxyzine (Atarax): Available as syrup, 10 mg/5 mL and tabs, 10, 25, 50, 100 mg
      a. Infants and children: 0.5 mg/kg/dose at bedtime for 5-7days
      b. Adolescents: 25-50 mg at bedtime for 5-7 days
      c. For both children and adolescents, TID use is safe, but patient should be warned about sedation and impaired psychomotor performance which could interfere with normal activities
      d. A better choice for daytime use is fexofenadine (Allegra): Children 12 and older, 60 mg BID; children 6-11 years, 30 mg BID; not recommended for children <6 years of age
   2. Sarna lotion, Prax lotion and Itch-X are available without prescription; instruct patient to use as directed on label
   3. Advise patient that pruritus may continue for up to 2 weeks after treatment because of the hypersensitivity reaction created by the mite

D. If secondary bacterial infection of lesions is present, prescribe topical or oral antibiotics (see section on IMPETIGO AND ECTHYMA for treatment recommendations)

VI. Control Measures

A. Prophylactic therapy recommended for household members; therefore all household members should be treated simultaneously to prevent reinfection
   1. Launder all clothing and bedding in hot water and hot drying cycle
   2. Clothing that cannot be laundered should be placed in plastic storage bags for at least a week; parasites cannot survive off the skin for longer than 3-4 days
   3. Children in daycare or school can return the day after treatment completed

B. Follow up
   1. Some experts recommend re-treatment after 1-2 weeks for patients who remain symptomatic
   2. Others recommend re-treatment only if live mites are observed
   3. Patients who do not respond to the recommended treatment should be re-treated with an alternative regimen

PEDICULOSIS

I. Definition: Infestation with one of the three species of lice that infest humans

    A. *Pediculus humanus* var. *capitis* (head louse)

    B. *Pediculus humanus* var. *corporis* (body louse)

    C. *Pthirus pubis* (pubic or crab louse)

II. Pathogenesis

    A. Transmission of head lice occurs by direct contact with infested persons or through hats, brushes, and combs; head lice cannot jump or fly and pets are not vectors

    B. Fomites play a major role in transmission of body lice, but almost no role in transmission of pubic lice, which are transmitted through sexual contact

    C. Ova hatch in a week; lice feed on human blood

    D. Incubation period from laying of eggs to hatching of first nymph is 6-10 days; mature lice (capable of reproducing) do not appear until 2-3 weeks later

III. Clinical Presentation

CLINICAL PRESENTATION OF LICE

Pediculosis capitis (head lice)
➡ Most common in girls between the ages of 5 and 11; all socioeconomic groups affected; rare in blacks
➡ Eggs are initially translucent and attached to a hair shaft close to scalp
➡ After hatching, the 1mm long empty egg cases (nits) become white and more visible; nits remain firmly attached to hair shaft, moving away from scalp as hair grows
➡ Distance of nits from scalp is measure of age (1 cm = 1 month)
➡ Additional information can be found at www.headlice.org

Most infestations involve fewer than 10 lice (mostly small nymphs 1-2 mm long); adults are about the size of a sesame seed (3-4 mm long)
➡ Lice most commonly seen in hair on back of the head near nape of neck
➡ Head lice can survive only 1-2 days away from the scalp
➡ Excoriation from scratching, secondary bacterial infections, and cervical adenopathy are common

Pediculosis corporis (body lice)
➡ Generally found on persons with poor hygiene; lice cannot survive away from blood source for longer than 10 days
➡ Body lice are vectors of disease including typhus, trench fever, and relapsing fever
➡ Excoriation and secondary bacterial infection are common
➡ Body lice and nits may be found in seams of clothing

Pediculosis pubis (pubic lice)
➡ Highly contagious; chance of acquiring from one exposure is about 90%
➡ Common in adolescents and young adults; African-Americans and other racial groups are affected with same frequency
➡ Pubic hair is most common site of infestation, but can also infest hair on chest, abdomen, and thighs
➡ Infested adults may spread pubic lice to eyelashes of children
➡ Eyelash infestation is seen almost exclusively in children
    • Acquired from other children or adult infested with pubic lice
    • May be a sign of sexual abuse in children
➡ Frequently coexists with other sexually transmitted diseases

---

IV. Diagnosis/Evaluation

    A. History
        1. Determine if nits or lice have been visualized and when they were first noticed
        2. Ask if itching present, especially nocturnal; determine if itching is generalized or localized

3. Question if nits, lice present in close contacts
4. If lice in eyelashes of child, explore with parent/caregiver how this might have occurred

B. Physical Examination
1. For head lice, the following approach is recommended

STEPS IN EXAMINING HAIR AND SCALP FOR LICE AND NITS

→ First, comb or brush hair to remove tangles
→ Using a fine-toothed "nit" comb (teeth of comb should be 0.2 to 0.3 mm apart to trap lice) insert the comb near the crown touching the scalp
→ Draw comb firmly down the length of the hair
→ Repeat the process with small sections of the hair until the entire head of hair has been systematically combed at least twice
→ After each stroke, examine the comb for lice
→ Usually takes approximately one minute to find the first louse
→ Combing wet hair is probably more sensitive than combing dry hair but is impractical for routine clinical use

---

Adapted from Roberts, F.J. (2002). Head lice. *New England Journal of Medicine, 346,* 1645-1650.

2. Check eyelashes closely
3. Examine skin of infested site for excoriation secondary to scratching
4. If body lice suspected, examine seams of clothing for lice

C. Differential Diagnosis: Scabies, neurotic excoriation

D. Diagnostic Tests
1. Identification of eggs, nymphs, and lice with naked eye or magnifying glass
2. Microscopic exam usually unnecessary

V. Plan/Management

A. The following products are recommended for the treatment of head lice; **select one**

TREATMENT OF HEAD LICE

Permethrin 1% cream rinse (Nix) OTC
→ Apply cream rinse to shampooed, rinsed, and towel dried hair (and scalp)
→ Leave on for 10 minute; rinse
→ A single treatment is usually adequate, but some experts recommend retreatment 7-10 days after the initial treatment

Malathion 0.5% lotion (Ovide) Rx
→ Apply to dry hair until scalp and hair are wet and thoroughly coated (bedtime application is most convenient)
→ Allow hair to dry naturally and after 8-12 hours, shampoo hair thoroughly
→ Repeat application is not routinely recommended; a second treatment may be given in 7 days if crawling lice are still found after treatment

Pyrethrins 0.33% shampoo or mousse (RID) OTC
→ Apply to area until thoroughly wet, massage in, wait 10 minutes, add water to form lather, shampoo, and rinse thoroughly

---

B. To remove nits for aesthetic reasons (not necessary to prevent spread)
1. Soak hair with white vinegar; then wrap damp towel soaked in the vinegar around head for 30-60 minutes
2. Use fine-tooth comb to mechanically remove nits
3. There are numerous nit removal aids available; product examples include Clear Lice Egg Remover, Pronto Crème, and Rid Lice Egg Loosener Gel
4. With heavy involvement, a haircut may be preferable to tedious nit removal (child should not be forced to have hair cut, however, if he/she would find it humiliating)

C. Children can return to daycare/school the next day after their first treatment for head lice; provide a note for school (exclusion of children from school based on the presence of nits is not recommended by the American Public Health Association)

D. Combs and brushes should be soaked in hot water with pediculicide shampoo for 15 minutes

E.   Treatment of pubic and body lice is described below

RECOMMENDED REGIMENS FOR TREATMENT OF PUBIC LICE AND BODY LICE

Pubic Lice:
Permethrin 1% creme rinse (Nix) [OTC] applied to affected areas and washed off after 10 minutes
OR
Lindane 1% shampoo (Kwell) [Rx] applied to the affected areas and then thoroughly washed off after 4 minutes; this regimen is not recommended for pregnant or lactating women
OR
Pyrethrins 0.33% shampoo, get (A-200, RID) [OTC] applied to the affected area and washed off after 10 minutes

Other management considerations: The recommended regimens should not be applied to the eyes. Sex partners within the last month should be treated. Patients who do not respond to one of the recommended regimens should be re-treated with an alternate regimen. Patients should be evaluated for other sexually transmitted diseases

For infestation of eyelashes or eyebrows, apply occlusive ophthalmic ointment (such as Lacri-Lube (OTC) which contains petrolatum and mineral oil) to the eyelid margins twice a day for 10 days

Body Lice
For the treatment of body lice, pediculocides are not necessary
✓   Treatment consists of improving hygiene and laundering clothing
✓   Infested clothing should be washed and dried at very hot temperatures to kill lice

---

F.   Children with infestation of eyelashes or eyebrows should be treated as in table above. Possibility of sexual abuse should be explored with the parent as pubic lice (which cause eyelash infection in most cases) are usually transmitted by sexual contact

G.   Household and other close contacts should be examined and treated if they have head or body lice; bed mates should be treated prophylactically (**Note:** Head lice do not live on pets; thus pets should not be treated!)

H.   Clothing, bedding should be laundered in hot soapy water and dried on hot cycle or dry cleaned; combs, brushes should be washed in hot (130 degree) soapy water; floor and furniture should be vacuumed

I.   Use of insecticides to disinfect furnishings is not recommended

J.   Provide patients with good written information such as the CDC Division of Parasitic Diseases fact sheet available at http://www.cdc.gov/ncidod/dpd/parasites/lice/

K.   Follow Up: Unnecessary unless treatment failure

CUTANEOUS LARVAE MIGRANS

I.   Definition: A skin disease caused by infected larvae of cat and dog hookworms with *Ancylostoma braziliense* and *Ancylostoma caninum* the usual causes; often referred to as creeping eruption

II.   Pathogenesis

A.   Ova of *A. braziliense* or *A. caninum* are deposited in cat or dog feces

B.   Larvae in soil or sand penetrate human skin that contacts soil

III.   Clinical Presentation

A.   A disease of persons likely to come into contact with sandy soil contaminated with cat/dog feces (e.g., children, gardeners, sunbathers, outdoor workers)

B.   Disease is most prevalent in the southeastern part of the US

C.   Classically presents as pruritic, erythematous, thread-like (or serpiginous) lesions that advance about one cm/day

D. Lesions are usually located on feet, hands, buttocks, or upper thighs; excoriation may obscure the otherwise typical serpiginous lesion

IV. Diagnosis/Evaluation

A. History
1. Inquire about location, onset, duration, and if pruritus is present
2. Ask if sitting or playing in soil/sand has occurred recently

B. Physical Examination: Examine skin for typical serpiginous, thread-like lesions; look for signs of scratching

C. Differential Diagnosis
1. Tinea
2. Urticaria
3. Erythema chronicum migrans
4. Scabies

D. Diagnostic Tests: None indicated

V. Plan/Management

A. Drugs recommended for treatment of hookworm infection for both children and adults (nonpregnant adults only) are the following: (**Note:** All three of the drugs listed are approved drugs, but considered investigational for this indication by the FDA)
1. Albendazole, 400 mg PO daily x 3 days for both children and adolescents **OR**
2. Ivermectin, 200 mcg/kg PO daily x 1-2 days for both children and adolescents **OR**
3. Thiabendazole suspension, apply topically to affected areas x 5-7 days

B. If itching is bothersome, prescribe hydroxyzine (Atarax) and/or recommend OTC topical products
1. Hydroxyzine: Children: 0.5mg/kg/dose (supplied as 10 mg/5 mL syrup); sedating so best used at bedtime
2. Hydroxyzine: Children >12: 25-50 mg/dose (supplied as 10, 25, 50 mg tabs)
3. Sarna lotion, Prax lotion, and Itch-X gel are all OTC

C. Patient Education: Should be advised not to sit, lie, or walk barefoot on wet soil or sand in areas where cats or dogs are likely to deposit feces

D. Follow Up: None indicated

PSORIASIS

I. Definition: A chronic, relapsing hyperproliferative inflammatory disorder of the skin of unknown cause

II. Pathogenesis

A. A complex cascade of events within the skin begins with antigen presentation and T-cell activation that result in the release of cytokines and chemoattractants; these local chemical mediators create a hyperproliferative state in the epidermis and increased vascularity in the dermis

B. In addition to the obvious genetic component, numerous initiating factors are postulated as causing the T-cell deficit including local trauma, infection, stress, and use of certain medications including β-blockers, lithium, and antimalarials

C. The classic pathologic features of psoriasis seen on skin biopsy denote inflammation associated with features of epidermal proliferation

III. Clinical Presentation

    A.   Fewer than 10% of patients with psoriasis have onset during childhood; nonetheless, the disorder has an annual prevalence of 3.1 per 1000 US children, making it one of the most common papulosquamous eruptions in childhood

        1.   The eruption consists of erythematous macular or papular lesions that develop a thick, silvery scale

        2.   Discrete scaly papules, called guttate lesions, may be evident, or several papules may coalesce to form raised, sharply demarcated, erythematous plaques

    B.   The most common clinical picture of psoriasis in childhood is involvement of the elbows, knees, and scalp, but the ears, eyebrows, gluteal fold, genitalia, and nails are also often affected

        1.   Approximately 44% of children with psoriasis have genital involvement (i.e., perineal area, penis, and gluteal cleft)

        2.   Involvement of the palms and soles is uncommon in children, but can occur

    C.   Guttate psoriasis, the form of psoriasis with multiple discrete papules, is more common in children than adults

        1.   Often begins on the trunk as multiple erythematous macules that mimic a viral exanthem—the macules progress to papules that develop a silvery scale

        2.   In addition to the trunk, the lesions are also commonly found on the upper extremities

        3.   Eruption often follows a sore throat, particularly streptococcal pharyngitis by 2-3 weeks

    D.   Koebner phenomenon, in which psoriatic lesions develop in sites of skin trauma (e.g., lacerations, abrasions, sunburn, insect bites) several days after the event, is a helpful diagnostic feature of psoriasis

    E.   The majority of children with psoriasis have scalp involvement—an accumulation of thick scales throughout the scalp, particularly along the frontal hairline and behind the ears; hair loss is not common

    F.   Nail signs in psoriasis include multiple tiny pits on the surface of the nails (pitting), yellowing of the distal nail, separation of the nail plate from the bed, and thickening of the distal nail

        1.   Nail changes occur in about 15% of children with psoriasis, but it is unusual for nail changes to be the presenting complaint

        2.   If there is nail involvement, all 20 nails are often involved

    G.   Itching is not a common complaint, but it sometimes occurs; appearance of the lesions may be altered by scratching or picking at the lesions

IV. Diagnosis/Evaluation

    A.   History

        1.   Inquire about location and appearance of lesions, onset, and duration; specifically ask about involvement of the elbows, knees, and scalp

        2.   Ask if nail pitting or other nail changes have occurred

        3.   Ask about past history of chronic dandruff, scaling of external ear and canal

        4.   Ask about recent streptococcal infection (pharyngitis)

        5.   Ask about treatments tried and results

        6.   Review past medical history

        7.   Assess the impact of the disease on the patient's quality of life

        8.   Ask about family history of psoriasis in first-degree relatives

    B.   Physical Examination

        1.   Complete examination of the entire cutaneous surface is necessary because lesions may be few in number

        2.   Look for characteristic lesions, particularly on elbows, knees, and scalp, the areas most often affected; observe for silvery scale on at least some of the lesions

        3.   Observe trunk for guttate lesions, drop-like papules that develop a silvery scale over time

        4.   Examine nails for pitting and other characteristic changes

    C.   Differential Diagnosis

        1.   Lichen planus (this disorder does involve the knees and elbows, but lacks the silvery scale feature and red color of psoriatic plaques)

        2.   Seborrheic dermatitis (this disorder is characterized by greasy scale—scaling of scalp in psoriasis is nongreasy)

3. Onychomycosis (this disorder is rare in children, and if it occurs, usually only involves 1-2 nails; pitting does not occur)
4. Candidiasis (this disorder can be differentiated from psoriasis by potassium hydroxide (KOH) examination and fungal culture

D. Diagnostic Tests
1. When diagnosis is uncertain, a biopsy should be performed
2. If guttate psoriasis is suspected (scaly papules on trunk), obtain throat swab for culture and antistreptolysin-O antibody titers

V. Plan/Management

A. Education of the patient and the family is the first step in management
1. Emphasize that psoriasis is a chronic condition that can certainly be controlled, but not cured
2. Reassure patient that the disorder is not contagious (patients are often treated as though it were by others, even family members and friends)
3. Most patients believe that psoriasis adversely affects their lives; provide patient with opportunities to discuss feelings in this area
4. Counsel patient regarding elements of a healthy lifestyle, including well-balanced diet, good skin care, frequent exercise, and avoidance of all tobacco products
5. Discuss the role of stress (from acute illnesses such as respiratory tract infections and from psychosocial sources such as family difficulties, school related problems)
6. Shaving (face in adolescent males, armpits and legs in adolescent girls) should be done very cautiously to avoid trauma to the skin; moisturizers should be applied afterwards
7. Provide patient with information about the National Psoriasis Foundation (NPF), a nonprofit organization that can be a major resource for patient education

| **National Psoriasis Foundation** |
| 6600 SW 92nd Avenue, Suite 300 |
| Portland, Oregon 97223-7195 |
| 800-723-9166 |
| http://www.psoriasis.org |

B. Good skin care, with an emphasis on keeping the skin well-hydrated, is one of the cornerstones in the treatment of psoriasis and can have a sustainable impact on the patient's well-being
1. Dry skin, the most common cause of itching, can cause much discomfort
2. Daily lubrication and moisturization of the skin is of paramount importance
3. See recommendations regarding care of dry skin in section CARE OF DRY AND OILY SKIN

C. Treatment for psoriasis is divided into three major categories: topical therapy, phototherapy, and systemic therapy

D. Children with psoriasis are best managed by a pediatric dermatologist; if this is not possible, management should be in consultation with a pediatric dermatologist; most of the recommended treatments are not FDA-approved for use in children

E. Follow Up: The pediatric dermatologist managing the patient should determine the follow-up schedule

PITYRIASIS ROSEA

I. Definition: A common, benign, often asymptomatic, self-limiting skin eruption of unknown etiology

II. Pathogenesis: Unknown, but some evidence suggests it is viral in origin

III. Clinical Presentation

A. Most commonly seen in children, adolescents and young adults (75% of cases are in persons 10-35 years of age)

B. May be preceded by a prodrome of pharyngitis, lymphadenopathy, headache, and malaise, but in most cases, no history of these symptoms is given

C. In its typical form, a 2-10 cm scaly, round-to-oval plaque (the herald patch) appears on the trunk
    1. Precedes the appearance of the generalized eruption by 7-14 days
    2. Herald patch, unlike the subsequent lesions, usually has central clearing

D. The herald patch is followed by a generalized eruption consisting of multiple, pink (in Caucasians) to dark brown (in African Americans) macules progressing to plaques which enlarge and become oval; a peripheral rim of fine scale is present

E. Long axes of oval lesions tend to run parallel to each other, creating a "Christmas tree" distribution on trunk

F. Lesions usually fade over 4-6 weeks and mild to intense itching is common

IV. Diagnosis/Evaluation

A. History
    1. Question regarding recent occurrence of herald patch and location and presence of other lesions
    2. Question regarding medications currently taking
    3. Question if symptoms such as pruritus are present

B. Physical Examination
    1. Examine skin for characteristic lesions; look specifically for herald patch which is usually on trunk
    2. Determine distribution of lesions, looking to see if long axes of oval-shaped lesions are parallel to each other
    3. Check the mucous surfaces, palms, and soles which are spared by pityriasis rosea

C. Differential Diagnosis
    1. Tinea corporis
    2. Tinea versicolor
    3. Viral exanthems
    4. Drug eruptions
    5. Syphilis

D. Diagnostic Tests: **Always** order VDRL or RPR as syphilis can mimic this disorder

V. Plan/Management

A. No therapy is required, but symptomatic management of pruritus may be indicated (see section on ATOPIC DERMATITIS for prescribing information)

B. Sunlight exposure to the point of minimal erythema will hasten disappearance of lesions and decrease itching; caution against sunburn

C. Follow Up: Usually unnecessary except for follow-up on syphilis serology

PITYRIASIS ALBA

I. Definition: A disorder of pigmentation which may be a form of atopic dermatitis, but it occurs without the features of atopic dermatitis

II. Pathogenesis

A. Cause of hypopigmentation is unknown

B. Likely related to inflammatory mediators that inhibit melanocyte function

III. Clinical Presentation

    A. Occurs primarily in children before puberty; up to 40% of children are affected

    B. Presents as multiple oval, scaly, hypopigmented patches on the face, extensor surfaces of upper arms, and on neck

    C. Lesions range in size from 5-10 mm in diameter with 10-20 lesions commonly seen

    D. Lesions are asymptomatic but are cosmetically bothersome to child and parents

IV. Diagnosis/Evaluation

    A. History
        1. Inquire about location, onset, duration, and any symptoms of lesions
        2. Ask about treatments tried and results

    B. Physical Examination: Examine skin for characteristic lesions

    C. Differential Diagnosis
        1. Tinea versicolor
        2. Vitiligo (dead white appearing; does not scale)

    D. Diagnostic Tests: KOH exam to exclude tinea versicolor

V. Plan/Management

    A. There is no satisfactory treatment for this skin disorder; emphasize the chronic, recurrent nature of this benign disorder; reassure patient/parent that condition gradually improves after puberty

    B. Triamcinolone acetonide, 0.025% (Aristocort A) cream applied BID x 7-10 days may be prescribed so long as the patient/parent understands that this treatment has limited efficacy and does not affect pigmentation

    C. After 7-10 day course of topical steroids, apply moisturizers such as Moisturel at bedtime to control scaling

    D. Emphasize the importance of good skin care (see information on managing dry skin in the section CARE OF DRY AND OILY SKIN)

    E. Use this opportunity to discuss sun avoidance, use of protective clothing, and use of sunscreen with an SPF >30

    F. Follow Up: None indicated

CAFÉ AU LAIT SPOTS

I. Definition: Uniformly brown macules with distinct borders found on any cutaneous surface

II. Pathogenesis

    A. Increased levels of melanin in melanocytes and in keratinocytes of the basal cell layer occur for unknown reasons

    B. There is no increase in the actual number of melanocytes

    C. Benign lesion in most cases, but also a cutaneous marker of type 1 neurofibromatosis (NF-1), an autosomal dominant disease

III. Clinical Presentation

A. Hyperpigmented (pale brown) macules with distinct borders ranging in size from 0.5-2.0 cm

B. Rarely present at birth, but increase in number with age through the teenage years; occur in 25-35% of children between the ages of 4 and 18 years and are usually of little significance

C. Six or more café-au-lait spots greater than 5 mm in diameter in prepubertal child or >1.5 mm in postpubertal child is a diagnostic criterion of NF-1 (there are several others and two or more of the criteria are needed to make the diagnosis of NF-1) [see diagnostic criteria in table under IV.B.]

IV. Diagnosis/Evaluation

A. History
1. Question about location, onset, and duration of lesions; ask if lesions were present at birth
2. Ask if lesions have increased in number or size
3. Ask about family history of neurofibromatosis, an autosomal dominant disease

B. Physical Examination
1. Examine skin surface for characteristic lesions
2. Carefully count and measure lesions, mapping location and size in chart
3. Using the criteria in the table below, determine if patient meets diagnostic criteria for neurofibromatosis

DIAGNOSTIC CRITERIA FOR NEUROFIBROMATOSIS TYPE 1
Two of more of the following must be present:
✓ Six or more café-au-lait spots as described under III.B. above
✓ Two of more neurofibromas of any type
✓ One plexiform neurofibroma
✓ Axillary freckling
✓ Inguinal freckling
✓ Two or more Lisch nodules (iris hamartomas)
✓ Distinctive osseous lesion
✓ First-degree relative with NF-1

Adapted from Westin, W.L,, Lane, A.T., & Morelli, J.G. (2002). *Color textbook of pediatric dermatology.* St. Louis: Mosby.

C. Differential Diagnosis: Freckles, lentigo

D. Diagnosis Tests: None indicated

V. Plan/Management

A. Any child who meets diagnostic criteria for NF-1 should be referred to an expert for further evaluation and management

B. Prepubertal child with <6 lesions that are <5 mm in diameter and without any of the diagnostic criteria for NF-1 (see table above) should be observed at yearly health maintenance visit for changes

C. Parent of child should be instructed to bring child to office if number or size of lesions increases, or if any of the other diagnostic criteria (see table above) are met

D. Postpubertal child with <6 lesions that are <1.5 mm in diameter and without any of the diagnostic criteria for NF-1 (see table above) should be observed at yearly health maintenance visit for changes

E. Parent or adolescent should be instructed to return to office if number or size of lesions increases, or if any of the other diagnostic criteria are met

F. Café au lait spots cannot be lightened by hydroquinone bleaching agents

G. Follow Up: Yearly to evaluate for change

HERPES SIMPLEX

I.   Definition: Cutaneous infections with herpes simplex viruses which are enveloped, double-stranded, DNA viruses of two types that have major genomic and antigenic differences

    A.   HSV-1 is usually associated with orolabial infections

    B.   HSV-2 is usually associated with genital infections (genital herpes is considered under SEXUALLY TRANSMITTED DISEASES)

II.   Pathogenesis

    A.   HSV-1 and HSV-2 are epidermotropic viruses with infection occurring within keratinocytes

    B.   Transmission is only by direct contact with active lesions, or by virus-containing fluid such as saliva or cervical secretions in persons with no evidence of active disease

    C.   Inoculation of the virus into skin or mucosal surfaces produces infection, with an incubation period of 2 days to 2 weeks

    D.   About 48 hours after entering the host, the virus transverses afferent nerves to find host ganglion
        1.   The trigeminal ganglia are the target of the oral virus—primarily HSV-1
        2.   The sacral ganglia are the target of the genital virus—most often HSV-2

    E.   Upon reactivation, the virus retraces its route, causing recurrence in the cutaneous area affected by the same nerve root, but not necessarily in the original site

    F.   Generally HSV-1 is associated with orolabial infection and HSV-2 with the genitalia (see SEXUALLY TRANSMITTED DISEASES section for a full discussion of this topic)

    G.   An increasing number of genital herpes cases are attributable to HSV-1

    H.   In neonates, Type 2 (HSV-2) is the most common cause of infection

III.   Clinical Presentation

    A.   Two clinical stages define the course of herpes viruses: primary infection after which the virus becomes established in a nerve ganglion, and recurrent infection

    B.   During the first stage—primary infection with HSV1 virus—the following usually occurs:
        1.   Lesions may appear 2-14 days following inoculation; lesions are typically grouped vesicles on an erythematous base, usually affecting the orolabial area (herpes labialis), and commonly known as "cold sores" or "fever blisters"
        2.   Vesicles rupture, leaving erosions that slowly form crusts; crusting signals the end of viral shedding; lesions are intraepidermal and usually heal without leaving a scar
        3.   There may be tenderness, pain, mild paresthesia, or burning prior to and during the eruption of lesions; person may also have fever, myalgia, malaise, or cervical lymphadenopathy
        4.   In addition to orolabial infection, other clinical variants of herpes simplex that commonly occur are herpetic whitlow which occurs in HSV-1 infected children due to thumb sucking, and herpes gladiatorum which can occur on the torso of wrestlers (or other athletes) with frequent skin-to-skin contact
        5.   Nearly 30% of infected persons are entirely asymptomatic during the primary infection state

    C.   During the primary infection stage, the virus enters nerve endings in the skin below the lesions and travels through peripheral nerves to the dorsal root ganglia, and remains dormant

D. During the recurrent infection, or second clinical stage, the virus is reactivated and travels down peripheral nerves to the site of the initial infection, causing the characteristic focal infection; recurrent infection is not inevitable and may be triggered by one or more of the following:
1. Local skin trauma
2. Sunlight exposure
3. Systemic changes such as menses, fatigue, or fever

IV. Diagnosis/Evaluation

A. History
1. Question regarding location, onset, duration, and appearance of lesions; ask if pain, burning, or paresthesia present prior to eruption
2. Ask about associated symptoms of fever, myalgia, malaise
3. Ask regarding previous occurrence of similar lesions, symptoms
4. Inquire about exposures to infected persons

B. Physical Examination
1. Examine lesions for characteristic location, distribution, and appearance
2. Check for cervical lymphadenopathy

C. Differential Diagnosis: Erythema multiforme, pemphigus

D. Diagnostic Tests
1. Premier type-specific HSV-1 IgG test (Meridian Diagnostics, Research Triangle Park, North Carolina) is a rapid ELISA test available for the diagnosis of HSV-seropositivity
2. Viral culture is also an option, but the results are not immediate
   a. Unroof vesicle and scrape the material with Dacron-tipped swab
   b. Place swab in viral transport media
   c. Viral detection usually requires 1-3 days after inoculation

V. Plan/Management

A. Reassure patient that infections resolve without treatment
1. Base treatment decisions on needs of each patient
2. Several oral antiviral drugs and topical agents are available for the treatment or primary and recurrent herpes orolabial infection in adolescents ≥18 years of age

TREATMENT OF HERPES LABIALIS IN ADOLESCENTS ≥ 18 YEARS OF AGE			
Oral Therapy (Therapy must be initiated within 48 hours of the onset of signs and symptoms)			
Primary/recurrent orolabial infections	Acyclovir (Zovirax)*	400 mg PO 5 times a day x 5 days **OR**	$52.81**
	Famciclovir (Famvir)*	500 mg PO BID x 7 days **OR**	$103.27
	Valacyclovir (Valtrex)	2 g PO Q 12 hrs x 1 day	$25.98
Topical Therapy (can also be used in lieu of oral antiviral agents, but oral treatment is usually more efficacious)			
✓ Penciclovir cream 1% (Denavir), applied every 2 hours while awake x 4 days reduces the duration of herpes labialis by about half a day			$23.09
✓ Docosanol cream 10% (Abreva), applied 5 x/day until healed and is available without a prescription			$13.75
✓ Tetracaine cream 1.8% (Cepacol Viractic Cream) reduces healing time of recurrent herpes labialis lesion by about 2 days and is available without a prescription			$12.50
✓ Lips should be protected from sun exposure with agents such as zinc oxide or with lip balm containing sun-blocking agents			
✓ Compresses with cool water decrease erythema and help to débride the lesion			

* Not FDA approved for this indication (Famvir is approved for use in HIV-infected patients)
** Cost of one course of treatment with oral drug or tube of cream

B. Immunocompromised patients ≥18 years of age with persistent intraoral or extralabial lesions
1. Acyclovir, 200 mg PO 5 x/day x 7 days OR
2. Valacyclovir, 500 mg PO BID x 5 days
3. If suppressive therapy is indicated, prescribe acyclovir, 200-400 mg PO BID

C. Follow Up: None indicated

MOLLUSCUM CONTAGIOSUM

I. Definition: A benign, usually asymptomatic viral disease of the skin characterized by discrete, flesh-colored to translucent dome-shaped papules

II. Pathogenesis

    A. Caused by a poxvirus (sole member of the genus Molluscipoxvirus) that induces epidermal cell proliferation

    B. Humans are the only known source of the virus and infectivity is relatively low

    C. Spreads by direct contact, including sexual contact, or by fomites such as towels

    D. Incubation period varies between 2-7 weeks and may be up to 6 months

III. Clinical Presentation

    A. More common in children and adolescents, but may affect any age group

    B. Tiny (2-5 mm), early lesions are shiny, flesh-colored to translucent, dome-shaped discrete papules with a firm, waxy appearance that often occur in groups
        1. As lesions mature, the centers become soft and umbilicated
        2. Usual number of lesions ranges from 2-20
        3. Commonly occur on the face, trunk, and extremities and in genital area in adults; an eczematous reaction may encircle the papules in about 10% of patients

    C. Self-limiting; usually spontaneously clears in 6-9 months

    D. A common, cutaneous manifestation of HIV infection

IV. Diagnosis/Evaluation

    A. History
        1. Inquire about location, appearance of lesions, onset and duration
        2. Ask about past medical history, determine if patient is immunocompromised

    B. Physical Examination
        1. Examine skin for characteristic lesions
        2. Magnification may assist in seeing central umbilication in more mature lesions
        3. Palpate the lesions to reveal their solid versus fluid-filled nature (wear gloves)

    C. Differential Diagnosis
        1. Basal cell carcinoma
        2. Epidermal cyst
        3. Wart
        4. Herpes simplex

    D. Diagnostic Tests: Usually based on clinical appearance of lesions; biopsy of lesion is recommended in persons who are immunocompromised

V. Plan/Management

    A. For small number of asymptomatic lesions that are stable (not spreading), observe for spontaneous resolution over next few months; advise patient that there is a small risk of scarring with all removal modalities

    B. Genital lesions should be treated to prevent spread via sexual contact (see D. below)

C. Removal using a curette works well when there are just a few lesions; removal of the umbilicated core (evisceration) can be done simply with the use of a hollow needle and this results in resolution of the lesion(s) when there are just a few

D. Liquid nitrogen therapy is also an option that is often used with genital lesions in adolescents
　　1. Papule is touched lightly with the nitrogen-bathed probe until the advancing, white, frozen border progresses down the side of the lesion to form a 1 mm halo on the normal skin surrounding the lesion
　　2. Process is very rapid (around 5 seconds)
　　3. Excessive freezing can cause scarring, hypopigmentation, or hyperpigmentation

E. Other options involve use of one of the following topical agents
　　1. Salicylic acid 17% (Duofilm liquid), available as 15 mL with applicator; apply thin layer daily up to 12 weeks (not FDA approved for this indication) OR
　　2. Podofilox 0.5% gel (Condylox topical gel), available as 3.5 g; apply BID x 3 days (not FDA approved for this indication) [not for use in children <18 years of age] OR
　　3. Imiquimod 5% cream (Aldara), available as 12 single use packets; apply a thin layer 3 times a week at bedtime and remove with soap and water after 6-10 hours for up to two weeks (not FDA approved for this indication) [not for use in children <18 years of age]
　　4. Tretinoin gel 0.01% (Retin-A-Gel), (available as 15 g); apply sparingly at bedtime for up to two weeks (not FDA approved for this indication) [not for use in children <18 years of age]
　　5. With all of these topical agents, protection of surrounding skin with petrolatum is recommended
　　6. Prescribe medications for off-label use cautiously!

F. Follow Up: In 2-4 weeks to evaluate treatment efficacy

WARTS

I. Definition: Virus-induced proliferation of keratinocytes resulting in tumors of the skin and mucous membranes

II. Pathogenesis

　　A. Human papillomaviruses (HPVs) produce epithelial tumors of the skin and mucous membranes

　　B. HPVs are members of the Papovaviridae family and are DNA viruses

　　C. More than 70 types have been identified; a small number of HPV types account for most warts

　　D. HPV types causing nongenital warts generally are distinct from those causing anogenital infections

III. Clinical Presentation

　　A. Cutaneous warts occur frequently among school-age children with prevalence rates as high as 50%

　　B. Warts are transmitted by touch and commonly appear at sites of trauma on the hands, periungual regions from biting, and on plantar surfaces from weight bearing

　　C. Most warts resolve in 12-24 months without treatment

　　D. Generally, warts are asymptomatic except for plantar warts which may be painful

　　E. Presentation is variable depending on type:
　　　　1. Common warts (*verruca vulgaris*) may arise anywhere on body (often on hands) and appear as solitary flesh-colored papules with scaly, irregular surface; usually are asymptomatic and multiple
　　　　2. Filiform warts are usually seen on face (lips, nose, eyelids) and appear as thin projections on a narrow stalk
　　　　3. Flat warts (*verruca plana*) are usually located on face and extremities and appear in groups as flat-topped, skin-colored papules

4. Plantar warts occur on weight-bearing areas of the feet; papule is pushed into skin and verrucous surface appears level with skin surface (characterized by marked hyperkeratosis and sometimes with black dots [black dots appear in warts when small dermal vessels become thrombosed])
5. Anogenital warts are considered under SEXUALLY TRANSMITTED DISEASES section

IV. Diagnosis/Evaluation

    A. History
        1. Question about location, onset, duration, and if any symptoms are present
        2. Ask about treatments tried and results

    B. Physical Examination
        1. Examine lesion looking for characteristic appearance
        2. Use hand lens to aid in visualizing surface characteristics

    C. Differential Diagnosis
        1. Calluses (have smooth rather than rough irregular surface)
        2. Lichen planus (look for Wickham's striae)
        3. Seborrheic keratosis (have stuck-on appearance with horn cysts visible on close inspection)

    D. Diagnostic Tests: Most are easily diagnosed based on clinical appearance

V. Plan/Management

    A. Counsel patient that most nongenital warts eventually regress without treatment but may persist for weeks or months

    B. Optimal treatment for warts that do not resolve spontaneously has not been identified; nonetheless, many patients desire treatment and some success has come from methods that rely on chemical or physical destruction of the infected epithelium

    C. Common wart: Topical salicylic acid preparations applied at bedtime for 6-8 weeks
        1. Examples of 17% concentrations are Occlusal HP, DuoPlant, Compound W, Duofilm, Wart-Off; all are OTC and in liquid form
        2. An example of a 15% solution in karaya gum base patches for use on isolated thicker lesions is Trans Ver Sal (40 patches of varying size with securing tapes and emery file)
        3. May use liquid nitrogen in cooperative patients (can be quite uncomfortable for young children)

    D. Filiform wart: Refer for removal by snip excision unless experienced in the procedure

    E. Flat wart: Refer for removal; these warts are resistant to treatment and are usually located in cosmetically important areas

    F. Plantar wart: Use 40% salicylic acid plasters; examples are Mediplast and Duofilm Patch
        1. Plaster is cut to size of wart and applied over wart
        2. Plaster is removed in 24-48 hours and pliable dead white keratin is removed with pumice stone
        3. Process is repeated every 24-48 hours until wart is removed (usually 6-8 weeks)
        4. Pain relief occurs early because a large part of wart is removed in first few days of treatment

    G. Follow Up: In 2-4 weeks to evaluate response to treatment (if any treatment was initiated)

REFERENCES

Abramowicz, M. (2002). Drugs for non-HIV viral infections. *The Medical Letter, 44,* 9-16.

Abramowicz, M. (2002). Desloratadine (Clarinex). *The Medical Letter, 44,* 27-28.

Abramowicz, M. (2002). Topical pimecrolimus (Elidel) for treatment of atopic dermatitis. *The Medical Letter, 44,* 48-50.

Abramowicz, M. (2002). Tazarotene (Tazorac) for acne. *The Medical Letter, 44,* 52-53.

American Academy of Pediatrics. (2000). Candidiasis. In L.K. Pickering (Ed.), *2000 red book: Report of the Committee on Infectious Diseases* (25th ed., pp. 198-201). Elk Grove Village, IL: Author.

American Academy of Pediatrics. (2000). Cutaneous larva migrans. In L.K. Pickering (Ed.), *2000 red book: Report of the Committee on Infectious Diseases* (25th ed., pp. 225-226). Elk Grove Village, IL: Author.

American Academy of Pediatrics. (2000). Herpes simplex. In L.K. Pickering (Ed.), *2000 red book: Report of the Committee on Infectious Diseases* (25th ed., pp. 309-318). Elk Grove Village, IL: Author.

American Academy of Pediatrics. (2000). Hookworm infections. In L.K. Pickering (Ed.), *2000 red book: Report of the Committee on Infectious Diseases* (25th ed., pp. 321-322). Elk Grove Village, IL: Author.

American Academy of Pediatrics. (2000). Molluscum contagiosum. In L.K. Pickering (Ed.), *2000 red book: Report of the Committee on Infectious Diseases* (25th ed., pp. 403-404). Elk Grove Village, IL: Author.

American Academy of Pediatrics. (2000). Pediculosis capitis (head lice). In L.K. Pickering (Ed.), *2000 red book: Report of the Committee on Infectious Diseases* (25th ed., pp. 427-429). Elk Grove Village, IL: Author.

American Academy of Pediatrics. (2000). Pediculosis corporis. In L.K. Pickering (Ed.), *2000 red book: Report of the Committee on Infectious Diseases* (25th ed., pp. 429-430). Elk Grove Village, IL: Author.

American Academy of Pediatrics. (2000). Pediculosis pubis. In L.K. Pickering (Ed.), *2000 red book: Report of the Committee on Infectious Diseases* (25th ed., pp. 430-431). Elk Grove Village, IL: Author.

American Academy of Pediatrics. (2000). Scabies. In L.K. Pickering (Ed.), *2000 red book: Report of the Committee on Infectious Diseases* (25th ed., pp. 506-508). Elk Grove Village, IL: Author.

American Academy of Pediatrics. (2000). Tinea capitis (ringworm of the scalp). In L.K. Pickering (Ed.), *2000 red book: Report of the Committee on Infectious Diseases* (25th ed., pp. 569-570). Elk Grove Village, IL: Author.

American Academy of Pediatrics. (2000). Tinea corporis (ringworm of the body). In L.K. Pickering (Ed.), *2000 red book: Report of the Committee on Infectious Diseases* (25th ed., pp. 570-572). Elk Grove Village, IL: Author.

American Academy of Pediatrics. (2000). Tinea cruris (jock itch). In L.K. Pickering (Ed.), *2000 red book: Report of the Committee on Infectious Diseases* (25th ed., pp. 572-573). Elk Grove Village, IL: Author.

American Academy of Pediatrics. (2000). Tinea pedis (athlete's foot). In L.K. Pickering (Ed.), *2000 red book: Report of the Committee on Infectious Diseases* (25th ed., pp. 573-574). Elk Grove Village, IL: Author.

American Academy of Pediatrics. (2000). Tinea versicolor. In L.K. Pickering (Ed.), *2000 red book: Report of the Committee on Infectious Diseases* (25th ed., pp. 574-576). Elk Grove Village, IL: Author.

American Academy of Pediatrics. (2000). Varicella-zoster infections. In L.K. Pickering (Ed.), *2000 red book: Report of the Committee on Infectious Diseases* (25th ed., pp. 624-637). Elk Grove Village, IL: Author.

Centers for Disease Control and Prevention. (2002). Sexually transmitted diseases treatment guidelines 2002. *MMWR, 51* (RR-6), 1-84.

Dahl, M.V. (2002). Contact dermatitis. In R.E. Rakel, & E. T. Bope (Eds.), *Conn's current therapy* (pp. 852-853). Philadelphia: Saunders.

Davis, K.J., Cokkinides, V.E., Weinstock, M.A., O'Connell, M.C., & Wingo, P.A. (2002). Summer sunburn and sun exposure among US youths ages 11 to 18: National prevalence and associated factors. *Pediatrics, 110,* 27-35.

Eichenfield, L.F., Lucky, A.W., Boguniewicz, M., Langley, R.G., Cherill, R., Marchall, K., Bush, C., et al. (2002). Safety and efficacy of pimecrolimus (ASM 981) cream 1% in the treatment of mild and moderate atopic dermatitis in children and adolescents. *Journal of the American Academy of Dermatology, 46,* 495-504.

Fradin, M.S., & Day, J.D. (2002). Comparative efficacy of insect repellents against mosquito bites. *New England Journal of Medicine, 347,* 13-18.

Habif, T.P., Campbell, J.L., Quitadamo, M.J., Zug, K.A. (2001). *Skin disease: Diagnosis and treatment.* St. Louis: Mosby.

Honig, P.J. (2002). Allergic contact dermatitis. In. F.D. Burg, J.R. Ingelfinger, R.A. Polin, & A.A. Gershon (Eds.), *Gellis and Kagan's current pediatric therapy* (pp. 857-858). Philadelphia: Saunders.

Hwogn, H., & Levy, M.L. (2002). Atopic dermatitis. In R.E. Rakel, & E. T. Bope (Eds.), *Conn's current therapy* (pp. 843-845). Philadelphia: Saunders.

Izakovic, J. & Schachner, L. (2002). Pediculosis. In. F.D. Burg, J.R. Ingelfinger, R.A. Polin, & A.A. Gershon (Eds.), *Gellis and Kagan's current pediatric therapy* (pp. 876-877). Philadelphia: Saunders.

Izakovic, J., & Schachner, L. (2002). Scabies. In. F.D. Burg, J.R. Ingelfinger, R.A. Polin, & A.A. Gershon (Eds.), *Gellis and Kagan's current pediatric therapy* (pp. 874-876). Philadelphia: Saunders.

Jackson, A.D. (2002). Warts and their management. In R.E. Rakel, & E. T. Bope (Eds.), *Conn's current therapy* (pp. 801-804). Philadelphia: Saunders.

Kazaks, E.L., & Lane, A.T. (2000). Diaper dermatitis. *Pediatric Clinics of North America, 47,* 909-918.

Kim, H. J. (2002). Atopic dermatitis. In. F.D. Burg, J.R. Ingelfinger, R.A. Polin, & A.A. Gershon (Eds.), *Gellis and Kagan's current pediatric therapy* (pp. 858-859). Philadelphia: Saunders.

Kristal, L., & Klein, P.A. (2000). Atopic dermatitis in infants and children: An update. *Pediatric Clinics of North America, 47,* 877-895.

Landau, J.W. (2002). Warts and molluscum contagiosum. In. F.D. Burg, J.R. Ingelfinger, R.A. Polin, & A.A. Gershon (Eds.), *Gellis and Kagan's current pediatric therapy* (pp. 873-876). Philadelphia: Saunders.

Lazarus, M.C., Baumann, L., & Schachner, L. (2002). Sun protection in the pediatric population. In. F.D. Burg, J.R. Ingelfinger, R.A. Polin, & A.A. Gershon (Eds.), *Gellis and Kagan's current pediatric therapy* (pp. 897-897). Philadelphia: Saunders.

Lebwohl, M., & Ali, S. (2001). Treatment of psoriasis. Part 1. Topical therapy and phototherapy. *Journal of the American Academy of Dermatology, 45,* 487-498.

Leyden, J.J. (1997). Therapy for acne vulgaris. *New England Journal of Medicine, 336,* 1156-1162.

Morelli, J.G., & Weston, W.L. (1987). Soaps and shampoos in pediatric practice. *Pediatrics, 80,* 634-637.

Pardasani, A.G., Feldman, S.R., & Clark, A.R. (2000). Treatment of psoriasis: An algorithm-based approach for primary care physicians. *American Family Physician, 61,* 725-736.

Roberts, F.J. (2002). Head lice. *New England Journal of Medicine, 346,* 1645-1650.

Rockwell, P.G. (2001). Acute and chronic paronychia. *American Family Physician, 63,* 1113-1116.

Rogers, P., & Bassler, M. (2001). Treating onychomycosis. *American Family Physician, 63,* 663-672.

Rostan, E.F., & Fitzpatrick, R.E. (2002). Fungal infections of the skin. In. F.D. Burg, J.R. Ingelfinger, R.A. Polin, & A.A. Gershon (Eds.), *Gellis and Kagan's current pediatric therapy* (pp. 869-872). Philadelphia: Saunders.

Schwetz, B.A. (2001). New treatment for eczema. *Journal of the American Medical Association, 285,* 1874-1876.

Shenefelt, P.D. (2002). Parasitic diseases of the skin. In R.E. Rakel, & E. T. Bope (Eds.), *Conn's current therapy* (pp. 824-827). Philadelphia: Saunders.

Urbatsch, A.M., & Elmets, C.A. (2002). Disorders of pigmentation. In. F.D. Burg, J.R. Ingelfinger, R.A. Polin, & A.A. Gershon (Eds.), *Gellis and Kagan's current pediatric therapy* (pp. 877-880). Philadelphia: Saunders.

Webster, G. (2002). Acne vulgaris and rosacea. In R.E. Rakel, & E. T. Bope (Eds.), *Conn's current therapy* (pp. 771-773). Philadelphia: Saunders.

Weinberg, J.M. (2002). Fungal diseases of the skin. In R.E. Rakel, & E. T. Bope (Eds.), *Conn's current therapy* (pp. 827-829). Philadelphia: Saunders.

Weston, W.L., Lane, A.T., & Morelli, J.G. (2002). *Color textbook of pediatric dermatology.* St. Louis: Mosby.

Wilkerson, M.D. (2002). Bacterial diseases of the skin. In R.E. Rakel, & E. T. Bope (Eds.), *Conn's current therapy* (pp. 815-817). Philadelphia: Saunders.

Zampogna, J.C., & Flowers, F.P. (2002). Viral diseases of the skin. In R.E. Rakel & E.T. Bope. *Conn's current therapy* (pp. 817-823). Philadelphia: Saunders.

Zic, J.A. (2002). Papulosquamous diseases. In R.E. Rakel, & E. T. Bope (Eds.), *Conn's current therapy* (pp. 784-788). Philadelphia: Saunders.

8 ▼ Problems of the Eyes

MARY VIRGINIA GRAHAM

AMBLYOPIA

I.   Definition: Marked decrease in visual acuity (most often in one eye) in the absence of organic disease; most likely due to lack of continuous use of one or both foveae for visual fixation occurring during a critical period in the first few years of life (before age 7)

II.   Pathogenesis

    A.   Exact mechanism is unknown, but there appears to be a microscopic defect in wiring of the retina-to-brain connections that results from nonuse of fixation reflex; fixation must be developed and used early in life

    B.   There are three different perceptual phenomena that are integral to the expression of single binocular vision: simultaneous perception, fusion, and stereopsis; they may function simultaneously or in decreasing degrees, with stereopsis being the most highly developed and simultaneous perception the least developed in normal eyes

    C.   There are three main causes of amblyopia, all of which affect one eye only: strabismic amblyopia, anisometropic (refractive) amblyopia, and deprivation amblyopia

III. Clinical Presentation

    A.   An important cause of permanent vision loss, affecting about 5% of the US population

    B.   Strabismic amblyopia is the most common type
        1.   Occurs most often in patients with esotropia (deviating eye turns in)
        2.   Also occurs, but less frequently, in exotropia (deviating eye turns out)
        3.   To avoid double vision (diplopia), patient inhibits the foveal region of the deviating eye, a compensation that results in strabismic amblyopia of disuse

    C.   Anisometropic or refractive amblyopia develops when there is marked disparity in the refractive error between the eyes
        1.   Child comes to rely on the sight of the more focused eye, suppressing the blurred image of the other eye
        2.   As a result, the unfocused eye loses its visual potential

    D.   Deprivation amblyopia is the most severe type in terms of vision loss in the child
        1.   Develops when the retina does not receive a clear image
        2.   Causes include unilateral or bilateral congenital cataracts, corneal or vitreous opacity, severe ptosis (droopy eyelid), or excessive patching

    E.   Condition is potentially reversible if identified before visual development is complete (by age 7 or earlier)

    F.   Typical presentation is a young child with an acuity difference between the eyes or with bilateral vision less than expected for the age of the child (isometropic amblyopia is type of amblyopia affecting both eyes in which there is a high refractive error in both eyes, leading to bilateral amblyopia due to bilateral blurred vision)

    G.   Child with amblyopia usually tests poorly on standard visual acuity charts using rows of letters or symbols because of difficulty in separating out individual letters/symbols (crowding phenomenon); vision testing is more accurate using single, isolated, letters or symbols

IV.   Diagnosis/Evaluation

    A.   History
        1.   Ask parents when symptoms were first noticed and what in particular was observed
        2.   In infant, ask parent if child can fixate on and follow objects
        3.   In infant, ask parent if fine motor coordination is at appropriate level based on age
        4.   Ask parent if child has abnormal face or head position (head turn or chin tilt may improve acuity or correct diplopia)

     5.   In older child, ask parent if developmental tasks were achieved at appropriate age

     6.   Inquire about other eye problems and their treatment

B.   Physical Examination

     1.   Test for visual acuity (testing both eyes separately) using the Snellen letters or numbers, HOTV, Lea symbols, or Tumbling E charts (see VISUAL IMPAIRMENT for how to test visual acuity in children)

     2.   Test for stereo vision. Stereopsis (perception of the third dimension) using the Random Dot E test may be the more effective than visual acuity testing in detecting amblyopia and strabismus. See VISUAL IMPAIRMENT for how to test for stereo vision in children

     3.   Inspect eyelids, conjunctiva, cornea, height and equality of the level of upper eyelids

     4.   Assess pupils for shape, size, equality, reaction to light

     5.   Assess extraocular movement using an interesting target

     6.   Perform cover test (see STRABISMUS for technique and interpretation of cover testing)

     7.   Perform corneal light reflex test. Shine penlight directly in eyes from a distance of about 24 inches; observe the position of the reflection of the light on each cornea with respect to the location of the pupil—the corneal surface of both eyes should reflect the examining light symmetrically

     8.   Assess for presence of red reflex (see section on VISUAL IMPAIRMENT for red reflex examination in children)

C.   Differential Diagnosis

     1.   Optic nerve hypoplasia

     2.   Abnormalities of the retina

     3.   Cortical blindness

     4.   Cataract

     5.   Anisometropia (unequal refractive error between the eyes)

     6.   Strabismus

D.   Diagnostic Tests: Additional testing will be done by pediatric ophthalmologist

V.   Plan/Management

A.   Referral to an ophthalmologist is necessary

B.   Recognition and treatment of underlying cause is the first step in treatment (e.g., if a cataract is interfering with vision, it needs to be removed)

C.   The second component of treatment by the ophthalmologist is to force the child to depend on the amblyopic eye for vision

     1.   Occlusion therapy with patching of the preferred eye has been the treatment of choice for many years

     2.   Other treatment options have been introduced in recent years and include the following:

          a.   Lens occlusion in which the lens of eyeglasses is occluded on side with preferred eye

          b.   Occluder contact lens is more frequently used in patients with high anisometropia

          c.   Atropinization of the preferred eye (use of atropine in the preferred eye to blur vision and force use of the amblyopic eye) is being increasingly used as an alternative to patching

D.   Follow Up: Make certain the patient keeps appointment with the ophthalmologist

BLEPHARITIS

I.   Definition: Inflammation of the eyelid margins

II.   Pathogenesis:

A.   Often due to colonization of eyelash follicles and the meibomian glands with staphylococci

B.   Allergic disorders and dermatologic diseases (usually seborrheic dermatitis or rosacea) are also common causes

III. Clinical Presentation

   A.   A common, chronic problem which often begins in childhood and continues throughout adulthood

   B.   Characterized by hypertrophy and desquamation of the epidermis near the lid margin which results in erythema and scaling of the lid border

   C.   Main complaint is redness of the eyelid margin but sensation of foreign body, burning, and eye discomfort may be additional symptoms

   D.   Severe and chronic cases may produce purulent discharge and over time permanent changes in the eyelid structure can occur (misdirection and lost eyelashes and distortion of lid contour)

   E.   Patient usually has a history of recurrent chalazia and hordeola

IV. Diagnosis/Evaluation

   A.   History
        1.   Determine onset and duration of symptoms
        2.   Ask about presence of flaking, crusting at lid margins, frequency of eye rubbing
        3.   Inquire about eye pain, visual disturbances, dry eyes and tearing
        4.   Obtain ocular history including prior eye disease, injuries, surgery, or other treatments and medications
        5.   Inquire about previous and present skin problems, particularly of the face and scalp
        6.   Ask about chronic exposure to irritants such as smoke, cosmetics, and chemicals

   B.   Physical Examination
        1.   Determine visual acuity
        2.   Perform a complete eye examination, paying particular attention to the following components:
             a.   Inspect eyelid margins (with magnifying glass if necessary) for crusting, scaling, erythema, and erosions
             b.   Examine sclera and conjunctiva for abnormalities
             c.   Palpate lid margins and lid for masses
        3.   Palpate for preauricular adenopathy
        4.   Examine skin of face and scalp for characteristic findings of seborrheic dermatitis and rosacea (see sections on SEBORRHEIC DERMATITIS)

   C.   Differential Diagnosis: Chalazion, hordeolum, conjunctivitis, and keratitis

   D.   Diagnostic Tests: None are usually indicated

V. Plan/Management:

   A.   If an underlying source of the lid irritation can be identified, it is important to treat the source as the first step in management: If seborrheic dermatitis of the scalp and face is present, institute appropriate treatment (see section on SEBORRHEIC DERMATITIS for treatment recommendations)

   B.   Treatment for blepharitis is outlined below
        1.   Instruct patient in lid hygiene as follows
             a.   Apply warm, wet facecloth compresses for two minutes, 2-4 times a day to the lids to increase circulation, mobilize meibomian secretions, and help cleanse crusting debris on lid margins
             b.   After a compress application, gently scrub eyelids once a day with fingertips (or cotton-tipped applicator) using baby shampoo diluted 1:1 with clean water (or commercial cleansing pads such as Eye Scrub or Lid Wipes SPF) in order to remove crusts and scale
             c.   Blepharitis associated with seborrhea is often improved by use of a dandruff shampoo on scalp and eyebrows
        2.   For flares, topical antibiotic therapy may also be helpful: Adolescents and children: Prescribe erythromycin 0.5% (Ilotycin or generic) ophthalmic ointment BID x 7 days OR sulfacetamide sodium 10% (Bleph-10) available as ophthalmic solution or ointment (solution: 1-2 drops Q3H during day; ointment: QID and at HS) x 7 days

C. Because most cases of blepharitis are chronic and require long-term therapy, they are best managed by an ophthalmologist

D. Follow Up
1. None needed for mild cases
2. Refer recurrent cases to ophthalmologist for management

CHALAZION

I. Definition: Focal chronic inflammation of a meibomian gland

II. Pathogenesis

A. Chronic granuloma from obstructed meibomian gland

B. May occur as a result of a chronic hordeolum (a focal acute infection of meibomian gland)

C. Secondary infection of the surrounding tissues may develop

III. Clinical Presentation

A. Usually hard, non-tender nodule is found on midportion of the tarsus, away from the lid border; may develop on lid margin if the opening of the duct is involved and can present with lid tenderness, pain, and swelling

B. Chalazia which become infected result in painful swelling of the entire lid

C. Small chalazia may resolve spontaneously without treatment

D. History of chronic hordeolum and prior excision of chalazia are often present

IV. Diagnosis/Evaluation

A. History
1. Determine onset and duration of symptoms
2. Inquire about pain or tenderness of the lid
3. Inquire about any changes in visual acuity level
4. Ask about past episodes and previous treatments

B. Physical Examination
1. Assess visual acuity
2. Perform a complete eye examination, paying particular attention to the following components
a. Inspect eyelids for inflammation and masses
b. Palpate eyelids for masses and tenderness
c. Evert the eyelid and examine inner surface for pointing
d. Inspect sclera and conjunctiva for abnormalities
3. Palpate for preauricular adenopathy

C. Differential Diagnosis
1. May be associated with a hordeolum and blepharitis
2. Sebaceous cell carcinoma is a rare condition which should be considered

D. Diagnostic Tests: None indicated

V. Plan/Management

A. Small, asymptomatic, chronic chalazia do not require treatment and usually disappear spontaneously within a few months

B. If chalazia are large or if there is secondary infection, treatment is needed
   1. Apply warm, moist compresses for several minutes throughout the day
   2. Prescribe erythromycin ointment 0.5% (Ilotycin or generic), small amount to affected eye, BID-QID x 7 days OR polymyxin B-trimethoprim drops (Polytrim), 1-2 drops to affected eye, BID-QID x 7 days

C. If the chalazion does not respond to conservative therapy, patient should be referred to an expert for injection of the lesion or incision and curettage

D. Follow Up
   1. Small chalazia do not require follow up
   2. Follow up for chalazia that do not respond to conservative therapy should be with ophthalmologist

CONGENITAL NASOLACRIMAL DUCT OBSTRUCTION

I. Definition: A congenital defect of the lacrimal drainage system in which a lack of patency affects drainage function

II. Pathogenesis: An imperforate membrane at the distal end of the nasolacrimal duct is the usual cause of occlusion

III. Clinical Presentation

   A. The most common congenital abnormality of the lacrimal apparatus in newborns

   B. As many as 30% of newborn infants may have closure of the duct at birth; in most cases, the obstruction is transient, and patency rapidly occurs

   C. Usually presents within the first few weeks of life with persistent tearing, crusting of the lashes, and mucopurulent discharge

   D. Tears spill over the lower lid and there is a persistent "wet look" in the involved eye or eyes

   E. Reflux of mucopurulent material from either punctum can be elicited by gently pressing over the nasolacrimal sac of the involved eye(s)

   F. Discharge is most evident after the infant awakens and parent must use a moistened cloth to loosen dried mucus on the lashes

   G. Most (almost 90%) congenital obstructions of the nasolacrimal duct clear spontaneously within one year

IV. Diagnosis/Evaluation

   A. History
      1. Ask parent when condition was first noticed, and if one or both eyes are affected
      2. Inquire regarding appearance of discharge, and if matting of lashes occurs
      3. Ask if condition is worse in mornings and after naps when child first awakens
      4. Ask about treatments tried and results
      5. Ask parent if child's vision seems normal

   B. Physical Examination
      1. Assess visual acuity (ability to fix and follow an interesting object) and elicit red reflex
      2. Examine the lids and adnexa for symmetry, swelling, abnormal discharge, erythema; examine sclera, cornea, and conjunctiva for signs of inflammation
      3. Palpate the soft tissue of the orbit, lids, and zygoma
      4. Inspect and palpate the lacrimal apparatus, including the lacrimal gland, superior and inferior puncta, canaliculi, and lacrimal sac
      5. Gently press over the nasolacrimal sac on the affected side to elicit material from the puncta
      6. Note appearance of discharge (if present) from affected eye(s)

C. Differential Diagnosis
 1. Conjunctivitis
 2. Blepharitis
 3. Dacryocystitis

D. Diagnostic Tests: None indicated

V. Plan/Treatment

A. Conservative treatment is the recommended approach to management of nasolacrimal duct obstruction in children less than 12 months of age

B. Instruct parent to massage the lacrimal sac several times a day in an effort to rupture the membrane at the lower end of the duct
 1. As illustrated, instruct parent to place index finger over the nasolacrimal sac and exert downward pressure
 2. Then slide finger downward toward the mouth
 3. Theoretically, fluid is trapped in the lacrimal sac, and then the downward motion breaks the obstruction in the lacrimal duct with hydrostatic pressure

C. The technique is shown in Figure 8.1

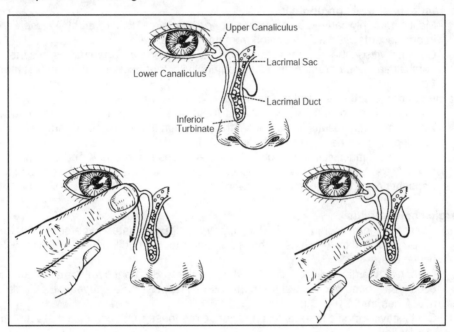

Figure 8.1. Nasolacrimal Duct Massage

D. If there is evidence of secondary conjunctivitis (conjunctiva is inflamed) or significant discharge that is purulent or mucopurulent, administration of topical antibiotics is indicated
 1. Sodium sulfacetamide 10% (Sulamyd) solution, 1-2 drops TID x 7 days
 2. Erythromycin ointment (Ilotycin) 0.5 cm strip of ointment in lower conjunctival sac QID x 7 days
 3. Advise parent that antibiotic drops or ointment reduce the infectious component of the discharge, but do not cure the blockage
 4. Aim of antibiotic therapy is to alter the character of the discharge so that it is mucoid
 5. Prolonged use of antibiotics for tearing without purulent or mucopurulent discharge is not indicated

E. Controversy exists regarding when to surgically treat the condition
 1. Some authorities recommend conservative treatment for a short time and then referral of the child for surgery at less than 6 months of age (early probing may be more successful and may obviate need for general anesthesia)
 2. Other experts recommend that conservative therapy be continued for almost the first year of life, and then referral for surgery at that time if the condition has not spontaneously resolved (late probing and irrigation [at 12-13 months of age] may reduce the number of unnecessary probings)

F. Follow Up: In 2 weeks if child placed on topical antibiotics to determine efficacy of treatment

CONJUNCTIVITIS

I. Definition: Inflammation of the conjunctiva characterized by vascular dilation, cellular infiltration, and exudation

II. Pathogenesis

    A. **Viral conjunctivitis**
        1. Usually caused by adenovirus
        2. May develop during or after an upper respiratory tract infection

    B. **Bacterial conjunctivitis**
        1. Caused by a wide range of gram-positive and gram-negative organisms, but gram-positive organisms predominate
        2. *Staphylococcus aureus* is probably the most common cause of bacterial conjunctivitis, particularly in adults
        3. *Streptococcus pneumoniae* (more commonly a causative organism in children rather than adults)
        4. *Haemophilus influenzae* (more commonly a causative organism in children rather than adults)

    C. **Hyperacute bacterial conjunctivitis**
        1. Most commonly caused by *Neisseria gonorrhoeae* and less often by *Neisseria meningitidis;* occurs in adolescents via autoinoculation from infected genitalia
        2. Conjunctivitis in the newborn caused by *Neisseria gonorrhoeae* represents the most serious type of ophthalmia neonatorum, defined as conjunctivitis that occurs during the first month of life

    D. **Chlamydial conjunctivitis**: Ocular chlamydial infections are of two types
        1. Trachoma is associated with serotypes A through C and causes a chronic keratoconjunctivitis which frequently results in blindness; this condition is rare in the US but occurs in rural areas of developing countries, particularly Africa, Asia, and the Middle East
        2. Inclusion conjunctivitis is associated with serotypes D through K and is a common, primarily sexually transmitted disease that occurs in both newborns and adolescents in the US; it is the most frequent cause of conjunctivitis in neonates

    E. **Allergic conjunctivitis**
        1. Seasonal allergic conjunctivitis (SAC), a type I, IgE-mediated hypersensitivity to certain allergens (e.g., grass and tree pollens in the spring and ragweed pollen in the fall) is most common form of ocular allergy
        2. Perennial allergic conjunctivitis (PAC), is similar to SAC but symptoms are less severe; tends to occur year round because of the nonseasonal nature of the antigens, e.g., animal dander, house mite feces, mold, and dust
        3. Conjunctivitis medicamentosa is an allergic response that occurs as a reaction to use of ocular medications

III. Clinical Presentation

    A. **Viral conjunctivitis** (presumably adenoviral)
        1. Leading cause of conjunctivitis in children; highly contagious
        2. Usual modes of transmission are contaminated fingers and swimming pool water
        3. Characterized by conjunctival hyperemia, edema, and a watery discharge; onset is usually acute
        4. Vision is unaffected; watery discharge can cause some transient blurring; photophobia is uncommon
        5. Usually self-limited but treatment with a topical antibiotic shortens its course

    B. **Bacterial conjunctivitis**
        1. Characterized by acute onset of ocular irritation and tearing
        2. Develops in one eye initially, and then spreads to the other eye within 48 hours
        3. Within one or two days, a mucopurulent or purulent discharge develops
        4. Eyelids are often edematous with a collection of debris at base of lashes and matting of the eyelashes upon awakening
        5. Diffuse hyperemia of the bulbar and tarsal conjunctiva is usually prominent
        6. Lymphadenopathy is generally minimal

C. **Hyperacute bacterial conjunctivitis**
   1. A severe, rapidly progressing sight-threatening ocular infection most often affecting sexually active young adults and newborn infants
      a. In adolescents/adults, organism is transmitted from genitalia to hands, and then to eyes
      b. In newborns, transmission is via vaginal delivery from an infected woman and symptoms are usually present at 3-5 days of age
   2. Characterized by an abrupt onset of copious yellow-green purulent discharge that is bilateral, with lid edema, erythema, and chemosis
   3. Preauricular adenopathy often present
   4. Because of rapid onset, progression, and severity of signs and symptoms, patient often seeks care before infection has spread to both eyes

D. **Chlamydial conjunctivitis** in adolescents and young adults
   1. Usually presents in young sexually active urban dwellers between the ages of 18 and 30, and is often initially unilateral
   2. Transmission occurs most often via autoinoculation from infected genital secretions
   3. Typically, an indolent infection which is characterized by a thin, mucoid discharge
   4. Patient may have photophobia and enlarged, tender preauricular nodes
   5. Subacute or chronic in nature, with patients presenting with symptoms that have been present for as long as 6 months

E. **Chlamydial conjunctivitis** in newborns
   1. By far the most common cause of conjunctivitis in newborn
   2. Usually presents 5 to 12 days after birth in infants exposed during vaginal delivery
   3. Presents with more mucopurulent discharge and inflammation than in adults

F. **Allergic conjunctivitis**
   1. Itching is the hallmark of this condition; often accompanied by tearing and nasal congestion, and mucoid discharge
   2. SAC symptoms are itchy, watery eyes, often with rhinitis or allergic pharyngitis; eye signs are mild lid edema, fine papillary hypertrophy, and bulbar conjunctival hyperemia; corneal involvement is rare
   3. PAC symptoms are itching, burning, and tearing in normal-appearing eyes (symptoms are less severe in PAC than in SAC)
   4. Conjunctivitis medicamentosa is characterized by bilateral dilatation of the conjunctival blood vessels, with eyelid edema, erythema, and scaling in a patient using a topical ophthalmic medication

IV. Diagnosis/Evaluation

   A. History
      1. Inquire regarding onset and duration of symptoms (is the condition acute, subacute, chronic, or recurrent?)
      2. Determine if condition is unilateral or bilateral; ask about the type and amount of discharge
      3. Determine if ocular pain, photophobia, or blurred vision (that fails to clear with a blink) are present
      4. Ask if itching and other symptoms of allergy are present
      5. Ask about contact with a person with "pink-eye"
      6. Inquire about personal and family history of hay fever, allergic rhinitis
      7. Obtain past medical and medication history, specifically asking about use of any ocular medications (including OTCs); ask about allergies

   B. Physical Examination
      1. Determine visual acuity, visual fields, pupillary function, and extraocular movements
      2. Examine eyelids for inflammation or tenderness
      3. Examine sclera and conjunctiva for hyperemia and edema; check cornea for clarity
      4. Determine type of discharge
      5. Palpate for regional lymphadenopathy

   C. Differential Diagnosis: Patients typically present with the main complaint of red eye; there is need to distinguish conjunctivitis from other conditions causing red eye
      1. In conjunctivitis, redness of the conjunctiva is diffuse, pain is minimal (except in hyperacute bacterial conjunctivitis), and vision, pupil size, and reactivity are normal

2. Lacrimal duct obstruction presents with pain, redness, and edema around lacrimal sac; pressure over lacrimal sac will express mucopurulent material from the upper and lower canaliculi

3. Blepharitis may have similar presentation as conjunctivitis with burning and itching of the conjunctiva, but with blepharitis there also is inflammation of lid margins and it is almost always a chronic, recurring condition

4. Corneal abrasions usually have a history of trauma with mild to moderate bulbar injection and a foreign-body sensation

D. Diagnostic Tests

In Most Cases
Culture of discharge is usually not recommended for mild conjunctivitis with a suspected viral, bacterial, or allergic origin

Exceptions
If there is severe inflammation as occurs with hyperacute conjunctivitis, or if the condition is unresponsive to initial treatment, culture and sensitivity are indicated

Sensitive and specific methods used to diagnose chlamydial ophthalmia in the neonate include both tissue culture and nonculture tests (e.g., direct fluorescent antibody tests, enzyme immunoassays, and nucleic acid amplification tests); specimens must contain conjunctival cells, not exudate alone, and must be obtained from the everted eyelid using a Dacron-tipped swab or the swab specified by the manufacturer's test kit

Nonculture tests for chlamydia can be used in older children

V. Plan/Management

A. **Viral conjunctivitis**
1. Usually self-limited, but some evidence indicates that treatment with a topical antibiotic shortens its course
2. One rationale for treatment is that it prevents bacterial superinfection
3. Children >2 months: Prescribe broad-spectrum topical eyedrops: Polymyxin B-trimethoprim combination (Polytrim), one or two drops QID x 7 days
4. Topical antiviral drugs are not administered
5. See Patient Education under V.H., below for recommendations regarding patient counseling

B. **Bacterial conjunctivitis**: If treatment is based on clinical evaluation alone (which occurs in the majority of cases), select a broad spectrum topical antibiotic such as ONE of the following, administered 4 times daily for 7-10 days
1. Gentamicin solution (0.3%) [Garamycin, Genoptic, generic]
2. Tobramycin solution (0.3%) [Tobrex, generic]
3. The topical fluoroquinolones, ciprofloxacin and ofloxacin, are also highly effective but should be reserved for severe infections
4. **Note:** Empiric treatment is highly effective and adverse consequences are infrequent

C. **Hyperacute bacterial conjunctivitis**: Immediate referral to an ophthalmologist is required for aggressive management to prevent serious complications; systemic antibiotics (as well as topical antibiotics) are required (systemic antibiotics given for the conjunctivitis will be effective against the genital reservoir of the disease)

D. **Chlamydial conjunctivitis** in adolescents: Prescribe systemic antibiotics—doxycycline (Vibramycin) 100 mg BID for 14 days
1. Once a diagnosis has been established, a genital work-up of the patient and sexual partner is indicated
2. Pregnant and lactating women: Use erythromycin 250 mg QID x 21 days
3. Diagnosis of chlamydial disease in an infant, child, or adolescent should prompt investigation for other sexually transmitted diseases, including syphilis, gonorrhea, hepatitis B, and HIV infection

E. **Chlamydial conjunctivitis** in newborns: Systemic erythromycin is the treatment of choice
1. Oral erythromycin 50 mg/kg/day in 4 divided doses for 14 days
2. Topical treatment of chlamydial conjunctivitis is ineffective and unnecessary
3. See V.D.3. above

F. **Allergic conjunctivitis**
   1. A simple and inexpensive treatment is to remove the offending allergen when possible or diluting it by instilling artificial tears every two or three hours during the acute phase
   2. Prescribe topical and systemic antihistamines to relieve itching
      a. **Topical agent:** Olopatadine HCL (0.1%) [Patanol] solution—combination antihistamine and mast cell stabilizer; children ≥3 years, one drop in affected eye(s) BID
      b. **Systemic agent:** Fexofenadine (Allegra) tabs, children ≥12 years, 60 mg BID; children 6-11 years, 30 mg BID; not recommended for children <6 years of age
   3. Consider prescribing a topical mast-cell stabilizer for chronic conditions such as perennial allergic conjunctivitis. Prescribe cromolyn sodium (Crolom) ophthalmic solution: Children >4 years, 1-2 drops 4 times a day

G. Refer the patient for emergent management by an expert if any of the following occur
   1. There is no improvement in 24 hours
   2. Patient has moderate to severe ocular pain, decreased visual acuity, abnormal eye exam
   3. Infection from herpes simplex virus
   4. Hyperacute bacterial conjunctivitis

H. Patient Education
   1. Instruct patient to instill medication in the inner aspect of the lower eyelid
   2. Teach patient that infection is easily spread to unaffected eye and to other household members
   3. The role of frequent handwashing in limiting the spread of ocular infections cannot be overemphasized
   4. Discuss with patient that eye secretions are contagious for 24 to 48 hours after therapy begins
   5. Patient with viral infection should be instructed that the ocular infection is contagious for at least 7 days after the onset

I. Follow Up
   1. If no improvement in 24 hours, or if condition worsens, patient should return for referral for expert care
   2. No follow up is indicated for mild cases which resolve without problems

HORDEOLUM (STYE)

I. Definition: Focal, acute infection of the eyelid margins

II. Pathogenesis: An acute infectious process involving the meibomian glands or other glands of the eyelid margins usually caused by *Staphylococcus aureus*

III. Clinical Presentation

A. More common in children and adolescents than adults

B. Patient often presents with sudden onset of localized tenderness, redness, and swelling of the eyelid

C. May occur in crops because the infecting pathogen may spread from one hair follicle to another

D. May point to the conjunctival side of the lid (posterior hordeolum involving the meibomian glands) or may involve the lid margin (anterior hordeolum involving the sebaceous or sweat glands)

IV. Diagnosis/Evaluation

A. History
   1. Determine onset and duration of symptoms
   2. Inquire about pain and visual disturbances
   3. Ask about past episodes and previous treatments

B. Physical Examination
   1. Assess visual acuity
   2. Inspect eyelids for inflammation, swelling, and discharge
   3. Palpate eyelids for induration and masses
   4. Evert the eyelid and examine inner surface for pointing
   5. Examine sclera and conjunctiva for abnormalities
   6. Palpate for preauricular adenopathy

C. Differential Diagnosis
   1. Chalazion
   2. Blepharitis

D. Diagnostic Tests: None indicated

V. Plan/Management

A. Apply warm, moist compresses for 15 minutes throughout the day

B. Children >2 months: Prescribe erythromycin 0.5% (Ilotycin or generic) ophthalmic ointment BID-QID x 7 days OR polymyxin B-trimethoprim (Polytrim) drops, 1-2 drops in affected eye BID-QID x 7 days

C. Cleanse eyelids daily with a neutral soap (e.g., Johnson's Baby Shampoo) in a 1:1 solution with clean water

D. If not responsive to medical therapy, refer to expert for incision and drainage

E. If crops of styes occur, diabetes mellitus must be excluded and patient should be told not to rub eyes; some authorities recommend a course of tetracycline to stop recurrences

F. Patient Education
   1. Advise patient that good lid hygiene may help prevent recurrence (see section on BLEPHARITIS for description)
   2. Advise female patients to abstain from wearing eye makeup until clear and disposing of all old make up as it may be contaminated

G. Follow Up: None indicated

STRABISMUS

I. Definition: A general term for abnormal ocular alignment

II. Pathogenesis

A. Abnormal ocular alignment may be due to extraocular muscle weakness, focusing difficulties, unilateral refractive error, nonfusion, or anatomical differences in the eyes

B. Because visual axes are not parallel, the brain receives two images thereby interfering with binocular vision

C. There are three different perceptual phenomena that are integral to the expression of single binocular vision: simultaneous perception, fusion, and stereopsis; they may function simultaneously or in decreasing degrees, with stereopsis being the most highly developed and simultaneous perception the least developed in normal eyes

D. When misalignment is present under binocular conditions, it is a manifest strabismus (tropia); when present under monocular conditions, it is a latent strabismus (phoria)

E. Familial tendencies toward strabismus have been well documented, but no clear-cut genetic mode of inheritance has been identified

III.   Clinical Presentation

A.   Occurs in about 3% of the population; the direction of deviation of the nonfixating deviated eye names the deviation
1.   Horizontal deviations include esotropia (inward deviation) and exotropia (outward deviation)
2.   Vertical deviations include hypertropia (upward deviation) and hypotropia (downward deviation)
3.   Torsional deviations include conditions in which the superior poles of the corneas are tilted either medially or temporally

B.   Whereas the eyes of newborn infants are rarely aligned during the first few weeks of life, by the age of three months, normal oculomotor behavior is usually established and an experienced examiner may be able to document the existence of abnormal alignment by that time

C.   Pseudostrabismus is one of the most common reasons a pediatric ophthalmologist is asked to evaluate an infant
1.   A false appearance of strabismus when visual axes are in reality aligned accurately
2.   Appearance may be due to flat, broad nasal bridge, prominent epicanthal folds, or narrow interpupillary distance
3.   Observer may see less white sclera nasally than expected due to above factors

D.   Esotropia is the condition of inward or convergent deviation of the eyes
1.   Most common type of strabismus and is characterized by nasal deviation of the nonfixating eye
2.   Infantile esotropia begins in infancy (during first 6 months of life) and whether it is congenital or has onset soon after birth is undetermined
3.   Accommodative esotropia (considered an acquired esotropia because it is detected beyond 6 months of age) begins when the child is 6 months to 7 years of age with an average age at onset of 2.5 years and may be intermittent or constant; based on the accommodation reflex
a.   Patients with no refractive error may have nearly perfectly aligned eyes during distance focusing, but develop an esotropia during near focusing because their normal accommodation efforts result in excessive convergence
b.   Patients who are hyperopic will have an esotropia during distance focusing that becomes larger during near focusing, again because of the additional accommodation required

E.   Exotropia is characterized by divergent misalignment of the eyes; occurs much less frequently than does esotropia and may be infantile or acquired; in addition, exotropia may be intermittent or constant
1.   Infantile (or congenital) exotropia has its onset in the first 6 months of life; occurs much less frequently than infantile esotropia
2.   Acquired exotropia refers to any exotropia with an onset after the child reaches 6 months of age; visual function must be assessed because strabismus that is exotropic versus esotropic is more likely to be secondary to a retinoblastoma
3.   Intermittent exotropia is the most common type of exotropia seen in children with an initial onset at about 2-3 years of age
a.   When eyes are aligned, binocular vision may be developing normally
b.   Careful observation by the parents can determine when binocular vision is deteriorating

F.   A discussion of vertical and cyclovertical deviations is beyond the scope of this book

V.   Diagnosis/Evaluation

A.   History
1.   Ask when symptoms were first noticed (age of onset) and what in particular was observed (description of deviation)
2.   Ask about frequency and duration of deviation, symptoms, and previous treatment
3.   Request that parents bring in unposed photos of the child at various ages to help evaluate deviation over time
4.   In infants, ask if child fixates on and follows objects
5.   In infants, ask if fine motor coordination is at appropriate level based on age
6.   Ask if child has abnormal face or head position (head turn or chin tilt may improve acuity or correct diplopia)
7.   Ask if child spontaneously closes one eye (squints) when looking at near or far objects/persons
8.   Ask about presence of eye deviations in blood relatives
9.   In older children, ask if developmental tasks have been achieved at appropriate age

B. Physical Examination
1. Observe for abnormal head posture and spontaneous closure of one eye (squint) when the child interacts with parent, examiner, or inanimate objects (toys)
2. Test for visual acuity (testing both eyes separately) using age-appropriate charts for preschoolers and school-age children and using fixation and following ability to test infants (See section on VISUAL IMPAIRMENT for information on testing)
3. Perform stereopsis testing using the Random Dot E (see section on VISUAL IMPAIRMENT for information on testing)
4. Inspect eyelids, conjunctiva, cornea, height and equality of the level of upper eyelids
5. Assess pupils for shape, size, equality, reaction to light
6. Perform corneal light reflex test. Shine penlight directly in eyes from a distance of about 24 inches; observe the position of the reflection of the light on each cornea with respect to the location of the pupil. Test is based on ability of cornea to reflect the examining light symmetrically
7. Assess extraocular movement using an interesting target that is age appropriate
8. Assess for presence of red reflex (see section on VISUAL IMPAIRMENT for red reflex examination)
9. Perform cover test which depends on the fixation reflex

TECHNIQUE AND INTERPRETATION FOR COVER TESTING

Overview
✓ A prerequisite to cover testing is the ability of each eye to focus when the fellow eye is covered; if organic disease (such as cataract) or functional conditions (for example, eccentric fixation) prevent central fixation, the test is invalid. Because the child begins the test with both eyes viewing, the cover test examines a binocular circumstance

Technique
✓ Have child look at fixation target with both eyes viewing (use interesting toy or picture at about a 24" distance)
✓ Place an occluder over one eye and assess the uncovered eye by answering the following questions:
 • Is fixation central (i.e., does the eye appear to be lined up with the target?)
 • Is fixation steady or did it shift when the other eye was covered?
✓ If fixation is central and steady (no shift occurred), the occluder may have been placed in front of the deviating eye, in which case the fellow eye would already have been fixed on the target
✓ Allow the child to return to binocular vision for several seconds, so that fusion (if it exists) can take place
✓ The second eye is then covered and the first eye is observed for movement

Interpretation
✓ If fixation is not maintained, the shift is evidence that the uncovered eye was not regarding the target with its fovea when both eyes were viewing
✓ This deviation is called a heterotropia, or a manifest deviation (i.e., it exists under normal seeing circumstances, both eyes viewing)

Summary: Sequence of Cover Test
✓ Child's attention is drawn to fixation target
✓ Cover one eye, observing the fellow eye
✓ Uncover that eye and wait for a few seconds to allow fusion (if it exists) to take place
✓ Cover the second eye while observing the first eye

C. Differential Diagnosis: Pseudostrabismus, cranial nerve palsies (III, IV, or V), and numerous strabismic syndromes

D. Diagnostic Tests: There are many diagnostic tests in strabismus; many of the tests involve eliciting diplopia or double vision as a means of evaluation. Additional diagnostic testing should be done by a pediatric ophthalmologist

V. Plan/Management

A. All children in whom strabismus is suspected must be evaluated by a pediatric ophthalmologist

B. Treatment varies with the type of deviation; interventions include correction of the refractive error, local botulinum A toxin injection, orthoptics (eye muscle exercises), use of prisms (more common in older children and adults), and surgery

C. Surgery typically involves recession or resection of the extraocular muscles; more than one procedure may be necessary to attain adequate alignment

D. Follow up is by an ophthalmologist

VISUAL IMPAIRMENT

I. Definition: A decline in vision in one or both eyes

II. Pathogenesis

A. Etiology of impaired vision can be divided into two general categories
   1. Refractive errors or those problems that can be improved by glasses (common causes: myopia, hyperopia, anisometropia, and astigmatism)
   2. Non-refractive errors (retinal abnormalities, glaucoma, cataract, retinoblastoma, eye muscle imbalance, neurological disorders, and systemic diseases with ocular manifestations) that cannot be corrected by glasses alone

B. For clear vision, light must focus precisely on the retina
   1. In nearsightedness, or myopia, light is focused in front of the retina and the person sees near objects best
   2. In farsightedness, or hyperopia, light is focused behind the retina and the person sees far objects best

C. **Myopia** is a condition in which objects can be seen clearly if held close enough to the eye (the person is "nearsighted"); person typically has no problem with reading or close work but distance vision is blurred

D. **Hyperopia** is called farsightedness, and means that the individual cannot see near objects; because children have strong focusing or accommodative mechanisms that enable them to overcome moderate amounts of hyperopia and still maintain clear vision, this condition is relatively uncommon in children

E. **Anisometropia** is a state in which there is a difference in the refractive error of the two eyes; condition may be congenital or acquired (due to asymmetric age changes or disease)

F. **Astigmatism** is a condition in which curvature variations of the optical system result in unequal light refraction and impaired vision

G. Pathophysiology of conditions causing non-refractive errors is dependent on the condition

III. Clinical Presentation

A. Refractive errors requiring the use of corrective lenses exist in almost 20% of the pediatric population

B. Children with refractive errors most often have difficulty with far vision. Typically, the child is unable to read the blackboard from back of the room, or see movie from back of the theater; squinting, which creates a pinhole aperture effect, suggests the presence of an uncorrected refractive error, most often myopia

C. **Myopia** is the most common clinically significant refractive error seen in childhood
   1. Condition is rarely present at birth
   2. Often begins to develop as the child grows and is usually detected by age 9 or 10 in school vision testing
   3. Usually stabilizes in mid-teens, at about 5 diopters or less

D. **Hyperopia** usually does not necessitate correction in children unless it causes the eyes to cross, or causes reduced vision

E. In **anisometropia,** the visual acuity differences between the two eyes may result in suppression strabismus or amblyopia

F. **Astigmatism** can begin in childhood and can be easily corrected if it causes blurred vision or eye discomfort

G. Children with non-refractive errors have impaired vision at both near and far distances
   1. Children with open-angle glaucoma are usually asymptomatic until neural damage has occurred; visual dysfunction in glaucoma is first expressed in the mid-peripheral field of vision (central vision functions such as acuity remain relatively intact until late in the disease process)
   2. Children with cataract may be observed to have nystagmus of the wandering or searching type (nystagmus of the blind)
   3. Young children with impaired vision from both refractive and non-refractive causes rarely complain but may rub the eye (if pain present) or may squint
   4. See STRABISMUS and AMBLYOPIA for more information on impaired vision due to these causes

H. A faulty visual system has a major impact on children's intellectual and physical development, since vision provides almost 80% of the sensory input during the first years of life

I. Visual acuity correctable by glasses or contact lenses to 20/200 or less in both eyes, or visual fields in both eyes less than 10 degrees centrally, constitutes legal blindness in the US

IV. Diagnosis/Evaluation

A. History
   1. Determine if vision in one or both eyes is impaired and if both near and far vision are affected
   2. Ask if there are associated symptoms of eye discomfort, increased tearing or cloudy vision
   3. In infants and toddlers, ask parent if vision seems normal
      a. Ask if there are any behaviors present that suggest vision is a problem (e.g., does he look at things at an unusually close distance? Does he squint?)
      b. Ask regarding achievement of developmental tasks particularly in the area of eye-hand (fine motor) coordination
   4. In school-age child, ask about school performance, reading ability, and teacher's observations about child's visual acuity
   5. Ask about chronic or past eye problems, previous treatments, and response
   6. Ask if there is a family history of eye disease

B. Physical Examination
   1. Examine external eye and lid for swelling, ptosis, injection of the conjunctiva, and corneal clarity
   2. Determine extraocular movement: In infants and young children, have them fixate on and follow a brightly colored or interesting object
   3. Measure peripheral vision (recognizing that this is only a very gross assessment of visual fields)
      a. Very young children can be tested by using a threatening gesture from the periphery and observing response
      b. Older children (even those as young as 3 years) can be tested by direct confrontation

---

Peripheral Visual Field Testing

✓ Test unilaterally (eye not being tested is covered with occluder)

✓ Continually tell child to look at examiner's nose, who is seated 3 feet in front of the child with eyes at the same level

✓ The examiner presents two closed hands in different visual field quadrants, thus the child is not automatically drawn to the quadrant to be tested

✓ Then, the examiner flashes 1, 2, or 5 fingers in the peripheral quadrant to be tested, more quickly than the child can shift the view into that quadrant (child is looking at examiner's nose)

✓ If the child correctly identifies the number of fingers presented in all quadrants, the visual field is recorded as full to finger counting (FTFC)

✓ An alternative for the younger child (if counting is too difficult) is to wiggle two fingers in the quadrant to be tested and ask the child to find the wiggly fingers

---

   4. Infants and young children, perform the cover test (described in detail under STRABISMUS)
   5. Perform corneal light reflex test (refer to Physical Exam section in STRABISMUS for more information)
   6. Elicit red reflex (see technique below) and perform ophthalmoscopic exam (ophthalmoscopy may be possible in very cooperative children as young as 3-4 years old who are willing to fixate on a toy while evaluation of the optic nerve and retinal vasculature in the posterior pole of the eye is completed)
   7. Perform visual acuity and stereoacuity testing (in preschool and school-aged children) as described in the tables that follow

KEY POINTS TO KEEP IN MIND IN THE ASSESSMENT OF VISUAL ACUITY

General Principles for Testing

- The child should be in good health and younger children (3-5 years) should be in a cooperative mood at the time of the examination
- Testing distance of 10 feet (except for the Allen cards—a test using flash cards) is recommended as this may result in better compliance due to closer interaction with the examiner
- Each eye must be tested independently, with the nontested eye occluded
- For older children and adolescents, use of a paddle occluder is usually satisfactory
- For young children, commercially available occluder patches provide complete occlusion necessary for appropriate testing
- Tell child to keep both eyes open (the nontested eye should be kept open beneath the occlusion)
- Children who wear corrective eyeglasses should be tested wearing the eyeglasses, unless the glasses were prescribed only for reading)

Recommended Tests

Tests are listed in decreasing order of cognitive difficulty; the highest test that the child is capable of performing should be used; in general, the Snellen letters or numbers should be used for children 6 years and older, the tumbling E or the HOTV test should be used for children 3-5 years of age

- ✓ Snellen letters
- ✓ Snellen numbers
- ✓ Tumbling E (works well for the 4 or 5 year old)
- ✓ HOTV (good test for 3 year old or 4-5 year old who is shy)

- ✓ Picture tests (best choice for the 3 year old)
  - Allen figures
  - Lea symbols

Children 6 Years and Older: Measure distance visual acuity using a Snellen Acuity Chart (letters or numbers)

- Test the right eye first by covering the left. Have the child read the practice line with the right eye; if the child fails the practice line, move up the chart to the next larger line
- If the child fails this line, continue moving up chart until a line is reached that the child can read
- Then, move down the chart, line by line, until the child fails to read a line
- To pass a line, the child must identify 4 of 6 symbols on the line correctly
- Repeat the procedure, testing the left eye, and covering the right eye

Referral Criteria for Children 6 Years and Older

Fewer than 4 of 6 correct on 15-ft line with either eye tested at 10 ft monocularly (i.e., less than 10/15 or 20/30) *or* two-line difference between eyes, even within the passing range (i.e., 10/10 and 10/15 or 20/20 and 20/30)

Children Ages 3-5 Years: Measure distance visual acuity using Tumbling E, HOTV, or Picture Tests (Allen or Lea)

- Prior to the exam, some preparation can be helpful in this age group; parents can demonstrate the anticipated testing procedures to the child as a way of preparing for the exam

Information for parents (and clinicians) about visual acuity testing in children is available from the following source:

American Academy of Ophthalmology
PO Box 7424, San Francisco, CA 94109
415-561-8500   http://www.aao.org

For specific information about the tumbling E and *Preschoolers Home Eye Test* (parents can obtain practice Es, and tumbling E wall chart):

Prevent Blindness America
500 East Remington Road, Schaumburg, IL 60173
847-843-2020   http://www.preventblindness.com

- Materials and methods for specific tests used in this age group vary, but in general, pretest is performed binocularly and is for the purpose of testing the child's ability to identify or match the symbols on a line that is expected to be suprathreshold (10/100 or greater); child must be able to identify or match 4 of 6 symbols in order to continue
- Testing procedure follows the same general format as described above for Snellen test

Referral Criteria for Children Ages 3-5

Fewer than 4 of 6 correct on 20-ft line with either eye tested at 10 ft monocularly (i.e., less than 10/20 or 20/40) *or* two-line difference between lines within the passing range (i.e., 10/12.5 and 10/20 or 20/25 and 20/40)

Children Ages 0 to 3 Years:

- In performing visual assessment in this age group, keep in mind that vision can be assessed no matter the age or cognitive ability of the child if age and cognitively appropriate testing is used
- From birth onward, infants prefer looking at the human face to looking at other objects; this preference can be helpful to the examiner who needs a visual target that attracts the infant
- Birth to 4 weeks of age, vision assessment is limited to uniocular reaction to light—either withdrawal, blinking, or pupil constriction
- At 4-6 weeks of age, a term infant will develop central fixation, followed very soon by visual tracking
- Thus, in children between 6 weeks of age and approximately 3 years, the quality of visual fixation, one eye at a time, is the best method for evaluating vision (many 2.5 year old children will cooperate for objective visual acuity testing if an age-appropriate test is utilized)
- Determine whether each eye can fixate on an object, maintain fixation, and then follow the object into various gaze positions
- Visual fixation patterns vary by age, and examiner experience based on examining many children in each age group is necessary in order to appreciate these pattern differences
- To illustrate, a normal 6-week-old can maintain fixation on an interesting object such as a face for just a few seconds before shifting focus; a one-year-old child will consistently gaze at an interesting object, attentively follow the object as it is moved in peripheral gaze, and even reach for the object
- The child's ability to perform these maneuvers are noted as fix and follow (F&F), or central, steady, and maintained (CSM) fixation

Referral Criteria for Children Ages 0-3 Years

A child's failure to perform these maneuvers (based on age-appropriate testing) indicates a need for immediate referral

Adapted from American Academy of Pediatrics. (2003). Eye examination in infants, children, and young adults by pediatricians. *Pediatrics, 111*, 902-907.

RED REFLEX TEST AND SIMULTANEOUS RED REFLEX TEST (BRUCKNER TEST)

Purpose: To detect (1) abnormalities of back of eye, (2) opacities in the visual axis (e.g., cataract, corneal opacity), and (3) amblyogenic conditions such as strabismus

Technique: To maximize pupil dilation in the child, the room should be darkened; the child should be comfortably seated
The direct ophthalmoscope is focused on **each pupil** individually approximately 12 to 18 inches away from the eye
Next, **both eyes** are viewed simultaneously through the direct ophthalmoscope at approximately 3 feet away with the child fixating on the ophthalmoscope light

Interpretation:
  ✓ When each eye individually is tested, the examiner should observe for dark spots in the red reflex, a blunted (dull) red reflex, lack of red reflex, or presence of a white reflex—any of which indicate a need for referral
      Note: False positive tests are common because of small pupils, uncooperative children, difficulties in interpretation of test, variation in color of the reflex due to normal variations in the color of the retinal pigmentation

  ✓ When the eyes are viewed together with the child focusing on the ophthalmoscope light (Bruckner test), the examiner should observe for any asymmetry in color, brightness, or size—all indications for referral for a possible amblyogenic condition

Examples of normal and abnormal Bruckner test appearances are available for purchase at http://www.aap.org/sections/ophthal.htm

Adapted from American Academy of Pediatrics. (2003). Eye examination in infants, children, and young adults by pediatricians. *Pediatrics, 111*, 902-907.

EVALUATION OF STEREOPSIS IN PRESCHOOL AND SCHOOL-AGE CHILDREN

Stereograms such as the Random Dot E (RDE) test are fundamentally different from the light reflex test or the cover test which detect physical misalignment of the eyes; stereopsis can be absent in patients with straight eyes

Testing Procedure
Child wears Polaroid glasses while viewing the test cards which are held about 16 inches from the child's eyes; all testing, including pretesting should be performed binocularly with the glasses on (if eyeglasses are worn, place the Polaroid glasses over them)

During the pretest, establish the child's ability to perform the test by having her identify the location of the legs on the 3-dimensional E on 4 of 6 trials (E on left, right, above, or below)

The test consists of having the child identify the location of the stereo E. Tester should use 6 presentations, varying a location in a nonsystematic manner

The child must correctly locate the stereo E on 4 of 6 presentations in order to pass the test

The actual test (not counting pretest time) takes about 1 minute
A more detailed test procedure is contained in the Random Dot E test kit

Adapted from American Academy of Pediatrics. (2003). Eye examination in infants, children, and young adults by pediatricians. *Pediatrics, 111*, 902-907.

    C.   Differential Diagnosis
        1.   Refractive errors
        2.   Non-refractive errors (common causes: strabismus and amblyopia)

    D.   Diagnostic Tests: None indicated other than those described under V.B. above

V.   Plan/Management

    A.   Infants and children who demonstrate any abnormality on the above testing should be referred for further evaluation (see table for "Referral Criteria" by age group and test)

    B.   Children with acute onset of impaired vision need immediate referral for emergency care

    C.   Follow Up: Variable depending on physical examination findings and need for referral

REFERENCES

American Academy of Pediatrics (2002). Policy statement: Red reflex examination in infants. *Pediatrics, 109,* 980-981.

American Academy of Pediatrics. (2000). Preschool vision screening: Summary of a task force report. *Pediatrics, 106,* 1105-1113.

American Academy of Pediatrics. (2003). Eye examination in infants, children, and young adults by pediatricians. *Pediatrics, 111,* 902-907.

Centers for Disease Control and Prevention. (2002). Sexually transmitted diseases treatment guidelines. *MMWR, 51* (No. RR-6): 1-82.

Curnyn, K.M., & Kaufman, L.M. (2003). The eye examination in the pediatrician's office. *Pediatric Clinics of North America, 50,* 25-40.

Friedman, L.S., & Kaufman, L.M. (2003). Guidelines for pediatrician referrals to the ophthalmologist. *Pediatric Clinics of North America, 50,* 41-53.

Goroll, A.H., & Mulley, A.G. (2002). *Primary care medicine recommendations.* Philadelphia: Lippincott Williams & Wilkins.

Green, M., & Palfrey, J.S. (Eds.). (2002). *Bright futures: guidelines for health supervision of infants, children, and adolescents* (2nd ed.). Arlington, VA: National Center for Education in Maternal and Child Health.

Greenberg, M.F., & Pollard, Z.F. (2003). The red eye in childhood. *Pediatric Clinics of North America, 50,* 105-124.

Jockin, Y.M. (2002). Strabismus and amblyopia. In F.D. Burg, J.R. Ingelfinger, R.A. Polin, & A.A. Gershon (Eds.), *Current pediatric therapy* (17th ed., pp. 915-916). Philadelphia: Saunders.

Katowitz, J.A. & Goldstein, J.B. (2002). Nasolacrimal duct stenosis. In F.D. Burg, J.R. Ingelfinger, R.A. Polin, & A.A. Gershon (Eds.), *Current pediatric therapy* (17th ed., pp. 900-901). Philadelphia: Saunders.

Lanternier, M.L. (2002). Ophthalmology. In M.A. Graber & M.L. Lanternier (Eds.), *University of Iowa: The family practice handbook* (pp. 699-711). St. Louis: Mosby.

Leibowitz, H.M. (2000). The red eye. *New England Journal of Medicine, 343,* 345-351.

McManaway, J.A. & Frankel, C.A. (2001). Red eye. In R.A. Hoekelman, H.M. Adams, N.M. Nelson, M.L. Weitzman, & M. H. Wilson (Eds.), Pediatric primary care (pp.1240-1246). St. Louis: Mosby.

McManaway, J.A. & Frankel, C.A. (2001). Strabismus. In R.A. Hoekelman, H.M. Adams, N.M. Nelson, M.L. Weitzman, & M. H. Wilson (Eds.), Pediatric primary care (pp.1253-1259). St. Louis: Mosby.

Pavan-Langson, D. (2002). Ocular examination techniques and diagnostic tests. In D. Pavan-Langson (Ed.), *Manual of ocular diagnosis and therapy* (pp. 1-20). Philadelphia: Lippincott Williams & Wilkins.

Pavan-Langson, D. & Azaar, N. (2002). Extraocular muscles, strabismus, and nystagmus. In D. Pavan-Langson (Ed.), *Manual of ocular diagnosis and therapy* (pp. 332-364). Philadelphia: Lippincott Williams & Wilkins.

Peterson, R.A., & Boger, W.P. (2002). Pediatric ophthalmology. In D. Pavan-Langson (Ed.), *Manual of ocular diagnosis and therapy* (pp. 286-331). Philadelphia: Lippincott Williams & Wilkins.

Rubin, P.A. (2002). Eyelids and lacrimal system. In D. Pavan-Langson (Ed.), *Manual of ocular diagnosis and therapy* (pp. 47-55). Philadelphia: Lippincott Williams & Wilkins.

Simon, J.W., & Kaw, P. (2001). Commonly missed diagnoses in the childhood eye examination. *American Family Physician, 64,* 623-628.

US Preventive Services Task Force. (1996). *Guide to clinical preventive services.* (2nd ed.). Baltimore: Williams & Wilkins.

Problems of the Ears, Nose, Sinuses, Throat, Mouth, and Neck

CONSTANCE R. UPHOLD

FOREIGN BODY IN EAR

I. Definition: Presence of object(s) in the external auditory canal

II. Pathogenesis

    A. Intentional placement of object into ear usually due to curiosity, boredom, or imitation of others

    B. Accidental entry of foreign body can occur during play; insects may fly into ear

III. Clinical presentation

    A. Children 2-4 years of age are most likely to have foreign bodies in the ear

    B. Symptoms depend on depth of object, nature and composition of object, and duration in the canal
        1. Nonreactive substances such as plastic do not usually cause any symptoms
        2. Insects usually cause discomfort, erythema, and sometimes drainage
        3. Vegetable matter may cause itching and minor pain
        4. Alkaline batteries may leak acid and result in pain, swelling, and discharge
        5. Decreased hearing may occur if the object is large or causes swelling

    C. Complications are uncommon; otitis media, perforation of tympanic membrane, and development of cholesteatoma may occur

IV. Diagnosis/Evaluation

    A. History
        1. Inquire about onset, duration, and character of symptoms
        2. Determine if there is a history of placing objects in ear

    B. Physical Examination; perform a thorough examination of the ear
        1. If foreign body is suspected, but cannot be visualized, instill water to fill the medial half of the external canal; this may allow visualization of the tympanic sulcus in which objects often become lodged
        2. Inspect auditory canal and tympanic membrane for signs of inflammation and injury

    C. Differential Diagnosis
        1. Otitis externa
        2. Otitis media

V. Plan/Management

    A. Removal of nonreactive foreign bodies
        1. Stabilize patient's head
        2. Use alligator forceps under direct visualization with an operating head otoscope to remove object; pulling the pinna superiorly and laterally will facilitate removal
        3. Gentle irrigation with warm water may also be used if tympanic membrane (TM) is intact and there is no inflammation in the external canal
        4. Direct stream around the object and position patient such that gravity will help drainage
        5. **Do not irrigate if foreign body is vegetable matter** as these objects tend to swell when water is applied
        6. Frazier tip suction can also be used to retrieve objects

    B. For round, smooth objects, place a curette with a curved end behind object and gently pull out

    C. Live insects should be killed by instilling mineral oil into ear before extraction with suction or alligator forceps

    D. Alkaline batteries should be removed immediately; magnets may facilitate removal

E. Following removal of object perform the following:
1. Carefully inspect tympanic ear and external auditory canal
2. If there are any signs of inflammation or injury and TM is intact; instill 2% acetic acid otic solution (VoSoL Otic) 5 drops QID X 5-7 days or polymyxin B sulfate, neomycin, hydrocortisone (Cortisporin Otic suspension); 3-4 drops in canal, QID x 7 days (use 3 drops in children)

F. Refer to otorhinolaryngologist if foreign body cannot be removed after several attempts, if moderate or severe injury to ear has occurred, if child has severe pain, or if child cannot remain still and needs general anesthesia for removal

G. Follow Up: Evaluate patient in 2-3 days if there are signs of inflammation or injury to the ear, otherwise no follow up is needed unless patient has problems

HEARING LOSS

I. Definitions: Reduction in a person's ability to perceive sound

A. Hearing loss is measured according to hearing thresholds (the softest tone heard by patient at a given frequency) during pure tone audiometric testing
1. Normal hearing: 0 to 25 dB
2. Mild impairment: 26 to 40 dB
3. Moderate impairment: 41 to 55 dB
4. Moderately severe: 56 to 70 dB
5. Severe: 71 to 90 dB
6. Profound: 91 dB and above

B. Conductive hearing loss occurs when sound is inadequately conducted through the external or middle ear to the sensorineural apparatus of the inner ear; conductive hearing loss occurs when there is interference with the mechanical reception or amplification of sound

C. Sensorineural hearing loss occurs when sound is normally carried through the external and middle ear but there is a defect within the inner ear or eighth cranial nerve which results in sound distortion

II. Pathogenesis

A. Common causes of conductive hearing loss
1. Impacted cerumen
2. Foreign bodies
3. Otitis externa
4. Benign tumors of middle ear
5. Carcinoma of external auditory canal and/or middle ear
6. Eustachian tube dysfunction
7. Otitis media
8. Perforation of the tympanic membrane
9. Serous otitis media with effusion
10. Otosclerosis
11. Cholesteatoma
12. Tuberculosis of the temporal bone

B. Common causes of sensorineural hearing loss
1. Congenital and neonatal hearing loss may be hereditary (albinism, Alport's syndrome, User's syndrome, or Waardenburg syndrome) or caused by maternal rubella, prematurity, traumatic delivery, or other infections during the perinatal period
2. Noise exposure
3. Ménière's disease (see DIZZINESS section)
4. Acoustic tumors (see DIZZINESS section), tumor of eighth cranial nerve
5. Opportunistic infections of the temporal bone may occur in patients with acquired immunodeficiency syndrome

6. Other diseases
    a. Syphilis
    b. Paget's disease
    c. Collagen diseases
    d. Endocrine disease such as diabetes mellitus or hypothyroidism
    e. Bacterial meningitis
    f. Tuberculosis of the temporal bone
7. Basilar migraines
8. Viral illnesses such as mumps, cytomegalovirus, and herpes zoster
9. Demyelinating processes such as multiple sclerosis
10. Drug ototoxicities
    a. Antibiotics such as streptomycin, neomycin, gentamicin, and vancomycin
    b. Diuretics such as ethacrynic acid and furosemide
    c. Salicylates
    d. Antineoplastic agents such as cisplatin
11. Trauma such as skull fracture or tympanic membrane perforation

III. Clinical presentation of common causes of hearing loss

A. Epidemiology and clinical consequences in children
    1. Approximately 1 of every 1000 infants has bilateral sensorineural hearing loss (SNHL)
    2. Diagnosis of congenital hearing loss is often delayed
        a. In infants, hearing loss of 30 dB and greater is important for speech recognition
        b. Hearing loss may delay development in language, learning, and speech; these delays lead to lifelong problems in school performance, and later, in work situations; early identification and appropriate treatment within the first 6 months can prevent these adverse consequences

B. In conductive hearing loss (most common), sensitivity to sound is diminished, but clarity is unchanged; if volume is increased to compensate for loss, the hearing is normal
    1. Serous otitis media
        a. Most frequent cause in children
        b. Patient usually has fullness and decreased hearing in one or both ears
    2. Otosclerosis is associated with slow, progressive hearing loss (usually bilateral) beginning in second or third decade of life
        a. Most common cause of progressive conductive hearing loss in young adults
        b. Hereditary condition of unknown etiology in which there is an irregular ossification in the bony labyrinth of the inner ear, particularly of the stapes
        c. Patients have tinnitus and hearing loss which may progress to deafness
        d. On physical examination, the tympanic membrane (TM) is normal
    3. Cholesteatoma
        a. Benign, slowly growing lesion in the middle ear or mastoid that destroys bone and normal ear tissue
        b. Chronic drainage that fails to resolve with antibiotics is typical presentation

C. Sensorineural hearing loss results in decreased sound sensitivity to high frequencies
    1. Noise-induced hearing loss (second most common cause) is due to excessive noise exposure in the workplace or during recreation
        a. Loss is permanent and not fully treatable, but is 100% preventable
        b. Early in condition there is isolated pure tone loss at 4000 Hz unilaterally or bilaterally
        c. Pure tone loss progresses to other frequencies with increased exposure
    2. Acoustic neuroma presents with tinnitus, unilateral unexplained hearing loss, and disequilibrium (see DIZZINESS section)
    3. Ménière's disease is characterized by episodic vertigo, fluctuating sensorineural hearing loss, and roaring tinnitus (see DIZZINESS section)

IV. Diagnosis/Evaluation

A. History (parental concern has good predictive value)
    1. For infants, ask parents:
        a. If child has inappropriate response to sound such as lack of eye blinking, startling, head turning, or eye widening
        b. If there was any birth trauma, anoxia, and prenatal or perinatal infections such as rubella or cytomegalovirus
        c. If infant babbles (absence of babbling by 6 months of age is abnormal)

2. Ask parents if child must watch television with increased volume and question about school performance and development
3. Question about nature of the hearing loss (unilateral vs bilateral; rapid or slow progression; acute vs. chronic; fluctuating vs. constant)
4. Determine what sounds the patient has most trouble hearing; difficulty understanding spoken words suggests sensorineural hearing loss
5. Inquire about associated symptoms such as fever, ear pain, discharge from ear, vertigo, tinnitus, and neurologic disturbances
6. Explore predisposing factors such as trauma, barotrauma (air plane travel or diving), antecedent infections, and medication use
7. Ask about excessive noise exposure; for employed adolescents, ask if patient must shout at work to converse with someone at arm's length (indicates a potentially harmful noise level)
8. Obtain a thorough past medical history
9. Ask about family history of hearing loss and neoplastic diseases
10. Inquire about the impact of the hearing loss on activities of daily living

B. Physical Examination
1. Examine the skin; abnormal pigmentation may be associated with hearing loss, as in Waardenburg syndrome
2. Carefully examine the head, neck, and cranial nerves; abnormalities are often present in children with congenital or hereditary hearing loss; the following findings are associated with hearing impairment:
   a. Heterochromia of the irises
   b. Malformation of the auricle or ear canal
   c. Dimpling or skin tags around the auricle
   d. Cleft lip or palate
   e. Asymmetry or hypoplasia of the facial structures
   f. Microcephaly
3. Examine the nasopharynx
4. Perform visual examination of TM and external auditory canal
5. Perform pneumatic otoscopy to determine mobility of TM
6. Perform clinical hearing test: whispered voice should be done with the patient using a finger to occlude the opposite ear to prevent crossover
7. For infants, clap hands and watch for response of child (eye blinking, head turning, etc.)
8. Perform Weber and Rinne tests (see table that follows)

TUNING FORK TESTS

	Weber Test	Rinne Test
Procedure	Strike fork and hold in middle of forehead or apex of skull and ask patient to localize sound	Strike fork, then place firmly on mastoid tip (measure of bone conduction [BC]); ask patient to raise hand when sound is no longer present; then move fork so that it resonates beside ear (measure of air conduction [AC])
Conductive Loss	Sound louder in ear in which patient perceives the hearing loss	In affected ear, sound is louder when on mastoid tip than beside ear (BC>AC)
Sensorineural Loss	Sound louder in unaffected ear	In normal ear and ear with sensorineural hearing loss, the sound is louder beside the ear than on the mastoid tip (AC>BC)

9. Complete head, neck, and cranial nerve examinations are often indicated; craniofacial and ophthalmic abnormalities are often present in children with congenital or hereditary hearing loss
10. Assess developmental level; determine whether child has attained the expected speech-language auditory-milestones (see table that follows)

EXPECTED SPEECH-LANGUAGE-AUDITORY MILESTONES	
Age	**Milestone**
Birth to 3 months	Awakens to sounds Startles to loud noises Blinks eyes reflexively to noises
3-4 months	Quiets to parents' voices Stops playing and listens and looks for sources of new sounds
6-9 months	Coos and gurgles with inflection Says "mama"
12-15 months	Follows simple commands Uses expressive vocabulary of 3-5 words Imitates some sounds
18-24 months	Knows body parts Uses expressive vocabulary of 2-word phrases
By 36 months	Uses expressive vocabulary of 4- to 5-word sentences Understands some verbs

C. Differential Diagnosis: See common causes of hearing loss under pathogenesis; important to determine the following:
  1. Is hearing loss acute versus chronic? (acute hearing loss almost always requires immediate intervention such as removal of cerumen or treatment with antibiotics for otitis media)
  2. Is hearing loss conductive versus sensorineural?

D. Diagnostic Tests
  1. Hearing screening prior to hospital discharge at birth:
    a. Joint Committee for Infant Hearing (JCIH) and the American Academy of Pediatrics (but not the United States Preventive Services Task Force [USPSTF]) recommend universal newborn hearing screening; for locations where newborn hearing screening programs are unavailable, the JCIH recommends referrals for hearing tests among infants with the following risk factors:
      (1) ICU admission of 48 hours or greater
      (2) Stigmata or other findings associated with a syndrome known to include sensorineural and/or conductive hearing loss
      (3) Family history of permanent childhood sensorineural hearing loss
      (4) Craniofacial anomalies
      (5) *In utero* infection such as cytomegalovirus, herpes, toxoplasmosis, rubella
    b. Infants who do not pass birth admission screen or other rescreening should have audiological and medical evaluations to confirm hearing loss before 3 months
  2. Hearing screening following hospital discharge; JCIH recommends that neonates and infants at risk for hearing loss who passed birth screen should receive audiologic monitoring every 6 months until age 3; following are risk factor indicators:
    a. Parental or caregiver concern about hearing, speech, language, or development (most important factor to consider)
    b. Family history of permanent childhood hearing loss
    c. Stigmata of other findings associated with syndrome known to include hearing loss (Down syndrome, Waardenburg syndrome)
    d. Ear and other craniofacial anomalies
    e. Low Apgar scores: 0-3 at 5 minutes; 0-6 at 10 minutes
    f. Postnatal infections associated with hearing loss such as bacterial meningitis
    g. *In utero* infections
    h. Neonatal indicators – specifically hyperbilirubinemia, persistent pulmonary hypertension associated with mechanical ventilation, and conditions requiring the use of extracorporeal membrane oxygenation
    i. Syndromes associated with progressive hearing loss (neurofibromatosis, osteopetrosis, and Usher's syndrome)
    j. Neurodegenerative disorders or sensory motor neuropathies

          k.   Head trauma
          l.   Recurrent or persistent otitis media with effusion for at least 3 months
          m.   Ototoxic medication

3. All newborns who receive routine care should ideally be evaluated for hearing loss before discharge from the hospital with one physiologic measure (otoacoustic emissions [OAEs] and/or auditory brainstem response [ABR])

    a. Both OAE and ABR are tests of auditory pathway structural integrity but are not true tests of hearing

    b. Even if ABR and OAE tests are normal, hearing cannot be definitely assessed as normal until child is old enough for audiometry

4. Behavioral pure tone audiometry is the gold standard of the hearing examination

    a. Children 9-12 months can be screened with conditioned oriented response (COR) or visual reinforced audiometry (VRA)

    b. Children 2-4 years can be tested with play audiometry

    c. Children >4 years can be tested with pure-tone audiometry

       (1) Pure-tone audiometry characterizes the extent of impairment; air-conduction and bone-conduction measurements are made for sounds of varying intensity (decibels) and frequency (Hertz or cps): Indicated for all cases of chronic hearing loss and in cases of acute hearing loss with uncertain etiology

       (2) Noise-induced hearing loss: high frequency loss, greatest at 4000 cycles and improvement at 8000 cycles

       (3) Conductive hearing loss: low frequency hearing loss (125-500 cycles)

5. Other tests used for diagnosis or to evaluate the extent of hearing loss:

    a. Behavioral tests can be performed in infants >6 months: common tests use sound generators and observation of the auropalpebral reflex, the startle reflex, and arousal

    b. Vestibular testing should be considered if there are symptoms of tinnitus and vertigo: electronystagmometry, rotational tests, and posturography are useful adjuncts

    c. Computerized tomography should be considered if tumors and bony lesions are suspected

    d. If acoustic neuroma is suspected, order magnetic resonance imaging

    e. Order fluorescent treponemal-antibody-absorption test if there is a possibility of late latent syphilis

    f. Tympanometry should be considered to assess TM stiffness

    g. Impedance audiometry evaluates middle ear function by testing tympanic membrane compliance and acoustic reflex thresholds

V. Plan/Management

A. Infants with hearing loss:

    1. Enroll in a family-centered early intervention program before 6 months

    2. Begin use of amplification when appropriate and agreed on by the family within one month of confirmation of hearing loss

    3. Enroll in program to achieve language development

B. Referral to otolaryngologist is needed for patients with acute hearing loss who do not have an apparent diagnosis or for patients with apparent treatable acute or chronic causes for hearing loss who do not improve with standard treatments

C. Referral to audiologist is needed for patients with chronic deficits who may benefit from a hearing device

D. Many patients with otosclerosis and congenital or acquired causes of conductive hearing loss can be helped by surgical procedures

E. Aural rehabilitation is often beneficial for patients with sensorineural hearing loss

    1. Hearing aids are the mainstay of therapy

    2. Inexpensive auditory amplifiers are available and include telephone receiver amplifiers and radio and television earphones

    3. Cochlear implants stimulate the eighth cranial nerve directly and can provide sound awareness for patients with severe hearing loss

    4. Lip reading and sign language may be helpful

    5. Tinnitus may be relieved by masking it with background music or with "tinnitus retraining therapy" (sound therapy such as hearing aids combined with skilled counseling)

F.   Patient education
1.   Discuss ways to enhance communication such as facing patient, obtaining his/her attention before speaking, speaking slowly, using gestures, and only speaking louder or moving closer if the patient states that it is helpful
2.   Some patients have difficulty in discriminating consonants; take time to carefully enunciate all words to patient
3.   Because many patients are embarrassed about wearing a hearing aid, emphasize that today's hearing aids are small, less noticeable, and more efficient
4.   Discuss prevention of hearing loss
a.   Ear plugs or fluid-filled ear muffs with tight seal may reduce noise by 10-30 dB
b.   People vary in their susceptibility to noise-induced trauma, but typically if sound causes pain, tinnitus, or temporary blocking of ear, extended exposure to this noise will cause permanent hearing loss
c.   Limit exposure to loud noise; prolonged or repeated exposure to any noise above 85 dB can cause hearing loss; most lawn mowers, motorcycles, chain saws, and powerboats produce noise >85 dB; personal stereos, rock concerts, and firecrackers may produce noise at 140 dB or more
5.   Sources of patient information (see following table)

WEBSITE RESOURCES ON HEARING LOSS AND TINNITUS	
Organization	Website
American Academy of Audiology	www.audiology.org
American Academy of Otolaryngology-Head & Neck Surgery	www.aao-hns.org
American Speech-Language-Hearing Association	www.asha.org
American Tinnitus Association	www.ata.org
National Campaign for Hearing Health	www.hearinghealth.net/pages/home
National Institute on Deafness and Other Communication Disorders (National Institutes of Health)	www.nidcd.nih.gov
Self Help for Hard of Hearing People, Inc.	www.shhh.org

G.   Follow up is dependent on the type and cause of the hearing loss

IMPACTED CERUMEN

I.   Definition: Obstruction of the ear canal by cerumen (earwax)

II.   Pathogenesis

A.   Cerumen is produced by the ceruminous glands in the outer portion of the canal and is a naturally occurring lubricant and protectant of the external ear canal

B.   While cerumen is normally cleared from the ears through the body's natural mechanisms, excessive accumulation may occur and partially or totally occlude the canal

III.   Clinical Presentation

A.   Ear pain may be present if cerumen hardens and touches the tympanic membrane, or if the external canal is irritated by build up of hardened cerumen

B.   Symptoms may include pain, itching, and sensation of fullness on the affected side; conductive hearing loss may also be present with total occlusion of the canal

IV. Diagnosis/Evaluation

    A. History
        1. Ask about onset, and if ear discomfort or a feeling of fullness is present
        2. Ask patient/parent how ears are usually cleaned (are cotton-tipped swabs used?)
        3. Ask if wax removal has been required in the past
        4. Determine if patient has history of previous ear surgery with resultant scarring and increased risk of perforation (procedure is **contraindicated** if patient responds positively)

    B. Physical Examination
        1. Examine both ear canals
        2. Attempt to visualize the tympanic membranes around the wax to ascertain intactness
        3. Test hearing to determine if the affected ear is the only hearing ear (if so, referral to a specialist is indicated)

    C. Differential Diagnosis
        1. Foreign body
        2. Otitis media
        3. Otitis externa

    D. Diagnostic Tests: None indicated

V. Plan/Management

    A. Removal of cerumen may be necessary in the following situations
        1. Accumulation is causing decreased hearing, tinnitus, feeling of fullness, vertigo, or ear discomfort
        2. Accumulation is obstructing the examiner's view of the tympanic membrane

    B. Contraindications to removal of impacted cerumen: large perforation of tympanic membrane; severe ear trauma; irregular, sharp foreign body; very hard wax; inability to fully immobilize the patient; cholesteatoma; tumors

    C. Removal of cerumen using either the curette or irrigation technique is usually successful (see tables that follow)

    D. The irrigation technique takes longer than the curette technique and is usually implemented when the curette technique fails or is poorly tolerated by patient; irrigation technique rarely fails

REMOVAL USING CURETTE TECHNIQUE	
Equipment needed/types of curette	Metal and plastic Metal curettes are either rigid or flexible Plastic are either the flex-loop ear curette or infant ear scoop
Positioning patient	For infant/young child, place in supine position and restrain head carefully
	For older children and adolescents, seat comfortably on exam table and explain procedure and the importance of remaining still
Visualize cerumen	Using otoscope, look into the canal using posterior traction on helix
Select the appropriate curette	Gently remove the impacted cerumen, working through the otoscope or by direct vision (after having identified where the impaction is and keeping in mind the anatomy of the external auditory canal)
If hard wax is encountered	Stop the procedure and instill a few drops of mineral oil into the canal to soften for 10 minutes and then resume removal
If wax appears to be adherent to the tympanic membrane itself	Removal must be via gentle irrigation
Immobilization	**Absolutely necessary** to avoid risk of perforation and trauma to the ear canal!
If removal is via direct vision	Use the otoscope to assess progress during procedure

REMOVAL USING IRRIGATION TECHNIQUE

Equipment needed	• Use a soft-tipped syringe such as a 22-gauge butterfly intravenous catheter tubing with needle and butterfly removed and a 20 to 50 cc syringe, or • A bulb syringe, or • A water jet device such as Water-Pik
Irrigate with lukewarm water	• **Caution**: Use of cold or hot water may lead to dizziness and nausea! • Squirt water on your wrist to verify that temperature is correct
Positioning patient	• Place in supine position, or seat comfortably on exam table • Cover the patient's shoulder with towel • Instruct the patient to tilt head toward side being irrigated and place a small kidney-shaped basin under the ear to catch water (patient can hold basin)
Visualize cerumen	• Use otoscope to determine location
Place the tip of the tubing or syringe just inside the canal	• Infuse the water with a moderately strong and steady force • If the water jet irrigator is used, set at **lowest** setting to reduce risk of perforation
Direct the jet of water superiorly toward the occiput; aim stream of water at the superior gap or interface between the wax plug and the canal wall	• Allow for space in the canal for the return of water and cerumen • **Do not** direct the stream of water onto the tympanic membrane • Try to direct the stream of water past the plug of cerumen so as to create outward pressure on it • Take care not to touch the canal as this can produce cough and pain
Evaluate the effluent	• Sometimes an intact plug of cerumen is expelled and at other times the effluent will be tinted yellow but no obvious plug will be seen
Reassess progress using the otoscope	• It will be necessary to dry the external canal with gauze for good visualization and to reduce risk of infection
If pain or bleeding occur	• **STOP!**
If the irrigation is not successful after a few minutes	• Terminate the procedure
Instruct the patient to	• Instill 1-2 drops of baby oil in the affected ear twice a week to soften wax, or • Use 3 drops of hydrogen peroxide and water solution (1:1 solution) in affected ear 2-3 times a week
Ask the patient to return	• In one week for evaluation and removal of cerumen

E.   Cerumen solvents that are commercially available are not recommended because they frequently make the condition worse

F.   If recurrences are a problem, instruct patient to apply 1 or 2 drops of baby oil in each ear once or twice weekly to help soften wax; patient may also use a squeeze bulb syringe filled with lukewarm water to gently irrigate canals every month or so (best to do about 10 minutes after oil has been instilled into canals)

G.   Patient education
1.   Instruct to avoid the use of cotton-tipped applicators that can impact cerumen
2.   Inform that cerumen is a normal bodily secretion that protects the ear canal and does not usually need removal

H.   Follow Up:
1.   None indicated unless cerumen removal fails
2.   Contact office if decreased hearing, vertigo, dizziness, drainage, or pain occurs

OTITIS EXTERNA

I.   Definition: Inflammation of the external auditory canal

II.   Pathogenesis

    A.   Predisposing factors
        1.   Frequent exposure to moisture (e.g., swimming; humid, warm climates), aggressive cleaning of the canal, or trauma
        2.   Allergies or skin conditions such as psoriasis or seborrhea

    B.   Pathogens
        1.   Bacterial: *Pseudomonas aeruginosa* (most common), *Staphylococcus aureus* (common), and less frequently *Proteus* species and anaerobes
        2.   Fungal (account for 9% of cases): *Candida* and *Aspergillus*

    C.   Secondary fungal otitis externa (OE) may develop following treatment of OE with topical antibiotics

III.   Clinical Presentation

    A.   Ear pain (occurs in approximately 85% of cases) may begin gradually or suddenly; increases when pressure is placed on the tragus or when the pinna is moved

    B.   Sensation of fullness or obstruction of the ear occurs early in the process

    C.   Itching may occur and it is the predominant symptom with fungal infections

    D.   Otorrhea (discharge in or coming from the external auditory canal) is common
        1.   Acute bacterial OE typically has white mucus that is usually scant but may be thick
        2.   Chronic bacterial OE often has a bloody discharge, particularly in the presence of granulation tissue
        3.   Fungal OE has fluffy, white discharge or discharge may be black, gray, bluish-green, or yellow

    E.   If there is sufficient swelling to occlude the external auditory canal, hearing loss may occur

    F.   Systemic symptomatology such as fever or chills is uncommon

    G.   An uncommon, serious complication is malignant or necrotizing external otitis which can lead to cranial neuropathies and infection of the temporal bone; characterized by deep-seated nocturnal pain and granulation tissue at the bony-cartilaginous junction

IV.   Diagnosis/Evaluation

    A.   History
        1.   Ask about the location of pain/discomfort and time of onset
        2.   Ask about the occurrence of itching and bleeding/purulent exudate
        3.   Question about hearing loss
        4.   Ask about location and frequency of swimming
        5.   Obtain history of recent ear trauma; ask type of ear cleaning method
        6.   Ask if there is a history of previous episodes and risk factors such as diabetes and immunosuppression

    B.   Physical Examination
        1.   Determine if febrile
        2.   Carefully inspect the skin as many dermatological conditions can cause OE
        3.   Assuming the ear is extremely tender, carefully examine the external canal with the otoscope; the following are signs of otitis externa:
            a.   Erythema and edema of the canal
            b.   Weeping secretions, purulent otorrhea, and exudate or crusting of the skin
        4.   Apply pressure to the tragus and move the pinna, noting degree of tenderness

5. If possible, observe the tympanic membrane which is usually normal; edema may impede observation
6. Palpate the infra-auricular cervical lymph nodes for signs of lymphadenitis and lymphadenopathy

C. Differential Diagnosis
1. Furunculosis
2. Otitis media
3. Mastoiditis
4. Foreign body

D. Diagnostic Tests: Culture should be performed if resistance to initial management occurs

V. Plan/Management

A. Referral is recommended whenever malignant otitis externa cannot be ruled out or for severe, recalcitrant infections, and recurrent otitis externa

B. Before treatment, remove all exudative and epidermal debris (meticulous clearing of the canal is the cornerstone of effective treatment) (see section CERUMEN REMOVAL)
1. Can use either curette or irrigation technique
2. Irrigation should not be done if perforation of tympanic membrane cannot be ruled out

C. If swelling prevents the passage of topical medications, insert cotton wick
1. Insert by gently twisting the wick into the canal
2. Place drops on wick for first two days, then remove wick and place drops directly in ear

D. If it is unknown whether the tympanic membrane (TM) is perforated or intact, prescribe a nonototoxic quinolone antibiotic such as ofloxacin 0.3% solution (Floxin Otic); dosage for children 1-12 years, instill 5 drops into ear BID for 7-10 days; for patients >12 years, instill 5-10 drops BID for 7-10 days

E. For routine cases of OE with intact TM, one of the following is recommended:
1. 2% acetic acid otic solution (VoSoL Otic) is usually effective; prescribe 5 drops QID for 5-7 days; also available with hydrocortisone (VoSoL HC Otic) to decrease inflammation, and with aluminum acetate (Otic Domeboro)
2. Polymyxin B sulfate, neomycin, hydrocortisone (Cortisporin Otic suspension); 3-4 drops in canal, QID x 7 days (use 3 drops in children)

F. For fungal infections prescribe one of the following otic medications for 7 days:
1. Acetic acid, aluminum acetate solution (Otic Domeboro) 5 drops QID
2. Propylene glycol solution of acetic acid (VoSoL) 5 drops QID
3. Clotrimazole (Lotrimin) solution 3 drops BID

G. Duration of treatment for all topical medications is three days beyond cessation of symptoms (typically 5-7 days); for more severe cases, duration is extended to 10-14 days

H. Systemic oral antibiotics are rarely needed, but should be used when OE is persistent, associated with acute otitis media, when patient has systemic symptoms such as fever and lymphadenopathy, or when patient is immunocompromised
1. For adolescents >18 years, prescribe Ciprofloxacin (Cipro) 500 mg BID
2. For children use a broad spectrum antimicrobial such as cefaclor (Ceclor) or amoxicillin-clavulanate (Augmentin)

I. Health education
1. Keep moisture out of ear for 4-6 weeks. May bathe or shower but plug ear with cotton impregnated with petroleum jelly. Swimming is not permitted for 7-10 days
2. When using topical medications, suggest the following:
   a. Particularly with ofloxacin, warm the bottle in hands before instilling to minimize dizziness
   b. Insert a small cotton plug moistened with drops if patient cannot lie still long enough to allow absorption
3. To prevent recurrence of infection, teach the following:
   a. Advise to instill 2-3 drops of 1:1:1 solution of vinegar/isopropyl alcohol/water after each contact with water; solution is also beneficial for patients with persistent OE
   b. Use ear plugs while swimming, showering, or shampooing
   c. Instruct in proper way to clean ears; avoid using cotton-tipped applicators or other devices such as hairpins

J.   Follow Up
1.   If properly treated, otitis externa should resolve in 7 days; mild cases do not require follow-up
2.   Moderate and severe cases should return to office in 3 days and 24 hours, respectively

OTITIS MEDIA, ACUTE

I.   Definitions: Otitis media is an inflammation in the middle ear without reference to etiology

A.   Acute otitis media (AOM): Presence of middle ear effusion in conjunction with rapid onset of one or more signs or symptoms of inflammation of the middle ear; other terms used in the past and synonymous with AOM include suppurative otitis media, acute bacterial otitis media, and purulent otitis media

B.   Persistent AOM: Persistence of symptoms and signs of middle ear infection following 1 to 2 courses of antibiotic therapy

C.   Recurrent AOM: Three or more separate episodes of AOM in a 6-month time span or 4 or more episodes in a 12-month time span

D.   Middle ear effusion (MEE) is liquid in the middle ear and can occur with AOM or otitis media with effusion

II.   Pathogenesis

A.   Most important factor is eustachian tube dysfunction that prevents effective drainage of middle ear fluid
1.   Typically, patient has an antecedent event such as an infection or allergy which results in edema and congestion of the mucosa of the nasopharynx, eustachian tube, and middle ear
2.   The congestion of the eustachian tube impedes the flow of middle ear secretions
3.   Negative pressure often increases, which further pulls fluid into the middle ear
4.   As middle ear secretions increase microbial pathogens grow, resulting in otitis media; common pathogens are as follows:
a.   *Streptococcus pneumoniae* (predominant)
b.   *Haemophilus influenzae*
c.   *Moraxella catarrhalis*
d.   Viruses
e.   Other bacteria such as *Streptococcus pyogenes* and *Staphylococcus aureus*
5.   Due to overuse and/or inappropriate use of antibiotics as a result of overdiagnosis of AOM, pathogens of this condition are becoming increasingly resistant
a.   Drug-resistant *S. pneumoniae* (DRSP) is becoming a major health problem (particularly in persistent and recurrent AOM)
b.   The rates of infections due to beta-lactamase producing organisms *(M. catarrhalis* and *H. influenzae)* are also increasing

B.   Risk factors for recurrent otitis media:
1.   An episode of AOM during first 6 months of life
2.   Parental smoking
3.   Male gender
4.   Congenital disorders such as cleft palate and trisomy 21
5.   History of enlarged adenoids, tonsillitis, or asthma
6.   Bottle feeding
7.   Use of soother or pacifier
8.   Family history of otitis media
9.   Birth in the fall
10.   Day care center attendance

III.   Clinical Presentation

A.   Occurs most frequently in winter months in children <7 years old, with highest incidence in children between 6 months and 3 years of age; commonly seen following a viral upper respiratory infection

B.   Symptoms (see table CONSENSUS DEFINITION OF ACUTE OTITIS MEDIA)

CONSENSUS DEFINITION OF ACUTE OTITIS MEDIA

AOM is defined as
1.   Presence of MEE as demonstrated by the actual presence of fluid in the middle ear as diagnosed by tympanocentesis or the physical presence of liquid in the external ear canal as a result of TM perforation or indicated by limited or absent mobility of the TM as diagnosed by pneumatic otoscopy, tympanogram, or acoustic reflectometry with or without the following:
     a.   opacification, not including erythema
     b.   a full or bulging TM
     c.   hearing loss
AND
2.   Rapid onset (over the course of 48 hours)
OF
3.   One or more of the following signs or symptoms:
     a.   otalgia (or pulling of the ear in an infant)
     b.   otorrhea
     c.   irritability in the infant or toddler
     d.   fever

Adapted from Rosenfeld, R.M., Casselbrant, M.L., and Hannley, M.T. (2001). Implications of the AHRQ evidence report on acute otitis media. *Otolaryngology-Head and Neck Surgery, 125*, 440-448.

C.   Complications are uncommon even in patients who do not receive antibiotics; infrequent events include hearing loss, perforation of eardrum, cholesteatoma, acute mastoiditis, bacteremia, meningitis, and epidural abscess

IV.   Diagnosis/Evaluation

    A.   History
       1.   Determine onset and duration of symptoms
       2.   Ask about ear pain, fever, irritability
       3.   Inquire about hearing loss, tinnitus, and dizziness
       4.   Ask about drainage from ear
       5.   Inquire about associated symptoms such as nasal congestion, headache, sore throat, or cough
       6.   Carefully document the number and, if possible, dates of previous occurrences; ask about successes and failures of previous treatments
       7.   Determine whether an upper respiratory infection preceded the fever or ear pain
       8.   Inquire about history of allergies and other risk factors such as active or passive smoking and congenital disorders such as cleft palate
       9.   In infants, inquire about manner of bottle feeding

    B.   Physical Examination
       1.   Measure vital signs
       2.   Inspect conjunctivae, pharynx, and nasal mucosa
       3.   Palpate sinuses
       4.   Palpate for auricular and cervical adenopathy
       5.   Examine auricle and external auditory canal
       6.   Carefully examine tympanic membranes (TM) bilaterally for position, color, degree of translucency, and mobility (important to remove cerumen if TM is partially occluded)
          a.   Position: Process of the malleus should be visible but not prominent through the membrane; retraction and bulging indicate effusion
          b.   Color: Normal TM is gray; an amber color often indicates an effusion; erythema may indicate infection but also may be due to crying, severe coughing, or vascular engorgement
          c.   Translucency: Middle ear or bony landmarks should be visible through the TM; air fluid level, bubbles, and inability to visualize middle ear landmarks suggest effusion
          d.   Mobility: Normal ear will move with pneumatic otoscopy; **to be diagnosed with AOM there must be presence of fluid in middle ear; this can only be detected with pneumatic otoscopy, tympanogram, or acoustic reflectometry**
          e.   Distorted light reflex and bullae between layers of TM are suggestive of AOM
       7.   Perform a lung examination
       8.   When a healthy adult has ear pain and the examination of the ear is completely normal, a more thorough evaluation of the head and neck is essential
          a.   Examine mouth and teeth for dental disorders
          b.   Assess functioning of temporomandibular joint
          c.   Assess nose and pharynx for nasopharyngeal carcinoma
          d.   Assess cranial nerves to detect neurological problems that could be associated with intracranial neoplasms

C. Differential Diagnosis (health care providers can generally detect OM 90% of time when it is present, but over diagnosis frequently occurs [as high as 40%])
    1. Otitis externa
    2. Transient middle ear effusion may result with flying or traveling in high altitudes (barotrauma) or with allergies
    3. Mastoiditis
    4. Furuncle
    5. Temporomandibular joint dysfunction
    6. Mumps
    7. Dental abscess
    8. Tonsillitis
    9. Foreign body
    10. Trauma

D. Diagnostic Tests
    1. Usually no diagnostic tests are ordered
    2. Tympanocentesis for culture and sensitivity of middle ear effusion is the gold standard for diagnosis of AOM and is recommended to guide choice of therapy in persistent and recurrent AOM
    3. Tympanometry is useful, particularly in recurrent cases and when there is suspicion of fluid behind the TM without clinical signs
    4. Acoustic reflectometry helps diagnose AOM by analyzing sound pressure and reflected sound in the eardrum
    5. Consider ordering sinus films in patients with recurrent otitis media
    6. Order CBC with differential and blood cultures in children who appear toxic, have a high fever, are not drinking and voiding, or are immunocompromised
    7. Consider audiometry post treatment

V. Plan/Management

A. General management concepts (see following table)

GENERAL CONCEPTS OF MANAGEMENT	
1. Be cautious	Remember favorable natural history of AOM (80% of cases resolve spontaneously)
2. Prescribe antibiotics sparingly	Antibiotics improve resolution by only about 15% Antibiotics increase risk of bacterial resistance

3. Modify risk factors	Improve odds of resolution:
	    Avoid passive smoking
	    Control food and inhalant allergies
	    Treat sinusitis
	    Limit pacifier use in day
	    Consider alternatives for group day care

4. Practice prevention	Encourage breast feeding Advise parents not to prop infant's bottle and to elevate infant's head when feeding Pneumococcal vaccine is recommended in children <2 years; consider for children >2 years who have recurrent, persistent infections Consider influenza vaccine, recommended whenever feasible for children age 6-23 months
5. Avoid unproven therapies	Antihistamines/decongestants Homeopathy and naturopathy Folk remedies such as "sweet oil"

B. Treatment with antibiotics
    1. Antibiotics for correctly diagnosed AOM provide a small benefit (reduce pain and the risk of developing contralateral AOM and mastoiditis); the following outcomes are not affected by antibiotic use: Tympanic membrane perforation, pain and fever resolution at 4-7 days, recurrent AOM
    2. Some experts recommend that patients who have AOM without bulging tympanic membranes should be managed with a delayed antibiotic-prescribing strategy; provide patient with prescription for antibiotic to be used only if otalgia or fever persist or there is no clinical improvement after 48-72 hours

3. Amoxicillin is the first line antibiotic (see following table)
   a. In patients with low risk for drug-resistant *S. pneumoniae* (DRSP) (>2 years with no antimicrobial exposure in preceding 1-3 months and no day care attendance) use dose of 40-45 mg/kg/day
   b. In patients at high risk for DRSP, increase dose to 80-90 mg/kg/day
4. For patients allergic to penicillins and cephalosporins, prescribe azithromycin or clarithromycin (for dosing, see table THIRD-LINE ANTIBIOTICS V.B.5.); increasing resistance to trimethoprim/ sulfamethoxazole and erythromycin/sulfisoxazole has been found, but in some areas these antibiotics may also be effective

RECOMMENDED FIRST-LINE ANTIBIOTIC FOR MEDICAL MANAGEMENT*

Generic (Trade) Name *Duration of treatment*	Dosing	Comment
Amoxicillin (Amoxil) *10 day treatment* OR	40-45 mg/kg/day in 3 divided doses (Available 125 mg/5 mL and 250 mg/5 mL liquid) **Adolescents:** 500 mg tabs BID	Use this lower dose in uncomplicated AOM and in patients at low risk for DRSP Inexpensive, few adverse effects Disadvantage: Ineffective against beta-lactamase producing organisms
Amoxicillin (Amoxil) 10 day treatment*	80-90 mg/kg/day in 2 or 3 divided doses	Use this increased dose in patients with high risk of DRSP

* Shortened courses of antibiotics may be acceptable for patients >2 years of age who have mild, uncomplicated AOM, no underlying medical condition, no history of chronic or recurrent otitis media, and whose symptoms improve within 72 hours

5. Use second-line antibiotics (see following table) for patients with following clinical features:
   a. Received antibiotics within one month of course of treatment (consider high dose amoxicillin or one of the second-line antibiotics)
   b. Failed to respond by third day of treatment with amoxicillin
   c. Have complicated infections
   d. Have ipsilateral conjunctivitis suggesting *H. influenzae* infection

RECOMMENDED SECOND-LINE ANTIBIOTICS FOR MEDICAL MANAGEMENT

Generic (Trade) Name *Duration of treatment*	Dosing	Comment
Amoxicillin-clavulanate (Augmentin) *10 day treatment* -OR- (Augmentin ES-600) *10 day treatment*	40 mg/kg/day in 2-3 divided doses (available 125 mg/5 mL and 250 mg/5 mL liquid) **Adolescents:** 250-500 mg tab TID -OR- 80-90 mg/kg/day in 2 divided doses (available 600 mg/5 mL)	- Broad spectrum - 15-20% patients have gastrointestinal upset
Cefuroxime (Ceftin) *10 day treatment*	Over 3 months: 30 mg/kg/day in 2 divided doses (available 125 mg/5 mL and 250 mg/5 mL) **Adolescents:** 250-500 mg cap BID	- Broad spectrum - Bitter taste (chocolate syrup, ice cream, or white grape juice chaser may disguise the taste) - Take with food
Ceftriaxone (Rocephin) *1-5 day treatment*	50-75mg/kg/day IM injection QD	- Good choice if patient is vomiting, has diarrhea, refuses oral medications, or is toxic

* Shortened courses of antibiotics may be acceptable for patients >2 years of age, who have mild, uncomplicated AOM, no underlying medical condition, no history of chronic or recurrent otitis media, and whose symptoms improve with 72 hours

6. Use third-line antibiotics for special cases; see following table

RECOMMENDED THIRD-LINE ANTIBIOTICS FOR MEDICAL MANAGEMENT

Generic (Trade) Name *Duration of treatment*	Dosing	Comment
Azithromycin (Zithromax) *5 day treatment**	Over 6 months: 10 mg/kg QD Day 1; 5 mg/kg QD Days 2-5 (available 100 mg/5 mL & 200 mg/5 mL); **Adolescents:** 500 mg tab QD Day 1; 250 mg Days 2-5	- Broad spectrum - Oral suspension: Take 1 hour before or 2 hours after meals
Cefprozil (Cefzil) *10 day treatment**	Over 6 months: 15-30 mg/kg/day in 2 divided doses (available 125 mg/5 mL & 250 mg/5 mL liquid); **Adolescents:** 500 mg tab BID	- Broad spectrum
Cefpodoxime (Vantin) *10 day treatment**	Over 2 months: 10 mg/kg in 2 divided doses (available 50 mg/5 mL & 100 mg/5 mL suspension) **Adolescents:** 200 mg tab BID	- Broad spectrum - Convenient dosing for children - For adults, take tabs with food
Ceftibuten (Cedax) *10 day treatment**	Over 6 months: ≤45 kg: 9 mg/kg QD; (available 90 mg/5 mL) **Adolescents & children >45 kg:** 400 mg cap QD	- Broad spectrum; convenient dosing - Take suspension on empty stomach; caps may be taken without regard for meals
Clarithromycin (Biaxin) *10 day treatment**	Over 6 months: 15 mg/kg/day in 2 divided doses (available 125 mg/5 mL & 250 mg/5 mL liquid); **Adolescents:** 250-500 mg cap BID	- Broad spectrum - Well tolerated
Loracarbef (Lorabid) *10 day treatment**	Over 6 months: 30 mg/kg/day in 2 divided doses (Available 100 mg/5 mL & 200 mg/5 mL liquid); **Adolescents:** 200-400 mg caps BID	- Broad spectrum - Must take on an empty stomach

*Shortened courses of antibiotics may be acceptable for patients >2 years of age who have mild, uncomplicated AOM, no underlying medical condition, no history of chronic or recurrent otitis media, and whose symptoms improve with 72 hours

C. Management of pain
    1. Usually, an analgesic such as acetaminophen or ibuprofen is all that is needed
    2. Topical pain relievers such as Auralgan Otic solution (fill ear canal and insert moistened cotton plug) every 1-2 hours may be beneficial; **do not use if TM is ruptured**

D. Treatment of persistent and recurrent AOM
    1. If no response in 2-3 days and patient is not toxic switch to a second-line or third-line antibiotic
    2. Tympanocentesis with culture of middle ear fluid can guide antibiotic selection and can be beneficial in draining the effusion and breaking the cycle of persistent and recurrent AOM
    3. Clindamycin is another possible choice, but is ineffective against *H. influenzae* and *M. catarrhalis*; consider if tympanocentesis confirms that pathogen is *S. pneumoniae*
    4. Consider consultation with specialist if 2-3 courses of recommended treatments fail
    5. If middle ear fluid cultures are not available, previous treatment and current symptoms may provide clues to likely pathogen (see following table)

CLUES TO ETIOLOGY OF PERSISTENT AND RECURRENT AOM

Clinical feature	Pathogen
Increased otalgia & fever Spontaneous perforation	More likely to be *S. pneumoniae*
Therapy in preceding month with amoxicillin, erythromycin-sulfisoxazole, azithromycin, antibiotic prophylaxis Epidemiological features: <2 years, day care attendance, history of recurrent AOM, contact with individuals treated with antibiotics	More likely to be resistant *S. pneumoniae*
Mild symptoms Preceding therapy was with high-dose amoxicillin	Less likely to be *S. pneumoniae*
Otitis-conjunctivitis syndrome	More likely to be *H. influenzae*
Preceding therapy was with amoxicillin	More likely to be β-lactamase-positive *H. influenzae*
Preceding therapy was with third-generation cephalosporin	Less likely to be *H. influenzae*

Adapted from Pichichero, M.E., Reiner, S.A., Brook, I., Gooch, W.M. III, Yamauchi, T., Jenkins, S.G., et al. (2000). Controversies in the medical management of persistent and recurrent acute otitis media: Recommendations of a clinical advisory committee. *Annals of Otology, Rhinology, and Laryngology, 109*, 2-12.

E.   Nasal and oral decongestants are usually ineffective in preventing or treating AOM, but may provide symptomatic relief of associated symptoms that often accompany AOM

F.   Antihistamines are not recommended unless the predisposing factor for developing AOM is an allergy; antihistamines may thicken the secretions and aggravate the problem

G.   Treatment of otitis-prone children
      1.   Defined as child who has had two episodes of AOM in 6-month period or more than three episodes in 12 months.
      2.   Always try preventive measures
            a.   See table (GENERAL CONCEPTS V.A.): Limit passive smoking, administer vaccines (see V.H.), etc.
            b.   Xylitol syrup and chewing gum were found to reduce incidence of AOM in some studies
      3.   Others recommend prophylaxis therapy with sulfisoxazole (Gantrisin) 30-50 mg/kg as single dose at bedtime or amoxicillin 13 mg/kg as a single dose at bedtime
            a.   Continue prophylactic treatment for approximately 3-6 months or until regimen fails
            b.   Evaluate children every 4 weeks to ensure that AOM is not overlooked
            c.   If acute infection occurs, treat with full dose of a different antimicrobial
            d.   When prophylaxis fails, consult specialist who will consider placement of tympanostomy tubes, myringotomy, adenoidectomy, or tonsillectomy

H.   Vaccination to prevent pneumococcal AOM
      1.   Although findings have been inconsistent, pneumococcal conjugate vaccine has been shown to prevent invasive disease, reduce frequency of AOM (particularly in children with a history of recurrent AOM), and reduce nasopharyngeal carriage of pneumococci
      2.   American Academy of Pediatrics recommends vaccination of all children <23 months
      3.   Vaccination may be beneficial for children 24-59 months old who have not previously received vaccine and who have a history of recurrent AOM or who have AOM complicated by placement of tympanostomy tube

I.   Treatment of tympanic membrane perforation involves prescription of oral antibiotic supplemented with topical antibiotic for maximum of 10 days; select one of the following topical antibiotics:
      1.   Ofloxacin otic solution 3% (Floxin Otic): For children 1-12 years instill 5 drops into ear BID; for patients >12 years: instill 5-10 drops BID
      2.   Combination of neomycin sulfate, polymyxin-B and hydrocortisone (Cortisporin Otic suspension) 3-4 drops (in children, use 3 drops) in each ear, 3-4 times a day

J.   Consult specialist in following cases:
      1.   Hearing loss bilaterally of 20 dB or more
      2.   Chronic or persistent infection with evidence of mastoid involvement
      3.   Cholesteatoma formation or chronic perforation
      4.   Children with febrile seizures, antibiotic intolerance, speech problems, or chronic otitis media with effusion
      5.   Infants <3 months because of possibility of AOM associated with bacteremia, meningitis, or pneumonia

K.   Follow Up
      1.   Assess patient in 48-72 hours for symptom improvement
      2.   Typically, return visits are scheduled several days after completion of drug therapy or recheck in 2-3 weeks from initial visit; some authorities recommend delaying follow-up for 4-6 weeks if the patient is older than 15 months, asymptomatic, and parents/patient report that the infection has resolved
      3.   For patients treated with prophylactic antibiotics, evaluate every 4 weeks

OTITIS MEDIA WITH EFFUSION

I. Definition: Accumulation of serous fluid in the middle ear **without signs and symptoms of acute infection** (previously referred to as serous otitis media [OM], nonsuppurative OM, or secretory OM)

II. Pathogenesis

   A. Loss of patency of the eustachian tube with subsequent negative pressure and effusion behind the tympanic membrane (TM)

   B. Risk factors are similar to those of acute otitis media (see section ACUTE OTITIS MEDIA)

III. Clinical Presentation

   A. Between 50-79% of children will develop otitis media with effusion (OME) after a course of antibiotics for treatment of AOM

   B. Effusion may occur in adults but is less common than in children

   C. Patient are often asymptomatic, but may have mild pain, sensation of stuffiness or fullness in ear, or popping and crackling sounds in ear with chewing, yawning, or blowing nose

   D. A small number of patients may experience vertigo or ataxia

   E. Tympanic membrane is often retracted, opaque, and has a diffuse light reflex
      1. Bubbles or a fluid level may be present behind the tympanic membrane
      2. Decreased tympanic membrane movement with insufflation (pneumatic otoscopy) is usually present

   F. Chronic effusion may result in the following:
      1. Hearing loss which, in children, may lead to a delay in language development
      2. Delay of gross motor skills in children

   G. Complications are rare, but may include chronic drainage and perforation, cholesteatoma, and facial nerve paralysis

IV. Diagnosis/Evaluation

   A. History
      1. Determine onset, duration, character of symptoms
      2. Inquire about rhinitis, cough, and fever
      3. Question about pain and decreased hearing acuity level
      4. Inquire about recent upper respiratory infection and allergies
      5. Inquire about past episodes of otitis media and treatments received
      6. Ask about family history of allergies

   B. Physical Examination
      1. Measure vital signs
      2. Examine nasal passages and pharynx
      3. Examine tympanic membranes (TM) for fluid level, retraction, diffuse light reflex and/or bubbles
      4. Assess TM mobility with pneumatic otoscopy (removal of cerumen is mandatory)
         a. Recommended for primary diagnosis
         b. Accuracy of diagnosis with pneumatic otoscopy is 70-79%
      5. Perform Rinne and Weber tests (see section on HEARING LOSS)
      6. Palpate neck and jaw for adenopathy
      7. Examine neck and head for anatomical abnormalities
      8. In children, assess language development

   C. Differential Diagnosis
      1. Nasopharyngeal carcinoma
      2. Anatomic abnormalities

   D. Diagnostic Tests

1. Tympanometry (indirect measure of tympanic membrane compliance and estimate of middle ear pressure)
   a. Often falsely positive due to impacted cerumen, foreign body, TM perforation, or improper placement of instrument tip on the ear canal wall
   b. Pneumatic otoscopy recommended for primary diagnosis, followed by tympanometry as confirmatory test
   c. Tympanogram is flat with an effusion
2. Audiometry
   a. Patients with fluid in both ears for three months should undergo hearing evaluation; prior to three months, audiometry is an option
   b. Hearing impairment is defined as equal to or worse than 20 decibels (dB) hearing threshold level in the better-hearing ear
3. Acoustic reflectometry; experts disagree about the value of this test

V. Plan/Management

A. For asymptomatic children (normal hearing, speech, school performance) watchful waiting with vigilant monitoring is usually recommended, but patients who do not have resolution of effusion within 2 months may be candidates for antibiotic therapy
   1. Watchful waiting is becoming the preferred approach due to accumulating evidence that antibiotic use increases the risk for both colonization and invasive disease with penicillin-resistant *Streptococcus pneumoniae*; additional rationale for this recommendation:
      a. The majority of cases spontaneously resolve without antibiotic treatment
      b. Effect of antibiotics is marginal and often short-lived; antibiotics increase short-term resolution by approximately 15%
      c. Incidence of delayed suppurative complications from effusion is small
   2. If antibiotic therapy is chosen, prescribe a beta-lactamase stable antibiotic such as the following:
      a. Amoxicillin-clavulanate (Augmentin) 40 mg/kg/day in three divided doses for 2-3 weeks. Available in 125 mg/5 mL and 250 mg/5 mL liquids
      b. Clarithromycin (Biaxin) 15 mg/kg/day in two divided doses for 2-3 weeks. Available in 125 mg/5 mL and 250 mg/5 mL liquids

B. Assess hearing status and structural integrity of TM with audiometry and pneumatic otoscopy every 3-4 months

C. Children with bilateral OME for greater than 3 months and hearing loss (defined as 20 dB hearing threshold level or worse in the better-hearing ear) should be referred to an ENT specialist for possible placement of tympanostomy tubes

D. Oral corticosteroids are sometimes recommended for children **>3 years old** as a last-resort alternative to surgery; although limited, most studies have found that steroid treatment does not improve outcomes
   1. Dangers of this approach: chickenpox exacerbation, immunosuppression and adverse effects such as insomnia, changes in behavior, weight gain
   2. Prescribe prednisolone (Pediapred) 1 mg/kg/day in one dose or two divided doses for 5-7 days, Available 5 mg/5 mL liquid (do not prescribe steroids if child has NOT had chickenpox or is not immunized for chickenpox and if there has been exposure to chickenpox in last 4 weeks)

E. For older children and adolescents, consider autoinflation of eustachian tube with plastic nasal cannula attached to balloon

F. Patient education, modification of risk factors, and controlling concurrent illnesses are important
   1. Limit passive smoke exposure and group day-care attendance (if possible) and bottle-feeding in infants
   2. Consider milk-free diet for several weeks as a diagnostic trial in children <2 years as allergy to milk proteins may cause middle ear inflammation
   3. Treat concurrent illnesses such as sinusitis and allergic rhinitis
   4. Emphasize importance of follow up
   5. Discuss with family the possibility of hearing loss due to this condition
   6. Children should be seated in front of the class until hearing is normal

G. Most studies indicate that decongestants and antihistamines are ineffective; the role of allergies in patients with effusions is still uncertain

H. Referral to speech therapist may be needed for language delay or a speech problem

I.	Nasopharyngeal cancer is a remote possibility in a healthy adult and consultation with an otolaryngologist is necessary if there is suspicion of this condition

J.	Follow Up
1.	Assess every 4-6 weeks or sooner if ear pain or other bothersome symptoms occur
2.	If effusion persists at 3-month follow-up visit, hearing evaluation is indicated

CARE OF PATIENT WITH TYMPANOSTOMY TUBES

I.	Definition: Middle ear ventilation tubes placed in tympanic membrane (TM) after myringotomy

II.	Procedure

A.	Tubes restore hearing to pre-effusion threshold, permit normal vibration of TM and middle ear bones, permit ventilation of middle ear tissues, equalize middle ear and atmospheric pressures, and prevent accumulation of fluid or mucus in middle ear

B.	Tubes are placed in pars tensa of the tympanic membrane, in any location except the posterosuperior quadrant, overlying the incus and stapes

C.	Generally, tubes are made of plastic, metal or Teflon and are designed for short-term placement (8-15 months) or long-term placement (>15 months)

D.	Possible candidates for tube placement:
1.	Patients with bilateral middle ear effusion and hearing deficiency for more than 3 months; recommended if condition existed for 4-6 months
2.	Patient with middle ear effusion and structural changes of tympanic membrane
3.	Experts consider earlier tube placement for patients with recurrent painful ear infections, language delay, and craniofacial anomalies

III.	Clinical Presentation

A.	Potential benefits in children include improvements in behaviors, sleep, communication, and hearing

B.	Potential Risks
1.	Auditory canal wall laceration, persistent otorrhea, granuloma formation, cholesteatoma, and permanent TM perforation
2.	Structural changes in TM such as flaccidity, retraction, and/or tympanosclerosis have occurred; long-term effects on hearing are unknown but estimated as small
3.	Risks associated with general anesthesia
4.	Intrusion of tube into middle ear cleft rather than normal extrusion through external ear canal
5.	Approximately 30% of children have repeat tympanostomy tube insertion within 5 years of initial surgery

IV.	Diagnosis/Evaluation

A.	History
1.	Question about pain and ear discharge
2.	Inquire about noticeable changes in hearing, speech, and/or development

B.	Physical Examination
1.	Inspect ear canal for possible tube extrusion and signs of ear discharge
2.	Inspect TM for placement of tube and color and degree of translucency (TM should be gray and translucent if tube is properly functioning)
3.	Assess for mobility with pneumatic otoscopy (TM should be immobile if tube is properly functioning)

C. Diagnostic tests
    1. If tube functioning is questionable, order tympanometry which should be flat if tube is properly functioning
    2. An audiologic evaluation should be performed postoperatively if normal hearing was not established prior to tube placement

V. Plan/Management

A. Initial postoperative follow-up examination should be performed by the otolaryngologist to ascertain that the tube is patent and functional; visit is usually within first month after placement of tube

B. After initial postoperative visit, follow-up examinations should be scheduled at intervals no longer than 6 months; interval examinations may be performed by the primary care clinician as long as there is documented communication between the otolaryngologist and the clinician

C. Refer back to an otolaryngologist children who have the following:
    1. Recurrent, chronic, or unresponsive tube otorrhea
    2. A documented medialized tube (tube has migrated into middle ear space)
    3. Documented tube obstruction from cerumen, dry secretions, or granulation tissue
    4. Ears that are difficult to examine because of external ear canal stenosis as seen in some children with Down syndrome and other craniofacial syndrome
    5. Decreased hearing acuity, balance difficulties, or persistent otalgia
    6. Suspicion of cholesteatoma, TM perforation, or other structural diseases of the TM
    7. Symptomatic children in whom a previously placed tube cannot be visualized
    8. An extruded tube that cannot be removed from the ear canal
    9. Retention of tube for more than 2 years; prolonged tube retention may increase occurrence of otorrhea, granulation tissue formation, and persistent TM perforation; children >7 years have more complications than younger children
    10. Pre-existing sensorineural hearing loss, documented language or developmental delay, or special needs in whom the additional conductive hearing compromise associated with a nonfunctional tube could be particularly debilitating

D. For tubes clogged with dried middle ear effusion, consider consultation with specialist and prescribe topical antibiotic such as Cortisporin otic suspension for 5-7 days; hydrogen peroxide and cerumolytics are usually contraindicated

E. Post-tube otorrhea occurs in 10-30% of patients
    1. Prescribe amoxicillin (Amoxil) 40 mg/kg/day PO in three divided doses. Available 125 mg/5mL and 250 mg/5mL liquid or a beta-lactamase stable antibiotic in areas with prevalence of resistant organisms (see second-line antibiotics under OTITIS MEDIA)
    2. If unresponsive to first course of antibiotics, consider the possibility of water contamination with *Pseudomonas aeruginosa* and *Staphylococcus aureus* and prescribe one of the following:
        a. Cortisporin drops are considered safe, but should not be overused because of risks of ototoxicity and maceration of canal; prescribe 3-5 drops only BID or TID for 5-7 days
        b. Ofloxacin otic solution 3% (Floxin Otic)
            (1) Dosage: for children 1-12 years instill 5 drops into ear BID for 7-10 days; patients >12 years: instill 5-10 drops BID for 7-10 days
            (2) To avoid dizziness, hold bottle in hand for 1-2 minutes to warm; after instilling drops pump tragus 4 times by pushing inward to enhance penetration of drops

F. Patient education
    1. Teach patient and family to watch for tube extrusion and possible complications such as discharge from ear and fever
    2. Emphasize importance of follow-up visits
    3. Wear fitted ear plugs when diving or swimming more than a foot below surface of water, especially in lakes, ponds, rivers
    4. Avoid prolonged soaking of head in bath water and direct shower stream on ear canal

G. Follow Up
    1. Initial postoperative examination should be performed by the otolaryngologist
    2. Other follow-up examinations should be scheduled at intervals no longer than 6 months and may be performed by the primary care clinician with communication with an otolaryngologist
    3. Return to office if otorrhea or clogged effusion occurs

ALLERGIC AND NONALLERGIC RHINITIS

I.   Definition of rhinitis: Inflammation of mucous membranes of the nose, usually accompanied by edema of mucosa and a nasal discharge. Rhinitis may be allergic or nonallergic

II. Pathogenesis

A.   Allergic rhinitis: An IgE-mediated inflammatory disease involving the nasal mucosa membranes
1.   When a person with a genetic predisposition to allergy is exposed to a strong allergic stimulus, antigen IgE-antibody molecules are produced and bind to mast cells in the respiratory epithelium
2.   Re-exposure to offending allergen causes a hypersensitivity to offending allergen and triggers the release of histamines and other mediators
3.   Histamine release results in immediate local vasodilation, mucosal edema, and increased mucous production
4.   A late-phase reaction sometimes occurs 4-8 hours after the original reaction in persons with severe disease; results in hyper-responsiveness to antigenic and nonantigenic stimuli and is linked to development of chronic disease
5.   Most common form is the seasonal pattern due to inhalant pollen allergens
6.   Year-round perennial type is difficult to diagnose and treat; usually related to house dust mites, mold, cockroaches, and animal dander; in adults, food allergies are a rare cause

B.   Nonallergic Rhinitis
1.   Vasomotor rhinitis or idiopathic perennial nonallergic rhinitis: Unknown etiology but possibly due to abnormal autonomic responsiveness or vascular dysfunction; unrelated to allergy, infection, structural lesions, systemic diseases, or drug use
2.   Chronic inflammatory diseases such as midline granuloma, Wegener's granuloma, and sarcoidosis present with chronic nasal congestion and rhinitis
3.   Rhinitis medicamentosus or rebound rhinitis is due to overuse of topical decongestant
4.   Rhinitis of pregnancy is due to hormonal increase (will not be discussed further)
5.   NARES syndrome (non-allergic rhinitis with eosinophilia syndrome) occurs infrequently in adults who have nasal eosinophils but negative skin and *in vitro* tests
6.   Gustatory rhinitis may be due to an overly sensitive cholinergic reflex that can be triggered by eating or cold air
7.   Other causes: infections (chronic rhinosinusitis), anatomic problems (adenoidal hypertrophy, nasal polyps, deviated nasal septum), trauma, foreign bodies, neoplasm, cocaine abuse, and rhinitis associated with systemic diseases such as hypothyroidism

III. Clinical Presentation of allergic rhinitis and vasomotor rhinitis

A.   Allergic rhinitis
1.   Prevalence is increasing worldwide
2.   Onset of symptoms is most common between ages 10-20; rarely begins before age 4 or after age 40
3.   Usually involves the triad of nasal congestion, sneezing, and clear rhinorrhea
4.   Nasal itching, nasal obstruction, nasal pain, post-nasal drip, coughing, sore throat, and itching and puffiness of eyes may occur
5.   Individuals with allergic rhinitis are more likely to develop asthma over time than other individuals
6.   There is an increased prevalence of acute and chronic bacterial sinusitis among patients with allergic rhinitis
7.   Signs include the following:
     a.   Pale, boggy nasal mucosa with clear thin secretions
     b.   Enlarged nasal turbinates which may obstruct airway flow
     c.   "Allergic shiners" or a dark discoloration beneath both eyes
     d.   Cobblestone appearance of the conjunctiva
     e.   "Dennie's lines" or extra wrinkles below the lower eyelids
     f.   Transverse nasal crease due to chronic upward wiping of the nose
     g.   Nasal salute
     h.   Mouth-breathing
     i.   Short upper lip
     j.   Enlarged tonsils and adenoids
8.   Associated with significant comorbidities and complications such as asthma, sinusitis, nasal polyposis, and otitis media with effusion (OME)

B. Vasomotor rhinitis
    1.   Onset is usually in adult life
    2.   Rapid onset of nasal congestion and a pronounced and noticeable postnasal drip are typical
    3.   Symptoms are similar to allergic rhinitis, but with less prominent nasal pruritus and conjunctival irritation
    4.   Triggers of attacks are the following: abrupt changes in temperature and barometric pressure, odors, smoke, and emotional stress
    5.   Negative family history of allergy
    6.   Nasal smear and skin tests are negative
    7.   Patients are usually unresponsive to environmental controls and medications

IV. Diagnosis/Evaluation

A. History
    1.   Question about onset, duration, and progression of symptoms
    2.   Explore relationship of symptoms to season, place, time of day, and activity
    3.   Question about contact with offending allergens and other triggers such as exposure to cold air, ingestion of spicy foods, odors, and changes in temperature and barometric pressure
    4.   Determine occupational exposure and obtain a detailed environmental history to identify precipitating factors
    5.   Question about nasal stuffiness or obstruction, sensation of pressure over and under the eyes, itching of the eyes, nose and pharynx, sneezing, color, consistency, and amount of nasal and postnasal discharges, and sensation of needing to constantly clear throat
    6.   Ask about mouth breathing, changes in hearing and smell acuity, snoring during sleep, and fatigue
    7.   Inquire about self-treatment, particularly duration and use of nasal sprays
    8.   Inquire about family history and past history of allergies
    9.   Assess impact on patient's quality of life

B. Physical Examination
    1.   Check pulse and blood pressure as sympathomimetic decongestants may increase both
    2.   Measure temperature which should be normal
    3.   Inspect eyes for allergic "shiners," tearing, conjunctival injection, lid swelling, and periorbital edema
    4.   Palpate for sinus tenderness
    5.   Examine ears to rule out otitis media and to check for serous otitis media
    6.   Assess for nasal obstruction and polyps
    7.   Inspect nasal mucosa noting color, edema, and type and color of nasal discharge
    8.   Assess pharynx for tonsillar enlargement and inflammation
    9.   Palpate lymph nodes
    10.   Always check breath sounds to rule out concurrent asthma

C. Differential Diagnosis; see pathogenesis (II.A.B.) for causes
    1.   Patients with persistent sinusitis, asthma, or OME need evaluation for presence of allergies
    2.   Suspect upper respiratory infections with a history of contagion, presence of fever, purulent nasal discharge, inflamed nasal mucosa, and absence of eosinophils on nasal smear
    3.   Suspect foreign body or an anatomical problem if rhinitis is unilateral

D. Diagnostic tests (diagnosis is usually made from the history and physical and no tests are required)
    1.   Skin testing for allergies is the gold standard test; compare results with the clinical history
        a.   Two types are available: epicutaneous (prick or scratch test) and intradermal (antigen is injected between skin layers)
        b.   Warn patients to avoid use of antihistamines, decongestants, and corticosteroids before testing as these may interfere with results
    2.   Nasal smear is often helpful; eosinophils are elevated with allergic rhinitis whereas an infection is likely if neutrophils predominate; peripheral eosinophil count is not useful
    3.   Nasal cytology helps in differentiating allergic rhinitis from other forms (e.g., vasomotor, infectious rhinitis)
    4.   Because serum IgE levels are elevated in 30-40% of patients with allergic rhinitis and increased levels occur in nonallergies, this testing has limited value
    5.   *In vitro* serum allergy tests (radioallergosorbent, fluoroallergosorbent, and multiple allergosorbent tests) are expensive and not as specific nor as sensitive as skin testing
    6.   If there is any question of an infectious process obtain a CBC
    7.   Fiberoptic nasal endoscopy and/or rhinomanometry may be needed to rule out associated diseases such as sinusitis and anatomical problems; consult specialist

V. Plan/Management

A. Allergic rhinitis
1. Effective long-term management may prevent or reduce general respiratory tract inflammation and lower airway hyper-reactivity, thereby decreasing incidence and worsening of asthma and other diseases (e.g., otitis media, sinusitis)
2. Patient Education: Allergen avoidance is the most effective form of treatment.
    a. The bedroom is considered the room that must be the most allergen-free
    b. Try to eliminate dust and allergen exposure in the household (see table that follows)

MEASURES OF ENVIRONMENTAL CONTROL IN THE HOME

✓ Vacuum weekly (some vacuums spread dust and mites, so the vacuum should be cleaned regularly) or perform damp mopping
✓ Dust furniture and all horizontal surfaces weekly with a damp cloth
✓ Encase mattress and pillow in allergen-impermeable cover; wash sheets and blankets in hot water weekly
✓ Remove carpets from bedroom; avoid lying on upholstered furniture; remove carpets laid on concrete
✓ Avoid rubber mattress
✓ Recommend keeping windows and doors closed to decrease influx of mold and pollen; may necessitate air conditioning in the summer (have AC unit professionally cleaned to clear mold/mildew off coils)
✓ Reduce indoor humidity to less than 50%
✓ Eliminate or restrict exposure to pets; use high efficiency particulate air (HEPA) filter or electrostatic air purifier if pets remain in house; wash pets weekly
✓ To control cockroaches, use poison traps or bait; do not leave food or garbage exposed
✓ Use clothes dryer rather than hanging clothes outside to air dry
✓ Wear high-efficiency mask and long-sleeved shirt when gardening; bathe and change clothes immediately after coming inside

---

3. Inform patients that they may access information such as pollen counts on TV weather stations as well as on the internet (see following table for Websites)

WEBSITES FOR PATIENT INFORMATION

Organization	Website
American Academy of Allergy, Asthma and Immunology	www.aaaai.org
American College of Asthma, Allergy and Immunology	www.acaai.org
Asthma and Allergy Foundation of America	www.aafa.org

4. Drug therapy is indicated when allergen avoidance is ineffective or impractical
    a. No recommended first-line drug of choice; choice of medication depends on the patient's symptoms, adverse drug reactions, adherence factors, risk of drug interactions, and cost (see table COMPARATIVE EFFICACY)
    b. Because of potentially dangerous side effects (sedation and performance impairment) of first generation antihistamines, second generation antihistamines or nasal corticosteroids for severe cases are often considered the first-line drugs

COMPARATIVE EFFICACY OF MEDICATIONS

	Pruritus	Rhinorrhea	Nasal Blockage	Eye Symptoms
Oral antihistamines	+++	++	±	+++
Oral decongestants	---	±	+++	---
Antihistamine/decongestant combinations	+++	++	+++	+++
Intranasal decongestants	---	---	+++	---
Intranasal corticosteroids	+++	+++	++(+)	+
Intranasal cromolyn	+	+	±	---
Intranasal ipratropium	---	+++	---	---

5. Second generation antihistamines (see table that follows)
   a. Advantages: Fewer adverse drug effects and simpler dosing schedule than first-generation antihistamines
   b. Disadvantages: No relief for rhinorrhea and nasal congestion; do not control underlying inflammatory response

COMPARISON OF SECOND GENERATION ANTIHISTAMINES			
	Cetirizine (Zyrtec)	Desloratadine (Clarinex)	Fexofenadine (Allegra)	Loratadine (Claritin and Claritin Reditabs*)
Formulation	tablets: 5 mg, 10 mg syrup: 1 mg/mL	tablets: 5 mg	tablets: 30 mg, 60 mg, 180 mg capsules: 60 mg	tablets: 10 mg syrup: 1 mg/mL
Dosage Patients >18 years	5 or 10 mg QD	5 mg QD (Initially 5 mg EOD**)	60 mg BID or 180 mg QD (Initially 60 mg QD)	10 mg QD (Initially 10 mg EOD**)
Dosage Children	2-5 years: 2.5 or 5 mg QD or 2.5 mg BID (initially 2.5 mg QD) 6-11 years: 5 or 10 mg QD	Not recommended	6-11 years: 30 mg BID ≥12 years: 60 mg BID or 180 mg QD	2-5 years: 5 mg QD 6-11 years: 10 mg QD (initially 10 mg EOD**) ≥12 years: 10 mg QD
Sedation	Yes	No	No	No
Dry mouth and urinary retention	Yes	No	No	No
Interactions	Potentiates CNS depression with alcohol and other CNS depressants	None known	Avoid aluminum or magnesium-containing antacids	None known

*Rapidly disintegrating tablets; dissolve on tongue; swallow with or without water
** EOD - every other day

6. First generation antihistamines (see table that follows)
   a. Advantages: Inexpensive; anticholinergic properties may reduce rhinorrhea; early onset of action is useful for intermittent symptoms
   b. Disadvantages: Numerous adverse effects such as drowsiness, impaired performance, anticholinergic effects such as dry mouth, urinary retention, and constipation; do not relieve nasal congestion; must be cautious when used in the elderly; may worsen asthma symptoms; do not control underlying inflammatory response
   c. Warn patients to avoid driving cars or operating heavy machinery when beginning therapy
   d. Avoid or use cautiously in patients with prostate hypertrophy and angle-closure glaucoma
   e. Rule of thumb is to use the smallest dose that is effective
   f. Slowly titrate drugs beginning with one dose at bedtime for several days, then add a small morning dose; tolerance to sedative effects occurs after 1-2 weeks of dosing
7. Azelastine HCl nasal spray (Astelin) is the first topical antihistamine
   a. Advantages: Effective in reducing allergic symptoms, has good safely profile, and is more beneficial in relieving nasal obstruction than oral antihistamines
   b. Disadvantages: Causes sedation and has a bitter taste
   c. Prescribe 2 sprays per nostril BID in patients ≥12 years
   d. Not recommended for children <5 years; 5-11 years: 1 spray per nostril BID

FIRST GENERATION ANTIHISTAMINES

	Patients >18 Years Dose (mg)	Child's Dose (liquid forms)
Ethanolamine		
Diphenhydramine (Benadryl)*†	25-50 TID/QID	5 mg/kg/day (12.5 mg/5 mL) in 3-4 doses
Clemastine (Tavist)†	1 BID	---
Alkylamine		
Chlorpheniramine (Chlor-Trimeton)†	4 QID or 8 BID	2-5 yrs: 1 mg QID; >6 yrs: 2 mg QID (2 mg/5 mL)
Piperazine		
Hydroxyzine (Atarax, Vistaril)	10-25 TID/QID	<6 yrs: 50 mg daily in divided doses (10 mg/5 mL) in divided doses ≥6 yrs: 50-100 mg daily
Piperidine		
Cyproheptadine (Periactin)	4 TID	2-6 yrs: 2 mg BID/TID; 7-14 yrs: 4 mg BID/TID (2 mg/5 mL)

*Benadryl may decrease cognitive function in elderly patients   †Over-the-counter medication

8. Oral decongestants are often combined with antihistamines to enhance effectiveness and/or counterbalance sedative side effects (see table that follows); products containing phenylpropanolamine are banned because of increased risk of stroke in young women

COMMON COMBINATION ANTIHISTAMINE/DECONGESTANT PRODUCTS

Antihistamine/Decongestant	Brand Name	Patients >18 Years Dose	Child's Dose
Chlorpheniramine 4 mg/ pseudoephedrine 60 mg	Deconamine	1 tab TID/QID	2-6 yrs, 2.5 mL TID/QID; >6 yrs, 2.5-5 mL TID/QID (chlorpheniramine 2 mg/- pseudoephedrine 30 mg per 5 mL)
Fexofenadine 60 mg/ pseudoephedrine 120 mg	Allegra-D	1 tab BID	Not recommended
Loratadine 10 mg/ pseudoephedrine 240 mg	Claritin-D 24 Hour	1 tab QD	Not recommended

9. For patients with significant nasal congestion, a topical decongestant may be needed first
   a. Minimal side effects but ineffective for pulmonary and ocular allergic symptoms
   b. Never use beyond 3-4 days
   c. For adolescents and children ≥6 years prescribe oxymetazoline (Neo-Synephrine 12-Hour Spray) 2-3 sprays in each nostril up to every 10-12 hours; not recommended for children <6 years
10. Steroid sprays are often drug of choice, particularly for severe cases, because they are the most effective and potent agents available for treatment (see table that follows)
   a. Advantages: Control nasal congestion and rhinorrhea; few adverse effects; control underlying anti-inflammatory response; steroid sprays were more efficacious than antihistamines in several studies
   b. Disadvantages: Expensive; slow onset of activity; do not relieve ocular symptoms; adverse effects are epistaxis, nasal irritation, and, very rarely, septal perforation; in children, may have suppressive effect on bone growth
   c. May be combined with antihistamines for enhanced effectiveness
   d. Steroid sprays have a slow onset of activity; warn patients they might <u>not</u> see effects for 2 weeks after initiating therapy
   e. Use on a regular basis and reduce dose when benefit is obtained

INTRANASAL CORTICOSTEROIDS	
Medication	**Dosing**
Beclomethasone (Beconase AQ)	1-2 sprays in each nostril BID (not approved for children <6 years)
Fluticasone propionate (Flonase)	1 spray in each nostril QD (not approved for children <4 years)
Mometasone furoate (Nasonex)	Patients ≥12 years: 2 sprays in each nostril QD; children 2-11 years: 1 spray per nostril QD (not approved for children <2 years)
Triamcinolone (Nasacort AQ)	Patients >6 years: 2 sprays in each nostril QD; reduce dose as condition improves (not approved for children <6 years)

11. Oral corticosteroids are reserved for short-term therapy for patients with severe disease
12. Mast cell stabilizers are usually reserved for patients with chronic or severe symptoms
    a. Advantages: Good safety profile, control underlying inflammatory response
    b. Disadvantages: Less effective than other therapies in relieving nasal obstruction; frequent dosing makes it difficult for patients to adhere; expensive
    c. Prevent symptoms from starting and are generally not beneficial once an attack has started; can use prophylactically (e.g., just before visiting a home with a cat)
    d. Recommend over-the-counter, intranasal cromolyn sodium (NasalCrom) 1 spray in each nostril every 4 to 6 hours; not approved for children <2 years
    e. Concomitant use of decongestants may be useful to relieve congestion
13. Intranasal ipratropium (do **not** prescribe to patients who have peanut allergies)
    a. Advantages: Excellent safety profile and few adverse reactions
    b. Disadvantage: Effective for only rhinorrhea; minimal effect on other symptoms
    c. Prescribe ipratropium bromide 0.03% aqueous solution (Atrovent nasal spray) 2 sprays in each nostril 2-3 times daily; not recommended for children <6 years
14. Application of saline to nasal mucosa acts as a mild decongestant and can liquify mucus and prevent crusting; administer 2-4 times a day
15. Allergic conjunctivitis which often accompanies allergic rhinitis may require flushing eyes with artificial liquid tears or use one of the following ophthalmic solutions
    a. Naphazoline HCl 0.025% and pheniramine maleate 0.3% (Naphcon A) 1-2 drops in each eye up to 4 times daily (not recommended children <6 years)
    b. Cromolyn sodium 4% (Crolom) 1-2 drops in each eye 4-6 times daily (not recommended children <4 years)
16. Leukotriene modifiers: Some research studies found that these drugs were effective in relieving symptoms; use montelukast (Singulair) for patients who don't benefit from or tolerate nasal steroids and/or antihistamines
17. For patients with nasal polyps, refer to specialist
18. Patient education
    a. Remind patients with perennial allergic rhinitis to take medications regularly rather than sporadically when symptoms occur
    b. Teach patients to read drug labels before taking over-the-counter medication as many cold products and sleep aids contain antihistamines
    c. Teach patient proper administration of intranasal medications (see following table)

INSTRUCTIONS FOR USE OF INTRANASAL MEDICATION
✓ Clear nasal passages or blow nose before administering medication
✓ Keep head upright and tilted slightly forward; breathe out slowly
✓ Squeeze the pump or press down the canister as you slowly breathe through nose
✓ Spray medication away from nasal septum
✓ Spray each nostril separately and wait at least 1 minute before second spray
✓ If possible, avoid sneezing or blowing nose for 5-10 minutes after spraying
✓ Cleanse medicine canister device after each use

19. Allergen immunotherapy (also see table that follows)
    a. Consider this therapy for patients who have demonstrable evidence of specific IgE antibodies to clinically relevant allergens after skin testing and who wish to avoid or reduce the long-term use of medications
    b. Immunotherapy is effective for pollen, fungi (molds), animal dander, dust mites, and cockroaches

        c.   Decision to begin therapy should depend on degree to which symptoms can be reduced by avoidance and medication, amount and type of medications needed for symptom control, and the adverse effects of medications

---

GUIDELINES FOR THE SAFE AND EFFECTIVE USE OF ALLERGEN IMMUNOTHERAPY

- Contraindications: Severe asthma uncontrolled by pharmacotherapy, significant cardiovascular disease, and use of beta-adrenergic blocking agents
- Use very cautiously in older adults with comorbid conditions
- Whenever possible, use standardized extracts to prepare vaccine treatment
- Efficacy of immunotherapy depends on achieving an optimal therapeutic dose of each of the clinically relevant constituents in the vaccine
- Routine periodic skin testing or in vitro IgE antibody testing of patients receiving immunotherapy is not recommended
- Only administer the vaccine in settings where prompt recognition and treatment of anaphylaxis are assured
- Inject agent subcutaneously into triceps muscle with a 26- or 27-gauge syringe with a 3/8- or 1/2–inch nonremovable needle
- Patients should remain in clinician's office at least 20-30 minutes after injection
- The usual frequency of vaccine administration is one to two injections per week, at least 2 days apart
- When the maintenance dose is reached, the interval between injections can be progressively increased as tolerated to 4-6 weeks
- Clinical improvement is usually seen within one year after a patient reaches maintenance dose
- Evaluate patients every 6-12 months during immunotherapy
- Carefully consider stopping immunotherapy after 3-5 years

Adapted from Li, J.T., Lockey, R.F., Bernstein, I.L., Portnoy, J.M., & Nicklas, R.A. (2003). Allergen immunotherapy: A practice parameter. *Annals of Allergy, Asthma, & Immunology*, 90, 1-40.

B.   Nonallergic rhinitis; difficult to relieve symptoms
    1.   Nonspecific broad-based therapy includes topical azelastine, topical corticosteroids, and cromoglycate
    2.   Symptomatic-specific therapy
         a.   Decongestants for patients whose symptoms are primarily obstructive
         b.   Topical ipratropium bromide for patients whose symptom is primarily rhinorrhea
         c.   A nasal spray of physiological saline solution or a more thorough cleansing of nose with powered irrigators such as the Grossan irrigator may be helpful for postnasal drainage, sneezing, and congestion
    3.   Patient education: increase water intake, decrease caffeine and alcohol intake (both have a diuretic effect), and consider adding humidity to bedroom

C.   Follow up of all types of rhinitis
    1.   Schedule visits in 2-3 weeks to review patient education topics and check therapy results
    2.   Schedule quarterly or biannual rechecks depending on patient's level of comfort and health

EPISTAXIS

I.   Definition: Nasal bleeding from any cause

II.   Pathogenesis

A.   The nose acts as a conduit to allow air into the lungs and has a very well vascularized mucosa with a complex interior surface composed of folds and irregularities

B.   The blood supply of the nose comes from both the internal and external carotid systems

C.   More than 90% of bleeds are related to local irritation and most occur in the absence of a specific underlying anatomic lesion

D. Bleeding is typically due to disruption of the nasal mucosa: dry nasal mucosa, infection, allergy, trauma (nose picking, forceful blowing, injury), foreign body, neoplasm, cocaine use

E. Epistaxis is infrequently due to systemic diseases: liver disease, hypertension (hypertension does not cause nasal bleeding but may exacerbate the problem), bleeding disorders (such as thrombocytopenia and problems related to chemotherapy for cancer), hereditary hemorrhagic telangiectasia (Rendu-Osler-Weber disease), granulomatous disease (Wegener's, sarcoidosis)

F. The following medications may be associated with bleeds: aspirin, warfarin, dipyridamole, antihistamines, nasal steroids, diuretics

G. Site of the bleeding helps to determine the cause
   1. Anterior bleeds usually involve the Kiesselbach's plexus (triangle of the anterior portion of the septum) and result from local irritation, cracks in dry nasal mucosa, or trauma
   2. Posterior bleeds are usually just superior or inferior to the posterior tip of inferior turbinate and are associated with systemic causes or facial trauma

III. Clinical Presentation

A. Approximately 10% of the population experiences at least one significant nosebleed

B. Commonly seen in children and episodes are typically infrequent, mild, and self-limiting

C. Over 90% of nosebleeds are anterior
   1. Generally less severe and easier to control than posterior nosebleeds
   2. Usually are unilateral, continuous, and have moderate bleeding

D. Posterior bleeds are often intermittent, severe, and difficult to treat
   1. Tend to occur in older persons
   2. Blood may flow into pharynx and lungs

IV. Diagnosis/Evaluation

A. History; quickly assess patient and, if stable, begin history
   1. Question about onset, duration, pattern, and severity (quantity) of bleeding
   2. Ask about an increase in nasal mucus; if yes, determine color, character, and quantity
   3. Ask if nasal obstruction is present, and if so, is it an acute or chronic occurrence
   4. Ask about bleeding into pharynx which commonly indicates a posterior bleed
   5. Ask about occupational exposure to irritating chemicals or dust; ask about dry, indoor environment
   6. Inquire about medication usage; ask about cocaine use if appropriate
   7. Inquire about previous episodes and treatments
   8. Ask about trauma (injury, nose picking, forceful blowing)
   9. Question about other medical conditions (infections, allergies, bleeding disorders, hypertension)
   10. Inquire about history of clotting problems (easy bruising, hematuria, melena, heavy menstrual flow)

B. Physical Examination; patient is best examined sitting and leaning forward
   1. Assess blood pressure and pulse
   2. Use gentle suction with a bulb syringe removing blood and secretions to make visualization of the involved vessels possible
   3. Locate bleeding site if possible; 90% are in the anterior septum; posterior site is indicated by persistent drainage of blood down the pharynx
   4. If systemic illnesses are likely assess the following:
      a. Skin for pallor, rash, purpura, petechiae, telangiectasias
      b. Lymph nodes for enlargement due to malignancy or other illnesses
      c. Percuss sinuses to assess for sinusitis

C. Differential Diagnosis (see Pathogenesis II.C.-G.)

D. Diagnostic Tests; history and physical examination should guide selection of tests
   1. Extensive evaluation should be reserved for cases that are recurrent or particularly severe
   2. Hemoglobin or hematocrit if significant blood loss has occurred
   3. CBC with differential, platelets, PT, and PTT if bleeding disorders are suspected

V.   Plan/Management

A.   Use the approaches outlined in the table below for anterior nose bleeds

<table>
<tr><td colspan="2" align="center">**MANAGEMENT OF ANTERIOR NOSE BLEEDS**</td></tr>
<tr><td>•</td><td>First, apply pressure to anterior nasal septum while head is tilted forward; continue pressure for 10-15 minutes (patient should be sitting and leaning forward)</td></tr>
<tr><td>•</td><td>Then, if clot formation and bleeding cessation do not occur, do the following
✓ Place a small piece of cotton soaked in 1:1000 epinephrine or a vasoconstricting nose drop such as phenylephrine (Neo-Synephrine) or oxymetazoline (Afrin) into the vestibule of the nose
✓ Press against the bleeding site for 10 to 15 minutes to promote vasoconstriction
✓ Remove to observe for bleeding (almost all venous types of anterior nosebleeds are stopped with this treatment)</td></tr>
<tr><td>•</td><td>If bleeding continues, but has slowed considerably
✓ Repeat treatment
✓ Apply ice pack over the nose as an additional therapy</td></tr>
<tr><td>•</td><td>If these remedies fail,
✓ Anesthetize the mucous membrane with 4% lidocaine or 4% cocaine (apply to cotton ball and hold in place for several minutes)
✓ Apply a silver nitrate stick to the bleeding site</td></tr>
<tr><td>•</td><td>Finally, if bleeding persists consider the following (consider consultation with a specialist)
✓ Use adherent materials such as oxidized cellulose (Oxycel, Surgicel), microfibrillar collagen (Avitene), or absorbable gelatin sponge (Gelfoam) placed at the bleeding site; these agents dissolve in a few days
✓ A compressed nasal tampon (Merocel) can also be placed in nares and left in place for 1-3 days; usually tampon is impregnated with antibiotic ointment and patient is treated with antistaphylococcal antibiotics</td></tr>
</table>

B.   Patients with anterior bleeds who do not respond to above treatments should be referred to emergency department for cautery and/or packing; refer recurrent and severe cases to specialist

C.   Patients with posterior bleeds should be immediately referred to otolaryngologic specialist; while awaiting consult, efforts to control bleeding should be limited to spraying nose with topical anesthetic or vasoconstricting substance such as 5% oxymetazoline or 4% cocaine

D.   Patient education
    1.   Instruct patient regarding management of simple nose bleeds at home
        a.   Sit up, lean forward, spray nose with over-the-counter nasal sprays (Afrin, Neo-Synephrine), then apply and press cotton soaked with nasal spray against bleeding area
        b.   Apply petrolatum-based ointment to septum to prevent further drying
        c.   Limit heavy lifting, straining, bending over, intake of spicy or hot foods, hot showers, and medications that might affect hemostasis
    2.   Teach about prevention of nosebleeds
        a.   Increase humidity in home through use of humidifier, especially during winter months
        b.   Advise liberal use of lubricant such a petrolatum in nares to promote hydration
        c.   Recommend trial of nasal saline drops, particularly at night
        d.   Teach to avoid traumatizing nose; in children, suggest keeping fingernails trimmed

E.   Follow Up: None indicated for cases due to local trauma or inflammation

FOREIGN BODY IN THE NOSE

I.   Definition: Presence of object(s) in the nasal cavity

II.   Pathogenesis: Intentional placement of an object in nose, or occasionally accidental placement of a foreign body while child is attempting to sniff or smell the object

III.   Clinical Presentation

A.   Child may insert object into nose as a result of boredom, curiosity, or acts of imitation; the most common underlying factor is a history of chronic rhinitis

B.   Typically, these objects are soft materials such as tissues, erasers, clay, or part of a toy

C.   The key feature is unilateral symptoms

1. Symptoms include unilateral obstruction, mild discomfort, sneezing, and occasionally epistaxis
2. Unilateral purulent, foul-smelling, nasal discharge can also occur over time
3. When an alkaline disk battery is lodged, the symptoms are more acute and may include electrical burns and necrosis

D. Complications include local infection, inflammation, chronic sinusitis, and rhinolith (occurs when foreign body remains in nose for long time and becomes calcified); aspiration can be avoided by prompt and skilled removal

IV. Diagnosis/Evaluation

A. History
1. Inquire about onset and duration of symptoms
2. Ask parent/child if this has occurred in the past
3. Determine type of foreign body by asking parents what objects the child was playing with; child will usually not confess to insertion of object

B. Physical Examination
1. Test both nares for patency
2. Examine both nares with nasal speculum; powerful illumination and adequate visualization is mandatory (see Plan/Management V.A. for strategies to improve visualization)

C. Differential Diagnosis; Unilateral nasal discharge in a young child should be considered evidence of a foreign body until proven otherwise
1. Suppurative rhinitis
2. Sinusitis
3. Adenoiditis
4. Nasal or nasopharyngeal tumors
5. Nasal polyps

D. Diagnostic Tests: X-rays may be helpful if the object is radiopaque or has become calcified, but usually no tests are needed

V. Plan/Management

A. Use topical decongestant such as Neo-Synephrine to reduce mucosal edema, remove secretions with a small suction tip, and then, visualize object with an endoscope; child may need sedation or general anesthesia

B. Method of removal depends on location and type of foreign body; consider the following:
1. For shallow objects, occlude the uninvolved nostril and have the child blow forcefully out or remove with a Frazier tip suction
2. For hard objects, a right-angle hook can be placed behind the object and pulled out slowly; insert instruments perpendicular to the plane of the face and avoid instrumenting the medial wall to prevent damage to the turbinates
3. Soft objects can be grasped with alligator forceps if the child is cooperative; instruments introduced into the nasal passage require a steady hand resting on the child's head
4. Some experts recommend removal with a Fogarty or small Foley catheter
   a. Catheter is placed beyond the foreign body and then inflated with 2-3 ml of saline solution
   b. Then gently draw catheter out, expelling the object
   c. Aspiration is a risk because foreign body may be pushed posteriorly into the nasopharynx

C. After removal of object if local irritation is present, use saline drops 2-3 times/day for 2-3 days or antibacterial ointment such as bacitracin or mupirocin; use sterile water if the foreign object was an alkaline battery

D. For uncooperative children, or when the nasal passage is completely occluded by an expanding foreign object such as plant materials, beans, or other seeds, or when there is marked edema and inflammation, referral to a specialist is indicated

E. Always refer to a specialist if the foreign body appears to be going deeper

F. Follow Up
    1. Advise to return if signs of retained foreign body develop (purulent discharge or epistaxis)
    2. Evaluate healing of mucosa in 2 days

RHINOSINUSITIS

I. Definition: Acute, subacute, or chronic inflammation of the mucous membranes that line the paranasal sinuses and concomitant inflammation of nasal mucosa

    A. Acute rhinosinusitis: Abrupt onset of infection with duration of symptoms of less than 4 weeks

    B. Subacute rhinosinusitis: Persistent occurrence of purulent nasal discharge despite therapy; epithelial damage is usually reversible; minimal to moderate symptoms last 4-12 weeks

    C. Chronic rhinosinusitis: Prolonged inflammation and/or repeated or inadequately treated acute infection; irreversible damage to the mucosa is present, symptoms last >12 weeks

    D. Recurrent acute rhinosinusitis: Four or more episodes per year with each episode of at least seven days' duration; absence of intervening signs and symptoms

II. Pathogenesis

    A. Etiological factors
        1. Main factor is obstruction of the sinus ostia (small opening in which the maxillary, frontal, ethmoid, and sphenoid sinuses all drain into nasal cavity) that leads to lower levels of oxygen within sinuses, decreased clearance of foreign material, and mucus stasis which creates a good environment for pathogens to grow; the following are predisposing factors:
            a. Recent upper respiratory infection
            b. Allergic rhinitis
            c. Environmental pollutants (smoke)
            d. Anatomic abnormalities such as a deviated septum or adenoidal hypertrophy
            e. "Aspirin triad" of aspirin sensitivity, asthma, and nasal polyps
            f. Medication side effects (antiosteoporosis agents, hormone replacement sprays, or rhinitis medicamentosa from abuse of topical decongestants and cocaine)
            g. Diving and swimming
            h. Extension of dental abscess
            i. Neoplasms
            j. Hormone-based turbinate edema as occurs during pregnancy
            k. Trauma
            l. Foreign body
        2. Other patients have problems with mucus stasis due to immune deficiency, immotile cilia syndrome, or cystic fibrosis

    B. Pathogens in acute sinusitis
        1. Common
            a. Viruses (viral rhinosinusitis occurs more often than bacterial rhinosinusitis)
            b. *Streptococcus pneumoniae*; penicillin-resistant *S. pneumoniae* is becoming common
            c. *Haemophilus influenzae* (may be ß-lactamase producing)
            d. *Moraxella catarrhalis* ([may be ß-lactamase producing]; prevalence greater among children than adults)
            e. *Streptococcus pyogenes*
        2. Less common
            a. Streptococcus species
            b. *Chlamydia pneumoniae*
            c. *Staphylococcus aureus*
            d. Fungi (e.g., *Aspergillus fumigatus*) (more common in patients who are immunosuppressed or have diabetes mellitus)

C. Pathogens in chronic or subacute sinusitis are usually polymicrobial but commonly include the following:
1. Anaerobic bacteria
2. *Staphylococcus aureus*

D. Anaerobes are common in sinusitis resulting from dental infections

III. Clinical Presentation

A. Most sinus disease in adults and children involves the maxillary and anterior ethmoidal sinuses

B. Once believed an adult disease, today acute sinusitis is considered a common pediatric problem, complicating 5-10% of upper respiratory infections and affecting all age groups, even infants
1. Younger children are at greater risk due to their small anatomic structures, frequency of viral infections, increased exposure to pathogens, allergens, and irritants, as well as their "immature" immune systems
2. Children, in contrast to adults, usually have more nonspecific complaints and symptoms are more difficult to distinguish from those of the common cold
   a. Typically children <5 years do not complain of headaches and facial pain
   b. The most common symptoms in children are cough and nasal discharge

C. Acute bacterial rhinosinusitis has the following characteristics (see following table):

DIAGNOSTIC PREDICTORS OF BACTERIAL RHINOSINUSITIS*	
Major factors	Facial pain or pressure (requires another major factor for diagnosis) Facial congestion or fullness Nasal obstruction Nasal purulence or discolored postnasal discharge Hyposmia or anosmia Fever (acute sinusitis only)
Minor factors	Headache Halitosis Fatigue Dental pain Cough Ear pain, pressure, or fullness Fever (nonacute sinusitis)

*Diagnosis of bacterial rhinosinusitis depends on the presence of at least 2 major factors or 1 major factor and 2 minor factors

Adapted from Lanza, D.C., & Kennedy, D.W. (1997). Adult rhinosinusitis defined. In J.B. Anon (Ed.). Report of the Rhinosinusitis Task Force Committee Meeting. *Otolaryngology–Head and Neck Surgery, 111*(Suppl), S1-S7.

1. Other clinical features include sore throat, early morning periorbital swelling, toothache, malaise, increased pain with coughing, bending over, or sudden head movement, and lack of response to decongestants
2. Signs and symptoms are prolonged for at least for 10 days

D. Subacute or chronic sinusitis has the following characteristics:
1. Nasal discharge, nasal congestion, or cough lasting >30 days
2. Hallmark is dull ache or pressure across midface or headache
3. Other symptoms include thick postnatal drip, "popping" ears, eye pain, halitosis, chronic cough, and fatigue

E. Chronic sinusitis is a relatively uncommon problem in children

F. Thick, tenacious, brown secretions are characteristic of fungal sinusitis

G. All types of sinusitis may exacerbate asthma

H. Diabetics and immunosuppressed patients often experience severe, invasive sinus disease

I. Complications include contiguous spread or hematogenous dissemination of infection and can result in life-threatening intraorbital (cellulitis, abscess) and intracranial suppuration (cavernous sinus thrombosis, meningitis, subdural empyema, brain abscess); patients with frontal headaches and associated frontal sinusitis are at greatest risk for intracranial complications

IV. Diagnosis/Evaluation

    A.   History
1. Question regarding onset, duration, and seasonality of symptoms
2. Ask whether symptoms are improving or worsening
3. Inquire about the laterality and quality (mucoid, purulent, serous) of nasal discharge; change in color or consistency is not a specific sign of bacterial infection
4. Ask about fever and systemic symptoms such as fatigue
5. Question about character (dry, productive) and timing (day, night, continual) of cough
6. Ask patient to describe pain and what aggravates it
7. Ask about timing and quality of headaches and morning puffiness about the eyes
8. Ask about past episodes and treatments
9. Inquire about past medical history such as allergies, diabetes mellitus, immunodeficiency, asthma
10. Question about smoking, recent trauma to the nose, recent upper respiratory infections
11. Inquire about family history of allergies, immunodeficiency, chronic respiratory complaints

    B.   Physical Examination
1. Determine vital signs
2. Examine eyes, noting peri-orbital swelling and presence of allergic shiners; if proptosis, impaired visual acuity, or impaired extraocular mobility are present, computerized tomography is needed to rule out suppurative complications
3. Examine nasal mucosa for erythema, edema, and discharge
4. Determine patency of both nasal nares
5. Anterior rhinoscopy (use of nasal speculum and otoscope) is important; use of topical decongestant before examination may facilitate inspection
      a. Does not allow visualization of middle meatus, but can view inferior turbinate and can evaluate quality of mucus within anterior nose
      b. Determine presence of polyps, septal deviation, and other anatomical deformities
6. Examine ears, throat, and mouth for signs of inflammation
7. Transilluminate and percuss frontal and maxillary sinuses (not reliable in young children)
8. Examine teeth and gingivae for caries and inflammation; tap maxillary teeth with tongue blade because 5% to 10% of maxillary sinusitis is due to dental root infection
9. Palpate neck and jaw for lymphadenopathy
10. Auscultate heart and lungs
11. Perform a neurological examination to rule out complications

    C.   Differential Diagnosis
1. Any condition that results in rhinitis (see Pathogenesis II.A.)
2. Differentiating viral from bacterial rhinosinusitis is difficult because viral infection frequently precedes bacterial infection
      a. Typically, in bacterial rhinosinusitis symptoms worsen after 5 days and persist for at least 10 days; persistence of respiratory symptoms without evidence that they are beginning to resolve suggests bacterial infection
      b. Symptoms are more severe and patients with bacterial infections often have purulent nasal discharge for 3-4 days and fever >102°F (39°C) (see table DIAGNOSTIC PREDICTORS OF BACTERIAL RHINOSINUSITIS, III.C.)

    D.   Diagnostic Tests
1. None indicated for typical presentation and for first episode of acute rhinosinusitis
2. Sinus aspiration with culture is the "gold standard" test (impractical in most primary care settings)
3. Radiologic studies are not routinely ordered and must be interpreted cautiously
      a. The common cold often includes radiologic evidence of sinus involvement (abnormal images only reflect inflammation, they do not pinpoint whether the inflammation is viral, bacterial or allergic in origin)
      b. Order radiographs to confirm clinical impression and in patients with frontal headaches, refractory cases, when complications are suspected, and when diagnosis is unclear
        (1) Sinus x-rays
          (a) Need antero-posterior, lateral, and occipitomental (Waters view) views
          (b) An air-fluid level or complete opacification of the sinuses and thickening of the mucosal lining are most diagnostic
          (c) X-rays are not recommended in children ≤6 years
          (d) Accuracy of diagnosing ethmoid disease is questionable with x-rays
        (2) Computerized tomography (CT scan) is gold standard of radiographic study, but is reserved for recalcitrant cases and patients in need of surgery

4. Flexible fiberoptic rhinoscopy, after the topical application of a vasoconstrictor and anesthetic, may be indicated
5. CBC with differential indicated for severely ill patients
6. Allergy testing when the history suggests an allergic disease
7. Consider ordering nasal cytology (diagnosis of allergic rhinitis, eosinophilia syndrome), a sweat chloride test (diagnosis of cystic fibrosis), and tests for immunodeficiency in recurrent cases

V. Plan/Management

A. Treatment of acute and subacute rhinosinusitis
   1. Antibiotics
      a. Although 40% of cases recover spontaneously without drugs, antibiotics are indicated for correctly diagnosed bacterial infections because they arrest progression to chronic sinusitis and concomitant permanent mucosal damage and also prevent complications
      b. Duration of treatment is controversial; 10-14 days is usually recommended; some experts suggest that antibiotics be continued until patient is free of symptoms and then for an additional 7 days
      c. First line drug is amoxicillin; but should not be drug of choice in certain patients (see table RISK FACTORS PROMPTING USE OF SECOND-LINE DRUGS)
         (1) Adolescents: Amoxicillin (Amoxil) 500 mg TID
         (2) Children: Amoxil 45 mg/kg/day PO in 2 divided doses (available in 125 mg/5 mL and 250 mg/5 mL strengths)
         (3) In areas with high resistance to *S. pneumoniae* double the dosage (90 mg/kg/per day)
      d. Trimethoprim-sulfamethoxazole and erythromycin-sulfisoxazole are sometimes recommended as first line drugs, however, because they have substantial resistance to *S. pneumoniae*, other antibiotics should be used

---

RISK FACTORS PROMPTING USE OF SECOND-LINE DRUGS

Antibiotic use in previous 4-6 weeks
Resistance common in community
Smoker in family
Child in day-care setting
Children <2 years of age
Allergy to penicillin or amoxicillin
Frontal or sphenoidal sinusitis
Complicated ethmoidal sinusitis
Possibly severe and protracted symptoms

Adapted from Brook, I., Gooch, W.M., III, Jenkins, S.G., et al. (2000). Medical management of acute bacterial sinusitis: Recommendations of a Clinical Advisory Committee on Pediatric and Adult Sinusitis. *Annals of Otology, Rhinology, and Laryngology, 109*, 2-20.

      e. Second line drugs
         (1) Amoxicillin/clavulanate (Augmentin); adolescents: 500-875 mg BID; children: 45 mg/kg/day in two divided doses (both based on amoxicillin content); or in adolescents Augmentin XR 2 tabs every 12 hours
         (2) Cefdinir (Omnicef); adolescents: 300 mg BID; children: 14 mg/kg/day in one or two divided doses
         (3) Cefuroxime axetil (Ceftin); adolescents: 250-500 mg BID; children: 30 mg/kg/day in two divided doses (available 125 mg/5 mL or 250 mg/5 mL liquid)
         (4) Cefpodoxime proxetil (Vantin); adolescents: 200-400 mg BID; children: 10mg/kg/day in one or two divided doses (available 50 mg/5 mL or 100 mg/5 mL liquid)
      f. Third line drugs (useful for patients who are penicillin and cephalosporin sensitive)
         (1) In persons >18 years, prescribe gatifloxacin, levofloxacin, or moxifloxacin
         (2) In children, prescribe clarithromycin or azithromycin
      g. Switch to another drug if there is lack of response at ≥72 hours; a good choice is high-dose amoxicillin/clavulanic acid; in adults use a total of 3-3.5 g/day and in children use 80-90 mg/kg/day of amoxicillin component and 6.4 mg/kg/day of clavulanate in two divided doses
      h. A single dose of ceftriaxone (50 mg/kg/day) IM or IV can be given if patient has difficulty taking oral antibiotics (e.g., vomiting)

2. Decongestants or saline nasal spray at the time of diagnosis of acute sinusitis and in acute episodes of subacute and chronic sinusitis can improve patency of ostiomeatal unit
   a. Topical decongestants should be used no longer than 3-4 days. For patients >6 years use oxymetazoline (Neo-Synephrine 12 hour spray 0.05%) 2-3 sprays in each nostril up to every 10-12 hours
   b. In children <6 years, use saline nasal drops, 2-3 drops in each nostril BID-QID (1/4 tsp of salt in 8 oz of boiled water)
   c. Oral decongestants are not as effective as topical agents but can be used for a longer time period; oral decongestants are not recommended in children
      (1) Use cautiously in patients with hypertension
      (2) Adolescents: pseudoephedrine hydrochloride (Sudafed) 60 mg every 4-6 hours
3. Nasal corticosteroids are not recommended for the treatment of acute rhinosinusitis

B. Treatment of chronic sinusitis
   1. Antibiotics: prescribe a β-lactamase stable antibiotic such as amoxicillin/clavulanate (Augmentin) or clarithromycin (Biaxin) and extend treatment for 2-4 weeks
   2. Topical nasal steroid sprays may be effective, but should not be used during acute episodes or exacerbations; prescribe one of the following:
      a. Beclomethasone (Beconase AQ) 1-2 sprays in each nostril BID (not approved for children <6 years)
      b. Fluticasone propionate (Flonase),1 spray in each nostril QD (not approved for children <4 years)
      c. Decrease dosages as symptoms improve

C. For acute sinusitis due to dental infection prescribe amoxicillin/clavulanate (Augmentin)

D. Treatment of fungal infections involves surgery and broad-spectrum antibiotics for intercurrent bacterial infections

E. Oral antihistamines should not be used unless patient has allergies as they tend to slow the movement of secretions out of the sinuses

F. Referral to a specialist is needed for the following:
   1. Recurrent, recalcitrant symptoms
   2. Exquisite pain with palpation or percussion of the face
   3. Possibility of cellulitis or other severe complications
   4. Periorbital swelling
   5. Uncontrolled asthma, nasal polyposis, or severe allergies

G. Functional endoscopic sinus surgery which removes only affected tissue has improved the surgical treatment of sinus disease

H. Patient Education
   1. Instruct patient to return for further evaluation if symptoms are not improved within 48 hours
   2. Teach patient about the complications of sinusitis, particularly the need to return if there is swelling in the periorbital area
   3. Humidify the air
   4. Increase fluid intake
   5. Steam inhalation and warm compresses often help relieve pressure
   6. Sleep with head of bed elevated
   7. Avoid allergens and excessively dry heat
   8. Avoid swimming/diving and air travel during acute period
   9. Avoid use of antihistamines unless there is an allergic basis to disease
   10. Encourage cessation of smoking
   11. Teach proper application of nasal sprays (see table on instructions for use of intranasal medications in ALLERGIC RHINITIS section)
   12. Patients who have recurrent sinusitis should be instructed to begin decongestants at the first sign of sinusitis to facilitate sinus drainage and decrease development of infection

I. Follow Up
   1. If no decrease in symptoms in 48-72 hours, patient should be re-evaluated; refer to specialist if symptoms are actually worsening
   2. Schedule return visit for 10-14 days
   3. Patients with chronic sinusitis who do not have marked improvement in four weeks with continuous medical therapy may require needle aspiration of a maxillary sinus or surgery

PHARYNGITIS

I. Definition: Inflammation of the pharynx and surrounding lymph tissue (tonsils)

II. Pathogenesis

    A. Viruses are the most common pathogens; the following are common viral infections:
        1. Infections due to rhinovirus, adenovirus, parainfluenza, coronavirus, echovirus, respiratory syncytial virus
        2. Herpangina due to Coxsackie virus and echovirus
        3. Hand, foot, and mouth syndrome due to Coxsackie virus
        4. Infectious mononucleosis caused by Epstein-Barr virus
        5. Human immunodeficiency virus (HIV) infection

    B. Bacteria (listed common to rare)
        1. Group A β-hemolytic streptococcus
        2. *Neisseria gonorrhoeae*
        3. *Corynebacterium diphtheriae*
        4. Streptococci of serogroups *C* and *G* (often associated with contaminated food or water)

    C. Other atypical agents that occur primarily in adults include *Mycoplasma pneumoniae* (uncommon) and *Chlamydia trachomatis* (rare)

    D. Fungus: *Candida albicans*

    E. Peritonsillar abscess: Often due to anaerobic bacteria, but may be due to Group A streptococci, *Haemophilus influenzae*, or *Staphylococcus aureus*

    F. Noninfectious causes
        1. Allergic rhinitis or post-nasal drip
        2. Mouth breathing
        3. Trauma from heat, alcohol, irritants such as marijuana or sharp objects
        4. Subacute thyroiditis in females

III. Clinical presentation of common causes of pharyngitis

    A. Pharyngitis due to respiratory viruses such as adenovirus, influenza, parainfluenza, respiratory syncytial virus
        1. Sore throat is often accompanied by conjunctivitis, coryza, cough, diarrhea
        2. Typically patient is afebrile and has gradual onset of symptoms

    B. Herpangina
        1. Small oral vesicles or ulcers may be on tonsils, pharynx, or posterior buccal mucosa
        2. Fever, headache, and malaise often accompany sore throat

    C. Hand, foot, and mouth syndrome: usually oral lesions and sore throat are accompanied by lesions on hands and feet; may have lesions on arms, legs, buttocks as well

    D. Infectious mononucleosis: Exudative tonsillitis with fever, fatigue, lymphadenopathy, and palatal petechiae (see section on INFECTIOUS MONONUCLEOSIS)

    E. Primary HIV infection resembles signs and symptoms of mononucleosis with sore throat, fever, malaise, myalgia, photophobia, lymphadenopathy, and rash; duration is few days to 2 weeks

F.   Pharyngitis due to Group A β-hemolytic streptococci; referred to as strep throat or GAS pharyngitis
   1.   Epidemiology
      a.   Mode of transmission is usually via direct projection of large droplets or physical transfer of respiratory secretions; rarely due to contaminated articles or ingestion of contaminated milk or other food
      b.   Prolonged carriage of streptococci may occur in the throat or upper respiratory tract for weeks to months
      c.   Incubation period usually ranges from 2-5 days
      d.   Period of communicability: During incubation period and clinical illness or approximately 10 days; after 24 hours of antibiotic therapy, person is no longer infectious
      e.   Predominantly a disease of children 5-15 years, but can occur in all age groups
      f.   Commonly seen in 15-30% of children and 5-10% of adults with pharyngitis
      g.   Occurs in winter or early spring
   2.   Children <3 years have unique presentation; they do no not have exudative pharyngitis and often have coryza and crusting of nares which is uncharacteristic in other age groups
   3.   Symptoms include sudden onset of fever >101°F, headaches, and sore throat with dysphagia and without cold-type symptoms such as nasal congestion
   4.   Erythema of tonsils and pharynx with white or yellow exudate occur
   5.   "Strawberry" tongue presents as a thick white coat with hypertrophied red papillae
   6.   Tender and enlarged anterior cervical lymph nodes are often present
   7.   Abdominal pain, vomiting, and headache may occur, whereas upper respiratory symptoms suggest other causes of pharyngitis
   8.   Without proper antimicrobial treatment, streptococcal pharyngitis can lead to serious suppurative (direct extension from pharyngeal infection) and nonsuppurative complications (arise from immune responses to acute infection)
      a.   Suppurative adenitis involving tender, enlarged nodes (see section CERVICAL ADENITIS)
      b.   Scarlet fever or scarlatina (suppurative)
         (1)   "Sandpaper" rash due to a vascular response to bacterial exotoxin occurs
         (2)   Exanthem appears 24-48 hours after infection and lasts 4-10 days
         (3)   Presents as fine, pin-head sized eruptions, often confluent, on an erythematous base which blanches on pressure
         (4)   Rash rapidly becomes generalized but is typically absent on the face which usually has a flushed appearance with circumoral pallor
         (5)   Petechiae may be present in a linear pattern along the major skin folds in the axillae and antecubital fossa (Pastia's sign)
         (6)   Rash fades 3-4 days after onset
         (7)   Desquamation of the skin usually occurs at the end of first week and disappears by end of 3 weeks
      c.   Peritonsillar abscess (suppurative) (see III.J.)
      d.   Glomerulonephritis (nonsuppurative) appears 1-3 weeks after pharyngeal infection (proper treatment with antimicrobials does not prevent)
      e.   Rheumatic fever (nonsuppurative); criteria for diagnosis is seen in table that follows
         (1)   Leading cause of cardiac death in individuals between 5 and 24 years; chronic cardiac valve disease and mitral regurgitation are the major complications
         (2)   Carditis is a new or changed murmur, a pericardial friction rub or effusion, and a recent or worsening heart enlargement with or without heart failure
         (3)   Polyarthritis, the most common major manifestation, is a benign condition involving the larger joints such as the knees, ankles, elbows, and wrists
         (4)   Sydenham's chorea, a benign sign, presents as purposeless, involuntary, rapid movements of the trunk and/or extremities
         (5)   Subcutaneous nodules are painless and freely movable; located under the skin over the extensor surfaces of joints (e.g., elbows, knees, and wrists)
         (6)   Rheumatic fever lasts an average of less than 3 months; fewer than 5% of the cases persist for more than 6 months

Adapted from Dajani, A.S., et al. (1993). Guidelines for the diagnosis of rheumatic fever: Jones criteria, updated 1992. *Circulation, 87,* 302-307.

        9.   Pediatric Autoimmune Neuropsychiatric Disorder Associated with Streptococcal Infection (PANDAS) has been linked to group A β-hemolytic streptococcal pharyngitis

           a.   Clinical features include abrupt onset and episodic course of obsessive-compulsive disorder, tic disorder, motoric hyperactivity, or choreiform movements in children

           b.   Children have rapid response to antibiotic treatment

    G.   Pharyngitis due to *Corynebacterium diphtheriae* (rare in US)
        1.   Grayish brown, adherent membrane on the nasal mucosa, tonsils, uvula, or pharynx
        2.   Bleeding occurs when membrane is removed

    H.   Pharyngitis due to *Neisseria gonorrhoeae* and *Chlamydia trachomatis*
        1.   Seen in those patients who practice orogenital sex and sexually abused children
        2.   Commonly presents as a chronic sore throat

    I.   Pharyngitis due to *Mycoplasma pneumoniae*
        1.   Uncommon in children <5 years of age, but seen in adolescents and adults
        2.   Signs and symptoms indistinguishable from streptococcal disease

    J.   Pharyngitis due to *Candida albicans*
        1.   Thin diffuse or patchy exudate on mucous membranes
        2.   Patients typically have history of antibiotic use or are immunosuppressed

    K.   Peritonsillar abscess
        1.   Most common in older children and adults following an episode of tonsillitis
        2.   Often presents with gradually increasing unilateral ear and throat pain
        3.   Dysphagia, dysphonia, drooling, and trismus (difficulty opening mouth) are common
        4.   Muffled "hot potato" voice may be present
        5.   The affected tonsil is usually grossly swollen medially and erythematous and may displace uvula and soft palate to contralateral side
        6.   Swelling and erythema of the soft palate are characteristic
        7.   Fluctuance may be felt with palpation of affected side
        8.   Enlarged and very tender lymph nodes are usually present

IV.   Diagnosis/Evaluation

    A.   History
        1.   Determine onset and duration of symptoms
        2.   Question about rhinorrhea and coughing (suggestive of viral agent)
        3.   Inquire about trismus, drooling and dysphagia (suggestive of peritonsillar abscess)
        4.   Ask about mouth lesions (suggestive of herpangina, hand, foot, and mouth syndrome, and thrush)
        5.   Inquire about skin changes and exanthems
        6.   Determine other associated symptoms such as abdominal pain, headache, and fatigue
        7.   Ascertain that sore throat is not significantly reducing intake of fluids

8. Inquire about possible streptococcal exposure
9. Inquire about immunization status
10. If applicable, inquire about sexual practices

B. Physical Examination
1. Do not attempt to examine the pharynx of a patient (particularly if the patient is between 3-7 years old) who has drooling, stridor, or trouble breathing (may have epiglottitis)
2. Measure vital signs
3. Observe appearance for signs of toxicity and distress
4. Inspect skin for color and exanthems
5. Palpate skin for texture and turgor, noting whether the skin has a "sandpaper" rash
6. Inspect mouth for lesions and thrush
7. Examine ears for concurrent otitis media or effusion
8. Visualize throat and pharynx for exudate and swelling (unilateral swelling occurs with peritonsillar abscess)
9. Palpate jaw and neck for adenopathy and nuchal rigidity
10. Perform complete heart and lung examinations
11. Depending on history of sexual activity, may need to perform genitourinary examination
12. Palpate abdomen

C. Differential Diagnosis
1. Stomatitis
2. Rhinitis or sinusitis with post nasal drip
3. Epiglottitis
4. Thyroiditis
5. Oropharyngeal anthrax (typically accompanied by ulcers at base of tongue and may have neck swelling and difficulty breathing)
6. Infectious diseases such as Kawasaki disease, rubella, rubeola

D. Diagnostic Tests
1. Diagnosis of GAS should be suspected on clinical presentation and epidemiological grounds (patient's age, the season, and family and community epidemiology) and then supported by results of a laboratory test
   a. Patients with acute onset of sore throat, fever, headache, pain on swallowing, anterior cervical node enlargement, and abdominal pain who do not have features suggestive of a viral syndrome (cold-type symptoms, conjunctivitis, diarrhea) should be tested
   b. A positive throat culture (sensitivity of 90-95%) or rapid antigen detection testing (RADT) (sensitivity 60-95%) provides confirmation of diagnosis
   c. A negative RADT should be confirmed with throat culture results
   d. Follow-up cultures are not routinely indicated for asymptomatic patients who complete their courses of antibiotics; patients with history of rheumatic fever or who develop pharyngitis during outbreaks of rheumatic fever or glomerulonephritis should have follow-up testing
   e. Testing of asymptomatic household contacts for GAS is not recommended except during outbreaks or when contacts have increased risk of developing complications; also test contacts who have rheumatic fever, glomerulonephritis, or symptoms suggestive of GAS
2. Consider heterophil agglutination, or mono spot test
3. Consider CBC with differential; expect WBC elevation with bacterial infection and WBC decrease with viral agent
4. Obtain culture on Thayer-Martin medium if gonococcal pharyngitis is suspected
5. If acute HIV infection is suspected, measure HIV RNA levels or obtain p24 antigen
6. Consider viral cultures of throat and mouth lesions
7. Tests for diagnosing peritonsillar abscess
   a. Consider ultrasonography or computed tomographic scanning
   b. Needle aspiration of abscess and culture; performed by trained clinician
8. To diagnose diphtheria, order culture of pseudomembrane in Loeffler's or tellurite selective medium

V. Plan/Management

A. For viral pharyngitis (i.e., herpangina, hand, foot, and mouth syndrome, and infectious mononucleosis), treatment is symptomatic, such as pain medication and use of hard candy, lozenges, or warm saline gargles to soothe throat

B. Streptococcal pharyngitis
1. Therapy is aimed at preventing suppurative complications such as rheumatic fever and decreasing infectivity
2. A delay of treatment as long as 9 days after acute onset does not increase risk of rheumatic fever
3. Treatment of choice is oral or intramuscular penicillin
   a. Persons >18 years: Penicillin V (Veetids) 500 mg BID or TID PO for 10 days (take on empty stomach)
   b. Children: Penicillin V (Veetids) 250 mg BID or TID PO for 10 days; available 125 mg/5 mL and 250 mg/5 mL liquid (take on empty stomach); amoxicillin may be alternative in young children because of its more acceptable taste of suspension
   c. Benzathine penicillin G (IM) 600,000 units for children <60 pounds (27 kg); 1,200,000 units for larger children and adults
      (1) Be familiar with signs, symptoms, and treatment of anaphylaxis and observe patient for 30 minutes after injection.
      (2) Bring medication to room temperature before injecting to reduce discomfort
4. Antibiotics for patients allergic to penicillin
   a. Because of the increase in macrolide-resistant group A streptococcus, always prescribe penicillin unless patient has a penicillin allergy
   b. Erythromycin: Persons >18 years- prescribe erythromycin stearate: 1 g per day, divided into 2 or 4 doses; Children - prescribe erythromycin ethyl succinate (EryPed): 40 mg/kg/day divided into 2 to 4 doses for 10 days; available 200 mg/5 mL and 400 mg/5 mL susp.
   c. First- and second-generation cephalosporins and azithromycin are acceptable alternatives to erythromycin; however, remember that 15% of penicillin-allergic persons also are allergic to cephalosporins
5. Treatment of patient who has recurrence of streptococcal pharyngitis shortly after completing recommended antibiotic therapy includes one of following:
   a. Retreat with same antibiotic
   b. Prescribe an alternative oral antibiotic such as amoxicillin-clavulanic acid (Augmentin) or clindamycin (Cleocin) every six hours; take with full glass of water
   c. Administer IM dose of benzathine penicillin G
   d. Administer benzathine penicillin G with rifampin PO (20 mg/kg/day in 2 divided doses for 4 days; maximum daily dose is 600 mg); addition of rifampin to benzathine penicillin may be helpful in eradicating streptococci from pharynx
   e. Also, rifampin 20 mg/kg/day PO once daily added during the final 4 days of a 10 day course of oral penicillin V might increase rate of eradication
6. Treatment of asymptomatic contacts is not recommended except in cases at increased risk of frequent infections or nonsuppurative streptococcal sequelae
7. Treatment of streptococcal pharyngeal carriers;
   a. Antibiotics are not indicated except for the following:
      (1) During outbreaks of acute rheumatic fever or poststreptococcal glomerulonephritis
      (2) During an outbreak of GAS pharyngitis in a closed or semi-closed community
      (3) Family history of rheumatic fever exists
      (4) Multiple episodes of documented, symptomatic GAS pharyngitis continue to occur within a family over weeks despite appropriate antibiotic therapy
      (5) Family has excessive anxiety of GAS pharyngitis
      (6) When tonsillectomy is considered due to chronic strep carriage
      (7) When a case of GAS toxic shock syndrome or necrotizing fasciitis has occurred in a household contact
   b. To eliminate carriage, prescribe clindamycin (Cleocin) 20 mg/kg/day (maximum 1.8 g/day) in three divided doses for 10 days; in adults prescribe 600 mg/day in 2-4 divided doses

C. Acute rheumatic fever (ARF)
1. Treatment of first attack of ARF depends on severity; consult with specialist
2. Prevention of recurrent attacks of ARF or secondary prevention
   a. Continuous prophylaxis is recommended for patients with a well-documented history of ARF
   b. Begin prophylaxis, after full course or antibiotics to eradicate residual Group A β-hemolytic streptococci even if throat culture is negative; promptly treat family members who have current or previous rheumatic fever
   c. Prescribe one of the following medication regimens (see following table)

SECONDARY PROPHYLAXIS OF ACUTE RHEUMATIC FEVER

Drug	Dose	Frequency
Benzathine penicillin G IM	1,200,000 units	Every 3-4 weeks
Penicillin V PO	250 mg	BID
Sulfadiazine PO	>60 pounds (27 kg): 1 gm	QD
	≤60 pounds (27 kg): 500mg	QD
Erythromycin PO*	250 mg	BID

*For patients allergic to penicillin and sulfadiazine

Adapted from Dajani, A., et al., 1995. Treatment of acute streptococcal pharyngitis and prevention of rheumatic fever: A statement for health professionals. *Pediatrics, 96*, 758-764.

        d.   Duration of continuous prophylaxis is controversial. Duration of treatment is dependent on risk of recurrence. Risk increases with multiple, previous attacks and in persons who have increased risk of exposure to streptococcal infections such as school teachers, health professionals, or military recruits; additional recommendations for therapy duration are as follows:

                (1)   ARF without carditis: 5 years or until age 21 years, whichever is longer

                (2)   ARF with carditis but without residual heart disease (no valvular disease): 10 years or well into adulthood, whichever is longer

                (3)   ARF with carditis and residual heart disease: at least 10 years since last episode and at least until age 40 years

    3.   Short-term antibiotic prophylaxis for bacterial endocarditis prior to certain procedures (including dental and surgical procedures) is needed for patients with rheumatic valvular heart disease (see pages 736-740 in *Red Book 2002, Report on the Committee on Infectious Diseases* for recommended regimens)

D.   Pharyngeal gonorrhea is usually treated with ceftriaxone (Rocephin) 250 mg IM or a single dose of oral quinolone (ciprofloxacin, 500 mg, or ofloxacin, 400 mg) plus either a single dose of azithromycin (1 g) or doxycycline (100 mg) BID for 7 days

E.   Diphtheria needs immediate consultation with a specialist and is usually treated with equine antitoxin and penicillin or erythromycin; notify public health department

F.   For pharyngitis due to *Mycoplasma pneumoniae* and *Chlamydia trachomatis*, treat with erythromycin (Ery-Tab) 500 mg BID for 10 days

G.   *Candida albicans* (see section on CANDIDIASIS)

H.   Peritonsillar abscess needs an immediate referral to a specialist

    1.   Initially, in outpatient setting, prescribe drug of choice, penicillin, and a pain medication

    2.   Needle aspiration, incision and drainage, or abscess tonsillectomy are current surgical approaches to management

I.   Patient Education

    1.   Teach parents and patients to immediately call office if the pain becomes more severe or if dyspnea, drooling, difficulty swallowing, and inability to fully open mouth develop

    2.   Advise increased fluid intake

    3.   Patients with streptococcal pharyngitis should not return to school or work until they have been on antibiotic therapy for a full 24 hours

    4.   Reinforce that patients will usually feel well in 24-48 hours, but that it is important to take full 10-day course of antibiotic to prevent complications, particularly rheumatic fever

    5.   Assure family that rheumatic fever does not occur with appropriate antibiotic therapy

J.   Follow Up

    1.   If no significant improvement in 3-4 days patient should return for re-evaluation

    2.   Patients with streptococcal pharyngitis: Post-treatment throat cultures are indicated only for patients who have high risk for rheumatic fever or who are still symptomatic after treatment

APHTHOUS STOMATITIS

I.   Definition: Chronic Inflammation of the oral mucosal tissue with ulcers often called canker sores

II.   Pathogenesis:

    A.   Etiology is uncertain, but heightened immunologic response to oral mucosal antigens probably plays a role
        1.   Common in persons with leukemia, neutropenia, and HIV infection
        2.   Increased prevalence in patients with autoimmune diseases such as Crohn's disease, Behçet's syndrome, Reiter's syndrome, and ulcerative colitis

    B.   Contributing factors include the following:
        1.   Allergies to coffee, chocolate, potatoes, cheese, figs, nuts, citrus fruits, and gluten
        2.   Stress
        3.   Generalized physical debility
        4.   Viral and bacterial pathogens
        5.   Trauma
        6.   Nutritional deficiencies such as vitamin B_{12}, folate, and iron
        7.   Hormones
        8.   Medications such as antihypertensives, antineoplastics, gold salts, and nonsteroidal anti-inflammatory drugs

    C.   Regardless of cause, when mucosal breakdown occurs, the lesions are invaded by mouth flora and become secondarily infected

III.   Clinical Presentation

    A.   Less prevalent in males and in chronic smokers

    B.   In approximately 1/3 of patients, recurrences continue for numerous years

    C.   Lesions divided into 3 categories
        1.   Minor
            a.   Most common type; often present initially in childhood or adolescence
            b.   Lesions are usually singular (but may be multiple), shallow, small (<1 cm), and painful
            c.   Lesions appear on labial or buccal mucosa, tongue, soft palate, and floor of mouth; rarely do lesions appear on attached gingiva and hard palate as occurs in herpes simplex
            d.   Prodromal burning or tingling may precede ulcers
            e.   Typically lesions heal in 7-14 days and tend to recur
        2.   Major
            a.   This severe form presents with lesions that are deep and large (>1 cm)
            b.   Lesions take 6 weeks or longer to heal with possible scarring
        3.   Herpetiform
            a.   Typically present as crops of small (1-5 mm) painful ulcers from 3 to >12
            b.   Lesions are initially round or oval and later coalesce to form large ulcers with irregular margins

IV.   Diagnosis/Evaluation

    A.   History
        1.   Ask about onset and duration of symptoms
        2.   Inquire about fever, rashes on other parts of body, and systemic symptoms
        3.   Question regarding nutritional deficiencies, stressors, allergies, recent mouth trauma, infections, and risk factors for sexually transmitted diseases
        4.   Obtain medication history
        5.   Inquire about systemic diseases
        6.   Ask about past episodes and previous treatments

B. Physical Examination
1. Determine vital signs
2. Assess hydration status; patients may not be drinking fluids due to mouth pain
3. Assess skin for lesions on other parts of body
4. Perform complete head, ears, eyes, nose, mouth, and throat examinations; note location, number and distribution of lesions
5. Palpate neck and jaw for adenopathy
6. Auscultate chest
7. May need complete physical examination if systemic disease is suspected

C. Differential Diagnosis
1. Oral cancer (consider if lesions are present for more than 6 weeks, are unresponsive to therapy, and have unusual presentations such as indurated or rolled borders)
2. Oral candidiasis (white patches in mouth) (see CANDIDIASIS section)
3. Hand-foot-and-mouth disease (papulovesicular lesions with erythematous halo on hands and feet as well as mouth)
4. Herpes simplex virus (see HERPES SIMPLEX section)
   a. Vesicles form before ulcers develop and are confined to pharynx, tonsils and soft palate in primary herpes and are on the vermilion borders of lip in secondary herpes
   b. Tzanck smear is positive for inclusion-bearing giant cells
5. Syphilis (risk factors, skin lesions on hands and feet and positive RPR/FTA tests are present)
6. Vincent's stomatitis (ulcers appear on gingivae and are covered by purulent, gray exudate)
7. Herpangina
   a. More common in children than adults
   b. Multiple distinctive papular, vesicular, and ulcerative lesions on anterior tonsillar pillars, soft palate, tonsils, pharynx, and posterior buccal mucosa
8. Behçet's syndrome (lesions are similar to aphthous stomatitis, but with this syndrome genital ulceration, uveitis, and retinitis are also present)
9. Reiter's syndrome (uveitis, conjunctivitis, and arthritis are present)
10. Acute necrotizing ulcerative gingivitis (history of periodontal disease is present)
11. Trauma due to dental appliances or rough surfaced teeth
12. Varicella (chickenpox)
13. Pemphigus (presence of bullous lesions in mouth and other parts of body and Tzanck smear from lesions reveals acantholytic cells)
14. Oropharyngeal anthrax (ulcers at base of tongue; initially edematous and hyperemic)

D. Diagnostic Tests
1. Usually none indicated
2. Order vitamin B_{12}, folate, and iron levels if nutritional deficiencies are suspected
3. Consider CBC with differential to assist in ruling out anemias
4. Consider Tzanck smear for distinguishing herpetic stomatitis from other causes
5. Consider HIV testing when ulcers are large and slow to heal
6. Biopsy is needed if cancer is suspected

V. Plan/Management

A. Pharmacologic treatment includes one of following:
1. Liquid antacids or 3% hydrogen peroxide/water solution, 1:1 as a gargle
2. Xylocaine (Lidocaine 2%) viscous solution. Adolescents: may apply to lesions every 3 hours or use 15 mL as a gargle or mouthwash and swallow every 3 hours (maximum 8 doses/day). Children <3 years: apply 1.25 mL to affected area with applicator every 3 hours (maximum 8 doses/day). Adjust dosage for older children
3. Diphenhydramine 5 mg/mL (Benadryl) elixir mixed 1:1 with attapulgite (Kaopectate) or aluminum hydroxide, magnesium hydroxide (Maalox). May be used as mouth rinse QID
4. Corticosteroid creams can provide pain relief and promote healing, but be cautious as they worsen viral infections; apply thin layer of triamcinolone acetonide 0.1% (Kenalog) in paste vehicle, Orabase, after meals and HS (moderate potency); not recommended for young children
5. Tetracycline syrup (Sumycin) 250 mg/10 mL syrup QID for 7-14 days; rinse for 2 minutes and then expectorate; contraindicated in pregnant women and children <8 years old
6. Dexamethasone elixir (Decadron) 0.5 mg/5 mL; rinse with 5 mL every 12 hours and then expectorate
7. Remind patient not to eat or drink for 20 minutes after this treatment

B. Treat severe, recurrent aphthous ulcers with one of following:
1. May require oral corticosteroids: Initially, in adults, prescribe prednisone 30-60 mg/day with tetracycline syrup QID for 5 days, then, decrease to 5-20 mg every other day for 10 days
2. Ask pharmacist to mix clobetasol propionate 0.05% (Temovate) ointment with an equal amount of Orabase; dry ulcer site lightly and apply sufficient paste to cover lesion three to six times daily

C. Alternative agents include zinc gluconate lozenges; oral vitamins (vitamin B, vitamin B complex, lysine), sage and chamomile mouthwash, and juices (carrot, celery, cantaloupe); limited research is available on the efficacy of these agents

D. Thalidomide (Thalomid) 200 mg once or twice a day for 3-8 weeks is used in HIV-infected patients who have severe, nonhealing ulcers; contraindicated in other patients because of risk of adverse effects and teratogenicity

E. Patient Education
1. Warn that using steroid pastes or elixirs could result in secondary fungal infection
2. Encourage good nutrition and increased fluid intake
3. Stress the importance of good oral hygiene, even for infants
4. Avoid spicy, salty, and acidic foods and drinks
5. Use soft-bristled toothbrush and avoid foods with sharp surfaces and talking while chewing
6. Aphthous ulcers are not contagious, so there is no danger in spreading

F. Follow Up
1. Immediately in infants and elderly persons not taking fluids
2. In severe cases, reschedule in 2-3 days
3. Consult specialist if not healed in 2-3 weeks

DENTAL CARIES AND TOOTHACHE (PULPITIS)

I. Definitions

A. Dental caries: Infectious disease resulting in decay of teeth

B. Pulpitis: A suppurative process that usually results from pulpal infection

II. Pathogenesis

A. Dental caries is a bacterial disease characterized by demineralization of tooth enamel and dentine
1. Caries result from overgrowth of organisms that are part of normally occurring human dental flora
2. Human dental flora is site specific; the infant is not colonized until around age 6 to 30 months of age when the eruption of the primary dentition occurs
3. The mother or another intimate care provider is the most likely source of inoculation of the infant's dental flora; inoculation may occur through shared utensils, etc.

B. Pulpitis
1. Inflammation involving pulp tissue, the central portion of the tooth containing vital soft tissue; usually occurs due to trauma
2. Diverse flora, including gram-positive anaerobes and bacteroides are the organisms most often involved in the infectious process

III. Clinical presentation

A. Dental caries may be the most prevalent infectious disease in US
1. Dental caries is the most frequent type of injury that causes pulpitis; pain does not occur until the decay impinges on the pulp and an inflammatory response develops
2. More than 40% of children have dental caries by the time they enter kindergarten
3. High caries rates run in families and are passed from mother to children from generation to generation
4. Largely a disease that can be prevented
5. Primary teeth decay can negatively impact on children's growth and development and can lead to malocclusion, pulpitis, and potentially life-threatening swelling

B. Pulpitis
   1. Constant, throbbing pain is the most frequent complaint
   2. Affected tooth is extremely sensitive to touch and pain is intensified with the application of heat or cold (thermal sensitivity)
   3. The affected area of the jaw is tender to palpation
   4. Systemic manifestations may or may not be present and are usually limited to regional lymphadenopathy, malaise, and fever
   5. Complications include periapical abscess and cellulitis

IV. Diagnosis/Evaluation

   A. History
      1. Children should begin to receive oral health risk assessments by a trained primary care clinician by 6 months of age
         a. The Caries Risk Assessment Tool is provided and updated by the American Academy of Pediatric Dentistry (available at http://www.aapd.org/members/referencemanual/pdfs/02-03/Caries%20Risk%20Assess.pdf)
         b. Ask questions to identify parents (usually mothers) and infants who are at high risk for caries; inquire about the following:
            (1) Dietary practices
            (2) Fluoride exposure
            (3) Oral hygiene
            (4) Visits to dental services
            (5) Number and location of mother's dental fillings
      2. To assess for pulpitis, ask about the following:
         a. Recent toothache
         b. Occurrence of fever and chill
         c. History of heart murmur or defect
         d. Type of medication taken for pain relief and when was it last taken

   B. Physical examination
      1. Determine if febrile
      2. Do a complete oral examination
         a. Inspect and gently percuss teeth to determine location of affected tooth
         b. Examine adjacent tissues for signs of inflammation
         c. Observe for facial symmetry and examine jaw in area for signs of cellulitis
      3. Examine for regional lymphadenopathy
      4. Auscultate heart (risk of sepsis and complications increase with valvular disease)
      5. Because the dental health of the mother has a direct correlation with dental health of infant, ask permission to perform oral examination of mother

   C. Differential Diagnosis
      1. Mumps
      2. Cellulitis
      3. Pericoronitis (painful wisdom teeth)
      4. Sinusitis
      5. Myofascial inflammation
      6. Migraine headache
      7. Neuralgia

   D. Diagnostic tests: Consider ordering x-rays

V. Plan/Management

   A. Refer child to dentist as early as 6 months of age and no later than 6 months after the first tooth erupts or 12 months of age for aggressive anticipatory guidance and an intervention program if child is at high risk for caries based on the Caries Risk Assessment Tool or has one the following:
      1. Special health need
      2. Mother with high caries rates
      3. Demonstrable caries, plaque, demineralization, and/or staining
      4. Habit of sleeping with bottles or breastfeeding throughout the night
      5. Member of low socioeconomic status family

B. Anticipatory guidance for the mother or other intimate caregiver before and during the colonization process is important (see following table)

PARENT EDUCATION

✓ Instruct parent to brush teeth thoroughly twice a day and to floss at least once every day

✓ Instruct parent to consume fruit juices only at meals and to avoid carbonated beverages during the first 30 months of infant's life

✓ Teach parents to use fluoride toothpaste approved by the American Dental Association and to rinse every night with an alcohol-free over-the-counter mouth rinse with 0.05% sodium fluoride

✓ Refer parents to dentist for examination and care of active decay

✓ Educate mothers to prevent early colonization of dental flora in their infants; avoid sharing utensils or transmitting their saliva to infants

✓ Discuss that xylitol chewing gum may have a significant impact on decreasing rates of caries

---

C. Anticipatory guidance for the child 0-3 years is found in the following table

---

ANTICIPATORY GUIDANCE FOR CHILD 0-3 YEARS

✓ Brush child's teeth (twice a day) as soon as they erupt and floss child's teeth every day as soon as teeth contact one another

✓ After eruption of teeth, emphasize that parents should provide fruit juices (not to exceed 1 cup per day) during meals only

✓ Teach to eliminate carbonated beverages from child's diet

✓ Instruct that infants should not be placed in bed with bottle containing anything other than water

✓ Remind to cleanse infant's teach with a damp cloth after feeding

✓ Assure that child has optimal exposure to topical and systemic fluoride

---

D. Encourage the family to establish a dental home for all children in the early toddler years

E. Treatment of pulpitis (see table that follows)

TREATMENT OF TOOTHACHE

Category 1: Patients who are afebrile, with no extraoral swelling (no facial asymmetry present) or intraoral swelling
✓ Prescribe analgesics:
  - **Adolescents:** Prescribe acetaminophen (300 mg) with codeine (30 mg) (Tylenol #3), 1-2 tabs, every 4 hours.
  - **Children:** Prescribe acetaminophen or ibuprofen. See PAIN MANAGEMENT section for dosing
✓ Recommend warm salt water rinses (swish and spit) every 3-4 hours
✓ Refer to dentist within 24 hours

Category 2: Patients who have either slight extraoral or intraoral swelling, or who have a low-grade fever
✓ Prescribe analgesics (as above) and
✓ Prescribe antibiotics: Treatment of choice is Penicillin V (Pen-Vee-K).
  - **Adolescents:** 250-500 mg Q 6 hours x 5-7 days.
  - **Children:** 40-60 mg/kg/day in 4 divided doses x 5-7 days
✓ Patients allergic to penicillin should be treated with erythromycin; consult PDR for dosing recommendations
✓ Recommend warm salt water rinses (swish and spit) every 3-4 hours
✓ Refer to dentist within 12-24 hours

Category 3: Patients who have fever ≥101°F (38.5°C) with intraoral and/or extraoral swelling (causing facial asymmetry)
✓ Emergency consultation and treatment by dentist is needed
✓ Management must be immediate because the consequences of delayed treatment can be serious and occasionally life threatening!

F. Treatment by the dentist for these three categories of toothache varies from extraction to root canal to incision and drainage, and to hospitalization for IV antibiotic therapy for patients with cellulitis

G. Follow Up
  1. Child should regularly visit dentist every 6 months
  2. Follow up for pulpitis should be done by dentist

CERVICAL ADENITIS

I. Definition: Acute pyogenic infection of a cervical lymph node

II. Pathogenesis

   A. Usually reactive or secondary to an upper respiratory tract infection or dental infection; less frequently due to trauma

   B. Pathogens:
       1. *Staphylococcus aureus* and *Streptococcus pyogenes* account for 80% of unilateral cervical adenitis
       2. Increasingly, anaerobic pathogens are being identified
       3. Less common pathogens: viruses and group B streptococci, *Mycobacterium avium* complex, and *M. scrofulaceum*

III. Clinical Presentation

   A. Most common in children 1-5 years

   B. Typically, patient is afebrile or has a low-grade fever, malaise, and an upper respiratory infection or dental infection

   C. Usually presents as tender, soft, warm, rapidly enlarging lymph node with erythema of the overlying skin and possibly with fistulas to the skin; node ranges from 2-6 cm

   D. Most common sites are the submandibular and anterior cervical areas

IV. Diagnosis/Evaluation

   A. History
       1. Ascertain duration and onset of node enlargement
       2. Ask if node is increasing in size and whether overlying skin has changed in color
       3. Ask about pain during eating which suggests parotid gland involvement
       4. Question about dysphagia, odynophagia, stridor, speech disorders, or a sensation of a lump in the throat
       5. Inquire about associated constitutional symptoms
       6. Question about recent infections, trauma, insect bites, pet scratches, tuberculosis contact, drug usage, and foreign travel

   B. Physical Examination
       1. Measure vital signs
       2. Observe for general state of health
       3. Carefully examine scalp and face for skin lesions
       4. Assess for facial-nerve weakness that can be caused by a parotid gland tumor
       5. Thoroughly examine ears, eyes, nose, throat, and mouth
       6. Carefully examine neck for other masses and nuchal rigidity
       7. Carefully palpate cervical mass to determine exact anatomic location, presence of tenderness, mobility, and consistency; examine skin overlying node for color
       8. Thoroughly examine areas of lymph nodes
       9. Inspect skin for lesions and rashes
       10. Assess respiratory status
       11. Palpate abdomen for organomegaly

   C. Differential Diagnosis (see Figure 9.1 for common location of masses of the neck)
       1. Congenital cysts (these conditions need referral and usually surgery)
           a. Thyroglossal duct cyst (located at midline and typically moves with swallowing or tongue protrusion)
           b. Brachial cleft cysts (small dimple or opening anterior to middle portion of the sternocleidomastoid muscle)
           c. Cystic hygromas (fluid-filled, compressible mass in the posterior triangle just behind the sternocleidomastoid muscle and in the supraclavicular fossa)

2. Salivary gland disorders; salivary glands are located in area of lymph nodes and enlarged glands may be confused as cervical adenitis; care must be taken to distinguish glands from nodes; for example, enlargement of the parotid gland obliterates the angle of the mandible
3. Cervical lymphadenopathy (see section on LYMPHADENOPATHY)
   a. Viral infections (most common)
      (1) Often due to herpesviruses, adenoviruses, enteroviruses, and Epstein-Barr virus
      (2) Nodes are typically bilateral, discrete, oval, soft, and minimally tender
   b. Bacterial infections of the upper respiratory tract and mouth
   c. Cat scratch disease (see CAT SCRATCH DISEASE section)
   d. Kawasaki disease (see KAWASAKI DISEASE section)
   e. Atypical mycobacterium
   f. Toxoplasmosis
   g. Systemic disorders such as lupus, rheumatoid arthritis, sarcoidosis, histoplasmosis

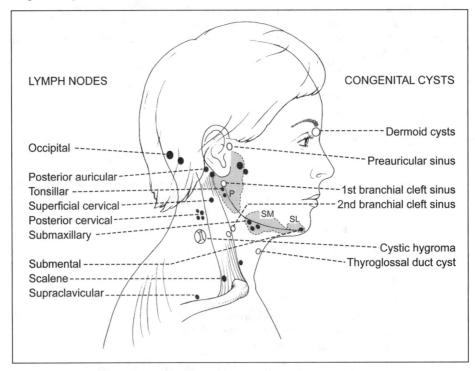

Figure 9.1. Common Location of Masses of the Face and Neck
P = Parotid gland; SM = Submandibular gland; SL = Sublingual gland

4. Abscesses, furuncles, and soft tissue tumors (arise from cutaneous or subcutaneous tissue)
5. Lipoma is a benign, subcutaneous tumor composed of fat cells and may be located in back of neck (other common sites are trunk and extremities); consistency is soft and rubbery
6. Malignancy
   a. Neck mass is usually persistent and enlarging
   b. Node is often supraclavicular, firm and fixated to skin and underlying tissue
   c. Patient often has persistent fever, weight loss, voice change, and hearing loss
   d. Patient may have lesion in oral cavity or pharynx or unilateral nasal obstruction
   e. Smokers, alcoholics, African Americans, and older individuals are at most risk
7. Generalized lymphadenopathy is usually caused by systemic disease (see LYMPHADENOPATHY section)
8. Thyroid nodules or goiters may be confused with enlarged nodes

D. Diagnostic Tests; often no tests are needed
   1. Ultrasound is helpful in establishing whether mass is solid, cystic, or fluctuant
   2. In moderately or severely ill patients, consider CBC, sedimentation rate, throat culture, and blood culture
   3. PPD should be considered if tuberculosis is suspected
   4. Heterophil tests or titers for Epstein-Barr virus, cytomegalovirus, and toxoplasma may be indicated to rule-out specific viral infections
   5. Consider aspiration and culture in patients who have large, fluctuant nodes which do not respond to initial therapy
   6. Biopsy of node is needed when malignancy is suspected

V.   Plan/Management

A.   For patient who appears well with minimal pain, close observation for 2-3 days and symptomatic treatment may be all that is needed
1.   Prescribe analgesic such as Tylenol or nonsteroidal anti-inflammatory agent
2.   Warm compresses every 4 hours

B.   For the patient with moderate to severe adenitis prescribe one of following antibiotics:
1.   Amoxicillin/clavulanic acid (Augmentin) 500 mg TID or 875 mg BID or in children, 40 mg/kg/day in 3 divided doses or 45 mg/kg/day in 2 divided doses. Available 125 mg/5 mL or 250 mg/5 mL suspension for 7-14 days
2.   Cephalexin (Keflex) 500 mg BID or in children, 75 mg/kg/day in 4 divided doses for 7-14 days

C.   Patient education
1.   Emphasize that patient should immediately return if difficulty swallowing or breathing occurs
2.   Reinforce that follow-up is important if symptoms persist

D.   Patients with lymph node enlargement persisting more than 2 weeks without regression with antibiotic therapy need further evaluation and possible referral to a specialist

E.   Follow Up
1.   Return to clinic if symptoms not resolved in 2-3 days
2.   For the patient who appears well and is treated only symptomatically, re-evaluate symptoms at 3-5 day intervals; some nodes take many weeks to regress but other nodes regress spontaneously within 2-3 weeks without pharmacological treatment
3.   Re-evaluate patients who are treated with antibiotics after completion of therapy
4.   Individualize follow-up for patients who are at risk for systemic or serious disorders

REFERENCES

Agency for Healthcare Policy & Research. (1999). *Diagnosis and treatment of acute bacterial rhinosinusitis. Summary, evidence report/technology assessment.* (AHCPR Publ. No. 99-E016). Rockville, MD.

Agency for Healthcare Policy & Research. (*2000). Diagnosis and treatment of uncomplicated acute sinusitis in children.* (AHCPR Publ. No. 01-E005). Rockville, MD.

Agency for Health Care Research & Quality. (2000). *Management of acute otitis media. Summary, evidence report/technology assessment.* (AHRQ Publ. No. 15), Rockville MD   http://ahrq.gov/clinic/epcsums./otitisum.htm

Agency for Health Care Research & Quality. (2002). *Management of allergic and nonallergic rhinitis. Summary, evidence report/technology assessment.* (AHRQ Publ. No. 54), Rockville MD. http://ahrq.gov/clinic/epcsums/rhinsum.thm

Agency for Health Care Research & Quality. (February 2003). *Management of Allergic Rhinitis in Working-Age Population.* Summary, Evidence Report/Technology Assessment: Number 67. AHRQ Publication No. 03-E013). Rockville, MD. http://www.ahrq.gov/clinic/epcsumsrhinworksum.htm

American Academy of Pediatrics. (1999). Newborn and infant hearing loss: Detection and intervention. *Pediatrics, 103,* 527-530.

American Academy of Pediatrics. (2002). Follow-up management of children with tympanostomy tubes. *Pediatrics, 109,* 328-329.

American Academy of Pediatrics. (2003). Oral health risk assessment timing and establishment of the dental home. *Pediatrics, 111,* 1113-1116.

American Academy of Pediatrics. (1995). Joint Committee of Infant Hearing 1994 position statement. *Pediatrics, 95,* 152-155.

American Academy of Pediatrics. (2000). Group A streptococcal infections. In Pickering, L.K. (Ed.) *2000 red book: Report of the Committee on Infectious Diseases* (25th ed.). Elk Grove Village, IL: Author.

American Academy of Pediatrics Committee on Infectious Diseases. (2000). Policy statement: Recommendations for the prevention of pneumococcal infections, including the use of pneumococcal conjugate vaccine (Prevnar), pneumococcal polysaccharide vaccine, and antibiotic prophylaxis. *Pediatrics, 106,* 362-366.

American Academy of Pediatrics Subcommittee on Management of Sinusitis and Committee on Quality Improvement. (2001). Clinical practice guideline: Management of sinusitis. *Pediatrics, 108,* 798-808.

American Pharmaceutical Association Pediatric Disorders Protocol Panel. (2000). American Pharmaceutical Association drug treatment protocols: Management of pediatric acute otitis media. *Journal of American Pharmacy Association, 40,* 599-608.

Bachur, R. (2001). Minor trauma. In C. Green-Hernandez, J.K. Singleton, & D.Z. Aronzon (Eds.). *Primary care pediatrics.* Philadelphia: Lippincott.

Balk, E.M., Zucker, D.R., Engels, E.A., Wong, J.B., Williams, J.W., & Lau, J. (2001). Strategies for diagnosing and treating suspected acute bacterial sinusitis. *Journal of General Internal Medicine, 16,* 701.

Bartnik, G., Fabijanska, A., & Rogowski, M. (2001). Effects of tinnitus retraining therapy (TRT) for patients with tinnitus and subjective hearing loss versus tinnitus only. *Scandinavian Audiology Supplement, 52,* 206-208.

Bisno, A.L. (2001). Acute pharyngitis. *New England Journal of Medicine, 344,* 205-211.

Bisno, A.L., Gerber, M.A., Gwaltney, J.M. Jr., Kaplan, E.L., & Schwartz, R.H. (2002). Practice guidelines for diagnosis and management of group A streptococcal pharyngitis. *Clinical Infectious Diseases, 35,* 113-125.

Bluestone, C.D., Gates, G.A., Klein, J.O., Lim, D.J., Mogi, G., Ogra, P.L., et al. (2002). Panel reports: 1. Definitions, terminology, and classification of otitis media. *Annals of Otology, Rhinology, and Laryngology, 111,* 8-18.

Bluestone, C.D., Klein, J.O., Rosenfeld, R.M., Berman, S., Casselbrant, M.L., Chonmaitree, T., et al. (2002). Panel reports: 9. Treatment, complications, and sequelae. *Annals of Otology, Rhinology, and Laryngology, 111,* 102-119.

Brook, I., Gooch, W.M., III, Jenkins, S.G., Pichichero, M.E., Reiner, S.A., Shar, L., et al. (2000). Medical management of acute bacterial sinusitis: Recommendations of a Clinical Advisory Committee on Pediatric and Adult Sinusitis. *Annals of Otology, Rhinology, and Laryngology, 109,* 2-20.

Buchman, C.A., & Wamback, B.A. (2002). Otitis externa. In R.E. Rakel & E.T. Bope (Eds.). *Conn's current therapy 2002.* Philadelphia: Saunders.

Casselbrant, M.L., Gravel, J.S., Margolis, R. H., Bellussi, L., Dhooge, I., Downs, M.P., et al. (2002). Panel reports: 8. Diagnosis and screening. *Annals of Otology, Rhinology, and Laryngology, 111,* 95-99.

Centers for Disease Control and Prevention. (1999). Acute otitis media: management and surveillance in an era of pneumococcal resistance. *Pediatric Infectious Disease Journal, 18,* 1-9.

Consensus Panel, Hannley, M.T., Denneny, J.C., III, & Holzer, S.S. (2000). Consensus Panel Report: Use of ototopical antibiotics in treating common ear diseases. *Otolaryngology–Head and Neck Surgery, 122,* 934-940.

Culpepper, L., & Froom, J. (1997). Routine antimicrobial treatment of acute otitis media: Is it necessary? *JAMA, 278,* 1643-1645.

Cunningham, M., Cox, E.O., the Committee on Practice and Ambulatory Medicine, and the Section on Otolaryngology and Bronchoesophagology or the American Academy of Pediatrics. (2003). Hearing assessment in infants and children. Recommendations beyond neonatal screening. *Pediatrics, 111,* 436-440.

Dajani, A.S., et al. (1993). Guidelines for the diagnosis of rheumatic fever: Jones criteria, updated 1992. *Circulation, 87,* 302-307.

Dajani, A., Taubert, K., Ferrieri, P., Peter, G., Shulman, S., and other committee members. (1995). Treatment of acute streptococcal pharyngitis and prevention of rheumatic fever: A statement for health professionals. *Pediatrics, 96,* 758-764.

Dajani, A.S., Taubert, K.A., Wilson, W., Bolger, A.F., Bayer, A., Ferrieri, P., et al. (1997). Prevention of bacterial endocarditis: Recommendations by the American Heart Association. *JAMA, 277,* 1794-1801.

Dolitsky, J.N., & Ward, R.F. (2001). Foreign bodies of the ear, nose, airway, and esophagus. In R.A. Hoekelman. *Primary pediatric care.* St. Louis: Mosby.

Douglass, A.B., & Douglass, J.M. (2003). Common dental emergencies. *American Family Physician, 67,* 511-516.

Ebell, M.H., Smith, M.A., Barry, H.C., Ives, K., & Carey, M. (2000). Does this patient have strep throat? *JAMA, 284,* 2912-2918.

El-Bitar, M.A., Pena, M.T., Choi, S.S., & Zaizal, G.H. (2002). Retained ventilation tubes: Should they be removed at 2 years? *Archives of Otolaryngology Head and Neck Surgery, 128,* 1357-1360.

Fireman, B. (2003). Impact of the pneumococcal conjugate vaccine on otitis media. *Pediatric Infectious Disease Journal, 22,* 10-16.

Flynn, C.A., Griffine, G., & Tudiver, F. (2002). Decongestants and antihistamines for acute otitis media in children (Cochrane review). *The Cochrane library, Issue 2.* Oxford: Update Software Ltd.

Forzley, G.J. (1994). Cerumen impaction removal. In J.L. Pfenninger, & G.C. Fowler (Eds.), *Procedures for primary care physicians.* St. Louis: Mosby.

Glasziou, P.P., Del Mar, C.B., Sanders, S.L., & Hayem. M. (2002). Antibiotics for acute otitis media in children (Cochrane review). *The Cochrane library, Issue 2.* Oxford: Update Software Ltd.

Giebink, G.S. (2001). The prevention of pneumococcal disease in children. *New England Journal of Medicine, 345,* 1177-1183.

Goroll, A.H., & Mulley, A.G., Jr. (2000). Approach to the patient with chronic nasal congestion and discharge. In A.H. Goroll, & A.G. Mulley, Jr. (Eds.), *Primary care medicine.* Philadelphia: Lippincott, Williams & Wilkins.

Goroll, A.H., & Mulley, A.G., Jr. (2000). Management of aphthous stomatitis. In A.H. Goroll, & A.G. Mulley, Jr. (Eds.), *Primary care medicine*. Philadelphia: Lippincott, Williams & Wilkins.

Gulya, A.J. (2000). Evaluation of hearing loss. In A.H. Goroll & A.G. Mulley, Jr. (Eds.), *Primary care medicine*. Philadelphia: Lippincott.

Hayden, M.L. (2001). Allergic rhinitis: A growing primary care challenge. *Journal of the American Academy of Nurse Practitioners, 13,* 545-551.

Haynes, J.H., & Newkirk, G.R. (1994). Removal of foreign bodies from the ear and nose. In J.L. Pfenninger, & G.C. Fowler (Eds.), *Procedures for primary care physicians*. St. Louis: Mosby.

Hayes, C.S., & Williamson, H., Jr. (2001). Management of group A beta-hemolytic streptococcal pharyngitis. *American Family Physician, 63,* 1557-1565.

Hendley, J.O. (2002). Otitis media. *New England Journal of Medicine, 347,* 1169-1174.

Herendeen, N.E., & Szilagyi, P.G. (2001). Cystic and solid masses of the face and neck. In R.A. Hoekelman et al., (Ed.). *Primary pediatric care,* St. Louis: Mosby.

Hoberman, A., Marchant, C.D., Kaplan, S.L., & Feldman, S. (2002). Treatment of acute otitis media consensus recommendations. *Clinical Pediatrics, 41,* 373-390.

Huovinen, P. (2002). Macrolide-resistant group A streptococcus–Now in the United States. *New England Journal of Medicine, 346,* 1243-1245.

Isaacson, G., & Rosenfel, R.M. (1996). Care of the child with tympanostomy tubes. *Pediatric Clinics of North America, 43,* 1183-1193.

Joint Committee on Infant Hearing. (2000). Year 2000 position statement: Principles and guidelines for early hearing detection and intervention program. *Pediatrics, 106,* 798-817.

Kleinegger, C.L. (2002). Diseases of the mouth. In R.E. Rakel & E.T. Bope, (Eds.). *Conn's current therapy 2002*. Philadelphia: Saunders.

Krouse, J.H., Mirante, J.P., & Christmas, D.A., Jr. (1999). *Office-based pediatric otolaryngology and audiology*. Philadelphia: Saunders.

Leberman, P. (2002). Nonallergic rhinitis. In R.E. Rakel, & E.T. Bope (Eds.). *2002 Conn's current therapy*. Philadelphia: Saunders.

Leibovitz, E., & Dagan, R. (2001). Otitis media therapy and drug resistance–Part 1: Management principles. *Infectious Medicine, 18,* 212-216.

Li, J.T., Lockey, R.F., Bernstein, I.L., Portnoy, J.M., & Nicklas, R.A. (2003). Allergen immunotherapy: A practice parameter. *Annals of Allergy, Asthma, and Immunology, 90,* 1-40.

MacLeod, D.K. (1999). Chronic dental and oral problems. In L.R. Barker, J.R. Burton, & P.D. Zieve (Eds.), *Principles of ambulatory medicine*. Baltimore: Williams & Wilkins.

Mandel, E.M., Casselbrant, M.L., Rockette, H.E., Fireman, P., Kurs-Lasky, M., & Bluestone, C.D. (2002). Systemic steroids for chronic otitis media with effusion in children. *Pediatrics, 110,* 1071-1080.

McBride, D.R. (2000). Management of aphthous ulcers. *American Family Physician, 62,* 149-154, 160.

McKenna, M.W. (2002). Epistaxis. In R.B. Taylor (Ed.). *Manual of family practice*. Philadelphia: Lippincott Williams & Wilkins.

Murphy, M.L., & Pichichero, M.E. (2002). Prospective identification and treatment of children with pediatric autoimmune neuropsychiatric disorder associated with group A streptococcal infection (PANDAS). *Archives of Pediatric Adolescent Medicine, 156,* 356-361.

Nudelman, J. (2001). How should we treat acute maxillary sinusitis? *American Family Physician, 63,* 837-838.

O'Brien, K.L., Dowell, S.F., Schwartz, B., Marcy, S.M., Phillips, W.R., & Gerber, M.A. (1998). Acute sinusitis--principles of judicious use of antimicrobial agents. *Pediatrics, 101,* 174-177.

O'Connor, J.M. (1999). Dentistry for the pediatrician. In R.A. Dershewitz (Ed.), *Ambulatory pediatric care*. Philadelphia: Lippincott.

Otitis Media with Effusion in Young Children Guideline Panel. (1994). *Otitis media with effusion in young children: Clinical practice guideline, No. 12*. (ACHPR Publication No. 94-0622) Rockville, MD.

Owens, T.P., Jr. (2000). Removal of impacted cerumen. In R.E. Rakel (Ed.). *Saunders manual of medical practice (2nd ed.)*. Philadelphia: Saunders.

Piccirillo, J.F., Mager, D.E., Frisse, M.E., Brophy, R.H., & Goggin, A. (2001). Impact of first-line vs second-line antibiotics for the treatment of acute uncomplicated sinusitis. *JAMA, 286,*1849-1856.

Pichichero, M.E. (2000). Acute otitis media: Part 1. Improving diagnostic accuracy. *American Family Physician, 61,* 2051-2056.

Pichichero, M.E. (2000). Acute otitis media: Part II. Treatment in an era of increasing antibiotic resistance. *American Family Physician, 61,* 2410-2416.

Pichichero, M.E., Reiner, S.A., Brook, I., Gooch, W.M. III, Yamauchi, T., Jenkins, S.G., et al. (2000). Controversies in the medical management of persistent and recurrent acute otitis media: Recommendations of a clinical advisory committee. *Annals of Otology, Rhinology, and Laryngology, 109,* 2-12.

Piglanski, L., Leibovitz, E., Raiz, S., Greenberg, D., Press, J., Leiberman, A., & Dagan, R. (2003). Bacteriologic and clinical efficacy of high dose amoxicillin for therapy of acute otitis media in children. *Pediatric Infectious Disease Journal, 22,* 405-412.

Rabinowitz, P.M. (2000). Noise-induced hearing loss. *American Family Physician, 61,* 2749-2756, 2759-2760.

Rosenfeld, R.M., Casselbrant, M.L., & Hannley, M.T. (2001). Implications of the AHRQ evidence report on acute otitis media. *Otolaryngology–Head and Neck Surgery, 125,* 440-448.

Sander, R. (2001). Otitis externa: A practical guide to treatment and prevention. *American Family Physician, 63,* 927-936, 941-942.

Schantz, N.V. (1994). Management of epistaxis. In J.L. Pfenninger, & G.C. Fowler (Eds.), *Procedures for primary care physicians.* St. Louis: Mosby.

Schwartz, B., Marcy, S.M., Phillips, W.R., Gerber, M.A., & Dowell, S.F. (1998). Pharyngitis--principles of judicious use of antimicrobial agents. *Pediatrics, 101,* 171-174.

Sheeler, R.D., Houston, M.S., Radke, S., Dale, J.C., & Adamson, S.C. (2002). Accuracy of rapid strep testing in patients who have had recent streptococcal pharyngitis. *Journal of the American Board of Family Practitioners, 15,* 261-265.

Sinus and Allergy Health Partnership. (2000). Antimicrobial treatment guidelines for acute bacterial rhinosinusitis. *Otolaryngology–Head and Neck Surgery, 123,* S1-S29.

Steyer, T.E. (2002). Peritonsillar abscess: Diagnosis and treatment. *American Family Physician, 65,* 93-96.

Takata, G.S., Chan, L.S., Shekelle, P., Morton, S.C., Mason, W., & Marcy, S.M. (2001). Evidence assessment of management of acute otitis media: I. The role of antibiotics in treatment of uncomplicated acute otitis media. *Pediatrics, 108,* 239-247.

United States Preventive Services Task Force (USPSTF). (2001). Newborn hearing screening: recommendations and rationale. *American Family Physician, 64,* 1995-1999.

Williams, J.W., Aguilar, C., Makela, M., Cornell, J., Hollman, D.R., Chiquette, E., & Simel, D.L. (2002). Antibiotics for acute maxillary sinusitis (Cochrane review). In *The Cochrane library.* Oxford: Update Software Ltd.

Windom, H.H. (2002). Allergic rhinitis caused by inhalant factors. In R.E. Rakel, & E.T. Bope (Eds.). *2002 Conn's current therapy.* Philadelphia: Saunders.

Wirtschafter, A., Cherukuri, S., & Benninger, M.S. (2002). Anthrax: ENT manifestations and current concepts. *Otolaryngology–Head and Neck Surgery, 126,* 8-13.

Problems of the Upper Airways, Lower Respiratory System

CONSTANCE R. UPHOLD & BETSY HERNANDEZ WARREN

ASTHMA

I. Definition: Chronic inflammatory disorder of the airways which causes bronchial hyper-responsiveness to stimuli and recurrent episodes of respiratory symptoms which are usually associated with reversible airflow obstruction

II. Pathogenesis

   A. Inflammation plays a central role
      1. Results from complex interactions among many cells and cellular elements (mast cells, eosinophils, T lymphocytes, macrophages, neutrophils, and epithelial cells)
      2. Inflammation is associated with airway obstruction, airway hyperresponsiveness, respiratory symptoms, and disease chronicity

   B. Airway obstruction leads to airflow limitation and is usually widespread, recurrent, variable, and reversible either with treatment or spontaneously; obstruction is due to the following:
      1. Acute bronchoconstriction results from airway hyperresponsiveness after exposure to a variety of stimuli such as allergens, drugs (aspirin, nonsteroidal anti-inflammatory drugs), stimuli (exercise, cold air, irritants) and possibly stress
      2. Airway wall edema and mucosal thickening are caused by increased microvascular permeability and leakage
      3. Chronic mucus plug formation sometimes occurs in severe, intractable cases
      4. Airway wall remodeling may develop in severe cases, causing persistent abnormalities in lung function which are unresponsive to treatment

   C. Factors contributing to asthma severity:
      1. Inhaled allergens such as animal allergens, house-dust mites, outdoor allergens, indoor fungi, and cockroaches
      2. Occupational exposures
      3. Irritants such as tobacco smoke and pollution
      4. Rhinitis/sinusitis
      5. Gastroesophageal reflux
      6. Sensitivity to aspirin, other nonsteroidal anti-inflammatory drugs, and sulfites
      7. Topical and systemic beta-blockers
      8. Viral respiratory infection

   D. In children, there usually is a strong history of atopy; allergy or family history of allergy is the factor most strongly related to continuing asthma throughout childhood

III. Clinical Presentation

   A. Underdiagnosis and inappropriate therapy are major factors in morbidity and mortality

   B. Symptoms typically begin in childhood or adolescence, but can develop in adulthood; 50-80% of asthmatic children develop symptoms before fifth birthday
      1. Most common, chronic illness of childhood; affects 5-10% of children <20 years
      2. In children, two general patterns of disease progression exist: remission of symptoms in preschool years or symptoms persist throughout childhood

   C. Clinical manifestations of asthma
      1. Wheeze or cough; typically cough accompanies wheeze
      2. Patient responds to bronchodilators or oral steroids in short-term or inhaled anti-inflammatory drugs in the long-term
      3. Typical history includes exacerbating factors such as irritant exposure, upper respiratory tract infection, exercise, or allergen exposure

   D. Exercise-induced bronchospasm occurs with loss of heat and/or water from lungs during exercise; cough, shortness of breath, chest pain or tightness, wheezing or endurance problems may develop during exercise

E. Spectrum ranges from few mild episodes in a lifetime to daily debilitating symptoms; classification of asthma severity is based on symptoms and lung function before treatment (see table CLASSIFICATION OF THE SEVERITY OF ASTHMA)

CLASSIFICATION OF THE SEVERITY OF ASTHMA*

Step/ Category	Symptoms**	Nighttime Symptoms	Lung Functions[+$]
STEP 4 Severe Persistent	• Continual symptoms • Limited physical activity • Frequent exacerbations	Frequent	• FEV_1 or PEF ≤60% predicted • PEF variability >30%
STEP 3 Moderate Persistent	• Daily symptoms • Daily use of inhaled short-acting beta$_2$-agonist • Exacerbations affect activity • Exacerbations are ≥2 times a week	>1 time a week	• FEV_1 or PEF >60%-<80% predicted • PEF variability >30%
STEP 2 Mild Persistent	• Symptoms >2 times a week but <1 time a day • Exacerbations may affect activity	>2 times a month	• FEV_1 or PEF ≥80% predicted • PEF variability 20-30%
STEP 1 Mild Intermittent	• Symptoms ≤2 times/week • Asymptomatic & normal PEF between exacerbations • Exacerbations brief (from a few hours to few days) • Intensity may vary	≤2 times a month	• FEV_1 or PEF ≥80% predicted • PEF variability <20%

*The presence of one of the features of severity is sufficient to classify patient in that category. A patient should be assigned to the most severe grade in which any feature occurs
**Patients at any level of severity can have mild, moderate, or severe exacerbations
[+]For individuals >5 years who can use a spirometer or peak flow meter
[$]$FEV_1$ = forced expiratory volume in one second; PEF = peak expiratory flow

Adapted from National Institutes of Health. National Heart, Lung, and Blood Institute. (1997). *The Expert Panel Report 2: Guidelines for the diagnosis and management of asthma.* National Asthma Education Program. NIH Publ. #97-4051. Bethesda, MD.

F. For infants and children aged <5 years, the use of spirometry to diagnose and classify asthma is not feasible; an expanded medical history and physical examination should be performed to look for the following factors associated with the development of chronic, persistent asthma (see box that follows)

Chronic, Persistent Asthma in Infants and Children <5 years

More than three episodes of wheezing in the past year that lasted more than one day & affected sleep
-AND-
Parental history of asthma or clinician-diagnosed atopic dermatitis
-OR-
Two of the following:
  *Clinical-diagnosed allergic rhinitis
  *Wheezing apart from colds
  *Peripheral blood eosinophilia

IV.   Diagnosis/Evaluation

   A.   History
       1.   Identify the symptoms likely to be due to asthma (see table KEY INDICATORS)

KEY INDICATORS OF ASTHMA

✓   Wheezing
✓   History of any of the following:
   - Cough worse at night or in early morning
   - Recurrent difficulty breathing
   - Recurrent tightness in chest
✓   Reversible airflow limitation and diurnal variation as measured by peak flow meter
✓   Symptoms occur or are worsened by any of the following:
   - Exercise, viral infection, animals, house-dust mites, mold, smoke, pollen, changes in weather, laughing, hard crying, airborne chemicals or dusts, menses
✓   Symptoms occur or worsen at night, awakening the patient

Adapted from National Institutes of Health. National Heart, Lung, and Blood Institute. (1997). *The Expert Panel Report 2: Guidelines for the diagnosis and management of asthma*. National Asthma Education Program. NIH Publ. #97-4051. Bethesda, MD.

       2.   Assess onset and duration of symptoms (number of days/nights per week/month)
       3.   Determine whether symptoms are seasonal, continuous, episodic, or diurnal
       4.   Determine profile of asthma attacks or exacerbations
       5.   Assess past and present management strategies and responses
       6.   Inquire about factors known to be related to asthma
       7.   Determine family history of asthma, allergy, sinusitis, rhinitis, or nasal polyps
       8.   Assess impact of disease on family, finances, school, work, activity, sleep, and behavior
       9.   Assess attainment of growth and developmental milestones
       10.   Assess patient's and family's knowledge level, understanding of treatments, and sociocultural beliefs
       11.   Inquire about number of sick days taken from school or work per month
       12.   At each follow-up visit assess whether the goals of therapy are being met

   B.   Physical Examination
       1.   It is especially important to determine pulse rate and respiratory rate (>40 respirations per minute is worrisome)
       2.   Assess for signs of dehydration such as delayed capillary refill, poor skin turgor, and dry mucous membranes
       3.   Observe for use of accessory respiratory muscles, retractions, nasal flaring, diaphoresis, and cyanosis
       4.   Observe for hyperexpansion of thorax (hunched shoulders or chest deformity)
       5.   Observe for flexural eczema or other manifestations of allergic skin conditions
       6.   Assess for nasal discharge, mucosal swelling, frontal tenderness, postnasal discharge, nasal polyps, and allergic shiners (dark discoloration beneath both eyes)
       7.   Auscultate and percuss lungs
           a.   Wheezing during forced exhalation is no longer believed to be a reliable indicator
           b.   In mild, intermittent asthma, wheezing may be absent between attacks; in severe asthma, wheezing may be absent due to diminished breath sounds
       8.   Perform a complete cardiac examination

   C.   Differential Diagnosis: Underdiagnosis of asthma, especially in children, is common; remember that recurrent episodes of coughing and wheezing are usually due to asthma; the following should be included in the differential diagnosis:
       1.   Vocal cord dysfunction can cause recurrent wheezing
       2.   Enlarged lymph nodes, tumors
       3.   Pulmonary infections such as pneumonia, tuberculosis, mycoplasma, and respiratory syncytial virus
       4.   Gastroesophageal reflux
       5.   Sinusitis
       6.   Pertussis
       7.   Bronchiolitis
       8.   Cystic fibrosis

9. Bronchopulmonary dysplasia
10. Heart disease
11. Laryngotracheomalacia, tracheal stenosis, or bronchostenosis
12. Foreign body
13. Vascular rings or laryngeal webs
14. Aspiration from swallowing dysfunction

D. Diagnostic Tests: regular monitoring of pulmonary function is essential, particularly for patients who do not perceive their symptoms until airways are severely obstructed
   1. Spirometry tests should be performed on individuals >5 years; most objective measure of lung function
      a. Recommended at following intervals:
         (1) Time of diagnosis
         (2) After treatment when symptoms and peak flow reading are stabilized to document attainment of normal airway function
         (3) Every 1-2 years to monitor maintenance of airway function
      b. More frequent testing is needed in the following cases: to check accuracy of peak flow, when precision is needed to determine treatment response, and when peak flow readings may be unreliable such as when patients are young, elderly, or have neuromuscular problems
   2. Peak expiratory flow (PEF) meters for individuals >5 years
      a. **Should be used to monitor lung function not to confirm diagnosis**
      b. Daily monitoring is not mandatory for all patients, but is important for patients after an exacerbation and for patients with moderate-to-severe persistent asthma
      c. Teach patients to determine their best PEF (see table PATIENT EDUCATION OF PEAK FLOW METER)
   3. Order an exercise challenge test to confirm exercised-induced bronchospasm
   4. Consider the following additional tests
      a. CBC or chest x-ray if infection is suspected
      b. Allergy skin testing (preferred) or *in vitro* testing for patients with persistent wheezing
      c. Sweat chloride testing for children with recurrent wheezing to rule out cystic fibrosis

---

PATIENT EDUCATION OF THE PEAK FLOW METER

1. Demonstrate and have return demonstration of use of peak flow meter
   - Stand, do not sit
   - Place indicator at bottom of numbered scale
   - Take deep breath
   - Close lips around mouthpiece
   - Blow out as hard and fast as possible in a single blow
2. Teach patient to repeat #1 two more times and record the best of the three blows
3. Instruct patients how to determine their personal best peak flow number
   - Take readings twice a day for 2-3 weeks: upon awakening or between 12 noon & 2:00 PM
   - Take readings before and after inhaling beta$_2$-agonist
4. Explain that personal best peak flow numbers are categorized into zones to help patients self-manage their illnesses and to assess progression of disease and need for additional therapy
   - Green Zone: 80% of patient's personal best and denotes good control
   - Yellow Zone: 50-<80% of patient's personal best and denotes caution and the need to take a short-acting inhaled beta$_2$-agonist
   - Red Zone: <50% of patient's personal best and denotes severe asthma exacerbation and the need to take short-acting inhaled beta$_2$-agonist and call health care provider or emergency room or go directly to hospital
5. Explain to patient that once their personal best peak flow is documented they may decrease peak flow readings to once a day in the morning. If morning reading is <80% of personal best, instruct patient to monitor more frequently
6. Teach parents of children with moderate-to-severe persistent asthma that determination of personal best readings should be done every 6 months due to changes that occur with growth

Adapted from National Institutes of Health. National Heart, Lung, and Blood Institute. (1997). *The Expert Panel Report 2: Guidelines for the diagnosis and management of asthma*. National Asthma Education Program. NIH Publ. #97-4051. Bethesda, MD.

V. Plan/Management

A. Referral to an asthma specialist is recommended in the following situations:
1. Life-threatening or severe persistent asthma (step 4) is present
2. Goals of asthma therapy are not fulfilled after 3 to 6 months of treatment, or earlier if clinician concludes asthma is not responding to current therapy
3. Signs and symptoms are atypical or diagnosis is uncertain
4. Other illnesses such as sinusitis, gastroesophageal reflux, or chronic obstructive pulmonary disease complicate the airway disease
5. The patient has a history suggesting that asthma is being provoked by occupational factors, an environmental inhalant, or an ingested substance
6. Initial diagnosis is severe, persistent asthma
7. Additional diagnostic testing is indicated
8. Immunotherapy is a treatment consideration
9. Continuous oral corticosteroids or high-dose inhaled corticosteroids or two bursts of oral steroids in 1 year are needed
10. Patient is <3 years and needs step 3 or step 4 care
11. Patient or family requires additional education or guidance in following the treatment plan or avoiding asthma triggers

B. Control of the factors contributing to asthma severity is important
1. Instruct patient to avoid the following:
a. Allergens (see table MEASURES OF ENVIRONMENTAL CONTROL in ALLERGIC AND NONALLERGIC RHINITIS section)
b. Environmental tobacco smoke
c. Exercise when levels of pollution are high
d. Beta-blockers
e. Foods containing sulfite and other foods to which they are sensitive
2. Caution patients with severe persistent asthma, nasal polyps, or a history of sensitivity to aspirin or nonsteroidal anti-inflammatory drugs that there is risk of severe and possibly fatal exacerbations when using these drugs
3. Treat patients for rhinitis, sinusitis, and gastroesophageal reflux if present
4. Recommend annual influenza vaccination

C. General pharmacological principles a stepwise pharmacological approach is recommended for infants, young children, and individuals >5 years: see tables: STEPWISE APROACH IN INDIVIDUALS >5 YEARS (V.C.8.) and STEPWISE APPROACH IN INFANTS AND YOUNG CHILDREN (V.H.5.)
1. The dose and dosing interval are dictated by the asthma severity with the goal of suppressing airway inflammation and preventing exacerbations
2. As needed, begin therapy at a high level (short course of systemic corticosteroids plus inhaled corticosteroids or use of medium-to-high dose of inhaled corticosteroids) to promptly control symptoms and then lower level
3. Cautiously and very gradually step down therapy after control is achieved and sustained for several weeks or months
a. Generally, the last medication added should be the first medication reduced
b. Inhaled corticosteroids may be reduced 25% every 2-3 months to the lowest dose possible to maintain control
4. Continual monitoring is imperative; control is indicated by the following:
a. Peak expiratory flow (PEF) less than 10-20% variability
b. PEF consistently greater than 80% patient's personal best
c. Minimal symptoms
d. Minimal need for short-acting inhaled $beta_2$-agonist
e. Absence of nighttime awakenings
f. No activity limitations
5. Other actions needed if control is not achieved and sustained at any step
a. Assess patient adherence and technique in using medication
b. Step up to next higher step of care or temporarily increase anti-inflammatory therapy such as with a burst of prednisone
c. Reassess for factors that diminish control
d. Consult a specialist
6. Long-term control drugs are used daily to maintain control of persistent asthma; quick-relief drugs treat acute symptoms and exacerbations

7. See next four tables for the STEPWISE APPROACH IN INDIVIDUALS >5 YEARS and for information and dosing of long-term control medications
8. Quick relief medications can be used at all steps to rapidly control symptoms (see table)

STEPWISE APPROACH FOR MANAGING ASTHMA IN INDIVIDUALS OLDER THAN 5 YEARS OF AGE

Preferred treatments are in bold print

Medications Needed to Maintain Long-Term Control

Daily Medications

STEP 4
Severe
Persistent

Preferred treatment:
- **High-dose inhaled corticosteroids AND Long-acting inhaled beta$_2$-agonists**

AND, if needed:
- Corticosteroid tablets or syrup long-term (2 mg/kg/day, generally do not exceed 60 mg/day). (Make repeat attempts to reduce systemic corticosteroids and maintain control with high-dose inhaled corticosteroids)

STEP 3
Moderate
Persistent

Preferred Treatment: (Listed alphabetically)
- **Low-to-medium dose inhaled corticosteroids and long-acting inhaled beta$_2$-agonists**

Alternative Treatment:
- Increase inhaled corticosteroids within medium-dose range

OR
- Low-to-medium dose inhaled corticosteroids and either leukotriene modifier or theophylline

If needed (particularly in patients with recurring severe exacerbations)
Preferred treatment:
- **Increase inhaled corticosteroids within medium-dose range and add long-acting inhaled beta$_2$-agonists**

Alternative Treatment:
- Increase inhaled corticosteroids within medium-dose range and add either leukotriene modifier of theophylline

STEP 2
Mild
Persistent

Preferred Treatment:
- **Low-dose inhaled corticosteroids**

Alternative Treatment: (Listed alphabetically)
- Cromolyn, leukotriene modifier, nedocromil, OR sustained release theophylline to serum concentration of 5-15 mcg/mL

STEP 1
Mild
Intermittent

- **No daily medication needed**
- Severe exacerbations may occur, separated by long periods of normal lung function and no symptoms. A course of systemic corticosteroids is recommended

QUICK RELIEF
All patients

- Short-acting bronchodilator: 2-4 puffs **short-acting inhaled beta$_2$-agonists** as needed for symptoms
- Intensity of treatment will depend on severity of exacerbation; up to 3 treatments at 20-minute intervals or a single nebulizer treatment as needed. Course of systemic corticosteroids may be needed
- Use of short-acting beta$_2$-agonists >2 times/week in intermittent asthma (daily, or increasing use in persistent asthma) may indicate the need to initiate (increase) long-term control therapy

Step down
Review treatment every 1 to 6 months; a gradual stepwise reduction in treatment may be possible

Step up
If control is not maintained, consider step up. First: review patient medication technique, adherence, and environmental control

Adapted from National Institute of Health. National Heart, Lung and Blood Institute. (2002). *NAEPP Expert Panel Report guidelines for diagnosis and management of asthma – update on selected topics 2002.* National Asthma Education and Prevention Program. NIH Publ. #02-5075, Bethesda, MD.

LONG-TERM CONTROL MEDICATIONS

1. Corticosteroids are the most potent and effective agents in adults and children
   - ✓ Oral/systemic form used for prompt control when initiating long-term therapy
   - ✓ Inhaled form is preferred for long-term control
   - ✓ Benefits outweigh risk of adverse effects; to reduce adverse effects, the following are recommended:
     - Use with spacers/holding chambers
     - Rinse mouth after use
     - Use lowest possible dose to maintain control
     - Consider a long-acting beta$_2$-agonist rather than a higher dose inhaled corticosteroid
     - In children, periodically monitor growth
     - Do not give varicella vaccine to patients receiving ≥2 mg/kg or 20 mg/day of oral prednisone
   - ✓ In children with episodic therapy with systemic corticosteroids who have not had clinical chickenpox give varicella vaccine

2. Cromolyn sodium and nedocromil are mild to moderate anti-inflammatory medications
   - ✓ May be initial choice for long-term therapy in children
   - ✓ Comparison of nedocromil and cromolyn
     - Nedocromil is more potent in inhibiting bronchospasm due to exercise, cold dry air, and bradykinin aerosol; more effective in nonallergic patients using inhaled corticosteroids
     - Nedocromil may help reduce dose requirements of corticosteroids

3. Long-acting beta$_2$-agonists are used with anti-inflammatory medications; helpful for nocturnal symptoms
   - ✓ Salmeterol and Formoterol are **not used for treatment of acute symptoms or exacerbations**
   - ✓ Daily use of these drugs should not exceed recommended amounts
   - ✓ Even if symptoms improve, patients should **not** stop anti-inflammatory medication

4. Methylxanthines (mainly sustained-release theophylline) are used as adjuvant to inhaled corticosteroids for prevention of nocturnal symptoms
   - ✓ Although not preferred, sustained-release theophylline may be alternative for long-term preventive therapy when cost or adherence in using inhaled medications is problematic
   - ✓ Essential to monitor serum concentration levels
   - ✓ Smoking increases metabolism of theophylline

5. Leukotriene modifiers are alternatives to low doses of inhaled corticosteroids or cromolyn or nedocromil for persons with mild persistent asthma (need more research and experience)
   - ✓ Zafirlukast (Accolate) has an interaction effect with warfarin; essential to closely monitor prothrombin times and adjust appropriately (not recommended for children <7 years old)
   - ✓ Zileuton (Zyflo) (not recommended for children <12 years old)
     - May infrequently cause liver toxicity; essential to monitor liver enzymes
     - May inhibit metabolism of terfenadine, warfarin, and theophylline
   - ✓ Montelukast sodium (Singulair)
     - Can be used in children ≥2 years old

USUAL DOSAGES FOR LONG-TERM-CONTROL MEDICATIONS

Medication	Dosage Form	Dose: Individuals >12 years	Child Dose*
Inhaled Corticosteroids (See table: *Estimated Comparative Daily Dosages for Inhaled Corticosteroids*)			
Systemic Corticosteroids (*applies to all three corticosteroids*)			
Methylprednisolone Prednisolone Prednisone	2, 4, 8, 16, 32 mg tablets 5 mg tablets, 5 mg/5cc, 15 mg/5 cc 1, 2.5, 5, 10, 20, 50 mg tablets; 5 mg/cc, 5 mg/5cc	▪ 7.5-60 mg daily in a single dose in AM or QOD as needed for control ▪ Short-course "burst" to achieve control: 40-60 mg/day as single or 2 divided doses for 3-10 days	▪ 0.25-2 mg/kg daily in a single dose in AM or QOD as needed for control ▪ Short-course "burst": 1-2 mg/kg/day, maximum 60 mg/day for 3-10 days
Long-Acting Inhaled Beta$_2$-Agonists (*Should not be used for symptom relief or for exacerbations. Use with inhaled corticosteroids*)			
Salmeterol	MDI 21 mcg/puff DPI 50 mcg/blister	2 puffs q 12 hours 1 blister q 12 hours	1-2 puffs q 12 hours 1 blister q 12 hours
Formoterol	DPI 12 mcg/single-use capsule	1 capsule q 12 hours	1 capsule q 12 hours
Combined Medication			
Fluticasone/Salmeterol	DPI 100, 250, or 500 mcg/50 mcg	1 inh BID; dose depends on severity of asthma	1 inh BID, dose depends on severity of asthma

(Continued)

USUAL DOSAGES FOR LONG-TERM-CONTROL MEDICATIONS (CONTINUED)

Medication	Dosage Form	Dose: Individuals >12 years	Child Dose*
Cromolyn and Nedocromil			
Cromolyn	MDI 1 mg/puff	2-4 puffs TID-QID	1-2 puffs TID-QID
	Nebulizer 20 mg/ampule	1 ampule TID-QID	1 ampule TID-QID
Nedocromil	MDI 1.75 mg/puff	2-4 puffs BID-QID	1-2 puffs BID-QID
Leukotriene Modifiers			
Montelukast	4 or 5 mg chewable tablet	10 mg QHS	4 mg QHS (2-5 years)
	10 mg tablet		5 mg QHS (6-14 years)
			10 mg QHS (>14 years)
Zafirlukast	10 or 20 mg tablet	40 mg daily (20 mg tablet BID)	20 mg daily (7-11 years) (10 mg tablet BID)
Zileuton	300 or 600 mg tablet	2,400 mg daily (give tablets QID)	

* Children ≤12 years of age

ESTIMATED COMPARATIVE DAILY DOSAGES FOR INHALED CORTICOSTEROIDS

Drug	Low Daily Dose		Medium Daily Dose		High Daily Dose	
	Individuals >12 years	Child*	Individuals >12 years	Child*	Individuals >12 years	Child*
Beclomethasone CFC 42 or 84 mcg/puff	168-504 mcg	84-336 mcg	504-840 mcg	336-672 mcg	>840 mcg	>672 mcg
Beclomethasone HFA 40 of 80 mcg/puff	80-240 mcg	80-160 mcg	240-480 mcg	160-320 mcg	>480 mcg	>320 mcg
Budesonide DPI 200 mcg/inh	200-600 mcg	200-400 mcg	600-1,200 mcg	400-800 mcg	>1,200 mcg	>800 mcg
Inhalation suspension for nebulization (child dose)		0.5 mg		1.0 mg		2.0 mg
Flunisolide 250 mcg/puff	500-1,000 mcg	500-750 mcg	1,000-2,000 mcg	1,000-1,250 mcg	>2,000 mcg	>1,250 mcg
Fluticasone MDI: 44, 110, or 220 mcg/puff	88-264 mcg	88-176 mcg	264-660 mcg	176-440 mcg	>660 mcg	>440 mcg
DPI: 50, 100, or 250 mcg/inh	100-300 mcg	100-200 mcg	300-600 mcg	200-400 mcg	>600 mcg	>400 mcg
Triamcinolone acetonide 100 mcg/puff	400-1,000 mcg	400-800 mcg	1,000-2,000 mcg	800-1,200 mcg	>2,000 mcg	>1,200 mcg

* Children ≤12 years of age

QUICK-RELIEF MEDICATIONS

1. Therapy of choice is a short-acting beta$_2$-agonist
   - ✓ Use of >1 canister in 1 month signifies poor control & need to begin or increase anti-inflammatory drug
   - ✓ Regularly scheduled, daily use of these drugs is **not** recommended

2. Anticholinergics (ipratropium bromide) may provide additive benefit to inhaled beta$_2$-agonist or may be alternative quick-relief drug for patients unable to tolerate inhaled beta$_2$-agonist

3. Oral/systemic corticosteroids are used for moderate-to-severe exacerbations and can speed resolution of airflow obstruction and reduce rate of relapse

Adapted from National Institutes of Health. National Heart, Lung, and Blood Institute. (1997). *The Expert Panel Report 2: Guidelines for the diagnosis and management of asthma.* National Asthma Education Program. NIH Publ. #97-4051. Bethesda, MD.

D. Treatment of **Step 1: Mild Intermittent Asthma in Individuals >5 years**

    1. No daily medicine needed; prescribe short-acting inhaled beta$_2$-agonist on an as-needed basis (see table)

DOSAGES FOR INHALED SHORT-ACTING BETA$_2$-AGONISTS

Medication	Dosage Form	Dose: Persons >12 years	Child Dose	Comments
	Metered-Dose Inhaler			
Albuterol (Ventolin) Albuterol HFA (Proventil HFA)	90 mcg/puff, 200 puffs	2 puffs TID-QID prn	2 puffs TID-QID prn	Increasing or regular use on a daily basis indicates the need for additional long-term-control therapy
Pirbuterol (Maxair Autohaler)	200 mcg/puff, 400 puffs			
	Dry Powder Inhaler			
Albuterol Rotacaps (Ventolin)	200 mcg/capsule	1-2 capsules Q 4-6 hours prn	1 capsule Q 4-6 hours prn	
	Nebulizer solution			
Albuterol (Ventolin)	5 mg/mL (0.5%)	1.25-5 mg (0.25-1 cc) in 2-3 cc of saline Q 4-8 hours	0.05 mg/kg (min 1.25 mg, max 2.5 mg) in 2-3 cc of saline Q 4-6 hours	May mix with cromolyn or ipratropium nebulizer solutions
Levalbuterol (Xopenex)	0.63 mg/3 mL 1.25 mg/3 mL	0.63 mg-1.25 mg in 3 cc TID Q 6-8 hours	>6 years: 0.31 mg TID	Advantage for patients who have significant side effects to albuterol
Bitolterol (Tornalate)	2 mg/mL (0.2%)	0.5-3.5 mg (0.25-1 cc) in 2-3 cc of saline Q 4-8 hours	Not established	May not mix with other nebulizer solutions

Adapted from National Institutes of Health. National Heart, Lung, and Blood Institute. (1997). *The Expert Panel Report 2: Guidelines for the diagnosis and management of asthma*. National Asthma Education Program, Office of Prevention, Education and Control. NIH Publication #97-4051. Bethesda, MD.

2. Treatment of **exercise-induced bronchospasm**; use one of following:
    a. Short-acting inhaled beta$_2$-agonist 1-2 puffs 5 minutes prior to exercise
    b. Inhaled cromolyn sodium (Intal) or nedocromil (Tilade) 2 puffs 10 minutes prior to exercise
    c. Formoterol (Foradil Aerolizer) is indicated for adolescents and children >12 years of age when administered on an occasional as needed basis for the acute prevention of exercise-induced bronchospasm (dose one capsule [one 12 microgram inhalation] inhaled at least 15 minutes prior to exercise; additional doses should not be used for 12 hours)
    d. Inhaled corticosteroids are recommended for long-term control

3. Treatment of **mild exacerbations** due to viral respiratory infections: prescribe short-acting beta$_2$-agonist every 4-6 hours for approximately 24 hours

4. Treatment of **moderate-to-severe exacerbations:**
    a. Use both of the following:
        (1) Give short-acting beta$_2$-agonist by nebulizer or MDI (with close supervision can give 3 treatments spaced every 20-30 minutes)
        (2) Also, prescribe systemic corticosteroid; patients with history of severe exacerbations should start corticosteroids at first sign of infection (see table USUAL DOSAGES FOR LONG-TERM CONTROL MEDICATIONS)
    b. Oxygen is recommended for most patients
    c. Careful, vigilant monitoring of patient's condition is paramount

5. Antibiotics are not recommended for treating acute exacerbations, except as needed for comorbid conditions (fever and purulent sputum, evidence of pneumonia, or suspected sinusitis)

E. Treatment of **Step 2: Mild Persistent Asthma in Individuals >5 years**: Use inhaled short-acting beta$_2$-agonist on an as-needed basis
    1. Prescribe inhaled corticosteroids at a low dose (see table DAILY DOSAGES OF INHALED CORTICOSTEROIDS); when taking several inhaled medications simultaneously, always use beta$_2$-agonist first to open airway and then use steroid inhaler for greater penetration of medication

2.   Alternative treatment (select one)
        a.   Cromolyn (Intal) or Nedocromil (Tilade): A trial of one of these drugs is recommended in children because of the safety profile
        b.   Sustained-release theophylline is an alternative, but is not preferred because of modest effectiveness and potential for toxicity; prescribe drug to achieve a serum concentration of between 5 and 15 mcg/mL (periodic monitoring is necessary to maintain a therapeutic level)
        c.   Leukotriene receptor antagonists (zafirlukast, zileuton, or montelukast sodium) are alternative drugs
3.   For exacerbations, see V.D.3.4. and V.L.

F.   Treatment of **Step 3: Moderate Persistent Asthma in Individuals >5 years:** Consultation with an asthma specialist is advised
1.   Preferred treatment is low-to-medium dose of inhaled corticosteroids and long-acting beta$_2$-agonists such as formoterol (Foradil) or salmeterol (Serevent); for patients on fluticasone (Flovent) when salmeterol is being added to regimen, fluticasone/salmeterol (Advair Diskcus) is an option
2.   Alternative treatment: Increase inhaled corticosteroid within medium-dose range – OR – low-to-medium dose inhaled corticosteroid and either leukotriene modifier or theophylline
3.   Additional plan: If symptoms are not optimally controlled with initial plan, either of the following two strategies is recommended
        a.   Increase inhaled corticosteroid within medium-dose range and add long-acting inhaled beta$_2$-agonist
        b.   Increase inhaled corticosteroid within medium-dose range and add either leukotriene modifier or theophylline (alternative)

G.   Treatment of **Step 4: Severe Persistent Asthma in Individuals >5 years:** Consult specialist
1.   Preferred treatment: High-dose inhaled corticosteroids AND long-acting inhaled beta$_2$-agonists
2.   Additionally, if needed, prescribe an oral systemic corticosteroid
        a.   Prescribe lowest possible dose (single daily dose on alternate days)
        b.   Do not exceed 60 mg/day
        c.   Carefully monitor for adverse side effects such as secondary infections, electrolyte imbalances, hypertension, peptic ulcers, dermal atrophy, carbohydrate intolerance, osteoporosis, cataracts, glaucoma, and psychological effects
        d.   Conscientiously try to reduce systemic corticosteroids once symptoms are controlled and maintain control with high-dose inhaled corticosteroids that have less adverse effects (euphoria, depression)
        e.   For exacerbations see V.D.3.4. and V.L.

H.   Treatment of **Infants and Young Children ≤5 Years** (see table STEPWISE APPROACH FOR MANAGING INFANTS AND YOUNG CHILDREN)
1.   Consultation with a specialist should be considered for infants and young children requiring step 2 care; consultation is recommended for all children requiring step 3 and step 4 care
2.   Consider beginning long-term control therapy; inhaled corticosteroids are the preferred therapies in infants and children who have the following:
        a.   Require symptomatic treatment more than two times per week
        b.   Experience severe exacerbations less than 6 weeks apart
        c.   Experience more than three episodes of wheezing in the past year that lasted more than one day and affected sleep – AND – parental history of asthma or clinician-diagnosed atopic dermatitis – OR – two of the following
            (1)   Clinical-diagnosed allergic rhinitis
            (2)   Wheezing apart from colds
            (3)   Peripheral blood eosinophilia
3.   In children <2 years, nebulizers may be preferred delivery system; children between 3-5 years may use MDI and spacer/holding chamber alone, but they may require a nebulizer or an MDI plus spacer/holding chamber and face mask (see table AEROSOL DELIVERY DEVICES)
4.   Regularly monitor and graph height and weight; ongoing studies indicate that treatment with inhaled corticosteroids has a potential but small risk of delayed growth; inhaled corticosteroids have no adverse effects on bone mineral density or the incidence of cataracts or glaucoma
5.   See V.C. for general pharmacological principles, as well as tables after V.C.8. on long-term control medications

STEPWISE APPROACH FOR MANAGING ASTHMA IN INFANTS AND YOUNG CHILDREN
(5 YEARS OF AGE AND YOUNGER)

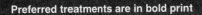

Preferred treatments are in bold print

Medications Required to Maintain Long-Term Control

Daily Medications

STEP 4
Severe
Persistent

Preferred treatment:
- **High-dose inhaled corticosteroids AND Long-acting inhaled beta₂-agonists**

AND, if needed,
- Corticosteroid tablets or syrup long term (2 mg/kg/day, generally do not exceed 60 mg per day). (Make repeat attempts to reduce systemic corticosteroids and maintain control with high-dose inhaled corticosteroids)

STEP 3
Moderate
Persistent

Preferred treatment:
- **Low-dose inhaled corticosteroids and long-acting inhaled beta₂-agonists**
    OR
- **Medium-dose inhaled corticosteroids**

Alternative treatment:
- Low-dose inhaled corticosteroids and either leukotriene receptor antagonist or theophylline

If needed (particularly in patients with recurring severe exacerbations):
Preferred treatment:
- **Medium-dose inhaled corticosteroids and long-acting beta₂-agonists**

Alternative treatment:
- Medium-dose inhaled corticosteroids and either leukotriene receptor antagonist or theophylline

STEP 2
Mild
Persistent

Preferred treatment:
- **Low-dose inhaled corticosteroid** (with nebulizer or MDI with holding chamber with or without face mask or DPI)

Alternative treatment:
- Cromolyn (nebulizer is preferred or MDI with holding chamber) OR leukotriene receptor antagonist

STEP 1
Mild
Intermittent

No daily medication needed

QUICK RELIEF*
All patients

Bronchodilator as needed for symptoms. Intensity of treatment will depend upon severity of exacerbation
- *Preferred treatment:* **Short-acting inhaled beta₂-agonists by nebulizer or face mask and space/holding chamber**
- *Alternative treatment:* Oral beta₂-agonist

With viral respiratory infection
- Bronchodilator q 4-6 hours up to 24 hours (longer with clinician consult); in general, repeat no more than once every 6 weeks
- Consider systemic corticosteroid if exacerbation is severe or patient has history of previous severe exacerbations

Use of short-acting beta₂-agonists >2 times/week in intermittent asthma (daily, or increasing use in persistent asthma) may indicate the need to initiate (increase) long-term control therapy

 Step down
Review treatment every 1 to 6 months; a gradual stepwise reduction may be possible

 Step up
If control is not maintained, consider step up. First: review patient medication technique, adherence, and environmental control

*In infants and children, antibiotics are not recommended for treatment of acute asthma except as needed for comorbid conditions: fever and purulent sputum, suspected pneumonia, or sinusitis

Adapted from National Institutes of Health. National Heart, Lung, and Blood Institute. (2002). N*AEPP Expert Panel Report guidelines for the diagnosis and management of asthma. Update on selected topics 2002.* National Asthma Education and Prevention Program. NIH Publ. #02-5075, Bethesda, MD.

I.   Special considerations in school-age children and adolescents
1.   Involve this age group in establishing goals and plans
2.   Active participation in physical activities should be encouraged
3.   A written asthma management plan should be given to the student's school

J.   Treatment of exercise-induced bronchospasm (EIB) (see V.D.2.)

K. Home management of exacerbations
    1. Increase inhaled beta$_2$-agonist (up to three treatments of 2-4 puffs by MDI at 20 minute intervals or a single nebulizer treatment)
        a. If good response: continue beta$_2$-agonist every 3-4 hours for 24-48 hours; patients on inhaled corticosteroids should double dose for 7-10 days; contact clinician for followup instructions
        b. If response is incomplete: Add oral corticosteroid and continue beta$_2$-agonist and contact clinician within the day
        c. If poor response: Add oral corticosteroid, repeat beta$_2$-agonist immediately; if distress is severe go to emergency department or call 911
    2. Continue more intensive treatment for several days as recovery from exacerbations is often slow

L. Route of administration: inhaled route more effectively delivers medication to lung, has reduced side effects, and the onset of action is shorter than oral medications (see following tables on descriptions and how to use various delivery devices)

AEROSOL DELIVERY DEVICES		
Device/Drugs*	**Population**	**Therapeutic Issues**
Metered-dose inhaler (MDI) Beta$_2$-agonists Corticosteroids Cromolyn sodium and Nedocromil Anticholinergics	>5 years	Takes coordination to actuate and inhale. Mouth washing is effective in reducing systemic absorption
Breath-actuated MDI Beta$_2$-agonists	>5 years	Best for patients unable to coordinate inhalation and actuation. Cannot be used with currently available spacer/ holding chamber devices
Dry powder inhaler (DPI) Beta$_2$-agonists Corticosteroids	May be used in children 4 years old; effects more consistent in children >5 years	Delivery may be ≥MDI depending on device and technique. Mouth washing is effective in reducing systemic absorption
Space/holding chamber	>4 years ≤4 years with face mask	Easier to use than MDI alone Decrease oropharyngeal deposition. Reduce potential systemic absorption of inhaled corticosteroid preparations that have higher oral bioavailability; recommended for all patients on medium-to-high doses of inhaled corticosteroids May be as effective as nebulizer in delivering high doses of beta$_2$-agonists during severe exacerbations
Nebulizer Beta$_2$-agonists Cromolyn Anticholinergics Corticosteroids	≤2 years	Method of choice for cromolyn in children and for high-dose beta$_2$-agonists and anticholinergics in moderate-to-severe exacerbations in all patients Less dependent on patient coordination or cooperation

*See additional tables for directions on how to use metered-dose inhaler, dry powder capsules, nebulizers, and Diskcus

Adapted from National Institutes of Health. National Heart, Lung, and Blood Institute. (1997). *The Expert Panel Report 2: Guidelines for the diagnosis and management of asthma*. National Asthma Education Program. NIH Publ. #97-4051. Bethesda, MD.

DIRECTIONS ON HOW TO USE AN INHALER*

- Remove the cap, hold the inhaler upright and shake it

- Tilt your head back slightly and slowly exhale

- Put the inhaler 1-2 inches from your mouth (open mouth technique) -- OR -- Enclose mouthpiece with your lips (closed mouth technique); do **not** use closed mouth technique for corticosteroids -- OR -- Use spacer/holding chamber** (slowly inhale or tidal breathe immediately after actuation; actuate only once into chamber per inhalation or if face mask is used, allow 3-5 inhalations per actuation)

- Press down on the plunger and take a full, deep, slow, even breath (breathe in through mouth, not through nose)

- Hold your breath for 10 seconds, then exhale slowly through your nose

- Wait one minute before taking next puff

- Rinse your mouth afterward to prevent possible fungal infection

- Keep mouthpiece clean

*Counsel regarding danger of overuse of inhaler. Patients should be using <u>no</u> more than 1 canister (200 metered dose inhalations of a beta$_2$-agonist) in a month

**Spacers/holding chambers are particularly recommended for young children and older adults and for patients using inhaled corticosteroids

Adapted from National Institutes of Health. National Heart, Lung, and Blood Institute. (1997). *The Expert Panel Report 2: Guidelines for the diagnosis and management of asthma*. National Asthma Education Program. NIH Publ. #97-4051. Bethesda, MD.

DIRECTIONS ON HOW TO USE DRY POWDER CAPSULES

- Close mouth tightly around mouthpiece
- Inhale deeply and rapidly
- Minimally effective inspiratory flow is device dependent

DIRECTIONS ON HOW TO USE A NEBULIZER

- Measure correct amount of normal saline solution and place into cup (if medicine is premixed, go to step 3)
- Measure correct amount of medicine and put into cup with saline solution
- Fasten mouthpiece to the T-shaped part and then fasten this unit to the cup OR fasten mask to cup (use mouthpiece for persons >2 years)
- Put mouthpiece in mouth and seal lips tightly around OR place mask on face
- Turn on the air compressor machine
- Take slow, deep breaths through mouth
- Hold breath 1-2 seconds before exhaling
- Continue until medicine is depleted from cup (approximately 10 minutes)
- Do not forget to clean nebulizer; cleaning removes germs and prevents infection as well as keeps nebulizer from clogging

Adapted from National Institutes of Health. (1992). *Teach your patients about asthma: A clinician's guide.* National Asthma Education Program, Office of Prevention, Education and Control. Publication #92-2737. Bethesda, MD.

DIRECTIONS ON HOW TO USE DISKCUS

- Hold device level with one hand
- With thumb of the other hand on the thumbgrip, push thumb away from you until you hear the mouthpiece snap into position
- With mouthpiece towards you, slide the lever away from you until you hear a click (each time the lever is pushed back a dose is available for inhalation)
- Breathe out as far as comfortable while holding device level and away from your mouth
- With the mouthpiece to your lips, breathe in deeply and steadily through the device
- Hold your breath for around 10 seconds, then breathe out slowly
- To close the device, slide the thumbgrip back towards you and click the device shut (the device will be reset and ready for next scheduled dose)
- Remember to never exhale into device
- Keep the device dry; never wash any part of the device

Adapted from GlaxoWellcome. (1995) Patient instructions for use of Serevent Diskcus (salmeterol xinafoate) inhalation powder. Research Triangle Park, NC.

M. Patient education: Establish a partnership with the patient and family and include them in developing goals and plan: <u>written action plans</u> should be part of patient education; important components include the following:
   1. Basic facts about asthma
   2. Roles of medications
   3. Discuss asthma triggers and ways to avoid or control them (see V.B.)
   4. Review techniques and ask patient to demonstrate use of inhaler, spacer, nebulizer, or Diskcus (many drug failures are due to improper use of equipment)
   5. Counsel regarding overuse of inhalers which could result in tachyarrhythmias and death
   6. Teach how to recognize symptom patterns that indicate poor asthma control and when to seek medical care; may need to keep a daily diary of symptoms, peak flow readings, and medications
   7. Develop a written action plan based on peak flow readings (see Expert Panel Report 2, 1997)
   8. Extensive teaching on exacerbation management is needed
      a. Discuss indicators of worsening asthma, specific recommendations for using $beta_2$-agonist rescue therapy, early administration of systemic corticosteroids, and directions on seeking medical care
      b. Patients at high risk of asthma-related death include those using >2 canisters per month of $beta_2$-agonists, difficulty perceiving airflow obstruction, comorbidity, severe psychiatric or psychosocial problems, low socioeconomic status, illicit drug use, and prior history of severe exacerbations, intubation, hospitalizations, frequent ER visits
   9. Good web site resources (see following table)

WEBSITE RESOURCES	
Organization	**Website**
Allergy and Asthma Network/Mothers of Asthmatics, Inc.	http://www.aanma.org
Asthma and Allergy Foundation of America	http://www.aafa.org
National Asthma Education and Prevention Program, National Heart, Lung, and Blood Information Center	http://www.nhlbi.nih.gov
Asthma in America	http://www.asthmainamerica.com

N. Follow Up
   1. Schedule first follow-up visit within one month after initial diagnosis
   2. For acute exacerbations with incomplete or poor responses see patient within 24 hours and then re-evaluate in 3-5 days
   3. After exacerbation has resolved completely, schedule follow up visits every 1-3 months
   4. For patients on theophylline, check serum drug levels after 2 weeks from initiation of therapy; then every 4 months; in children, need more frequent monitoring during growth spurts
   5. Follow up for other patients depends on symptom severity, symptom control, knowledge level, social support and other resources; for new asthmatics, frequent visits are important to monitor disease as well as for patient education; routine visits are scheduled every 1-6 months

BRONCHIOLITIS

I. Definition: Inflammation of the bronchioles resulting in small airway obstruction

II. Pathogenesis

A. Due to necrotizing desquamation and subsequent deposition of debris along epithelium of bronchioles, lumina become partially obstructed resulting in air trapping and hyperinflation of lungs

B. Usually caused by one of the following viruses: respiratory syncytial virus (RSV) (majority of cases), parainfluenza type III, adenovirus, and enterovirus; *Mycoplasma pneumoniae* is less common pathogen but may occur in older children

C. RSV is transmitted by direct contact or in aerosolized nasal secretions; eyes and nose are common sites of inoculation; fomite transmission is also possible
    1. Virus may be shed for three to eight days but may continue to shed for as long as three to four week; infants shed for longest time period
    2. Incubation period is approximately three to five days

III. Clinical Presentation

A. Most common lower respiratory tract infection in infants
    1. Most infants have mild forms and can be managed as outpatients
    2. Some infants require hospitalization; rates of hospitalization have markedly increased since 1980

B. Factors contributing to increased risk include male gender, low socioeconomic status, crowded living conditions, passive cigarette smoke exposure, attendance in day care, presence of older siblings in home, and lack of breastfeeding

C. Yearly epidemics usually occur in late winter and early spring

D. Criteria which are helpful for diagnosing bronchiolitis include the following:
    1. First episode of wheezing
    2. Infant 24 months of age or younger
    3. Associated physical findings of viral infection such as coryza, cough, and low-grade fever
    4. Elimination of atopy or pneumonia as cause of wheezing

E. Although wheezing is the prominent sign, child may have diffuse crackles and rhonchi

F. Child may have respiratory distress with flaring nares, intercostal and subcostal retractions, and may use accessory muscles of respiration; because of hyperinflated lungs, liver and spleen may be pushed down and palpable; dehydration may occur with increased respiratory effort

G. Most children improve substantially within several days; upper respiratory symptoms gradually improve over 1-2 weeks

H. Mortality rate is less than 1%
    1. Emergent cases may have cyanosis, listlessness, apnea or decreased breath sounds
    2. Infants, children with underlying cardiopulmonary disease, those born prematurely, and immunodeficient children are at increased risk for complications

I. Children with RSV bronchiolitis have increased risk of persistent bronchial reactivity and asthma

IV. Diagnosis/Evaluation

A. History
    1. Determine activity level and presence of any breathing problems
    2. Explore fluid/food intake
    3. Question about number of wet diapers, or frequency of voiding in older child
    4. Question about onset and characteristics of URI symptoms (especially describe cough and wheeze)
    5. Inquire about duration of any temperature elevation
    6. Ask about any periods of apnea or cyanosis
    7. Question about gastroesophageal reflux, choking, and vomiting
    8. Explore family history of asthma and allergies
    9. Explore past history of previous respiratory distress, cyanosis, weight loss, and fatigue
    10. Explore history of other cardiac or pulmonary diseases as these conditions predispose children to dangerous sequelae from bronchiolitis

B. Physical Examination
    1. Determine respiratory rate and color (an increasing respiratory rate is the sign best correlated with poor oxygenation); tachypnea is a constant finding; respiratory rate is usually between 45-80 breaths per minute
    2. Observe for nasal flaring, accessory muscle use, intercostal or subcostal retractions

3. Observe chest wall and abdominal motion (an ominous sign is failure of abdomen to move outward with inspiration)
4. Assess degree of alertness and fatigue (eye contact with mother, crying, ability to suck or drink)
5. Assess hydration status: capillary refill time, skin turgor, moisture of mucous membranes
6. Auscultate lungs (children with bronchiolitis may have fine crackles, wheezes, and prolonged expiratory phase)
7. Ascertain that breath sounds are equal bilaterally
8. Percuss chest (usually has a hyperresonant ring with bronchiolitis)
9. Auscultate heart and determine pulse; tachycardia often accompanies tachypnea
10. Palpate for organomegaly

C. Differential Diagnosis
1. Asthma is difficult to differentiate from bronchiolitis; asthma usually has the following:
   a. Strong family history of asthma
   b. Marked positive response to bronchodilators
   c. Symptoms which are episodic and precipitated by exercise, allergens, weather changes, or irritant exposure
   d. Wheezes occurring without predisposing viral respiratory infection
   e. Fine inspiratory crackles are usually NOT present as in bronchiolitis
2. Pneumonia
3. Cystic fibrosis is characterized by the following:
   a. Frequent respiratory infections
   b. Failure to thrive
   c. Chronic cough
   d. Malabsorption; symptoms include diarrhea and foul-smelling bowel movements
4. Anatomic abnormalities such as tracheomalacia
   a. Hypercompliant tracheal cartilage that collapses during expiration and may vibrate during inspiration
   b. Symptoms are continuous and do not go away
5. Gastroesophageal reflux (chronic symptoms)
6. Aspiration of foreign body (unilateral wheezing)
7. Congenital heart disease
8. α_1-antitrypsin deficiency, immunodeficiency, dysmotile cilia syndrome
9. Croup (prolonged inspiratory stridor, hoarseness, and barky cough)

D. Diagnostic Tests: Disease is clinically defined using well-accepted criteria; empirical data do not support the usefulness of any testing to diagnose disease
1. Pulse oximetry may be used to determine degree of hypoxemia
2. Gold standard for detecting RSV infection is cell culture but it is rarely recommended because it is costly, requires technical expertise and facilities, and takes at least 2-21 days to detect virus
3. Rapid antigen tests using enzyme-linked immunosuppressive assay or rapid fluorescent antibody studies are acceptable alternatives for cell culture; these tests have an average sensitivity and specificity of 80-90%
   a. Usually not performed except when confirmation of diagnosis will change clinical management
   b. Nasopharyngeal wash specimens are superior to nasal or pharyngeal swabs
4. Collection of urine for determination of specific gravity may be helpful in determining hydration status
5. Order chest x-ray if diagnosis is unclear; suspect bronchiolitis if x-ray reveals the following:
   a. Hyperinflation
   b. Increased anterior-posterior diameter of chest
   c. Flat or depressed diaphragm
   d. Scattered areas of atelectasis and interstitial infiltrates which may be difficult to differentiate from pneumonia
6. Arterial blood gases may be needed in severe cases

V. Plan/Management

A. Children with respiratory distress need immediate transport to hospital for oxygen and ventilatory support; hospitalization is not required unless child is small infant or has underlying cardiac or pulmonary disease

B. Carefully and frequently observe child's respiratory rate and status

C.   If oxygen saturation measures <95% with pulse oximetry, humidified oxygen with nasal prongs, face mask, or via a hood is recommended

D.   Treatment for uncomplicated cases is supportive and symptomatic
    1.   Encourage parents to frequently offer clear fluids or diluted milk
    2.   Vigorous and frequent suctioning of nasal secretions is important, particularly in infants who become easily fatigued when breathing through a mucous obstruction
    3.   Mist treatment with vaporizer is no longer recommended
    4.   Administer antipyretics if necessary

E.   Pharmacological treatment is controversial; in 2003 evidence is insufficient to recommend any drug therapy over good supportive care; however, the following therapies show some potential for being efficacious (consultation with a specialist is recommended)
    1.   Nebulized epinephrine (Wainwright, et al. [2003] found this therapy was ineffective)
    2.   Nebulized salbutamol plus ipratropium bromide
    3.   Nebulized ipratropium bromide
    4.   Oral or parenteral corticosteroids (preferably dexamethasone)
    5.   Inhaled corticosteroids (preferably budesonide); however, due to potential for adverse effects, these drugs warrant caution in their use
    6.   The following two therapies are recommended ONLY for the most severely ill children
        a.   Inhaled helium-oxygen
        b.   Surfactant for ventilated children

F.   Ineffective medications include decongestants, antihistamines, antibiotics, aerosolized ribavirin, nebulized furosemide, nebulized recombinant human deoxyribonuclease (rhDNase), and inhaled alpha-interferon

G.   Two products are available for prophylaxis and should be considered for children 6-24 months who are in high risk groups such as premature infants (<35 weeks gestation) and children with bronchopulmonary dysplasia; do not prescribe for high-risk infants with cyanotic cardiac disease
    1.   Palivizumab (Synagis) 15 mg/kg IM once a month during RSV season; does not interfere with the response to vaccines
    2.   Respiratory Syncytial Immune Globulin (RSV-IGIV) (RespiGam) 15 mL/kg (750 mg/kg) intravenously (IV) once per month just before and monthly throughout RSV season (in most areas of US, RSV season begins October to December and ends March to May)
    3.   Do not administer measles-mumps-rubella vaccine and varicella vaccine within 9 months of last dose of RSV-IGIV
    4.   Palivizumab is preferred due to ease of administration, low incidence of adverse effects, and increased efficacy; however in the RSV-IGIV trial, immunoprophylaxis decreased overall rate of non-RSV respiratory infections; this may be of value for infants/children who are not eligible for influenza vaccinations or those with severe pulmonary disease

H.   Patient Education
    1.   Teach parents to assess child for signs of respiratory distress and changes in level of activity and signs of dehydration
    2.   Remind parents about the highly contagious nature of viral infections
        a.   Family members need good handwashing techniques
        b.   Eliminate exposure of other small children to ill patient
    3.   Teach ways to possibly prevent episodes: avoid tobacco smoke and air pollutants such as wood stoves

I.   Although trials of an effective vaccine to prevent bronchiolitis are under way, no safe vaccines are currently available

J.   Follow Up: Close monitoring of child's condition is needed
    1.   Phone call to child's home in 2-8 hours often is warranted
    2.   Consider return visit next morning
    3.   After this initial follow up, schedule return visit for 10-14 days or sooner if symptoms have not improved

BRONCHITIS, ACUTE

I.   Definition: Infection of the tracheobronchial tree that causes reversible bronchial inflammation

II. Pathogenesis

    A.   Mucous membrane of tracheobronchial tree becomes hyperemic, edematous, with increased bronchial secretions and destruction of epithelium and impaired mucociliary activity

    B.   Pathogens
        1.   In >90% of cases, the infection has a nonbacterial cause; the viruses most frequently associated with lower respiratory tract disease include influenza B, influenza A, parainfluenza, respiratory syncytial virus
        2.   *Bordetella pertussis, Mycoplasma pneumoniae, Chlamydia pneumoniae* as a group are associated as the nonviral causes in 5-10% of cases
        3.   Secondary bacterial invasion by *Streptococcus pneumoniae, Moraxella catarrhalis* and *Haemophilus influenzae* type B usually occur in patients with underlying lung disease

III. Clinical Presentation

    A.   Cough, with or without sputum, particularly at night, is hallmark symptom; sputum may be clear or purulent

    B.   Most patients are afebrile with mild symptoms

    C.   Symptoms such as fever, substernal pain, and possibly mucoid sputum production, dyspnea, or bronchospasm with wheezing occur occasionally (fever is a common sign especially the first 48 hours but often resolves over a few days)

    D.   Symptoms typically last 7-14 days but may continue for 3 weeks (cough lasting longer than 3 weeks exceeds case definition for acute bronchitis)

    E.   Smokers have more frequent, longer, and more severe episodes than nonsmokers

    F.   Some patients with acute bronchitis have an underlying predisposition to bronchial reactivity which may turn into more chronic bronchial inflammation which characterizes asthma

    G.   Older children and adolescents with acute bronchitis due to pertussis typically have a chronic cough which is often paroxysmal and may or may not have the typical "whooping"; adults with unrecognized pertussis may transmit pathogen to nonimmune children (limit suspicion and treatment unless there are documented outbreaks)

IV. Diagnosis/Evaluation

    A.   History
        1.   Determine onset, duration and characteristics of cough, particularly ask about night coughing
        2.   Inquire about frequency and pattern of previous episodes of coughing
        3.   Ask about associated symptoms such as fever, pharyngitis, dyspnea, chest pain
        4.   Questions about the appearance of the sputum are not considered helpful as purulent sputum occurs when inflammatory cells are present and neither the character or production of sputum is predictive of a bacterial etiology
        5.   Inquire about infectious illnesses of other household members
        6.   Always ask if patient or household members smoke
        7.   Inquire about past medical history, particularly respiratory diseases
        8.   Determine immunization history of patient and household members

    B.   Physical Examination
        1.   Assess eyes, ears, nose, and throat for signs of inflammation
        2.   Palpate and transilluminate sinuses
        3.   Perform a heart examination

4. Perform a complete lung examination; inspect, palpate, percuss, and auscultate
5. Palpate for lymph nodes

C. Differential Diagnosis
1. Pneumonia and acute bronchitis are extremely difficult to differentiate. The following characteristics are more consistent with <u>pneumonia</u> than bronchitis in adults:
   a. Fever >100.4°F oral body temperature (>38°C)
   b. Increased respiratory rate (>24 breaths/minute)
   c. Increased heart rate (>100 beats/minute)
   d. Rigors and constitutional symptoms
   e. Pleuritic chest pain
   f. Rusty/bloody sputum
   g. Focal consolidation with rales, egophony, fremitus
   h. X-ray abnormalities
2. Upper respiratory infection and sinusitis
3. Tuberculosis
4. Asthma should be considered in patients who have repetitive episodes of acute bronchitis
5. Allergies
6. Cystic fibrosis
7. Nonpulmonary causes of cough such as congestive heart failure, reflux esophagitis, and bronchogenic tumors

D. Diagnostic Tests: acute bronchitis is a diagnosis of exclusion
1. Order a chest x-ray if the patient has severe symptoms to confirm or rule out the diagnosis of pneumonia
2. Consider PPD if patient is at risk for tuberculosis
3. Consider diagnostic pulmonary function testing or provocative testing with a methacholine challenge test when asthma is suspected; to diagnose asthma, abnormalities in tests must persist after the acute phase
4. If a diagnosis of pertussis is suspected, consult local public health officials concerning appropriate diagnostic tests (culture or polymerase chain reaction)
5. CBC and sputum cultures are not necessary unless diagnosis is uncertain

V. Plan/Management

A. Antibiotic treatment is NOT recommended in uncomplicated acute bronchitis, as most cases of acute bronchitis are viral; even patients who have a persistent cough (>10 days) usually do not need antibiotics; empiric antibiotic therapy should be avoided
1. Children with cystic fibrosis and underlying severe chronic lung disease and a persistent cough (>10 days) may benefit from antibiotic treatment; treatment must be tailored to each child
2. Consider prescribing erythromycin for 14 days for patients in frequent contact with nonimmunized infants due to risk of pertussis infection; however, careful surveillance of infant is probably more beneficial than treating contagious patient

B. Consider a trial of inhaled albuterol (Ventolin) 2 puffs every 6 hours for 7 days for patients with troublesome cough and evidence of bronchial hyperresponsiveness; the effect of anticholinergic bronchodilator treatment in acute bronchitis is unknown

C. Only symptomatic treatment is needed in most cases

D. Patient Education
1. Antihistamines should be avoided because they dry out secretions; expectorants have not been found to relieve symptoms
2. Cough suppressants should be avoided except if patient is unable to sleep due to irritating cough
3. Encourage smoking cessation
4. Website resources
   a. American Thoracic Society (http://www.thoracic.org)
   b. National Heart, Blood and Lung Information Center (http://www.nhlbi.nih.gov)

E. Follow Up
1. Return to clinic if symptoms persist longer than 7-14 days or if condition worsens; although previously patients with symptoms lasting over one week were treated with antibiotics for a bacterial etiology; today it is recognized that even viral infections may persist for 3 weeks
2. Patients who do not improve after 4 to 6 weeks need further evaluation (see section on COUGH)

COMMON COLD

I.   Definition: An acute, mild, and self-limiting syndrome caused by a viral infection of the upper respiratory tract mucosa

II.   Pathogenesis

    A.   Inflammation of all or part of the mucosal membranes from the nasal mucosa to the bronchi

    B.   Etiology is usually rhinoviruses, coronaviruses, or other viruses; respiratory syncytial virus (RSV) is common pathogen in older children

    C.   Incubation period averages 48 hours with a range of 12 hours to 5 days; maximum viral shedding occurs in first 2-4 days

    D.   Transmission occurs through direct contact with infectious secretions on skin and environmental surfaces and air-borne droplets

III.   Clinical Presentation

    A.   Children average 3-8 colds per year

    B.   Characterized by one or more of the following symptoms:
        1.   General malaise with low grade or no fever
        2.   Nasal discharge, obstruction or congestion
        3.   Sneezing, coughing, sore throat and hoarseness
        4.   Conjunctivae may be watery and inflamed

    C.   Usually self-limited (lasting approximately 5-7 days), but can predispose patient to bacterial infections such as otitis media, sinusitis, pneumonia and exacerbation of chronic conditions such as asthma

IV.   Diagnosis/Evaluation

    A.   History – Question about the following:
        1.   Respiratory distress (wheezing, dyspnea, stridor), inability to swallow, drooling and severe headaches which indicate the need for immediate evaluation
        2.   Fever, chills, anorexia, nausea, vomiting, and diarrhea
        3.   Duration, character, and timing (day and/or night) of cough
        4.   Facial, head, ear, throat, or chest pain
        5.   Number and seasonal pattern of previous colds within 1 year
        6.   Exposure to others with similar symptoms
        7.   Medication use
        8.   Past medical and family history; particularly history of allergies, asthma, or other respiratory problems
        9.   History of tobacco use and passive tobacco exposure

    B.   Physical Examination
        1.   Measure temperature, pulse and blood pressure
        2.   Examine conjunctivae, ears, nose and throat
        3.   Sinus percussion and transillumination
        4.   Palpate cervical lymph nodes for enlargement and tenderness
        5.   Perform a complete lung examination

    C.   Differential Diagnosis
        1.   Allergic rhinitis (nasal mucosa may be pale and boggy rather than erythematous and swollen as in common cold)
        2.   Foreign body (especially if nasal discharge is unilateral, purulent and malodorous)

3. Sinusitis
   a. Thick, opaque, and discolored nasal discharge are typical of the common cold and do not indicate a more severe, sinus infection
   b. Symptoms persisting or worsening for >10-14 days with facial swelling and tenderness and mucopurulent sputum are suggestive of sinusitis
4. Influenza (arthralgias are usually present)
5. Streptococcal pharyngitis
6. Otitis media
7. Pneumonia

D. Diagnostic Tests
1. Usually none are indicated
2. Throat culture or quick strep test if symptomatic or history of streptococcal exposure

V. Plan/Management

A. Decongestants cause vasoconstriction and reduce nasal secretions and congestion; topical decongestants are effective for short-term therapy and provide rapid decrease in airway resistance whereas oral decongestants are best when treatment is needed for more than 3-4 days
1. Topical decongestants should be used no longer than 3-4 days because of potential for rebound congestion; suggest one of the following:
   a. Children over 6 years of age and adolescents: Oxymetazoline hydrochloride 0.05% (Afrin 12-Hour Nasal Spray) 2-3 sprays each nostril BID or phenylephrine hydrochloride 1% (Neo-Synephrine Spray) 1 spray each nostril every 3-4 hours as needed
   b. Children 2-6 years: Oxymetazoline hydrochloride (Afrin 12-hour Children's Nasal Spray) 2-3 sprays each nostril every 12 hours
   c. Children <2 years should not use topical decongestant; instead, use nasal saline drops
2. Oral decongestants (not as effective); suggest one of the following:
   a. In adolescents, prescribe pseudoephedrine hydrochloride (Sudafed) 60 mg, 1 tablet every 4-6 hours or pseudoephedrine sulfate (Afrin 12-Hour Tablets) 120 mg, 1 tablet every 12 hours.
   b. In children 2-6 years, prescribe pseudoephedrine hydrochloride (Sudafed) 5 mL every 4-6 hours (available 15 mg/5 mL liquid); 6-12 years, 30 mg tablets or 10 mL liquid every 4-6 hours (maximum 4 doses per day)
   c. In infants less than 4 months of age, oral decongestants are not recommended. For older infants, can cautiously prescribe pseudoephedrine hydrochloride 7.5 mg/0.8 mL dropperful (Triaminic Infant Oral Decongestant): 12-17 lbs, 1 dropper; 18-23 lbs, 1½ droppers; 24-35 lbs, 2 droppers; every 4-6 hours; maximum 4 doses per day

B. Intranasal ipratropium bromide 0.06% (Atrovent) 2 sprays per nostril TID or QID reduces nasal discharge, severity of rhinorrhea and sneezing; not recommended as first-line agent for these symptoms but may prove useful in patients with disease-state contraindications to oral decongestants such as severe hypertension or angle-closure glaucoma (not recommended for children <12 years of age)

C. Equivocal research is available on the benefits of zinc acetate or zinc gluconate lozenges
1. Therapy should be initiated within 24 hours of symptom onset
2. Adverse effects of bad taste and nausea limit use of lozenges
3. Zinc is not safe in pregnancy
4. Dosages of zinc
   a. Zinc acetate lozenges (12.8 mg elemental zinc) 1 every 2 to 3 hours while awake
   b. Zinc gluconate lozenges (Hall's Zinc Defense) 1 every 2 hours for 4 days while awake

D. Although controversial, some researchers found a decrease in the duration and severity of cold symptoms with the use of Vitamin C 1 gram daily

E. Symptomatic treatment of cough (choose one of the following options)
1. Dexbrompheniramine 6 mg/pseudoephedrine sulfate 120 mg (Drixoral Cold & Allergy) one tab BID for 1 week (not recommended for children)
2. Naproxen (Naprosyn) 500 mg loading dose then 500 mg TID for 5 days (not recommended for treatment of cough in children)
3. Ipratropium (Atrovent) 0.06% nasal spray (42 µg per spray) 2 sprays per nostril TID for 4 days for adolescents and children ≥5 years

F. Acetaminophen or nonsteroidal anti-inflammatory agents (NSAIDs) such as ibuprofen are effective in relieving fever and headaches

G. Nonpharmacologic approaches to relieve symptoms
  1. Saline nose drops or sprays: 2-3 drops in each nostril BID to QID of commercial products (Ocean, Salinex) or homemade solution (1/4 tsp salt in 8 oz boiled water)
  2. Steamy showers or inhalation of steam
  3. Fluids or hydration help loosen secretions and prevent upper airway obstruction; warm fluids such as tea and chicken soup can increase the rate of mucus flow
  4. Salt-water gargle for sore throat
  5. Hard candy or throat lozenge for sore throat and cough

H. Treatments that are not recommended
  1. Antihistamines are ineffective because nasal congestion in colds is not mediated by histamine receptors; antihistamines may increase upper airway obstruction by impairing flow of mucus
  2. With exception of increased water intake, expectorants such as guaifenesin provide no benefit in cold management

I. Patient Education
  1. Review the etiology, course, and proper treatment of the common cold
    a. Explain that colds are caused by viruses which are not eradicated with antibiotics
    b. Reinforce that the indiscriminate use of antibiotics can cause adverse effects such as diarrhea, yeast infection, and drug resistance
  2. Emphasize that cold remedies are to relieve symptoms and prevent complications rather than cure infection
  3. Demonstrate use of nasal bulb syringe and saline drops to help clear nasal discharge in infants
  4. Advise rest and increased oral fluid intake
  5. Increase humidity of the air at home; place a cool-mist humidifier in the child's room
  6. Discuss ways to prevent the spread of colds
    a. All household members should frequently wash hands
    b. Since complications are more common in children during the first year of life, try to avoid undue exposure of infants to other people with colds and limit visits to areas with large crowds such as shopping malls

J. Follow Up: none indicated unless symptoms worsen after 3-5 days, new symptoms develop, or symptoms do not improve or resolve after 10-14 days

COUGH, PERSISTENT

I. Definition: Host defense mechanism to clear airway of secretions and inhaled particles which lasts at least 3 weeks or longer

II. Pathogenesis

A. In infancy, persistent cough is often abnormal and may be due to any of the following: congenital malformations (e.g., tracheoesophageal fistula or tracheobronchomalacia), cystic fibrosis, tuberculosis, infections (e.g., bronchiolitis, chlamydial pneumonia or HIV infection), gastroesophageal reflux, or congestive heart failure

B. In toddlers and preschool children, the most common causes are viral bronchitis, hyperactive airway disease such as asthma, foreign body aspiration, or laryngotracheobronchitis

C. In school age children, mycoplasma infection may be the etiology

D. In adolescents, the most common causes are postnasal drip or clearing of the throat due to rhinitis or tracheobronchitis, bacterial sinusitis, asthma, gastroesophageal reflux, chronic bronchitis due to cigarette smoking or environmental irritants

E. Other causes have no age predilection such as physical irritants, foreign body aspiration, tuberculosis, and psychogenic factors

F. Worrisome causes of coughing include mediastinal or pulmonary masses such as tumors or nodes

G. Greater than 90% of patients with chronic cough have postnasal drip syndrome, asthma, gastroesophageal reflux or a combination of these conditions

III. Clinical presentation of important causes of persistent cough

A. Cystic fibrosis
1. Genetic disorder usually occurring in Caucasian children
2. Cough is often productive, purulent, and paroxysmal
3. Associated symptoms include recurrent respiratory infections, poor weight gain, large and foul-smelling, steatorrheic bowel movements

B. Tuberculosis
1. Initially cough is minimally productive of yellow or green mucus which is worse upon arising in morning
2. As disease progresses, cough becomes more productive
3. Associated symptoms include fatigue, night sweats, dyspnea, and hemoptysis

C. Gastroesophageal reflux
1. May have history of heartburn, dysphagia, sour or bitter taste in mouth, and frequent use of antacids
2. Symptoms are often aggravated by meals and relieved by sitting up

D. Asthma
1. Often occurs at night or after exercise, laughing, or exposure to cold air
2. May be seasonal in occurrence and have a strong family history
3. Cough may be nonproductive or productive but not purulent
4. Associated symptoms include wheezing and intercostal retractions

E. Aspirated foreign body
1. Cough may persist for weeks or even months
2. Fixed, localized wheezing audible when chest is auscultated

F. Viral infections
1. Infrequently last beyond 2 weeks
2. Often occur during the winter
3. Cough is often nonproductive
4. Usually accompanying symptoms are mild and include rhinitis and nasal congestion

G. Bacterial infections such as pneumonia
1. Cough may be productive and purulent but this is not always the case
2. Associated symptoms may include fever and respiratory distress

H. Postnasal drip syndrome
1. Usually related to chronic sinusitis or allergic rhinitis
2. Patient often complains of clear nasal discharge, nasal congestion, tickle in throat, and frequent throat clearing

I. Chronic bronchitis
1. Often dry, hacking cough
2. Worse in the morning

J. Carcinoma of the lung
1. Cigarette smoking accounts for the majority of cases
2. Characteristic of the cough depends on location of the primary tumor

K. Cough related to psychogenic factors (rare)
1. Disappears during sleep; worsens when attention is drawn to it and during times of emotional stress
2. Lacks other associated physical symptoms

L.   Pertussis is a diagnosis of exclusion
1.   Characteristic but infrequently heard whoop with coughing and vomiting; fever is absent or minimal
2.   History of contact with known case
3.   Striking more teenagers and young adults; speculation is that pertussis vaccination given during infancy may lose its effectiveness as one ages
4.   Duration of symptoms is 6-10 weeks
5.   Complications include seizures, encephalopathy and death; infants have most severe disease

M.   Diseases associated with intentional release of biologic agents
1.   Inhalation anthrax caused by inhalation of infectious spores
a.   Incubation period of 1-6 days
b.   First phase is a nonspecific illness characterized by nonproductive cough, mild fever, malaise, myalgias, and mild chest or abdominal pain
c.   Within 2-3 days, the second phase abruptly begins and involves fever, acute dyspnea, diaphoresis, and cyanosis
(1)   Stridor may be present due to obstruction of trachea by enlarged lymph nodes, mediastinal widening, and subcutaneous edema of chest and neck
(2)   In about half of patients meningitis develops with obtundation and nuchal rigidity
(3)   Within 24-36 hours of the second stage, shock, associated hypothermia, and death occurs
2.   Pneumonic plague occurs when *Yersinia pestis* infects lungs
a.   Cough with mucopurulent sputum, hemoptysis, and chest pain are clinical features along with nonspecific symptoms such as fever, headache, and weakness
b.   Chest radiograph shows evidence of bronchopneumonia
c.   Pneumonia progresses for 2-4 days and without treatment, patients may have respiratory failure, shock, and eventual death
3.   Inhalational tularemia can occur alone from exposure via aerosol or can be spread hematogenously from other forms of tularemia
a.   Three to five days after exposure, patient has abrupt onset of nonspecific febrile illness such as dry cough, headaches, myalgias, and weakness
b.   In subsequent 7 days, pleuropneumonitis develops in many cases

IV.   Diagnosis/Evaluation

A.   History
1.   Determine duration of cough
2.   Determine characteristics of cough
a.   Productive (white, purulent, bloody) or nonproductive
(1)   Productive cough may suggest infection
(2)   Thick, tenacious sputum in children may indicate cystic fibrosis
b.   Quality (raspy, barking, harsh, wet)
(1)   Barking cough suggests croup
(2)   Paroxysms of cough occur in pertussis, cystic fibrosis, and foreign body aspiration
(3)   Loud, brassy cough is associated with cough tic (habit cough) or tracheomalacia
c.   Temporal occurrence (night, morning, or seasonal)
(1)   Nighttime cough suggests asthma, sinusitis with postnasal drip
(2)   Cough when awakening suggests postnasal drip or sinusitis
(3)   Cough associated with exercise may indicate asthma, cardiac disease (rare), and bronchiectasis
3.   Ask about associated symptoms such as fatigue, rhinitis, epistaxis, tickle in throat, pharyngitis, night sweats, dyspnea, fever, heartburn, hemoptysis, weight loss
a.   Hemoptysis signals concern for tuberculosis, cancer, or foreign body (see section on HEMOPTYSIS)
b.   Weight loss and fever suggest tuberculosis or HIV infection
4.   Ask if the cough occurs during or after feeding or eating (signals aspiration, vascular ring, gastroesophageal reflux, tracheoesophageal fistula, food allergy [especially if accompanied by rhinitis, hives, or wheezing])
5.   Ask if the cough is preceded by feeding or choking episodes
6.   Inquire about precipitating factors such as exercise, cold air, laughing
7.   Explore environmental and occupational exposure
8.   Inquire about infectious illness of other household members
9.   Always ask about smoking or the exposure to passive smoking

10. Ask about medications, particularly angiotensin-converting enzyme (ACE) inhibitors
11. Explore family history of cystic fibrosis, malabsorption, asthma, and allergies
12. Inquire about past medical history such as allergies, frequent infectious diseases, obstructive airway disease, cardiac disease

B. Physical Examination
   1. Observe patient for signs of respiratory distress such as cyanosis, shortness of breath on ambulating, intercostal retractions, accessory muscle use
   2. Observe general appearance, noting whether patient appears robust or fatigued and wasted
   3. Consider reproducing the cough in the office by having the child exercise or watching the infant feed
   4. In children always plot height and weight, noting any growth changes
   5. Listen for the quality of spontaneous coughing during the interview
   6. Assess eyes, ears, nose, and throat
      a. Conjunctivitis, rhinitis, and pharyngitis suggest infection
      b. Cobblestoning in oropharynx suggests allergies or chronic sinusitis but may not always be present in postnasal drip syndrome
   7. Check for tenderness of sinuses
   8. Palpate lymph nodes
   9. Observe for tracheal deviation which suggests mediastinal mass or foreign body aspiration
   10. Perform a complete lung exam including inspection, palpation, percussion, and auscultation
   11. Perform a complete cardiac exam as chronic cardiovascular problems may present with persistent cough

C. Differential Diagnosis: see pathogenesis section

D. Diagnostic Tests
   1. Order tuberculin skin test (PPD) and chest x-ray for unexplained persistent cough
   2. If diagnosis is unclear after PPD and chest x-ray, order spirometry to detect airway obstruction as in asthma
   3. In young children, consider ordering a sweat chloride test to rule out cystic fibrosis
   4. Consider a CBC with differential if infection, anemia, carcinoma are likely possibilities
   5. Cough that is productive should have Gram's stain of sputum as well as cultures
   6. If asthma is suspected, a methacholine challenge should be considered
   7. To determine pertussis, culture nasopharyngeal mucus (obtained by aspiration or with a Dacron or calcium alginate swab)
   8. To detect pathologic gastroesophageal reflux, 24-hour pH probe monitoring may be needed
   9. Oximetry may be helpful to quickly evaluate the patient's respiratory status and later may be used to assess response to treatment
   10. Other possible tests to order depend on characteristics of patient and include sinus x-rays, immunologic testing, allergy testing, or a barium swallow for detecting structural lesions
   11. More invasive tests such as bronchoscopy may be needed
   12. At first suspicion of patients exposed to intentional release of biologic agents, notify local or state health department, local hospital epidemiologist, and local or state laboratory; definitive tests can be arranged through a reference laboratory

V. Plan/Management

A. Treat all known causes: antibiotic therapy for bacterial infections, bronchodilators for asthma, and antihistamines for allergies

B. Treatment of pertussis
   1. Infants <6 months of age require hospitalization
   2. Drug of choice is erythromycin 40-50 mg/kg per day orally in 4 divided doses for 14 days

C. Treatment for diseases associated with intentional release of biologic agents: consult infectious disease specialist immediately and obtain information from national sources (see table WEBSITES: RESPONDING TO BIOTERRORISM); usual treatment is the following:
   1. Inhalation anthrax
      a. Persons >18 years: Ciprofloxacin 400 mg every 12 hours (begin with IV treatment and switch to oral therapy); alternatively use doxycycline 100 mg every 12 hours and one or two additional drugs such as rifampin, vancomycin, penicillin, ampicillin, chloramphenicol, imipenem, clindamycin, and clarithromycin

386

    b.   Children: Ciprofloxacin 10-15 mg/kg every 12 hours (begin with IV and switch to oral therapy); alternatively use doxycycline >8 years and >45 kg: 100 mg every 12 hours and one or two additional antimicrobials; <8 years and/or <45 kg: doxycycline 2.2 mg/kg every 12 hours and one or two antimicrobials (see adult treatment)

    2.   Pneumonic plague
        a.   Antibiotics must be given within 24 hours of first symptoms
        b.   Streptomycin, gentamicin, the tetracyclines, and chloramphenicol are effective agents

    3.   Inhalational tularemia: drugs of choice are doxycycline and ciprofloxacin

WEBSITES: RESPONDING TO BIOTERRORISM	
Agency	**Website**
Centers for Disease Control and Prevention	http://www.bt.cdc.gov
US Army Medical Research; Research Institute of Infectious Diseases	http://www.usamriid.army.mil/education/bluebook.html
Association for Infection Control Practitioners	http://www.apic.org
The Johns Hopkins Center for Civilian Biodefense	http://www.hopkins-biodefense.org

D.   Discuss need to stop cigarette smoking and avoid environmental irritants

E.   Air humidification and keeping the throat moist are simple suggestions that may be beneficial; adequate hydration with at least 1500 mL of fluid daily

F.   Cough suppressants such as dextromethorphan or codeine may be beneficial in improving sleep and rest (use only at bedtime)

G.   Expectorants and mucolytic agents are ineffective

H.   For parents who hear wheezing in their children at night, encourage a visit to the emergency department for documentation

I.   A stepwise approach may be beneficial by progressing from simple to more aggressive diagnostic tests and treatments in older children and adults with persistent, mild-to-moderate coughing of unknown etiology
    1.   Initial screen: Eliminate environment irritants (smoking, cough-producing medications, etc.)
    2.   Step 1: Treat empirically for postnasal drip with antihistamine-decongestant combination (post nasal drip syndrome is non-histamine mediated and second generation antihistamines do not appear to be effective); add nasal steroids or order CT of sinuses if symptoms persist
    3.   Step 2: Evaluate and treat possible asthma with inhaled cromolyn, steroids, and bronchodilators
    4.   Step 3: Order chest radiographs and CT of sinuses if asthma is not confirmed; treat specific, identified disease
    5.   Step 4:
        a.   Treat for GERD if no abnormalities found in Step 3: Antireflux measures and high-dose proton-pump inhibitor (may take 2 to 3 months of intensive therapy before cough starts to improve)
        b.   Order endoscopy or 24-hour esophageal pH monitoring
    6.   Step 5:
        a.   Perform bronchoscopic examination if no abnormalities are found and previous treatments are unsuccessful
        b.   Repeat course of antihistamine-decongestant combination
        c.   Consider less common diagnoses such as cancer, tuberculosis, congestive heart failure, sarcoidosis, bronchiectasis, etc.

J.   In undiagnosed patients with risk factors for cancer such as smoking or occupational exposure, consider referral to specialist

K.   Follow Up
    1.   Frequency of return visits will depend on patient's condition
    2.   Patients who have a complete work-up with no abnormalities should be seen at least every 1-3 months if their coughing persists

CROUP, ACUTE LARYNGOTRACHEOBRONCHITIS

I.   Definition

        A.   Clinical syndromes characterized by laryngeal obstruction caused by subglottic edema

        B.   Two most common croup syndromes are spasmodic croup and laryngotracheobronchitis
                1.   Differentiation of the two syndromes is difficult and is of questionable value because the
                        management of the syndromes is similar
                2.   Typically, patients with spasmodic croup improve quickly whereas patients with
                        laryngotracheobronchitis have a longer course; an allergy may be a predisposing factor in
                        spasmodic croup

II.   Pathogenesis

        A.   Pathogens
                1.   Parainfluenza is most common agent in all age groups
                2.   Younger children may be infected with *Respiratory syncytial virus*
                3.   Influenza virus and *Mycoplasma pneumoniae* are common pathogens in children >5 years

        B.   Symptoms are due to inflammation and narrowing of the subglottic region of the larynx

III.   Clinical Presentation

        A.   Epidemiology
                1.   Most common in children 3 months to 5 years with a peak at 2 years
                2.   Higher incidence in males than females
                3.   Occurs in fall and winter months

        B.   Symptoms are usually preceded by coryza, cough, nasal congestion, low-grade fever for 12-72 hours

        C.   Characterized by inspiratory stridor, a barking cough, and hoarseness which are usually worse at night;
                prolonged inspiration and coarse rales are often present

        D.   Respiratory rate is increased but not usually >50 breaths per minute (in contrast to bronchiolitis in which
                respirations may be between 80-90 breaths per minute)

        E.   Most children have mild symptoms and look ill but not toxic; those with cyanosis, hypoxemia, rales, and
                retractions may require hospitalization

        F.   Child can usually lie comfortably in a recumbent position and can handle oral secretions without difficulty

IV.   Diagnosis/Evaluation

        A.   History
                1.   Determine if child has any change in activity level, alertness, fluid intake, and voiding
                2.   Explore whether child has had episodes of apnea or difficulty with breathing
                3.   Question about duration and onset of any upper respiratory infection
                4.   Ask parents to describe the cough
                5.   Determine what helps or worsens the symptoms
                6.   Explore family medical history, particularly asking about allergies or asthma
                7.   Inquire about *Haemophilus influenzae* immunization status to eliminate a diagnosis of epiglottitis

        B.   Physical Examination
                1.   Measure respiratory rate and observe for signs of respiratory distress such as cyanosis, nasal
                        flaring, accessory muscle use, and retractions
                2.   Assess for hydration status such as capillary refill time, skin turgor, and moisture of mucous
                        membranes

3. Assess degree of alertness and fatigue
4. Observe for signs of drooling or difficulty swallowing
5. Assess ears, nose, throat, and sinuses (do not examine throat with tongue blade; do not place in supine position until epiglottitis can be ruled out as a diagnosis)
6. Perform complete heart and lung examinations

C. Differential Diagnosis
1. Epiglottitis, a pediatric emergency, is characterized by inspiratory and expiratory stridor, drooling, and a toxic appearance; child cannot lie recumbent comfortably
2. Bacterial tracheitis, a pediatric emergency, is characterized by respiratory stridor, high fever, and frequently copious purulent secretions; caused by infection secondary to streptococcus species, staphylococcus species, or *Haemophilus influenzae* type B pathogens
3. Congenital subglottic stenosis presents as prolonged or recurrent episodes of croup
4. Aspirated foreign body presents with unequal breath sounds
5. Laryngeal edema can occur from an allergic reaction
6. Diphtheria is characterized by gray, exudative, pharyngeal membrane and acute dysphagia
7. Retropharyngeal or peritonsillar abscess presents with severe sore throat, drooling, and unilateral tonsillar swelling

D. Diagnostic Tests
1. Usually diagnosis is made on clinical presentation without diagnostic tests
2. Pulse oximetry may be beneficial in determining degree of hypoxemia
3. In cases where the diagnosis is questionable, consider ordering a lateral inspiratory and expiratory chest x-ray and a posteroanterior x-ray of the neck which may reveal a steeple sign due to subglottic swelling if diagnosis of croup is correct
4. If brachial tracheitis is suspected, a sputum culture is helpful

V. Plan/Management

A. Consider hospitalization for children with severe symptoms such as dehydration, fatigue, increasing respiratory rate, retractions, nasal flaring, and use of accessory muscles

B. Outpatient management is acceptable for children with moderate symptoms who have reliable families and available transportation to the hospital if needed

C. Drug therapy for outpatients is controversial
1. No therapy is recommended for children with mild symptoms and there is no evidence supporting the effectiveness of mist therapy
2. Consider treatment with corticosteroids for child who demonstrates increased work of breathing (see V.C.3.b.) to prevent complications
3. For children with moderate symptoms, epinephrine plus corticosteroids or corticosteroids alone are recommended with close follow up and comprehensive health education (see V.F.)
   a. Nebulized racemic epinephrine is often recommended but recent studies have found nebulized L-epinephrine to be equally effective but less expensive
      (1) Administer nebulized racemic epinephrine (0.25-0.5 mL of 2.25% racemic epinephrine hydrochloride in 3-5 mL of normal saline) or nebulized L-epinephrine (5 mL of 1:1000 solution)
      (2) Action of epinephrine lasts approximately 2 hours and children may have rebound mucosal vasodilation and dyspnea; **observe patients in outpatient setting for 3 hours after administration**
      (3) Children requiring two epinephrine treatments need hospitalization
   b. Because of rebound phenomena, corticosteroids that are longer acting are often given alone, concurrently or after epinephrine; administer one of the following:
      (1) A single dose of dexamethasone (Decadron) given orally or in an intramuscular injection is recommended
         (a) Oral dexamethasone may be given 0.15, 0.3, or 0.6 mg/kg (0.6 mg/kg dose has been most widely studied)
         (b) IM dexamethasone is given 0.6 mg/kg; available 4 mg/mL
         (c) Avoid giving if child has been exposed to varicella in the preceding 3 weeks or if child has received varicella virus vaccine in preceding 2 weeks
         (d) Avoid giving if child has tuberculosis unless receiving appropriate anti-tuberculous therapy
         (e) Medication may increase child's appetite and aggressiveness

    (2) Nebulized budesonide 2 mg (4 mL) may be used in mild to moderate croup; in moderate to severe croup, dexamethasone offers greater improvement

 D. Antibiotics are usually not indicated because secondary bacterial infection is unusual

 E. Symptomatic treatment for outpatients
  1. Administer oxygen if oximetry results are less than 88% to 92%
  2. Cool-mist humidifier or breathing of cool, dry, night air
  3. Control of fever with acetaminophen 5-15 mg/kg/dose
  4. Encourage fluids (offer fluids every 5-10 minutes)

 F. Patient Education
  1. For the child with moderate symptoms, explain to parents that any disturbance may result in hyperventilation and respiratory distress so they should remain calm and hold and comfort their child
  2. Teach parents to count respirations, to assess child's levels of alertness and fatigue, monitor fluid intake and output, and degree of respiratory distress such as observing for retractions, use of accessory muscles and nasal flaring; explain that if symptoms intensify, they should go to emergency room or health care provider

 G. Follow Up
  1. For children with moderate croup who are discharged to home, contact parents by phone in 8-24 hours; frequent monitoring is needed thereafter
  2. Return visit is needed if there is no improvement in symptoms within 48 hours

EPIGLOTTITIS (SUPRAGLOTTITIS)

I. Definition: Inflammation of the soft tissues above the glottis

II. Pathogenesis

 A. Caused primarily by *Haemophilus influenzae* type B

 B. Involves rapid and pronounced inflammation of the epiglottis and surrounding areas which results in edema and subsequent mechanical obstruction to the flow of air

 C. The swollen epiglottis may be pulled down into the larynx during inspiration and create complete airway obstruction

 D. The inflammation may also result in increased secretions and exudate which can compound the airway obstruction

III. Clinical Presentation

 A. *Haemophilus influenzae* type B (HIB) vaccine can prevent invasive *H. Influenzae* infections such as epiglottitis and meningitis

 B. Previous to current vaccine era, primarily a disease in ages 2 to 4 years; anticipate change in age distribution as epiglottitis can occur in older unimmunized children and adults

 C. Classic symptoms are an abrupt onset of severe sore throat, fever, and toxicity in a previously active child

 D. Children do not have hoarseness and brassy cough as with croup; instead their voice sounds muffled

 E. Usual appearance is a child in sitting position, leaning forward with head extended, jaw thrust forward, mouth open, tongue protruding, and drooling

F.   As the condition progresses may have dysphagia, stridor, respiratory distress, anxiety and later exhaustion and limpness with diminished breath sounds

G.   Signs include cyanosis, chest retractions, and a "beefy red" pharynx with copious secretions

IV.   Diagnosis/Evaluation

    A.   History: Quickly question parents about onset and characteristics of symptoms and level of alertness

    B.   Physical Examination
        1.   Quickly assess vital signs and respiratory status such as respiratory rate, cyanosis, retractions, use of accessory muscles, nasal flaring
        2.   Quickly auscultate lungs; may have inspiratory stridor and expiratory rhonchi
        3.   If epiglottitis is suspected, do **NOT** attempt to examine pharynx with a tongue depressor because occlusion of airway may result

    C.   Differential Diagnosis
        1.   Croup
        2.   Bacterial tracheitis
        3.   Aspiration of foreign body
        4.   Diphtheria
        5.   Peritonsillar abscess
        6.   Angioneurotic edema

    D.   Diagnostic Tests
        1.   Tentative diagnosis must be made quickly on the basis of the history and clinical presentation
        2.   After admission to hospital the following are performed:
            a.   Laryngoscopy to visualize epiglottis; performed in operating room in case of airway obstruction and need for intubation
            b.   Lateral neck radiography is important when direct laryngoscopy is unavailable; "thumb sign" (swelling of epiglottis) and the vallecular sign (decrease in the vallecular air space) confirm the diagnosis
            c.   Computed tomography of the neck is recommended when diagnosis cannot be confirmed and when complications are suspected
            d.   Blood and surface cultures are obtained after intubation to confirm the presence of *H. influenzae*

V.   Plan/Management

    A.   Immediate transport to the hospital as this is a medical emergency; airway must be established by endotracheal tube or tracheostomy

    B.   Attempt to keep patient calm

    C.   Initial in-hospital treatment is cefotaxime sodium (Claforan), ceftizoxime sodium (Cefizox), or ceftriaxone sodium (Rocephin)

    D.   Chemoprophylaxis of child and household contacts is recommended with rifampin (Rifadin) when there is invasive *H. influenzae* type B infection and there is a child unimmunized, incompletely immunized, or immunocompromised
        1.   Infant 0-1 month: 10 mg/kg/day QD for 4 days
        2.   Child >1 month to adult: 20 mg/kg/day QD for 4 days (maximum of 600 mg/day QD for 4 days)

    E.   Follow up after discharge from the hospital will depend on the child's condition

HEMOPTYSIS

I.   Definition: Spitting or coughing of blood that originates from the thorax; involves expectoration of both blood-tinged and grossly bloody sputum

II.   Pathogenesis

    A.   Hemoptysis is an uncommon occurrence in children; see following table for possible causes

POSSIBLE CAUSES OF HEMOPTYSIS IN CHILDREN		
Clinical Condition	**Common/Uncommon**	**Cause**
No preexisting medical condition	Common	Pneumonia
	Common	Foreign-body aspiration
	Uncommon	Tuberculosis
	Uncommon	Autoimmune disorders
	Uncommon	Congenital malformations
	Rare	Heiner syndrome
	Rare	Primary pulmonary neoplasm
Preexisting medical condition	Common	Cystic fibrosis
	Common	Bronchiectasis
	Common	Congenital heart lesions
	Uncommon	Sickle cell anemia
	Uncommon	Aspergillosis
	Rare	Pulmonary embolism
	Rare	Idiopathic pulmonary hemosiderosis
	Rare	Primary pulmonary neoplasm

    B.   Hemoptysis may result from any of the following:
        1.   Inflammation of the tracheobronchial mucosa
        2.   Injury to the pulmonary vasculature
        3.   Elevations in pulmonary capillary pressure
        4.   Bleeding disorders and excessive anticoagulant therapy
        5.   Chest trauma
        6.   Intentional release of biologic agents (pneumonic plague)

III.   Clinical presentation of important causes of hemoptysis

    A.   Blood that is coughed is bright red, frothy, has an alkaline pH, and is mixed with sputum rather than hematemesis that is darker brown, has an acid pH, and may be mixed with food particles

    B.   Blood-streaked sputum is common, usually occurs with nonthreatening conditions, and often arises from the nasal mucosa and oropharynx rather than the lower respiratory tract

    C.   Pneumonia
        1.   Sputum appears red-brown or red-green and is mixed with pus
        2.   May have fever, pleuritic chest pain, and malaise

    D.   Foreign body aspiration
        1.   For many children the initial choking episode when the foreign body is aspirated is not observed or not remembered
        2.   There may be paroxysmal coughing after the initial event, but often the body adapts and the coughing subsides
        3.   Approximately 40% of children have classic triad of wheezing, coughing, and decreased breath sounds distal to the site of obstruction
        4.   Many foreign bodies are not radiopaque and will not be visualized on x-ray
        5.   A diagnostic clue is localized wheezing that does not respond to medical therapy

    E.   Tuberculosis is associated with systemic manifestations such as anorexia and weight loss

F. Children with autoimmune disorders such as systemic lupus erythematosus present with pulmonary hemorrhage and associated manifestations such as weight loss, joint pain, etc.

G. Infants who have a variety of congenital defects can develop hemoptysis and diffuse pulmonary hemorrhage; typically these conditions are diagnosed in the newborn period

H. Heiner syndrome
   1. Intake of milk causes multisystem damage; elimination of milk from diet results in dramatic improvement
   2. Symptoms include failure to thrive, vomiting, and upper respiratory tract congestion

I. Cystic fibrosis is the most common chronic disease associated with hemoptysis
   1. Approximately half of children with cystic fibrosis present with cough and wheezing
   2. Hemoptysis typically begins in second or third grade
   3. Hemoptysis may range from blood-tinged sputum to massive bleeding
   4. Bronchiectasis occurs in most patients and is progressive with age

J. Bronchiectasis
   1. Occasional foul-smelling, blood-tinged sputum Is characteristic
   2. Patient usually has chronic, productive cough which may be worse when lying down
   3. Dyspnea, fever, pleurisy may be present

K. Hemoptysis is a well-recognized complication of congenital heart disease; child has associated signs and symptoms of dyspnea, cyanosis, and clubbing

L. Aspergillosis is associated with cystic fibrosis or asthma; peripheral eosinophilia and fungi are seen on Gram's stain of sputum

M. Pulmonary infarction secondary to pulmonary emboli
   1. Characterized by a sudden onset of pleuritic pain in conjunction with hemoptysis
   2. Diaphoresis and syncope are often present
   3. Signs include tachypnea, tachycardia, rales, fever, shock, fourth heart sound, pleural rub, or cyanosis
   4. Frequently patient has a history of phlebitis, calf pain, immobilization of the legs, oral contraception use, or recent abortion

N. Idiopathic pulmonary hemosiderosis (IPH) occurs in children before age 7 and after 16 years of age; clinical manifestations include respiratory distress, bilateral alveolar infiltrates, and iron-deficiency anemia

O. Primary pulmonary neoplasms are rare in children; the most frequent clinical manifestations are fever, recurrent cough, and pneumonitis

IV. Diagnosis/Evaluation

A. History
   1. Inquire about onset and whether hemoptysis is a recurrent problem
   2. Explicitly determine that the bleeding is originating from the lungs rather than from vomiting blood or expectorating blood from nasopharyngeal bleeding
   3. Ask patient to describe the color, consistency, and characteristics of sputum
      a. Pink sputum is suggestive of pulmonary edema fluid
      b. Putrid sputum suggests a lung abscess
      c. Currant-jelly-like sputum may indicate necrotizing pneumonia
      d. Copious amounts of purulent sputum mixed with blood points toward bronchiectasis
   4. Ask patient to quantify amount of bleeding or if possible collect the sputum
   5. Inquire about associated symptoms such as recent weight loss, fatigue, persistent cough, dyspnea, wheezing, fever, night sweats, excessive bruising, hematuria
   6. Determine whether patient has had recent respiratory inflammation or infection
   7. Inquire about past medical history; particularly ask about previous lung, cardiac, hematological, and immunological problems
   8. Inquire about exposure to tuberculosis
   9. Ask about patterns of cigarette smoking
   10. Inquire about history of chest trauma

11. Ask about use of anticoagulant drugs
12. Explore environmental exposure to such things as asbestos
13. Ask about family history of hemoptysis, respiratory, cardiac, and hematological problems
14. Inquire about date of last chest x-ray and tuberculin skin test

B. Physical Examination
1. Assess vital signs, particularly noting fever and tachypnea
2. Observe skin for pallor, ecchymosis, telangiectasis, and nails for clubbing; clubbing is consistent with neoplasm, bronchiectasis, lung abscess and other severe respiratory problems
3. Examine nose, sinuses and pharynx for source of bleeding
4. Inspect neck for jugular venous distention which is suggestive of heart failure
5. Palpate for lymph nodes; lymphadenopathy is associated with TB, sarcoidosis, and malignancy
6. Perform a complete lung and cardiovascular exam
7. Check for ankle edema

C. Differential Diagnosis: hemoptysis is a symptom; see pathogenesis for possible causes
1. Most cases of blood-tinged sputum are upper-respiratory in nature and do not need extensive workup
2. Differentiate hemoptysis from epistaxis, hematemesis, and bleeding from nasopharyngeal sources
3. Determine whether hemoptysis is from a localized site or due to diffuse alveolar hemorrhage (presenting sign in collagen-vascular or immunological disorders)

D. Diagnostic Tests
1. Order chest x-ray; inspiratory and expiratory films may demonstrate local air trapping if foreign body aspiration is suspected
2. Computed tomography and magnetic resonance imaging may detect additional abnormalities unrecognized on chest x-ray
3. Administer tuberculin skin test (PPD) unless there has been a positive PPD in the past
4. Consider Gram's stain of sputum for suspected infections, an acid-fast stain for suspected tuberculosis, and cytologic examination of three sputum samples for malignant cells
5. Urinalysis and specific serological markers are helpful in determining whether child has an immunological disorder
6. Consider bronchoscopy in the following patients:
   a. Smokers
   b. Patients with persistent, recurrent hemoptysis
   c. Patients with massive bleeding
   d. Patients in whom the diagnoses are unclear
   e. Patients who do not respond to therapy
7. Consider ventilation-perfusion scanning or angiography when pulmonary embolization is suspected
8. PT, PTT, platelet count, and bleeding time are necessary when more than one site of bleeding is present

V. Plan/Management

A. Children's clinical conditions and abilities to clear airways rather than the amount of blood expectorated are more important in determining need for urgent care; greatest danger to the child is asphyxiation from aspirated blood

B. Consider consultation with a specialist for patients who are at increased risk for malignancy and patients in whom bronchoscopies are indicated

C. Foreign body aspiration
1. Emergency care for complete airway obstruction:
   a. For individuals >12 months deliver 6-10 abdominal thrusts (Heimlich maneuver) until foreign body is expelled; if unsuccessful deliver 4 sharp blows to back
   b. For infants <12 months, support in prone position with head lower than trunk and deliver 5 back blows; if unsuccessful, turn to supine position and give 4 chest thrusts
2. Refer to specialist patients who have partial obstructions or if foreign body aspiration is suspected as airway endoscopy is usually performed; removal of object is usually curative and corticosteroids and bronchodilators are not needed; antibiotics are prescribed if bacterial infection has occurred

B. Treat any underlying illness or infection

C. Patient Education
   1. Instruct patient to record episodes of hemoptysis and collect all blood that is expectorated
   2. Instruct patient to return to clinic or emergency room if bleeding increases, has clots, or if patient has respiratory distress, diaphoresis, chest pain, or tachypnea

D. Follow Up
   1. For mild blood-streaking of sputum with respiratory infection, all blood streaking should resolve in 2-3 days. If blood-streaking of sputum persists, patient needs a reevaluation
   2. Patients with hemoptysis which involves expectoration of blood, not just minimal amounts of blood-streaked sputum, should have follow up visit within 12-48 hours

PNEUMONIA

I. Definition: Acute respiratory infection of the lung parenchyma including the interstitial tissue and the alveolar spaces

II. Pathogenesis

   A. Mainly results from aspiration of pathogens into the lower respiratory tract from oropharyngeal contents

   B. Less commonly, pathogens spread to lungs hematogenously from distant foci such as bacterial endocarditis or from aerosolized particles

   C. Aspirated pathogens are usually cleared before infection develops unless there are alterations in the normal protective mechanisms such as depressed mucociliary transport by obstruction of bronchus by mucus or tumors, or preexisting clearance abnormalities such as bronchopulmonary dysplasia or cystic fibrosis

   D. Bacterial pneumonia is often aided by concurrent viral infection that may suppress the immune system and disrupt the respiratory tract mucosa

   E. In infants from birth to 20 days, Group B streptococci, gram-negative enteric bacteria, and cytomegalovirus are common pathogens

   F. In infants 3-11 weeks of age, suspect infection due to *Chlamydia trachomatis*; in addition, infants less than three months of age may have infection from respiratory syncytial viruses, genital mycoplasmas, although bacterial pneumonia such as *Bordetella pertussis* must also be considered

   G. In the older infant (3 months) to the young child (4-5 years), viruses are the most common cause with respiratory syncytial being the most common virus, peaking at 2-5 months of age; parainfluenza and influenza viruses also play important roles; one third of children in this group have bacterial infection usually due to *Streptococcus pneumoniae* or *Haemophilus influenzae* type B

   H. In children older than 5 years and adolescents, *Mycoplasma pneumoniae, Streptococcus pneumoniae, Chlamydia pneumoniae*, and viruses are most common causes

   I. Children with congenital or acquired immunodeficiency may have cytomegalovirus infection or *Pneumocystis carinii.*

III. Clinical Presentation

   A. Even though pneumonia accounts for only 10-15% of respiratory infections in children, it causes significant morbidity and mortality

   B. Chlamydial infection in the infant is characterized by a staccato cough, rales, wheezes, and possibly a history of conjunctivitis in the first 2 weeks of life

   C. Viral infections often begin gradually with rhinorrhea, low-grade fever, cough, wheezing followed by progressive increase in respiratory rate and intercostal retractions

D.   Bacterial pneumonia is characterized by acute onset of fever, productive cough, pleural pain, rales or diminished breath sounds, tachypnea and toxic appearance
    1.   Infants and young children may not have these classic findings and may present with lethargy, vomiting, diarrhea and poor feeding; often rales are not present when initially examined
    2.   Abdominal pain may be associated with acute lower respiratory tract infection

E.   In pneumonia due to *Mycoplasma pneumoniae*, cough and fever, but not coryza, are usually the first symptoms, followed by malaise, headache, rales, pharyngitis, and wheezing

F.   The older child and adolescent with pneumonia due to *Chlamydia pneumoniae* have symptoms and disease course similar to pneumonia due to *M. pneumoniae*

G.   Children with underlying pulmonary obstruction such as cystic fibrosis, cleft palate, and anatomic abnormalities are at increased risk for developing bacterial pneumonia and complications of pneumonia

H.   Empyema, lung abscess, and bacteremia are complications of bacterial pneumonia; death occurs almost exclusively in patients with underlying diseases

IV.   Diagnosis/Evaluation

A.   History
    1.   Determine whether onset was gradual involving mild upper respiratory symptoms or abrupt with rapid onset of fever and cough
    2.   Inquire about attentiveness and consolability
    3.   Question about fluid intake and number of wet diapers or voiding patterns
    4.   Inquire about associated symptoms such as conjunctivitis, rhinorrhea, fever, chills, myalgias, pharyngitis, nausea, and diarrhea
    5.   Ask patient or parents to describe cough and any sputum that is produced; infants rarely produce sputum
    6.   Inquire about recent infectious illnesses in the patient's household
    7.   Ascertain that child has not missed any immunizations which may indicate susceptibility to measles, pertussis or *Haemophilus influenzae* type B infection
    8.   Question about choking which may indicate foreign body aspiration
    9.   Ask about birth history in infants and whether mother had a history of sexually transmitted diseases during pregnancy
    10.   Inquire about past medical history such as acquired immunodeficiency, asthma, tuberculosis, cystic fibrosis
    11.   Ask about prior episodes of chest symptoms because recurrence may suggest reactive airway disease

B.   Physical Examination
    1.   Observe general appearance as well as attentiveness to the environment, ability to drink, ability to sustain sucking, vocalization, color, and consolability
    2.   Assess vital signs, paying particular attention to respiratory rate and hydration status (see table on normal respiratory rates in section FEVER WITHOUT LOCALIZING SOURCE)
    3.   Observe for respiratory distress such as cyanosis, tachypnea, intercostal retractions, accessory muscle use, nasal flaring, and grunting
    4.   Auscultate lungs; typical findings are the following:
        a.   Localized diminished breath sounds
        b.   Rales and tubular breath sounds
        c.   Egophony (changes child's "ee" to what sounds like "ay")
        d.   Bronchophony (voice sounds are louder and clearer than usual)
        e.   Whispered pectoriloquy (whispered sounds are louder and clearer than normal)
    5.   Palpate chest for tactile fremitus (palpate for increased areas of vibration as child cries or says "ninety-nine")
    6.   Percuss chest for dullness which is typical over consolidated lung tissue
    7.   Perform a cardiac examination

C. Differential Diagnosis: The best individual sign for ruling out pneumonia is absence of tachypnea; chest indrawing and other findings of increased work of breathing increases the likelihood of pneumonia
   1. Upper respiratory infections (URI); pneumonia can usually be distinguished from URIs by presence of lower respiratory tract signs (tachypnea, cyanosis, rales, hypoxemia) and area of infiltration on chest x-ray
   2. Differentiating viral and atypical pneumonias from bacterial pneumonia is difficult; typically, patients with viral and atypical pneumonias have fever less than 40°C., gradual onset of symptoms, and nonproductive cough; WBCs are normal or slightly elevated and chest x-ray may reveal an interstitial infiltrate in a diffuse or perihilar distribution
   3. Bronchiolitis
   4. Asthma
   5. Croup
   6. Bronchitis
   7. Diseases associated with intentional release of biologic agents: Inhalational anthrax, pneumonic plague, and inhalational tularemia
   8. Tuberculosis
   9. Noninfectious diseases: gastroesophageal reflux, aspiration, tracheoesophageal fistula with aspiration

D. Diagnostic Tests
   1. Order PA and lateral chest x-ray; although not always present, in bacterial pneumonia, x-ray often reveals hyperaeration with alveolar infiltrate in a patchy or consolidated lobar or subsegmental distribution
   2. Order CBC; elevated WBCs with left shift in bacterial pneumonia
   3. Consider ordering serum cold agglutinins for diagnosing *M. pneumoniae*
   4. Gram stain of sputum is helpful but difficult to obtain in young children
   5. Enzyme-linked immunosorbent assay (ELISA), latex agglutination, or counterimmunoelectrophoresis are being used more frequently to detect antigens
   6. Blood and sputum cultures should be ordered for patients with severe symptoms
   7. Urine cultures should be obtained on all seriously ill children with fever
   8. Administer purified protein derivative (PPD) if tuberculosis is suspected

V. Plan/Management

A. Consider hospitalization for infants <6 months old or if child appears toxic, has underlying deficiencies in host defenses, has concomitant chronic cardiac or pulmonary disease, is in respiratory distress, or is dehydrated

B. Refer to specialist, patients who fail to recover from first episode of pneumonia or who have recurrent disease; patients should begin to respond to antibiotics within 48-72 hours

C. Treatment for viral pneumonia is usually symptomatic
   1. Hospitalized child may be prescribed ribavirin therapy
   2. If the likely diagnosis is influenza A or B pneumonia consider one of the following:
      a. Zanamivir (Relenza) 5 mg/blister; prescribe 2 oral inhalations twice daily (at least 2 hours apart) on first day; then 2 inhalations every 12 hours for the next 4 days (5 days total); not indicated for <7 years of age
      b. Oseltamivir (Tamiflu) available in 75 mg capsules and 12 mg/mL liquid; begin within 2 days of symptom onset and treat for 5 days; In children ages 1-13 years use suspension; children ≤15 kg: 30 mg twice daily; children 15-23 kg: 45 mg twice daily; children 23-40 kg: 60 mg twice daily; children >40 kg: 75 mg twice daily
      c. Amantadine (Symmetrel) 50 mg/5 ml syrup: children aged 1-9 years give 4.4-8.8 mg/kg/day in two or three divided doses for maximum of 150 mg/day; children aged 9-12 years 100 mg caps BID; continue dose for 24-48 hours after all symptoms have subsided

D. Empiric drug therapy for pneumonia not caused by viruses is based on age of child, clinical presentation, and x-ray findings (modifications in antibiotics should be made when susceptibility profile is known)
   1. Neonates are usually treated in a hospital with ampicillin plus an aminoglycoside
   2. In infants 3 weeks to 3 months prescribe one of the following for a 10 day course:
      a. Erythromycin ethylsuccinate (EES) available in 200 mg/5 mL, 400 mg/5 mL liquid; 40 mg/kg/day in divided doses every 6 hours

     b.   Clarithromycin (Biaxin) available in 125 mg/5 mL, 250 mg/5 mL liquid; prescribe 15 mg/kg/day in divided doses every 12 hours (not recommended <6 months old)

     c.   Azithromycin (Zithromax) available in 100 mg/5 mL, 200 mg/5 mL liquid; prescribe 10 mg/kg once daily for 1 day; then 5 mg/kg once daily for 4 days (not recommended if <6 months old); Suspension must be taken 1 hour before or 2 hours after meals

     d.   Admit patient if fever or hypoxia is present

3.   For children 4 months to 4 years or children with suspected bacterial infection from *Streptococcus pneumoniae* and *Haemophilus influenzae* type B prescribe one of the following for a 10 day course:

     a.   Amoxicillin (Amoxil), available in 125 mg/5 mL, 200 mg/5 mL, 250 mg/5 mL, 400 mg/5mL liquid or 125 mg, 200 mg, 250 mg, 400 mg chewable tablets; 45 mg/kg/day in divided doses every 12 hours or 40 mg/kg/day in divided doses every 8 hours

     b.   If suspect infection due to ß-lactamase producing organism or if child has severe infection, prescribe amoxicillin/clavulanic acid (Augmentin), available in 125 mg/5 mL, 200 mg/5 mL, 250 mg/5mL, 400 mg/5 mL liquid or 125 mg, 200 mg, 250 mg, 400 mg chewable tablets: base dose on amoxicillin component 45 mg/kg/day in divided doses every 12 hours or 40 mg/kg/day in divided dosages every 8 hours. To avoid side effect of diarrhea suggest that child eat cultured yogurt

4.   For children 5 to 15 years or children who have suspected mycoplasma pneumonia or chlamydial pneumonia prescribe one of the following:

     a.   Erythromycin ethylsuccinate (EES) available in 200 mg/5 mL, 400 mg/5 mL liquid; 40 mg/kg/day in divided doses every 6 hours for 10 days. Also available as (EryPed) 200 mg chewable tablets for older children. For adolescents, prescribe erythromycin (E-Mycin) 250 mg TID or QID

     b.   Clarithromycin (Biaxin) available in 125 mg/5 mL, 250 mg/5 mL liquid or 250 mg and 500 mg tablets: 15 mg/kg/day in divided doses every 12 hours for 7-14 days (maximum 500 mg twice daily)

     c.   Azithromycin (Zithromax) available in 100 mg/5 mL, 200 mg/5 mL liquid or 250 mg scored tablets:

         (1)   Adolescent ≥16 years: 500 mg daily for 1 day, then 250 mg daily for 4 days

         (2)   Children 6 months to <16 years: 10 mg/kg once daily for 1 day; then 5 mg/kg once daily for 4 days (oral suspension but not tablets must be taken one hour before or two hours after meals)

     d.   In children >8 years, consider oral doxycycline (4 mg/kg/day) in 2 divided doses

E.   Prevention

1.   Routine immunizations for pertussis, measles, and *Haemophilus influenzae* type B have reduced the incidence of pediatric pneumonia

2.   Consider vaccines for influenza and streptococcus pneumonia in children with enhanced susceptibility

3.   Administer palivizumab or Respiratory Syncytial Immune Globulin for infants with chronic lung diseases (see section on BRONCHIOLITIS for dosing and discussion)

F.   Patient Education

1.   Teach parents to watch for signs of respiratory distress such as changes in level of activity and signs of dehydration

2.   Increase child's fluid intake

3.   Avoid giving child cough medications, particularly cough suppressants

G.   Follow Up

1.   Evaluate patient within 48-72 hours or sooner if condition is not improving

2.   Consider hospitalization if child fails to respond to therapy in 48-72 hours

3.   After initial follow up, schedule return visit for 2 weeks

4.   Repeat chest-rays are needed for children with recurrent pneumonia; after acute pneumonia x-rays can remain abnormal for 4-6 weeks

TUBERCULOSIS

I.   Definition: Necrotizing bacterial infection most commonly infecting the lungs; other important definitions include the following:

   A.   Positive tuberculin skin test: applies to a person who has likely infection with *Mycobacterium tuberculosis*, an acid-fast bacillus

   B.   Exposure: applies to a person who has recent contact with an individual with suspected or confirmed, contagious pulmonary tuberculosis (TB) and whose tuberculin skin test is non-reactive, physical examination is normal, and chest x-ray is normal; some exposed persons have infection (and eventually develop a positive tuberculin skin test) whereas some do not

   C.   Latent TB infection: applies to a person who has a positive tuberculin skin test, absent physical findings of disease, and a chest x-ray which is either normal or has only granulomas or calcifications in lung and/or regional lymph nodes

   D.   TB disease: applies to a person with infection who has signs, symptoms, and x-ray manifestations that appear to be caused by *M. tuberculosis*; disease may be pulmonary or extrapulmonary

II.   Pathogenesis

   A.   Primary or initial infection occurs by inhalation of the etiologic agent, *Mycobacterium tuberculosis*; it is dispersed as droplet nuclei (small airborne particles) from persons who have infectious pulmonary or laryngeal TB when they cough, sneeze, speak, or sing

   B.   The duration of infectivity is variable, but the majority of adolescent patients are noncontagious within a few weeks of starting appropriate therapy; children <12 years are usually not contagious because their lesions are small and cough is minimal

   C.   Incubation period from infection to development of a positive reaction to tuberculin skin test is 2-10 weeks

   D.   Close contacts of persons who have infectious TB are at the highest risk of becoming infected; infection rates range from 21%-23% for the contacts of infectious TB patients

   E.   Approximately 90% of primary TB infections remain in a latent or dormant infection stage:
   1.   Persons in this stage are not infectious
   2.   Persons with latent TB infection may develop active clinical disease after periods of stress or at times when the body is undergoing change or fighting an infection

   F.   The most common site for clinical TB (73% of cases) is the lungs; however, TB is a systemic disease which can result in disseminated TB (miliary TB) or infections in the bones and joints as well as in the lymphatic, genitourinary, and central nervous systems

   G.   Current classification system (see table CLASSIFICATION SYSTEM) is based on pathogenesis

CLASSIFICATION SYSTEM FOR TB*		
Class	**Type**	**Description**
0	No TB exposure Not infected	No history of exposure Negative reaction to tuberculin skin test
1	TB exposure No evidence of infection	History of exposure Negative reaction to tuberculin skin test
2	TB infection No disease	Positive reaction to tuberculin skin test Negative bacteriologic studies (if done) No clinical, bacteriological, or radiographic evidence of TB
3	TB, clinically active	*M. tuberculosis* cultured (if done) Clinical, bacteriological, or radiographic evidence of current disease
4	TB Not clinically active	History of episode(s) of TB **or** Abnormal but stable radiographic findings Positive reaction to the tuberculin skin test Negative bacteriologic studies (if done) **and** No clinical or radiographic evidence of current disease
5	TB suspected	Diagnosis pending

*All persons with class 3 or class 5 TB should be reported promptly to state and local health departments

Source: US Department of Health and Human Services, Centers for Disease Control and Prevention. (2000). *Core curriculum on tuberculosis* (4th ed.). Atlanta, GA.

III.   Clinical Presentation

A.   Of the estimated 10-15 million persons in the U.S. who are infected with *M. tuberculosis*, about 10% of those with normal immune systems will develop TB disease if there is no intervention

B.   Although the number of TB cases has declined since 1993, the incidence of drug-resistant tuberculosis is increasing

C.   Outbreaks of multidrug-resistant TB (MDR-TB) -- resistant to both isoniazid (INH) and rifampin (RIF) -- are a serious concern; these outbreaks have been associated with a high prevalence of HIV infection among the outbreak cases, a high mortality rate, and a high transmission rate of MDR-TB to heath-care and correctional facility workers
1.   Transmission of drug-resistant TB is the same as drug-susceptible TB
2.   Two types of drug resistance
a.   Primary resistance occurs in persons who are initially infected with resistant organisms
b.   Secondary resistance or acquired resistance occurs during TB therapy because the regimen was inadequate or the regimen was not taken appropriately

D.   Presenting symptoms of TB in adolescents and young adults are often vague
1.   Productive, prolonged cough over 3 weeks' duration
2.   Chest pain
3.   Hemoptysis
4.   Increased fatigue, malaise, anorexia, weight decrease
5.   Periodic fever, night sweats

E.   Children are usually asymptomatic with normal chest x-rays; the infection is usually self-limited but clinical manifestations can occur 1-6 months after the initial infection
1.   Fever, weight loss, cough, night sweats, chills
2.   Lymphadenopathy of hilar, mediastinal, cervical, or other lymph nodes
3.   Atelectasis or pleural effusion
4.   Extrapulmonary disease occurs in approximately 25% of children <15 years who are not treated in early stages of disease
5.   Infants are more likely than others to develop disseminated TB if the infection is not treated aggressively and early in the course of the disease

F.   Symptoms of extrapulmonary TB depend on the site affected; hematuria may occur in TB of the kidney, and back pain may occur in TB of the spine

G.   Certain persons are at higher risk for exposure to or infection with *M. tuberculosis*
    1.   Close contacts of person known or suspected to have TB
    2.   Foreign-born persons from areas where TB is common
    3.   Residents and employees of high-risk congregate settings
    4.   Health care workers who serve high-risk patients
    5.   Medically underserved, low-income populations
    6.   High-risk racial or ethnic minority populations
    7.   Children exposed to adults in high-risk categories
    8.   Persons who inject illicit drugs

H.   Certain persons are at higher risk of developing TB disease once infected (see table INDIVIDUALS AT RISK FOR TB DISEASE)

INDIVIDUALS AT RISK FOR DEVELOPING TB DISEASE ONCE INFECTED

- HIV infection

- Anyone with associated diabetes, silicosis, prolonged corticosteroid therapy, other immunosuppressive therapy, cancer of the head and neck, hematologic and reticuloendothelial disease, end-stage renal disease, intestinal bypass or gastrectomy, chronic malabsorption syndromes, low body weight (10% or more below the ideal)

- Recent infection with *M. tuberculosis* (within the past 2 years), chest radiograph findings suggestive of previous TB (in a person who received inadequate or no treatment)

- Substance abuse (especially drug injection)

Source: U.S. Department of Health & Human Services, Centers for Disease Control and Prevention. (2000). *Core curriculum on tuberculosis* (4th ed.). Atlanta, GA.

IV.   Diagnosis/Evaluation

    A.   History
        1.   Inquire about onset and duration of weight loss, fatigue, fever, night sweats, anorexia, cough, hemoptysis, chest pain, as well as localized symptoms in other body organs such as hematuria, enlarged lymph nodes
        2.   Consider risk factors (country of origin, age, occupation, ethnic or racial group, HIV, substance use)
        3.   Ask about history of TB exposure, infection, or disease
        4.   Ask about results and dates of TB skin tests and chest x-rays
        5.   Determine whether patient has had previous TB treatment; may need to contact the local health department to confirm
        6.   Assess medical conditions that increase risk for TB disease (see III.H., table INDIVIDUALS AT RISK FOR TB DISEASE)
        7.   Inquire about travel to developing countries where TB is common

    B.   Physical Examination
        1.   Observe for skin pallor
        2.   Palpate for lymphadenopathy
        3.   Inspect, palpate, percuss, and auscultate chest (rales in upper posterior chest, bronchovesicular breathing, and whispered pectoriloquy are often positive findings in patients with TB)
        4.   Complete physical exam is needed if disseminated TB is suspected

    C.   Differential Diagnosis
        1.   Malignancy
        2.   Silicosis
        3.   Chronic obstructive pulmonary disease
        4.   Asthma
        5.   Bronchiectasis
        6.   Pneumonia

D.   Diagnostic Tests
    1.   Screening is recommended routinely for children and adolescents (see following table)

REVISED TUBERCULIN SKIN TEST RECOMMENDATIONS FOR CHILDREN AND ADOLESCENTS*

Immediate Skin Testing
- Contacts of persons with confirmed or suspected infectious tuberculosis in the last 5 years
- Children with radiographic or clinical findings suggesting tuberculosis
- Children immigrating from countries where TB is endemic
- Children with travel histories to endemic countries and significant contact with indigenous persons from such countries

Annual Skin Testing**
- Children infected with HIV
- Incarcerated adolescents

Skin Testing Every 2-3 Years**
- Children exposed to the following individuals: HIV-infected, homeless, residents of nursing homes, institutionalized adolescents or adults, users of illicit drugs, incarcerated adolescents or adults, and migrant farm workers; this would include foster children with exposure to adults in the above high-risk groups

Consider for Tuberculin Skin Testing at Ages 4-6 and 11-16 Years
- Children whose parents immigrated from endemic areas; continued potential exposure by travel to the endemic areas and household contact with persons from the endemic areas
- Children without specific risk factors who reside in high-prevalence areas

Risk for Progression to Disease
- Children with other medical risk factors, including diabetes mellitus, chronic renal failure, malnutrition, and congenital or acquired immunodeficiencies deserve special consideration; initial histories of potential exposure to tuberculosis should be included in all these patients; if these histories or local epidemiologic factors suggest a possibility of exposure, immediate and periodic tuberculin skin testing should be considered in these patients

---

*BCG immunization is not contraindication to tuberculin skin testing.
**Initial tuberculin skin testing initiated at the time of diagnosis or circumstance.
Adapted from American Academy of Pediatrics. (1996). Committee on Infectious Diseases: Update on tuberculosis skin testing of children. *Pediatrics, 97,* 282.

    2.   Testing is performed to identify infected individuals at higher risk for TB exposure or infection and to identify individuals at higher risk for TB disease once infected; regular tuberculin testing of high risk groups is recommended (no need to repeat PPD on person with a known positive tuberculin skin test)
        a.   Preferred method of testing is the Mantoux tuberculin skin test 5 TU-PPD
            (1)   The skin test is the only way to diagnose TB infection before the infection has progressed to TB disease; generally, takes 2 to 10 weeks after infection for person to react positively to skin test (persons who recently had contact with someone with TB and have a negative tuberculin skin test should be re-tested 10-12 weeks after last exposed to infectious TB)
            (2)   Administer intradermal injection of 0.1 mL of purified protein derivative (PPD) tuberculin containing 5 tuberculin units (TU) into inner surface of forearm; should produce a discrete pale wheal 6-10 mm in diameter
                (a)   Monitor for reactions 48-72 hours after application
                (b)   Measure only the area of induration and record in millimeters
            (3)   Interpretation of PPD (see table POSITIVE PPD)

POSITIVE PPDs

- ≥5 mm if patient is one of the following: known HIV+, recent contacts of infectious TB case, chest x-ray with fibrotic changes or findings suggestive of previous TB, organ transplant and other immunosuppressed patients (receiving the equivalent of >15 mg/day of prednisone for >1month)

- ≥10 mm if patient is one of the following: recent arrival (<5 years) from high-prevalence country, injection drug users, residents and employees of high-risk congregate settings, mycobacteriology laboratory personnel, person with medical risk factors, children <4 years of age, or children and adolescents exposed to adults in high-risk categories

- ≥15 mm: all persons with no known risk factor for TB

Source: U.S. Department of Health and Human Services, Centers for Disease Control and Prevention. (2000). *Core curriculum on tuberculosis* (4th ed.). Atlanta, GA.

(4) Anergy testing

    (a) Does **not** rule out diagnosis of TB based on a negative skin test; persons may have a condition known as anergy in which the tuberculin reactions are decreased or disappear

    (b) Although routine anergy testing is no longer routinely recommended, consider anergy on an individual basis in persons with negative skin tests who have the following: HIV infection, severe or febrile illness, immunosuppressive therapy, live-virus vaccinations, viral infections or overwhelming TB infection

    (c) Determine anergy by administering two delayed-type hypersensitivity antigens such as mumps or *Candida* by the Mantoux technique; persons with a reaction ≥3 mm are not anergic

    (d) If anergy is present, probability of infection should be evaluated and persons judged at high risk of exposure should be considered for preventive therapy

(5) Two-step testing is used to differentiate boosted reactions from reactions due to new infection; should be performed in individuals who will be retested periodically, such as health care workers

    (a) Some individuals with TB infection may have a negative skin test when tested several years after an infection; however, the skin test may stimulate their ability to react to tuberculin and cause positive reactions to subsequent tests (boost) which may be misinterpreted as new infections

    (b) To distinguish a boosted reaction from a new infection when the first test is negative, administer a second skin test 1-3 weeks after first test

        (i) If second test is negative: person is uninfected and any subsequent positive test should be classified as a new infection

        (ii) If second test is positive: person is infected and should be treated accordingly

b. Chest radiograph or sputum smears may be the recommended first screening test in populations where risk of transmission is high and difficulties in administering and reading tests exist, such as jails or homeless shelters

3. Diagnosis of active disease

    a. Order three sputum specimens for **both** smear examination and culture in patients suspected of pulmonary or laryngeal TB

    (1) A presumptive diagnosis of TB can be made with detection of acid-fast bacilli (AFB); results can usually be obtained in 24 hours

    (2) A positive sputum culture for *M. tuberculosis* is essential to confirm diagnosis but often takes several weeks for results to be obtained

    (3) Drug susceptibility testing should be done on the initial *M. tuberculosis* isolate; testing should also be performed on additional isolates from patients whose cultures fail to convert to negative within 2 months of beginning therapy or if there is clinical evidence of failure to respond to therapy

    (4) Aerosol induction to stimulate sputum production, bronchoscopy, or gastric aspiration should be done if the patient cannot produce a sputum specimen and there is suspicion of TB

    b. A tuberculin skin test is helpful in making diagnosis and should be applied, but absence of a reaction to the test does not exclude diagnosis; see anergy testing IV.D.1.a.(4)

    c. Order posterior-anterior chest x-ray

    (1) Abnormalities are suggestive but are not diagnostic of TB; x-rays may rule out possibility of pulmonary TB in an asymptomatic person with a positive skin test

    (2) In pulmonary TB, abnormalities are often present in apical or posterior segments of upper lobes or superior segments of lower lobes; in HIV infected persons, other abnormalities are often present

4. Baseline laboratory testing is ordered after TB is diagnosed (also see V.C. for specific baseline laboratory tests that should be ordered when patients are prescribed specific medications)

    a. For latent TB infection, baseline testing is not routinely recommended for all patients at the start of treatment; obtain baseline hepatic measurements for the person whose initial evaluation suggests liver disease, patients with HIV infection, women who are pregnant or within 3 months postpartum, and persons with a history of chronic liver disease

b. For TB disease, baseline testing includes measurements of hepatic enzymes, bilirubin, serum creatinine, blood urea nitrogen (BUN), CBC, and platelet count; measure serum uric acid if pyrazinamide is used; test visual acuity if ethambutol is used; test hearing function if streptomycin is used

V. Plan/Management

A. Latent TB infection (LTBI) therapy reduces the risk that TB infection will progress to actual disease; children usually have latent TB, rather than active disease

   1. LTBI therapy is indicated for persons who would benefit from treatment (see table CANDIDATES FOR TREATMENT OF LTBI)

CANDIDATES FOR TREATMENT OF LTBI

❧ Positive skin test result ≥5 mm:
- ✓ HIV-positive persons
- ✓ Recent contacts of a TB case
- ✓ Persons with fibrotic changes on chest radiograph consistent with old TB
- ✓ Patients with organ transplants and other immunosuppressed patients

❧ Positive skin test result ≥10 mm:
- ✓ Recent arrivals (<5 years) from high-prevalence countries
- ✓ Injection drug users
- ✓ Residents and employees of high-risk congregate settings
- ✓ Mycobacteriology laboratory personnel
- ✓ Persons with high-risk clinical conditions
- ✓ Children younger than 4 years of age, or children and adolescents exposed to adults in high-risk categories

❧ Positive skin test result ≥15 mm:
- ✓ Persons with no known risk factors for TB may be considered

❧ Other candidates:
- ✓ Persons who are close contacts with infectious cases and have a negative TB skin test reaction (<5 mm) should be considered for LTBI treatment (after TB disease has been ruled out); children <4 years, immunosuppressed persons, and others who may develop TB disease quickly after infection; close contacts with negative initial reaction should be retested 10-12 weeks after last exposure to TB

- ✓ Infants exposed to person with TB should be given a skin test and chest x-ray and started on preventive therapy even if tests are negative because infants <6 months may be anergic; retest again in 10-12 weeks after last exposure to TB (LTBI treatment may be discontinued if **all** the conditions are met: infant is at least 6 months of age, second TB test is also negative, second test was performed at least 10 weeks after the child was last exposed to infectious TB)

❧ Consult specialist for pregnant women

Source: U.S. Department of Health and Human Services, Centers for Disease Control and Prevention. (2000). *Core curriculum on tuberculosis* (4th ed.). Atlanta, GA.

   2. Before initiating treatment for LTBI:
      a. Exclude possibility of TB disease as this would require multiple drug therapy
      b. Question history of previous treatment for LTBI or disease
      c. Explore characteristics of person (preventive therapy might **not** be indicated in the following persons: persons at high risk for adverse reactions to isoniazid (INH) such as those with acute or active liver disease, persons who cannot tolerate INH, persons likely to be infected with drug-resistant *M. tuberculosis*, persons who are highly unlikely to complete course of preventive therapy)
      d. Recommend HIV testing if there are risk factors
   3. There are several drug treatment regimens available for the treatment of LTBI (see table REGIMEN OPTIONS FOR LTBI)
      a. Dispense only a 1-month supply of drug at a time (2 weeks only if taking rifampin and pyrazinamide)
      b. Monthly question for the following: compliance, symptoms of neurotoxicity (paresthesias of hands and feet), signs of hepatitis, signs and symptoms of active TB disease (if taking rifampin and pyrazinamide must be reassessed every 2 weeks)
      c. In patients prone to developing neuropathy, pregnant women, and persons with seizure disorders prescribe pyridoxine (vitamin B_6) 10-50 mg/day

d.   New, short-course preventive treatment regimens are currently being investigated; however 9-month Isoniazid is considered optimal and the only option for children <15 years

REGIMEN OPTIONS FOR TREATMENT OF LTBI	
Type of Patient	**Dosage***
⚕ All infants and children (with or without HIV infection)	Isoniazid (INH) 10-15 mg/kg (maximum 300 mg) QD for 9 months (minimum of 270 doses within 12 months)
⚕ Persons >15 years (without HIV infection)	INH 300 mg QD for 6 months or 9 months** (minimum of 180 doses within 9 months for the 6 month regimen; minimum 270 doses within 12 months for 9 month regimen); four months of daily rifampin is an acceptable alternative; because of the risks of liver injury, the two-month rifampin and pyrazinamide combination should be used with caution, especially if the patient is taking other medications associated with liver injury or those with alcoholism
⚕ Persons >15 years with HIV infection	INH 300 mg QD for 9 months *OR* Rifampin 10 mg/kg/day QD (maximum dose of 600 mg) and pyrazinamide 15-30 mg/kg/day QD (maximum dose of 2 grams) for 2 months*** (minimum of 60 doses in 3 months); available data do not show excessive risk for severe hepatitis associated with this RIF-PZA treatment in HIV-infected adults
⚕ Persons >15 years with positive skin test, chest x-ray demonstrating old fibrotic lesions, no evidence of active disease, no history of treatment for TB	INH 300 mg QD for 9 months *OR* 4 months of rifampin (with or without isoniazid) *OR* 2 months of rifampin plus pyrazinamide cautiously
⚕ Persons >15 years with close contacts of infectious patients who have INH-resistant TB	<u>HIV negative persons</u>: 4 month regimen of daily rifampin *OR* 2 months with a rifamycin and pyrazinamide cautiously <u>HIV positive persons</u>: 2 month regimen with a rifamycin and PZA
⚕ Children with close contacts of infectious patients who have INH-resistant TB	Rifampin 10 mg/kg/day QD for 4 months
⚕ Pregnancy and Breast-feeding	INH daily or twice weekly (dosages as above) Pyridoxine supplementation Breast-feeding not contraindicated

*INH can also be given 2 times weekly in dose of 15 mg/kg when compliance is doubtful and direct observation is needed (minimum of 76 doses administered within 12 months)

9-month regimen is considered optimal; twice-weekly 6 month regimen should have a minimum of 52 doses within 9 months; 2-month RIF-PZA treatment regimen should be used with **caution due to risk of severe liver injury

***Twice-weekly regimens should consist of at least 16 doses in 2 months or 24 doses in 3 months; PZA dose for twice weekly regimen 4 grams (50-70 mg/kg/day)

Source: US Department of Health and Human Services, Centers for Disease Control and Prevention. (2000). *Core curriculum on tuberculosis* (4th ed.). Atlanta, GA.

B.   Treatment of active disease (uncomplicated, intrathoracic TB): initial treatment should include four drugs: isoniazid (INH), rifampin (RIF), pyrazinamide (PZA), and either ethambutol (EMB) or streptomycin (SM)
    1.   See tables that follow for regimens and dosages of initial drug therapy in children and adolescents and in patients with special considerations; when drug susceptibility results are available, the regimen should be altered as appropriate

REGIMEN OPTIONS FOR INITIAL TREATMENT OF PULMONARY AND EXTRAPULMONARY TB AMONG CHILDREN AND ADOLESCENTS

TB without HIV Infection

Option 1	Option 2	Option 3
Administer daily INH, RIF, PZA, and EMB or SM for 8 wks, followed by 16 weeks* of INH and RIF daily for 2-3 times/ week;** EMB or SM should be continued until susceptibility to INH and RIF is demonstrated. In areas where the INH resistance rate is <4%, EMB or SM may not be necessary for patients with no individual risk factors for drug resistance. Consult a TB medical expert if the patient is symptomatic or smear or culture positive after 3 months.	Administer daily INH, RIF, PZA, and SM or EMB for 2 weeks followed by 2 times/week** administration of the same drugs for 6 weeks (by DOT#), and subsequently, with 2 times/week** administration of INH and RIF for 16 weeks (by DOT).** After the 8-week induction phase, continue EMB or SM until susceptibility to INH and RIF is demonstrated, unless drug resistance is unlikely. Consult a TB medical expert if the patient is symptomatic or smear or culture positive after 3 months.	Treat by DOT, 3 times/week** with INH, RIF, PZA, and EMB or SM for 6 months.*** Consult a TB medical expert if the patient is symptomatic or smear or culture positive after 3 months. This regimen has been shown to be effective for INH-resistant TB.

*For infants and children with miliary TB, bone and joint TB, or TB meningitis, treatment should last 12 months; for adults with these forms of extrapulmonary TB, response to therapy should be closely monitored and treatment should be altered accordingly

**All regimens administered 2 times/week or 3 times/week should be monitored by DOT for the duration of therapy

***The strongest evidence from clinical trials is the effectiveness of all 4 drugs given for the full 6 months. There is weaker evidence that SM can be stopped after 4 months if the isolate is susceptible to all drugs. The evidence for stopping PZA before the end of 6 months is equivocal for the 3 times/week regimen, and there is no evidence on the benefit of this regimen with EMB for less than the full 6 months

#DOT = Directly observed therapy

OPTIONS FOR INITIAL TREATMENT OF PULMONARY AND EXTRAPULMONARY TB AMONG CHILDREN AND ADOLESCENTS IN SPECIAL CIRCUMSTANCES

Smear-and culture negative pulmonary TB in adults	Pulmonary and extrapulmonary TB in adults and children when PZA is contraindicated
Administer INH, RIF, PZA, and EMB or SM following option 1, 2, or 3 for initial therapy in table above for 8 weeks followed by INH, RIF, PZA, and EMB or SM daily or 2-3 times per week (DOT) for 8 weeks. If drug resistance is unlikely, EMB or SM may be unnecessary and PZA may be discontinued after 2 months	Administer INH, RIF, and EMB or SM daily for 4-8 weeks followed by INH and RIF daily or 2 times per week (DOT) for 28-32 weeks. EMB or SM should be continued until susceptibility to INH and RIF is demonstrated. If drug resistance is unlikely, EMB or SM may be unnecessary

DOSAGE RECOMMENDATION FOR FIRST-LINE DRUGS IN INITIAL TREATMENT OF TB AMONG CHILDREN* AND ADOLESCENTS

Drugs	Dosage					
	Daily		2 times/week		3 times/week	
	Children	Adolescents	Children	Adolescents	Children	Adolescents
Isoniazid	10-20 mg/kg Max 300 mg	5 mg/kg Max 300 mg	20-40 mg/kg Max 900 mg	15 mg/kg Max 900 mg	20-40 mg/kg Max 900 mg	15 mg/kg Max 900 mg
Rifampin**	10-20 mg/kg Max 600 mg	10 mg/kg Max 600 mg	10-20 mg/kg Max 600 mg	10 mg/kg Max 600 mg	10-20 mg/kg Max 600 mg	10 mg/kg Max 600 mg
Pyrazinamide**	15-20 mg/kg Max 2 gm	15-30 mg/kg Max 2 gm	50-70 mg/kg Max 4 gm	50-70 mg/kg Max 4 gm	50-70 mg/kg Max 3 gm	50-70 mg/kg Max 3 gm
Ethambutol#	15-25 mg/kg	15-25 mg/kg	50 mg/kg	50 mg/kg	25-30 mg/kg	25-30 mg/kg
Streptomycin	20-40 mg/kg Max 1 gm	15 mg/kg Max 1 gm	25-30 mg/kg Max 1.5 gm	25-30 mg/kg Max 1.5 gm	25-30 mg/kg Max 1.5 gm	25-30 mg/kg Max 1.5 gm

* Children ≤12 years of age.

** Dispense no more than a 2-week supply of RIF-PZA at a time to facilitate periodic clinical assessments due to the risk of severe liver injury

Ethambutol is generally not recommended for children whose visual acuity cannot be monitored (<6 years of age); however, ethambutol should be considered for all children with organisms resistant to other drugs, when susceptibility to ethambutol has been demonstrated, or susceptibility is likely. No maximum doses. Calculate dosage on lean body weight in obese patients

Source: US Department of Health and Human Services, Centers for Disease Control and Prevention. (2000). *Core curriculum on tuberculosis* (4th ed.). Atlanta, GA.

2.   Second-line TB drugs may be prescribed after consulting a specialist: capreomycin, kanamycin, ethionamide, para-aminosalicylic acid, cycloserine, ciprofloxacin, levofloxacin, ofloxacin, amikacin, clofazimine

3.   Treatment of persons with additional medical conditions must be individualized
   a.   For patients with impaired renal function avoid streptomycin, kanamycin and capreomycin
   b.   In patients with HIV infection, duration of treatment is the same as HIV-negative adults; HIV positive adults should be aggressively assessed for response to treatment and treatment should be prolonged if response is slow or suboptimal

4.   Treatment of children and infants
   a.   Treat with same regimens as adults; avoid EMB in children too young to be monitored for visual acuity
   b.   In infants, treat as soon as diagnosis is suspected because disseminated TB is more likely

5.   Treatment of drug-resistant TB
   a.   In patients with documented INH resistance during initial four-drug therapy, discontinue INH and continue RIF, PZA, and EMB or SM for entire 6 months *OR* treat with RIF and EMB for 12 months
   b.   Consult specialist for multidrug-resistant TB

6.   Directly observed therapy (DOT) is one method to ensure adherence
   a.   DOT requires that a health-care provider or other designated person observe patient while ingesting anti-TB medications
   b.   All patients with TB caused by organisms resistant to either INH or RIF and all patients receiving intermittent therapy should receive DOT

C.   Monitoring of patients on drug therapy includes the following:
1.   Obtain baseline measurements of hepatic enzymes, bilirubin, serum creatinine or BUN, CBC, and platelet count; measure serum uric acid if pyrazinamide is used; test visual acuity if EMB is used; test hearing function if SM is used

2.   At minimum, assess patients monthly and evaluate for adverse drug reactions

3.   Drug interactions: current literature and package inserts should be consulted

4.   Specific guidelines for drug monitoring
   a.   INH: baseline hepatic enzymes; repeat tests if abnormal or risks for adverse reactions
   b.   Rifampin: baseline CBC, platelets, hepatic enzymes; repeat as needed
   c.   PZA: baseline uric acid and hepatic enzymes; repeat as needed (asymptomatic hyperuricemia is not an indication for discontinuing the drug)
   d.   RIF-PZA combination therapy: serum aminotransferase (AT) and bilirubin at baseline and at 2, 4, and 6 weeks of treatment; stop treatment if AT >5 times the upper limit of normal in an asymptomatic person, AT greater than normal range when accompanied by symptoms of hepatitis, or a serum bilirubin greater than normal range
   e.   Ethambutol: baseline and monthly visual acuity and color vision tests
   f.   Streptomycin: baseline hearing test and kidney function; repeat as needed

5.   Monitoring response to therapy includes the following:
   a.   Sputum exam at least monthly until conversion to negative; then, at least one sputum at completion of therapy; most important response to treatment is culture conversion
   b.   For patients with multi-drug resistant TB, monthly sputum evaluation should continue for entire course of treatment
   c.   Chest radiographs are less important than sputums but chest film at completion of treatment provides a baseline for future comparisons
   d.   Patients with sputum that remains culture positive beyond 3 months should be evaluated for disease due to drug-resistant organisms
   e.   When waiting for drug susceptibility results, continue the original drug regimen or augment regimen with at least three new drugs; **never** add one drug to a failing regimen

D.   BCG vaccination should be undertaken only after consultation with health department; vaccination is used in many countries but is not generally recommended in US

E. Patient Education: teach about possible reactions to medicines
   1. INH
      a. Hepatic toxicity is the most common adverse reaction
      b. Instruct patient to immediately report nausea, loss of appetite, vomiting, unexplained fever over 3 days, abdominal tenderness (all hepatitis-suggesting symptoms)
      c. Peripheral neuropathy may be prevented by taking daily 10-50 mg of pyridoxine (vitamin B_6)
   2. Rifampin
      a. GI upset, hepatitis, bleeding problems, flu-like symptoms, and rash
      b. Warn patient that tears, urine, saliva, etc., may turn orange-red; may permanently stain contact lenses
   3. Pyrazinamide: hyperuricemia, gout (rare), hepatitis, joint aches, rash, and GI upset
   4. Ethambutol: Optic neuritis and rash
   5. Streptomycin: Hearing and balance changes and renal toxicity

F. Additional patient education also includes discussion of mode of transmission and need to cover nose and mouth when coughing or sneezing; no sharing of eating utensils

G. A good website resource is the CDC National Center for HIV, STD, and TB Prevention, Division of Tuberculosis Elimination (http://www.cdc.gov/nchstp/tb/default.htm)

H. Follow Up (see V.C.4.-5. for follow-up guidelines for drug and response monitoring)

REFERENCES

Agency for Healthcare Research and Quality. (2003). Management of bronchiolitis in infants and children. Summary, evidence report/technology assessment: Number 69. AHRQ Publication Number 03-E009, http://www.ahrq.gov/clinic/epcsums/broncsum.htm.

Allen, D.B. (2002). Inhaled corticosteroid therapy for asthma in preschool children: Growth Issues. *Pediatrics, 109*, 373-380.

American Academy of Pediatrics. (2000). In L.K. Pickering (Ed.). *Red Book: Report of the Committee on Infectious Disease.* (25th ed.). Elk Grove Village, IL: Author.

American Academy of Pediatrics, Committee on Infectious Diseases and Committee on Fetus and Newborn. (1998). Prevention of respiratory syncytial virus infections: Indications for the use of palivizumab and update on the use of RSV-IGIV. *Pediatrics, 102*, 1211-1216.

American Academy of Pediatrics, Committee on Infectious Diseases. (2000). Policy statement: Recommendations for the prevention of pneumococcal infections, including the use of pneumococcal conjugate vaccine (Prevnar®), pneumococcal polysaccharide vaccine, and antibiotic prophylaxis. *Pediatrics, 106*, 362-366.

Ampofo, K.K. & Saiman, L. (2002). Tuberculosis. In F.D. Burg, J.R. Ingelfinger, R.A. Polin, & A.A. Gershon. *Gellis & Kagan's current pediatric therapy:* Saunders: Philadelphia.

Bisgaard, H. (2001). Leukotriene modifiers in pediatric asthma management. *Pediatrics, 107,* 381-390.

Blumberg, M.Z. (2001). Chronic cough in children: Determining the cause. *Consultant,* 795-801.

Busse, W.W., & Lemanske, Jr, R.F. (2001). Asthma. *New England Journal of Medicine, 344,* 350-362.

Cain, W.A. (2002). Tularemia. *American Journal for Nurse Practitioners, 5,* 24-26.

Centers for Disease Control and Prevention. (2001). Recognition of illness associated with the intentional release of a biologic agent. *MMWR, 50(41),* 893-897.

Centers for Disease Control and Prevention. (2001). Update: Fatal and severe liver injuries associated with rifampin and pyrazinamide for latent tuberculosis infection, and revisions in American Thoracic Society/CDC recommendations-United States, 2001. *MMWR, 50(34),* 733-735.

Centers for Disease Control and Prevention. (2003). Key clinical activities for quality asthma care. Recommendations of the National Asthma Education and Prevention Program. *MMWR, 52(RRO6),* 1-8.

Drazen, J M., Israel, E., & O'Byrne, P.M. (1999). Treatment of asthma with drugs modifying the leukotriene pathway. *New England Journal of Medicine, 340,* 197-206.

GlaxoWellcome. (1995). Patient instructions for use of Serevent Diskcus® (salmeterol xinafoate) inhalation powder. Research Triangle Park, NC.

Gonzales, R., Bartlett, J.G., Besser, R.E., Cooper, R.J., Hickner, J.M., Hoffman, J.R., & Sande, M.A. (2001). Principles of appropriate antibiotic use for treatment of uncomplicated acute bronchitis: Background. *Annals of Internal Medicine, 134,* 521-529.

Gonzales, R., & Sande, M.A. (2000). Uncomplicated acute bronchitis. *Annals of Internal Medicine, 133,* 981-991.

Guthrie, R. (2001). Community-acquired lower respiratory tract infections: Etiology and treatment. *Chest, 120,* 2021-2034.

Hall, C.B. (2001). Respiratory syncytial virus and parainfluenza virus. *New England Journal of Medicine, 344,* 1917-1928.

Hall, C.B., & Hall, W.J. (2001). Bronchiolitis. In R.A. Hoekelman, (Ed.), *Primary pediatric care* (4th ed.). St. Louis: Mosby.

Hall, C.B., & Hall, W.J. (2001). Croup. In R.A. Hoekelman, (Ed.), *Primary pediatric care* (4th ed.). St. Louis: Mosby.

Hall, C.B., & Hall, W.J. (2001). Epiglottitis. In R.A. Hoekelman, (Ed.), *Primary pediatric care* (4th ed.). St. Louis: Mosby.

Harris, J.S. (2001). Pneumonia in kids. *Contemporary Pediatrics* (Suppl. 1), 15-18.

Hueston, W.J., & Mainous, A.G. (1998). Acute bronchitis. *American Family Physician, 57,* 1270-1276.

Inglesby, T.V., O'Toole, T., Henderson, D.A., et al. (2002). Anthrax as a biological weapon 2002: Updated recommendations for management. *JAMA, 287,* 2236-2252.

Irwin, R.S., & Madison, J.M. (2000). The diagnosis and treatment of cough. *New England Journal of Medicine, 343,* 1715-1721.

Irwin, R.S., & Madison, J.M. (2001). Symptom research on chronic cough: A historical perspective. *Annals of Internal Medicine, 134,* 809-814.

Jaffe, D.M. (1998). The treatment of croup with glucocorticoids. *New England Journal of Medicine, 339,* 553-555.

Kacker, A., & Keller, J.L. (2002). Acute laryngotracheobronchitis, bacterial tracheitis, and acute epiglottitis/supraglottitis. In F.D. Burg, J.R. Ingelfinger, R.A. Polin, & A.A. Gershon. *Gellis & Kagan's current pediatric therapy:* Saunders: Philadelphia.

Kemp, J.P., & Kemp, J.A. (2001). Management of asthma in children. *American Family Physician, 63,* 1341-1348, 1353-1354.

Klassen, T.P. (1999). Croup: A current perspective. *Pediatric Clinics of North America, 46,* 1167-1178.

Kormos, W. A. (2000). Approach to the patient with acute bronchitis or pneumonia in the ambulatory setting. In A.H. Goroll & A.G. Mulley, Jr. (Eds.), *Primary care medicine: Office evaluation and management of the adult patient* (4th ed.). Philadelphia: Lippincott, Williams and Wilkins.

Kormos, W.A. (2000). Management of the common cold. In A.H. Goroll & A.G. Mulley, Jr. (Eds.), *Primary care medicine: Office evaluation and management of the adult patient* (4th ed.). Philadelphia: Lippincott, Williams and Wilkins.

Lowenthal, D. (2001). Approach to the child with a cough. In C. Green-Hernandez, J.K. Singleton, & D.Z. Aronzon. *Primary care pediatrics.* Lippincott: Philadelphia.

McIntosh, K. (2002). Community-acquired pneumonia in children. *New England Journal of Medicine, 346,* 429-437.

Merino, J.M., Alvarez, T., Marrero, M., Anso, S., Elvira, A., Iglesias, G., & Gonzalez, J. B. (2001). Microbiology of pediatric primary pulmonary tuberculosis. *Chest, 119,* 1434-1438.

Mysliwiec, V., & Pina, J.S. (1999). Bronchiectasis: The 'other' obstructive lung disease. *Postgraduate Medicine, 106*(1), 123-31.

National Institutes of Health. National Heart, Lung, and Blood Institute. (1997). *The Expert Panel Report 2: Guidelines for the diagnosis and management of asthma.* National Asthma Education Program, Office of Prevention, Education and Control. NIH Publication #97-4051. Bethesda, MD.

National Institutes of Health. National Heart, Lung, and Blood Institute. (2002). N*AEPP Expert Panel Report Guidelines for the diagnosis and management of asthma.* Update on selected topics 2002. National Asthma Education and Prevention Program. NIH Publ. #02-5075, Bethesda, MD.

Naureckas, E.T., & Solway, J. (2001). Mild asthma. *New England Journal of Medicine, 345,* 1257-1262.

Niederman, M.S. (1998). Community-acquired pneumonia: A North American perspective. *Chest, 113,* 179S-182S.

Novartis Pharmaceuticals Corporation. (2001). Foradil® Aerolizer (formoterol fumarate inhalation powder) package insert. East Hanover, NJ.

O'Brien, K.L., Dowell, S.F., Schwartz, B., Marcy, S.M., Phillips, W.R., & Gerber, M.A. (1998). Cough illness/bronchitis--principles of judicious use of antimicrobial agents. *Pediatrics, 101,* 178-181.

Prasad, A.S., Fitzgerald, J.T., Bao, B., Beck, F.W.J., & Chandrasekar, P.H. (2000). Duration of symptoms and plasma cytokine levels in patients with the common cold treated with zinc acetate. *Annals of Internal Medicine, 133,* 245-252.

Rittichier, K.K. & Ledwith, C.A. (2000). Outpatient treatment of moderate croup with dexamethasone: Intramuscular versus oral dosing. *Pediatrics, 106,* 1344-1348.

Rosenstein, N., Phillips, W.R., Gerber, M.A., Marcy, M., Schwartz, B., & Dowell, S.F. (1998). The common cold--principles of judicious use of antimicrobial agents. *Pediatrics, 101,* 181-184.

Schroeder, S.A. (2001). Hemoptysis. In R.A. Hoekelman, (Ed.), *Primary pediatric care* (4th ed.). St. Louis: Mosby.

Scott, J., & Orzano, A.J. (2001). Evaluation and treatment of the patient with acute undifferentiated respiratory tract infection. *Journal of Family Practice, 50,* 1070-1077.

Skoner, D.P. (2002). Balancing safety and efficacy in pediatric asthma management. *Pediatrics, 109,* 381-392.

Slovis, B.S., Plitman, J.D., & Haas, D.W. (2000). The case against anergy testing as a routine adjunct to tuberculin skin testing. *JAMA, 283,* 2003-2007.

Small, P.M., & Fujiwara, P.I. (2001). Management of tuberculosis in the United States. *New England Journal of Medicine, 345,* 189-200.

Strunk, R.C. (2002). Defining asthma in the preschool-aged children. *Pediatrics, 109,* 357-361.

US Department of Health and Human Services, Centers for Disease Control and Prevention. (2000). *Core curriculum on tuberculosis* (4th ed.). Atlanta, GA.

Wainwright, C., Cheney, L., Cheney, J., Barber, S., Price, D., Moloney, S., et al. (2003). A multicenter, randomized, double-blind, controlled trial of nebulized epinephrine in infants with acute bronchiolitis. *New England Journal of Medicine, 349,* 27-35.

Williamson, H.A., Jr. (2003). What is the best treatment for bronchiolitis? *The Journal of Family Practice, 52,* 69-70.

Cardiovascular Problems

JEAN E. DEMARTINIS & CONSTANCE R. UPHOLD

CHEST PAIN

I. Definition: Chest discomfort or a sensory response to noxious stimuli associated with actual or potential tissue damage involving the chest wall, thoracic organs, and adjacent structures; cardiac chest pain is uncommon in children

II. Pathogenesis

 A. Chest wall pain may be caused by irritation, trauma, and/or compression of the muscles, cartilaginous structures, nerves, or bones comprising the chest wall area

 B. Pain originating from the lungs or adjacent structures may be caused by the following:
  1. Irritation/inflammation of the lung tissue, pleura (called pleurisy), or diaphragm secondary to inflammation, infection, chronic disease, and/or neoplasm
  2. Reactive airway/bronchospasm due to irritation or inflammation of the bronchi

 C. Cardiac pain may be associated with the following:
  1. A low-flow state to the myocardium causing spasm, tissue hypoxia, anaerobic metabolism, lactic acidosis, and increased prostaglandin secretion
  2. Other causes involve the irritation of structures of the mediastinum near the heart, such as in pericarditis

 D. Pain due to gastrointestinal problems results from structural defects (luminal laxity, obstruction, or distention) and/or mucosal or organ tissue irritation, inflammation, or infection involving the esophagus and abdominal organs

 E. Pain related to psychogenic disorders may be secondary to anxiety, depression, anxiety-tension syndromes, illicit drug use, or neuroses or other psychiatric disorders

III. Clinical Presentation: Only 1% to 3% of all complaints of chest pain in children and adolescents is caused by heart disease, however much of the evaluation and teaching surrounding chest pain in children is focused on convincing families that the heart is normal

 A. Young children most frequently present with chest pain from a musculoskeletal injury generally related to overexercise (overuse, misuse, or abuse injury)
  1. Chest pain resulting from musculoskeletal or nerve origins is variable and may last from a few seconds to several days or even a month or more and may be sharp, dull, or aching and may be aggravated by deep inspiration and cough; the chest is tender on palpation (called point-tenderness) or along the dermatome
  2. Musculoskeletal pain tends to occur with movement, stretching, or palpation of the inflamed muscle/tendon
  3. Bone pain is usually well localized and described as intensely tender
  4. Costochondritis is characterized by sharp, usually well localized pain (but may radiate across anterior chest and down the arms) that worsens with deep breath or coughing
   a. Pain is most intense at the costochondral junction (junction of the anterior ribs and sternum)
   b. Pain is often accompanied with warmth, erythema, and swelling at junction
  5. Nerve irritation or compression results in pain and motor and sensory deficits (numbness or tingling) in the neck, chest, upper arms or legs; symptoms follow the dermatomes

 B. Pleural causes of chest pain typically present as pain worsened by deep inspiration and coughing or spasm secondary to cold weather and increased activity
  1. In children, exercise-induced bronchospasm and asthma are the most common causes of pleuritic pain
  2. Bacterial pneumonia is characterized by abrupt onset of fever, chills, leukocytosis, and purulent sputum
  3. Pulmonary embolus (PE) is an uncommon event in children
   a. Characterized by a sudden onset of dyspnea, tachypnea, tachycardia, hypotension, and possibly hemoptysis
   b. Remember, however, that many patients with PE may be asymptomatic
   c. Rales and a pleural friction rub may be present; may exhibit decreased or absent breath sounds distal to PE

        d.   May progress to pulmonary hypertension, acute right heart failure, or respiratory arrest

        e.   Typically associated with risk factors:

             (1)   Immobility, surgery, pregnancy, oral contraceptives, pelvis or lower extremity trauma (fat embolus)

             (2)   Children with a history of large bone fracture, malignancy, deep venous thrombosis, previous pulmonary embolus, congestive heart failure, obesity, and hypercoagulability conditions are more prone to developing a PE

    4.   Spontaneous pneumothorax or hemothorax secondary to trauma or disease

        a.   Causes acute, unilateral, stabbing pain with dyspnea

        b.   Typically, auscultation reveals decreased breath and voice sounds

        c.   Be on the alert for mediastinal shift and cardiopulmonary compromise

C.   Chest pain due to cardiac diseases may be mild to severe, transient (generally exertional and relieved by rest) or constant (often radiating to neck, jaw, or arms; sometimes the back)

    1.   Pericarditis

        a.   Presents with one of two types of pain:

             (1)   Pleuritic pain resulting from spread of the inflammation from the relatively insensitive pericardium to the pain-sensitive parietal pleura

             (2)   Steady substernal or left precordial pain that resembles angina (aggravated by swallowing and deep breathing with radiation to the left shoulder, upper back and neck)

        b.   Pain is paroxysmal and decreases upon sitting and leaning forward

        c.   Characterized by a friction rub

        d.   Associated signs are fever, tachycardia, pulsus paradoxus, tamponade, elevated sedimentation rate, and leukocytosis

        e.   Classic sign if accompanied by tamponade is narrowed pulse pressure

        f.   Risk factors include infection, autoimmune disease, cardiac surgery for congenital heart anomaly, malignancy, and uremia

    2.   Mitral valve prolapse (MVP)

        a.   Children are often asymptomatic, but chest pain, fatigue, palpitations (especially when lying supine on left side), lightheadedness, dizziness, shortness of breath, headaches, and mood swings may be present

        b.   Pain is sharp, fleeting, localized over mid or left chest wall; rarely radiates

        c.   Pain is not relieved by nitroglycerin; usually pain is unrelated to exertion

        d.   Pain may be brief or last for several days

        e.   MVP can progress to mitral insufficiency with enlargement of left atrium and left ventricle, and congestive heart failure

        f.   Hallmark diagnostic sign is a mid-systolic click and late systolic murmur

        g.   Echocardiogram will reveal extent of regurgitation and may reveal abnormally thickened, billowing mitral valve leaflets

    3.   Cocaine-induced chest pain

        a.   May present with severe, sharp, pressure-like or squeezing substernal pain

        b.   Associated symptoms include euphoria, mydriasis, hyperstimulation, paranoia, delusions, followed by depression, nausea, and muscle twitching

        c.   Complications include myocardial ischemia and infarction, arrhythmias, respiratory failure, and circulatory collapse

D.   Pain from disorders of the gastrointestinal system can mimic cardiovascular symptoms, however, visceral pain is mostly characterized by deep, poorly localized pain that radiates to the back, shoulder blades, or up into the shoulders or neck

    1.   Gastroesophageal reflux (see section on GASTROESOPHAGEAL REFLUX DISEASE)

        a.   Presents with burning and substernal pain that starts in the epigastrium and radiates upward toward the throat

        b.   Pain is related to consuming a large meal, lying down, or bending over

        c.   Pain is usually relieved by ingestion of antacid or food

    2.   Esophageal spasm

        a.   Presents as an intense, substernal, sharp pain radiating to interscapular region

        b.   Unfortunately, also relieved by nitroglycerin as with true angina; but unlike angina, it may persist as a dull ache long after the acute attack

    3.   Other gastrointestinal problems such as cholecystitis and peptic ulcer disease resemble cardiac pain, but their association with eating and their relief with antacids can distinguish them

E. Chest pain may be due to psychiatric or mental health disorders
1. Children with psychogenic problems often describe pain as generalized, constantly present, and aggravated by any effort, particularly at times of family or school stress
2. Typically a family history of chest pain exists
3. Associated symptoms include dyspnea, fatigue, headache, hyperventilation, and other somatic symptoms
4. Pain absent on weekends and at non-stress times indicates an anxiety-tension syndrome
5. Children with panic disorders often have chest pain that is accompanied by intense fear, tachypnea, palpitations, diaphoresis, trembling, nausea, dizziness, syncope or near syncope, and chills or hot flashes

F. Chest pain in children, not associated with any abnormal finding in the history or physical examination, is often termed idiopathic; symptoms are usually self-limited and resolve within two years; rule out psychogenic causes before making this diagnosis

IV. Diagnosis/Evaluation

A. History (length of history will depend on patient's clinical presentation); perform a rapid history for any patient with a suspected emergent condition
1. Determine the pattern and whether onset was sudden, gradual, recurrent, or new
2. If possible, children should describe the nature, quality, and character of the pain in their own words and should be asked what they think is causing the pain
3. Determine the quantity of pain, use the visual analog scale from 0 to 10 (10 is the worst pain ever experienced and 0 indicates no pain)
   a. Cardiac chest pain should never be allowed to persist greater than 0, as is allowable for skeletal muscle pain
   b. Young children and toddlers should be shown a visual analog scale or a instrument containing faces with variable expressions that they can point to and match how they are feeling
4. Inquire about aggravating factors such as exercise or activity, stress, food intake, movement, coughing, emotional experiences, or cold temperatures
5. Inquire about relieving factors -- rest, antacids, food intake
6. Ask about associated symptoms such as fatigue, dyspnea, hemoptysis, fever, chills, cough, sputum production, exanthem, diaphoresis, dizziness, syncope or near syncope, nausea, diarrhea, cyanosis, pallor, leg pain, or edema
7. Ask if a coexistent illness is present or if other members of the household are sick
8. Explore stress-related factors in school, work, or home environments
9. Questions to rule out trauma should always be asked even if a traumatic event occurred months before; the pain could represent a posttraumatic pericardial effusion----sharp pain that decreases when the child leans forward is characteristic of pericardial inflammation
10. Ask about risk factors for ischemic heart disease
11. Explore past medical history
12. Obtain a complete family history
    a. Particularly inquire about cardiovascular disease
    b. Children who have a family history of Turner's or Marfan syndrome, as well as those who have a history of Kawasaki disease or congenital heart disease, warrant referral to a pediatric cardiologist

B. Physical Examination
1. Observe general appearance of patient, assessing for level of distress and anxiety
2. Measure vital signs
   a. Take blood pressure in both arms and both legs—coarctation of the aorta is exhibited by a discrepancy in arm and leg pressures
   b. If unable to detect, use Doppler and/or take thigh pressure to assess presence and compare with arm pressures
   c. Obtain postural pressures; lying, sitting, and standing measurements are best
3. Measure height & weight (growth delays suggest organic problems)
4. Inspect skin for pallor, cyanosis, jaundice, or herpetic rash
5. Examine eyes, including funduscopy
6. Assess neck for lymphadenopathy, thyromegaly, tracheal shift, or jugular venous distention
7. Examine chest wall for signs of trauma, lifts, or heaves
8. Palpate chest wall, noting tenderness and swelling or the presence of thrills

9.	Perform a complete examination of the heart
	a.	Note extra heart sounds, murmurs, clicks, hums, rubs, S_3 or S_4 sounds, or irregular irregularities
	b.	Findings that point toward a possible cardiac cause for the pain include clicks, rubs, and systolic murmurs; a third heart sound, although generally a normal finding in some children, may also indicate that myocarditis or congestive heart failure is present or developing
10.	Auscultate lungs for equal breath sounds, a pleural rub, crackles, or wheezes
11.	Auscultate abdomen for bowel sounds and bruits
12.	Palpate abdomen for tenderness and masses (particularly in the right upper quadrant and epigastrium), organomegaly, bounding pulses, and ascites
13.	Palpate for femoral pulses
14.	Assess lower extremities for cyanosis, diminished pulses, unilateral swelling, and other signs of phlebitis
15.	Children who present with pain that changes with movement should have a musculoskeletal and neurological exam performed, focusing on focal tenderness, muscular weakness, and motor and sensory deficits

C.	Differential Diagnosis: (see following table)

CHEST PAIN: DIFFERENTIAL DIAGNOSIS

Cardiac	Gastrointestinal	Pulmonary
Ischemic Syndromes	Biliary colic	Bronchitis/bronchospasm
• Variant angina	Esophageal spasm	Empyema
Congenital heart defects	Esophagitis/gastritis	Pleural effusion
Myocarditis	Gastric/duodenal ulcer	Pleuritis
Pericarditis	Gastroesophageal reflux disorder	Pneumonia
Valvular Disease		Pneumothorax
• Aortic stenosis	Neurologic	Pulmonary edema
• Mitral valve prolapse	Nerve root compression	Pulmonary embolism
• Hypertrophic obstructive cardiomyopathy		Pulmonary hypertension
	Vascular	
Musculoskeletal	Aortic dissection	
Cervical radiculopathy	Pulmonary embolism	
Costochondritis	Pulmonary hypertension	
Muscle strain/spasm		

1.	A detailed history (if condition allows) is extremely important in assisting the clinician in ruling in and ruling out potential diagnoses
2.	Age and sex of the child can also help narrow the differential diagnoses
3.	Risk factors provide important information to arrive at a diagnosis
4.	Quality, location, radiation, and intensity of pain are nonspecific symptoms and are usually not helpful in arriving at a diagnosis

D.	Diagnostic Tests are based on data collected in the history and physical examination
	1.	Order pulse oximetry to assess for oxygen desaturation and order cardiac-specific troponins, highly sensitive C-reactive protein (hsCRP), and brain natriuretic peptide (BNP) in patients with suspected cardiac or cardiopulmonary problems
	2.	Order an electrocardiogram (ECG) for patients with suspected cardiac chest pain, when a cardiac diagnosis cannot be ruled out immediately, or when significant risk factors exist
	3.	Echocardiography is helpful in diagnosing mitral valve prolapse or other valvular abnormalities, pericarditis, and to assess for wall motion and ejection fraction
	4.	Computed tomography (CT) with contrast, transesophageal echocardiography (TEE), and aortic angiography are diagnostic tests for coarctation of the aorta and congenital abnormalities
	5.	Consider exercise stress echocardiogram and radionuclide scans using thallium or Cardiolite with treadmill for ruling in or ruling out a cardiac diagnosis
	6.	Order a complete metabolic profile including liver enzymes and a CBC; include amylase and lipase if pancreatitis is suspected
	7.	Consider ordering a chest x-ray when there is suspicion of following: Chest trauma (rib fractures), pulmonary diseases (pneumonia or tuberculosis, pneumothorax, pulmonary embolus) or a widened mediastinum (dissecting abdominal aneurysm)
	8.	Consider a lung CT scan or ventilation/perfusion scan for children with suspected pleural problems
	9.	Consider Gram's stain of sputum for suspected pulmonary infections
	10.	An acid perfusion (Bernstein) test or more invasive tests such as esophageal manometry, barium x-ray studies, and endoscopy may be helpful in diagnosing specific gastrointestinal problems

V. Plan/Management

A. Relief of pain is based on the etiology; remember cardiac pain must be relieved to level 0

B. Treatment of musculoskeletal problems such as costochondritis is usually symptomatic; recommend use of pain medications such as nonsteroid anti-inflammatory drugs or acetaminophen and local ice and heat applications (see chapter on MUSCULOSKELETAL PROBLEMS)

C. Treatment of pulmonary problems
    1. Pneumonia, bronchitis, asthma, bronchospasm (see RESPIRATORY chapter)
    2. Pulmonary embolus requires hospitalization and intravenous anticoagulation
    3. Carefully assess vital signs and watch for mediastinal shift in patients with a pneumothorax
        a. A small, stable pneumothorax without evidence of respiratory compromise requires only observation for several days until stabilization and resolution
        b. Hospitalization and insertion of chest tubes is needed for a large, expanding pneumothorax or tension pneumothorax

D. Treatment of cardiac pain
    1. Hospitalization and immediate referral to a pediatric cardiologist is required for myocardial abnormalities
    2. Pericarditis is treated with aspirin, non-steroidal anti-inflammatory drugs, or, for severe cases, corticosteroids; hospitalization is required for patients with signs of cardiac tamponade
    3. Mitral valve prolapse
        a. No specific treatment is indicated for most patients, except for reassurance about a good prognosis
        b. The major therapeutic dilemma is whether to recommend antibiotic prophylaxis against infective endocarditis when certain invasive procedures are performed; prophylaxis is often recommended for patients who have the following:
            (1) Moderate to severe mitral regurgitation and/or thickened leaflets
            (2) Murmur of mitral regurgitation, but not in those who have only a click
            (3) If there is uncertainty about the diagnosis of mitral regurgitation refer to cardiologist
        c. Patients with severe mitral regurgitation may require valve surgery

E. Treatment of abdominal problems (see chapter on GASTROINTESTINAL PROBLEMS)

F. Treatment of psychogenic problems
    1. Reassure patient that pain does not have a cardiac etiology
    2. Counseling and psychotherapy may be helpful

G. Patient Education
    1. Refer to specialist if acute cardiac or serious conditions are identified; otherwise, educate patient and family about the diagnosis and treatment and how best to comply with the prescribed regimen
    2. To avoid panic, carefully explain to parents and the child that the history, physical exam, and diagnostic results revealed no cardiac abnormality
    3. Educate patients and families about problems other than cardiac that can cause "chest pain," how to recognize them, and when to seek medical attention
    4. Allow time for the parents and child to express concerns and ask questions
    5. Teach about risk factors for cardiac disease and strategies to reduce risks that the entire family can work on together

H. Follow up is variable depending on diagnosis and child's condition

HYPERTENSION

I. Definitions:

    A. Normal blood pressure (BP): Systolic and diastolic BP <90th percentile for height, age, and sex

    B. High-normal or borderline BP: Average systolic or diastolic BP ≥90th percentile but <95th percentile

    C. Hypertension: Persistent elevation in BP with average systolic or diastolic BP ≥95th percentile for height, age, and sex measured on at least three separate occasions

    D. Severe hypertension: Persistent elevation in BP >99th percentile for all categories

II. Pathogenesis: Dysfunctions of the arterial baroreceptors and chemoreceptors, disturbance of vascular autoregulation, overstimulation of the renin-angiotensin system, and/or faulty regulation of body fluid volume alter peripheral vascular resistance, heart rate, or stroke volume creating a rise in systemic arterial blood pressure

    A. Primary or essential hypertension has no identifiable cause; it is a syndrome rather than a disorder with a single etiology and over time definitive diagnoses may be deduced
        1. A familial influence on BP occurs early in life
        2. Mild to moderate hypertension in children >6 years is usually essential hypertension, but always rule out secondary causes immediately

    B. Secondary hypertension is the usual cause of high BP in children younger than 10 years
        1. Approximately 80% of cases are due to renal disorders (renal parenchymal disease, renal artery disease); another 5-10% of cases are due to coarctation of the aorta (COA)
        2. The other 5-10% are associated with endocrine disorders (hyperthyroidism, adrenal dysfunction, hyperaldosteronism), neurogenic disorders (increased intracranial pressure, sleep apnea), or drugs/chemicals (sympathomimetic drugs, oral contraceptives, steroids, NSAIDs, amphetamines, cocaine, heavy metal poisoning) and miscellaneous causes (hypercalcemia, hypervolemia, hypernatremia)

    C. Transient hypertension or an acute, short-lived elevation of blood pressure is often related to acute illness or ingestion of oral contraceptives or anabolic steroids

    D. Labile hypertension occurs predominantly in adolescents and is due to stressful events

    E. Severe, abrupt onset of elevated blood pressure is usually a result of poor control of the chronically hypertensive patient but can be due to head trauma, drug reactions, acute glomerulonephritis, pregnancy, and pheochromocytoma

III. Clinical Presentation

    A. Hypertension (HTN) in childhood is a risk factor for the development of true HTN in adulthood; also associated with left ventricular hypertrophy

    B. A direct relationship between weight and BP has been documented as early as 5 years of age; obesity is recognized as an important independent risk factor for HTN in children
        1. Most children and adolescents with HTN are overweight and have family histories of HTN
        2. Obesity in children of all ages, but particularly in adolescents, has been increasing markedly

C.   Height is independently related to BP at all ages

D.   African-American and Asian-American children have higher BPs than Caucasian children

E.   Primary hypertension is often asymptomatic and detected through routine screening

F.   Secondary hypertension occurs most frequently during infancy and late childhood; symptoms include dizziness, headaches, and changes in vision; occasionally neurological manifestations, chronic heart failure, renal dysfunction, or stroke may be the presenting problem

G.   Severe, abrupt onset of elevated blood pressure is a medical emergency and can lead to encephalopathy, cardiac failure, acute renal failure, and loss of vision if not corrected immediately

IV.   Diagnosis/Evaluation

A.   History
1.   Inquire about associated symptoms such as headaches, dizziness, nausea, vomiting, irritability, visual changes, and personality changes
2.   Explore risk factors for developing cardiovascular disease such as family history, obesity, diet, smoking, and physical inactivity
3.   In adolescents, explore use of oral contraceptive, anabolic steroids, alcohol, cocaine, or other addictive substances
4.   Obtain a complete medical history focusing on cardiac, renal, endocrine, and genetic disorders; list all medications including prescription, over-the-counter, and herbal; antihistamines, decongestants, nasal sprays, antiasthmatic drugs can cause elevated BP
5.   Obtain a complete family history of both first- and second-degree relatives
6.   Explore psychosocial and environmental factors that might affect BP control

B.   Physical Examination
1.   Screening for HTN should begin at age 3 years with annual BP measurements
2.   Measure blood pressure in all extremities; measure BP lying, sitting, and standing (in infants and very young children use automated devices for measurement)
    a.   For consistency and comparison use the right arm for measurement
    b.   When BP is taken in seated position, child's arm should rest on solid supporting surface at heart level
    c.   Use the appropriate cuff size: Choose a cuff with a width that is approximately 40% of arm circumference midway between the olecranon and the acromion; cuff bladder should cover 80-100% of the arm circumference and approximately 2/3 of the length of the upper arm
    d.   Measure BP in controlled environment, after 3-5 minutes of rest, in seated position with antecubital fossa supported at heart level
    e.   Record at least twice on each occasion and arrive at an average of each of the systolic and diastolic BP measurements
    f.   Inflate cuff 20-30 mm Hg above systolic BP and deflate cuff at 2-3 mm Hg/s
    g.   The fifth Korotkoff sound (K5), or the disappearance of Korotkoff sounds is used as the definition of diastolic pressure
    h.   Compare arm and leg pressures

3. Ambulatory BP monitoring devices may be beneficial for evaluating diurnal patterns of BP and persistence of BP elevation
4. Electronic BP devices should be used in interpretation of BP very cautiously
5. Measure height and weight and plot on growth charts
6. Assess skin; observe for neurocutaneous lesions of neurofibromatosis or tuberous sclerosis; pallor suggests anemia; edema may be related to chronic kidney disease
7. Do a complete eye exam, including funduscopy
8. Assess the neck for thyromegaly, bruits, and distended veins
9. Palpate, percuss, and auscultate the heart
10. Auscultate the lungs
11. Assess for abdominal bruits
12. Palpate abdomen for hepatomegaly, splenomegaly, and enlarged kidneys or masses
13. Inspect and palpate extremities, noting edema, decreased femoral and pedal pulses, and temperature and color changes
14. Perform a complete neurological exam; observe for Bell's palsy (a heralding sign of marked hypertension)
15. For neonates and infants determine BP level percentiles (see table that follows)

NEONATES AND CHILDREN <1 YEAR: BLOOD PRESSURE CLASSIFICATION

Age Group	Significant Hypertension (mm Hg)	Severe Hypertension (mm Hg)
Newborn - 7 days	Systolic BP ≥96	Systolic BP ≥106
Neonate - 8 days -30 days	Systolic BP ≥104	Systolic BP ≥110
Infant (<1 year)	Systolic BP ≥112 Diastolic BP ≥74	Systolic BP ≥118 Diastolic BP ≥82

Adapted from National, Heart, Lung, and Blood Institute. (1987). Report of the Second Task Force on Blood Pressure Control in Children--1987. *Pediatrics, 79,* 1-19.

16. For children >1 year old determine BP level percentiles: after documenting height percentile from standard growth charts, child's measured systolic and diastolic BPs are compared with numbers in the following tables (boys or girls) for age and height percentiles (see following tables)

BOYS AGED 1-17 YEARS: BLOOD PRESSURE LEVELS FOR THE 90TH AND 95TH PERCENTILES OF BLOOD PRESSURE BY PERCENTILES OF HEIGHT

Age, y	Blood Pressure Percentile	Systolic Blood Pressure by Percentile of Height, mm Hg							Diastolic Blood Pressure by Percentile of Height, mm Hg						
		5%	10%	25%	50%	75%	90%	95%	5%	10%	25%	50%	75%	90%	95%
1	90th	94	95	97	98	100	102	102	50	51	52	53	54	54	55
	95th	98	99	101	102	104	106	106	55	55	56	57	58	59	59
2	90th	98	99	100	102	104	105	106	55	55	56	57	58	59	59
	95th	101	102	104	106	108	109	110	59	59	60	61	62	63	63
3	90th	100	101	103	105	107	108	109	59	59	60	61	62	63	63
	95th	104	105	107	109	111	112	113	63	63	64	65	66	67	67
4	90th	102	103	105	107	109	110	111	62	62	63	64	65	66	66
	95th	106	107	109	111	113	114	115	66	67	67	68	69	70	71
5	90th	104	105	106	108	110	112	112	65	65	66	67	68	69	69
	95th	108	109	110	112	114	115	116	69	70	70	71	72	73	74
6	90th	105	106	108	110	111	113	114	67	68	69	70	70	71	72
	95th	109	110	112	114	115	117	117	72	72	73	74	75	76	76
7	90th	106	107	109	111	113	114	115	69	70	71	72	72	73	74
	95th	110	111	113	115	116	118	119	74	74	75	76	77	78	78
8	90th	107	108	110	112	114	115	116	71	71	72	73	74	75	75
	95th	111	112	114	116	118	119	120	75	76	76	77	78	79	80
9	90th	109	110	112	113	115	117	117	72	73	73	74	75	76	77
	95th	113	114	116	117	119	121	121	76	77	78	79	80	80	81
10	90th	110	112	113	115	117	118	119	73	74	74	75	76	77	78
	95th	114	115	117	119	121	122	123	77	78	79	80	80	81	82
11	90th	112	113	115	117	119	120	121	74	74	75	76	77	78	78
	95th	116	117	119	121	123	124	125	78	79	79	80	81	82	83
12	90th	115	116	117	119	121	123	123	75	75	76	77	78	78	79
	95th	119	120	121	123	125	126	127	79	79	80	81	82	83	83
13	90th	117	118	120	122	124	125	126	75	76	76	77	78	79	80
	95th	121	122	124	126	128	129	130	79	80	81	82	83	83	84
14	90th	120	121	123	125	126	128	128	76	76	77	78	79	80	80
	95th	124	125	127	128	130	132	132	80	81	81	82	83	84	85
15	90th	123	124	125	127	129	131	131	77	77	78	79	80	81	81
	95th	127	128	129	131	133	134	135	81	82	83	83	84	85	86
16	90th	125	126	128	130	132	133	134	79	79	80	81	82	82	83
	95th	129	130	132	134	136	137	138	83	83	84	85	86	87	87
17	90th	128	129	131	133	134	136	136	81	81	82	83	84	85	85
	95th	132	133	135	136	138	140	140	85	85	86	87	88	89	89

Source: National High Blood Pressure Education Program Working Group on Hypertension Control in Children and Adolescents. (1996). *Pediatrics, 98*, 649-658.

GIRLS AGED 1-17 YEARS: BLOOD PRESSURE LEVELS FOR THE 90TH AND 95TH PERCENTILES OF BLOOD PRESSURE BY PERCENTILES OF HEIGHT

Age, y	Blood Pressure Percentile	Systolic Blood Pressure by Percentile of Height, mm Hg							Diastolic Blood Pressure by Percentile of Height, mm Hg						
		5%	10%	25%	50%	75%	90%	95%	5%	10%	25%	50%	75%	90%	95%
1	90th	97	98	99	100	102	103	104	53	53	53	54	55	56	56
	95th	101	102	103	104	105	107	107	57	57	57	58	59	60	60
2	90th	99	99	100	102	103	104	105	57	57	58	58	59	60	61
	95th	102	103	104	105	107	108	109	61	61	62	62	63	64	65
3	90th	100	100	102	103	104	105	106	61	61	61	62	63	63	64
	95th	104	104	105	107	108	109	110	65	65	65	66	67	67	68
4	90th	101	102	103	104	106	107	108	63	63	64	65	65	66	67
	95th	105	106	107	108	109	111	111	67	67	68	69	69	70	71
5	90th	103	103	104	106	107	108	109	65	66	66	67	68	68	69
	95th	107	107	108	110	111	112	113	69	70	70	71	72	72	73
6	90th	104	105	106	107	109	110	111	67	67	68	69	69	70	71
	95th	108	109	110	111	112	114	114	71	71	72	73	73	74	75
7	90th	106	107	108	109	110	112	112	69	69	69	70	71	72	72
	95th	110	110	112	113	114	115	116	73	73	73	74	75	76	76
8	90th	108	109	110	111	112	113	114	70	70	71	71	72	73	74
	95th	112	112	113	115	116	117	118	74	74	75	75	76	77	78
9	90th	110	110	112	113	114	115	116	71	72	72	73	74	74	75
	95th	114	114	115	117	118	119	120	75	76	76	77	78	78	79
10	90th	112	112	114	115	116	117	118	73	73	73	74	75	76	76
	95th	116	116	117	119	120	121	122	77	77	77	78	79	80	80
11	90th	114	114	116	117	118	119	120	74	74	75	75	76	77	77
	95th	118	118	119	121	122	123	124	78	78	79	79	80	81	81
12	90th	116	116	118	119	120	121	122	75	75	76	76	77	78	78
	95th	120	120	121	123	124	125	126	79	79	80	80	81	82	82
13	90th	118	118	119	121	122	123	124	76	76	77	78	78	79	80
	95th	121	121	123	125	126	127	128	80	80	81	82	82	83	84
14	90th	119	120	121	122	124	125	126	77	77	78	79	79	80	81
	95th	123	123	125	126	128	129	130	81	81	82	83	83	84	85
15	90th	121	121	122	124	125	126	127	78	78	79	79	80	81	82
	95th	124	125	126	128	129	130	131	82	82	83	83	84	85	86
16	90th	122	122	123	125	126	127	128	79	79	79	80	81	82	82
	95th	125	126	127	128	130	131	132	83	83	83	84	85	86	86
17	90th	122	123	124	125	126	128	128	79	79	79	80	81	82	82
	95th	126	126	127	129	130	131	132	83	83	83	84	85	86	86

Source: National High Blood Pressure Education Program Working Group on Hypertension Control in Children and Adolescents. (1996). *Pediatrics, 98,* 649-658

C. Differential Diagnosis
1. Goal is to differentiate essential or primary hypertension from elevated blood pressure due to secondary causes; see II.B. for list of differential diagnoses
2. The younger the child and the higher the blood pressure, the greater the possibility of secondary hypertension

D. Diagnostic Tests: Initial laboratory tests should be directed to detecting or ruling out renal parenchymal disease, renovascular disease, and coarctation of the aorta
1. Most children should have a general laboratory screening for possible renal etiologies that includes a urinalysis, complete blood count, electrolytes, blood urea nitrogen, serum creatinine
    a. Usually a urine culture and renal ultrasound are ordered; always order if proteinuria is detected on urinalysis
    b. If screening tests and ultrasound are normal, renal scan (DTPA radionuclide) and arteriography should be ordered to further test for renovascular HTN
2. Order an echocardiogram and possibly an electrocardiogram (ECG); in children and adolescents an echocardiogram is more sensitive for detecting early cardiac effects of HTN than ECG
3. Order a lipid profile, particularly if there is a family history of hyperlipidemia
4. Consider ordering a chest x-ray
5. Thyroid function tests and catecholamines are needed if thyroid problems or pheochromocytoma are suspected
6. Less frequently ordered are renin levels, 24-hour urine collection for creatinine clearance and protein, 3-D computerized tomography, drug studies, magnetic resonance angiography, hormone studies, and exercise stress testing
7. Genetic types of hypertension such as glucocorticoid-remediable aldosteronism can be detected from blood sent to centers that perform genetic testing
8. Ambulatory Blood Pressure Monitoring (ABPM), providing round-the-clock BP measurements, is increasingly recognized as a useful tool; delineates patterns over time and is more accurate diagnostically than a single office BP measurement that may fluctuate with time of day, physical activity, emotional excitement, posture, or level of wakefulness

V. Plan/Management

A. Treat all causes of secondary hypertension immediately and aggressively, usually with consultation with a pediatric cardiologist and other specialists

B. Life style modifications should be introduced and used as initial therapy in children with essential hypertension; lifestyle modification should be a "**family affair**" – it is particularly hard for children and adolescents to follow strict rules for diet, exercise, and/or weight management if family support, encouragement, and participation are not present
1. Dietary recommendations
    a. Weight reduction in obese children
    b. Increase fresh fruits and vegetables in diet
    c. Eliminate added salt to home-cooked meals and reduce foods with high sodium content
    d. Decrease fat in diet; decrease access to "fast food" restaurants
    e. Entire family would benefit from following the DASH diet (see table that follows)
2. Regular exercise is recommended; uncomplicated, primary hypertension should not prevent asymptomatic children from participating in physical activities
3. Identification and reduction of stressors are important
4. Counsel about other risk factors for cardiovascular disease such as smoking
5. Strongly counsel against use of anabolic steroids

DASH Diet*

Food/Servings	Food Examples
Grains & grain products--7 to 8 daily	Whole wheat breads, English muffins, pita bread, bagels, cereals, oatmeal, grits
Fruits & vegetables--4 to 5 fruit servings daily; 4 to 5 vegetable servings daily	Apricots, bananas, grapes, oranges, grapefruit, melons, strawberries, tomatoes, peas, carrots, potatoes, broccoli, squash, leafy greens
Dairy foods (low-fat or nonfat)--2 to 3 daily	Skim or 1% milk, nonfat or low-fat yogurt, nonfat or part-skim cheese
Meats, poultry & fish--2 or fewer daily	Lean meats only; trim visible fat, remove skin from poultry; broil, roast or boil
Nuts, seeds & legumes--4 to 5 a week	Almonds, peanuts, mixed nuts, sunflower seeds, kidney beans, lentils

*For DASH diet details visit the following website: nhlbi.nih.gov/health/public/heart/hbp/dash/

Adapted from Joint National Committee on Detection, Evaluation, and Treatment of High Blood Pressure. (1997). The sixth report of the Joint National Committee on Detection, Evaluation, and Treatment of High Blood Pressure (JNV VI). *Archives of Internal Medicine, 157*, 24-14-2446.

C. Pharmacologic therapy (consultation with a specialist is recommended)
1. Medications are generally warranted for the following children:
   a. Those with persistent severe hypertension (BP levels above the 99th percentile)
   b. Those with high risk for organ injury such as patients with diabetes and renal disease with BP ≥90th percentile
2. Decision to begin medications should also take into consideration other risk factors for cardiovascular disease, evidence of end-organ damage, and family history; guidelines for drug therapy are not well established in children
3. Goal is to reduce BP to below the 95th percentile
4. Angiotensin-converting enzyme (ACE) inhibitors, calcium channel blockers (CCB), beta blockers, and diuretics are usually prescribed first; angiotensin receptor blockers (ARB) may be beneficial, but further research is needed in children
5. Individualize therapy based on level of BP, degree of response, occurrence of adverse effects, and child's medical history (see following table)

ANTIHYPERTENSIVE MEDICATIONS IN CHILDREN

Medication	Dose mg/kg/day	Dosing Interval	Route
Diuretics			
Hydrochlorothiazide	1-3	Q 12 hours	Oral
Furosemide	0.5-4	Q 6-12 hours	Oral
Metolazone	0.05-0.5	Q 12-24 hours	Oral
Spironolactone	1-3	Q 6-12 hours	Oral, intravenous
Adrenergic Blocking			
β Adrenergic blockers			
Metoprolol	1-4	Q 12-24 hours	Oral
Propranolol	0.5-5	Q 6-12 hours	Oral
Atenolol	1-2	Q 12-24 hours	Oral
α Blocker, Prazosin	0.05-0.5	Q 6-8 hours	Oral
α/β Blocker, Labetalol	1-3	Q 6-12 hours	Oral, intravenous
α-Agonist, Clonidine	5-25 µg/kg/day	Q 6 hours	Oral
Angiotensin-Converting Enzyme Inhibitor			
Captopril			
Neonates	0.03-2	Q 8-24 hours	Oral
Children	0.05-6	Q 8 hours	Oral
Enalapril	0.15-0.5	Q 12-24 hours	Oral
Ramipril[†]	1.25*-20**	Q 12-24 hours	Oral

(Continued)

ANTIHYPERTENSIVE MEDICATIONS IN CHILDREN (CONTINUED)

Medication	Dose mg/kg/day	Dosing Interval	Route
Calcium Channel Blockers			
Nifedipine	0.25-3	Q 12-24 hours	Oral
Isradipine	2.5*-20**	Q 8-12 hours	Oral
Amlodipine[†]	2.5*-10**	Q 24 hours	Oral
Vasodilators			
Hydralazine	0.75-7.5	Q 12-24 hours	Oral, intravenous
Minoxidil	0.1-1	Q 12 hours	Oral

* Total initial dose in milligrams
** Total daily dose in milligrams
[†] Pediatric dose is under investigation

Adapted from Adapted from Bonilla-Felix, M, Portman, R.J., & Falkner, B. (2002). Systemic hypertension. In F.D. Burg, J.R. Ingelfinger, R.A. Polin, & A.A. Gershon (Eds.). *Gellis & Kagan's current pediatric therapy.* Saunders: Philadelphia.
-AND-
National High Blood Pressure Education Program Working Group on Hypertension Control in Children and Adolescents. (1996). Update on the 1987 Task Force Report on High Blood Pressure in Children and Adolescents. *Pediatrics, 98,* 649-658.

6.   Choice of first drug also depends on specific cause of HTN (see table that follows)

INDICATIONS FOR ANTIHYPERTENSIVE DRUGS

Drug	Recommended For	Not Recommended For
Angiotensin-converting enzyme inhibitors	Diabetes mellitus Chronic glomerulonephritis Reflux nephropathy Unilateral renal artery stenosis Neonatal hypertension Congestive heart failure	Bilateral renal artery stenosis Post-transplant hypertension
Calcium channel blockers	Post-transplant hypertension Raynaud's disease Reactive airway disease	Congestive heart failure
Beta blockers	Essential hypertension Mitral valve prolapse	Reactive airway disease Diabetes mellitus Raynaud's disease
Diuretics	Acute glomerulonephritis Chronic renal failure Post-transplant hypertension Use with vasodilators	Athletes
α-Adrenergic antagonists	Pheochromocytoma	
Central α-agonists	Athletes Adolescents (transdermal)	Depression
Vasodilators	Neonatal hypertension Acute glomerulonephritis Congestive heart failure	

Adapted from Bonilla-Felix, M, Portman, R.J., & Falkner, B. (2002). Systemic hypertension. In F.D. Burg, J.R. Ingelfinger, R.A. Polin, & A.A. Gershon (Eds.). *Gellis & Kagan's current pediatric therapy.* Saunders: Philadelphia.

7.   Diuretics and beta-blockers were recommended as first-line drugs in the first Task Force Report and these drugs continue to be appropriate first line choices
8.   However, ACE inhibitors and calcium channel blockers have been gaining favor as drugs of first choice as they are often better tolerated in children
9.   ACE inhibitors
    a.   Do not prescribe in patients with bilateral renal artery stenosis or renal artery stenosis in a solitary or transplanted kidney
    b.   ACE inhibitors (and angiotensin II receptor blockers) have teratogenic risks with fetal exposure; use with extreme caution in adolescent girls who may be sexually active
10.   Calcium channel blockers (CCB) work well in children and adolescents
    a.   Short acting dihydropyridines, particularly nifedipine, should no longer be used because of increased risk of cardiac events as with adults
    b.   Extended release forms of the dihydropyridines are still used effectively in BP management and are better agents at reducing BP than the non-dihydropyridine derivatives

11. Beta-blockers may cause fatigue, an important problem for adolescent athletes, and cannot be taken by patients with reactive airway disease and those with fluid overload

12. Diuretics can cause deleterious effects of potassium, sodium, and water depletion and abnormalities in lipid and glucose metabolism

D. Acute hypertensive therapy consists of one of the following medications: IV sodium nitroprusside, IV labetalol, IV esmolol, IV diazoxide, IV hydralazine, oral minoxidil; IV nicardipine has replaced oral nifedipine as CCB of choice; consult specialist in pediatric hypertension for selection and dosage

E. Follow Up
1. Children with elevated blood pressure detected on screening should have blood pressure measured 2 more times before the diagnosis of hypertension is made
2. Ambulatory blood pressure monitoring (ABPM) may be more appropriate for initial work-up and early follow-up
3. Frequency of follow up is variable depending on patient characteristics, degree of BP elevation, etiology, and physiologic status
4. Generally, when BP is well-controlled, patient should be evaluated at least every 6 months; consider lowering doses or discontinuing medications at each visit depending on BP levels and clinical manifestations

INNOCENT HEART MURMURS

I. Definition: Vibrations of physiologic structures within the normal heart at rest that occur in the absence of structural or pathological cardiac disease

A. Murmur reflects the normal ejection pattern of blood from the ventricles; there is no obstruction in the outflow tract

B. Other synonymous terms are normal, functional, benign, innocuous, or physiological murmurs

II. Pathogenesis: Since the murmur is caused by turbulent blood flow in the normal heart under resting conditions, it is representative of a normal physiologic variance and no pathology is present

III. Clinical Presentation

A. Innocent heart murmurs occur in almost 50% of all school-aged children

B. Approximately 80% of all children with murmurs have one of the following innocent murmurs:
1. Classic vibratory murmur (Still's)
    a. Most common functional murmur heard in children 3-6 years old; uncommon before age 2 years, but heard in 50% of healthy children by age 3 or 4
    b. Characteristic feature is the vibratory, buzzing, twanging string quality
    c. Nonradiating, midsystolic, nonregurgitant, low-pitched murmur
    d. Heard best with the bell of the stethoscope when child is supine along the lower, left sternal edge, at the third to fourth left interspace; diminished in upright position
    e. When child holds breath or performs a Valsalva maneuver the murmur usually disappears
    f. Accompanied by normal first and second heart sounds and no extra sounds or other cardiac abnormalities
2. Venous hum
    a. Commonly occurs between 3 and 6 years of age
    b. Continuous murmur with a humming quality; heard loudest in diastole
    c. Maximally audible above and sometimes below the clavicle on one or both sides; only heard in sitting or standing position
    d. Can be obliterated by having child turn head to side, compressing external jugular vein, or assuming of supine position
    e. Normal second heart sound

3. Pulmonary flow murmur/pulmonary ejection murmur in childhood
   a. Common between ages 8-14 years but most frequent in adolescents
   b. Short, early to midsystolic murmur with 1-3/6 intensity and rough sound heard best at upper left sternal border
   c. Normal second heart sound and no associated thrill or click
4. Pulmonary flow murmur of newborn
   a. Frequently present in newborns, especially those with low birth weight; usually disappears by 3-6 months of age
   b. Only grade 1-2/6 intensity, but vibratory quality aids in assessment
   c. Heard best in pulmonic area but radiates to both axilla and back
5. Carotid bruit
   a. Found in children of any age
   b. Early systolic ejection murmur, grade 2-3/6 intensity, and although rare, a faint thrill (palpable sensation) may be palpable over carotid artery
   c. Heard best above clavicles or over carotid arteries
   d. Normal second heart sound
6. Pulmonary soufflé or mammary arterial soufflé
   a. Occurs in adolescence and in young adult females who are pregnant or lactating
   b. Soft, blowing, early to midsystolic murmur heard best in the pulmonic area
   c. Heard in high cardiac output states such as fever, anemia, or hyperthyroidism

IV. Diagnosis/Evaluation

A. History
   1. Key question: Time of first appearance and circumstances of its discovery
   2. Ask about symptoms related to cardiovascular dysfunction such as failure to thrive, syncope, chest pain, palpitation, and shortness of breath
   3. Question regarding child's activity level and endurance; in an infant, question about ability to vigorously suck when feeding
   4. Carefully take comprehensive prenatal and perinatal histories
   5. Obtain a complete medical history including past hospitalizations, frequency of infections, and previous illnesses
   6. Inquire about family history, particularly explore history of hypertrophic cardiomyopathy, congenital cardiac disease, and unexplained death at any age

B. Physical Examination
   1. Observe general appearance and nutritional status, assessing skin for temperature, turgor, and moisture
   2. Inspect skin for color; differentiate central from peripheral cyanosis
      a. Central cyanosis denotes an elevated percentage of reduced hemoglobin in arterial blood and usually requires referral to cardiologist; observe for cyanosis in inner portion of lips, tongue, and nail beds
      b. Peripheral cyanosis or acrocyanosis is related to a normal level of reduced hemoglobin and normal oximetry readings; cyanosis may be present in healthy children around mouth and on hands and feet
   3. Measure temperature, pulse rate, and respiratory rate
   4. Measure blood pressure in both arms and legs
   5. Examine neck for thyromegaly and distended veins
   6. Auscultate neck for bruits; palpate the cardiac apex while simultaneously listening to bruit to differentiate a bruit from a murmur; a radiating murmur will be synchronous with apical impulse whereas a bruit will occur later
   7. Inspect chest for precordial bulge and observe for asymmetry of chest which reflects long-standing enlargement of the heart
   8. Palpate chest for thrill or heave and locate point of maximal impulse (PMI)
   9. Auscultate heart
   10. Perform techniques to elicit murmurs
      a. Compare murmur when patient is standing versus sitting
      b. Listen to murmur when child squats for 30 seconds and then when child quickly rises to a standing position
      c. Listen in both the sitting position with child leaning forward and in the left lateral position; both positions bring the heart closer to the chest wall
      d. Ask child to perform Valsalva maneuver by exhaling and holding breath midway through cycle
      e. In young children, passive raising of the legs to about 45° is helpful

11. Assess the murmur for following characteristics (see table below)

CHARACTERISTICS OF CARDIAC MURMURS	
Characteristic	**Examples**
Timing	Relative position within cardiac cycle; relationship to S_1 and S_2 (systolic, diastolic, continuous)
Quality	Presence of harmonics and overtones (harsh, soft, vibratory, musical)
Intensity	Loudness; (see table below on grades of murmurs): Systolic graded on scale of I to VI (1-6) Diastolic graded on scale of I to IV (1-4)
Duration	Length (midsystolic, holosystolic)
Location	Anatomic landmarks; loudest at site of origin (mitral, tricuspid, aortic, pulmonic areas)
Radiation of sound	Direction of murmur; use anatomic landmarks (to axilla, to right neck, to apex)
Pattern	Dynamic shape (crescendo/decrescendo, square, or plateau)
Pitch	Frequency range (low, medium, high)

12. Grade the murmur based on degree of loudness and presence of a thrill

GRADES OF HEART MURMURS	
Grade I	Very faint; may not be heard in all positions
Grade II	Quiet, but clearly audible
Grade III	Moderately loud, but not associated with a thrill
Grade IV	Loud and may be associated with a thrill
Grade V	Very loud and associated with an easily palpable thrill
Grade VI	Heard with stethoscope off the chest; accompanied with audible and visible thrill

13. Perform a complete lung exam
14. Palpate abdomen for organomegaly
15. Examine extremities for pulses, edema, color, and clubbing of nails

C. Differential Diagnosis:
   1. Crucial to distinguish a pathological murmur from an innocent murmur; quality and characteristics of murmur do not always provide reliable criteria for diagnosis
      a. Atrial septal defects, hypertrophic cardiomyopathy, and coarctation of aorta produce relatively unimpressive murmurs yet indicate significant pathology
      b. It is more likely a pathology requiring a cardiac consultation if one or more of the following are present with the murmur: Symptoms, abnormal cardiac size or silhouette or abnormal pulmonary vasculature, abnormal ECG, diastolic murmur, a particularly loud systolic murmur, cyanosis, abnormally strong or weak pulses, abnormal heart sounds or extra sounds
   2. Patient's age at onset of murmur and physical findings help to differentiate pathological murmurs from innocent murmurs
      a. Consider all murmurs in infants less than one year as pathological until proven otherwise
      b. In first year of life, poor feeding, excessive irritability, tachypnea, and central cyanosis are signs suggestive of cardiovascular instability

3.   The following table illustrates the differential diagnosis of abnormal murmurs

DIFFERENTIAL DIAGNOSIS OF ABNORMAL MURMURS*		
Timing of Murmur	**Pathology**	**Characteristics**
Systolic		
Midsystolic	Pulmonic stenosis	Variable click, radiates to left sternal border, left neck
	Aortic stenosis	Loud, harsh, crescendo/decrescendo, radiates to right neck, apex
	Atrial septal defect	Systolic ejection murmur with diastolic rumble, wide fixed S_2, radiates to left lower sternal border
	Ventricular septal defect (VSD) (small)	Blowing, radiates to left lower sternal border
	Coarctation	Weak femoral pulses
Late systolic	Mitral valve prolapse (MVP)	Murmur may or may not be present, variable apical click
	Hypertrophic obstructive cardiomyopathy (HOCM)	Crescendo/decrescendo; biphasic carotid pulse
Holosystolic	Ventricular septal defect (VSD)	Regurgitant systolic, well localized at left lower sternal border, thrill often present
	Mitral regurgitation	Blowing murmur, radiates to left axilla, heard best in apex
Diastolic		
Early diastolic	Tricuspid stenosis	Decrescendo; radiates to apex and xiphoid area
	Aortic regurgitation	Decrescendo; radiates to apex and left sternal border
	Pulmonary regurgitation	Decrescendo; radiates to apex
Mid-diastolic	Mitral stenosis	Crescendo, no radiation
Continuous	Patent ductus arteriosus (PDA)	Bounding pulses, systolic-diastolic murmur, localized below left clavicle, may be associated with a thrill

* Patients with abnormal murmurs are usually referred to a cardiologist

D.   Diagnostic Tests: Innocent heart murmurs often do not need diagnostic tests. If there is any question about the type of murmur consider the following:
1.   Echocardiogram is ordered if child is thought to have cardiac disease or if diagnosis is uncertain (American Academy of Pediatrics recommends that all echocardiograms be evaluated by a pediatric cardiologist)
2.   Electrocardiogram and chest x-ray; all innocent heart murmurs are associated with normal ECG and x-ray findings
3.   In some cases, consider hemoglobin level to determine anemia or polycythemia which is a sensitive indicator for chronic hypoxemia
4.   Once diagnosis of innocent murmur is made, no further diagnostic tests are needed

V.   Plan/Management

A.   If murmur type or suspicion of physiological versus pathological origin is uncertain, studies have found that the most cost-effective approach is referral to a pediatric cardiologist

B.   Emphasize to parents that the child does not have heart disease and that nearly half of all children have an innocent murmur; inform parents that the murmur may become louder when the child has a fever or strenuously exercises; stress that the child does not need antibiotic prophylaxis against endocarditis when visiting the dentist nor should child limit activities due to risk of sudden death

C.   Follow Up: Assess child at each health maintenance visit, carefully documenting the characteristics of the murmur over time
1.   Re-assess for changes in intensity, timing, location, transmission, and quality from that of baseline assessment, indicating need for referral
2.   Continued assessment as child ages is necessary to determine whether the murmur follows its projected course as discussed in section III.B. -- if not, referral to pediatric cardiologist is needed

PRESYNCOPE/SYNCOPE

I.   Definitions:

    A.   Presyncope or Near Syncope: Sensation of dizziness, lightheadedness and an impending loss of consciousness

    B.   Syncope: Sudden transient loss of consciousness and loss of postural tone and motor control with spontaneous recovery

II.   Pathogenesis

    A.   Usually due to any mechanism that decreases cerebral blood flow; results in decreased delivery of oxygen and nutrients to brain

    B.   Pathophysiologic abnormalities underlying presyncope/syncope
        1.   Neurocardiogenic types of syncope are associated with a reflex-mediated, vasomotor instability resulting from a decrease in vascular resistance and/or venous return causing peripheral venous and arterial pooling and subsequent decreased cerebral perfusion.
            a.   Conditions are usually benign and include vasovagal episodes, situational crises, orthostatic hypotension, drugs, and carotid sinus disorders
            b.   Simple faint (also referred to as vasovagal or vasodepressor syncope is the most common cause of presyncope/syncope
                (1)   Accounts for 20-40% of all syncopal episodes
                (2)   Due to psychological activation of the stress-mediated autonomic system that causes an intense vagal drive and transient decrease in cardiac output
        2.   Cardiac causes are associated with decreased cardiac output or obstruction of blood flow within the heart or pulmonary circulation
            a.   Electrical etiology such as arrhythmias and heart block are possible causes
            b.   Mechanical etiology such as idiopathic hypertrophic subaortic stenosis (IHSS) now referred to as hypertrophic obstructive cardiomyopathy (HOCM), valvular diseases, and, although rare, myocardial ischemia or infarction secondary to congenital anomalies or acquired disease (Kawasaki's disease) of the coronary artery may cause syncope
        3.   Neurologic, vascular, or psychogenic causes include cerebrovascular diseases (due to hypoperfusion of the vertebrobasilar vascular system), subclavian steal syndrome, seizures, migraines, and psychiatric illnesses
        4.   Metabolic causes such as hypoglycemia and hypoxia may result in syncope, however, these disorders usually lead to somnolence and coma rather than syncope

    C.   In contrast to adults, in whom most cases are due to vascular or cardiovascular problems, in children and adolescents, most incidents of syncope are benign, resulting from vaso-vagal episodes (most common), orthostatic syncope, hyperventilation, and breath holding

    D.   The prevalence of syncope and near syncope in children is unknown, but may be as high as 3% of emergency room visits

    E.   Recurrent episodes of unexplained syncope may cause functional impairment and possible serious injury to the child and may produce tremendous psychological stress for the child and the family

III. Clinical Presentation of important causes of presyncope/syncope

    A.   Vasovagal or vasodepressor syncope
        1.   Often precipitated by trigger events that include noxious stimuli, unpleasant sights or smells, fear, anxiety, anticipated pain, alcohol, a large meal, micturition, defecation, cough, sneezing, or swallowing
        2.   Symptoms occur in the standing or seated position
        3.   Typically child has prodromal symptoms such as nausea, warmth, lightheadedness, weakness, diaphoresis, constriction of visual fields, epigastric discomfort, and a sensation of impending faint
        4.   At first, child has increased heart rate, but then becomes bradycardic; combination of tachycardia followed by bradycardia (overdrive suppression) produces the syncope

5. Unconsciousness is usually brief (seconds to minutes once the child reaches the supine position) and in the recovery stage the child may have weakness, lightheadedness, or fatigue, but no confusion or signs of injury; usually after the episode, the child remembers the event and does not have loss of bowel and bladder control
6. Occasionally, hypotension and hypoperfusion are so profound that cerebral hypoxia and seizure activity occur, but there is no loss of consciousness or only a brief loss of consciousness

B. Orthostatic hypotension is common
   1. Reflex vasoconstriction and increase in heart rate fail to occur when the child stands, leading to inadequate cerebral perfusion
   2. Defined as systolic blood pressure fall of 20 mm Hg or more on standing
   3. Possible etiologic factors:
      a. Condition may be idiopathic; often this type occurs after the child has been exposed to a warm environment
      b. Medications such as diuretics or bronchodilators
      c. Blood loss often due to a gastrointestinal bleed
      d. Dehydration

C. Drug-induced syncope is most likely when adolescents are taking vasodilators, β-blockers, analgesics, and central nervous system antidepressants, or illicit drugs

D. Carotid sinus hypersensitivity is associated with pressure on carotid sinus that can occur with tumors and tissue scars in neck causing marked reflex bradycardia

E. Typical presentation of syncope due to cardiac disease
   1. Symptoms often worsen on standing and improve with lying down; however, patients with arrhythmias may have symptoms when supine
   2. May have generalized weakness, fatigue, and pallor; some children are asymptomatic
   3. Sudden onset without warning, sensation of rapid heart action without aura, or seizure may occur
   4. Exertional or effort syncope are common manifestations with valvular aortic stenosis; patients with HOCM may also experience effort syncope

F. Syncope from arrhythmias is rare in children
   a. Although uncommon, certain children with apparently normal hearts may have syncope due to arrhythmias from the following causes: Long QT syndrome, Wolff-Parkinson-White (WPW), right ventricular dysplasia (right ventricular cardiomyopathy)
   b. Children with congenital and acquire heart conditions may also have arrhythmias that result in syncope
   c. If arrhythmias occur the child presents with brief loss of consciousness, lack of prodrome, and palpitations

G. Subclavian steal syndrome --a child who has had surgery that sacrificed a subclavian artery, such as Blalock-Taussig shunt and subclavian flap aortoplasty for coarctation repair, may develop the syndrome during adulthood.
   1. Occurs as a result of an occlusion of proximal subclavian artery leading to reversal of flow in the adjacent vertebral artery during arm exercise
   2. Blood flow is redirected from brain and ischemic symptoms develop
   3. Syncope occurs with arm exercise

H. Syncope from cerebrovascular occlusive disease is extremely rare in children

I. Seizures
   1. May have signs and symptoms of blue face, frothing at mouth, myoclonic jerks, tongue biting, tonic spasms, staring, or repetitive facial grimacing which are not common with other types of syncope
   2. Commonly associated with warning symptoms (auras) such as certain smells, sounds or visual cues; these warning *symptoms* differ from the *triggers* that can initiate a sudden vasovagal/vasodepressive syncopal episode
   3. After seizure, postictal symptoms such as disorientation and headache are common

J. Psychological distress often involves circumoral numbness and digital paresthesia
   1. History of generalized anxiety disorder, panic disorder, somatization, or depression is common
   2. Estimated that up to 20% of patients presenting with syncope have psychiatric illness

3. Hysteria, a form of conversion reaction, may result in apparent loss of consciousness, especially if an audience is present, and is characterized by a graceful fainting to the floor while exhibiting otherwise normal vital signs and physical findings

IV. Diagnosis/Evaluation (see also section on DIZZINESS)

A. History; important to determine whether child has serious disorder (e.g., cardiac disease, gastrointestinal bleeding, intracranial tumor) or a benign condition
1. Ask child to briefly describe in own words the sensation he/she experiences
2. If possible obtain a description of the episode and events preceding the episode from a witness
3. Differentiate feelings of fainting from vertigo, imbalance, fatigue, weakness, or anxiety; specifically ask the following types of questions:
    a. Is there a sensation of movement or rotation? (vertigo)
    b. Is the sensation similar to when you get out of bed too quickly? (orthostatic hypotension)
    c. Does it feel like you can't keep your balance? (disequilibrium)
4. Ask about frequency of syncopal or near syncopal episodes, even though frequency does not correlate well with specific causes
5. Ask about duration of episode; brief duration is more common with vestibular disorders
6. Inquire about associated symptoms such as hearing loss, heart palpitations, neurological problems
7. Determine if sensation occurs after exertion or when one arises to a sitting or standing position
    a. Disequilibrium occurs primarily when one is standing or walking
    b. Benign positional vertigo often occurs with a change of position or when lying down
8. Determine precipitants such as cough with loss of consciousness (post-tussive syncope), emptying of distended bladder (postmicturition syncope), warm, crowded environment (simple faint), or shaving or tight collar (carotid sinus hypersensitivity)
9. Ask about symptoms occurring after episode; disorientation after an event is most common in children who have seizures
10. Inquire about past medical history including history of cardiac disease or risk factors, trauma, infection, seizures, thyroid disease, metabolic problems, anxiety, and medication/drug use

B. Physical Examination
1. Vital signs should include check for orthostatic hypotension (see following table)

DETERMINING ORTHOSTATIC HYPOTENSION

✓ Measure in lying (ideally) or sitting position first

✓ Measure immediately after standing and then, after patient stands for 2-5 minutes, measure again

✓ Normally, systolic pressure falls no more than 10 mm Hg, diastolic pressure rises 2-5 mm Hg, and heart rate increases 5-20 beats (if there is no increase in heart rate, consider a cardiac problem). A drop in systolic pressure of 20 mm Hg or more indicates orthostasis

---

2. Measure blood pressure in both arms and both legs; differences in pulse intensity and blood pressure (more than 20 mm Hg) in arms versus legs coarctation of the aorta
3. Perform cardiac examination noting forceful left ventricular impulse, murmurs, or arrhythmias
4. Perform a thorough neurological examination
5. Perform dizziness simulation tests such as following:
    a. Valsalva maneuver
    b. Carotid sinus massages help to determine autonomic impairment; tests should be done cautiously in facilities where cardiac monitoring and emergency equipment are available; if child has history of cardiac or cardiovascular disease, massage should be performed by a specialist
6. Determine if hyperventilation evokes symptomatology by asking child to breathe rapidly for 1-3 minutes
7. Complete psychological examination may be helpful

C. Differential Diagnoses
1. Epilepsy
2. Convulsive syncope
3. Dizziness: one way to sort out the various etiologies of dizziness is to differentiate the sensations the child experiences into 3 categories:
    a. Presyncope: Feeling of lightheadedness or feeling that one is about to faint
    b. Vertigo: Sensation of abnormal movements of the body or surroundings

       c.   Disequilibrium or imbalance due to multiple sensory deficits: Sensation of feeling drunk, seasick, or unsteady on one's feet; subtle, enduring symptom that one cannot keep balance and might fall; child will have frequent falling, near-falling, or bumping into things from a combination of visual, hearing, sensory, and/or motor impairment

    4.   Hypoglycemia
    5.   Hyperventilation
    6.   Hysteria

D.   Diagnostic Tests; routine laboratory testing is not recommended; instead, laboratory testing should be done based on results of history and physical examination
    1.   Electrocardiogram (ECG) should be core of the workup for most patients
    2.   Consider pregnancy testing in adolescent females of child-bearing age, especially those for whom tilt table or electrophysiologic testing is being considered
    3.   Tilt-testing may be frightening to the child
        a.   Upright tilt testing at 60-80° for at least a 15 minute baseline tilt or for 45 minutes is ordered in patients in whom cardiac causes of syncope have been excluded and who have infrequent syncopal episodes
        b.   Tilt-table testing with isoproterenol is recommended for patients with negative results on passive tilt-table test who have a high pretest probability of neurally mediated syncope; it is not clear whether prolonged tilt procedures of 45-60 minutes offer better specificity or sensitivity compared with shorter tilt periods and the addition of isoproterenol or adenosine
    4.   Order 24-hour Holter monitor or prolonged ambulatory continuous-loop ECG recordings using an Event monitor (patient activates system when a syncopal episode occurs) in patients who have the following:
        a.   Normal heart and frequent episodes of syncope
        b.   Heart disease or an abnormal ECG or symptoms suggestive of arrhythmias
    5.   Echocardiogram is useful for detecting suspected heart disease such as valve dysfunction or congenital anomaly
    6.   Exercise stress testing is important in adolescents experiencing exertional syncope
    7.   Intracardiac electrophysiologic studies are needed when symptoms are suggestive of cardiac syncope, but no abnormality is uncovered with noninvasive tests
    8.   Computerized tomography (CT) scan or magnetic resonance imaging (MRI) is warranted if intracranial abnormalities (patient has focal neurologic signs) are suspected
    9.   Electroencephalogram (EEG) may be indicated to detect seizure disorders
    10.   Lung ventilation-perfusion is reserved for patients with suspected pulmonary embolism
    11.   Consider other tests such as fasting blood glucose, hematocrit/hemoglobin, electrolytes, toxicology screens, and stool for occult blood based on child's symptomatology

V.   Plan/Management

A.   Placing child in supine position until circulatory crisis resolves may be all that is indicated; if child feels the prodrome to a faint, he or she should be told to lie down and raise feet above the chest; usually aborts the syncope

B.   Admit to hospital children with known serious cardiovascular anomalies; consider hospitalization for patients with disabling episodes of syncope, patients who have symptoms suggestive of pulmonary embolus, patients who have sudden loss of consciousness with injury, rapid pulses, or exertional syncope

C.   Depending on etiological factors, consultation with a specialist is often needed

D.   The following medications are sometimes successful in preventing syncope: Pseudoephedrine, metoprolol (Lopressor), fludrocortisone (Florinef), disopyramide (Norpace), or scopolamine; consult specialist for specific drug indications and dosage

E.   Questionable beneficial effects of an implanted pacemaker for intractable syncope: some investigators have reported positive results, but results have not been corroborated by others---it seems that even though the pacemaker maintains heart rate, blood pressure drops and symptoms still occur

F.   Patients with recurrent, disabling episodes of vasovagal syncope may benefit from the following medications (consult specialist for dosages):
    1.   Medications such as β-blockers (metoprolol [Lopressor or Toprol XL], atenolol [Tenormin] or anticholinergic agents [transdermal scopolamine, one patch every 2-3 days])

2. If symptoms are not relieved by first-line drugs, consider the following:
   a. Fludrocortisone acetate (Florinef); contraindicated in patients with congestive heart failure
   b. Midodrine (ProAmatine) is specific for orthostatic hypotension; may use in combination therapy with Florinef
   c. Fluoxetine (Prozac)
3. Measures to expand volume include increased salt intake and custom-fitted counter pressure support garments from ankle to waist
4. Atrioventricular pacing can be considered in patients with clinically important bradycardia in response to upright tilt testing or in variable tachy-brady syndromes

G. Orthostatic hypotension
   1. Prevention
      a. Wear elastic stockings, only if patient feels they help; there are no randomized control trials to date that indicate compression stockings add a statistically significant beneficial effect
      b. Change positions slowly
      c. Sleep with head of bed elevated
      d. Exercise legs before standing
      e. Eat multiple small meals
      f. Avoid alcohol
      g. Avoid hot environments and hot showers or baths
      h. Stay well hydrated
   2. Treatment: Medications in section V.D. may be prescribed if symptoms are more disabling

H. Advise patient not to drive automobiles until symptoms are resolved; refer to laws in each state for clinician's responsibilities in reporting condition

I. Follow up is variable depending on diagnosis

REFERENCES

Advani, N., Menahem, S., & Wilkinson, J.L. (2000). The diagnosis of innocent murmurs in childhood. *Cardiology in the Young, 10,* 340-342.

Alexson, C.G., Manning, J. A., & Fioravanti, J.L. (2001). Heart murmurs. In R.A. Hoekelman (Ed.) *Primary pediatric care* (4th ed.), St.Louis: Mosby

ALLHAT Officers and Coordinators for the ALLHAT Collaborative Research Group. (2002). Major outcomes in high-risk hypertensive patients randomized to angiotensin-converting enzyme inhibitor or calcium channel blocker vs. diuretic: The antihypertensive and lipid-lowering treatment to prevent heart attack trial (ALLHAT). *JAMA, 288,* 2981-2997.

Biffi, M., Boriani, G., Bronzetti, G., Frabetti, L., Picchio, F.M., & Branzi, A. (2001). Neurocardiogenic syncope in selected pediatric patients—natural history, long-term follow-up, and effect of prophylactic pharmacological therapy. *Cardiovascular Drugs & Therapy, 15,* 161-167.

Bonilla-Felix, M., Portman, R.J., & Falkner, B. (2002). Systemic hypertension. In F.D. Burg, J.R. Ingelfinger, R.A. Polin, & A.A. Gershon. (Eds.). *Gellis & Kagan's current pediatric therapy,* (17th ed.). Philadelphia: Saunders.

Buzzard, C.J., & Lipshultz, S.E. (2001). High blood pressure in infants, children, and adolescents. In R.A. Hoekelman (Ed.) *Primary pediatric care* (4th ed.), St.Louis: Mosby

Chobanian, A.V., Bakris, G.L., Black, H.R., Cushman, W.C., Green, L.A., Izzo, J.L., Jr., et al. (2003). The seventh report of the Joint National Committee on Prevention, Detection, Evaluation, and Treatment of High Blood Pressure: The JNC 7 report. *JAMA, 289,* 2560-2572.

Cohn, H.E. (1999). Chest pain. In R.A. Dershewitz (Ed.), *Ambulatory pediatric care* (3rd ed.). Philadelphia: Lippincott-Raven.

Daniels, S.R. (2002). Cardiovascular sequelae of childhood hypertension. *American Journal of Hypertension, 15*(Suppl.), 61S-63S.

Driscoll, D., Allen, H.D., Atkins, D.L., Brenner, J., Dunnigan, A., Franklin, W., Gutgesell, P., et al. (1994). Guidelines for evaluation and management of common congenital cardiac problems in infants, children, and adolescents: A statement for healthcare professionals from the Committee on Congenital Cardiac Defects of the Council on Cardiovascular Disease in the Young, American Heart Association. *Circulation, 90,* 2180-2188.

Epperly, T.D., & Fogarty, J.P. (2001). Syncope. In M.B. Mengel & L.P. Schwiebert (Eds.). *Ambulatory medicine: The primary care of families* (3rd ed.). New York: Lange Medical Books/McGraw-Hill.

Evangelista, J.A., Parsons, M., & Renneburg, A.K. (2000). Chest pain in children: Diagnosis through history and physical examination. *Journal of Pediatric Care, 14*, 3-8.

Feit, L.R. (1997). The heart of the matter: Evaluating murmurs in children. *Contemporary Pediatrics, 14*(10), 97-122.

Flynn, J.T. (2002). Pharmacologic management of childhood hypertension: Current status, future challenges. *American Journal of Hypertension, 15*(Suppl.), 30S-33S.

Frazier, J.P., Yetman, R.J., & Huang, D. (2001). Syncope in adolescent girls. *Clinical Pediatrics, 40*, 457-460.

Goroll, A.H., May, L.A., & Mulley, A.G. (2000). Evaluation of chest pain. In A.H. Goroll & A.G. Mulley, Jr. (Eds). *Primary care medicine.* Philadelphia: Lippincott/Williams & Wilkins.

Gutgesell, H.P., Barst, R.J., Humes, R.A., Franklin, W.H., & Shaddy, R.E. (1997). Common cardiovascular problems in the young: Part I. Murmurs, chest pain, syncope, and irregular rhythms. *American Family Physician, 56,* 1825-1830

Kalayoglu, M.V., Libby, P., & Byrne, G.I. (2002). *Chlamydia pneumoniae* as an emerging risk factor in cardiovascular disease. *JAMA, 288,* 2724-2731.

Kay, J.D., Sinaiko, A.R., & Daniles, S. R. (2001). Pediatric hypertension. *American Heart Journal, 142,* 422-32.

Kenny, K. (2000). Heart murmurs in children: A systematic approach to cardiac evaluation. *Advance for Nurse Practitioners, 8,* 26-31.

Killeen, P. (2002). Practical evaluation of pediatric heart murmurs. *Journal of the American Academy of Physician Assistants, 15,* 24-26, 31-32, 35-36.

Kris-Etherton, P.M., Harris, W.S., Appel, L.J. for Nutrition Committee. (2002). Fish consumption, fish oil, omega-3 fatty acids, and cardiovascular disease. *Circulation, 106,* 2747-2757.

Kushner, I., & Sehgal, A.R. (2002). Is high-sensitivity C-reactive protein and effective screening test for cardiovascular risk? *Archives of Internal Medicine, 162,* 867-869.

Lagi, A., Cencetti, S., Corsoni, V., Georgiadis, D., & Bacalli, S. (2001). Cerebral vasoconstriction in vasovagal syncope: any link with symptoms? A transcranial Doppler study. *Circulation, 104,* 2694-2698.

Lam, J.C., & Tobias, J.D. (2001). Follow-up survey of children and adolescents with chest pain. *Southern Medical Journal, 94,* 921-924.

Lehrer, S. (2002). *Understanding pediatric heart sounds.* Philadelphia: W.B. Saunders.

Meyer, K., Galler, A., Lietz, R., & Siekmeyer, W. (2001). Neurocardiogenic syncope in a 10-year-old boy. *Pediatric Cardiology, 22,* 415-416.

Meyer, T.E., Chung, E.S., & Gaasch, W.H. (2001). Evaluation and management of patients with heart failure in clinical practice. In R. Becker & J. Alpert (Eds.), *Cardiovascular medicine: Practice and management.* New York: Arnold.

Morris, J.A., Blount, R.L., Brown, R.T., & Campbell, R.M. (2001). Association of parental psychological and behavioral factors and children's syncope. *Journal of Consulting & Clinical Psychology, 69,* 851-857.

National Cholesterol Education Program (NCEP), National Institutes of Health, National Heart, Lung, and Blood Institute. (2001). *Executive summary of the third report of the National Cholesterol Education Program (NCEP) Expert Panel on Detection, Evaluation, and Treatment of High Blood Cholesterol in Adults (Adult Treatment Panel III).* NIH Publication No. 01-3305. Bethesda, MD: US Government Printing Office.

National High Blood Pressure Education Program Working Group on Hypertension Control in Children and Adolescents. (1996). Update on the 1987 task force report on high blood pressure in children and adolescents: A working group report from the National High Blood Pressure Education Program. *Pediatrics, 98,* 649-658.

National High Blood Pressure Education Program, National Institutes of Health, National Heart, Lung, and Blood Institute. (1997). *The Sixth Report of the Joint National Committee on Detection, Evaluation, and Treatment of High Blood Pressure* NIH Publication No. 98-4080. Bethesda, MD: US Government Printing Office.

Nehal, U.S., & Ingelfinger, J.R. (2002). Pediatric Hypertension: Recent literature. *Current Opinions in Pediatrics, 14,* 189-196.

Nutrition Committee of the AHA. (2000). AHA dietary guidelines: Revision 2000: A statement for healthcare professionals from the nutrition committee of the American Heart Association. *Circulation, 102,* 2284-2299.

Ockene, J.K., & Ockene, I.S. (2001). Primary prevention of cardiovascular disease: Helping patients change lifestyle behaviors. In R. Becker & J. Alpert (Eds.), *Cardiovascular medicine: Practice and management.* New York: Arnold.

Park, M.K. (2002). *The pediatric cardiology handbook.* St. Louis, Mosby.

Park, M.K., & Troxler, R.G. (2002). Syncope. In M.K. Park & R.G. Troxler (Eds.), *Pediatric cardiology for practitioners* (4th ed.). St.Louis: Mosby.

Park, M.K., & Troxler, R.G. (2002). Systemic hypertension. In M.K. Park & R.G. Troxler (Eds.), *Pediatric cardiology for practitioners* (4th ed.). St.Louis: Mosby.

Pelech, A.N. (1998). The cardiac murmur: When to refer? *Pediatric Clinics of North America, 45,* 107-122.

Sacks, F.M., Svetkey, L.P., & Vollmer, W.M. (2001). Effects on blood pressure of reduced dietary sodium and the dietary approaches to stop hypertension (DASH) diet. *New England Journal of Medicine, 344,* 3-10.

Schroeder, S.A. (2001) . Chest pain. In R.A. Hoekelman (Ed.). *Primary pediatric care* (4th ed.), St.Louis: Mosby.

Sheldon, R., Rose, S., Ritchie, D., Connolly, S.J., Koshman, M., & Lee, M.A. (2002). Historical criteria that distinguish syncope from seizures. *Journal of the American College of Cardiology, 40,* 142-143.

Sloane, P.D., Coeytaux, R.R., Beck, R.S., & Dallara, J. (2001). Dizziness: State of the science. *Annals of Internal Medicine, 134,* 823-832.

Sorof, J.M. (2002). Prevalence and consequence of systolic hypertension in children. *American Journal of Hypertension,* 15(Suppl.), 57S-60S.

Swenson, JM., Fischer, DR., Miller, SA., et al. (1997). Are chest radiographs and electrocardiograms still valuable in evaluating new pediatric patients with heart murmurs or chest pain? *Pediatrics, 99,* 1-3.

Talner, N.S., & Carboni, M.P. (2000). Chest pain in the adolescent and young adult. *Cardiology in Review, 8,* 49-56.

Umbereen, S., Nehal, M.D., Ingelfinger, J.R. (2002). Pediatric hypertension: Recent literature. *Current Opinion in Pediatrics, 14,* 189-196.

US Preventive Services Task Force (USPSTF). (2003). Screening for high blood pressure: Recommendations and rationale. Rockville, MD: Agency for Healthcare Quality (AHRQ). Available at http://www.guideline.gov/summary

Wells, T.G. (2002). Antihypertensive therapy: Basic pharmacokinetic and pharmacodynamic principles as applied to infants and children. *American Journal of Hypertension,* 15(Suppl.), 34S-37S.

Whelton, P.K., He, J., Appel, L.J., Cutler, J.A., Havas, S., Kotchen, T.A., et al. (2002). Primary prevention of hypertension: Clinical and public health advisory from the National High Blood Pressure Education Program. *JAMA, 288,* 1882-1888.

Williams, C.L., Hayman, L.L., Daniels, S.R., Robinson, T.N., Steinberger, J., Paridon, S., et al. (2002). Cardiovascular health in childhood: A statement for health professionals from the Committee on Atherosclerosis, Hypertension, and Obesity in Young (AHOY) of the Council on Cardiovascular Disease in the Young, American Heart Association. *Circulation, 106,* 143-160.

Gastrointestinal Problems

MARY VIRGINIA GRAHAM

Viral Hepatitis

<u>Parasitic Infections of the Intestine</u>
Ascariasis (Roundworm Infection)

Enterobiasis (Pinworm Infection)

ACUTE AND RECURRENT ABDOMINAL PAIN IN CHILDREN

I.   Definition: Acute pain is defined as recent onset of severe abdominal pain; recurrent pain is three or more discrete episodes of abdominal pain in children between the ages of 4-16 years, which persists for greater than a three-month period

II.   Pathogenesis

      A.   Viral gastroenteritis is the most common cause of acute abdominal pain in any age group beyond the neonatal period

      B.   Other common causes of acute pain for different age groups
            1.   Children <2 years of age: Trauma, intussusception, incarcerated hernia, urinary tract infection, and intestinal malrotation
            2.   Children 2-5 years of age: Right lower lobe pneumonia, constipation, urinary tract infection, and sickling syndromes
            3.   Children >5 years: Appendicitis (peak incidence is between 10-15 years) and constipation
            4.   Adolescents: Appendicitis, mittelschmerz (ovulatory pain), ectopic pregnancy, tubo-ovarian pathologic conditions
            5.   Less common occurrences in all age groups: Pancreatitis, cholecystitis, renal stones, peptic ulcer disease

      C.   Common causes of recurrent pain
            1.   Chronic constipation is the most common cause
            2.   Dysmenorrhea
            3.   Musculoskeletal pain
            4.   Lactose intolerance
            5.   Peptic ulcer disease
            6.   Functional abdominal pain (recurrent abdominal pain syndrome)

      D.   In over 90% of cases of recurrent abdominal pain in children, no organic basis for the symptoms can be found

III. Clinical Presentation

      A.   Approximately 15% of school-age children present to primary care settings each year because of abdominal pain

      B.   Viral gastroenteritis is characterized by crampy pain with associated symptoms of diarrhea, vomiting, malaise, and sometimes fever (see section on DIARRHEA)

      C.   Intussusception presents as paroxysmal, colicky pain and the infant often has currant jelly stools, a palpable right upper quadrant abdominal mass, and ultimately distention

      D.   Incarcerated hernias do not have to be strangulated to cause discomfort; a tender abdominal mass at any of the hernia orifices may be present

      E.   Urinary tract infection (UTI) can cause abdominal pain and often the child with a UTI does not complain of dysuria and frequency as adults typically do (see section on URINARY TRACT INFECTION)

      F.   Intestinal malrotation must be considered when a healthy infant suddenly refuses to eat, vomits, becomes inconsolable, and develops abdominal distention

      G.   Appendicitis
            1.   Often begins with symptoms of dull, steady epigastric or periumbilical pain and anorexia
            2.   After approximately 4-6 hours, the pain shifts to the right lower quadrant
            3.   Pain that awakens a previously well child from sleep is a common presentation

4. Vomiting and diarrhea present after the pain whereas with gastroenteritis the vomiting and diarrhea occur before the pain

5. May cause urinary frequency, urgency, and pyuria, making appendicitis difficult to distinguish from a UTI

H. Mittelschmerz is characterized by sudden onset of localized right or left lower quadrant pain at the midpoint of the menstrual cycle which persists for <24 hours

I. Girls with ruptured ectopic pregnancies have acute onset of unilateral lower quadrant pain which usually is continuous and crampy with some degree of vaginal bleeding and a low-grade fever

J. Chronic stool retention
1. Child may have history of stool withholding and abdominal pain is usually left-sided or suprapubic
2. Pain is most likely to occur in the evening or during dinner
3. See section on CONSTIPATION IN INFANTS AND CHILDREN

K. Lactose intolerance
1. If child is genetically programmed to become lactase deficient, the symptoms usually begin around 4-6 years of age, but can begin in infancy; prevalence is highest in African-Americans, Native Americans, and Asians
2. Symptoms include intestinal dilatation, bloating, increased flatulence, pain, and eventually diarrhea
3. Symptoms often do not appear until 2 hours after ingestion of milk or milk products; sometimes symptoms do not occur until as long as 12 hours after ingestion of lactose
4. Lactose intolerance is often confused with cow's milk protein allergy which occurs in infancy and has symptoms of blood in the stools and often manifestations of allergies such as eczema, hives or asthma

L. Inflammation of the upper gastrointestinal tract as occurs with gastritis and peptic ulcer disease commonly presents with epigastric pain and vomiting; the pain most often occurs during eating or in the immediate postprandial period

M. Musculoskeletal pain is usually sharp and triggered by various activities or body movements

N. Recurrent abdominal pain syndrome
1. Two distinct peaks of frequency-first peak occurs between 5 and 7 years of age, with equal frequency in boys and girls; the second peak occurs between 8 and 12 years of age and is far more prevalent in girls
2. Pain is vague and involves the periumbilical area; a general principle is that the further the pain is from the umbilicus, the more likely it is to have an organic cause
3. Pain is often irregular in timing, duration, and intensity, and is severe enough to disrupt the child's activities
4. Child may have pallor, nausea, vomiting, headache, and perspiration
5. On examination, the child may complain of tenderness, but there should be no muscle guarding or rebound tenderness
6. Child should be growing and developing normally and the abdominal pain should not be explainable by any structural or biochemical abnormalities

IV. Diagnosis/Evaluation

A. History
1. Determine onset and course of pain, including location, character, timing (time of day or night that pain occurs), radiation, and severity of pain; see section on PAIN for information regarding how to help younger children quantify pain using the "Faces" diagrams/scale
2. Determine whether pain awakens child from sleep
3. Ascertain whether pain is related to food or milk ingestion
4. Ask about other aggravating or relieving factors such as pain with micturition which suggests a urogenital cause
5. Inquire about associated symptoms such as fever, jaundice, change in stool pattern, nausea, vomiting, anorexia, weight loss; ask about reflux and satiety
6. Inquire about history of abdominal trauma, previous abdominal surgery, or recent excessive exercise; determine if there has been any recent travel
7. Explore history of predisposing disease such as diabetes, sickle cell disease, hemophilia, inflammatory bowel disease, recurrent pneumonia, or urinary tract infections

8. In adolescent females, always ask dates of last two normal menstrual periods, whether sexually active, condom use, and type of contraceptive use
9. Obtain past medical history, family history, and medication history
10. Ask how pain interferes with school, play, peer relations, and family dynamics
11. Screen for abuse (see section on CHILD HEALTH SUPERVISION) for how to approach this sensitive issue)
12. In adolescents, ask about sexual activity (without parent present, if possible) and unprotected intercourse

B. Physical Examination
1. Observe general appearance: Resisting movement or lying still on one side with legs flexed suggests acute, emergent abdominal pain
2. Assess vital signs to determine if child is febrile and to assess for volume depletion/impending shock; measure height and weight and compare with previous measurements to determine if growth patterns are within normal range
3. Complete abdominal exam is essential (position child with hips flexed) and make sure child has as much privacy as possible in terms of gown/draping)
   a. Inspect for scars and shape of abdomen
   b. Inspect the inguinal and femoral areas for evidence of hernia or (in males) testicular torsion
   c. Auscultate for decreased bowel sounds which suggest intestinal obstruction or possibly appendicitis
   d. Percuss abdomen, beginning in nonpainful region, and note gastric distention with intestinal obstruction, tympany with fluid accumulation, or a solid mass
   e. Palpate abdomen, evaluating for organomegaly, masses (including retained stool), tenderness, rebound tenderness, and guarding
4. Check for peritonitis which is marked by a tense, hard abdomen
   a. Evaluate for rebound tenderness

ASSESSING FOR REBOUND TENDERNESS

After thorough exam of the abdomen, evaluate for peritoneal irritation as follows

➡ Using the flat of your hand, press on the area identified by the patient as most painful
➡ Press sufficiently to depress the peritoneum. The patient will experience pain with this maneuver
➡ Keep pressing with a constant pressure and, as the patient adjusts to the constant pressure over a 30 to 60 second period, the pain lessens in intensity and may even subside
➡ Then, without warning, remove your hand suddenly to just above skin level
➡ Observation of the patient's face may be the best index of a complaint of pain and peritoneal irritation

---

   b. May additionally check for obturator and psoas signs

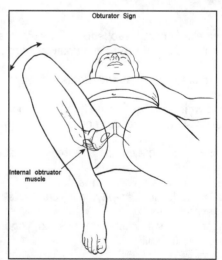

Figure 12.1. Obturator Sign.
Passively flex the right hip and knee and internally rotate the leg at the hip, stretching the obturator muscle. Right-sided abdominal pain is a positive sign, indicating irritation of the obturator muscle by an inflamed appendix

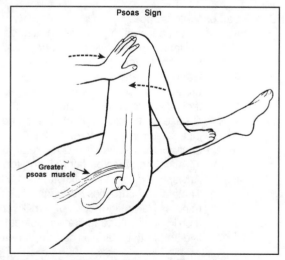

Figure 12.2. Psoas Sign.
With the patient in the supine position, instruct him/her to lift the right thigh against the resistance of the examiner's hand, which is placed just above the patient's knee. Increased pain with the maneuver is a positive test, indicating irritation of the psoas by an inflamed appendix

5. Check back for costovertebral angle (CVA) tenderness
6. Consider a pelvic exam in adolescent females who are sexually active
7. Rectal exam with stool testing for occult blood is recommended
8. Because abdominal pain is often referred pain, examination of the heart, lungs and other body systems should always be done

C. Differential Diagnosis
1. Rule out all emergent conditions such as appendicitis, volvulus, bowel obstruction, ruptured ectopic pregnancy, trauma, ovarian hernia, and torsion which require surgical intervention
2. Pain which is progressive, localized, steady for >6 hours with rebound tenderness and guarding suggests an emergent condition
3. The irritable bowel syndrome occurs infrequently before late adolescence
4. Functional recurrent abdominal pain is a diagnosis of exclusion

D. Diagnostic Tests: If the history and physical examination do not clarify the diagnosis, laboratory and radiologic evaluations may be helpful
1. Basic laboratory tests include
   a. CBC with differential
   b. Urinalysis and urine culture
2. Other laboratory tests individualized according to indication include
   a. Pregnancy test and testing for sexually transmitted diseases
   b. Stool testing and tests for polymorphonuclear leukocytes, parasites, *Giardia* antigen
   c. Serum chemistry profile, amylase level
   d. Breath hydrogen test is a simple method of determining whether lactose malabsorption may be present
   e. Serologic testing for amoebae, *Helicobacter pylori*
3. Imaging studies individualized according to indication
   a. Abdominal and pelvic ultrasonography
   b. Abdominal computed tomography

V. Plan/Management for common causes of abdominal pain

A. Consultation with a specialist is recommended if diagnosis is unclear and/or patient is unstable

B. Emergency transport and hospitalization are required when child has acute abdominal pain related to an emergent condition

C. Chronic stool retention problems or if child has overflow of liquid stool: See sections on CONSTIPATION or ENCOPRESIS

D. Lactose Intolerance
1. Teach parents to give child a lactose-free diet for 2 weeks (if pain disappears suspect lactose intolerance); gradually introduce regular diet noting emergence of symptoms (instruct parents to go through 2 cycles)
2. Remind parents that cake mixes, milk chocolate, salad dressings, canned meats, pancakes, breads, and cereals often contain lactose
3. If child is intolerant to lactose, teach parents and child which foods are high in lactose such as soft cheeses with exception of cream cheese; hard cheeses such as cheddar and Swiss are low in lactose and may be tolerated
4. Lactose intolerance is a dose-related phenomenon so children may be able to tolerate gradual introduction of lactose-containing foods after several weeks of a lactose-free diet
5. Advise child to drink milk with meals to minimize the occurrence of symptoms
6. Tablets and capsules containing lactose-digesting enzyme (Dairy Ease, Lactaid) can be taken 30 minutes before ingestion of a milk product to reduce symptoms
7. If child is unable to tolerate most lactose-containing foods, give calcium supplements; yogurt with live and active cultures can provide an excellent substitute for milk

E. Functional/recurrent abdominal pain
1. Consider asking parents to keep a diary or calendar of the child's pain to help uncover possible triggers (this strategy may have negative consequences because it focuses the family's attention on the pain; use cautiously and discontinue if the symptom diary seems to make the problem worse)
2. Provide support to parents, explaining that child's pain is real and that child is not fabricating pain

3. Explain that a thorough exam was done and no serious organic disease exists; emphasize that the child is in no physical danger
4. Explain that recurrent abdominal pain is common in children and that many different causes exist
5. Explain that child may have many reoccurrences of pain and will need to learn ways to cope with symptoms just as adults with recurrent headaches must learn to function at work and perform activities of daily living
6. Encourage normalization of the family's life-style with immediate return to school and try to minimize the importance of the pain episodes
7. During severely painful episodes, teach parents to allow child to rest; medications are usually not indicated
8. Teach parents to assess child for signs of emergent abdominal problems such as fever, pallor, sweating, vomiting, diarrhea, rigid and tender abdomen
9. Re-evaluate child periodically to provide support and assess for other problems
10. Consider referral to mental health specialist if underlying stress or family difficulties are suspected

F. Management and follow up of other causes of abdominal pain is variable depending on diagnosis
1. Children diagnosed with functional recurrent abdominal pain need regular follow up for support and to evaluate treatment plan
2. Referral to an expert is indicated in children whose recurrent abdominal pain continues to interfere with school, activities, and relationships with peers and family members

ACUTE DIARRHEA

I. Definition: Abrupt onset of increased fluid content of the stool above the normal value of approximately 10 mL/kg/day, that resolves in less that 14 days; implies an increased frequency of bowel movements also which can range from 4 to 5 to more than 20 per day

II. Pathogenesis

A. Increased water content of the stools results from an imbalance in the function of the small and large intestinal processes involved in the absorption of organic substrates and water

B. Imbalance in the intestinal handling of water and electrolytes involves one or a combination of four basic mechanisms
1. Osmotic: Occurs when poorly absorbed, osmotically active substances are ingested, creating an osmotic gradient that encourages movement of water into the lumen and subsequently into the stool–examples are ingestion of lactose in a lactase-deficient person, sorbitol, mannitol, magnesium-containing antacids in excess
2. Secretory: There is increased small intestinal secretion or reduced absorption–cholera has been the prototype of secretory diarrhea; in recent years, however, a growing number of infectious agents such as enterotoxigenic *Escherichia coli* have been associated with this mechanism; a number of noninfectious causes exist as well
3. Exudative: Intestinal mucosa becomes inflamed, causing mucus, blood, and pus to leak into the lumen; examples are invasive infections of small and/or large intestine by bacterial agents as well as non-infectious conditions such as inflammatory bowel disease
4. Motility disturbances: Contact time with bowel mucosa is limited which interferes with reabsorption of fluids–examples are irritable bowel syndrome and medications such as erythromycin

III. Clinical Presentation

A. In the US, there are 1-2 episodes of diarrhea per child each year in children <5 years; about 10% of all hospital admissions for children in this age group are for acute diarrheal illnesses

B. Acute gastroenteritis is usually benign and self-limited, subsiding within a few days

C. Most cases of acute diarrhea are due to infection of the gastrointestinal tract by a variety of pathogens; by far, the most common pathogens are **viral**
1. In infectious diarrhea, the clinical presentation and the course of the illness are greatly influenced by the host and by the infecting organism

2. Age and nutritional status appear to be the most important host factors—the younger the child, for example, the higher is the risk for severe dehydration as a result of the high body water turnover and limited renal compensatory capacity of very young children
3. Characteristics of the infecting organism also result in a variable pattern of clinical features—for example, children with viral diarrhea tend to have dehydration, vomiting, and watery stools. On the other hand, fever, cramping abdominal pain, and blood mixed with stools are more common in patients with invasive pathogens such as *Salmonella, Shigella*, and *Campylobacter*

D. Relative frequency of occurrence of diarrheal illnesses by specific infectious agents is outlined below
1. Viral pathogens—rotavirus, astrovirus, and noroviruses (formerly known as Norwalk-like viruses)—cause a watery diarrhea without leukocytes or blood in the stools. All three agents are **very** common causes of diarrhea (noroviruses infect children but are much more common in adults)
2. Diarrhea caused by S*higella*, S*almonella*, and *Campylobacter* share certain inflammatory features (an inflammatory etiology can be suspected on the basis of fever, tenesmus, or bloody stools and can be confirmed by microscopic examination for fecal polymorphonuclear leukocytes or immunoassay for the neutrophil marker lactoferrin [Leukotest by TechLab]). All three agents are common causes of diarrhea
3. *Clostridium perfringens* and *Staphylococcus aureus* also are common causes of diarrhea; enterotoxigenic *Escherichia coli* (ETEC) is also common, but only among travelers to developing countries
4. *Giardia lamblia* is a relatively uncommon cause of diarrhea

E. Distinguishing features as well as clinical presentation of commonly occurring infectious causes of acute diarrhea are summarized in the table that follows

COMMONLY OCCURRING INFECTIOUS CAUSES OF ACUTE DIARRHEA: DISTINGUISHING FEATURES

Infectious Agent	Mode of Transmission	Incubation Period	Associated Signs and Symptoms	Characteristics of Stool	Laboratory Examination of Stool	Important to Remember
Viral						
Rotavirus and norovirus	Fecal-oral; fomites may have a role	24-72 hrs	Nausea, vomiting, abdominal cramps Fever	Watery No occult or gross blood	No WBCs in stool	Rotavirus is by far the most common cause of acute diarrhea in children (norovirus occurs less often in children than in adults) Vomiting most prominent symptom in children
Astrovirus	Fecal-oral; contaminated food outbreaks have also been reported	3-4 days	Nausea, vomiting, abdominal cramps Fever	Watery No occult or gross blood	No WBCs in stool	Most infections have been detected in children <4 years of age Episodes have a winter seasonal peak Outbreaks tend to occur in closed populations (e.g., in day care centers and nursing homes)
Bacterial						
Staphylococcus aureus	Ingestion of food containing a preformed toxin produced by enterotoxicogenic staphylococci Food products most commonly involved are ham, poultry, filled pastries, egg/potato salads Contamination is via food handlers Not transmissible from person-to-person	Very short--30 minutes to 6 hours	Nausea, vomiting, abdominal cramps Fever is uncommon	Soft, but not watery No occult or gross blood	No WBCs in stool	Onset is abrupt Look for a common source pattern
Clostridium perfringens	Ingestion of food contaminated by the organism Once ingested, an enterotoxin is produced in the lower intestine of the host, producing symptoms Beef, poultry, Mexican-style foods are common sources Not transmissible from person-to-person	8-12 hours	Nausea, vomiting, moderate-to-severe mid-epigastric pain Fever is uncommon	Watery No occult or gross blood	No WBCs in stool	Onset is not as abrupt as in staphylococcal food poisoning because enterotoxin is not preformed, but is produced in host's intestine Look for a common source pattern Look for recent ingestion of foods served from steam tables
Campylobacter jejuni	Ingestion of contaminated food, including unpasteurized milk and untreated water OR by direct contact with fecal material from infected persons/animals Main vehicles of transmission: Improperly cooked poultry, untreated water, unpasteurized milk Person-to-person spread is not common	1-7 days	Nausea, vomiting, abdominal pain, malaise Fever	Watery Occult and gross blood	WBCs in stool Positive culture	Abdominal pain can mimic that produced by appendicitis Mild infection lasts 1-2 days with most patients recovering in <7 days Outbreaks in child care centers are uncommon

(continued)

COMMONLY OCCURRING INFECTIOUS CAUSES OF ACUTE DIARRHEA: DISTINGUISHING FEATURES (CONTINUED)

Infectious Agent	Mode of Transmission	Incubation Period	Associated Signs and Symptoms	Character-istics of Stool	Laboratory Examination of Stool	Important to Remember
Salmonella	Major modes: Ingestion of food of animal origin, including poultry, red meat, eggs, and unpasteurized milk Other modes: Ingestion of contaminated water, contact with infected animals such as pet turtles/reptiles Direct person-to-person transmission (fecal-oral) are less common than other modes	6-72 hours; usually <24 hours	Nausea, vomiting, abdominal cramping Fever	Watery Occult and gross blood	WBCs in stool Positive culture	Most likely to occur in children <5 (peaks in first year of life) Outbreaks of this infection are rare in day care centers Report all confirmed cases to local public health department
Shigella	Fecal-oral transmission is most common route in children Ingestion of contaminated food or water and homosexual transmission most common routes in adults Feces of infected humans are source of infection No animal reservoir known	1-7 days; usually 2-4 days	Abdominal pain Fever	Watery Occult and gross blood	WBCs in stool Positive culture	Most common in children 1-4 years of age Important problem in child care centers in US Report all confirmed cases to the local health department
Enterotoxigenic *Escherichia coli* (ETEC)	One of at least 5 different groups of diarrhea-producing strains of *E. coli* Most commonly from food or water contaminated with human or animal feces Most common cause of "travelers' diarrhea," acquired by travelers to developing countries	10 hours to 6 days	Abdominal cramps Usually no fever	Watery No occult or gross blood	No WBCs (usually); can be present Positive culture	The enterotoxin that is produced by the organism promotes fluid secretion in the small bowel which results in a watery diarrhea History of recent travel to a developing country is important epidemiologic information Causes travelers diarrhea in all ages
Protozoal *Giardia*	Main route of spread is fecal-oral transfer of cysts from feces of an infected person Many common source outbreaks are traced to contaminated drinking water Humans are principle reservoir but organism can infect animals such as dogs, cats, beavers	1-4 weeks	Abdominal pain associated with flatulence, distention, and anorexia Passage of foul-smelling stools No fever	Soft, watery No occult or gross blood	Positive stool for O & P	Most often represents an acute presentation of chronic or recurrent diarrhea

F. Medications such as laxatives and antibiotics can also cause acute diarrhea

G. Dietary causes of acute diarrhea include nonabsorbable sugar substitutes such as sorbitol, food intolerance or allergy, and excessive caffeine

H. Extra-intestinal infections–for example, middle ear, lung, and urinary tract infections can result in acute diarrhea via an unknown mechanism; the diarrhea is usually mild and self-limited

I. Chronic diarrhea (lasting at least 2 weeks or frequent recurrences after initial attack) also often presents in primary care settings; some of the more common causes of chronic diarrhea along with their associated signs and symptoms are listed here:
    1. Irritable bowel syndrome: recurrent abdominal pain, diarrhea alternates with constipation; the most common of the motility disorders causing chronic diarrhea (see IRRITABLE BOWEL SYNDROME section for a discussion of this condition)
    2. Inflammatory bowel diseases: destruction of the bowel wall compromises absorption of electrolytes; characterized by bloody stools, abdominal pain, fever, and extraintestinal manifestations involving skin, joints, liver, and heart
    3. Malabsorptive syndrome is characterized by abnormal fecal excretion of fat and variable malabsorption of fats, fat-soluble vitamins, other vitamins, proteins, carbohydrates, minerals, and water

---

- Carbohydrate and fat malabsorption are much more common than protein malabsorption
  - ✓ Carbohydrate malabsorption occurs in such circumstances as pancreatic insufficiency and lactase deficiency
  - ✓ Lipid malabsorption occurs in a variety of circumstances including rapid gastric emptying and improper mixing, pancreatic insufficiency, and cholestasis
  - ✓ Protein malabsorption occurs in pancreatic insufficiency, short-bowel syndrome, and celiac disease
- Clinically, all of the malabsorption syndromes resemble each other more than they differ; especially common are weight loss, anorexia, abdominal distention, borborygmi, muscle wasting, and passage of abnormally bulky, frothy, greasy, yellow or gray stools
- More specific manifestations are seen in particular categories

---

    4. Chronic laxative abuse can also cause diarrhea; occurs often in patients with bulimia; substances appear in the stool and the stool can be tested if laxative abuse is suspected

IV. Diagnosis/Evaluation

    A. History: Important to assess both clinical and epidemiological features

---

Relevant Clinical Features: Determine the Following

- When (duration) and how the illness began (e.g., was onset abrupt or gradual)
- Stool characteristics–whether watery, bloody, mucous-containing, purulent, greasy
- Frequency of bowel movements and relative quantity of stool produced
- If dysenteric symptoms are present–fever, tenesmus, blood and/or pus in stool
- If symptoms of volume depletion are present–thirst, tachycardia, orthostasis, decreased urine output, lethargy, decreased skin turgor
- If associated symptoms are present–nausea, vomiting, abdominal pain, cramps, headache, myalgias, altered sensorium–and gauge their severity
- In infants, ask about feeding, irritability, activity level, number of wet diapers, and if general behavior is significantly changed since onset of diarrhea

---

Relevant Epidemiological Risk Factors for Particular Diarrheal Illnesses and Their Spread: Determine the Following

- Recent travel to developing countries
- Day-care attendance or employment
- Consumption of unsafe foods (e.g., raw meats, eggs, shellfish, unpasteurized milk)
- Swimming in or drinking untreated surface water from a lake or stream
- Recent visit to a petting zoo or recent contact with reptiles or pets with diarrhea
- Knowledge of other ill persons (such as in households, dormitories, at social functions, or on cruise ships)
- Recent or regular medications (antibiotics, antacids)
- Underlying medical conditions predisposing to infectious diarrhea (AIDS, prior gastrectomy)
- Sexual practices that include receptive anal intercourse or oral-anal sexual contact
- Occupation as a food handler

B. Physical Examination
    1. Determine if patient is febrile and assess cardiovascular status (pulse, blood pressure; check for postural changes, a reflection of significant volume depletion)
    2. Weigh patient and determine if there has been a weight loss (especially an issue in infants and in chronic diarrhea)
    3. In infants and young children, assess hydration status based on criteria in ASSESSMENT OF DEHYDRATION IN INFANTS AND CHILDREN table below
    4. Examine abdomen for tenderness, rigidity, abnormal tympany, bowel sounds, liver/spleen enlargement
    5. Perform rectal exam for tenderness, masses; obtain stool for occult blood
    6. Look for extraintestinal infections such as otitis media and urinary tract infection which often are associated with diarrhea in children through an unknown mechanism

ASSESSMENT OF DEHYDRATION IN INFANTS AND CHILDREN			
Indicator	Mild, 3-5%	Moderate, 6-9%	Severe, ≥10%
Blood pressure	Normal	Normal	Normal to reduced
Quality of pulses	Normal	Normal or slightly decreased	Moderately decreased
Heart rate	Normal	Increased	Increased (bradycardia may occur also)
Skin turgor	Normal	Decreased skin elasticity	Decreased with tenting
Fontanelle	Normal	Somewhat depressed	Depressed
Mucous membranes	Sl dry lips, thick saliva	Dry lips, buccal mucosa	Very dry lips, buccal mucosa
Eyes	Normal	Sunken orbits	Deeply sunken orbits
Capillary refill time (In seconds)	Normal (<1.5)	Delayed (1.5-3.0)	Delayed (>3.0)
Mental status	Normal	Normal to listless	Normal to lethargic or comatose
Urine output	Slightly decreased	<1 mL/kg/h	<<1 mL/kg/hr
Thirst	Slightly increased	Moderately increased	Very thirsty or too lethargic to indicate

Adapted from Duggan, C., Santosham, M., & Glass, R.I. (1992). The management of acute diarrhea in children: Oral rehydration, maintenance, and nutritional therapy. *MMWR, 41*(RR-16), 1-20.

C. Differential Diagnosis: Diarrhea is a symptom. Refer to common causes of acute and chronic diarrhea under section III. above

D. Diagnostic Tests
    1. Any diarrheal illness lasting >24 hours, especially if accompanied by fever, bloody stools, systemic illness, dehydration, recent use of antibiotics, or day-care attendance should prompt evaluation of a fecal specimen
    2. Additional diagnostic testing such as complete blood cell count and serum chemistries may also be indicated in selected cases, depending on the clinical findings

V. Plan/Management

    A. Acute diarrhea is almost invariably a benign, self-limited condition, subsiding within a few days–age and the nutritional status of the patient are important factors in determining risk for severe dehydration with infants being the most vulnerable

    B. Appropriate management of acute dehydration, electrolyte status, and nutrition remains the cornerstones of therapy
        1. Whether or not the cause of the diarrhea is determined, supportive therapy must be instituted immediately to rehydrate (if necessary) and maintain hydration status and to maintain adequate nutrition through refeeding as soon as possible
        2. Because infants are at higher risk for development of **dehydration and malnutrition, the two major consequences of diarrhea**, management must be very aggressive in this age group (see TREATMENT OF DIARRHEA IN INFANTS > ONE MONTH AND CHILDREN ≤5 YEARS table)
        3. Breastfed infants should be continued on breast milk without any need for interruption as breastfeeding promotes faster recovery and provides improved nutrition when compared with formula feeding

4. Neonates (infants ≤1 month of age) who present with diarrhea should be referred to a specialist for management because of the greater likelihood of severe infection in this age group

C. Treatment of infants >one month of age and children ≤5 years of age with acute diarrhea is determined by the degree of dehydration that is present; management of children in this age group based on degree of dehydration is outlined in the table that follows

TREATMENT OF INFANTS >ONE MONTH OF AGE AND CHILDREN ≤ 5 YEARS OF AGE	
Degree of Dehydration	**Management**
Infants and children who have mild diarrhea and who are not dehydrated	✧ Continue to feed age-appropriate diet (including breast milk in breastfeeding infants) ✧ Children in this category do not require glucose-electrolyte solutions (oral rehydration therapy [ORT]) but they should be given more fluids than usual during episode of diarrhea
Children who are mildly dehydrated (3-5%)	✧ Give 50 mL/kg of ORT plus replacement of continuing losses during a 4-hour period; appropriate oral replacement solutions are listed at the end of this table ◆ Replacement of continuing losses from stool is achieved by providing 10mL/kg for each stool ◆ Emesis volume should also be estimated and replaced each time the child vomits ◆ At least every 2 hours, the hydration status of the child should be reevaluated and replacement of losses should occur ◆ Children who require rehydration should be fed age-appropriate diet as soon as they have been rehydrated ◆ Special diets such as the **BRAT are no longer recommended** as such diets are not calorie dense enough and lack adequate amounts of protein and fat
Children who are mildly dehydrated and who have vomiting	✧ Can be successfully treated with ORT with the administration of small volumes of the solution on a frequent basis ◆ Administer 5 mL every 2-3 minutes ◆ Using this technique, 100/150 mL/h can be given ◆ Once dehydration and electrolyte imbalance are corrected, vomiting often decreases and ends ◆ When rehydration is achieved, age appropriate diet should be reinstated
Infants and children who are moderately dehydrated (6-9%)	✧ Give 100 mL/kg of ORT plus replacement of continuing losses during a 4-hour period ◆ Every hour during the period of rehydration, hydration status should be assessed; continuing stool and emesis losses should be calculated with the total added to the amount remaining to be given over the 4-hour period ◆ These children are best managed in an emergency department or urgent care facility ◆ Children who require rehydration should be fed age-appropriate diet as soon as they have been rehydrated
Infants and children who are severely dehydrated (≥10%)	✧ **Require immediate emergency management**
Solutions Appropriate for Oral Rehydration Therapy (ORT) for Infants and Children ≤5 Years	
✓ Pedialyte ✓ Infalyte ✓ WHO ORS packets* ✓ Rehydralyte ✓ Pedialyte-RS ✓ CeraLyte	

* World Health Organization oral rehydration solution packets are not readily available in the US but can be obtained from Jianas Brothers Co., 2533 Southwest Blvd., Kansas City, MO 64018-2395, phone 816-421-2880, or www.rehydrate.org/resources/jianas.htm

Adapted from American Academy of Pediatrics, Provisional Committee on Quality Improvement, Subcommittee on Acute Gastroenteritis. (1996). Practice parameter: The management of acute gastroenteritis in young children. *Pediatrics, 97*, 424-433.

D. Supportive therapy for older children and adolescents should focus on attaining and maintaining adequate hydration status through appropriate fluid intake. Water or sports drinks may be used for hydration as well as the commercial rehydration products such as those listed in the table above
1. Children may also like products such as Pedialyte Freezer Pops
2. Normal diet should be resumed as soon as the patient can tolerate it; special diets such as the BRAT are no longer recommended as they are not calorie dense enough, and lack adequate amounts of protein and fat

E. The decision to treat patients with suspected bacterial or parasitic enteritis must be based on stool culture or testing for specific organisms
1. Keep in mind that any consideration of antimicrobial therapy must be carefully weighed against unintended and potentially harmful consequences
2. Unintended consequences include development of antimicrobial-resistant infections, side effects of treatment, and suprainfections when normal flora are eradicated

3. Situations in which empirical antibiotics are commonly recommended without obtaining a fecal specimen are the following
   a. Travelers' diarrhea, in which enterotoxigenic *E. coli* or other bacterial pathogens are likely causes and prompt therapy can reduce duration from 3-5 days to <1-2 days
   b. When giardiasis is suspected, based on patient's history of travel or water exposure, empirical treatment of diarrhea that has lasted longer than 10-14 days may also be considered
4. In addition, patients with febrile diarrheal illnesses, particularly when moderate to severe invasive disease is suspected, should be considered for empirical treatment (prior to treatment, a fecal specimen should be obtained for testing)

F. Counseling and control measures for patients with identified infectious agents as the cause of acute diarrheal illness as well as recommended pharmacologic management are contained in the table below

TREATMENT OF ACUTE DIARRHEA CAUSED BY COMMONLY OCCURRING INFECTIOUS AGENTS		
Infectious Agent	**Pharmacologic Management**	**Counseling and Control Measures**
Viral Rotavirus norovirus, and Astrovirus	✓ No specific antiviral therapy is available	✓ Emphasize importance of good hand washing ✓ Advise to clean all surfaces where diapering is done with chlorine-based disinfectants ✓ Infected children should be excluded from child-care centers until diarrhea resolves
Bacterial *Staphylococcus aureus*	✓ Antibiotics are not recommended	✓ Proper cooking and refrigeration of food helps prevent the disease ✓ Persons with staphylococcal infections should be excluded from handling food
Clostridium perfringens	✓ Antibiotics are not recommended	✓ *C. perfringens* should not be allowed to proliferate in food (beef, poultry, gravies, and Mexican-style foods are common sources) ✓ Foods should never be held at room temperature to cool, but should be refrigerated promptly, and reheated thoroughly before serving ✓ Foods should not be kept in warming devices or serving tables for long periods of time
Campylobacter infections	✓ Erythromycin (Ery-Tab), given early in the course of infection, shortens duration of illness and prevents relapse • Adolescents: 250 mg PO QID x 5-7 days • Children: 50 mg/kg/day divided into 4 doses for 5-7 days	✓ Persons who prepare food should practice frequent handwashing, wash surfaces that have been exposed to raw poultry, and thoroughly cook poultry ✓ Pasteurization of milk and chlorination of water supplies are essential ✓ Infected food handlers who are asymptomatic need not be excluded from work if proper personal hygiene measures are maintained ✓ Outbreaks are uncommon in child care centers
Salmonella infections (non-typhi species)	✓ Antimicrobial therapy is not routinely recommended for uncomplicated gastroenteritis caused by non-typhi species of *Salmonella* because it can prolong excretion of the organism ✓ Treatment is recommended for patients at an increased risk of invasive disease such as persons with valvular heart disease, uremia, or HIV infection. Consult specialists for treatment recommendations	✓ Emphasis should be on good hand-washing and personal hygiene ✓ There must be proper sanitation in food processing and preparation; **infected persons should be excluded from handling food** ✓ Eggs and other foods of animal origin should be cooked thoroughly before ingestion ✓ Raw eggs as well as food containing raw eggs should not be eaten ✓ Handwashing when handling pet turtles and other reptiles is important ✓ Outbreaks of *Salmonella* infection are rare in child care centers ✓ Vaccination for typhoid is recommended only for international travelers ✓ Report all cases of *Salmonella* infection to local public health department so that proper investigation of outbreak can be conducted

(Continued)

TREATMENT OF ACUTE DIARRHEA CAUSED BY COMMONLY OCCURRING INFECTIOUS AGENTS
(CONTINUED)

Infectious Agent	Pharmacologic Management	Counseling and Control Measures
Shigella	✓ To shorten course and prevent further spread, may treat with trimethoprim-sulfamethoxazole • Adolescents: 1 DS tab BID x 3-5 days • Children: 1 mL/kg/day in two divided doses (Q 12 hours) x 3-5 days (Available as Bactrim suspension 200 mg sulfamethoxazole and 40 mg trimethoprim per 5mL) ✓ Intestinal motility patterns are considered important in recovery from infection, therefore anti-diarrhea drugs should not be given	✓ Emphasis should be on good hand-washing and personal hygiene, particularly among workers in group care settings such as child care and group living facilities ✓ There must be proper sanitation in food processing and preparation; **infected persons should be excluded from handling food** ✓ Prevention of contamination of food by flies during preparation and serving is required ✓ Insuring that water supply is not contaminated is important ✓ Outbreak of Shigella infection must be reported to the local health department for investigation
Escherichia coli infection (entero-toxigenic) [ETEC], major cause of **Travelers' Diarrhea**	✓ May treat with trimethoprim-sulfamethoxazole • Adolescents: 1 DS tab, BID x 3 days • Children: 1 mL/kg/day in two divided doses (Q 12 hours) x 3 days (Available as Bactrim suspension 200 mg sulfamethoxazole and 40 mg trimethoprim per 5 mL) • Ciprofloxacin is an alternative agent for adolescents ≥18 years: 500 mg BID x 3 days	✓ When traveling in developing countries or in any area where water supply is questionable, drink only bottled water ✓ Avoid all raw fruits and vegetables that may not have been properly washed (unless can peel and eat)
Protozoal *Giardia*	✓ Drug of choice is metronidazole • Adolescents: 250 mg TID x 5 days • Children: 15 mg/kg/day in 3 doses x 5 days ✓ Alternative drug is furazolidone • Adolescents: 100 mg QID x 7-10 days • Children: 6 mg/kg/day in 4 divided doses x 7-10 days ✓ In pregnant women, paromomycin is recommended for treatment of symptomatic infections. Consult PDR for dosing recommendations	✓ Emphasize sanitation and personal hygiene, especially in group care settings ✓ Hand washing after diaper changes and after personal toilet use by workers cannot be overemphasized; persons with diarrhea (both workers and children) should be excluded from day care until problem resolves ✓ Adequate filtration of municipal water supply prevents water-borne outbreaks in metropolitan areas ✓ Boiling of water by campers, backpackers will eliminate cysts; drinking from streams is risky ✓ Treatment of asymptomatic carriers is not recommended except for prevention of household transmission by toddlers to pregnant women ✓ Outbreaks in day care centers require reporting to local public health department for epidemiological investigation

G.   Several products are available to provide some symptomatic relief to patients during a diarrheal illness; these agents do not alter the course of the illness or reduce fluid loss

H.   The following anti-diarrheal agents are available and may be used in selected cases of diarrheal illnesses in older children and adolescents for no longer than 3 days where there are no contraindications; use of these agents have not been shown to be beneficial in the management of acute diarrhea and patients should be advised of this

ANTI-DIARRHEAL AGENTS FOR ACUTE DIARRHEA		
Agents	**Medication**	**Dosage**
Antimotility agents	Imodium A-D (OTC), available as 1 mg/5mL syrup and 2 mg caplets	Adolescents: ≥12 years, 4 mg initially, then 2 mg after each unformed stool. Maximum 8 mg/day; use for 2 days Children: 6-8 years (48-59 lbs), 2 mg initially, then 1 mg after each loose stool Maximum 4 mg/day for 2 days Children: 9-11 years (60-95 lbs), 2 mg initially, then 1 mg after each loose stool Maximum 6 mg/day for 2 days
	Lomotil, available as 2.5 mg tabs and liquid, 2.5 mg/5 mL	Adolescents: ≥18 years of age, 2 tabs QID (maximum 20 mg/day) for 2-3 days only Children: Not recommended
Adsorbents	Kaolin-pectin mixture (Kaopectate) liquid	Adolescents: 30-120 mL after each loose stool Children: ≥6 years of age, see label for dosing
Antisecretory agents	Bismuth subsalicylate (Pepto-Bismol) available as 262 mg chewable tabs and 262 mg/15 mL liquid	Adolescents: >12 years of age, 2 tabs or 30 mL Q 30-60 minutes (Maximum 8 doses/day) Children: 6-9 years of age, 2/3 tab or 10 mL Q 30-60 minutes (Maximum 8 doses/day) 9-12 years of age, 1 tab or 15 mL Q 30-60 minutes (Maximum 8 doses/day)

I. Patients with chronic diarrhea require treatment of the underlying cause
  1. Refer to sections on HIV/AIDS and IRRITABLE BOWEL SYNDROME for management of patients with these conditions
  2. If *Giardia* is suspected, obtain appropriate diagnostic tests and treat as described in the table above–TREATMENT OF ACUTE DIARRHEA CAUSED BY COMMONLY OCCURRING INFECTIOUS AGENTS
  3. If a medication that the patient is taking is producing the diarrhea, change medication if possible
  4. If inflammatory bowel disease or a malabsorption syndrome such as sprue or lactase deficiency is suspected, refer to a specialist for management

J. Public health considerations
  1. Food handlers in food service establishments should be tested for bacterial pathogens if they have diarrhea because of their potential to transmit infection to large numbers of persons
  2. Workers in day-care centers, attendees of day-care centers, and residents in institutional facilities such as nursing homes and prisons who have a diarrheal illness should be evaluated for bacterial or parasitic infection because gastrointestinal illnesses in such settings may indicate that a disease outbreak is occurring
  3. When a disease outbreak is suspected due to an observed increased incidence of diarrheal illness among a particular group, diagnostic testing to facilitate identification of the etiologic agent and to define the extent of the outbreak should be undertaken; the suspected outbreak should be reported to public health authorities

K. Disease reporting to appropriate public health officials is the cornerstone of public-health surveillance, outbreak detection, and control and prevention efforts

Disease Reporting
✓ Reporting requirements and procedures differ by jurisdictions ✓ Requirements for the reporting of disease can be obtained from the state or local health department ✓ Can also be obtained at the Web site of the Council of State and Territorial Epidemiologists at http://www.cste.org

L. General counseling and patient education (in addition to that contained in the table above–TREATMENT OF ACUTE DIARRHEA CAUSED BY COMMONLY OCCURRING INFECTIOUS AGENTS) includes the following
  1. Hand-washing with soap after toileting and before food preparation is very effective
  2. Human feces must always be considered potentially hazardous and should be handled as hazardous waste

3. Select populations (such as food handlers and day-care attendants) require additional education about food safety and these persons should be referred to appropriate resources for education
4. Immunocompromised persons (e.g., HIV-infected, cancer chemotherapy recipients, persons receiving long term oral steroids or immunosuppressive agents) are more susceptible to infection from a variety of enteric pathogens and can reduce their risk through safe food-handling and preparation practices
5. General educational information on food safety is available from the following Web sites

Websites
http://www.cdc.gov/ncidod/dbmd/diseaseinfo/foodborneinfections_g.htm
http://www.fightbac.org
http://www.foodsafety.gov
http://www.healthfinder.gov
http://www.nal.usda.gov/fnic/foodborne/foodborn.htm

M. Follow Up
1. Infants and small children: In 24 hours
2. Older children and adolescents: In 48 hours if diarrhea has not resolved
3. In certain situations such as those involving food-handlers, daycare workers, and healthcare workers with laboratory-confirmed bacterial or parasitic diarrheal disease, confirmation that the disease has been cured or that the person is no longer a fecal carrier must be obtained; consult local public health officer to find out more about regulations pertaining to persons in these categories before the patient is allowed to return to work

NAUSEA AND VOMITING

I. Definition

A. Nausea: An unpleasant sensation of the throat or epigastric region alerting one that vomiting is imminent

B. Vomiting: The forceful oral expulsion of gastric contents

II. Pathogenesis

A. Three consecutive phases of emesis include nausea, retching, and vomiting
1. Nausea is entirely subjective and is commonly described as a sensation immediately preceding vomiting; may or may not lead to the act of vomiting
2. When vomiting does occur, it is preceded by retching which is repetitive active contractions of the abdominal musculature which generate the pressure gradient that leads to evacuation of the stomach
3. Vomiting is a highly specific physical event that results in the rapid, forceful evacuation of gastric contents in a retrograde way from the stomach and up to and out of the mouth

B. Vomiting is triggered by afferent impulses received in the vomiting center (VC) believed to be located in the medulla

C. Sensory centers such as the cerebral cortex, visceral afferents from the pharynx and gastrointestinal tract, and the chemoreceptor trigger zone (CTZ) are responsible for sending the impulses to the vomiting center

D. Once the VC is stimulated, efferent pathways to the salivation center, respiratory center, and the pharyngeal, gastrointestinal, and abdominal musculature work in concert to produce vomiting

III. Clinical Presentation

A. Nausea and vomiting are among the most common symptoms that children experience and may be associated with a variety of clinical presentations

B. May be evoked by a broad range of both pathologic and physiologic conditions; only the most common causes are listed in the box below

> *Toxic etiologies and medications*
> - Acute gastroenteritis, both viral and bacterial
> - Nongastrointestinal infections including otitis media and urinary tract infection
> - Numerous medications including hormonal preparations (e.g., oral contraceptives); antibiotics/antivirals, (e.g., erythromycin, acyclovir); analgesics (e.g., aspirin, NSAIDs); cancer chemotherapy (e.g., methotrexate)
>
> *Disorders of the gut and peritoneum*
> - Mechanical obstruction, e.g., small bowel obstruction, gastric outlet obstruction
> - Functional disorders, e.g., gastroparesis, irritable bowel syndrome
> - Organic disorders, e.g., peptic ulcer disease, pancreatitis, hepatitis
>
> *CNS causes*
> - Migraine
> - Labyrinthine disorders, e.g., motion sickness
>
> *Endocrinologic and metabolic causes*
> - Pregnancy
> - Uremia, diabetic ketoacidosis, hyperthyroidism
>
> *Postoperative nausea and vomiting*
>
> *Iatrogenic, as occurs in bulimia*

IV.   Diagnosis/Evaluation

A.   History
1. Question about onset, duration, quantity and quality of vomitus (undigested food, yellow-green bilious material, blood)
2. Determine if this is an acute (few days) or chronic (> 4 weeks) problem
    a. Acute onset of nausea and vomiting suggests gastroenteritis or a medication-related side effect
    b. A more insidious onset of nausea, without vomiting, should raise suspicion of gastroparesis, a drug-related side effect, or metabolic disorders
3. Ask about timing of vomiting and relation to meals
    a. Vomiting that occurs in the morning before meals is typical of that related to pregnancy, uremia, alcohol ingestion, and increased intracranial pressure
    b. Vomiting that occurs more than 1 hour after meal ingestion suggests gastroparesis or gastric outlet obstruction
4. Ask about associated symptoms such as abdominal pain, diarrhea, dizziness, headache
    a. Abdominal pain preceding vomiting usually indicates an organic lesion such as an obstruction
    b. With small bowel obstruction, pain is typically prominent, severe, and colicky; may temporarily improve after a vomiting episode
5. Ask if systemic symptoms of fever and malaise are present
6. Ask about past medical history and medication history
7. In infants, ask about feedings, activity level, irritability, lethargy, number of wet diapers (vomiting rapidly produces dehydration in infants and young children)
8. Ask if others in household are ill to identify a common source cause

B.   Physical Examination
1. Observe general appearance for pallor, perspiration, restlessness, signs of peritonitis, toxicity; determine if febrile
2. Assess hydration status: Check for dry mucous membranes, decreased skin turgor, tachycardia, and oliguria
3. Assess cardiovascular status (pulse, blood pressure; check for postural hypotension)
4. Examine abdomen for tenderness, rigidity, abnormal tympany, bowel sounds, liver and spleen size
5. Perform rectal exam for tenderness, masses; stool for occult blood

C.   Differential Diagnosis: Vomiting is a symptom; see Pathogenesis for possible causes

D. Laboratory Tests: Selection of laboratory studies should be directed by findings from history and physical examination
   1. Goals of testing are twofold: To assist in identifying cause and to evaluate the consequences of vomiting
   2. Basic laboratory tests include the following
      a. Complete blood count and erythrocyte sedimentation rate
      b. Serum chemistries to document acid-base, electrolyte status
      c. Pregnancy test in adolescent females
      d. Drug levels, if indicated

V. Plan/Management

A. Patients suspected of having an emergent condition involving the gastrointestinal tract, such as mechanical obstruction, perforation, or peritonitis should be immediately transported to the emergency department for evaluation and management

B. If central nervous system symptoms are present (headache, vertigo, neck stiffness, and focal neurologic deficits), refer the patient for emergent evaluation and management

C. If medications are believed to be the cause and can safely be switched, consider this option (nausea frequently subsides with many medications over time)

D. All underlying causes detected in history, physical examination, and laboratory testing should be either treated or referred for management

E. Most acute episodes of nausea and vomiting are caused by viral gastroenteritis or (less commonly) motion sickness, and are self-limiting; supportive therapy is all that is indicated

F. Nonpharmacologic interventions to promote hydration

NONPHARMACOLOGIC INTERVENTIONS	
Infants >1 month and children ≤5 years of age	• Almost all children with vomiting and mild dehydration can be treated with oral rehydration therapy (see section on ACUTE DIARRHEA which contains very specific and detailed guidelines for managing rehydration in infants and small children as well as guidelines for refeeding)
Children >5	• Discontinue solid foods • Encourage clear liquids only (not milk) until at least 4 hours have passed without vomiting • Start with 1 tbsp (15 cc) every 10 minutes • If vomiting does not occur, double the amount each hour • If vomiting does occur, allow stomach to rest briefly and then start again • Key is to gradually increase amount of fluid until taking 8 oz every hour • May use glucose-electrolyte solutions developed for infants/small children such as Pedialyte or Rehydralyte (may combine with flavored gelatin to make more palatable) or sports drinks such as Gatorade which contain salt and sugar in addition to water • Goal is to ingest 1000 to 1500 mL/day • Resume normal diet as soon as tolerated (usually, 4 hours after vomiting ceases)

G. Pharmacologic therapy is usually not indicated; however, for selected patients (for example, those with electrolyte disturbances, severe anorexia/weight loss, motion sickness, pregnancy, or with chemotherapy-induced nausea and vomiting) antiemetic therapy may be indicated

> **Emetrol** (OTC): Do not dilute or take fluids 15 minutes before or after. Can be used in pregnancy
> - ✓ Adolescents: 15-30 mL at 15 minute intervals as needed
> - ✓ Children: 5-10 mL, same time interval as adolescents
>
> **Promethazine** (Phenergan) is the agent of choice for n/v from gastroenteritis: Available as 12.5, 25, 50 mg tabs and rectal supp; also available as syrup (6.25 mg/5 mL and 25 mg/5 mL)
> - ✓ Adolescents: 25 mg Q 8-12 hrs
> - ✓ Children >2: 12.5-25 mg Q 12 hrs
> - ✓ Children <2: Not recommended
>
> **Prochlorperazine** (Compazine): Available 5, 10 mg tabs; 10, 15, 30 mg spansules; 5 mg/5 mL syrup; 2.5, 5, 25 mg rectal supp
> - ✓ Adolescents: Tabs/5-10 mg 3-4 times day; spansules/10 mg Q 12 hrs; rectal supp/25 mg bid
> - ✓ Children: >2: Syrup or rectal supp, dose by weight: 20-29 lbs/2.5 mg 1-2 x d (max 7.5 mg/day); 20-39 lbs/2.5 mg 2-3 x d (max 10 mg/day); 40-85 lbs/5mg 2 x d (max 15 mg/day)
> - ✓ Children <2: Not recommended
>
> **Trimethobenzamide** (Tigan) works well for gastroenteritis and motion sickness: Available as 100, 300 mg caps and rectal supp—adult/100, 200 mg; pediatric/100 mg
> - ✓ Adolescents: 300 mg caps OR 200 mg rectal supp 3-4 x day
> - ✓ Children: 30-90 lb: Use 100 mg rectal supp 3-4 x day
>
> **Scopolamine** (Transderm Scop) works well for prevention and treatment of motion sickness: Available as 0.33 mg patch
> - ✓ Adolescents ≥18 years of age: Apply one patch in hairless area behind ear 4 hours prior to when antiemetic effect is needed
> - ✓ Replace after 3 days
> - ✓ Children: Not recommended

H.   The 5-HT$_3$ antagonist drugs have dramatically reduced vomiting associated with chemotherapy treatment (these drugs have been unsuccessful in controlling chemotherapy-induced nausea, however); examples of these drugs are Ondansetron (Zofran) and Dolasetron (Anzemet) [patients receiving chemotherapy will have these medications prescribed by the oncologist]

I.   Follow Up: None needed unless failure to respond to nonpharmacologic or pharmacologic therapy

CONSTIPATION

I.   Definition: Subjective complaint of passage of abnormally delayed or infrequent passage of dry, hardened feces, often accompanied by straining and/or pain

II.   Pathogenesis

A.   In normal defecation, stool is propelled from the colon into the anorectum where it is stored until it can be eliminated at a convenient time
1.   The mechanism of storage and elimination of stool relies on the complex interaction between muscles of the pelvic floor, the autonomic and somatic nervous systems, and the group of muscles controlling the anal sphincters
2.   Once the bolus of stool reaches the anorectum, distention of the wall results in a temporary reflex relaxation of the internal anal sphincter which permits the stool to come into contact with sensitive receptors of the anal canal
3.   The external sphincter simultaneously contracts, and the person has time to decide if the time is convenient for defecation
a.   When the person elects to defecate, increased intrarectal pressure from straining moves the stool towards the anal canal, the puborectalis muscle relaxes which allows the pelvic floor to descend; descent of the pelvic floor straightens the anorectal angle, the external anal sphincter relaxes, and the stool is expelled
b.   When the person elects to defer defecation, voluntary contraction of the puborectalis muscle and the external anal sphincter muscle decreases the anorectal angle to less than the usual 85 to 105° which prevents defecation; the rectum accommodates to its contents

B.   In young infants, the role played by the cerebral cortex in terms of delaying defecation is nonexistent; thus, defecation occurs when the internal sphincter relaxes

C. Difficulties with defecation may occur when there is dysfunction in any element of the normal mechanism of defecation; however, the final common pathway is likely to be a reduction in propulsive forces, defective rectal sensation, or a functional outlet obstruction

D. Whereas all of the above mechanisms could lead to chronic constipation in children, most childhood constipation results from intentional or subconscious withholding of stool, and is called idiopathic or functional constipation
   1. Precipitating events vary based on the age of the child–for example, the breastfed infant who is switched to cow's milk at 1 year of age may experience stools which are firmer and produce anal irritation leading to a pattern of withholding; the toddler may initiate a pattern of stool retention over struggles with parents over toileting; the school-age child may develop a retentive pattern because of discomfort with school toileting facilities
   2. A cycle of retention develops as increasingly larger volumes of stool must be expelled, often causing pain in the child who stiffens the body and tightens the gluteal muscles in an effort to prevent stooling

III. Clinical Presentation

A. Constipation is the most common digestive complaint in the US; the exact prevalence is unknown, but the complaint accounts for approximately 3% of visits to general pediatric practices and 10 to 25% of visits to pediatric gastroenterologists

B. A normal pattern of stooling is believed to be a sign of well-being in children of all ages and parents pay close attention to frequency and other characteristics of their child's defecation patterns, particularly in the first months of life

---

PATTERN OF STOOLING IN INFANTS AND YOUNG CHILDREN

➡ During the first week of life, infants have an average of 4 stools per day
➡ Frequency gradually declines to an average of 1.7 stools per day at 2 years of age
➡ By 4 years of age, an adult pattern of stooling (1.2 stools per day) is achieved
➡ Greater variability occurs among breastfed infants than in formula fed infants; some breastfed infants have a stool after every feeding (this occurs mainly during the first few weeks only) and others have infrequent passage of stool; as long as the stools are soft and the infant is content and growing normally, there is no cause for concern
➡ Parents should keep in mind that stooling patterns vary in children just as they do in adults
➡ Parents should be aware of their child's normal bowel pattern and typical size/consistency of stools

---

Adapted from Baker, S.S., Liptak, G.S., Colletti, R.B., Croffle, J.M., DiLorenzo, C., Ector, W., et al. (1999). Constipation in infants and children: Evaluation and treatment. *Journal of Pediatric Gastroenterology and Nutrition, 29,* 612-626.

C. Idiopathic constipation represents a complex interaction between parental expectations, the child's gastrointestinal physiology, development, and food and fluid intake

D. In infants who are constipated, the infant typically screams with the urge to pass stool, stiffens the body, and tightens the gluteal muscles while making an effort to resist the urge; the face may become flushed during the process, a sign misinterpreted by parents as an extreme effort to pass the stool

E. In toddlers and older children who are constipated, the child typically crosses his legs, stands upright (versus sitting), rocks back and forth on tiptoes, and holds onto furniture while waiting for urge to pass (which occurs as the rectum accommodates to its contents); the "dance" that the child performs is often misinterpreted by the parent as the child's straining in an attempt to defecate

F. Over time, for both infants and children, retentive behavior becomes an automatic reaction

G. After several days without a bowel movement, the child may exhibit irritability, abdominal distension, cramps, and decreased interest in eating

IV. Diagnosis/Evaluation

A. History
   1. Determine what the parent (or child in older children) means by constipation (Is it small stools, infrequent stools, or difficulty/pain with passing stools?) [for most parents, frequency is usually the issue, as frequency is the characteristic that is easiest to set standards for]

2. Ask about consistency and size of stools, whether defecation is painful, whether blood has been present on the stool or toilet paper, and if the child experiences abdominal pain

3. Ask about associated symptoms and signs such as fever, abdominal distention, anorexia, nausea, vomiting, weight loss or poor weight gain (presence of any of these suggests an organic cause)

4. Determine how long the condition has been present; ask if there is a history of stool withholding behavior and of fecal soiling–often mistaken by parent for diarrhea; (a history of stool withholding virtually excludes an organic cause for constipation)

5. Ask about dietary intake and activity level (intake that is low in fiber and fluids may contribute to problem)

6. Determine if there have been any recent changes in child's life (e.g., travel, change in school)

7. In school-age children, ask if the child uses the school restrooms and if the response is "no," determine why not

8. In infants, ask about feeding patterns including content of diet; inquire about timing after birth of the first bowel movement (most patients with Hirschsprung's disease fail to pass meconium within the first 48 hours of life)

9. Ask about current medications and laxative use

10. Obtain psychosocial history, including the family structure, number of people living in household and their relationship to child, interaction of child with peers, and the possibility of abuse

B. Physical Examination
1. Measure child's height and weight and plot on growth chart; determine if child is following her own growth curve

2. Assess abdomen for tenderness, masses

3. Examine the perineum and perianal area; at least one digital examination of the anorectum is recommended–anorectal examination is to assess perianal sensation, anal tone, size of the rectum, and presence of an anal wink (also determines amount and consistency of stool and its location in rectum)

4. A test for occult blood in the stool should be performed in all infants with constipation, as well as in any child who also has abdominal pain, failure to thrive, intermittent diarrhea, or a family history of colon cancer

C. Differential Diagnosis
1. Functional causes such as low fiber diet, poor fluid intake, coercive toilet training, or school bathroom avoidance

2. Structural abnormalities such as imperforate anus or anal stenosis

3. Endocrine and metabolic conditions such as hypothyroidism or gluten enteropathy

4. Intestinal nerve or muscle disorders such as Hirschsprung disease or visceral neuropathies

5. Drugs such as antacids and drugs that may affect the central nervous system

D. Diagnostic Tests:
1. A thorough history and physical examination is usually sufficient to establish whether the child has idiopathic constipation or requires referral to an expert for further evaluation

2. Refer to IV.B.4. above for recommendation regarding stool for occult blood

3. In selected children, an abdominal x-ray can be useful in diagnosing fecal impaction

V. Plan/Management

A. Infants and children with simple, acute constipation usually respond well to the following measures
1. Infants who are exclusively breastfed are less likely to develop constipation than are their formula-fed counterparts; if the only parental complaint is infrequent stools in an otherwise healthy breastfed infant who is growing normally and whose stools are soft, the problem is most likely related to the almost complete absorption of breast milk leaving very little residue for stool formation; if stools are hard, 5 to 10 mL of malt soup extract (Maltsupex) may be offered in water (or juice in infants >6 months) twice a day

2. Formula fed infants can have 5 to 10 mL of malt soup extract (Maltsupex) or dark Karo syrup added to a feeding, two or three times a day (**Note**: Light and dark corn syrups are not considered to be potential sources of *C. botulinum* spores)

3. For older infants (>6 months), increasing intake of fluids containing sorbitol such as apple juice, prune juice, or pear juice may be helpful; an osmotic laxative such as lactulose or sorbitol may also be prescribed (for both drugs, dosing is 1-3 mL/kg/day in divided doses)

4. Infants older than 6 months who are consuming solid foods should be offered water several times a day to increase fluid intake; prunes, apricots, plums, peas, and beans (pureed at 6 months and progressing to chopped by 12 months of age) increase fiber intake and can help with stool softening

5.   Advise parents to promptly treat any anal fissures with an ointment such as Vaseline; such treatment reduces the likelihood that infant will withhold stool

B.   Toddlers and older children with simple, acute constipation usually respond well to increasing fluids, particularly sorbitol-containing fruit juices, and encouraging increased dietary fiber intake; an osmotic laxative such as lactulose may also be prescribed
1.   See section on NUTRITION for latest recommendations on fiber intake
2.   If anal irritation/fissure is present, treat as under V.A.5. above

C.   Management of children with idiopathic constipation that is chronic is more complicated as these children are voluntary stool-withholders (**Note:** Encopresis is not discussed here; instead, for the child who has encopresis, see the section on ENCOPRESIS); management of children with chronic constipation includes the following
1.   Provide parental education
2.   Determine if impaction is present; if present, treat the impaction before proceeding further
3.   Initiate treatment with an oral medication to correct constipation and recommend measures to promote healthy bowel habits
4.   Follow-up at regular intervals and adjust medications as necessary

D.   Educate parents about constipation, including pathogenesis, and ways in which patterns of withholding often develop in children
1.   Assure parents that child does not have a physical problem which is very reassuring to most parents
2.   Encourage parents to maintain a consistent, positive, and supportive attitude for all aspects of treatment

E.   Disimpaction, if needed, may be carried out according to the following recommendations based on the age of the child and the preferences of the parent and child
1.   In infants, rectal disimpaction can be performed with glycerin suppositories; enemas should be avoided
2.   In toddlers and older children, disimpaction can be carried out with either oral or rectal medications, or a combination of the two
      a.   Example of oral medication–polyethylene glycol electrolyte solution (GoLYTELY), 10 mL/kg/dose x 1-2 doses, depending on extent of impaction (children dislike the taste, making this option difficult to implement)
      b.   Example of rectal medication–hypertonic sodium phosphate enema (Fleet), children 2-12 years, 2.5 oz; >12 years, 4.5 oz, x 1-3 days

F.   Once the impaction has been removed (and for children presenting without impaction), maintenance therapy should be initiated–cornerstone of maintenance therapy is behavior modification, dietary interventions, and use of medications to assure that bowel movements occur at normal intervals and with a good evacuation

G.   Dietary interventions include recommending a balanced diet that includes whole grains, fruits, and vegetables (see section on NUTRITION for more detailed dietary recommendations including recommended dietary intake of fiber); child should be encouraged to drink 4-6 ounces of prune juice/day and to drink water frequently throughout the day

H.   All children should engage in 60 minutes of physical activity each day; many children lead sedentary lifestyles which predispose to constipation

I.   Behavior modification for the older, toilet-trained child includes the following recommendations
1.   Retrain the already toilet-trained child in proper bowel habits
      a.   Encourage child to not ignore urge to defecate, even though it may be inconvenient
      b.   Child should sit on toilet, with proper foot support to allow for hip flexion and to help leverage for 5 to 10 minutes after breakfast and the evening meal to take advantage of the gastrocolic reflex
2.   Child should be rewarded with stickers and given positive reinforcement such as having parent play a game or read a story as a reward for proper toileting

J.   Older, toilet-trained children should also be given a maintenance medication that will overcome their tendency to withhold stool and prevent reimpaction; mineral oil, magnesium hydroxide or lactulose are equally efficacious and the choice among these should be based on cost, the child's preference, ease or administration, and the clinician's experience
1.   Lactulose, 10 g/15mL, 1-3 mL/kg/day in divided doses (well tolerated long-term), OR
2.   Mineral oil, 1-3 mL/kg/day, OR
3.   Magnesium hydroxide, 1-3 mL/kg/day of 400 mg/5mL (inexpensive)
4.   Adjust dose to induce a daily bowel movement for 1-2 months, before attempting to wean child from drug
5.   Drug should be promptly reinstated if relapse occurs
6.   All 4 drugs are safe for long term use (but not FDA-approved for long-term use)
7.   Maintenance therapy is usually necessary for many months
8.   Relapses are common and difficulty with bowel movements may continue into adolescence

K.   Treatment of toddlers and preschoolers who are not yet toilet-trained (or who are only recently toilet trained) should focus on overcoming the child's tendency to withhold stool; a good choice is lactulose; dosing is 1-3 mL/kg/day in divided doses
1.   Behavior modification such as toilet-sitting after meals to take advantage of the gastrocolic reflex should be used with caution in this age group as toilet-sitting may be viewed as punishment and may cause power struggles relating to toilet-training
2.   The first step is to correct the withholding behavior; the next step is to resume toilet training
3.   Lactulose is safe for long term use; maintenance therapy is usually needed for many months
4.   Dose should induce daily bowel movement; after 1-2 months, parent should attempt to wean child from drug
5.   Drug should be reinstated if relapse occurs

L.   Follow-Up
1.   No follow up is needed for children with acute constipation unless the problem continues to recur
2.   Children with chronic constipation need follow-up in 2-4 weeks to determine efficacy, and then every 3-6 months
3.   Children who fail therapy should be referred to an expert for evaluation and management

IRRITABLE BOWEL SYNDROME

I.   Definition: Chronic, benign gastrointestinal disorder characterized by abdominal pain, bloating, and disturbed defecation that cannot be explained by structural or biochemical abnormalities

II.   Pathogenesis:

A.   A complex interaction of bio-psycho-social factors are believed to generate the symptoms of irritable bowel syndrome (IBS) in children and adolescents by a combination of intestinal motor, sensory, and central nervous system activity

B.   Little is known regarding these factors in childhood compared with adulthood; preliminary research, however, indicates that IBS in children is very similar to that in adults; thus the mechanisms involved must be similar and are summarized here
1.   **Altered bowel motility**: Changes in the contractility of the colon and small bowel. Such factors as psychological or physical stress, ingestion of food, ingestion of a high fat meal, and fasting have all been implicated in altering bowel motility in patients with IBS
2.   **Visceral hypersensitivity**: Differences in the way that the brain of affected persons modulates afferent signals from the dorsal-horn neurons through the ascending pathways suggest a primary central defect of visceral pain processing (an alternative hypothesis is that rather than true visceral hypersensitivity, hypervigilance may be responsible for the low pain threshold of IBS patients)
3.   **Psychosocial factors**: Psychological stress including a history of abuse in childhood can alter motor function in the small bowel and colon; one theory is that experiences early in life may affect the central nervous system in such a way as to confer a predisposition to a state of hypervigilance
4.   **Neurotransmitter imbalance**: Serotonin as well as a number of other neurotransmitters are known to influence bowel contractility and visceral sensitivity and may well provide links between the enteric and central nervous systems

5.   **Infection and inflammation**: Much evidence points to a role for infection in the initiation of (or a contribution to) activation of peripheral sensitization or hypermotility in affected persons

C.   Presently, no single conceptual model can explain all cases of the irritable bowel syndrome

III.   Clinical Presentation

A.   Fifteen percent of school-age children have episodes of recurrent abdominal pain that affect their daily activities; an organic cause can be found in only about 10% of cases, and the remainder are thought to be functional gastrointestinal disorders (FGIDs)

B.   Irritable bowel syndrome is a major disorder associated with functional abdominal pain in childhood
1.   Most common presentation is that of abdominal pain and bloating along with altered bowel habits with either diarrhea or constipation predominating
2.   Pattern of symptoms varies from person to person but symptoms are generally mild to moderate with little disability
3.   Symptoms are most often intermittent, though some patients have daily problems and a small percentage of patients are refractory to treatment, with pain that is disabling
4.   The syndrome can be divided into four subcategories according to the predominance of the symptom experienced by the patient: abdominal pain, diarrhea, constipation, or constipation alternating with diarrhea

C.   The Rome II criteria are a symptom-based classification system of FGIDs associated with recurrent abdominal pain; the Rome II criteria for irritable bowel syndrome are contained in the table that follows

ROME II CRITERIA FOR DIAGNOSIS OF IRRITABLE BOWEL SYNDROME
The child must be old enough to provide an accurate history of the pain
Presence for at least 12 weeks (not necessarily consecutive) in the preceding 12 months of abdominal discomfort or pain that cannot be explained by structural or biochemical abnormalities and that has at least 2 of the following 3 features: • Pain relieved with defecation; and/or   • Onset is associated with a change in frequency of stooling (diarrhea or constipation); and/or   • Onset is associated with a change in consistency or form of stool (loose, watery, or pellet-like)

Adapted from Thompson, W.G., Longstreth, C.F., Drossman, D.A., Heaton, K.W., Irvine, K.J., Muller-Lissner, S.A. (1999). Functional bowel disorders and functional abdominal pain. *Gut, 45* (Suppl2), 1143-1147.

D.   Additional features which support a diagnosis of IBS include abnormal stool frequency (>3 bowel movements per day or <3 bowel movements per week), abnormal stool form (lumpy/hard, loose/watery), abnormal stool passage (straining, urgency, or feeling of incomplete evacuation), passage of mucus, or bloating or feeling of abdominal distension

IV.   Diagnosis/Evaluation

A.   History
1.   Ask about onset, duration, location, and severity of abdominal pain and changes over time
2.   Is timing of pain related to meals or to the ingestion of certain foods?
3.   Ask questions relating to Rome II diagnostic criteria and the additional features outlined above

> • Has the abdominal pain/discomfort been present for at least 12 weeks during the last 12 months?
>   ✓ Is pain relieved with defecation?
>   ✓ Is pain associated with a change in frequency of stool?
>   ✓ Is pain associated with change in consistency of stool?
> • Determine which of 4 symptoms is predominant–abdominal pain, diarrhea, constipation, or constipation alternating with diarrhea

4.   If diarrhea is present, question about blood in diarrhea, awakening in night because of diarrhea (if positive response to either question, points to inflammatory bowel disease rather than IBS)
5.   Determine if alarm markers are present to rule out the possibility of a disease process causing the problems

6. Inquire if psychological stress occurred at about time the disorder appeared or intensified
7. Obtain diet history to determine usual diet and eating patterns
8. Ask about drug/alcohol use/present medications used
9. Ask detailed questions about previous diagnostic evaluations by other healthcare providers; determine outcomes of previous treatments
10. In adolescent females in whom menarche has occurred, take menstrual history

B. Physical Examination
   1. Determine if weight loss or delayed linear growth has occurred by performing measurements and comparing with previous weight and height
   2. Perform abdominal exam for general appearance, tenderness, guarding, rigidity, abnormal bowel sounds, masses, liver or spleen enlargement
   3. Perform rectal exam for tenderness, masses; stool for occult blood
   4. Assess sexual maturity (Tanner stages) **Note:** The physical exam serves mainly to exclude other diagnoses and to reassure the patient; mild left lower quadrant tenderness can be present in patients with IBS

C. Differential Diagnosis
   1. Lactase deficiency
   2. Urinary tract infection
   3. Inflammatory bowel disease
   4. Parasitic infection (Giardia)

D. Diagnostic Tests
   1. Complete blood count, erythrocyte sedimentation rate
   2. Stool for ova and parasites
   3. More selective testing, such as breath hydrogen analysis for carbohydrate malabsorption, can be done on a case-by-case basis

V. Plan/Management

A. For patients with typical presentation who meet the Rome II criteria and who demonstrate no abnormalities on physical examination or laboratory testing (and if alarm markers are not present), diagnosis of irritable bowel syndrome, a diagnosis of exclusion, can be made

B. Establishment of an effective relationship based on education and reassurance of the child and parents is important in order to maximize the efficacy of treatment and is fundamental to any treatment plan
   1. Clinician validation of the symptoms can be very beneficial to the child and parents
   2. The pathophysiology of the disorder should be explained in simple terms
   3. Asking the patient and family about their concerns and fears is a good beginning point to any discussion

C. The most reasonable approach to treating IBS is to use the patient's predominant symptom as a guide
   1. Based on the history, determine which subcategory best describes the patient: Is the predominant symptom abdominal pain, diarrhea, constipation, or constipation alternating with diarrhea?
   2. Implement a treatment plan based on the predominant symptom as a beginning point

D. For patients in all subcategories–abdominal pain, diarrhea, constipation, or alternating constipation and diarrhea–use of a food intake and symptom diary can be helpful. This approach serves the purpose of helping the patient take responsibility for his/her own care and also helps to identify whether exacerbation of symptoms occurs after consuming certain foods, or if certain events (exercise, menses, stressful situations) make condition worse

1. For a two week period, ask patient to record symptom, date/time of occurrence, description of severity (scale of 0-10), factors associated with symptom (diet, activity, menses, stressful event, etc.); emotional responses (what person feels); thoughts and cognition (what person thinks)
2. Review the symptom diary with the patient on return visit as a way of evaluating his/her progress in "gaining control" of the condition; decide with the patient if the symptom diary approach is helpful and worthwhile to continue on subsequent visits

E. **For patients in whom the predominant symptom is abdominal pain**, the following approach can be used
   1. Elimination of gas-forming foods may be helpful (legumes, broccoli, cauliflower, cabbage, onions, cucumbers); if symptoms improve, these foods can be gradually reintroduced
   2. Lactose should not be restricted unless laboratory tests document lactose malabsorption
   3. Prescribe an antispasmodic agent—dicyclomine hydrochloride or hyoscyamine sulfate—refer to table below for dosage guidelines; these drugs reduce abdominal pain or bloating through anticholinergic pathways
   4. Consider prescribing a secondary tricyclic amine such as nortriptyline or desipramine (refer to table below for dosage guidelines) which may be helpful in some patients

F. **For patients in whom the predominant symptom is diarrhea**, the following approach can be used
   1. Use of fiber supplements to add bulk to the stool may occasionally improve diarrhea (Note: Insoluble fiber such as methylcellulose [Citrucel] works well for persons with IBS because, unlike soluble fiber such as psyllium husk [e.g., Metamucil products], it is non gas-producing)
      a. Unfortunately, insoluble fiber—unlike soluble fiber—has no role in lowering cholesterol or normalizing blood sugar in persons who could benefit from such effects
      b. Dietary fiber may also be recommended (see fiber recommendations in section on NUTRITION)
   2. Advise patient to avoid foods that exacerbate symptoms (based on food diary experience); common foods that increase symptoms are those that contain sorbitol such as sugarless gum and dietetic candy
   3. Use of antidiarrheal agents such as loperamide or bismuth subsalicylate may help decrease the frequency of bowel movements and improve consistency of stool (refer to table below for dosage guidelines)

G. **For patients in whom the predominant symptom is constipation**, the following approaches can be used
   1. Increase dietary fiber as above under V.F.1.
   2. Prescribe use of a laxative such as milk of magnesia or lactulose; these medications are generally considered safe for long-term use although no laxative is approved for chronic use
      a. Milk of magnesia may be the best choice for many patients because it is inexpensive and effective—dosing is 15-45 mL PO once daily at bedtime
      b. Nonabsorbable sugars such as lactulose (Kristalose) are generally well-tolerated but may have side effects of bloating and flatulence (refer to table below for dosage guidelines)
      c. Patients should be advised to titrate dose of laxative until stool is soft, but not liquid
   3. Tegaserod maleate (Zelnorm) has been approved by the FDA for short-term treatment of women ≥18 years of age with irritable bowel syndrome with constipation as the predominant symptom
      a. Activates $5-HT_4$ receptors on neurons in GI tract thereby promoting motility and also decreasing visceral sensation
      b. Recommended duration of treatment is 4-6 weeks with an additional 4-6 weeks as an option for responders; cost of 60 2-mg or 6-mg tabs is approximately $150
      c. Dose at 6 mg orally BID before meals; consult PDR for contraindications, interactions, and precautions
      d. IBS is a chronic disease–long term efficacy and safety of this drug have not been established and is best reserved for use in a specialty setting

H. **For patients in whom there is constipation alternating with diarrhea**, the patient should be advised to self-monitor condition and to respond appropriately (based on recommendations in V.F. and G. above for management of diarrhea and constipation), depending on whether the symptom at the time is diarrhea or constipation

DOSAGE GUIDELINES FOR DRUGS COMMONLY USED TO TREAT IRRITABLE BOWEL SYNDROME

Drug	Dosing in Children
Anticholinergic agents	
Hyoscyamine sulfate (Levsin and Levsin Elixir) Available as scored tabs (0.125 mg) and elixir (0.125 mg/5mL)	40-49 kg: 3.75 mL Q 4 hrs PRN ≥50 kg: 5 mL or one tab Q 4 hrs PRN
Antidiarrheal agents	
Loperamide (Imodium) Available as A-D caplets (2 mg) and liquid (1 mg/5mL) [both OTC]	60-95 lbs (9-11 years): Initially 2 mg, then 1 mg after each loose stool (max 6 mg/day x 2 days) >12 years, initially 4 mg, then 2 mg after each loose stool (max 16 mg/day x 2 days)
Bismuth subsalicylate (Pepto-Bismol) Available as chewable tabs (262 mg) and liquid (262 mg/15 mL)	9-12 years, 1 caplet or 15 mL >12 years, 2 caplets or 30 mL For all, repeat Q 30-60 minutes if needed (max 8 doses/day)
Osmotic laxatives	

Lactulose
   Available as 10 g and 20 g packets
   10 g packet dissolved in 4 oz of water = 15 mL liquid lactulose
	1-3 mL/kg/day in divided doses (off-label use)

I.   Discuss with all patients and their parents–whether their predominant symptom is abdominal pain, diarrhea, constipation, or diarrhea alternating with constipation–that modifications in lifestyle are well recognized for their potential benefit on symptom management

    1.   Stress reduction is important, and can be accomplished via the use of relaxation tapes, books, or meditation taught by behavioral therapists or others in group settings

    2.   Biofeedback can sometimes help decrease stress and reduce gut hypersensitivity

    3.   Regular exercise can reduce stress and increase feelings of well-being; current recommendations are for adults to engage in 60 minutes of moderate intensity physical activity each day

J.   Follow Up

    1.   Frequent follow up is important; first follow up visit should be in 2 weeks, then monthly, then every 3-6 months

    2.   Patients who fail to respond to therapy after an adequate trial should be referred to an expert in the diagnosis and management of functional bowel disorders for evaluation and management

GASTROESOPHAGEAL REFLUX IN INFANTS

I.   Definition: Effortless regurgitation of a portion of the feeding without a definable anatomic, metabolic, infectious, or neurologic etiology

II.   Pathogenesis

    A.   There are three main physiological barriers for preventing reflux of gastric contents into the esophagus:

        1.   Functional esophageal sphincter

        2.   Normal distal esophageal motility

        3.   Efficient gastric emptying

    B.   Reflux in infants is considered to be a normal physiologic event, and appears to be caused by a delay in maturation of one or more of the three barriers and is considered a multifactorial disorder

III.   Clinical Presentation

    A.   Reflux is a common condition; estimates are that at least one episode of regurgitation a day occurs in 50% of 0- to 3-month old infants, with the incidence peaking at 4 months in most infants

    B.   Self-limited; resolves rapidly with time. Many affected infants have normal function by 6 months; by 12 months almost all have improved or resolved; over 90% have complete resolution by 18 months

    C.   Most often occurs during or soon after feeding

D. Infants with physiologic reflux are otherwise healthy with appropriate growth and development

E. Choking during feedings (except on a very occasional basis) should not be attributed to reflux

F. Infants with significant regurgitation or vomiting might be responding to disease process outside the gastrointestinal tract

G. Gastroesophageal reflux disease (GERD) is a pathologic process in infants and is usually accompanied by poor weight gain, signs of esophagitis, persistent respiratory symptoms, and, occasionally, changes in neurobehavior

IV. Diagnosis/Evaluation

A. History
1. Question regarding type, amount, and frequency of feeding; timing, frequency, and amount of reflux
2. Ask if coughing or frequent choking during feedings occurs
3. Question regarding bloody or bilious vomiting, regurgitation of entire feedings
4. Question about signs or symptoms such as fever, irritability, poor feeding, or diarrhea that might be associated with an infectious, metabolic, or neurologic cause for the reflux
5. Question regarding attainment of developmental milestones
6. Ask about any illnesses or hospitalizations since birth
7. Ask about family history of dietary protein allergy

B. Physical Examination
1. Measure length, weight, and head circumference and compare with previous serial measurements to document normal growth
2. Perform a complete head-to-toe exam, making sure to check gag and sucking reflexes
3. Observe child being fed; determine if developmental milestones are being achieved (see section on CHILD HEALTH SUPERVISION)

C. Differential Diagnosis
1. Partial upper-intestinal obstruction
2. Infections such as otitis media, pneumonia, urinary tract infection

D. Diagnostic Tests: None indicated if history and physical exam are normal and infant is growing and developing normally

V. Plan/Management

A. Uncomplicated GER in infants is usually self-limiting and resolves spontaneously by 12 months of age

B. Rationale for the indiscriminate treatment of reflux with pharmacologic therapy in infants under 2 years of age has received little justification in the medical literature and is therefore discouraged

C. Management should be aimed at reassuring the parents and counseling them about postural placement and feeding techniques

D. Recommended postural placement: Instruct parents to hold infant upright after feeding for 15-30 minutes
1. Although there is good evidence that the prone sleeping position reduces acid exposure, this position it is not recommended for infants because of its association with sudden infant death syndrome; therefore, it should not be used
2. Furthermore, once the infant reaches 3-4 months of age and can turn over, it is almost impossible to maintain infant in any specific position when placed in a crib

E. Dietary measures: Instruct parent in these feeding techniques
1. Avoid overfeeding and provide smaller, more frequent feedings to decrease stomach distention and reduce the volume available for reflux

2. Use of thickening agents such as rice cereal may be helpful, but there is not much research to support its use
3. For formula fed infants, the addition of 1 to 1.5 teaspoons of dry rice cereal per ounce of milk that thickens the formula but still allows for flow through a normal or slightly cross-cut nipple is reasonable; the added cereal results in a formula that is about 25 kcal/ounce instead of 20 kcal/ounces and is especially appropriate in infants whose weight gain is on the low normal side
4. Breastfed infants can be spoon-fed, mixed with breast milk in the same proportions as with formula (see above)
5. Use of hypoallergenic formula can also be considered in formula-fed infants, but there is no evidence that formula plays a role in most cases of infantile GER

F. With postprandial regurgitation of a small amount of feeding, no specific treatment other than reassurance to parent is indicated

G. Refer the patient to a specialist if abnormalities of the upper gastrointestinal tract are suspected, if there is failure to gain weight at an appropriate rate, or if developmental delays are noted

H. Follow Up: In 2-4 weeks to evaluate if reflux is resolving

COLIC

I. Definition: Episodes of intense fussing and crying in an otherwise healthy infant lasting for several hours a day, most often in the early evening

II. Pathogenesis: Possible etiologies include normal variant, discomfort between parent and infant, family tensions, immaturity of the gastrointestinal tract, stimulus sensitivity (infant easily startled and awakened), temperamental disposition in the infant, protein or carbohydrate intolerance

III. Clinical Presentation

A. Affects up to 30% of infants worldwide and occurs equally in breastfed and formula fed infants of both genders

B. Onset is usually at 2-4 weeks of age and condition resolves by about 3 months of age; most 4 month old infants are symptom-free

C. The most frequently used diagnostic criterion is the "rule of threes"–crying more than 3 hours per day, more than 3 days per week, for more than 3 weeks; crying is not random but tends to cluster in the late afternoon and early evening hours

D. During the attack, infant appears hypertonic with entire body stiffened, hands clenched, and legs flexed rigidly over abdomen; crying is paroxysmal—begins and ends without warning and unrelated to environmental events

E. Infants with colic resist soothing, lack the ability to self-calm, and have crying episodes that are difficult to terminate, once initiated

IV. Diagnosis/Evaluation

A. History
1. Determine age at onset and pattern of crying (time of day, duration, and so on); type, quantity, and frequency of feeding, satisfaction with feeding, and elimination patterns
2. Inquire about interventions tried and their effectiveness
3. Ask how the infant is doing otherwise in terms of behavior and activity

B. Physical Examination
1. Take vital signs; measure and plot length, weight, and head circumference to determine growth patterns
2. Assess for developmental milestones

3. Look for conditions that would increase irritability
4. Use exam to reassure parents

C. Differential Diagnosis
  1. Colic is a diagnosis of exclusion used to explain recurrent, prolonged crying episodes in healthy appearing infants
  2. Must exclude acute causes of infant crying such as infection, cow's mild protein intolerance, obstruction/gastrointestinal dysfunction, and injury

D. Diagnostic Tests: None indicated if child is gaining weight, achieving developmental milestones, has a normal physical exam, and nothing in the history indicates a need for further evaluation

V. Plan/Management

A. Intervention should focus on reducing the infant's crying and allaying the stress experienced by caregivers

FOUR AREAS OF INTERVENTION FOR COLIC	
Educate parents	Regarding infant colic and the self-limited nature of the condition; crying may be reduced temporarily by various interventions but is unlikely to disappear for several weeks
Provide support	To the family through empathic listening and assurance to the family that there will be follow up (allows parents to know that they are not alone in dealing with this)
Emphasize normality	Baby is growing and developing as expected (based on history and physical exam)
Suggest interventions	That parents may try with recognition that such treatments are of questionable value and may fail

B. To provide a focus for parental anxiety and to help parents recognize that the infant is growing normally in spite of the crying, consider suggesting that a diary of the crying bouts as well as a record of weight gain be kept (**Note**: Use this strategy selectively as some parents are already focusing too much on the crying bouts and this approach may not help)
  1. Based on information relating to episodes of crying, parents may be able to see a pattern in the infant's behavior and can anticipate periods during the day when more time may need to be spent in soothing the infant
  2. Infant weight gain will reassure parents that the crying is not associated with organic disease (in the absence of other symptoms and signs)

C. Interventions that **may** work with some babies are summarized in the table below

ADVICE TO PARENTS ON HOW TO SOOTHE A CRYING BABY
➡ Use rhythmic rocking motions, such as infant swing, car ride, carrying baby in body carrier
➡ Try continuous monotonous noise such as a fan, vaporizer, or fish tank aerator (warn parents **not to place infant on top of washer or clothes dryer** as serious injury from falls could occur)
➡ Encourage sucking using pacifier
➡ Try slow feedings with infant held in vertical position during feeding
➡ Burp infant in upright position after every 1-2 ounces of formula or 5-10 minutes of breastfeeding
➡ Place infant face down across knees with tummy on warm hot water bottle (wrapped in towel) and rub gently on back; pressure on abdomen may relieve discomfort
➡ Use swaddling, cuddling, and soothing methods to create restful environment
➡ Advise parent to have someone else look after baby every few days for a few hours if parent is feeling very tense and anxious
➡ Caution parent to never shake the baby!
➡ Finally, parents should understand that none of these strategies may work, and that putting a crying infant in her crib is permissible for short periods of time (<10 minutes); leaving infant to cry it out so that she learns to control her crying is not effective and should be strongly discouraged

D.	Watchful waiting may be the best approach
1.	There is no available safe medication with proven efficacy
2.	Formula changes have not been shown to be an effective remedy for colic and may suggest to the parents that the infant has a medical problem when none exists
a.	Allergy to cow's milk protein during infancy is very uncommon
b.	Infants who have dietary protein allergy present with persistent vomiting and/or diarrhea, weight loss, blood in stool
3.	Change to soy formulas is not usually helpful and about 25% of infants with a true allergy to cow's milk protein are also allergic to soy formula
4.	If mother is breastfeeding, she should continue

E.	Follow up by telephone in a few days and again in a week or two to determine progress

HYPERBILIRUBINEMIA IN THE HEALTHY TERM INFANT

I.	Definition: Elevations in bilirubin in the circulating blood, resulting in clinically apparent icterus or jaundice that occurs in infants ≥37 weeks of gestation who are otherwise healthy

II.	Pathogenesis

A.	Newborn hyperbilirubinemia results from a predisposition to the production of bilirubin in newborn infants and their limited ability to excrete it

B.	Nonpathologic causes of hyperbilirubinemia in the neonate are physiologic jaundice and jaundice associated with breastfeeding
1.	Physiologic jaundice results from the interaction of a number of complex factors that results in an overproduction of bilirubin as well as delayed conjugation of bilirubin
a.	Newborns, especially those who are preterm, have higher rates of bilirubin than adults because their red cells have a shorter life span and a higher turnover
b.	Unconjugated bilirubin is not readily excreted, and the ability to conjugate bilirubin is limited
c.	These limitations lead to physiologic jaundice–that is, high serum bilirubin concentrations in the first days of life in full-term infants, followed by a decline during the next several weeks to values commonly found in adults
2.	Jaundice associated with breastfeeding most likely results from the following mechanisms
a.	Predominant source of bilirubin is the breakdown of hemoglobin in red cells; heme is degraded by heme oxygenase, resulting in the release of iron and formation of carbon monoxide and biliverdin; biliverdin is further reduced to bilirubin by biliverdin reductase
b.	Bilirubin then enters liver where it is modified to an excretable conjugated form that enters the intestinal lumen
c.	Exclusively breastfed infants have low levels of the intestinal bacteria that are capable of converting bilirubin to nonresorbable derivatives in the intestinal lumen
d.	In these infants, the enterohepatic circulation of bilirubin may be increased

C.	There are numerous pathologic causes of neonatal jaundice including hemolysis from Rh/ABO incompatibility, hemoglobinopathies, erythrocyte membrane defects, sepsis, hypoxia, and Gilbert's syndrome

III.	Clinical Presentation

A.	Over the past decade, the trend to discharge newborns from the hospital sooner after birth, limiting the opportunity to detect jaundice during the period when the serum bilirubin concentration is likely to rise, has been a factor in delaying the early identification and treatment of hyperbilirubinemia; in recent years, there have been case reports of kernicterus in the US

B.	The average full-term newborn infant has a peak serum bilirubin concentration of 5 to 6 mg/dL;
1.	Exaggerated physiologic jaundice occurs at values above this threshold (7 to 17 mg/dL)
2.	Serum bilirubin concentrations higher than 17 mg/dL in full-term infants are not considered physiologic; a cause of pathologic jaundice can usually be identified in such infants

C. Physiologic jaundice is a self-limited clinical state that usually appears on the second or third day of life and resolves in 7-10 days in the full-term infant (pattern in preterm infant is different)
   1. Peak rise in bilirubin occurs at 3 days of age and rarely exceeds 10 mg/dL
   2. Presently, it remains unclear as to what level of bilirubin concentration or under what circumstances significant risk of brain damage occurs or when the risk of damage exceeds the risk of treatment

D. Jaundice associated with breastfeeding occurs in about 1% of breast-fed infants, usually appearing between the 6th and 8th days of life in otherwise healthy infants
   1. Frequently recurs in siblings
   2. The serum concentration of unconjugated bilirubin is usually ≤15 mg/dL
   3. Approximately 30% of healthy breastfed infants have persistent jaundice
   4. Breast milk jaundice has never been known to cause kernicterus

E. A mild, gradual caudal progression of yellow skin discoloration is the usual presentation in a neonate with physiologic jaundice or jaundice associated with breastfeeding
   1. Dermal icterus is apparent first in the face and progresses caudally to the trunk and extremities
   2. As the total serum bilirubin (TSB) rises, the extent of cephalocaudal progression may be helpful in quantifying the degree of jaundice; the use of an icterometer or transcutaneous jaundice meter may be helpful
   3. Skin color of the infant may alter the clinical presentation of jaundice but the sclera, mucous membranes, and palmar aspects of the hands and feet are good indicators of the degree of jaundice

IV. Diagnosis/Evaluation

A. History
   1. Question parent about onset of jaundice; ask when was jaundice first noticed and what part of the body was involved initially
   2. Obtain complete feeding history including whether bottle or breast fed, type of formula (if bottle-fed), number and amount of feedings, and how infant tolerates feedings
   3. In addition to jaundice, question parent if other signs and symptoms are present such as poor feeding, vomiting, lethargy, irritability, abnormal stooling, decrease in number of wet diapers
   4. Inquire about the course of pregnancy, including history of maternal illnesses, exposure to infection, drug use during pregnancy, and any medications taken during the pregnancy; obtain complete birth history including any maternal complications, weight and Apgar scores of infant at birth
   5. Obtain detailed family history including presence of familial forms of jaundice, whether jaundice was present in sibling (or patient), and whether there have been infant deaths of patient's siblings

B. Physical Examination
   1. Determine if fever is present, and weigh infant to assess weight gain (or loss) since birth
   2. A well-lighted room is essential for a proper clinical assessment of jaundice
   3. Observe overall appearance, looking for congenital malformations and dysmorphism
   4. Observe skin color which may be yellowish; observe conjunctiva for icterus
   5. Blanch the skin using digital pressure to reveal the underlying color of the skin and the subcutaneous tissue (experts in the diagnosis and management of neonatal jaundice may use noninvasive measurement instruments such as an icterometer or transcutaneous jaundice meter to help quantify the degree of jaundice)
   6. Perform complete physical exam, focusing on the abdominal exam; determine size, firmness, and texture of the liver

C. Differential Diagnosis: Pathologic versus physiologic/breastmilk jaundice
   1. Factors that suggest the possibility of hemolytic disease are listed in the following table

FACTORS SUGGESTING HEMOLYTIC DISEASE IN THE NEWBORN
✓ Family history of significant hemolytic disease
✓ Onset of jaundice prior to age 24 hours
✓ A rise in serum bilirubin levels of more than 0.5 mg/dL/hour
✓ Pallor, hepatosplenomegaly
✓ Rapid increase in the TSB level after 24-48 hours
✓ Ethnicity suggestive of inherited disease
✓ Failure of phototherapy to lower the TSB level

2. Factors that suggest the possibility of other disease such as sepsis or galactosemia are listed in the following table

FACTORS SUGGESTING OTHER DISEASES
✓ Vomiting, poor feeding, lethargy
✓ Apnea, tachypnea
✓ Hepatosplenomegaly
✓ Weight loss, temperature instability

D. Diagnostic Tests
1. A direct Coombs' test, a blood type, and an Rh(D) type on the infant's cord (preferably) or venous blood are recommended when the mother has not had prenatal blood grouping or is Rh-negative
2. Measure infant's total serum bilirubin (TSB) with follow up measurements as indicated
3. If pathologic jaundice is suspected based on history and physical examination, additional testing will be done by the specialist to whom the infant is referred

V. Plan/Management

A. All newborn infants who are discharged 48 hours or less after delivery should meet the criteria of the American Academy of Pediatrics for early discharge and should be examined for jaundice within 2 to 3 days after discharge

B. All infants suspected of having pathologic jaundice, or who have difficulty feeding, behavior changes, apnea, fever, or temperature instability must be referred immediately to an expert for management

C. Management of hyperbilirubinemia in the healthy term newborn has been outlined in a practice parameter issued by the American Academy of Pediatrics (AAP) and provides the basis for the recommendations contained here

D. The practice parameter is based on the underlying belief that therapeutic interventions for hyperbilirubinemia in the healthy term infant may carry significant risk relative to the uncertain risk of hyperbilirubinemia in this population and that there are no simple solutions to management of neonates who are jaundiced

E. Management decisions are based on age of the infant in hours and the total serum bilirubin levels (**Note**: Keep in mind that this discussion involves management of the healthy term infant with physiologic or breast-feeding jaundice only!)
1. Four options are recommended and are detailed in the four tables that follow: Consider phototherapy, order phototherapy, order exchange transfusion, and order both exchange transfusion and phototherapy
2. Recommendations are for infants initially seen with elevated TSB levels as well as infants who are being followed up for clinical jaundice
3. The TSB level is relied on as the relevant criterion; because direct bilirubin measurements vary substantially among various laboratories, it is recommended that the direct bilirubin measurement NOT be subtracted from the TSB level
4. There is continuing uncertainty regarding what specific TSB levels warrant exchange transfusion

F.   Infants ≤24 hours old are excluded from the practice parameter because jaundice occurring before the age of 24 hours is considered pathologic and always requires further evaluation

G.   Treatment of jaundice associated with breastfeeding should follow the same guidelines as those outlined in the tables below with the following special considerations
    1.   Breastfeeding in healthy term newborns should not be interrupted; continued and frequent breastfeeding (8-10 times every 24 hours) is recommended (increasing the number of oral feedings allows for more rapid excretion of bilirubin)
    2.   Supplementing breastfeeding with water or dextrose water does not lower the bilirubin level in jaundiced, healthy, breastfed infants and is therefore unnecessary
    3.   However, depending upon the mother's preference and the clinician's judgment, several options are available; breastfeeding can be continued or interrupted and phototherapy administered if indicated based on age of infant in hours and TSB level

INFANTS IN THE FOLLOWING CATEGORY SHOULD BE CONSIDERED* FOR PHOTOTHERAPY	
Age in Hours	TSB Level, mg/dL (pmol/L)
25-48	>12 (170)
49-72	>15 (260)
>72	>17 (290)

*This means that treatment with phototherapy is a clinical option that is available and should be used according to the judgment of the clinician in consultation with experts and with the parents

INFANTS IN THE FOLLOWING CATEGORY SHOULD RECEIVE PHOTOTHERAPY	
Age in Hours	TSB Level, mg/dL (pmol/L)
25-48	>15 (260)
49-72	>18 (310)
>72	>20 (340)

INFANTS IN THE FOLLOWING CATEGORY SHOULD RECEIVE EXCHANGE TRANSFUSION IF INTENSIVE PHOTOTHERAPY FAILS*	
Age in Hours	TSB Level, mg/dL (pmol/L)
25-48	>20 (340)
49-72	>25 (430)
>72	>25 (430)

* Intensive phototherapy should produce a decline of TSB of 1-2 mg/dL within 4-6 hours and the TSB level should continue to fall and remain below the threshold level for exchange transfusion--if this does not occur, phototherapy is considered a failure

INFANTS IN THE FOLLOWING CATEGORY SHOULD RECEIVE EXCHANGE TRANSFUSION AND INTENSIVE PHOTOTHERAPY	
Age in Hours	TSB Level, mg/dL (pmol/L)
25-48	>25 (430)
49-72	>30 (510)
>72	>30 (510)

Source for preceding four tables: American Academy of Pediatrics, Provisional Committee for Quality Improvement and Subcommittee on Hyperbilirubinemia. (1994). Management of hyperbilirubinemia in the healthy term newborn. *Pediatrics, 94*, 558-562.

Follow Up
       1.   Infants requiring phototherapy and exchange transfusion are best managed by experts
       2.   Many issues must be managed such as selection of method for delivery of phototherapy,
             intermittent versus continuous phototherapy, role of intensive phototherapy, requirements for
             hydration and fluid supplementation, and criteria for discontinuation of phototherapy
       3.   Follow up should be with the specialist to whom the infant was referred

ABDOMINAL HERNIA (INGUINAL AND UMBILICAL)

I.   Definition: Protrusion of an abdominal viscus or part of a viscus through the abdominal wall

   A.   Inguinal hernias are classified as direct (portions of the bowel and/or omentum protrude directly through
         the floor of the inguinal canal and emerge at the external inguinal ring) or indirect (pass through the
         internal abdominal ring, traverse the spermatic cord through the inguinal canal and emerge at the external
         inguinal ring) [see Figure 12.3]

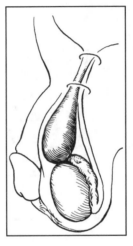

Figure 12.3. Hernia

   B.   Umbilical hernias are protrusion of bowel and/or omentum through the umbilical ring

   C.   Incarcerated hernias are hernias that cannot be reduced and the contents of the hernial sac cannot be
         returned to the peritoneal cavity

   D.   Strangulated hernias are hernias which occur when the blood supply to the viscera lying within the hernial
         sac is obliterated or cut off

II.   Pathogenesis

   A.   As a prelude to testicular descent in the male (and at the same gestational stage in females), a diverticular
         process of peritoneum, and the processus vaginalis, extends through the internal inguinal ring along the
         inguinal canal
       1.   In males, this is followed by the normal downward migration of the testicle, which acquires a portion
             of its covering—the tunical vaginalis—from the peritoneal process just described
       2.   In both sexes, the patent processus vaginalis undergoes obliteration at or shortly after birth; if this
             obliteration is incomplete, the potential for abdominal contents to enter the inguinal canal remains,
             constituting an indirect inguinal hernia

   B.   An umbilical hernia results from failure of closure of the fascial ring of the abdominal wall around the
         umbilicus

   C.   Thus, both umbilical hernias and indirect inguinal hernias are congenital

   D.   The direct inguinal hernia is acquired and is not considered here as it rarely occurs in pediatric patients

III.   Clinical Presentation

   A.   **Indirect inguinal hernia:** Approximately 5% of boys develop inguinal hernias, with a higher incidence in preterm infants
      1.   Hernias are up to 15 times more common in boys than in girls, but in children <1 year of age, the gender disparity is much less
      2.   More than 30% of all hernias are diagnosed before 6 months of age, and 50% are diagnosed by the time the child is 12 months old
      3.   A hernia is present on only one side in most cases (>75%), and is twice as likely to be on the right side as on the left
      4.   Most common finding in groin hernias is a bulge or lump in child's groin that is noticed by parent; mass may be transient or may be present constantly
      5.   A major risk with inguinal hernia is incarceration that occurs in up to 15% of patients, with approximately 60% occurring in infants <1 year of age (very high rates occur in those <2 months of age). When incarceration occurs, child is very fussy and abdomen becomes distended over several hours
      6.   Except with incarceration and strangulation, a hernia usually occurs without pain

   B.   **Umbilical hernia:** More frequent in African-American children than whites; in contrast with inguinal hernias, umbilical hernias occur equally in males and females
      1.   Typically become apparent in the first few weeks of life; produce a conspicuous bulge, stretching the overlying skin—the size of the skin-covered bulge bears little relationship to the size of the fascial defect
      2.   Often spontaneously close and rarely present with incarceration
      3.   Best predictor of spontaneous closure is the diameter of the defect at 3 months of age
         a.   If the defect is <0.5 cm, 96% usually spontaneously close
         b.   If >1.5 cm at 3 months, spontaneous closure is unlikely
      4.   Most umbilical hernias will have closed by 5 or 6 years of age; after that point there is little hope of spontaneous closure

IV.   Diagnosis/Evaluation

   A.   History
      1.   **Groin hernia:** Obtain an accurate description by the parents of where they saw the lump or bulge
         a.   Ask if the bulge is persistent or transient (comes and goes)
         b.   If infant, ask parent if bulge seems to cause the infant pain
         c.   In older child, ask the child if there is pain in area
         d.   Determine if there are associated symptoms of vomiting, inconsolable crying
         e.   Ask about aggravating and alleviating factors (is the bulge more pronounced with standing, crying, straining, coughing?)
      2.   **Umbilical hernia**
         a.   Determine if there are any associated signs and symptoms such as skin breakdown, redness, or warmth in the area
         b.   In infant, ask parent if hernia seems to cause the infant pain
         c.   In older child, ask the child if there is pain in the area

   B.   Physical Examination
      1.   **Groin hernia**
         a.   Determine if the child is in acute distress based on general appearance
         b.   Inspect the groin to determine whether obvious mass is present above the inguinal ligament and if it is symmetrical (on both sides) or unilateral (a visible swelling in the inguinal canal, scrotum, or both may be present—sometimes, however, despite a clear history given by the parents, no abnormality is visible on inspection)
         c.   Ascertain that the testes are in their normal position (undescended testis can appear as groin mass)
         d.   Inverting the upper portion of the scrotal skin into the inguinal canal with the examining finger to feel for a bulge when patient increases intra-abdominal pressure (as occurs with crying/coughing) is not recommended in infants and young children as it may cause unnecessary pain and yields little additional information
         e.   Perform abdominal exam for distension

2. **Umbilical hernia**
   a. Inspect the umbilicus
   b. With the tip of the index finger, gently compress the skin overlying the hernia, and estimate the size of the hernia—as the contents of the hernia are pushed gently back into the abdomen there is often a palpable "squish" as the small bowel loops are restored into the abdominal cavity

C. Differential Diagnosis
   1. Hydrocele: Swelling is transient or persistent, but occurs in the scrotum alone; parents of toddlers/young children describe the boy's scrotum a being normal in size when he awakens, but during the day size increases (see section on HYDROCELE)
   2. Undescended testis: Testis cannot be palpated in the scrotum (see section on UNDESCENDED TESTICLE)
   3. Testicular torsion: Causes acute pain and is an emergent condition (see TESTICULAR TORSION)
   4. Umbilical hernia as an isolated finding in an otherwise healthy child should be a straightforward diagnosis; however, umbilical hernias may be associated with a variety of conditions including chromosomal anomalies, metabolic disorders, and dysmorphic syndromes

D. Diagnostic Tests
   1. Ultrasound examination is the test of choice for the diagnosis of inguinal hernia
   2. None needed for umbilical hernia

V. Plan/Management

A. **Inguinal hernia**
   1. Major risk associated with an inguinal hernia is incarceration, a complication that occurs in up to 15% of patients; if incarceration is suspected, emergent referral to a pediatric urologist is indicated for immediate reduction
   2. In all other cases (incarceration is not suspected), referral for surgical repair is needed because the hernia does not resolve spontaneously

B. **Umbilical hernia**
   1. In the majority of cases (those in which the defect is 0.5 cm or less), all that is needed is parental reassurance that these hernias rarely produce any pain or develop incarceration and that closure will most likely occur over time
   2. If closure does not occur by the time the child is 5 or 6 years of age, surgical repair is generally indicated; spontaneous closure after this age will probably not occur
   3. Patients with very large defects (>1.5 cm) in whom spontaneous closure is unlikely should be referred for surgical repair; however, children <1 year of age are usually not considered for this procedure until they are older

C. Follow Up
   1. Umbilical hernias should be assessed at each well child visit to determine if closure has occurred and to reassure the parent
   2. Follow-up for patients with inguinal hernia should be with surgeon to whom the patient was referred

ABNORMAL LIVER-ENZYME RESULTS

I. Definition: Elevated liver-enzyme levels in asymptomatic patients

II. Pathogenesis:

A. **Aminotransferases**: Both aminotransferases–aspartate aminotransferase and alanine aminotransferase–are normally present in serum in low concentrations; elevations in normal levels are sensitive indicators of liver cell injury and are important in identification of hepatocellular diseases such as hepatitis
   1. Aspartate aminotransferase (AST) is found primarily in the liver, cardiac muscle, skeletal muscle, and kidneys
   2. Alanine aminotransferase (ALT) is found in highest amounts in the liver making this enzyme a more specific indicator of liver injury than AST

3. Both enzymes are released into the blood when the liver cell membrane is damaged; however, there is poor correlation between the degree of liver-cell damage and the level of aminotransferases as necrosis of liver cells is not required for the release of aminotransferases

4. The most common causes of elevated aminotransferase levels are the following: alcohol-related liver injury, chronic hepatitis B and C, autoimmune hepatitis, hepatic steatosis (fatty infiltration of the liver), nonalcoholic steatohepatitis, hemochromatosis, Wilson's disease, alpha$_1$-antitrypsin deficiency, and celiac sprue

B. **Alkaline phosphatase**: Levels most often become elevated from two sources–liver and bone and can indicate a pathologic, and sometimes, a physiologic process

1. Pathologic conditions that cause elevations in alkaline phosphatase levels include liver disorders such as chronic cholestatic or infiltrative liver diseases and bone diseases

a. Cholestatic diseases or conditions include partial obstruction of bile ducts, primary biliary cirrhosis, primary sclerosing cholangitis, adult bile ductopenia, and cholestasis induced by the use of substances such as anabolic steroids

b. Infiltrative diseases include sarcoidosis, other types of granulomatous diseases, and, less often, unsuspected metastasis of cancer to the liver

2. An influx of placental alkaline phosphatase into the circulation of women in their third trimester of pregnancy commonly occurs

3. Persons with blood type O or B may experience increases in serum alkaline phosphatase levels after eating a fatty meal because of an influx of intestinal alkaline phosphatase

4. Alkaline phosphatase levels also vary with age; adolescents in a growth spurt can have serum alkaline phosphatase levels two times as high as healthy adults due to the leakage of bone alkaline phosphatase into the blood

5. In adults, age is a factor in defining normal levels of this enzyme; for example, levels normally begin to gradually increase between 40 and 65 years, especially in women so that the normal alkaline phosphatase level in an otherwise healthy woman at age 65 is more than 50 percent higher than the level in her 30 year old counterpart

C. **γ-Glutamyltransferase**: Levels are a very sensitive indicator of the presence or absence of hepatobiliary disease; however, lack of specificity makes elevations difficult to interpret because increased levels can also occur in a wide variety of clinical conditions

1. Elevated levels can occur in pancreatic disease, myocardial infarction, renal failure, chronic obstructive pulmonary disease, diabetes, and alcoholism

2. In addition, elevated levels are also found in patients on medications such as phenytoin and barbiturates

3. Whereas the use of serum γ-glutamyltransferase measurements has been recommended by some to identify patients with unreported alcohol use, the lack of specificity of the test makes its use of questionable value

4. The best use of serum γ-glutamyltransferase may be to evaluate the meaning of elevations in other serum enzyme levels (see IV.E.4. below)

III. Clinical Presentation

A. Patients are asymptomatic and abnormal liver-enzyme results were unanticipated
1. As many as 6% of normal asymptomatic persons may have abnormal liver-enzyme levels
2. The overall prevalence of liver disease in the general population is about 1%
3. The normal range for any laboratory test is the average (mean) value in a group of healthy persons ±2 standard deviations; thus, 5% of results obtained from the norm group falls outside the defined "normal" range (2.5% below and 2.5% above)

B. Variable presentation depending on the underlying cause if one is eventually identified

IV. Diagnosis/Evaluation

A. The first step in the evaluation of patients with elevated liver-enzyme levels but no symptoms is to repeat the test to confirm the results
1. If the results of the repeat test are normal, no further evaluation is indicated; however, repeating the test again in 3 months is probably a good option
2. If the results of the repeat test remain abnormal, further evaluation is indicated beginning with a complete history and physical examination in an effort to identify the most common causes of liver-enzyme elevations

B.   History
1.   Inquire about any symptoms such as anorexia, weight loss, malaise
2.   Ask about alcohol and drug use; ask patient, "Do you ever drink alcohol?" If yes, continue with frequency and amount questions. Do the same with drug use keeping in mind that many patients conceal information about alcohol and drug use
3.   Obtain detailed medication history; a listing of medications, herbs, and drugs or substances of abuse reported to cause elevations in liver-enzyme levels are contained in the table below
4.   Determine if the initiation of a medication (prescription or over-the-counter), or other substance use could be associated with the increase in liver-enzyme levels
5.   Ask about previous medical history including any previous acute illnesses that could have been hepatitis, surgical history for any gastrointestinal problems, history of blood transfusions prior to 1990
6.   Obtain detailed sexual history
7.   Question patient about household/work /recreational exposures to chemicals such as carbon tetrachloride, vinyl chloride; ask about recent participation in strenuous exercise

MEDICATIONS, HERBS, AND DRUGS OR SUBSTANCES OF ABUSE REPORTED TO CAUSE ELEVATIONS IN LIVER-ENZYME LEVELS	
Medications *Antibiotics* ➡ Synthetic penicillins ➡ Ciprofloxacin ➡ Nitrofurantoin ➡ Ketoconazole and fluconazole ➡ Isoniazid *Antiepileptic drugs* ➡ Phenytoin ➡ Carbamazepine *Statins* ➡ Simvastatin ➡ Pravastatin ➡ Lovastatin ➡ Atorvastatin *Nonsteroidal anti-inflammatory drugs* *Sulfonylureas for hyperglycemia* ➡ Glipizide	**Herbs and homeopathic treatments** ➡ Chaparral ➡ Alchemilla (lady's mantle) ➡ Senna ➡ Shark cartilage ➡ Scutellaria (Skullcap) *Chinese herbs* ➡ Ji bu huan ➡ Ephedra (Ma-huang) **Drugs and substances of abuse** ➡ Anabolic steroids ➡ Cocaine ➡ MDMA ("Ecstasy") ➡ Phencyclidine ("Angel dust") *Glues and solvents* ➡ Glues containing toluene ➡ Trichloroethylene

Adapted from Pratt, D.S. (2000). Evaluation of abnormal liver-enzyme results in asymptomatic patients. *New England Journal of Medicine, 342,* 1268.

C.   Physical Examination: Focus should be on searching for evidence of liver disease
1.   Skin exam for spider angioma, palmar erythema, jaundice
2.   Sclera for icterus
3.   Abdominal exam, checking for ascites, right upper quadrant tenderness, hepatomegaly, splenomegaly
4.   Complete other parts of the exam as necessary

D.   Differential Diagnosis: Many conditions/diseases cause liver-enzyme elevations

E.   Additional Diagnostic Testing (once repeat testing has confirmed the liver-enzyme elevation)
1.   A cause for the persistent elevation should be sought
2.   If elevations in aminotransferase levels are persistent, evaluate for the most common causes, based on patient history (**Note:** Only two of the most common causes are discussed here–patients in whom other causes are suspected [see II.A. above, should be referred to an expert for evaluation and management])
a.   **Alcohol-related liver injury:** A γ-glutamyltransferase level that is two times the normal level in patients with an aspartate aminotransferase:alanine aminotransferase ratio of at least 2:1 strongly suggests a diagnosis of alcohol abuse. Use of γ-glutamyltransferase level as a single test to diagnose alcohol abuse is not recommended because of its lack of specificity
b.   **Hepatitis B or C:** Presence of hepatitis B surface antigen and core antibody indicates chronic hepatitis B infection; presence of hepatitis C antibody indicates chronic hepatitis C

3.   If elevations in alkaline phosphatase levels are persistent in a patient with no other symptoms, determination of the source of the evaluation–whether bone or liver–is the first step in the evaluation

    a.   Levels of γ-glutamyltransferase and alkaline phosphatase are usually elevated in parallel in patients with liver disorders; thus such a pattern should prompt an evaluation for liver disorders such as cholestatic diseases or infiltrative liver diseases (see II.B. above)

    b.   In bone disorders, an elevated serum alkaline phosphate level but a normal γ-glutamyltransferase level should prompt an evaluation for bone diseases

    c.   Referral to an expert at this point is appropriate

4.   Elevations in γ-glutamyltransferase levels are difficult to interpret because of the lack of specificity of such elevations

    a.   The value of this test is its role in evaluating the meaning of elevations in other serum enzyme levels

    b.   For example, it can be used to confirm the hepatic origin of elevated alkaline phosphatase levels and to support the diagnosis of alcohol abuse in patients with elevated aminotransferase levels

V.   Plan/Management

A.   Diagnostic testing (including repeat testing of the initial test) as outlined above is the first step in management

B.   If alcohol abuse is found to be the underlying problem, manage patient according to recommendations in the section on ALCOHOL PROBLEMS and consult with a hepatologist; refer patients with drug abuse for management

C.   If chronic hepatitis (B or C) is diagnosed, refer patient to a hepatologist for further evaluation and management

D.   If medications are suspected to be the cause of elevated aminotransferase levels, the easiest way to determine whether a medication is responsible is to stop its use and see whether the test results return to normal (obviously, some medications, e.g., antiepileptic drugs cannot be abruptly discontinued but must be tapered; therefore, discontinuation of a medications must be done using caution and judgment)

E.   Patients whose underlying cause for the persistent elevations in liver-enzymes remains unclear should be referred to an expert for further evaluation and management

F.   Follow up: Variable depending on whether patient is being managed in a primary care setting (as may be the case when a medication has caused the elevations in aminotransferase levels) or by the specialist to whom patient was referred

VIRAL HEPATITIS

I.   Definition: An inflammatory process of the liver caused by infection by one of six distinct viruses (A, B, C, D, E, and G); other causes of hepatitis are not considered here

II.   Pathogenesis

A.   Hepatitis A (HAV): RNA virus which is classified as a member of the picornavirus group; replication appears to be limited to the liver; only one serotype of HAV has been recognized in humans

B.   Hepatitis B (HBV): DNA-containing hepadnavirus; important components include HBsAg, hepatitis B core antigen, and hepatitis B e antigen (HBeAg)

C.   Hepatitis C (HCV): Small, single-stranded RNA virus that belongs to the family of flaviviruses; the most closely related human viruses are hepatitis G virus, yellow fever virus, and dengue virus; natural targets of HCV are hepatocytes

D.   Hepatitis D (HDV): Small particle consisting of an RNA genome and a delta protein antigen, both of which are coated with hepatitis B surface antigen; requires HBV as a helper virus and cannot produce infection in absence of HBV

E.   Hepatitis E (HEV): Single-stranded RNA virus that is presently classified as an unassigned genus of "hepatitis E-like" viruses

F.   Hepatitis G (HGV): Single-stranded RNA virus that is included in the Flaviviridae family and shares a 27% homology with HCV

III.   Clinical Presentation

A.   Hepatitis A
  1.   In US, hepatitis A is one of the most frequently reported vaccine-preventable diseases; highest rates occur in children 5 to 14 years of age and lowest rates among adults >40 years of age; reported cases have had an unequal geographic distribution in the US with the highest rates occurring in a limited number of states and communities; prevalence rates in these areas consistently remain higher than average
  2.   Incidence displays a cyclic pattern, and most disease occurs in the context of community-wide outbreaks during which a large proportion of persons do not have a recognized risk factor but become infected nonetheless
  3.   **Mode of transmission** is primarily through fecal-oral route; spreads readily in households and child care centers, with risk of spread in such centers increasing with the number of children who wear diapers; young children, frequently asymptomatic when infected, play an important role in HAV transmission
  4.   Other identified sources of infection include international travel, foodborne or waterborne outbreak, male homosexual activity, and injection-drug use; in approximately 50% of reported cases, the source cannot be determined
  5.   Unlike other infectious diseases that spread in child care centers, children who are infected are either asymptomatic or have very mild, nonspecific symptoms; adult contacts of infected children who themselves become infected, on the other hand, usually are symptomatic
  6.   Illness is self-limited and includes jaundice, anorexia, nausea, vomiting, malaise, and fever
  7.   When acquired during infancy and early childhood, infections are likely to be mild without jaundice; adult infections are likely to be quite severe
  8.   Viral shedding and the contagious period last 1-3 weeks, with the infected person being **most** contagious 1-2 weeks before the onset of illness; risk of transmission diminishes and is minimal in the week after onset of jaundice (if present)
  9.   **Incubation period** is 15-50 days, with an average of 25-30 days
  10.   **Chronic infection does not occur**
  11.   **Diagnosis**: Anti-HAV IgM appears early in the disease, and usually disappears after four months, but may persist for 6 months or longer. Presence of serum IgM indicates current or recent infection. Anti-HAV IgG develop shortly after the appearance of IgM; the presence of total anti-HAV without IgM anti-HAV indicates past infection and immunity

B.   Hepatitis B
  1.   The number of new infections per year has declined from an estimated 260,000 in the 1980s to about 78,000 in 2001
    a.   Highest rate of disease occurs in 20-49 year olds
    b.   Greatest decline has happened among children and adolescents due to routine hepatitis B immunization
  2.   **Transmission** occurs via contact with infected blood or body fluids such as semen, cervical secretions, wound exudates, and saliva (blood and serum contain the highest concentrations of virus and saliva contains the lowest)
  3.   **Modes of transmission** include
    a.   Transfusion of blood or blood products (uncommon in US today; estimated to be 1 in 63,000)
    b.   Needle-sharing
    c.   Percutaneous or mucous membrane exposures to blood or body fluids
    d.   Heterosexual and homosexual activity
    e.   Person-to-person spread of HBV can occur in settings involving close (nonsexual) contact over extended period which occurs when a chronically ill person resides in a household
    f.   Vertical transmission (during perinatal period)
    g.   More than 30% of infected persons do not have a readily identifiable risk factor
    h.   Not transmitted via fecal-oral route

4. The primary reservoir for infection is the HBV chronic carrier (defined as person with serum HBsAg-positive for 6 months or who is immunoglobulin [Ig] M anti-HBc [antibody to hepatitis B core antigen] negative and HBsAg-positive)
5. Hepatitis B causes a spectrum of illness ranging from an asymptomatic seroconversion, to acute illness with anorexia, nausea, malaise, and jaundice, to fatal hepatitis
6. Arthralgias, arthritis, and a macular skin eruption can also occur as part of the illness
7. Asymptomatic infection is most common in young children
8. Age of the person at initial HBV infection is the major determinant of chronicity; chronic HBV infection is much more likely to develop after prenatal or perinatal exposure than after exposure later in life
9. To illustrate the effect of age on chronic disease, chronic HBV infection develops in
   a. Up to 90% of infants infected by perinatal transmission
   b. Thirty percent of children 1-5 years of age
   c. Six percent of older children, adolescents, and adults
10. There are an estimated 1.25 million chronically infected persons in the US; 20-30% of that number acquired their infection in childhood
11. **Incubation period** is 45-160 days, with an average of 90 days
12. **Diagnosis**: Diagnostic tests are described in the table below

INTERPRETATION OF THE HEPATITIS B PANEL		
Tests	Results	Interpretation
HBsAg anti-HBc anti-HBs	negative negative negative	susceptible
HBsAg anti-HBc anti-HBs	negative positive positive	immune due to natural infection
HBsAg anti-HBc anti-HBs	negative negative positive	immune due to hepatitis B vaccination
HBsAg anti-HBc IgM anti-HBc anti-HBs	positive positive positive negative	acutely infected
HBsAg anti-HBc IgM anti-HBc anti-HBs	positive positive negative negative	chronically infected
HBsAg anti-HBc anti-HBs	negative positive negative	four interpretations possible*

* 1. May be recovering from acute HBV infection
   2. May be distantly immune and test not sensitive enough to detect very low level of anti-HBs in serum
   3. May be susceptible with a false positive anti-HBc
   4. May be undetectable level of HBsAg present in the serum and the person is actually a carrier

Source: Centers for Disease Control and Prevention. National Center for Infectious Diseases.(2002). Viral hepatitis B. Retrieved October 21, 2002, from http://www. cdc.gov/ncidod/diseases/hepatitis/b/Bserology.htm.

C. Hepatitis C
   1. Prevalence of HCV infection varies throughout the world, with the highest number of infections reported in Egypt; in the US 1.8% of the population is positive for HCV antibodies; given that 3 of every 4 seropositive persons also have viremia, an estimated 2.7 million persons in the US have active HCV infection
   2. **Mode of transmission** is primarily through injection drug use and receipt of a blood transfusion prior to 1990; in some cases, no risk factors can be identified
   3. Until the last decade, blood transfusion was a major risk of HCV infection in developed countries such as the US; with the introduction of improved blood-screening measures (in 1990 and 1992) based on detection of HCV antibodies, the risk of transfusion-associated HCV infection has dramatically declined (**Note**: Current risk from blood that is negative for HCV antibodies is less than 1 in 103,000 transfused units, with the residual risk a consequence of blood donations that occur in the interval between infection and the development of detectable antibodies (estimated to be less than 12 weeks)

4. Sexual transmission of the virus is an inefficient means, much less efficient than is the case for HIV-1 infection; reasons for this may be the low levels of the virus in genital fluids and tissues (of HCV infected persons) or to a lack of appropriate target cells in the genital tract; coinfection with HIV-1 appears to increase the risk of sexual transmission

5. Casual household contact and contact with the saliva of infected persons also appear to be very inefficient modes of transmission; nosocomial transmission has been documented (from patient to patient by a colonoscope, during dialysis, and during surgery)

6. Prevalence of HCV infection is not higher among healthcare workers than among the general population, but needle-stick injuries in the healthcare setting continue to result in nosocomial transmission

7. Estimate of the comparative risks of transmission through a needle stick based on the rule of threes
   a. HBV is transmitted in 30% of exposures
   b. HCV is transmitted in 3% of exposures
   c. HIV-1 is transmitted in 0.3% of exposures

8. Maternal-fetal transmission occurs infrequently and is most often associated with coinfection in HIV-1 in the mother

9. Signs and symptoms of acute infection are often indistinguishable from those of hepatitis A or B infection–jaundice, malaise, and nausea

10. HCV infection is infrequently diagnosed in the acute phase; the majority of persons have either no symptoms or only mild symptoms

11. Acute infection leads to chronic infection in the majority of persons; spontaneous clearance of the viremia once chronic infection has been established is rare

12. Most chronic infections result in hepatitis; cirrhosis of the liver occurs in 15-20% of those with chronic disease; in addition to hepatic disease, extrahepatic manifestations of HCV infection include autoimmune or lymphoproliferative states

13. The course of HCV infection is greatly accelerated by coinfection with HIV-1 or HBV; further, superinfection with hepatitis A virus in HCV persons can result in severe acute or fulminant hepatitis

14. All persons with HCV antibody and/or HCV-RNA in their blood are considered to be contagious

15. **Incubation period** ranges from 2 to 26 weeks with an average of 7 to 8 weeks

16. **Diagnosis**: Two types of tests are available for diagnosis of HCV

DIAGNOSTIC TESTS FOR HCV

Serologic assays for antibodies
⇨ Screening assays based on antibody detection have greatly reduced risk of transfusion-related infection; once persons seroconvert, they usually remain positive for HCV antibodies
⇨ Primary serologic screening assay for HCV is the enzyme immunoassay which has been greatly improved in sensitivity over the past few years; can detect antibodies within 4 to 10 weeks after infection
  ◆ Positive results are confirmed by a recombinant immunoblot assay (RIBA)
  ◆ With the availability of improved enzyme immunoassays and better RNA-detection assays, confirmation by recombinant immunoblot assay may become less important in the future

Molecular tests for viral particles
⇨ Qualitative HCV RNA tests are based on the PCR technique and have a lower limit of detection of fewer than 100 copies of HCV RNA per mL
⇨ Appropriate use for these tests include the following
  ◆ In patients with negative results on enzyme immunoassay in whom acute infection is suspected
  ◆ In patients who have hepatitis with no identifiable cause
  ◆ In patients with known reasons for false negative results on antibody testing
  ◆ For the confirmation of viremia and the assessment of treatment response

INTERPRETING ANTIBODY TO HEPATITIS C VIRUS (ANTI-HCV) TEST RESULTS		
Anti-HCV-Positive	**Anti-HCV-Negative**	**Anti-HCV-Indeterminate**

An anti-HCV-positive result is defined as 1) anti-HCV screening-test-positive* and recombinant immunoblot assay (RIBA)- or nucleic acid test (NAT)-positive; or 2) anti-HCV screening-test-positive, NAT-negative, RIBA-positive
 	
• An anti-HCV-positive result indicates past or current HCV infection
   An HCV RNA-positive result indicates current (active) infection, but the significance of a single HCV-RNA-negative result is unknown; it does not differentiate intermittent viremia from resolved infection
• All anti-HCV-positive persons should receive counseling and undergo medical evaluation, including additional testing for the presence of virus and liver disease
   Anti-HCV testing usually does not need to be repeated after a positive anti-HCV result has been confirmed
	An anti-HCV-negative result is defined as 1) anti-HCV screening-test-negative*; or 2) anti-HCV screening-test-positive, RIBA-negative; or 3) anti-HCV screening-test-positive, NAT-negative, RIBA-negative
	
	• An anti-HCV-negative person is considered uninfected
	• No further evaluation or follow-up for HCV is required, unless recent infection is suspected or other evidence exists to indicate HCV infection (e.g., abnormal liver enzyme levels in an immunocompromised person or a person with no other etiology for their liver disease)
		An indeterminate anti-HCV result is defined as anti-HCV screening-test-positive, RIBA-indeterminate
		
		• An indeterminate anti-HCV result indicates that the HCV antibody status cannot be determined.
		  • Can indicate a false-positive anti-HCV screening test result, the most likely interpretation among those at low risk for HCV infection; such persons are HCV RNA-negative
		  • Can occur as a transient finding in a recently infected person who is in the process of seroconversion; such persons usually are HCV RNA-positive
		  • Can be a persistent finding among persons chronically infected with HCV; such persons are HCV RNA-positive
		• If NAT is not performed, another sample should be collected for repeat anti-HCV testing (≥1 month later)

* Interpretation of screening immunoassay test results based on criteria provided by the manufacturer

Source: Centers for Disease Control and Prevention. (2003). Hepatitic C: Recommendations and reports. *MMWR 52* (No. RR-3), p. 3.

D. Hepatitis D
   1. Occurs as either a **coinfection** with HBV (e.g., following inoculation with blood or secretions that contain both agents) or as a **superinfection** in established chronic HBV infection
   2. **Mode of transmission** is via blood or blood products, injection drugs, or sexual contact providing HBV also is present
   3. Transmission from mother to newborn is uncommon
   4. Hepatitis D resembles hepatitis B in terms of when symptoms appear and period of infectivity
   5. Hepatitis D can cause hepatitis only in persons with acute or chronic HBV infection
   6. **Incubation period** for HDV superinfection is approximately 2-8 weeks; when both viruses (B and D) infect simultaneously, incubation period averages 90 days and ranges from 45-160 days
   7. **Diagnosis**: Radioimmunoassay and enzyme immunoassay for anti-HDV antibody are available (methods for detection of HDV RNA area also available)

E. Hepatitis E
   1. Occurs predominantly in India, South Central Asia, and the Middle East, but also occurs in the Western Hemisphere, including the US (rare)
   2. There is a possibility of a zoonotic reservoir for HEV
   3. **Mode of transmission** is the fecal-oral route
   4. Causes an acute illness with jaundice, malaise, anorexia, abdominal pain, arthralgias, and fever
   5. Occurs more commonly in adults than children and is most serious when it occurs in pregnant women
   6. **Period of communicability** is unknown, but probably continues for at least 2 weeks after the acute phase
   7. **Chronic infection does not seem to occur**
   8. **Incubation period** ranges from 15-60 days, with an average of 40 days
   9. **Diagnosis**: Serologic and PCR-based assay for the diagnosis of acute HEV infection are available in research and commercial laboratories

F. Hepatitis G
   1. Reported in adults and children throughout the world; found in about 1.5% of blood donors in US
   2. Infection with the virus causes mild, if any, disease; no treatment is indicated
   3. Infection has been reported in up to 20% of adults with chronic HBV or HCV infection, indicating that coinfection is a common occurrence
   4. **Mode of transmission** is through transfusions; also can be transmitted by organ transplantation

5. Other important risk factors include injection drug use, hemodialysis, and homosexual and bisexual contacts, indicating that sexual transmission can occur
6. Transplacental transmission seems to be rare
7. **Incubation period** is unknown
8. No evidence that HGV causes fulminant or chronic disease
9. **Diagnosis**: No serologic test is available; currently, can be diagnosed only by use of polymerase chain assay which is not readily available

G. The following table contains a comparison of viral hepatitis, A to E

COMPARISON OF VIRAL HEPATITIS, A TO E			
Form	Primary Route of Transmission	Incubation Period	Chronicity
Hepatitis A	Fecal-oral, contaminated food/water	15-50 days	None
Hepatitis B	Blood/body fluids	45-160 days	Yes
Hepatitis C	Blood/blood products	2 - 26 weeks	Yes
Hepatitis D	Blood/body fluids	2 - 8 weeks	Yes
Hepatitis E	Fecal-oral	(?) 2 - 9 weeks	None

H. Viral hepatitis, A to E, are similar in their clinical expression and therefore cannot be readily distinguished by clinical features

I. Clinical features include the following:
1. Fatigue, lassitude, anorexia, nausea, dark urine, low grade fever, right upper abdominal discomfort, myalgia, and arthralgias
2. Only a minority of persons who are infected develop jaundice
3. Many infected persons are asymptomatic

J. The characteristic laboratory abnormalities are elevated aminotransferase levels that are high early in the prodromal period, peak before jaundice is maximal, and fall slowly during the convalescent period
1. Aspartate aminotransferase (AST) and alanine aminotransferase (ALT) levels are typically 500-2000 IU/L
2. ALT is usually higher than AST (in alcoholic hepatitis, the reverse is usual)
3. Alkaline phosphatase is only modestly elevated
4. Degree of hyperbilirubinemia is variable
5. Urinary bile usually precedes jaundice
6. Increase in prothrombin time is uncommon; if present suggests severe illness
7. WBC count is usually low-normal, and blood smear may show a few atypical lymphocytes

K. Serologic testing determines the specific etiologic diagnosis

IV. Diagnosis/Evaluation

A. History
1. Question about onset and duration of symptoms (usual symptoms are general fatigue, malaise, joint and muscle pain, loss of appetite, nausea, vomiting, diarrhea, and low-grade fever; tenderness of right upper quadrant and jaundice may also occur)
2. Ask about darkened urine, light-colored stools
3. Inquire about similar illness in household contacts
4. Ask about sexual behaviors and similar illness in sexual partners
5. Ask about history of blood transfusions, IV drug use, alcohol abuse
6. Inquire about occupation
7. Obtain travel history, especially travel to Asia or Africa where hepatitis B is especially common
8. Obtain past medical history and medication history

B. Physical Examination
1. Examine skin, mucous membranes, and sclera for jaundice
2. Perform abdominal exam to determine size, surface characteristics, and tenderness of liver; determine if spleen is enlarged

C. Differential Diagnosis: Noninfectious causes of hepatitis including medications, acute alcohol induced injury

D. Diagnostic Tests
1. If acute viral hepatitis is suspected, order appropriate diagnostic tests recommended above based on type of hepatitis that is suspected (many insurance carriers will not pay for "hepatitis panels")
2. Serologic features of viral hepatitis (A to E) are summarized in the following table:

SEROLOGIC FEATURES OF VIRAL HEPATITIS		
Form of Infection	**Serologic Markers**	**Interpretation**
Hepatitis A	IgM anti-HAV	Acute disease
	IgG anti-HAV	Remote infection and immunity
Hepatitis B		See Interpretation of the Hepatitis B Panel above
Hepatitis C	Anti-HCV	Acute, chronic, or resolved disease
	HCV RNA	Qualitative tests to detect presence or absence of virus and quantitative tests to detect amount of virus
Hepatitis D	HBsAg and anti-HDV	Acute disease
	• IgM anti-HBc positive	Co-infection
	• IgG anti-HBc positive	Superinfection
Hepatitis E	IgM anti-HEV	Acute disease
	IgG anti-HEV	Remote infection and immunity
IgM, immunoglobulin M; anti-HAV, antibody to hepatitis A virus; IgG, immunoglobulin G; anti-HCV, antibody to hepatitis C virus; anti-HDV, antibody to hepatitis D virus; HBsAg, hepatitis B surface antigen; anti-HBc, antibody to hepatitis B core antigen; anti-HEV, antibody to hepatitis E virus		

3. If HBsAg is present, testing for HBeAg is needed to determine whether active viral replication is present
4. Testing for anti-HDV should be done in all persons with chronic hepatitis B to rule out coexisting hepatitis D
5. If all test results are negative, follow up testing for anti-HCV is appropriate because of delay in appearance of antibody
6. CBC, total and direct bilirubin, prothrombin time, liver enzymes, urinalysis should be obtained also
7. All persons with chronic hepatitis should have liver biopsy to determine extent of disease

V. Plan/Management

A. Hepatitis usually resolves spontaneously over 4-8 weeks

B. For acute infections for viral hepatitis (A, B, C, D, E), provide symptomatic treatment for symptoms such as myalgia, nausea, vomiting, and pruritus

C. Bed rest, special diets, vitamin supplements are not required; patient should abstain from alcohol and should not engage in strenuous activities or contact sports

D. If patient on hepatotoxic drugs, those should be discontinued until recovery has occurred

E. FDA-approved therapeutic options for treatment of chronic hepatitis B infection are interferon alfa-2b (Intron A), the nucleoside analog lamivudine (Epivir-HBV), and the nucleotide analog, adefovir (Hepsera)
1. Adefovir and lamivudine are given PO in a once daily dose, and the cost for a one month supply is $528 and $156, respectively
2. Interferon alfa-2b is given either SC or IM and the cost for a one month supply of a daily dose is $2,131, and for a 3x/week dose is $1,739 (based on AWP listings in *Drug Topics Red Book Update*, December 2002)
3. Patients should be referred to an expert for management

F. All patients with chronic HCV infection are potential candidates for antiviral therapy but the risks and benefits of treatment must be assessed individually, especially given the typically slow course of natural infection
1. Only a subgroup of persons with chronic infection will have a clear indication for therapy; patients with detectable levels of HCV RNA who have elevated alanine aminotransferase levels that are persistent and who have a liver biopsy positive for fibrosis or at least moderate necrosis and

inflammation have a high risk of disease progression and should be treated provided there are no contraindications

2. Combination therapy with interferon and ribavirin has proven to be very effective
3. Patients with persistently normal alanine aminotransferase levels and no histologic evidence of pathologic changes in the liver have a very good prognosis without therapy
4. Patients should be immediately referred to an expert for management

VI. Control measures: Hepatitis A

A. Improved sanitation and personal hygiene (especially good hand washing) are the keys to controlling spread of the virus

B. Postexposure prophylaxis for household and sexual contacts: Give 0.02 mL/kg of immune globulin (IG) as soon as possible after exposure (use of IG more than 2 weeks after last exposure in not indicated) **and** give HAV vaccine in dosage and schedule as described in table under VI.D. below

C. Newborn infants of infected mothers: If mother's symptoms began 2 weeks before or 1 week after delivery, some experts recommend that infant be given IG (0.02 mL/kg); efficacy has not been established and the best course of action is to consult an expert in this situation (**Note:** Perinatal transmission is rare)

D. Hepatitis A vaccine: Havrix and Vaqta, both with pediatric and adult formulations are available in the US; these are inactivated vaccines prepared from cell culture-adapted HAV; Havrix contains a preservative and Vaqta is formulated without a preservative
1. Currently, vaccination is recommended for adults with certain risk factors and for children who live in communities where the reported annual incidence exceeds two times the average annual rate in the US (high risk regions or states include the following–AK, AZ, CA, ID, NV, NM, OK, OR, SD, UT, WA)
2. There is disagreement among the experts regarding whether to extend routine hepatitis A immunization to children outside these areas

RECOMMENDED DOSES AND SCHEDULES FOR INACTIVATED HEPATITIS A VACCINES*				
Age (years)	Vaccine	Volume per Dose	No. of Doses	Schedule
2-18	Havrix	0.5 mL	2	Initial and 6-12 mos later
2-17	Vaqta	0.5 mL	2	Initial and 6-18 mos later
19 and older	Havrix	1.0 mL	2	Initial and 6-12 mos later
18 and older	Vaqta	1.0 mL	2	Initial and 6 mos later

* Havrix is manufactured b SmithKline Beecham Biologicas, Rixensart, Belgium, and distributed by SmithKline Beecham Pharmaceuticals, Philadelphia, PA; Vaqta is manufactured and distributed by Merck & Co, Inc, West Point, PA

E. Hepatitis A vaccine should be given routinely to persons ≥2 years of age in the following groups
1. International travelers
2. Children living in communities with high endemic rates/periodic outbreaks (see D. 1. above)
3. Patients with chronic liver disease
4. Homosexual and bisexual men
5. Users of injection and noninjection illegal drugs
6. Persons with clotting-factor disorders
7. Persons with risk of occupational exposure
8. Any healthy person at least 2 years of age at discretion of health care provider (examples, child care center staff/attendees, custodial care workers, hospital workers, food handlers)

VII. Control measures: Hepatitis B

A. **All infants** should receive hepatitis B vaccine as part of their routine immunizations in childhood (series of 3 doses is required for optimal antibody response); all children who have not received the vaccine previously should be immunized by or before 11 or 12 years of age [see IMMUNIZATIONS section]
1. Susceptibility testing before vaccination is not recommended in children and adolescents
2. Testing for previous infection should be considered in adults in high-risk groups

B. Prenatal screening for HBsAg can prevent perinatal transmission (for care of infant whose mother is HBsAg-positive, consult *Red Book* [2000] pp. 298-300, as these infants require special care including HBIG within 12 hours after birth)

C. Prevention of HBV transmission to medical personnel is possible through use of universal precautions for blood and body fluids; nonetheless, all health care workers and others with occupational exposure to blood are at high risk and should be immunized

D. Consult *Red Book* (2000) for complete listing of other high-risk groups who should receive pre-exposure hepatitis B immunization

E. Recommendations for Hepatitis B prophylaxis after percutaneous or permucosal exposure are contained in the following table

RECOMMENDED POSTEXPOSURE PROPHYLAXIS FOR EXPOSURE TO HEPATITIS B VIRUS			
Vaccination and Anti-body Response Status of Exposed Workers	Treatment When Source Is		
	HBsAg Positive	HBsAg Negative	Source Not Tested or Status Unknown
Unvaccinated	HBIG x 1; initiate HB vaccine series	Initiate HB vaccine series	Initiate HB vaccine series
Previously vaccinated: Known responder*	No treatment	No treatment	No treatment
Known non-responder**	HBIG x 2 or HBIG x 1 and initiate re-vaccination†	No treatment	If known high-risk source, treat as if source were HBsAg positive
Antibody response unknown	Test exposed person for anti-HBs 1. If adequate,* no treatment 2. If inadequate,** HBIG x 1 and vaccine booster	No treatment	Test exposed person for anti-HBs 1. If adequate,* no treatment 2. If inadequate,** administer vaccine and booster and recheck titer in 1 to 2 months

HBsAg = hepatitis B surface antigen; HBIG = hepatitis B immune globulin; HB = hepatitis B; anti-HBs = antibody to HBsAg
* Responder is defined as a person with adequate levels of serum antibody to hepatitis B surface antigen (i.e., anti-HBs ≥10 mIU/mL)
**A non-responder is a person with inadequate response to vaccination (i.e., anti-HBs <10 mIU/mL)
† The option of giving one dose of HBIG and reinitiating the vaccine series is preferred for non-responders who have not completed a second 3-dose vaccine series; for persons who previously completed a second vaccine series but failed to respond, 2 doses of HBIG are preferred
Adapted from Centers for Disease Control and Prevention. (2001). Updated US Public Health Service guidelines for the management of occupational exposures to HBV, HCV, and HIV and recommendations for postexposure prophylaxis. *MMWR, 50*, No. RR-11, p. 22.

VIII. Control measures: Hepatitis C

A. Should be managed with the universal precautions for blood and body fluids as in hepatitis B

B. Immunoprophylaxis is not available

IX. Control measures: Hepatitis D

A. Transmission is similar to that of HBV, so universal precautions for blood and body fluids should be observed

B. Cannot be transmitted in the absence of HBV, so prevention of HBV is key to prevention

C. Immunoprophylaxis not available; because HDV cannot be transmitted in the absence of HBV infection, hepatitis B immunization protects against HDV infection and thus should be obtained

X. Control measures: Hepatitis E

A. Immunoprophylaxis not available

B. Prevention through good sanitation and hygiene

XI. Control measures: Hepatitis G

A. Immunoprophylaxis not available

B. Should be managed with universal precautions for blood and body fluids as in hepatitis B

XII. Follow Up

    A. Variable depending on type of hepatitis

    B. Hepatitis A does not have a chronic stage, so generally resolves without any long-term effects (Hepatitis E only found in developing countries and rarely in the US at this time)
        1. Make sure post-exposure prophylaxis for household and sexual contacts as described under VI.B. above is given; contacts should then be appropriately immunized with HAV vaccine (see VI.D. above)
        2. Emphasize control measures to prevent spread
        3. Recheck patient after 2 weeks to evaluate condition

    C. Hepatitis B, C, D should be referred for management because of development of high rate of chronic hepatitis

ASCARIASIS (ROUNDWORM INFECTION)

I. Definition: An intestinal parasitic infection caused by *Ascaris lumbricoides*, a large roundworm of humans

II. Pathogenesis

    A. Adult worms live in small intestine of humans
        1. Female worms produce 200,000 eggs per day which are excreted in the stool
        2. Stool must be excreted into the soil and eggs must incubate in soil for 2-3 weeks in order for embryo to form and become infectious
        3. Ingestion of infective eggs from soil that is contaminated leads to infection

    B. Larvae hatch in the small intestine, penetrate the mucosa, and are transported by portal blood to liver and subsequently to the lungs
        1. From the lungs, they ascend through the tracheobronchial tree to the pharynx, and are swallowed
        2. Once swallowed, the worms mature into adults in the small intestine and the cycle is repeated
        3. If infection is untreated, adult worms can live for 12-18 months, resulting in daily excretion of large numbers of eggs

    C. Ingestion occurs from eating food that is unwashed or drinking water contaminated by human feces; in children, ingestion frequently occurs by playing in the soil infected with the eggs via hand-mouth behavior

    D. Interval from ingestion of eggs and development of egg-laying adult worms is about 8 weeks

III. Clinical Presentation

    A. Most commonly occurs in the tropics, in areas of poor sanitation, and in areas where human waste is used for fertilizer

    B. Worldwide, most common intestinal roundworms of humans; in US, second only to pinworms in prevalence

    C. Most infections are either asymptomatic infections or so mild that the infected person does not present for treatment

    D. May cause nausea, vomiting, anorexia, weight loss, fever, irritability, diarrhea, and abdominal cramping; acute intestinal obstruction may occur in patients with heavy worm loads; most likely to occur in children because of the smaller diameter of the intestinal lumen

    E. Larvae in the lungs may cause cough, wheezing, and an acute transitory pneumonia

    F. Adult worms may be vomited or passed in the stool

IV. Diagnosis/Evaluation

    A. History
        1. Question about anorexia, nausea, vomiting, weight loss, fever, irritability
        2. Ask about pica, toilet facilities, use of human feces for fertilizer in gardens
        3. Inquire if cough, fever (lung migration) present
        4. Ask if adult worm found in stool

    B. Physical Examination
        1. Measure weight
        2. Perform abdominal exam for tenderness, masses
        3. Obtain stool for occult blood

    C. Differential Diagnosis: Asthma, pneumonia, poor nutrition, *Giardiasis*

    D. Diagnostic Tests: If worms are visualized, none needed; if not, 3 stool specimens for ova and parasites

V. Plan/Treatment

    A. Consult the following table for treatment recommendations

DRUGS FOR TREATMENT OF ASCARIASIS (ROUNDWORM)		
Drug of Choice	**Adult Dosage**	**Pediatric Dosage (≥2 years)**
Mebendazole OR	100 mg BID x 3 days	100 mg BID x 3 days
Pyrantel pamoate OR	11 mg/kg x 1 dose (maximum 1 g)	11 mg/kg x 1 dose (maximum 1 g)
Albendazole	400 mg x 1 dose	400 mg x 1 dose
In pregnant women and children <2 years, benefits and risks should be considered		

Adapted from: American Academy of Pediatrics. (2000). Drugs for treatment of parasitic infections. In L.E. Pickering (Ed.), *2000 red book: Report of the Committee on Infectious Diseases* (25th ed., p. 696). Elk Grove Village, IL: Author.

    B. In cases of partial or complete intestinal obstructions by worms, piperazine citrate solution (75 mg/kg/day, not to exceed 3.5 g) may be given through a gastrointestinal tube; consult with an expert before administering this treatment for more details

    C. Importance of maintaining a clean play area for children and sanitary disposal of human feces should be emphasized; vegetables grown in soil fertilized with human feces must be thoroughly cooked or soaked in a dilute iodine solution before eating; household bleach is ineffective

    D. Follow Up: None indicated

ENTEROBIASIS (PINWORM INFECTION)

I. Definition: An intestinal parasitic infection caused by *Enterobius vermicularis*, a nematode, or roundworm

II. Pathogenesis

    A. A white, threadlike worm for which humans are the only hosts (cats and dogs do not harbor *E. vermicularis*; worms live primarily in the cecum and adjacent bowel)

    B. Adult gravid females, which are about 1 cm in length, migrate to perianal area to deposit eggs on perianal skin and then die

    C. Infection would be self-limited at that point were it not for reinfection through ingestion of worm eggs that occurs primarily via autoinfection or (less commonly), reinfection acquired from others in the household through ingesting worm eggs that they have shed

D.	Transmission occurs via various routes, but primarily through fecal-oral route; worm eggs are also transmitted via fomites such as toys, bedding, and toilet seats

E.	Incubation period from ingestion of egg until an adult worm migrates to perianal area is about 1-2 months

F.	Eggs are fairly hardy and can remain infective in an indoor environment for 2-3 weeks

III.	Clinical Presentation

A.	Occurs worldwide and commonly in family clusters; incidence appears to have declined over past few decades

B.	Prevalence rates are highest in preschoolers, in school-age children, in mothers of infected children, and in the institutionalized

C.	Perianal pruritus with secondary excoriation and dermatitis is common; rarely, pruritus vulvae occurs

D.	Many clinical problems such as bruxism (grinding of teeth at night), appendicitis, weight loss, and enuresis have been attributed to pinworm infections, but proof of a causal relationship is lacking

E.	Urethritis, vaginitis, salpingitis, or pelvic peritonitis may rarely occur from aberrant migration of the adult worm from the perineum

IV.	Diagnosis/Evaluation

A.	History
1.	Inquire about time of and circumstances surrounding onset of symptoms
2.	Ask if anal pruritus is present
3.	In females, question about genital irritation
4.	Ask if others in household have similar symptoms

B.	Physical Examination
1.	Focus on exam of anus; may be excoriated from scratching
2.	In females, also examine for genital irritation

C.	Differential Diagnosis
1.	Poor hygiene
2.	Chemical irritants, such as bubble bath

D.	Diagnostic Tests: There are two techniques for detection
1.	Parent may be able to visualize the adult worm in the perianal region by examining the region 2 to 3 hours after the child is asleep; visualization of the worm is diagnostic
2.	Alternatively, the transparent adhesive tape technique can be used

---

USING TRANSPARENT TAPE TO DETECT PINWORM EGGS

Instruct parents in the following technique that should be **repeated for 3 consecutive days**
- First thing in the morning, either immediately before or immediately after arising, is the best time to obtain specimen
- Using cellophane tape that is transparent, apply the tape to the perianal skin
- Cover tape with specimen with a second piece of tape and place in plastic bag for transport to office/lab
Technician affixes specimen to slide (using more tape if necessary)
- Slide is then scanned under low power for eggs (eggs are 50 x 30 μg, oval, flat on one side, and thin-shelled)
  - ✓ A single specimen usually detects 50% of infestations
  - ✓ Three tests will detect 90%; five tests will detect almost 100%

V.   Plan/Treatment

A.   Consult the following table for treatment recommendations

DRUGS FOR TREATMENT OF PINWORM INFECTION		
Drug of Choice	**Adult Dosage**	**Pediatric Dosage (2 years and older)**
Pyrantel pamoate OR	11 mg/kg x 1 dose (maximum 1 g) Repeat in 2 weeks	11 mg/kg x 1 dose (maximum 1 g) Repeat in 2 weeks
Mebendazole OR	100 mg x 1 dose Repeat in 2 weeks	100 mg x 1 dose Repeat in 2 weeks
Albendazole	400 mg x 1 dose Repeat in 2 weeks	400 mg x 1 dose Repeat in 2 weeks
In pregnant women and children <2 years, benefits and risks should be considered		

Adapted from: American Academy of Pediatrics. (2000). Drugs for treatment of parasitic infections. In L.E. Pickering (Ed.), *2000 red book: Report of the Committee on Infectious Diseases* (25th ed., p. 696). Elk Grove Village, IL: Author.

B.   No unusual cleaning or hygienic measures are required, but the following common sense recommendations should be followed
    1.   Keep nails trimmed short as eggs may lodge under nails with scratching; avoid nail biting to reduce risk of autoinfection
    2.   Wash hands frequently, and always on arising, before eating or preparing food, and after toileting
    3.   Morning showers will wash away any eggs deposited during the night
    4.   Changing the infected person's underclothes, bedclothes, and bed sheets on a frequent basis may reduce egg contamination of the environment and risk of reinfection
    5.   Application of bland ointment such as petroleum jelly to the perianal area may help reduce dispersion of eggs

C.   There is a high incidence of reinfections particularly in child care centers and schools; repeated infections should be treated the same as initial one

D.   Families may need to be treated as a group; in institutionalized settings, mass and simultaneous treatment, repeated in 2 weeks, can be effective

E.   Follow Up: None indicated

REFERENCES

Abramowicz, M. (2002). Adefovir (Hepsera) for chronic hepatitis B infection. *The Medical Letter, 44*, 105-106.

Abramowicz, M. (2002). Alosetron (Lotronex) revisited. *The Medical Letter, 44*, 67-68.

Abramowicz, M. (2002). Tegaserod maleate (Zelnorm) for IBS with constipation. *The Medical Letter, 44*, 79-80.

Ahluwalia, J.P., Graber, M.A., & Silverman, W.B. (2002). Gastroenterology and hepatology. In M.A. Graber & M.L. Lanternier (Eds.), *University of Iowa: The family practice handbook* (pp. 151-204). St. Louis: Mosby.

American Academy of Pediatrics, Provisional committee for Quality Improvement and Subcommittee on Hyperbilirubinemia. (1994). Practice parameter: Management of hyperbilirubinemia in the healthy term newborn. *Pediatrics, 94*, 558-562.

American Academy of Pediatrics. (2000). *Ascaris lumbricoides* infections. In L.E. Pickering (Ed.), *2000 red book: Report of the Committee on Infectious Diseases* (25th ed., pp. 176-178). Elk Grove Village, IL: Author.

American Academy of Pediatrics. (2000). Pinworm infection. In L.E. Pickering (Ed.), *2000 red book: Report of the Committee on Infectious Diseases* (25th ed., pp. 448-450). Elk Grove Village, IL: Author.

American Academy of Pediatrics. (2000). Drugs for treatment of parasitic infections. In L.E. Pickering (Ed.), *2000 red book: Report of the Committee on Infectious Diseases* (25th ed., pp. 693-717). Elk Grove Village, IL: Author.

American Academy of Pediatrics. (1996). Practice parameter. The management of acute gastroenteritis in young children. *Pediatrics, 97*, 424-633.

American Gastroenterological Association. (1999) AGA medical position statement: Guidelines for the evaluation and management of chronic diarrhea. *Gastroenterology, 116*, 1461-1463.

American Gastroenterological Association. (1999). AGA technical review on the evaluation and management of chronic diarrhea. *Gastroenterology, 116*, 1464-1486.

American Gastroenterological Association. (2001). AGA technical review on nausea and vomiting. *Gastroenterology, 120*, 263-286.

American Gastroenterological Association. (2001). AGA medical position statement: Nausea and vomiting. *Gastroenterology, 120*, 261-262.

Anand, C.A. (2002). Amebiasis. In R.E. Rakel & E.T. Bope (Eds.). *Conn's current therapy* (pp. 57-61). Philadelphia: WB Saunders.

Andres, J.M., & Francisco, M.P. (2001). Jaundice. In R.A. Hoekelman, H.M. Adams, N.M. Nelson, M.L. Weitzman, & M.H. Wilson (Eds.), *Pediatric primary care* (pp. 1170-1181). St. Louis: Mosby.

Ansdell, V. (2002). Intestinal parasites. In R.E. Rakel & E.T. Bope (Eds.). *Conn's current therapy* (pp. 537-544). Philadelphia: WB Saunders.

Arce, D.A., Ermocilla, C.A., & Costa, H. (2002). Evaluation of constipation. *American Family Physician, 65,* 2283-2290.

Armstrong, G.L., & Bell, B.P. (2002). Hepatitis A virus infections in the United States: Model-based estimates and implications for childhood immunizations. *Pediatrics, 109*, 839-845.

Averhoff, F., Shapiro, C.N., Bell, B.P., Hyams, I., Burd, L., Deladisma, A., et al. (2001). Control of hepatitis A through routine vaccination of children. *Journal of the American Medical Association, 286*, 2968-2973.

Baker, S.S., Liptak, G.S., Colleti, R.B., Croffie, J.M., DiLorenzo, C., Ector, W., et al. (1999). Constipation in infants and children: Evaluation and treatment: A medical position statement of the North American Society for Pediatric Gastroenterology and Nutrition. *Journal of Pediatric Gastroenterology and Nutrition, 29*, 612-626.

Bloom, M.D. (1997). Jaundice. In J. C. Gartner, Jr., & B.J. Zitelli (Eds.). *Common and chronic symptoms in pediatrics*. St. Louis: Mosby.

Borkowsky, W. (2002). Viral hepatitis. In F.D. Burg, J.R. Ingelfinger, R.A. Polin, & A.A. Gershon (Eds.). *Gellis & Kagan's current pediatric therapy* (pp. 116-121). Philadelphia: WB Saunders.

Broderick, A., & Kleinman, R.E. (2002). Constipation. In F.D. Burg, J.R. Ingelfinger, R.A. Polin, & A.A. Gershon (Eds.). *Gellis & Kagan's current pediatric therapy* (pp. 623-626). Philadelphia: WB Saunders.

Bromberg, D.I. (2001). Colic. In R.A. Hoekelman, H.M. Adams, N.M. Nelson, M.L. Weitzman, & M.H. Wilson (Eds.), *Pediatric primary care* (pp.815-818). St. Louis: Mosby.

Burkhart, D.M. (1999). Management of acute gastroenteritis in children. *American Family Physician, 60*, 2555-2563.

Bytzer, P., & Talley, N.J. (2001). Dyspepsia. *Annals of Internal Medicine, 134*, 815-822.

Centers for Disease Control and Prevention. (2001). Diagnosis and management of foodborne illnesses: A primer for physicians. *Morbidity and Mortality Weekly Report, 50*(No. RR-02), 1-69

Centers for Disease Control and Prevention. (2001). Updated US Public Health Service guidelines for the management of occupational exposures to HBV, HCV, and HIV and recommendations for postexposure prophylaxis. *Morbidity and Mortality Weekly Report, 50*(No. RR-11), 1-44.

Dennery, P.A., Seidman, D.S., & Stevenson, D.K. (2001). Neonatal hyperbilirubinemia. *New England Journal of Medicine, 344*, 581-590.

Drossman, D.A. (1995). Diagnosing and treating patients with refractory functional gastrointestinal disorders. *Annals of Internal Medicine, 123,* 688-697.

Duggan, C., Santosham, M., & Glass, R.I. (1992). The management of acute diarrhea in children: Oral rehydration, maintenance, and nutritional therapy. *Morbidity and Mortality Weekly Report*, (RR-16), 1-20.

Etzkorn, K.P., & Rodriquez, L. (2002). Constipation. In R.E. Rakel & E.T. Bope (Eds.). *Conn's current therapy* (pp. 18-21). Philadelphia: WB Saunders.

Faubion, W.A., & Zein, N.N. (1998). Gastroesophageal reflux in infants and children. *Mayo Clinical Proceedings, 73,* 166-173.

Goepp, J.G. (2001). Dehydration. In R.A. Hoekelman, H.M. Adams, N.M. Nelson, M.L. Weitzman, & M.H. Wilson (Eds.), *Pediatric primary care* (pp. 1925-1929). St. Louis: Mosby.

Goroll, A.H., & Mulley, A.G. (2002). *Primary care medicine recommendations*. Philadelphia: Lippincott Williams & Wilkins.

Goroll, A.H., & Mulley, Jr., A.G. (2000) Approach to the patient with an external hernia. In A.H. Goroll & A.G. Mulley, Jr. (Eds.), *Primary care medicine* (pp. 431-434). Philadelphia: Lippincott.

Graber, M.A. (1998). Dealing with acute abdominal pain: Part 1: Clues to the diagnosis. *Emergency Medicine, 30*, 74-100.

Guandalini, S. (2000). Acute diarrhea. In W.A. Walker, P.R. Durie, J. R. Hamilton, J.A. Walker-Smith, & J.B. Watkins (Eds.), *Pediatric gastrointestinal disease* (pp. 28-38). Lewison, NY: BC Decker.

Heillemeier, A.C. (2000). Gastroesophageal reflux. In W.A. Walker, P.R. Durie, J. R. Hamilton, J.A. Walker-Smith, & J.B. Watkins (Eds.), *Pediatric gastrointestinal disease* (pp. 289-302). Lewison, NY: BC Decker.

Horwitz, B., & Fisher, R.S. (2001). The irritable bowel syndrome. *New England Journal of Medicine, 344*, 1846-1850.

Infectious Diseases Society of America. (2001). Practice guidelines for the management of infectious diarrhea. *Clinical Infectious Diseases, 32*, 331-350.

Koch, K.L. (2002). Nausea and vomiting. In R.E. Rakel & E.T. Bope (Eds.). *Conn's current therapy* (pp. 6-9). Philadelphia: WB Saunders.

Lauer, G.M., & Walkers, B.D. (2001). Hepatitis C infection. *New England Journal of Medicine, 345*, 41-52.

Marion, R.W. (2001). Umbilical anomalies. In R.A. Hoekelman, H.M. Adam, N.M. Nelson, M.L. Weitzman, & M.H. Wilson (Eds.), *Primary pediatric care* (pp. 1889-1893). St. Louis: Mosby.

McColl, I. (1998). More precision in diagnosing appendicitis. *New England Journal of Medicine, 338*, 190-191.

Milla, P.J. (2001). Irritable bowel syndrome in childhood. *Gastroenterology, 120*, 287-307.

Mitchell, D.K. (2002). Campylobacter infections. In F.D. Burg, J.R. Ingelfinger, R.A. Polin, & A.A. Gershon (Eds.). *Gellis & Kagan's current pediatric therapy* (pp. 58-60). Philadelphia: WB Saunders.

Morris, J.G. (2002). Food-borne illness. In R.E. Rakel & E.T. Bope (Eds.). *Conn's current therapy* (pp. 77-82). Philadelphia: WB Saunders.

North American Society for Pediatric Gastroenterology and Nutrition. (2001). Guidelines for evaluation and treatment of gastroesophageal reflux in infants and children. *Journal of Pediatric Gastroenterology and Nutrition, 32*(Suppl 2), S1-S28.

Pickering, L.K., & Hotez, P.J. (2002). Giardiasis. In F.D. Burg, J.R. Ingelfinger, R.A. Polin, & A.A. Gershon (Eds.). *Gellis & Kagan's current pediatric therapy* (pp. 178-179). Philadelphia: WB Saunders.

Porter, M.L., & Dennis, B.L. (2002). Hyperbilirubinemia in the term newborn. *American Family Physician, 65*, 599-606, 613-614.

Pratt, D.S. & Kaplan, M.M. (2000). Evaluation of abnormal liver-enzyme results in asymptomatic patients. *New England Journal of Medicine, 342*, 1266-1271.

Rivkina, A., & Rybalov, S. (2002). Chronic hepatitis B: Current and future treatment options. *Pharmacotherapy, 22*, 721-737.

Sack, D.A. (2002). Acute infectious diarrhea. In R.E. Rakel & E.T. Bope (Eds.). *Conn's current therapy* (pp. 12-18). Philadelphia: WB Saunders.

Smith, J.C. (2001). Abdominal pain. In R.A. Hoekelman, H.M. Adams, N.M. Nelson, M.L. Weitzman, & M.H. Wilson (Eds.), *Pediatric primary care* (pp.965-970). St. Louis: Mosby.

Steele, R.W. (2002). Hepatitis A vaccine: Time for universal immunization. *Clinical Pediatrics, 41*, 1-3.

Thompson, W.G., Longstreth, G.F., Drossman, D.A., Heaton, K.W., Irvine, E.J., & Muller-Lissner, S.A. (1999). Functional bowel disorders and functional abdominal pain. *Gut, 45*(Suppl II), II43-II47.

Ulshen, M.H. (2001). Vomiting. In R.A. Hoekelman, H.M. Adams, N.M. Nelson, M.L. Weitzman, & M.H. Wilson (Eds.), *Pediatric primary care* (pp. 1298-1302). St. Louis: Mosby.

Weissbluth, M. (2002). Colic. In F.D. Burg, J.R. Ingelfinger, R.A. Polin, & A.A. Gershon (Eds.). *Gellis & Kagan's current pediatric therapy* (pp. 1626-629). Philadelphia: WB Saunders.

Yuan, Q., Pappa, H., & Russell, G.J. (2002). Gastroesophageal reflux. In F.D. Burg, J.R. Ingelfinger, R.A. Polin, & A.A. Gershon (Eds.). *Gellis & Kagan's current pediatric therapy* (pp. 583-585). Philadelphia: WB Saunders.

Zeiter, D.K., & Hyams, J.S. (2002). Recurrent abdominal pain in children. *Pediatric Clinics of North America, 49*, 53-73.

Genitourinary Problems

CONSTANCE R. UPHOLD

HEMATURIA

I. Definition: Presence of red blood cells (RBCs) in urine; hematuria may be either gross or microscopic

 A. Gross hematuria occurs when there are so many RBCs that they can be detected by the naked eye

 B. Microscopic occurs when a chemical test for hemoglobin (dipstick) or microscope is needed to detect the RBCs

 1. More than 3 RBCs per high-power field on microscopic evaluation of the urinary sediment from two of three properly collected urinalysis specimens is the diagnostic criteria for hematuria

 2. However, in patients at risk for significant disease (see following table), 1 or 2 RBCs are suspicious and deserve further evaluation

RISK FACTORS FOR SIGNIFICANT DISEASE IN PATIENTS WITH MICROSCOPIC HEMATURIA
✓ Analgesic abuse such as acetaminophen, aspirin compounds
✓ Cigarette smoking
✓ Male gender
✓ Occupational exposures: Individuals working in printing, leather, rubber, and dye industries
✓ Cyclophosphamide use
✓ History of gross hematuria
✓ History of urologic disorder or disease
✓ History of irritative voiding symptoms
✓ History of urinary tract infection
✓ Pelvic irradiation
✓ Family history of urologic cancer

II. Pathogenesis

 A. RBCs can enter the genitourinary tract at any site from the glomerulus to the urethral meatus and the causes can be categorized as prerenal, renal, postrenal, or false (see table)

CAUSES OF HEMATURIA ORGANIZED BY LOCATION

Prerenal Renal
Trauma
Arteriovenous malformations
Thrombocytopenia
Malignant hypertension
Coagulopathy such as hemophilia or
   thrombocytopenic purpura
Drugs such as warfarin sodium, heparin sodium,
   or aspirin
Sickle cell disease or trait
Collagen vascular disease such as systemic
   lupus erythematosus
Wilm's tumor

Renal
Nonglomerular
  Pyelonephritis
  Polycystic kidney disease
  Granulomatous disease such as tuberculosis
  Nephrocalcinosis
  Hydronephrosis
  Malignant neoplasm
  Congenital and vascular anomalies
Glomerular
  Glomerulonephritis
  IgA glomerulonephritis
  Henoch-Schönlein Purpura
  Goodpasture's disease
  Hemolytic uremic syndrome
  Berger's disease
  Systemic lupus erythematosus
  Benign familial hematuria
  Vascular abnormalities such as vasculitis
  Alport's syndrome (familial nephritis)

Postrenal
Renal calculi
Ureteritis
Cystitis
Prostatitis
Hypercalciuria
Obstruction/reflux
Epididymitis
Urethritis
Malignant neoplasm

False
Menstrual bleeding
Hemoglobinuria
Intake of certain foods such as beets, rhubarb,
   blackberries, fava beans
Intake of certain medications such as quinine
   sulfate, phenazopyridine, phenytoin,
   phenindione, phenothiazine, rifampin,
   sulfasalazine
Excretion of porphyrins

Miscellaneous causes
  Strenuous exercise
  Fever
  Trauma
  Viral infections
  Schistosomiasis (travel)

B. Causes of hematuria may also be categorized as gross or microscopic
1. Gross hematuria
   a. Common causes: Trauma, infection, irritation or ulceration of the perineum or urethral meatus, renal calculi, glomerulonephritis, sickle cell disease, arteriovenous malformations, and coagulopathies
   b. Occurs uncommonly; most often is caused by abnormalities of the lower urinary tract
2. Microscopic hematuria: Causes are similar to the causes of gross hematuria, but microscopic hematuria occurs more frequently
   a. Common causes of asymptomatic microscopic hematuria: Infection/inflammation, hypercalciuria, perineal trauma, exercise-induced hematuria, benign familial hematuria
   b. Common causes of symptomatic microscopic hematuria: Postinfectious glomerulonephritis, IgA nephropathy, systemic lupus erythematosus

C. Hematuria may be a complaint in patients with factitious hematuria such as narcotic seekers complaining of kidney stones or individuals in families with Munchausen syndrome

D. Essential hematuria occurs when no definable cause can be found

III. Clinical Presentation

A. Clinical presentation of common causes of hematuria
1. Urinary tract infection presents with urinary frequency, urgency, and dysuria
2. Irritation or ulceration of the perineum or urethral meatus; often occurs in healthy, male infants and is discovered by parents on the children's diapers
3. Trauma
   a. Blunt abdominal injuries cause the majority of renal injuries in children
   b. Renal injury may be present even if the child is asymptomatic and the physical examination is negative
4. Hypercalciuria may occur with or with renal stones
   a. Hematuria is typically microscopic, but gross hematuria can occur
   b. Positive family history is common

       c.   If stones are present, patient typically has renal colic and abdominal pain

       d.   In hypercalciuria without renal stone, symptoms include urinary frequency, dysuria, and abdominal or flank pain

  5.   Glomerulonephritis

       a.   Respiratory infection typically precedes or occurs concurrently; if due to a streptococcal infection, history of rash is common

       b.   Often presents with acute onset of edema and tea-colored urine

       c.   Patient may be asymptomatic or complain of malaise, headache, abdominal pain, and oliguria

       d.   Elevated blood pressure is common

       e.   Urinalysis often reveals RBC casts and proteinuria; BUN and creatinine may or may not be elevated

  6.   Sickle cell disease

       a.   Marked by recurrent episodes of gross hematuria

       b.   Hematuria is often painless and may be mild or severe

B.   Neoplasms are uncommon in children, but should be considered in the differential diagnosis

  1.   Patients with Wilms tumor typically have an abdominal mass

  2.   Patient may have only microscopic hematuria, but gross hematuria is the most common presentation

  3.   Painless hematuria is most often associated with neoplasms

IV.   Diagnosis/Evaluation

A.   History

  1.   Question about timing and appearance of hematuria

       a.   Hematuria seen at onset of urination often indicates bleeding in the urethra

       b.   Terminal hematuria seen in the last few drops of urine often indicates the bladder neck or prostate as the source

       c.   Hematuria seen throughout urination suggests that a lesion could be located anywhere from the upper urinary tract to the bladder

  2.   Ask about associated symptoms:

       a.   Colicky flank pain radiating to groin suggests a kidney stone

       b.   Dysuria and frequency suggest cystitis, especially in females

       c.   Hemoptysis, hematuria, and acute renal failure in an anemic patient suggest Goodpasture's syndrome

       d.   Loin-pain and hematuria in a young woman taking oral contraceptives may indicate small-vessel occlusive vascular disease

       e.   In a systemic disease, fever, joint pains, and rash are typical manifestations

  3.   Inquire about color of the urine

       a.   Pink or red urine usually indicates bladder or urethral bleeding

       b.   Brown or greenish urine usually indicates upper tract or renal parenchymal bleeding

  4.   Ask patient to describe any blood clots that have occurred

       a.   Large, thick clots suggest the bladder as the bleeding source

       b.   Specks or thin, stringy clots suggest the upper urinary tract as the source

  5.   Ask if symptoms are generalized or localized

       a.   Localized symptoms (frequency, dysuria) suggest lower tract urinary system disorders

       b.   Generalized symptoms (fever, edema, arthralgias, rash suggest a more extensive illness

  6.   Determine whether hematuria is transient or persistent; in children and adolescents, transient hematuria is common and seldom secondary to significant disease

  7.   Determine pattern of hematuria

       a.   Hematuria at each voiding suggests infection or parenchymal disease

       b.   Hematuria that is intermittent suggests hypercalciuria and/or renal stones

  8.   Ask whether the patient bruises easily or has extended bleeding after a minor cut or dental work (coagulopathy or bleeding dyscrasia may be present)

  9.   In females, inquire about the last menstrual period

  10.   Obtain a complete medication history

  11.   Inquire about a history of pharyngitis with an impetiginous skin rash followed by hematuria, edema and hypertension (presentation of glomerulonephritis)

  12   Ask about recent trauma and strenuous exercise

  13.   Question about risk factors for developing uroepithelial cancer (see preceding table I.B.)

  14.   Explore previous medical history, making certain to inquire about sickle cell disease and trait, previous urinary tract infections, metabolic and endocrine diseases, and surgeries

15. Inquire about exposure to tuberculosis
16. Explore patient's family history; kidney stone disease, Alport's syndrome, benign familial hematuria, and familial nephritis are common across generations of families

B. Physical Examination
1. Measure vital signs; elevated temperature suggests infection, neoplasm, or systemic disease; elevated blood pressure suggests glomerulonephritis or renal parenchymal disease
2. Measure height and weight; compare to norms
3. Observe skin for signs of exanthems, pallor, ecchymosis, purpura, or birth marks
4. Examine for systemic infection such as tonsillar enlargement, lymphadenopathy, and exanthems
5. If Alport's syndrome is suspected, perform a hearing test, as this syndrome is associated with hearing defects
6. Auscultate heart
7. Perform complete abdominal exam, noting tenderness, organomegaly, bladder distention, masses, or bruits
8. Assess for costovertebral angle tenderness which suggests pyelonephritis or urinary tract obstruction
9. Examine extremities for edema which may be associated with glomerulonephritis
10. In males:
    a. Examine testes, spermatic cord, and vas deferens for tenderness and masses
    b. Examine penis for condyloma acuminatum, meatal stenosis, foreign body
11. In females:
    a. Inspect perineum, vulva, and urethral meatus, noting signs of urethral carbuncle, irritation, or ulcerations
    b. In sexually active females, consider performing a pelvic examination

C. Differential Diagnosis
1. Essential hematuria is a diagnosis of exclusion
2. The majority of cases of hematuria will present with symptoms, signs, or laboratory test results that pinpoint a specific diagnosis
3. For those patients with asymptomatic, isolated hematuria for whom a cause cannot be identified always consider neoplasm (see table RISK FACTORS I.B.)

D. Diagnostic Tests
1. Always obtain a urinalysis (UA) and a subsequent culture to confirm findings on the UA (best to obtain a freshly voided, morning specimen and examine it within 30 minutes)
    a. Dipstick can give false-positive results and should always be used in conjunction with a microscopic examination
    b. Most experts recommend at least 2 or 3 urinalyses be abnormal over 2-3 weeks before further evaluation be performed unless there are significant associated symptoms or hematuria is severe
    c. Alkaline pH and positive nitrite and leukocyte esterase reactions suggest urinary tract infections
    d. Hematuria with pyuria but no bacteria suggest a sexually transmitted disease (chlamydia, gonorrhea), viral infection, or, less commonly, tuberculosis
    e. Protein suggests glomerulonephritis
    f. If the dipstick test is negative for RBCs but the urine appears red, pigmenturia caused by endogenous substances that change color of urine is the likely cause
    g. Microscopic examination of urinary sediment can help determine the site of bleeding
        (1) RBC casts suggest glomerulonephritis
        (2) Crystals suggest renal calculi
    h. If exercise hematuria is suspected, patient should refrain from active participation in sports for at least 48 hours prior to urinalysis
2. If bacterial infection is detected, treat patient and repeat urinalysis in 6 weeks (see sections on CYSTITIS and PYELONEPHRITIS)
3. Serum creatinine should be ordered if there is isolated microscopic hematuria in absence of bacterial infection
4. Complete evaluation for primary renal disease (see table that follows) or referral to a nephrologist is needed in the following patients:
    a. Patients whose microscopic hematuria is accompanied by significant proteinuria (+1 or greater on dipstick urinalysis should prompt 24-hour collection to quantify degree of proteinuria), dysmorphic red blood cells, red cell casts, or elevated serum creatinine levels
    b. Patients who have risk factors for significant disease (see table RISK FACTORS, I.B.)

I. Imaging Tests (order one of the following):

                             Advantages

    A. Intravenous urography   First choice; inexpensive; widely available

    B. Ultrasonography   Good for detection of renal cysts

    C. Computed tomography   Highest efficacy for the range of possible underlying pathologies and shortens diagnostic work-up

II. Cystoscopy to visualize bladder mucosa, urethra, and urethral orifices to exclude bladder cancer

III. Cytology to detect urothelial cancers; three first-morning voiding urine specimens should be obtained on three separate days

---

5. Order additional tests depending on clinical presentation of the patient
   a. If history of abdominal trauma is present, order abdominal computerized tomography (CT)
   b. Flat plate and upright films of abdomen to assess renal size and detect renal calculi
   c. Complete blood count to document blood loss and presence of systemic involvement
   d. 24-hour urine specimen for determination of the concentration of calcium, uric acid, and creatinine
   e. African American patients should be screened for sickle cell disease or trait
   f. Clotting studies (i.e., prothrombin time, partial thromboplastin time, platelet count, bleeding time) if a coagulopathy or a bleeding disorder is suspected
   g. Administer a purified protein derivative (PPD) and order urine culture for acid-fast bacillus when tuberculosis is a possibility
   h. In patients who have proteinuria in addition to hematuria order a 24-hour collection of creatinine and protein
   i. Order erythrocyte sedimentation rate (ESR) for patients with suspected secondary glomerular disease such as endocarditis and systemic lupus erythematosus
   j. An immunologic survey consisting of titers of IgG, IgA, IgM, and IgE are helpful if Schönlein-Henoch purpura or glomerular disease is suspected
   k. Voiding cystourethrography can reveal congenital anomalies, stone formation, or foreign bodies
   l. Angiography is not usually performed, but is the only test to detect arteriovenous malformations and may be considered in patients with gross, painless hematuria after other studies have excluded carcinoma and other renal disease
6. A renal biopsy is performed when no cause is apparent

V. Plan/Management

    A. Refer patients who have the following to a specialist:
   1. Gross, painless hematuria throughout the voiding process
   2. Risk factors for malignancy such as smoking
   3. Urologic trauma
   4. Microscopic hematuria accompanied with significant proteinuria, red blood cells, red cell casts, or elevated serum creatinine levels
   5. Recurrent urinary tract infections
   6. Suspected glomerulonephritis
   7. Thrombocytopenia and/or azotemia
   8. Suspected renal calculi

    B. Treat infections with appropriate antibiotics (see section on URINARY TRACT INFECTIONS)

    C. Exercise-induced hematuria and benign familial hematuria require no treatment, as they are self-limited conditions

    D. Treatment of infants with urethral irritation: Apply petroleum jelly to meatus and leave infant undiapered for short periods of time

    E. Treatment of renal calculi
   1. Once ureteral obstruction is excluded and the acute episode has passed, small stones which can be passed may be managed with hydration (maintain urine flow rate of 3-4 L/day) and analgesia; refer patients with large stones to specialist
   2. Patients can be considered for lithotripsy
   3. A low-purine diet and uricosuric agents may prevent recurrence of uric acid stones

F. Follow Up is variable depending on severity of diagnosis
   1. Reassure patient and family that microscopic hematuria without other significant findings is usually benign
   2. For patients with microhematuria perform annual screening urinalysis
   3. Instruct patient and family to call clinician if gross hematuria occurs as this is typically associated with uropathology
   4. Further evaluation or referral to a nephrologist is recommended if hematuria persists and either hypertension, proteinuria or evidence of glomerular bleeding develops

CYSTITIS AND PYELONEPHRITIS IN ADOLESCENTS

I. Definition: Bacteria in urine that have the potential to injure tissues of the urinary tract and adjacent structures. Urinary tract infections (UTIs) are often classified as upper and lower tract infections

   A. Cystitis, infection of the bladder, is an example of a common lower tract infection

   B. Pyelonephritis is the main upper tract infection and involves infection of the renal parenchyma

II. Pathogenesis of cystitis and pyelonephritis

   A. In females, the major cause is invasion of the urinary tract by bacteria that ascend the urethra from the introitus. Females have a short urethra that is in close proximity to the perirectal area making colonization possible

   B. Currently, researchers are exploring whether there is a genetic link for females who are prone to frequent UTIs; studies are underway to develop a blood test to identify high-risk females

   C. In males, cystitis and pyelonephritis are uncommon; in adolescent and young adult males, isolated cystitis may be due to endogenous bacteria without an underlying abnormality or related to a subclinical case of prostatitis

   D. Pathogens in community-acquired infections: Bacteria adhere to uroepithelial cells
      1. Gram negative bacilli are most common; 75-90% of infections are due to *Escherichia coli*
         a. Other gram negative bacilli organisms include *Klebsiella pneumoniae* or *Proteus mirabilis*
         b. A wide range of gram-negative bacilli and other microorganisms may be causative agents in men; particularly in older men
      2. Gram-positive cocci account for 5-15% of infections; *Staphylococcus saprophyticus* is the second most common pathogen and often occurs in young, sexually active females
      3. Rates of ampicillin resistance among pathogens is approximately 40%, whereas rates of trimethoprim-sulfamethoxazole resistance range from 10-20%

   E. In hospital settings, *E. coli* is less prevalent with Proteus, Klebsiella, Enterobacter, Pseudomonas, Staphylococci, and Enterococci species being more common

   F. Risk factors in both genders
      1. Diabetes mellitus: Not necessarily an increased risk for developing infection but often there is a disorder of bladder emptying which makes UTI more difficult to eradicate
      2. Urinary instrumentation and catheterization
      3. Obstruction of normal flow of urine resulting from calculi, tumors, urethral strictures
      4. Neurogenic bladder disease from strokes, multiple sclerosis, spinal cord injuries
      5. Vesicoureteral reflux as a result of a congenital abnormality or more often from bladder overdistention from obstruction

   G. Risk factors in females
      1. Increased sexual activity, diaphragm and spermicide use, and failure to void after intercourse
      2. Pregnancy
      3. History of recent urinary infection
      4. Postponing urination or incomplete voiding in women
      5. Tampons and wiping from back to front after a bowel movement are **not** risk factors

H. Risk factors in males
   1. Homosexuality
   2. Lack of circumcision
   3. Having a sexual partner with vaginal colonization by uropathogens
   4. HIV infection with CD4+ T-lymphocyte counts of less than 200/mm^3
   5. Obstruction of normal flow resulting from prostatic hypertrophy and urethral strictures

III. Clinical Presentation

A. Epidemiology: After puberty, the prevalence of UTIs increases significantly in females, but remains low in males

B. Cystitis
   1. Some adolescents may be asymptomatic
   2. Typical symptoms include abrupt onset of dysuria, urgency, frequency, nocturia, suprapubic heaviness or discomfort; fever is uncommon

D. Pyelonephritis
   1. Acute onset of chills, fever, flank pain, headache, malaise, costovertebral angle tenderness, and possibly hematuria
   2. Often occurs concurrently or after a lower urinary tract infection
   3. May be associated with renal calculi, ureteral obstruction, or neurogenic bladder.

IV. Diagnosis/Evaluation

A. History
   1. Determine onset and duration of urinary symptoms
   2. Ask about strength and character of urine stream when voiding
   3. Determine whether dysuria occurs during urination or after urine begins to pass over inflamed labia as with herpes simplex infections
   4. Inquire about associated symptoms such as fever, chills, nausea, vomiting, diarrhea, constipation, abdominal and back pain, hematuria
   5. Ask about onset, duration, and characteristics of vaginal or urethral discharge
   6. Always query females about recent sexual activity, method of birth control, and date of last menstrual period
   7. Past medical history should include drug allergies, chronic diseases such as diabetes mellitus or multiple sclerosis, previous genitourinary problems
   8. Ask patient to count number of previous UTIs and discuss results of previous treatments

B. Physical Examination
   1. Assess vital signs, particularly noting elevated temperature and signs of orthostatic hypotension
   2. Perform a complete abdominal exam to detect tenderness, a distended bladder, or a mass
   3. Palpate back for costovertebral tenderness
   4. In females may need to inspect perineum and do complete pelvic, speculum, and rectal exams
   5. In males inspect and palpate external genitalia and scrotum; perform prostate and rectal exams
   6. Consider performing a neurologic examination to detect diseases such as multiple sclerosis

C. Differential Diagnosis
   1. Males
      a. Gonococcal and nongonococcal urethritis in males (often asymptomatic, but may have mucoid or purulent urethral discharge)
      b. Prostatitis (a tender prostate on rectal exam is usually present)
      c. Epididymitis (testicular tenderness and erythema are present)
      d. Prostatodynia (presents with perineal or back pain accompanied by unilateral testicular pain or dysuria; urinalysis and urine culture are negative)
   2. Females
      a. Dysuria without accompanying symptoms is a poor indicator of UTI; four symptoms (dysuria, frequency, hematuria, and back pain) and one sign (costovertebral angle tenderness) increase the probability of UTI
      b. Interstitial cystitis is characterized by suprapubic pain that is relieved by bladder emptying
      c. Urethral syndrome
         (1) Patient has irritative voiding symptoms with an absence of objective findings
         (2) There is no cure; treatment is symptomatic
      d. Vulvovaginitis (external dysuria, vulvar erythema, and vulvar lesions are often present)

500

        e.   Vaginitis
              (1)   Patients deny urinary urgency and frequency
              (2)   Usually there are no bacteria in the urine unless vaginal discharge contaminates urine
                     specimen
              (3)   Vaginal discharge, odor, and pruritus may be present
        f.   Cervicitis (cervix will be abnormal on pelvic exam)
        g.   Urethral trauma due to sexual intercourse, physical activity (horseback riding, bicycling), and
              sensitivity to scented creams, bath products, and toilet paper
  3.   Both genders
        a.   Urinary calculi (usually patient has severe pain and hematuria)
        b.   Bladder outlet obstruction (changes in urinary stream occur)
        c.   Renal tuberculosis (hematuria is common)
        d.   Tumors and carcinoma (hematuria is common)

D.   Diagnostic Tests
  1.   Urine collection
        a.   Clean catch voided specimens are usually acceptable for adolescents
              (1)   First morning specimen is the best voided specimen
              (2)   If urine specimen is obtained later in the day, bladder should not be emptied for at
                     least 2 hours and patients should avoid high fluid intake which would dilute sample
        b.   Single in-and-out catheterization of the bladder should be done on patients who are unable
              to give a clean midstream urine specimen
  2.   Urinalysis
        a.   Dipstick urinalysis; findings of UTIs are the following:
              (1)   Leukocyte esterase test is positive and denotes pyuria or WBCs in the urine; false
                     positive esterase tests occur with kidney stones, tumors, urethritis, and poor
                     collection techniques; false negative test may occur early in course of UTI
              (2)   Nitrites are positive with gram negative infections; false negatives occur with use of
                     diuretics early in course of UTI, and inadequate levels of dietary nitrate or presence of
                     bacteria that do not produce nitrate reductase (*Staphylococcus saprophyticus,
                     Enterococcus, Pseudomonas*)
        b.   Microscopic analysis: Examine urine sediment under high power (40X) to count WBCs and
              perform gram stain to identify type of bacteria
              (1)   Significant pyuria is >2-5 leukocytes per high power field or if using a counting
                     hemocytometer, 10 or more white blood cels/mm^3 are used as the criterion
              (2)   Gram stain is done to identify whether bacteria are gram negative or positive and the
                     shape and pattern of bacteria; it is not helpful to count bacteria on a gram stain
  3.   Urine culture and sensitivity (urine C&S)
        a.   The traditional standard for significant bacteriuria was 10^5 colony-forming units (cfu) of a
              uropathogen per mL of urine; today the criterion that is used is 10^2 in symptomatic females
              or 10^3 in symptomatic males
        b.   Bacterial identification and determination of antibiotic susceptibilities or urine C&S is not
              necessary in most uncomplicated UTIs
        c.   Bacterial identification or urine C&S is important in infections in males, females who have
              complicated UTIs, and females who are symptomatic but pyuria is absent
  4.   With systemic symptoms order CBC with differential and in severely ill patients order blood cultures;
        consider ordering erythrocyte sedimentation rate
  5.   In females with symptoms associated with sexually transmitted disease (STD), perform wet mount
        of vaginal secretions and order *N. gonorrhoeae* (GC) cultures and chlamydia test; also gram stain
        cervical secretions
  6.   In a male with a possible STD, gram stain urethral secretion and order GC culture and chlamydia
        tests
  7.   Other studies are usually not needed; consider additional tests such as renal ultrasound, voiding
        cystourethrogram, intravenous pyelogram (IVP), renal scan, renal biopsy, or cystoscopy in patients
        with repeat infections, slow resolution of symptoms, and atypical features such as persistent
        hematuria

V.   Plan/Management

  A.   Acute uncomplicated bacterial cystitis in females (see table ANTIBIOTICS FOR TREATING CYSTITIS)
        1.   In females with uncomplicated UTIs (immunocompetent, nonpregnant, non-diabetic women without
              structural problems, previous UTIs, or history of indwelling urinary catheter or urinary tract
              instrumentation), urine cultures are not indicated before treatment or post-treatment

2. Trimethoprim-sulfamethoxazole for 3 days is considered the current standard therapy; shorter courses of therapy are not recommended
3. Trimethoprim alone is equivalent to trimethoprim-sulfamethoxazole
4. For individuals ≥18 years, fluoroquinolones may be prescribed, but they are more expensive and, to postpone emergence of resistance to these drugs, they should be used as initial empirical therapy only in communities with high resistance to trimethoprim-sulfamethoxazole; some experts also recommend a fluoroquinolone as first choice when the female has used trimethoprim-sulfamethoxazole within the past 6 months or for females who have been recently hospitalized
5. Nitrofurantoin and fosfomycin tromethamine (Monurol) may become more useful if resistance to trimethoprim-sulfamethoxazole increases; not recommended for patients <18 years
6. β-lactams are less effective in treatment of cystitis
7. Phenazopyridine HCl (Pyridium) may be prescribed 100 mg TID for three days if the patient is experiencing bladder spasms; warn patient that urine will turn orange

ANTIBIOTICS FOR TREATING CYSTITIS			
Trimethoprim/sulfamethoxazole (Bactrim)	160 mg/800 mg	1 DS tab	BID
Trimethoprim (Trimpex)	100 mg	1 tab	BID
Ofloxacin (Floxin)*†ᴵ	200 mg	1 tab	BID
Norfloxacin (Noroxin)*†ᴵ	400 mg	1 tab	BID
Ciprofloxacin (Cipro)ᴵ	100-250 mg	1 tab	BID
Ciprofloxacin extended release (Cipro XR)ᴵ	500 mg	1 tab	QD
Nitrofurantoin (Macrodantin)§ᴵ	100 mg	1 tab	QID
Fosfomycin tromethamine (Monurol)ᴵ	3 g	1 sachet with 3-4 oz. of H_2O	Single dose

*Take on an empty stomach
†Take with full glass of water
§Take with food
ᴵ Not recommended for children <18 years

B. Complicated bacterial cystitis in females
1. For females ≥18 years treat with an oral fluoroquinolone for 14 days (see table above) or if the organism is known to be susceptible, trimethoprim-sulfamethoxazole
2. If a gram-positive bacterium is the likely pathogen, prescribe amoxicillin (Amoxil) or amoxicillin/clavulanic acid (Augmentin); for both drugs, prescribe 875 mg every 12 hours or 500 mg every 8 hours
3. Order pretreatment and post-treatment urinalyses and urine culture and sensitivities

C. Recurrent infections in females (must repeat urine culture and sensitivity each time patient has symptoms)
1. Relapse (uncommon and caused by original infecting pathogen)
   a. Occurs within two weeks of completion of therapy
   b. Treat for 2-6 weeks longer
   c. Seek occult source of infection or urologic abnormality; consider renal function tests (BUN & creatinine), an intravenous pyelogram (IVP), and referral to a specialist
2. Reinfection (cystitis): Most recurrent UTIs are due to reinfection with a new organism rather than a relapse of the same initial infection; risk factors are history of UTI in earlier childhood, sexual intercourse, and spermicide exposure
   a. If patient has ≤2 UTIs in one year:
      (1) Recommend patient-initiated therapy for symptomatic episodes (give patient a written prescription which she may fill when symptoms occur)
      (2) Prescribe 3-day regimen (see preceding table on ANTIBIOTICS) based on patient's past culture results and clinical success
   b. If patient has ≥3 UTIs in one year
      (1) If UTIs occur only after intercourse recommend a single-dose antibiotic after coitus such as trimethoprim/sulfamethoxazole 160 mg/800 mg (2 double strength tablets) or nitrofurantoin (Macrodantin) 200 mg if patient ≥18 years
      (2) If UTIs are not related to intercourse, prophylactic antimicrobials should be used for 6 months after the infection has been eradicated
         (a) Urine cultures should be done every 1-2 months
         (b) Extend prophylactic therapy to 1-2 years if reinfection occurs at end of 6-month period

        (c)   One of the following prophylactic antimicrobials should be prescribed for 6 months (may take daily or thrice weekly): Nitrofurantoin (Furadantin) 50 mg tablet HS; trimethoprim/sulfamethoxazole (Bactrim) 40/200 mg tablets, half tablet of regular strength at HS; cephalexin (Keflex) 250 mg tablet at HS

   c.   Explore whether patient is using diaphragms, spermicides, and not voiding after intercourse which may be causing reinfections

D. Pyelonephritis in females (consider consultation with a specialist)

   1.   Urine cultures are always indicated to definitively identify the invading organism and its antimicrobial sensitivity before treatment

   2.   Hospitalization and intravenous antibiotics are recommended for certain cases:

        a.   Females with signs and symptoms suggestive of bacteremia (high fever, high WBC count), vomiting, dehydration

        b.   Females who are pregnant, have a chronic disease, have abnormal urinary tracts, who have a history of nonadherence to therapies, and who fail to improve during the initial outpatient period

   3.   Recommended treatment is parenteral fluoroquinolone (for patients ≥18 years), an aminoglycoside with or without ampicillin, or an extended-spectrum cephalosporin with or without an aminoglycoside

   4.   Milder cases can be treated on an outpatient basis but close monitoring is needed

        a.   Recommended treatment is an oral fluoroquinolone for 14 days (see table ANTIBIOTICS FOR TREATING CYSTITIS, V.A.) or if the organism is known to be susceptible, trimethoprim-sulfamethoxazole

        b.   If a gram-positive bacterium is the likely pathogen, prescribe amoxicillin (Amoxil) or amoxicillin/ clavulanic acid (Augmentin); for both drugs, prescribe 875 mg every 12 hours or 500 mg every 8 hours or

   5.   If the 2-week regimen fails, a longer course of 4-6 weeks should be considered because renal parenchymal disease is more difficult to eradicate than bladder mucosal infections

   6.   Patient's symptoms should improve within 12-48 hours; if not, consider consultation with a specialist and look for deeper infections (imaging studies are often done to exclude obstruction, calculi, and formation of intrarenal abscesses)

   7.   Schedule return visits or contact patient by phone in 12-24 hours

   8.   Follow up cultures should be ordered at 2 weeks and 3 months post-treatment

   9.   Consult specialist for patients with recurrences of pyelonephritis (recommended that these patients need further urologic investigation such as an excretory urography)

E. Treatment of uncomplicated bacterial cystitis in healthy males

   1.   In the past all cases of bacterial cystitis in males were believed to be due to underlying structural problems such as prostatic hypertrophy; today, some, but not all experts, recommend that the first UTI can be treated with 7-14 day regimen of fluoroquinolone (first choice for men), trimethoprim-sulfamethoxazole, or trimethoprim (see table ANTIBIOTICS FOR TREATING CYSTITIS, V.A.) for doses

   2.   Shorter treatments are not recommended

   3.   Pretreatment and post-treatment urine cultures are recommended

   4.   Some authorities recommend reculturing urine at 4-6 weeks as prostatitis may be a related cause

F. Persistent or recurrent bladder infections in males: Consult urologist

G. Pyelonephritis in males (consultation with a specialist is recommended)

   1.   In males, pyelonephritis usually suggests a structural problem and is an indication for hospitalization, parenteral antibiotic therapy, and an IVP

   2.   Close follow up is essential

   3.   Occasionally, outpatient therapy is an acceptable alternative In healthy males; outpatient treatment is similar to that in the adult woman

H. Patient education may help prevent future recurrent infections

   1.   Avoid a full bladder

   2.   Do not postpone urinating or rush during urination

   3.   Increase fluid intake at first signs of infection

   4.   Void after intercourse

   5.   For females, consider other types of birth control if using a diaphragm or spermicides

   6.   Call clinician if symptoms are not resolved at end of therapy or if new symptoms develop

I.   Catheter-associated UTI
    1.   Diagnosis can be made when the urine culture shows 100 or more cfu per ml
    2.   Infections are usually polymicrobic
    3.   For mild to moderate infections, treat with an oral fluoroquinolone for 10-14 days (not recommended for persons <18 years)
    4.   For severe infections, treat with an oral or parenteral fluoroquinolone for 14-21 days (not recommended for persons <18 years)
    5.   Patients with asymptomatic bacteriuria do not need treatment except for following cases: Patients who are immunosuppressed after organ transplant, patients at risk for bacterial endocarditis, and patients who are scheduled for urinary tract instrumentation

J.   Asymptomatic bacteriuria
    1.   Defined as reproducible growth of at least 10^5 cfu of the same species of bacteria per milliliter of urine in a patient who has no signs or symptoms of UTI (need 2 positive urine specimens)
    2.   Routine screening and treatment are not recommended; treatment is recommended for pregnant females and adults prior to invasive procedures and for renal transplant recipients
        a.   Order pretreatment and 2-week post-treatment urinalyses and urine cultures and sensitivities
        b.   Treat with seven-day course of antibiotics based on culture and sensitivity results
    3.   If bacteriuria is found by chance, further investigation to exclude predisposing structural and functional abnormalities of the urinary tract may be beneficial

K.   Referral
    1.   In females, consider referral for upper tract illness, recurrent multiple infections, and infections with unusual organisms
    2.   Consider referring all males with UTIs with exception of healthy males who do not have recurrent infections

L.   Follow up is variable depending on age, gender, and condition of patient
    1.   For uncomplicated cystitis in treated females no follow-up or urine testing is needed; for complicated cystitis in treated women, follow-up urine culture is needed
    2.   For cystitis in males, follow up urine culture is needed after treatment; some recommend following these patients with repeat urine testing and a segmented urine collection to detect prostatitis in 4-6 weeks
    3.   Reinfections need close follow up with urine cultures every 1-2 months
    4.   Patients with pyelonephritis should be contacted within 12-24 hours after treatment is begun; then, reschedule visits 2 weeks and 3 months post-treatment for urine cultures

CYSTITIS AND PYELONEPHRITIS IN CHILDREN

I.   Definition: Bacteria in urine which have the potential to injure tissues of the urinary tract and adjacent structures. Urinary tract infections (UTIs) are often classified as upper and lower tract infections

    A.   Cystitis or bladder infection is an example of a lower tract infection

    B.   Pyelonephritis is the main upper tract infection and involves infection of the renal parenchyma

II.   Pathogenesis of cystitis and pyelonephritis

    A.   In neonates, UTIs result from hematogenous spread of infection to the kidney, congenital urinary anomalies, and possibly immature kidneys that allow easier passage of bacteria through the renal filtration barrier than mature kidneys

    B.   The ascending route of infection is most common in older children.
        1.   In females, bacteria can ascend the urethra from the introitus. Females have a short urethra which is in close proximity to the perirectal area making colonization possible
        2.   In males, the prepuce may be the main source of the bacteria in ascending infections

C. Bacterial virulence factors such as bacterial adherence are related to the development of UTIs; some bacteria have p-fimbriae which are hair-like structures that have the ability to adhere to uroepithelial cells and produce an inflammatory response; these p-fimbriae are more common on *E. coli* strains and have a major role in the pathogenesis of pyelonephritis

D. Pathogens
    1. Gram negative bacilli are most common; 75-80% of community-acquired infections are due to *Escherichia coli*; other gram negative bacilli include *Klebsiella, Proteus,* or *Enterobacter*
    2. *Enterococcus* and *Staphylococcus saprophyticus* (typically occurs in young, sexually active females) are common gram-positive organisms

E. The prevalence and etiology of urinary tract infections (UTIs) vary with age and gender
    1. In infants <3 months of age, infections are often associated with bacteremia; infections are more common in premature or low-birth weight infants
    2. During the first year of life, incidence in UTIs is higher in girls than boys; the majority of infected boys are uncircumcised
    3. Infants and young children are at highest risk for incurring acute renal injury with UTI; vesicoureteral reflux occurs more often and is more severe in these age groups
    4. Prevalence increases in the preschool years, with infections predominant in females; infections in males are usually due to congenital abnormalities
    5. During the school years and before puberty, prevalence is about 1-5% of females; UTIs are rare in males
    6. After puberty, the prevalence of UTIs increases significantly in females, but remains low in males

F. Any factor that causes incomplete urinary drainage and/or stasis can predispose children to UTIs:
    1. Vesicoureteral reflux (VUR), a structural abnormality, can result in renal damage
        a. Occurs from an incompetent functional sphincter at the vesicoureteral junction or a defect in the valve-like mechanism at the junction of the ureter and bladder which enables organisms in bladder urine to be directly transmitted to the kidney
        b. VUR is the single most important risk factor in the development of pyelonephritis
        c. Approximately 50% of children <5 years of age who have UTIs and fevers also have VUR; more common in Caucasian children than African American children; common in young girls with dysfunctional voiding
        d. When VUR and infected urine are present, progressive loss of renal function often occurs; however, in the absence of infection, VUR does not result in renal scarring which highlights the importance of preventing infection in children with VUR
    2. Constipation
    3. Voiding dysfunction
    4. Behavioral factors such as voluntary deferral of micturition or defecation
    5. Poor hygiene, urethral irritation from soaps, pinworms, and presence of foreign body in introitus
    6. Noncircumcision in male infants
    7. Urinary tract obstruction such as urinary lithiasis, urethral strictures, retroperitoneal fibrosis, and neurogenic bladder
    8. Nonobstructive renal malformations such as renal hypoplasia, dysplasia, and polycystic kidney disease
    9. Urinary instrumentation and catheterization
    10. Neurogenic bladder disease from strokes, multiple sclerosis, spinal cord injuries, myelomeningocele (spina bifida), or other spinal anomalies
    11. Conditions such as hypokalemia, vitamin A deficiency, diabetes mellitus, and uremia

III. Clinical Presentation

A. UTIs in children can result in renal scarring and permanent renal damage and thus warrant greater attention and more aggressive management than UTIs in adults

B. Cystitis
    1. In infants, signs and symptoms may be fever, irritability, decreased appetite, vomiting, diarrhea, constipation, dehydration, jaundice, diapers that are constantly wet, and crying during urination
    2. Toddler and preschool children often present with nonspecific complaints such as anorexia and abdominal discomfort; may also have fever, changes in voiding pattern, and enuresis if they are toilet trained
    3. School-aged children and adolescents have signs and symptoms typical of adults such as dysuria, frequency, urgency, and suprapubic pain

C. Pyelonephritis is important to rapidly diagnose and treat as a delay in treatment increases the risk of renal damage
    1. Accurate diagnosis of pyelonephritis based on clinical symptoms is difficult as children may not have typical findings of fever and flank pain as seen in adults
    2. In infancy, sepsis is a greater possibility and there is increased likelihood of bladder obstruction marked by abdominal distention, weak urinary stream, infrequent voiding, and discolored and malodorous urine
    3. Older children sometimes have an acute onset of chills, fever, flank pain, costovertebral angle tenderness, and possibly hematuria
    4. Often occurs concurrently or after a lower urinary tract infection

D. Recurrent infections are common and are often associated with severe vesicoureteral reflux and concomitant progressive renal scarring
    1. Many children, typically girls, have a voiding dysfunction whereby residual volumes of urine are left in the bladder after voiding and daytime enuresis (often with small amounts of urine) occurs
    2. Chronic constipation and poor bowel habits are also correlated with recurrent UTIs and voiding dysfunction

E. Asymptomatic bacteriuria occurs in children with culture-proven bacteriuria who do not have symptoms; often this condition spontaneously resolves within a few months

IV. Diagnosis/Evaluation

A. History
    1. Inquire about child's degree of listlessness and ability to retain oral intake
    2. Determine onset and duration of urinary symptoms; ask about strength and character of urinary stream when voiding; for infants ask about constant wetting of diapers and odor (+/-)
    3. Explore normal voiding patterns and frequency of voids
    4. Determine whether dysuria occurs during urination or after urination begins to pass over inflamed labia as with herpes simplex infections
    5. Inquire about associated symptoms such as irritability, lethargy, fever, chills, anorexia, nausea, vomiting, diarrhea, abdominal, back pain, hematuria, and perianal itching
    6. Ask about specific "holding of urine" maneuvers such as squatting, curtsying, sitting on heels, or squirming
    7. Question about daytime enuresis or leaking of urine before child reaches toilet
    8. Ask about history of constipation and encopresis
    9. In older children ask about onset, duration, and characteristics of vaginal or urethral discharge
    10. Past medical history should include drug allergies, chronic diseases such as diabetes mellitus or multiple sclerosis, previous genitourinary problems (by history or chart)
    11. Count number of previous UTIs and discuss success and failure of previous treatments
    12. Family history of VUR and recurrent UTIs is important

B. Physical Examination
    1. Observe general appearance noting degree of toxicity, dehydration, pallor, diaphoresis, and listlessness
    2. Assess vital signs, particularly noting elevated temperature and signs of orthostatic hypotension or hypertension
    3. Assess for signs of sepsis and dehydration
    4. Perform an abdominal exam, assessing for distention, tenderness, and masses
    5. Palpate back for costovertebral angle tenderness
    6. Inspect genitalia for anomalies, irritation, trauma, and in females, vaginitis and labial adhesions; in males, document circumcision status
    7. Perform rectal examination for fecal impaction if there is a history of bowel problems
    8. In children with history of voiding dysfunction or associated constipation or encopresis, a neurologic examination should be performed; assess perineal sensation, peripheral reflexes of lower extremities, and examine lower back for sacral dimpling or cutaneous abnormalities suggestive of underlying spinal abnormalities
    9. Consider observing urinary stream when voiding

C. Differential Diagnosis
    1. Epididymitis and gonococcal and nongonococcal urethritis in older male children
    2. Urethral syndrome or dysuria-pyuria syndrome in older female children
    3. Abnormalities such as bladder outlet obstruction, previously undiagnosed posterior urethral valves in males, or tumors and carcinoma

4. Urinary calculi
5. Renal tuberculosis
6. Sexual abuse
7. Encopresis
8. Irritation from pinworm infestation, diaper dermatitis, bubble baths, or soap
9. Foreign body in urethra and vagina
10. Vaginitis

D. Diagnostic Tests: Any child 2 months to 2 years with an unexplained fever should be evaluated for UTI; consider evaluation for UTI of any child, regardless of age, who has unexplained fevers or recurrent abdominal pain
   1. Diagnosis of UTI in children requires a culture of the urine
      a. In children 2 months to 2 years of age, a urine specimen should be obtained by suprapubic aspiration of the bladder or transurethral bladder catheterization; diagnosis of UTI **cannot** be established by culture of urine collected in a bag
         (1) Suprapubic aspiration is "gold standard" for detecting bacteria in urine (see following table for performing suprapubic aspiration)

STEPS IN PERFORMING A SUPRAPUBIC ASPIRATION

- Ascertain that child has not voided within one hour of procedure; do not perform on a child with an empty bladder
- Restrain child in a supine, frog-legged position
- Cleanse suprapubic region with alcohol and povidone-iodine
- Find puncture site which is 1-2 cm above the symphysis pubis in the midline
- With a 22-gauge, 1½-inch needle attached to a 3-mL syringe, make a puncture at a 10°-20° angle of the true vertical, aiming toward the head
- Exert gentle suction while advancing needle until urine enters the syringe. Continue to aspirate urine with gentle suction. If no urine is obtained, attempt procedure again, but this time aim needle in a caudal direction. If both attempts fail, further attempts are unlikely to be successful

---

         (2) Transurethral catheterization is also acceptable; use a 5-French feeding tube in neonates, infants, and toddlers or an 8-French in older children (a Coudé tip or curved tip catheter may be helpful in males who have tight sphincters)
      b. Clean catch urine specimens are usually acceptable for older children (first morning specimen is the best); may be helpful for girls to sit in reverse position on the toilet seat before voiding to spread labia away from urethral meatus
      c. Criteria for the diagnosis of UTI by urine culture (see following table)

CRITERIA FOR DIAGNOSIS OF URINARY TRACT INFECTIONS BY URINE CULTURE

Method of Collection	Suprapubic Aspiration	Catheterization	Boy: Clean-Catch Void	Girl: Clean-Catch Void
Colony Count	Any gram-negative bacilli - or - > few thousand gram-positive cocci	$<10^3$ unlikely $>10^3$ suspicious* $>10^4$ likely	$>10^4$ likely	$<10^4$ unlikely $>10^4$ suspicious*[†] $>10^5$ likely (80% probability)

*Repeat culture
[†] If symptomatic, clinician should be suspicious of infection; if asymptomatic, infection is less likely

   2. Urinalysis can be valuable in selecting children for prompt initiation of treatment; remember, however, that it is **not** a substitute for urine culture
      a. If the child (particularly the child 2 months to 2 years old), with unexplained fever is assessed as not being toxic or not so ill to require immediate antimicrobial therapy; do one of the following:
         (1) Obtain a urine specimen by most convenient method and perform urinalysis; if urinalysis suggests UTI obtain a culture; if urinalysis does not suggest UTI, follow the child's clinical course without initiating antimicrobial therapy
         (2) Obtain urine culture by suprapubic aspiration or catheterization

b. Any of following are suggestive of UTI
(1) Dipstick with a positive leukocyte esterase test (denotes white blood cells or pyuria)
(2) Dipstick with positive nitrite test (denotes bacteria)
(3) More than 5 white blood cells per high power field determined with microscopic analysis in which specimen is spun and the urine sediment is examined under high power (40X)
(4) Bacteria detected on an unspun Gram-stained specimen

3. Traditional voiding cystourethrogram (VCUG) or radionuclide cystography (RNC) is recommended for detecting reflux; early detection of an anatomical abnormality may prevent recurrent infections and subsequent renal damage
a. Consider ordering in all children less than 16 years with a documented UTI, **always** order in the following children:
(1) All children <5 years of age
(2) Boys of any age
(3) Girls >5 years of age who have pyelonephritis
(4) Children with recurrent UTIs
(5) Children who have an infection which is not responsive to antibiotics
b. VCUG is better than RNC for detecting urethral or bladder abnormalities and is recommended for assessing boys and girls who have symptoms of voiding dysfunction
c. Children should continue antimicrobial treatment of prophylaxis until the imaging studies are completed (see V.B.8.)
d. Inform parents/patients that VCUG is invasive

4. Ultrasonography should be ordered when the child has a UTI and his/her rate of clinical improvement is slower than anticipated (i.e., no clinical response within 2 days of antimicrobial therapy)
a. Ultrasonography should be performed immediately to search for cause such as obstruction or abscess
b. Ultrasonography does not exclude VUR and is not as sensitive as VCUG and RNC but is noninvasive, does not expose child to radiation, and can detect dilation associated with obstruction

5. Although the role is uncertain, renal cortical scintigraphy (with 99 m Tc-DMSA or 99 m Tc-glucoheptonate) is a sensitive test to detect acute changes from pyelonephritis or renal scarring

6. Urodynamic testing should be considered in patients with suspected neurogenic disorders or in children suspected of dysfunctional voiding who fail behavioral therapy and treatment with medications

7. With systemic symptoms or children with suspected pyelonephritis and infants order CBC and blood cultures; consider ordering erythrocyte sedimentation rate

8. Spinal magnetic resonance imaging is recommended if there is suspicion of spinal abnormality

9. With symptoms associated with sexually transmitted disease, perform wet mount of vaginal and urethral secretions and order gonococcal (GC) cultures and chlamydial test; also, can Gram's stain urethral and cervical secretions

V. Plan/Management

A. First objective is to identify treatable anatomic abnormalities that may predispose the patient to renal injury; other objectives are to quickly eradicate infection and prevent recurrent infections

B. Treatment of UTI
1. Children who are assessed as toxic, dehydrated, or unable to retain oral intake should be hospitalized and given parenteral antibiotics; also consider hospitalization for children with high fevers, vomiting, poor compliance with medications, and symptoms of pyelonephritis
2. Order a urine culture and sensitivity on children suspected of UTI. However, begin treatment prior to obtaining the results if they are symptomatic and have a positive urinalysis
3. If treated as outpatient, close monitoring is essential
4. For outpatients, prescribe any of the following for 7-14 days
a. Trimethoprim/sulfamethoxazole (Septra) in children 2 months of age or older; prescribe 8-10 mg/kg/day of trimethoprim component in 2 divided doses. Available 40 mg trimethoprim, 200 mg sulfamethoxazole per 5 mL.
b. Cefixime (Suprax) in children >6 years: 8 mg/kg/day in 2 divided doses; available 100 mg/5 mL liquid
c. Cefpodoxime (Vantin): 10 mg/kg/day in 2 divided doses; available 50 mg/5 mL or 100 mg/5 mL

5. Avoid the following antibiotics:
   a. Quinolones in children because of potential arthropathy
   b. Nalidixic acid or nitrofurantoin because they do not achieve therapeutic concentrations in bloodstream and should not be used in children with renal involvement
   c. Ampicillin and amoxicillin because of their emerging resistance to *E. coli*
6. Children who do **not** demonstrate clinical response within 2 days of antibiotics should have another urine culture performed and ultrasonography ordered promptly; VCUG or RNC should be ordered at the earliest convenient time
7. If expected clinical response occurs, order ultrasonography and VCUG or RNC at earliest convenient time for all children <5 years of age, boys of any age, children with pyelonephritis and recurrent infection; consider VCUG or RNC for any child <16 years
8. After 7-14 day course of antibiotics, children who need imaging studies (see V.B.6.7.) should receive antibiotics in therapeutic or prophylactic doses; prescribe trimethoprim sulfamethoxazole 2 mg of trimethoprim, 10 mg of sulfamethoxazole per kg as single bedtime dose
9. Urine should be recultured 2-3 days after starting on therapy and after completion of therapy; followed by a reculture in 1 month, then every 3 months for a year; and then annually for 2-3 years to screen for recurrent infection (some authorities recommend monthly recultures in the first year after an infection)

C. Treatment of vesicoureteral reflux (VUR) (consult specialist)
   1. Mild to moderate reflux (grades I, II, and III) can be medically managed with prophylactic antibiotics (see V.B.8.) and yearly evaluation of VUR with VCUG, renal ultrasound, and/or DMSA renal scan to monitor renal growth and/or damage as long as VUR persists
   2. Referral to pediatric urologist is needed for children with high grade VUR (usually surgery is recommended)
   3. Siblings <5 years of age of children with VUR should have diagnostic tests because of the high familial incidence

D. Recurrent infections in children are usually relapses of the same initial infection, rather than reinfection with a new pathogen as is usually the case in adults
   1. Prophylactic antibiotic therapy is needed for children with recurrent infections (defined as 3 in 6 months or 4 in 1 year) as well as those with VUR, those waiting for further diagnostic tests, and in young children with non-reflux pyelonephritis with acute or chronic renal damage
   2. Duration of treatment depends on condition
      a. Children with VUR need treatment until reflux spontaneously resolves
      b. Children with recurrent infections and young children with pyelonephritis should remain on prophylaxis a minimum of 6-12 months with periodic urine specimens for cultures at 3-6 months; medications should be restarted for additional 12 months if infection recurs within 3 months of discontinuation of above therapy
      c. Prescribe one of the following:
         (1) Nitrofurantoin 1-2 mg/kg BID in children >2 months
         (2) Trimethoprim/sulfamethoxazole: 2-3 mg/kg/day(trimethoprim) in children >2 months
   3. Teach patient to double void (void, wait 3 minutes, void again) if post voiding residual (PVR) is present
   4. Many children with recurrent infections have constipation, stasis of urine, and voiding dysfunction; implement the following four-point program
      a. Correct constipation (i.e., fiber supplements, bowel stimulant as last resort)
      b. Improve voiding by using timed voiding every 2-3 hours; also work to improve flow of urine by teaching child to void with continuous rather than staccato voiding pattern
      c. Increase fluid intake
      d. Encourage hygiene awareness and improvement such as avoiding bubble baths and frequent changes of soiled diapers and underwear

E. Asymptomatic bacteriuria
   1. Although controversial, most authorities recommend no treatment unless the child has urinary tract abnormalities
   2. Voiding cystourethrogram at 1 month and a dimercaptosuccinic acid scan 6 months later is recommended

F. Follow Up
    1. In children with cystitis and pyelonephritis a reculture of urine should be obtained 2-3 days after treatment is initiated, possibly after treatment is completed, and then in 1 month, followed by every 3 months for a year; and then annually for 2-3 years to screen for recurrent infection (some authorities recommend monthly recultures in first year)
    2. Ultrasonography should be done immediately if child does not have expected clinical response within 2 days of antibiotics; if VCUG or RNC is needed, schedule at earliest convenient time
    3. Children with recurrent infections should have cultures every 3-6 months

PROBLEMS OF THE PENIS

I. Definition: Any of the following abnormalities of the penis:

    A. Balanitis: Inflammation/infection of the glans penis

    B. Balanoposthitis: Inflammation/infection of the foreskin of glans penis

    C. Balanitis xerotica obliterans (BXO): Inflammatory lesion of the glans and foreskin; synonymous with lichen sclerosus et atrophicus (LSA); starts as a erythematous lesion and subsequently forms a thickened white plaque that may erode into the urethral meatus causing meatal stenosis or a distal urethral stricture

    D. Penile foreskin adhesions: Adhesions between the penile foreskin and glans

    E. Meatal ulceration: Superficial ulceration of the male urethral meatus

    F. Phimosis: Loss of foreskin suppleness with resultant nonretractable foreskin over the glans penis

    G. Paraphimosis: Abnormality that occurs when foreskin is retracted over glans and becomes trapped behind it

    H. Hypospadias: Abnormality in which the urethral meatus opens on the ventral surface of the penis

    I. Epispadias: Abnormality in which the urethral meatus opens on the dorsum of the penis

II. Pathophysiology

    A. Balanitis
        1. Damp, moist environment causes inflammatory changes that lead to secondary opportunistic bacterial and fungal infiltration
        2. Urine and smegma sometimes become trapped under a foreskin that is long, tight, and not easily retracted, thus leading to bacterial overgrowth
        3. Inflammation may occur from trauma (zipper injury, masturbation), irritants (diaper dermatitis, allergies), poor hygiene, and infection (sexually transmitted disease)

    B. Balanoposthitis similar to balanitis (see II.A.)

    C. Balanitis xerotica obliterans
        1. Chronic inflammatory process of unknown etiology
        2. Associated with autoimmune disease, trauma, allergies, and infection

    D. Penile foreskin adhesions
        1. Soft adhesions between the glans and foreskin are normal in the small boy
        2. Sometimes hard adhesions develop if foreskin is prematurely and forcibly retracted

    E. Meatal ulceration: Inflammation occurs to the urethral meatus from trauma, primarily due to diaper contact and from the ammonia of the urine

F. Phimosis: Occurs in uncircumcised boys; typically the foreskin is scarred and loses its suppleness as a result of one of the following:
1. Trauma from forcible retraction of foreskin
2. Recurrent infections
3. Irritation from soiled diapers and poor hygiene
4. Improperly performed circumcision
5. Congenital anomalies

G. Paraphimosis:
1. Occurs in uncircumcised boys when the foreskin is not returned to its normal position
2. Typically related to one of following:
    a. Phimosis, a snugly fitting foreskin, or a foreskin that has a partially scarred tip
    b. May occur following masturbation or sexual abuse

H. Hypospadias: Unknown etiology but may be genetically transmitted or due to medications mother ingested during pregnancy

I. Epispadias: Similar to hypospadias (see II.H.)

III. Clinical presentation

A. Balanitis
1. Infection occurs most frequently in uncircumcised boys
2. Erythematous, edematous, tender glans penis is typical
3. Discharge from urethra, prepuce, and glans usually occurs
4. Dysuria, urinary frequency, and difficulty voiding are often present; fever may or may not occur
5. Secondary infection with *Staphylococcus aureus,* groups A and D streptococci, *Pseudomonas aeruginosa, Candida albicans,* and *Trichomonas vaginalis* is possible
6. Recurrent balanitis often occurs in diabetics, immunocompromised males, and adolescents with frequent sexually transmitted diseases
7. Complications include scarring, subsequent phimosis, penile shaft cellulitis, or abscess formation

B. Balanoposthitis
1. Erythematous, edematous, tender foreskin and glans penis
2. Clinical manifestations are similar to balanitis

C. Balanitis xerotica obliterans
1. Occurs most frequently in uncircumcised males with severe phimosis and balanitis
2. Begins with a lesion that subsequently develops into a thickened plaque that may result in meatal stenosis or distal urethral stricture
3. Symptoms include itching and loss of sensations of glans penis with painful erections, decreased urinary stream and/or dysuria; may have urethral discharge
4. In advanced cases, urinary retention may occur due to distal urethral obstruction
5. May predispose male to squamous cell carcinoma

D. Penile adhesions
1. In small boys, the adhesions usually release spontaneously
2. Sometimes adhesions may lead to smegma collection and the foreskin becomes inseparable from glans even when manual traction is applied

E. Meatal ulceration
1. Occurs primarily in circumcised boys
2. Dysuria is common, but patient may also be asymptomatic
3. Due to dysuria, boy may voluntarily retain urine
4. Subsequent meatal crusting may lead to involuntary urine retention
5. Recurrent cycles of ulceration and crusting may result in scarring, narrowing of the meatus, and stenosis with narrowing and upward direction of the urinary stream

F. Phimosis
1. Occurs in uncircumcised boys, with an incidence range of 2% to 10%
2. Until around age 5 years it is normal for the boy to a tight pinpoint opening of the foreskin and to have a minimally retractable foreskin, but by age 5 years, the foreskin should be retractable
3. Clinical manifestations include dysuria, hematuria, poor urinary stream, and tenderness of the foreskin

4. If the foreskin is severely scarred and the foreskin opening is stenotic, the boy's foreskin will "balloon" during urination
5. Complications include hydronephrosis and renal failure; phimosis is one of the primary causes of paraphimosis

G. Paraphimosis is a medical emergency
   1. The trapped foreskin obstructs venous return to the tip of the penis which results in edema and ischemia
   2. If foreskin is not released immediately, it can lead to necrosis of the glans penis

H. Hypospadias
   1. One of the most common penile abnormalities
   2. Boys may have various deformities
      a. Typically the urethral meatus is located on the distal half of the penile shaft with about 60% of cases located on the glans penis
      b. Less commonly the urethral meatus is located on the proximal section of the penile shaft, or scrotum, or perineum
   3. Chordee or a downward curving of the penis is often present
   4. In about 10% of cases, an associated unilateral or bilateral cryptorchism is present, suggesting the possibility of an intersex anomaly

I. Epispadias
   1. Uncommon abnormality
   2. Urethral meatus may be anywhere along the dorsum of penis even as far back as the symphysis pubis; dorsal chordee (upward bend of penis) may be present
   3. Urinary incontinence may be associated with the more proximal deformities

IV. Diagnosis/Evaluation

A. History
   1. If the boy is circumcised, determine age at which circumcision was performed and if there were any complications
   2. If the boy is not circumcised, ask if his foreskin can be easily retracted
   3. Inquire about use of topical allergens/irritants
   4. Ask about history of sexual contacts, sexually transmitted diseases, and systemic diseases such as HIV infection, diabetes, malignancies, and trauma
   5. Question about voiding symptoms such as dysuria, hesitancy, and frequency; determine if patient has voluntary urinary or involuntary urinary retention
   6. Ask about painful erections
   7. Inquire about urethral discharge
   8. Ask about force and direction of urinary stream
   9. Explore hygiene techniques
   10. Investigate for possibility of sexual abuse
   11. Explore previous medical history, especially history of immune, genitourinary, and endocrine problems
   12. If intersex abnormality is suspected, ask whether any family members have abnormal genitalia; obtain a pregnancy history of the mother, including medication use

B. Physical examination
   1. Perform a complete genital examination
      a. Inspect and locate urethral meatus
      b. Assess prepuce, glans penis, foreskin, scrotum, perineum (look for deformities [chordee], ulcers, discoloration, edema, lesions, discharge); palpate for tenderness, induration, and masses
      c. Carefully palpate and locate both testes
   2. Inspect and palpate the bilateral inguinal nodes

C. Differential diagnosis
   1. Balanitis and balanoposthitis
      a. Drug eruption
      b. Contact dermatitis
      c. Squamous cell carcinoma of penis
      d. Psoriasis

2. Balanitis xerotica obliterans
   a. Leukoplakia
   b. Bowen disease
   c. Squamous cell carcinoma
3. Penile foreskin adhesions: Phimosis
4. Meatal ulceration
   a. Balanitis and balanoposthitis
   b. Insect bites
   c. Trauma
   d. Condylomata acuminata
   e. Gonorrheal and nonspecific urethritis
   f. Syphilitic chancre
   g. Urethral malignancy (rare)
   h. Contact dermatitis, herpes, scabies, drug eruption
5. Phimosis: Penile foreskin adhesions
6. Paraphimosis: Condition is usually obvious from assessment
7. Hypospadias and epispadias: Intersex abnormalities

D. Diagnostic testing
   1. Balanitis and balanoposthitis
      a. Swab glans/foreskin for viral, bacterial, and fungal cultures; if sexual abuse is a possibility, diagnostic testing for sexually transmitted diseases is needed
      b. Biopsy of lesion is needed in selected cases
      c. Obtain either a urinalysis or a blood glucose test to rule-out diabetes
   2. Balanitis xerotica obliterans
      a. Order urinalysis and urine culture and sensitivity
      b. Consider retrograde urethrogram and voiding urethrogram
      c. In severe cases, biopsy of the glans is often warranted
      d. Occasionally urethroscopy is recommended
   3. Penile adhesions: None needed
   4. Meatal ulceration: Consider urinalysis and urine culture and sensitivity to rule out urinary tract infection
   5. Phimosis and paraphimosis: None usually needed
   6. Hypospadias and epispadias: In severe cases, renal and pelvic sonography are recommended; in severe cases a voiding cystourethrogram (VCUG) and blood karyotyping are required

V. Plan/Management

A. Balanitis and balanoposthitis
   1. Hospitalize if patient has severe systemic infection, vascular compromise of glans, severe dysuria, or inability to void
   2. Oral antibiotics may be needed pending the results of diagnostic tests; if yeast is identified, prescribe topical nystatin; if *T. vaginalis* is detected, metronidazole is indicated
   3. To reduce edema, elevate the penis and recommend Sitz baths and warm soaks to penis
   4. Referral is needed for patients with recurrences, balanitis xerotica obliterans, or vascular compromise to glans
   5. Carefully review proper hygiene and teach parents to observe for development of phimosis
   6. Circumcision can prevent recurrences if proper penile hygiene cannot be maintained or if phimosis occurs

B. Balanitis xerotica obliterans: Referral is required
   1. Explain to parents that this condition may be premalignant or may lead to urethral stricture disease; close follow up is important
   2. Local application of triamcinolone cream, estrogen cream, or testosterone cream may be beneficial
   3. Circumcision is usually needed, particularly if patient has phimosis
   4. Meatotomy or other surgical procedures are sometimes required

C. Penile adhesions
   1. Prevention is important; instruct parents in proper hygiene
      a. Teach to gently retract foreskin; never forcibly retract foreskin
      b. Carefully cleanse the area
   2. In most cases, clinician can easily lyse adhesions by applying gentle traction
   3. Surgical excision and repair are needed in more severe cases

D.   Meatal ulceration
    1.   Prevention is important
        a.   In newly circumcised infant provide good hygiene, frequent diaper changes, and if wearing cloth diapers properly rinse diapers to avoid ammoniacal dermatitis
        b.   Apply a protective ointment (e.g., A and D ointment) to glans for a week or two after circumcision to avoid irritation
    2.   If ulcers are present, cleanse with soap and water and apply a protective ointment
    3.   If adherent crusts are on meatus, mechanical debridement may be needed
    4.   If meatal stenosis has occurred, referral is needed and a meatotomy is required
        a.   After the procedure, cover meatus with ointment
        b.   Instruct parents to spread the meatal lips several times a day for the next 10-14 days to avoid recurrent stenosis

E.   Phimosis
    1.   Hospitalize if patient is unable to urinate, has renal failure, or has severe dysuria
    2.   In mild cases, normal cleansing and gentle stretching of foreskin to point of resistance is often effective
    3.   Consider lysis of adhesions and stretching the prepuce
    4.   If initial management fails to retract foreskin, a referral is needed and circumcision may be required

F.   Paraphimosis is an emergency; severe paraphimosis needs immediate surgical consultation
    1.   Manually try to reduce by applying gentle outward traction on foreskin while pushing glans inward
    2.   Other techniques to reduce
        a.   Iced-glove technique
            (1)   Lubricate and anesthetize foreskin with application of lidocaine jelly for 2 minutes
            (2)   Foreskin is retracted and the glans and shaft are put into the thumb of a glove that is sealed and filled with ice water
            (3)   Remove iced glove and slip foreskin over glans
        b.   Multiple puncture technique
            (1)   Anesthetize foreskin using a penile ring block with 20-30 punctures in foreskin with a 20- to 25-gauge needle
            (2)   Exudate should seep out and foreskin can then be reduced
    3.   If manual reduction fails or if blood supply to glans is severely compromised, boy should have general anesthesia and have manual reduction or a dorsal slit of foreskin
    4.   To prevent future recurrences, elective circumcision is recommended

G.   Hypospadias
    1.   Immediately consult urologist
    2.   If there is concern about an intersex anomaly or if the hypospadias is severe or accompanied with other genital abnormalities, also consult an endocrinologist
    3.   Surgery is required and is usually performed around 1 year of age
    4.   A circumcision should not be performed

H.   Epispadias
    1.   Consult pediatric urologist and an endocrinologist if abnormality is severe or associated with other problems
    2.   Similar to the treatment of hypospadias, surgery is warranted and circumcision should be avoided

I.   Follow Up
    1.   Balanitis and balanoposthitis: After treatment is initiated, patient's condition should be reassessed within 4-6 weeks, unless inflammation does not resolve or problems develop
    2.   Balanitis xerotica obliterans: Close follow up is required because this condition may represent a premalignant lesion or lead to urethral stricture disease
    3.   Penile adhesions: In most cases no follow-up is required unless adhesions recur or if problems develop
    4.   Meatal ulceration: Schedule return visit within 4-6 weeks, unless condition is severe or symptoms worsen
    5.   Phimosis, paraphimosis, hypospadia, and epispadia: Follow up is variable and depends of medical or surgical treatment that is initiated

EPIDIDYMITIS

I. Definition: Inflammation of the epididymis

II. Pathogenesis:

    A.   Pathogens apparently reach the epididymis through the lumen of the vas deferens from infected urine, the posterior urethra, or seminal vesicles
        1.   In postpubertal boys and males under 35 years, infection is often sexually transmitted
        2.   Most often caused by *Chlamydia trachomatis* or *Neisseria gonorrhoeae*
        3.   *Escherichia coli* may be a pathogen in men who are the insertive partner during anal intercourse

    B.   Epididymitis may be nonsexually transmitted
        1.   Typically caused by coliform bacteria that usually cause urinary tract infections
        2.   Usually associated with urinary tract infections in older males with urinary tract instrumentation, surgery, or anatomical abnormalities

    C.   Uncommon causes are due to trauma, tuberculous epididymitis, systemic fungal infections; antiarrhythmic drug, amiodarone, may cause infection confined to the head of the epididymitis

III. Clinical Presentation

    A.   Most common cause of acute scrotal pain in postpubertal males
        1.   Usually patients have a history of sexual activity
        2.   Sexually transmitted epididymitis usually is associated with urethritis

    B.   Commonly, there is a gradual onset of unilateral testicular pain and tenderness, dysuria, and urethral discharge

    C.   Fever occurs in approximately 50% of patients; nausea and vomiting is unusual

    D.   Scrotum is tender on palpation and usually accompanied with a hydrocele and palpable swelling of the epididymis

    E.   Uncommon complications include testicular necrosis, testicular atrophy, and infertility

IV. Diagnosis/Evaluation

    A.   History
        1.   Determine onset, duration, and course of symptoms
        2.   Ask about scrotal pain, dysuria, urinary frequency and urgency, and color, amount, and consistency of urethral discharge
        3.   Inquire about possible associated symptoms such as fever, nausea, and vomiting
        4.   Explore sexual history and condom use; ask about new sexual partners and if sexual partners have complained of dysuria or urinary frequency
        5.   Question about previous urinary tract infections and treatments
        6.   Inquire about previous genitourinary surgery, urinary tract instrumentation, and anatomic abnormalities
        7.   Inquire about recent trauma to testes

    B.   Physical Examination
        1.   Inspect scrotum, noting edema and erythema which are typical
        2.   Palpate scrotum
            a.   In epididymitis, testes are tender but the position, size, and consistency of testes is entirely normal
            b.   Palpable swelling of epididymis is usually present
        3.   Passive elevation of testis may relieve pain in epididymitis (Prehn's sign)
        4.   Perform rectal exam (this exam may elicit prostatic tenderness and result in expression of urethral discharge)

C. Differential Diagnosis
1. Must differentiate testicular torsion, which is an emergent condition, from epididymitis (see following table)

DIFFERENTIATION OF EPIDIDYMITIS AND TESTICULAR TORSION		
	Epididymitis	**Testicular Torsion**
History		
Onset of pain	Gradual	Acute
Nausea and vomiting	Rare	50%
Voiding symptoms	50%	No
Urethral discharge	50%	No
Physical Examination		
Epididymal swelling only	Early	10%
Scrotal edema	Most	Most
Scrotal erythema	Most	Most
Fever	50%	Rare

2. Orchitis (patient usually has recently had parotitis or mumps)
3. Testicular tumor (usually presents with painless swelling)
4. Trauma (usually elicited on history)
5. Skin pathology such as insect bites or folliculitis

D. Diagnostic Tests
1. Emergency testing for testicular torsion may be necessary when the onset of pain is sudden and severe or if there is uncertainty about the diagnosis; consult a specialist and consider ordering one of the following: Doppler ultrasound, scrotal ultrasound (operator-dependent), or radionuclide scrotal imaging (not operator-dependent)
2. Obtain urinalysis (in about 20-95% of epididymitis cases there is pyuria compared to 0-30% in cases with testicular torsion)
3. Collect urine culture and sensitivity and gram-stained smear of uncentrifuged urine for gram-negative bacteria
4. In postpubertal males who may have a sexually transmitted disease obtain the following:
   a. Gram-stained smear of urethral exudate or intraurethral swab specimen to detect urethritis ($\geq$5 polymorphonuclear leukocytes per oil immersion field) and for presumptive diagnosis of gonococcal infection
   b. Culture of urethral exudate or intraurethral swab specimen or nucleic acid amplification test (either by first-void urine or intraurethral swab) for *N. gonorrhoeae* and *C. trachomatis*
   c. Collect first-void urine and examine for leukocytes if the urethral Gram stain is negative; culture and Gram-stained smear of uncentrifuged mid-stream urine specimen should be collected
   d. Syphilis serology and HIV counseling and testing
5. In older men, a culture of expressed prostatic secretions should be obtained and a search should be made for an obstruction at the bladder outlet with tests such as an intravenous pyelography

V. Plan/Management

A. Most patients can be treated on outpatient basis; consider hospitalization for men with severe pain suggesting other diseases (i.e., torsion, abscess), or when men are febrile, or noncompliant

B. For active heterosexual males, most likely cause is a sexually transmitted disease
1. For epididymitis most likely due to gonococcal or chlamydial infection, treat empirically before culture results are available with the following: doxycycline (Vibramycin) 100 mg PO BID for 10 days and ceftriaxone (Rocephin) 250 mg IM in a single dose
2. For epididymitis most likely caused by enteric organisms or in patients allergic to tetracyclines and/or cephalosporins, treat empirically with ofloxacin (Floxin) 300 mg PO BID for 10 days or levofloxacin (Levaquin) 500 mg QD for 10 days
3. Treat sexual partners if their contact with the index patient was within 60 days preceding onset of symptoms in the patient
4. Instruct patients to avoid sexual intercourse until they and their sex partners are cured or until treatment is completed and patients and partners are asymptomatic

C. Symptomatic treatment of bed rest, scrotal support, scrotal elevation, sitz baths, pain medication, and ice packs may be beneficial

D. Follow Up
1. For patients whose symptoms fail to improve within 3 days, re-evaluate both the diagnosis and treatment
   a. Swelling and tenderness that persist after antimicrobial therapy require comprehensive evaluation
   b. Differential diagnosis includes tumor, abscess, infarction, testicular cancer, and tuberculosis or fungal epididymitis
2. For postpubertal males, no follow up or test of cure is needed if symptoms resolve
3. In older men, repeat urine cultures are needed after completion of the therapy and further diagnostic tests can also be scheduled at this time

TESTICULAR TORSION

I. Definition: Twisting of spermatic cord which results in compromised testicular blood flow

II. Pathogenesis

A. Occurs when the free-floating testis rotates on the spermatic cord and occludes its blood supply

B. May occur spontaneously (may occur in sleep) or after activity or trauma

III. Clinical Presentation

A. Commonly occurs between 6-12 years, but a significant number of patients are newborns, adolescents, and over the age of 21 years

B. If not surgically treated, there will be ischemic injury and necrosis of the testis
1. Many patients have an anatomic defect known as "bell-clapper" deformity
2. Typical history is sudden onset of testicular pain which radiates to groin; but in some cases there is minimal swelling and little or no pain
3. May also have lower abdominal pain which leads to erroneous diagnosis of appendicitis or gastroenteritis
4. Nausea and vomiting occur in about half of the patients; usually there is no fever, urethral discharge, or dysuria
5. Degree of injury is determined by the severity of the arterial compression and the interval between the onset and surgical intervention (for severe torsion, must intervene within 4-8 hours to salvage the testis)

IV. Diagnosis/Evaluation

A. History: Testicular torsion is a urological emergency so rapidly gather a focused history
1. Ask about onset and circumstances surrounding onset
2. Ask about accompanying symptoms such as nausea, vomiting, fever, dysuria, urethral discharge
3. Determine any occurrence of trauma or unusual physical activity
4. To rule out epididymitis, question about recent change in sexual partners and symptoms of dysuria and urethral discharge

B. Physical Examination: Perform a rapid but systematic exam
1. Observe general appearance (patients with testicular torsion are in acute distress, have pain on ambulation, and prefer to lie quietly on the examination table)
2. Inspect scrotal skin (often skin is erythematous, taut, and without normal rugae with torsion)
3. Palpate testes (testis may be located high in the scrotum as a result of shortening of the cord by twisting)
4. Palpate the epididymis which normally is located on the posterolateral surface of the testis and is smooth, discrete, and nontender (with testicular torsion the epididymis will not be in this typical position as a result of cord twisting and will be extremely tender)

5.　Palpate vas deferens from the testicle to the inguinal ring (normally vas deferens is smooth, discrete and nontender)
6.　Try to elicit the cremasteric reflex; positive reflex is testicular retraction when the upper, medial thigh is stroked (usually absent in torsion, but present in epididymitis)
7.　Perform a complete abdominal exam

C.　Differential Diagnosis
1.　Epididymitis is the most difficult condition to differentiate (see table in section on EPIDIDYMITIS, differentiating epididymitis from torsion)
2.　Torsion of the testicular appendage
   a.　More common in pre-pubertal males
   b.　Pain is usually less severe than with torsion of the entire testis; pain and swelling develop gradually
   c.　"Blue dot" sign at superior aspect of testis is diagnostic of this problem
   d.　Management is bedrest and scrotal elevation
   e.　With appropriate management, symptoms resolve within a week
3.　Epididymo-orchitis or orchitis
   a.　Often associated with diffuse swelling and pain along with fever, systemic signs, and possibly dysuria, urinary frequency and pyuria
   b.　Prehn's sign (relief of pain with elevation of testis) and elevated white blood cells may occur
4.　Incarcerated inguinal hernia
5.　Vasculitis
6.　Tumor
7.　Trauma
8.　Henoch-Schönlein purpura is a systemic vasculitic syndrome characterized by nonthrombocytopenic purpura, arthralgia, renal disease, gastrointestinal pain, and bleeding
9.　Idiopathic scrotal edema
10.　Varicoceles (see section VARICOCELE)

D.　Diagnostic Tests: When clinical presentation is typical, surgical exploration is usually carried out without further testing. When torsion is unlikely, but confirmation of clinical diagnosis is sought, consider ordering the following:
1.　Doppler ultrasound (absent testicular artery pulsations with torsion); the development of color Doppler imaging with pulsed Doppler has improved accuracy of this test
2.　Nuclear testicular scanning allows evaluation of blood flow to the scrotal contents (decreased perfusion with torsion)
3.　Scrotal ultrasonography can be ordered; does not distinguish torsion from epididymitis but is helpful in evaluating scrotal masses and trauma
4.　Urinalysis (will be normal in 90% of patients with testicular torsion, but will often be abnormal in epididymitis)

V.　Plan/Management:

A.　Immediate consultation and surgical intervention; this is a urological emergency; salvage of endocrine function requires detorsion within 4-8 hours

B.　Manual detorsion may be successful when performed by an experienced clinician, but surgical exploration is still needed to confirm complete detorsion

C.　Follow Up: Surgeon should arrange follow up to determine response to operation

HYDROCELE

I. Definition: Collection of peritoneal fluid trapped in a patent processus vaginalis which is beginning to undergo obliteration

II. Pathogenesis

A. Basic facts of the anatomy and embryology of the inguinal region are helpful in understanding the pathogenesis of a hydrocele
1. During the last months of gestation the testes migrate down from the internal inguinal region to the base of the scrotum
2. During this descent, the lining of the abdominal cavity (processus vaginalis) also descends with the testes
3. Normally, after the testicular descent, the processus vaginalis begins to close which leaves only the most distal portion of the processus, the tunica vaginalis that surrounds the testis

B. Noncommunicating hydroceles are most common and result when residual peritoneal fluid remains after closure of the processus vaginalis

C. In communicating hydroceles there is still a connection between the peritoneal cavity and the tunica vaginalis and peritoneal fluid can descend through the patent processus vaginalis; abdominal contents (hernia) can also descend

D. Hydroceles may form secondary to testicular pathology such as testicular tumors

III. Clinical Presentation

A. Noncommunicating and communicating hydroceles with and without hernias usually occur at birth or in the neonatal period; they infrequently occur later in life and are then usually associated with underlying pathology such as a testicular neoplasm, torsion, injury, or infection

B. Noncommunicating hydroceles
1. Scrotal sac appears full, fluctuant, tense, and clear if transilluminated
2. Fluid gradually absorbs during the first year of life
3. Since the processus vaginalis is closed off, there is no danger of a hernia developing

C. Communicating hydroceles
1. History reveals a flat scrotum in the morning with a gradual increase in fluid during the day
2. Rarely resolve and have the potential for herniation of the intestine

D. Trauma to the scrotum may cause hemorrhage into the hydrocele sac

IV. Diagnosis/Evaluation

A. History
1. Determine onset and course of the hydrocele
2. Ask patient/parents if the size of the scrotum remains the same or if enlarges from morning to evening
3. Ask patient/parents about intermittent bulges in scrotum or abdomen which increase when child cries
4. Ask about scrotal pain, heaviness, and symptoms of intestinal obstruction such as colicky abdominal pain and hyperperistalsis

B. Physical Examination
1. Inspect scrotum for size, shape, symmetry, swelling, lesions, and color
2. Any swelling should be assessed further with transillumination
    a. In a darkened room a beam of light is directed from behind the scrotum
    b. The light will appear as a red glow with serous fluid but not with blood or tissue
3. Palpate inguinal area and scrotum, checking for an inguinal hernia or other lesions such as varicocele or spermatocele

4. Palpate testes with thumb and first 2 fingers
   a. Normally testes are sensitive to compression but not tender and feel smooth, rubbery, and free of nodules; size in infant is 1 cm
   b. If mass is felt, carefully palpate to determine whether the mass is separate from the testis as occurs with a hernia or whether it cannot be delineated from testis as occurs with a tumor
5. Palpate epididymis on posterolateral surface of testis which should feel smooth, discrete, and nontender
6. Palpate vas deferens from testicle to inguinal ring (normally feels smooth and discrete)
7. Perform a complete abdominal exam

C. Differential Diagnosis (see Figure 13.1): Normal scrotum and hydrocele (see Figure 13.1A and 13.1B).
   1. Spermatocele is a cyst containing sperm that presents as circumscribed mass that can be separated from the testis, does not transilluminate, and persists when patient is supine (see Figure 13.1C); often found during adolescence
   2. Testicular tumor is the most important disorder to rule out (see Figure 13.1D)
      a. Most common tumor in males between the ages of 15-30
      b. Commonly occurs after age 15, but there is a small peak in incidence at 2 years of age
      c. Tumor is firm, painless mass that gives a sensation of heaviness in the testis
      d. Mass cannot be delineated from substance of testis; does not transilluminate
   3. Epididymitis (see Figure 13.1E) (see section on EPIDIDYMITIS)
   4. Orchitis (see Figure 13.1F) is associated with viral parotitis (mumps)
      a. Difficult to distinguish from testicular torsion
      b. Presents with sudden onset of pain, and red, warm, and tender testis or testes
   5. Hernia (see section on HERNIAS, ABDOMINAL)
   6. Varicocele (see section on VARICOCELE)
   7. Undescended testes (see section on UNDESCENDED TESTES)
   8. Folliculitis
   9. Sebaceous cyst
   10. Local trauma

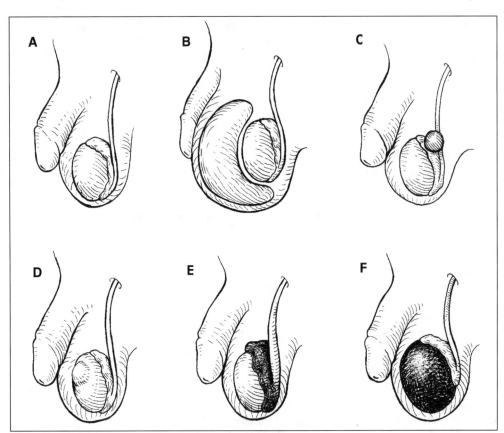

Figure 13.1. Scrotal Lesions.
A. Normal.   B. Hydrocele   C. Spermatocele   D. Testicular Tumor   E. Epididymitis   F. Orchitis

D. Diagnostic Tests
  1. Diagnostic tests are often not ordered if the clinician is confident that a hydrocele exists without pathological lesions
  2. Occasionally an abdominal roentgenogram is helpful because presence of air below the inguinal ligament indicates a hernia
  3. Ultrasound of the inguinal region and scrotum can differentiate a true hernia or another mass (tumor) from a hydrocele with peritoneal fluid

V. Plan/Management

A. Noncommunicating hydrocele in children
  1. Assure the parents that the scrotum is just enlarged with fluid which will absorb over the next year
  2. No surgical or medical treatment is necessary

B. Communicating hydrocele in children
  1. Usually refer to urologist/surgeon
  2. Because of the potential for herniation of the intestine, these hydroceles often are repaired
  3. Boys under 2 years of age should have bilateral exploration because of high incidence of contralateral patent processus vaginalis

C. Hydrocele with inguinal hernia in children
  1. Refer to urologist/surgeon for surgery
  2. If the hernia is incarcerated and cannot be reduced of if vomiting or signs of intestinal obstruction occur, emergency surgery is indicated

D. Referral to specialist is needed for adolescents with new hydroceles; usually adolescents do not require therapy unless complications exist or there is discomfort from the bulky mass or a tense hydrocele is present that may reduce the circulation and lead to atrophy

E. Follow Up
  1. For patients with noncommunicating hydroceles, closely monitor size of scrotum at each health maintenance visit or at least every 6 months and record findings
  2. Confer with urologist/surgeon about follow up for patients with communicating hydroceles and hernias

VARICOCELE

I. Definition: Dilated plexus of scrotal veins situated above the testis in the scrotum

II. Pathogenesis: Due to valvular incompetence of the spermatic vein

A. Varicoceles on left side in adolescents are usually of unknown etiology

B. Varicoceles on the right side may represent acute venous obstruction from a tumor or intra-abdominal pathology

III. Clinical Presentation

A. Typically varicoceles are clinically detectable between ages 10-15; once present, varicoceles persist into adulthood

B. Approximately 15% of all adult males have a varicocele

C. Varicoceles occur almost exclusively on the left side; a unilateral right varicocele is rare; bilateral varicoceles are more common than previously thought

D. Testis resembles a bag of worms with a bluish discoloration that is visible through the scrotum (see Figure 13.2)

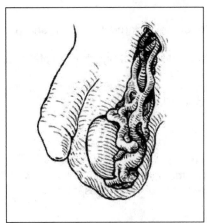

Figure 13.2. Varicocele

E. Varicocele is most prominent when the patient is standing; tends to collapse when the patient is sitting or supine

F. Patient is usually asymptomatic and testis is nontender, but may have mild pain or a feeling of heaviness in the scrotum

G. Varicoceles are associated with a time-dependent decline in testicular function; decreased sperm counts, infertility, and testicular atrophy are associated in about 65%-75% of patients with varicoceles

IV. Diagnosis/Evaluation

A. History
    1. Ask when patient first noticed varicocele
    2. Determine the rate the scrotum is enlarging
    3. Ask if the varicocele collapses upon sitting or standing
    4. Inquire about testicular pain or discomfort
    5. Question about problems with infertility

B. Physical Examination
    1. Assess Tanner stage in adolescents to determine normal growth and development of testes
    2. Ask patient to stand and perform a Valsalva maneuver
    3. Palpate testes, epididymis, and vas deferens first in standing then supine positions
    4. Perform a rectal examination to assess prostate size since the prostate may shrink with testosterone deficiency that may occur with varicoceles
    5. If possible, measure the volume of both testes with a standard orchidometer

C. Differential Diagnosis
    1. Hydrocele
    2. Spermatocele
    3. Testicular tumor
    4. Epididymal cyst

D. Diagnostic Tests
    1. In adolescents, consider ordering a testicular ultrasound to assess testicular volume and significant testicular size variations between testes with and without varicocele
    2. For right-sided varicoceles, suddenly appearing left-sided varicoceles, new onset varicoceles in adults, consult specialist about ordering the following:
        a. Venography is the gold standard for diagnosing varicoceles in adults; also used to detect venous obstruction or renal carcinoma associated with varicoceles
        b. Doppler ultrasound, thermography, and scrotal scintigraphy are nonspecific for diagnosing varicoceles, but may be beneficial in some cases
    3. Order annual semen analysis
        a. Infertile young men with varicoceles and abnormal semen analyses should be offered the option of varicocele repair
        b. Young men with normal semen analyses should be followed with semen analyses every one to two years
    4. Consult specialist about other tests for assessing reproductive function such as testis biopsy and fine needle aspiration with flow cytometry

V. Plan/Management

    A. Refer patients with the following manifestations to a surgeon:
        1. Right-sided varicoceles
        2. Large varicocele that is increasing in size or does not disappear in sitting and supine positions
        3. Pain
        4. Evidence of testicular atrophy, defined as two standard deviations in testicular size when compared with normal testicular growth curves
        5. Greater than a 2 mL difference in testicular volume as noted on serial ultrasonography examination
        6. Evidence of deteriorating semen patterns

    B. If surgery is not recommended, explain that patient needs to monitor the growth and symptoms related to the varicocele

    C. Follow Up
        1. Follow-up if surgery is not performed
            a. Explain to patient the need to return to clinic if he experiences increasing discomfort or if scrotum changes in size and shape
            b. Perform annual testicular examination in patients with moderately large and large varicoceles or when venous enlargement is greater than 2 cm
        2. If surgery is performed, follow recommendations of surgeon

UNDESCENDED TESTICLE (CRYPTORCHIDISM)

I. Definition: Failure of the testicle to descend into the scrotum

II. Pathogenesis:

    A. Most undescended testes are a result of a mechanical factor, a hernia sac, or a shortened spermatic artery which impedes the testicle's descent into the scrotum

    B. Failure of testes to descend may be partially due to a lack of gonadotropic and androgenic hormones during fetal development or an inability of the testes to respond to these hormones

III. Clinical Presentation

    A. Risk factors
        1. Because the testes descend into the scrotum around the 36th week of fetal life, the incidence is higher in the premature infant than in the full-term infant; about 3% of male term newborns and 20-30% of premature male infants have undescended testes at birth
        2. Low birth weight
        3. Family history of undescended testes
        4. Complicated pregnancies (e.g., toxemia) and deliveries including cesarean section
        5. Hypospadias
        6. Congenital subluxation of the hip
        7. Endocrine disorders, genetic abnormalities, or genitourinary anatomic abnormalities

    B. Testes that are undescended may stop their descent within the canal, in the abdomen (more likely to be abnormal), or descend through the inguinal canal, pass through the inguinal canal, and end in a position in the superficial inguinal space, thigh, or perineum

    C. Occasionally, descended testes can ascend spontaneously and occupy a permanent extrascrotal position; thus, it is important to examine the testes on all health maintenance visits, even in those boys who were previously found to have descended testes

    D. About 75% of boys with cryptorchidism have a hernia sac associated with the testis and cord structures

    E. If testes are undescended by 3 months of age, they are unlikely to spontaneously descend

F. Complications:
1. Deterioration of the undescended testes begins around 1 year of age and may ultimately correlate with poor semen quality and subsequent infertility
2. The risk of developing a testicular malignancy is higher in an undescended testicle than a normal testicle
3. Testicular torsion, emotional stress, hernia, and greater vulnerability to stress may occur

IV. Diagnosis/Evaluation

A. History
1. Determine whether the child was born prematurely
2. Ask about family history of cryptorchidism
3. Ask parents if they have noticed whether the child's testes are in the scrotum during baths or when he is relaxed

B. Physical examination
1. Inspect genitalia for hypospadias
2. Inspect scrotum; with cryptorchidism the scrotum is not fully developed on the affected side and may lack normal rugae
3. Gently palpate and ascertain that the testis is truly undescended (warm hands before examination); an overactive cremasteric reflex makes palpation difficult
   a. May avoid retraction by placing two fingers over both inguinal rings before examining scrotum
   b. Place child in supine position; sweep hand from the anterior-superior iliac spine over the inguinal canal and toward the pubis, attempting to palpate a testis. Try milking the testis into the scrotum; the older child can help by coughing or straining
   c. Soap or talcum powder on hands may facilitate massage of inguinal canal
   d. Placing a warm compress on inguinal region may relax the cremasteric muscle
   e. If still unable to locate testis in a supine position, ask the child to assume a tailor position (sitting cross-legged), kneeling position, or standing position; in infants, induction of crying and holding child in squatting position may cause testicle to descend
   f. If unable to locate testis with above methods, search beyond the scrotum and the inguinal canal, palpating as far distant as the inner thigh
   g. Note position, consistency, and size of testis in comparison to the contralateral testis as well as to boys of similar ages
4. Check for inguinal hernias and hydroceles as they are often associated with cryptorchidism; if a hernia is present, the impalpable hernia usually lies just inside the internal inguinal ring
5. Even if there are documented descended testes on previously visits, continue to regularly examine testes because re-ascent is possible

C. Differential Diagnosis
1. Anorchia or the complete absence of a testis; commonly occurs on the right side
2. Retractile testis which is a physiologic variation of normal (see physical examination IV.B.3. for how to examine a patient with a retractile testis)
   a. Due to an overactive cremasteric muscular reflex and the incomplete attachment of the testis to the scrotum by the gubernaculum
   b. Usually bilateral
   c. Less of a problem as the child gets older and the cremasteric reflex is less active and the testes become large
3. Newborns with bilaterally impalpable testes have high prevalence of chromosomal and endocrine disorders
4. Newborns with undescended testes and hypospadias often have an intersex disorder such as virilizing congenital adrenal hyperplasia

D. Diagnostic Tests are ordered when the testes are impalpable
1. Ultrasound is helpful to detect inguinal undescended testes, particularly in overweight boys; however, in a recent study ultrasound was unnecessary in most cases (Elder, 2002)
2. Computed tomography has many false positives, exposes the child to radiation, and requires sedation but is sometimes recommended in older boys
3. Magnetic resonance imaging is sometimes recommended, particularly in adolescents and adult males
4. Laparoscopy is recommended as the initial diagnostic test by some experts
5. A therapeutic trial of human chorionic gonadotropin (hCG) may also be helpful (see V.B.)

6.   Children with bilateral nonpalpable testicles need consultation with a specialist and the following tests are usually ordered: Ultrasound of pelvic structures, karyotyping, electrolytes, testosterone, müllerian-inhibiting hormone, adrenal hormones, and 17-hydroxyprogesterone

V.   Plan/Management

A.   Refer all children with cryptorchidism to a pediatric urologist
1.   Surgical repair, orchidopexy, should be done at 1 year or shortly thereafter to prevent infertility, diminish the possibility of testicular torsion, provide accessible examination (particularly in the event of malignant change), and prevent emotional trauma that often accompanies the disorder
2.   Patient education after orchidopexy
a.   Parents are usually anxious; inform parents that after orchidopexy the rate of fertility in these children is about 80% to 90%
b.   Discuss importance of regular self-examination of testes because of possible increased risk of testicular malignancy in this patient population

B.   If the location of the testis is uncertain, the potential for natural descent can be explored with a therapeutic trial of human chorionic gonadotropin (hCG) (consult urologist)

C.   Follow Up:
1.   The optimal timing of follow-up visits after birth is at 3 months, at which time most testicles descend in response to the postnatal testosterone surge
2.   If orchidopexy is performed, long-term follow-up should include regular testicular examinations through puberty to ensure the testicle remains in place

REFERENCES

American Academy of Pediatrics. (1999). The diagnosis, treatment, and evaluation of the initial urinary tract infection in febrile infants and young children (AC9830). *Pediatrics, 103,* 843-852.

American Urological Association. (2001). Evaluation of asymptomatic microscopic hematuria in adults: The American Urological Association best practice policy. Parts I and II. *Urology, 57,* 599-610.

Anderson, J.E. (1997). Hematuria. In L. Dornbrand, A.J. Hoole, & R.H. Fletcher (Eds.). *Manual of clinical problems in adult ambulatory care* (3rd ed.). Philadelphia: Lippincott-Raven.

Bass, P.F., Jarvis, J.A.W., & Mitchell, C.K. (2003). Urinary tract infections. *Primary Care Clinical Office Practice, 30,* 41-61.

Bellinger, M.F. (2001). Scrotal swelling. In R. A. Hoekelman (Ed.). *Pediatric primary care.* St. Louis: Mosby.

Bellinger, M.F. (2001). Meatal ulceration. In R.A. Hoekelman (Ed.). *Pediatric primary care.* St. Louis: Mosby.

Bent, S., Nallamothu, B.K., Simel, D.L., Fihn, S.D., & Saint, S. (2002). Does this woman have an acute uncomplicated urinary tract infection? *JAMA, 287,* 2701-2710.

Bock, G.H. (2001). Urinary tract infections. In R. A. Hoekelman (Ed.). *Pediatric primary care.* St. Louis: Mosby.

Chon, C.H., Lai, F.C., & Shortliffe, L.M.D. (2001). Pediatric urinary tract infections. *Pediatric Clinics of North America, 48,* 1441-1459.

Docimo, S.G., Silver, R.I., & Cromie, W. (2000). The undescended testicle: Diagnosis and management. *American Family Physician, 62,* 2037-2044, 2047-2048.

Elder, J.S. (2002). Ultrasonography is unnecessary in evaluating boys with a nonpalpable testis. *Pediatrics, 110,* 748-751.

Fang, L.S-T. (2000). Evaluation of the patient with hematuria. In A.H. Goroll, & A.G. Mulley, Jr. (Eds.). *Primary care medicine: Office evaluation and management of the adult patient* (4th ed.). Philadelphia: Lippincott.

Foglia, R.P. (1999). Groin hernias and hydroceles. In R.A. Dershewitz (Ed.). *Ambulatory pediatric care* (3rd ed.). Philadelphia: Lippincott.

Foglia, R.P. (1999). Undescended testes. In R.A. Dershewitz (Ed.). *Ambulatory pediatric care* (3rd ed.). Philadelphia: Lippincott.

Gearhart, J.P. (2001). Hypospadias, epispadias, and cryptorchism. In R.A. Hoekelman (Ed.). *Pediatric primary care.* St. Louis: Mosby.

Gomella, L.G., (Ed.). (2000). *The 5-minute urology consult.* Philadelphia: Lippincott.

Gupta, K., Hooton, T.M., & Stamm, W.E. (2001). Increasing antimicrobial resistance and the management of uncomplicated community-acquired urinary tract infections. *Annals of Internal Medicine, 135,* 41-50.

Hebel, S.K. (Ed.). (1996). *Drug facts and comparisons.* St. Louis: Facts and Comparisons, Inc.

Hellerstein, S., & Nickrell, E. (2002). Prophylactic antibiotics in children at risk for urinary tract infection. *Pediatric Nephrology, 17,* 506-510.

Jepson, R.G., Mihaljevic, L., & Craig, J. (2002). Cranberries for preventing urinary tract infection (Cochrane Review). *The Cochrane Library, Issue 2.*

Junnila, J., & Lassen, P. (1998). Testicular masses. *American Family Physician, 57,* 685-692.

Kass, E.J. (2001). Adolescent varicocele. *Pediatric Clinics of North America, 48,* 1559-1568.

Keren, R., & Chan, E. (2002). A meta-analysis of randomized, controlled trials, comparing short- and long-course antibiotic therapy for urinary tract infections in children. *Pediatrics, 105,* E70-E100.

Kogan, S.J., & Colbert-Kogan. (2001). Acute urology. In C. Green-Hernandez, J.K. Singleton, & D.Z. Aronzon. *Primary care pediatrics.* Philadelphia: Lippincott.

Langman, C.B. (1999). Hematuria. In R.A. Dershewitz (Ed.). *Ambulatory pediatric care* (3rd ed.). Philadelphia: Lippincott.

McKenna, P.H., & DeCambre, M. (2002). Bacterial infections in the urinary tract in girls. In R.E. Rakel & E.T. Bope (Eds.). *2002 Conn's current therapy.* Philadelphia: Saunders.

Patel, H.P., & Bissler, J.J. (2001). Hematuria in children. *Pediatric Clinics of North America, 48,* 1519-1537.

Ruley, E.J. (2001). Hematuria. In R.A. Hoekelman (Ed.). *Primary pediatric care.* St. Louis: Mosby.

Super, D.M. (2001). Phimosis. In R.A. Hoekelman (Ed.). *Pediatric primary care.* St. Louis: Mosby.

Van Haarst, E.P., van Andel, G., Heldeweg, E.A., Schlatmann, T.J.M., & van der Horst, H.J.R. (2001). Evaluation of the diagnostic workup in young women referred for recurrent lower urinary tract infections. *Urology, 57,* 1068-1072.

Ware, J.E., & Sherbourne, C.D. (1992). The MOS 36-item short-form health survey (SF-36): A conceptual framework and item selection. *Medical Care, 30,* 473-483.

Warren, J.W., Abrutyn, E., Hebel, J.R., Johnson, J.R., Schaeffer, A.J., & Stamm, W.E. (1999). Guidelines for antimicrobial treatment of uncomplicated acute bacterial cystitis and acute pyelonephritis in women. *Clinical Infectious Diseases, 29,* 745-758.

Weiss, R.A. (2001). Acute nephrology. In C. Green-Hernandez, J.K. Singleton, & D.Z. Aronzon. *Primary care pediatrics.* Philadelphia: Lippincott.

Winkler, W.H. (2001). The undescended testicle: What to do and when. *Family Practice Recertification, 23,* 57-63.

Workowski, K.A., & Levine, W.C. (2002). Sexually transmitted diseases treatment guidelines — 2002. *MMWR, 51*(RR06), 1-80.

Gynecology

MARY VIRGINIA GRAHAM & SYLVIA WORDEN

ABNORMAL PAPANICOLAOU (PAP) SMEAR

I.   Definition: Cervical cytological abnormalities interpreted and reported by cytologists using the 2001 Bethesda System

II.   Pathogenesis

   A.   Evidence linking human papillomavirus (HPV) with cervical cancer and its precursors is very strong
      1.   Oncogenic strains include HPV types 16, 18, 31, 33, 35, 39, 45, 51, 52, 56, and 58; types 16 and 18 are present in more than 80% of cervical cancers
      2.   Incidence of infection with HPV is directly related to sexual activity; the greater the number of partners, the greater the risk of HPV infection
      3.   Infection with an oncogenic strain does not mean that a woman will inevitably develop intraepithelial lesions

   B.   Other cofactors that have a role in development of cervical neoplasia include smoking, sexual behavior (early onset and multiple partners), and immunological status of the woman

III. Clinical Presentation

   A.   Approximately 13,000 women in the US develop cervical cancer each year, and about 4,500 women die of the disease

   B.   Most women who develop cervical cancer have never had a Pap smear or have not had one in the past 5 years

   C.   Of the more than 50 million women who undergo Pap testing in the US each year, approximately 3.5 million (7%) are diagnosed with a cytological abnormality requiring additional follow-up or evaluation

IV. Diagnosis/Evaluation/Plan/Management

   A.   Cervical cytology is primarily a screening test that in some instances may serve as a medical consultation by providing an interpretation that contributes to a diagnosis

   B.   The 2001 Bethesda System for reporting the results of cervical cytology is in the table below

BETHESDA SYSTEM 2001
SPECIMEN TYPE: *Indicate conventional smear (Pap smear) versus liquid-based versus other*
SPECIMEN ADEQUACY
• Satisfactory for evaluation *(describe presence or absence of endocervical/transformation zone component)*
• Unsatisfactory for evaluation *(specify reason)*
❖ Specimen rejected/not processed *(specify reason)*
❖ Specimen processed and examined, but unsatisfactory for evaluation of epithelial abnormality because of *(specify reason)*
GENERAL CATEGORIZATION *(optional)*
• Negative for Intraepithelial Lesion or Malignancy
• Epithelial Cell Abnormality: See Interpretation/Result *(specify 'squamous' or 'glandular' as appropriate)*
• Other: See Interpretation/Result *(e.g. endometrial cells in a woman ≥40 years of age)*
AUTOMATED REVIEW
• *If case examined by automated device, specify device and result*
ANCILLARY TESTING
• *Provide a brief description of the test methods and report the result so that it is easily understood by the clinician*
INTERPRETATION/RESULT
• ***NEGATIVE FOR INTRAEPITHELIAL LESION OR MALIGNANCY*** *(when there is no cellular evidence of neoplasia, state this in the General Categorization above and/or in the Interpretation/Result section of the report, whether or not there are organisms or other non-neoplastic findings)*
❖ **ORGANISMS:**
➤ *Trichomonas vaginalis*
➤ Fungal organisms morphologically consistent with *Candida* spp
➤ Shift in flora suggestive of bacterial vaginosis
➤ Bacteria morphologically consistent with *Actinomyces* spp
➤ Cellular changes consistent with Herpes simplex virus

(continued)

- ❖ OTHER NON-NEOPLASTIC FINDINGS *(Optional to report; list not inclusive)*:
  - ➢ Reactive cellular changes associated with
    - • inflammation (includes typical repair)
    - • radiation
    - • intrauterine contraceptive device (IUD)
  - ➢ Glandular cells status post hysterectomy
  - ➢ Atrophy
- • **OTHER**
  - ❖ Endometrial cells *(in a woman ≥40 years of age) (Specify if 'negative for squamous intraepithelial lesion')*
- • **EPITHELIAL CELL ABNORMALITIES**
  - ❖ SQUAMOUS CELL
    - ➢ Atypical squamous cells
      - • of undetermined significance (ASC-US)
      - • cannot exclude HSIL (ASC-H)
    - ➢ Low grade squamous intraepithelial lesion (LSIL) encompassing: HPV/mild dysplasia/CIN 1
    - ➢ High grade squamous intraepithelial lesion (HSIL) encompassing: moderate and severe dysplasia, CIS/CIN 2 and CIN 3
    - ➢ Squamous cell carcinoma
  - ❖ GLANDULAR CELL
    - ➢ Atypical
      - • endocervical cells (NOS *or specify in comments*)
      - • endometrial cells (NOS *or specify in comments*)
      - • glandular cells (NOS *or specify in comments*)
    - ➢ Atypical
      - • endocervical cells, favor neoplastic
      - • glandular cells, favor neoplastic
    - ➢ Endocervical adenocarcinoma *in situ*
    - ➢ Adenocarcinoma
      - • endocervical
      - • endometrial
      - • extrauterine
      - • not otherwise specified (NOS)
- • **OTHER MALIGNANT NEOPLASMS**: *(specify)*

EDUCATIONAL NOTES AND SUGGESTIONS *(optional)*
  Suggestions should be concise and consistent with clinical follow-up guidelines published by professional organizations (references to relevant publications may be included)

C. Components of the 2001 Bethesda System are further described in the following tables to assist in clinical decision-making

D. An explanation of **Specimen Type/Specimen Adequacy** is contained in box below

---

Specimen Type: In this first section of the report, the type specimen that was submitted is identified—conventional smear (Pap smear) versus liquid-based versus other

Specimen Adequacy: In the second section of the report, specimen adequacy is addressed; considered by many to be the single most important quality assurance component of the report, there are **two** mutually exclusive categories that are possible (**one** will be checked)

- • First category is *Satisfactory for evaluation*
  - ❖ A notation is made regarding the presence or absence of an endocervical/transformation zone component for specimens with adequate squamous cellularity
  - ❖ Further comments on quality indicators may be added to the *Satisfaction for evaluation* designation such as when the specimen is "partially obscured" (50-75% of epithelial cells cannot be visualized)
- • Second category is *Unsatisfactory for evaluation* (reason is specified; there are **two** possibilities)
  - ❖ Specimen rejected/not processed (reason will be specified, and includes such things as an unlabelled specimen; specimens in this category will not have been evaluated microscopically)
  - ❖ Specimen processed and examined, but unsatisfactory for evaluation of epithelial abnormality because of (reason will be specified here, and includes such things as ">75% of epithelial cells obscured")

E.   A description of **General Categorization** is contained in the box below

> **General Categorization:** The third section of the report is an **optional** component of the Bethesda System and its aim is to allow clinicians/office staff to triage reports easily
>
> Three mutually exclusive categories in this section
> - *Negative for Intraepithelial Lesion or Malignancy*
>   ❖   Specimens for which no epithelial abnormality is identified are reported here
> - *Epithelial Cell Abnormality*
>   ❖   Abnormality was detected and clinician is directed to "See Interpretation/Result"
> - *Other*
>   ❖   This category is for cases in which there are no morphological abnormalities in the cells per se, but the findings may indicate some increased risk (e.g., benign-appearing "endometrial cells in a woman ≥40 years of age")
>
> Note that because the categories are mutually exclusive, selection of the general category is based on the **most** clinically significant result when several findings are present

F.   The Automated Review/Ancillary Testing components are summarized in the box below

> **Automated Review:** The fourth section of the report. For slides scanned by automated computer systems, the instrumentation used and review results are included in the cytology report
>
> **Ancillary Testing:** If ancillary molecular test was performed, the type of assay as well as the results are reported here in the fifth section of the report

G.   **Interpretation/Result:** In this category, the sixth section of the report, there are three possibilities (1) *Negative for Intraepithelial Lesion or Malignancy*; (2) *Other*, and; (3) *Epithelial Cell Abnormalities* (**Note:** In the 2001 Bethesda System the term "diagnosis" has been replaced by "interpretation" or "result" to convey that cervical cytology provides an interpretation of findings that must be interpreted within the context of clinical findings)

H.   **Interpretation/Result:** *Negative for Intraepithelial Lesion or Malignancy* is the first reporting category and is described in the box below

> ***Negative for Intraepithelial Lesion or Malignancy***
>
> In this first category, specimens for which no epithelial abnormality is identified are reported here
>
> In addition, if certain non-neoplastic conditions are present, a notation is made regarding the presence of such conditions here. Non-neoplastic conditions that are identified are under two headings: (1) Organisms, and (2) Other non-neoplastic findings (optional to report)
>
> Organisms that are listed here include the following:
> > *Trichomonas vaginalis*
> > Fungal organisms morphologically consistent with *Candida* spp
> > Shift in flora suggestive of bacterial vaginosis
> > Bacteria morphologically consistent with *Actinomyces* spp
> > Cellular changes consistent with Herpes simplex virus
>
> Other non-neoplastic findings (optional to report; list not inclusive)
> > Reactive cellular changes associated with
> > > Inflammation (includes typical repair)
> > > Radiation
> > > Intrauterine contraceptive device (IUD)
> > Glandular cells status post-hysterectomy
> > Atrophy
>
> **Note:** Findings of non-neoplastic condition causing reactive changes does not alter the status of a specimen that has been reported as *Negative for Intraepithelial Lesion or Malignancy*

I. **Interpretation/Result:** *Other* is the second reporting category and is described in the box below

---

Other

In this second category, endometrial cells are noted if the woman is ≥40 years of age, regardless of the date of the LMP, because menstrual/menopausal status, exogenous hormone therapy, and other clinical risk factors are often unknown

Identification of endometrial cells if not associated with menses or after menopause may indicate risk for an endometrial abnormality, although most often this is a benign finding

Note: Cervical cytology, primarily a screening test for squamous epithelial lesions and squamous cancer, is unreliable for detection of endometrial lesions and should not be used to evaluate suspected endometrial abnormalities

---

J. **Interpretation/Result:** *Epithelial Cell Abnormalities* is the third reporting category and is described in the box below

---

Epithelial Cell Abnormalities

Epithelial cell abnormalities are of two types: Squamous Cell and Glandular Cell

- **Squamous Cell**
    - ❖ Atypical squamous cells (ASC) are subdivided into two categories: atypical squamous cells of undetermined significance (ASC-US) and atypical squamous cells, cannot exclude high-grade squamous intraepithelial lesion (ASC-H)
    - ❖ Squamous intraepithelial lesions (SIL) are defined by a two-tiered system using the terms low-grade squamous intraepithelial lesion (LSIL), and high-grade intraepithelial lesion (HSIL) to refer to cervical cancer precursors. Further, a two-tiered terminology for the histopathological classification of cervical intraepithelial neoplasia (CIN) has also been adopted with CIN 1 referring to low-grade precursors and CIN 2,3 denoting high-grade precursors. Current emphasis in the US has shifted to detection and treatment of histologically confirmed high-grade disease; thus it is logical for the ASC category qualifiers to emphasize the importance of detecting high-grade SIL (HSIL)
        - ➢ Dichotomous division of SIL is based on evidence that LSIL is generally a transient infection with HPV while HSIL is more often associated with viral persistence and higher risk for progression
        - ➢ Detection of HSIL has emerged as the central purpose of screening
- **Glandular Cell**
    - ❖ The classification of glandular abnormalities has been substantially revised in the 2001 Bethesda System. Glandular cell abnormalities are classified into three categories: (1) *Atypical glandular cells, either endocervical, endometrial, or "glandular cells" not otherwise specified [AGC NOS]*; (2) *Atypical glandular cells, either endocervical cells or "glandular cells" favor neoplasia [AGC "favor neoplasia"]*; and (3) *endocervical adenocarcinoma in situ (AIS)*
    - ❖ In a majority of cases, morphological features permit differentiation between atypical endometrial and endocervical cells. The finding of atypical glandular cells (AGC) is important clinically because the percentage of cases associated with underlying high-grade disease is higher than for ASC-US

K. Recommended management of women with squamous cell and glandular cell abnormalities are contained in the tables below

---

RECOMMENDED MANAGEMENT OF WOMEN WITH ATYPICAL SQUAMOUS CELLS OF UNDETERMINED SIGNIFICANCE (ASC-US)

There are three acceptable approaches to management of women with ASC-US: (1) A program of repeat cervical cytological testing; (2) Colposcopy; or (3) DNA testing for high-risk types of HPV. **(Note:** HPV-DNA testing is the preferred approach when liquid-based cytology is used at the initial screening visit; called "reflex testing," HPV DNA testing of the original sample is initiated only if the cytology test yields an interpretation of ASC-US)

- When a program of repeat cervical cytological testing is used to manage women with ASC-US
    - ❖ Patients should have repeat testing (using either conventional or liquid-based cytology) at 4- to 6-month intervals until 2 consecutive "negative for intraepithelial lesion or malignancy " results are obtained; at that point, patient can return to routine screening program
    - ❖ Women diagnosed with ASC-US or greater cytological abnormality on the repeat tests should be referred for colposcopy
- When immediate colposcopy is used to manage women with ASC-US
    - ❖ Women who are found not to have cervical intraepithelial neoplasia (CIN) should be followed up with repeat cytological testing at 12 months
    - ❖ Women who are found to have biopsy confirmed CIN should be referred without delay for treated by a specialist
- When DNA testing for high-risk types of HPV using a sensitive molecular test is used to manage women with ASC-US
    - ❖ Women who test positive for high-risk HPV DNA should be referred for colposcopic evaluation
    - ❖ Women who test negative for high-risk HPV DNA can be followed up with repeat cytological testing at 12 months

RECOMMENDED MANAGEMENT OF WOMEN WITH ASC-US IN SPECIAL CIRCUMSTANCES—POSTMENOPAUSAL, IMMUNOSUPPRESSED, PREGNANT

- Postmenopausal women
  - ➢ Provide a course of intravaginal estrogen (if evidence of genital atrophy and no contraindications to estrogen use)
  - ➢ Repeat cervical cytology test approximately one week after completing regimen; if the first repeat test is "negative for intraepithelial lesion or malignancy" a second repeat test should be done in 4 to 6 months; if this second repeat test is also "negative," patient can return to routine screening
  - ➢ If either repeat test is reported as ASC-US or greater, the patient should be referred for colposcopy
- Immunosuppressed women
  - ➢ Refer for colposcopy
- Pregnant women
  - ➢ Manage in the same manner as nonpregnant women

RECOMMENDED MANAGEMENT OF WOMEN WITH ATYPICAL SQUAMOUS CELLS, CANNOT EXCLUDE HIGH-GRADE SQUAMOUS INTRAEPITHELIAL LESION (ASC-H)

All women with ASC-H obtained using either conventional or liquid-based cervical cytology must be referred for colposcopic evaluation

RECOMMENDED MANAGEMENT OF WOMEN WITH LOW-GRADE SQUAMOUS INTRAEPITHELIAL LESION (LSIL)

Women with LSIL should be referred for colposcopy; subsequent management options depend on whether a lesion is identified, whether the colposcopic exam is satisfactory, and whether the patient is pregnant

Rationale: Whereas the majority of women with LSIL have either no cervical lesion or CIN 1 (which regress in most cases without treatment or are completely excised with biopsy); management of these women with repeat cytological studies is problematic for the following reasons

  - ➢ Rates of loss to follow-up for repeat testing are usually very high
  - ➢ There is a 53% to 76% likelihood of abnormal follow-up cytology results requiring eventual colposcopy
  - ➢ There is a small risk of delaying identification of invasive cancers

RECOMMENDED MANAGEMENT OF WOMEN WITH LISL IN SPECIAL CIRCUMSTANCES—POSTMENOPAUSAL, ADOLESCENT, PREGNANT

- Postmenopausal women
  - ➢ Follow-up without an initial colposcopy is an acceptable option when one of the two protocols below are used
    - ❖ May follow-up with repeat cytological testing at 6 and 12 months with a threshold of ASC-US or greater for referral for colposcopy (see MANAGEMENT OF WOMEN WITH ASC-US IN SPECIAL CIRCUMSTANCES—POSTMENOPAUSAL, IMMUNOSUPPRESSED, PREGNANT above)
    - ❖ A second option is to follow up with HPV DNA testing at 12 months with referral for colposcopy if testing is positive for high-risk HPV DNA
- Adolescents
  - ➢ Follow-up without initial colposcopy is an acceptable option; if this option is chosen, select one of the following approaches:
    - ❖ Repeat cytological testing at 6 and 12 months with a threshold of ASC for referral for colposcopy, OR
    - ❖ Follow up with HPV DNA testing at 12 months with referral for colposcopy if testing is positive for high-risk HPV DNA
- Pregnant women
  - ➢ See MANAGEMENT OF WOMEN WITH HISL IN SPECIAL CIRCUMSTANCES section below

RECOMMENDED MANAGEMENT OF WOMEN WITH HSIL

Colposcopy with endocervical assessment is the recommended management of women with HSIL; subsequent management options depend upon whether a lesion is identified, whether the colposcopic examination is satisfactory, whether the patient is pregnant, and whether immediate excision is appropriate

Rationale: A cytological diagnosis of HISL is **not common**; women with a cytological diagnosis of HSIL have about a 70-75% chance of having biopsy confirmed cervical intraepithelial neoplasia (CIN) 2 or 3 and a 2% chance of having invasive cervical cancer

RECOMMENDED MANAGEMENT OF WOMEN WITH HISL IN SPECIAL CIRCUMSTANCES— PREGNANT, YOUNG WOMEN OF REPRODUCTIVE AGE

- Pregnant women
  - ➤ Refer for colposcopic evaluation by clinicians who are experienced in the evaluation of colposcopic changes characteristic of pregnancy
- Young women of reproductive age
  - ➤ Refer for colposcopic evaluation and biopsy of lesions suspicious for high-grade disease or cancer; when biopsy-confirmed CIN 2, 3 is not identified in a young woman with cytology-confirmed HSIL, observation with colposcopy and cytology at 4- to 6-month intervals for 1 year is acceptable, provided colposcopic findings are satisfactory, endocervical sampling is negative, and the patient accepts the risk of occult disease

RECOMMENDED MANAGEMENT OF WOMEN WITH ATYPICAL GLANDULAR CELLS (AGC) OR ADENOCARCINOMA IN SITU (AIS)

- ➤ Women with all subcategories of AGC should be referred for colposcopy with endocervical sampling, with the exception of women with atypical endometrial cells, who should initially be evaluated with endometrial sampling; endometrial sampling should be performed in conjunction with colposcopy in women >35 years with AGC and in younger women with AGC who have unexplained vaginal bleeding
- ➤ Women with a cytological test result of AIS should also be referred for colposcopy with endocervical sampling
- ➤ Management of women with initial AGC or AIS using a program of repeat cervical cytological testing is **unacceptable**

L.   **Educational Notes and Suggestions:** This is the final section of the 2001 Bethesda System and is optional. In this section, written comments regarding the validity and significance of a cytology result are directed to the clinician who requested the test. If used, the format and style may vary depending on preferences of the laboratory and its clinicians and must be based on follow-up guidelines published by professional organizations (e.g., American College of Obstetricians and Gynecologists, American Society for Colposcopy and Cervical Pathology)

M.   For more detailed information, consult the 2001 Bethesda System dedicated web site (http://bethesda2001.cancer.gov) or download the guidelines at www.ama-assn.org

ABNORMAL UTERINE BLEEDING

I.   Definition: Bleeding not associated with normal menses, i.e., deviations in the amount, duration, or frequency of bleeding

   A.   During adolescence, menstrual cycle norms include a cycle interval of 21-40 days, and a cycle duration of 2-7 days.
      1.   Polymenorrhea refers to an abnormally shortened cycle with bleeding occurring every 21 days or sooner
      2.   Oligomenorrhea refers to an abnormally lengthened cycle with bleeding occurring every 35 days or later

B. Blood loss during normal menses totals about 60 mL over a maximum of 7 days (mean duration of flow is 4 days)
   1. Menorrhagia refers to total blood loss of >80 mL and bleeding for >7 days, occurring at regular intervals
   2. Hypomenorrhea refers to blood loss of <60 mL

C. Other abnormal bleeding patterns are the following:
   1. Intermenstrual bleeding is bleeding that occurs between regular menstrual periods
   2. Metrorrhagia is bleeding that is frequent and irregular
   3. Menometrorrhagia is a pattern of frequent and irregular bleeding that becomes prolonged

II. Pathogenesis

A. In adolescent girls, anovulation is the most common cause of abnormal bleeding patterns, and dysfunctional uterine bleeding (DUB) secondary to hypothalamic-pituitary-gonadal (HPG) immaturity is the underlying cause in most cases; the mechanism of DUB in anovulatory cycles is described in the box below

---

Menstrual Function in the Adolescent, Anovulatory Cycles, and DUB

- The median age of menarchal onset is 12.66 years in the US with African-Americans undergoing menarche a few months earlier than white females
  ✓ Most (about 65%) US females experience menarche during Tanner 4 stage of development
  ✓ Ovulation, accompanied by an LH surge at midcycle with resultant elevated progesterone levels and formation of the corpus luteum, is a later occurring maturational event and is not a prerequisite for menstrual bleeding
  ✓ Only about 18% to 45% of cycles are ovulatory during the first 2 years after menarche; that percentage increases to about 80% after 4-5 years

- In order to successfully stimulate the release of the two gonadotropins, follicle-stimulating hormone (FSH) and luteinizing hormone (LH) from the anterior pituitary, gonadotropin-releasing hormone (GnRH) must be released from the hypothalamus in a pulsatile fashion
  ✓ This pulsatile release of GnRH is modulated by neurotransmitters in the central nervous system. Dopamine, serotonin, and beta-endorphins inhibit GnRH, thereby decreasing the levels of FSH and LH released while norepinephrine exerts a stimulatory effect
  ✓ Many factors including stress, body composition, body mass, and exercise can interfere with GnRH release, and the consequence is inadequate secretion of the gonadotropins—FSH and LH, which are responsible for follicular development, estrogen production, and the LH surge required for ovulation

- The LH surge has two requirements: (1) an estradiol concentration >200 pg/mL and (2) maintenance of that level for approximately 48 hours
  ✓ Estrogen levels not meeting these requirements can lead to a negative feedback to the higher centers, resulting in decreased secretion of gonadotropins, and a subsequent reduction in estrogen levels that then halts endometrial proliferation and results in a withdrawal bleed—these anovulatory bleeding episodes are usually described as painless (unlike ovulatory cycles that often produce symptoms of bloating, lower abdominal cramps, and breast tenderness)
  ✓ The absence of an LH surge can also lead to a continuation of endometrial growth to a point where the lining is eventually unable to support itself, resulting in asynchronous tissue loss, or dysfunctional uterine bleeding

---

B. Reproductive tract disorders frequently cause abnormal vaginal bleeding
   1. Abnormal pregnancy (e.g., threatened, incomplete, missed abortions; ectopic pregnancies; trophoblastic disease; abnormalities of placental location)
   2. Anatomic abnormalities of the uterus (e.g., polyps, uterine myomas, adenomyosis, endometriosis)
   3. Trauma or presence of foreign body
   4. Infection of the lower or upper genital tract
   5. Malignancies involving the cervix, endometrium, vagina, vulva, or ovaries (rare)

C. Systemic diseases, including coagulation defects, platelet dysfunction, liver failure, prolactinemia, and thyroid dysfunction, can manifest as abnormal vaginal bleeding

D. Iatrogenic causes include medications that contain estrogen and progesterone, phenytoin, anticoagulants, corticosteroids, and spironolactone

III. Clinical Presentation

A. Most cases (up to 75%) of heavy and prolonged menstruation during adolescence are due to DUB
   1. Patients with DUB present with a history of heavy and prolonged bleeding, that may be associated with irregular cycle intervals; patients describe these irregular bleeding episodes as painless

2. Patients often also report that some periods are normal in terms of bleeding amount, duration, and that symptoms of bloating, menstrual cramps, and breast fullness occur with these normal periods (indicating that ovulatory and anovulatory cycles are intermixed, which is very common)
3. DUB is a diagnosis of exclusion, and other causes must be considered

B. A very common cause of menstrual irregularity (including both amenorrhea and irregular bleeding) in adolescence is pregnancy; therefore, the possibility of an abnormal pregnancy must always be ruled out, regardless of history

C. Patients with systemic diseases such as thyroid dysfunction or coagulation defects can also have abnormal vaginal bleeding
1. Patients with hypothyroidism may complain of weight gain, fatigue, cold intolerance, and constipation
2. Patients with coagulopathies usually bruise easily and may have had bleeding episodes involving nose, gingiva, or urinary tract in the past

D. Infection of the genital tract may produce abnormal bleeding, and patients typically present with pelvic and lower abdominal pain, fever, chills, dyspareunia, and mucopurulent vaginal discharge

E. Bleeding may be caused by trauma or presence of a foreign body (most often a tampon or object used for sexual pleasure); with a retained tampon, there is usually a foul odor and the bleeding is minimal

F. Menstrual disturbances may be associated with use of certain pharmacologic agents by the patient
1. Patients who take oral contraceptives may experience breakthrough bleeding
2. Long-acting contraceptives such as depot medroxyprogesterone acetate and levonorgestrel-releasing implants commonly cause irregular menses and eventually amenorrhea in patients who use these medications for longer than 6 months
3. Other drugs such as phenytoin, anticoagulants, corticosteroids, and psychopharmacologic agents can also cause menstrual disturbances

IV. Diagnosis/Evaluation

A. History
1. **Menstrual history**: Determine age at menarche. Inquire about timing and duration of last **normal** menses and ask if she has kept a menstrual calendar
2. **Patterns of menstrual flow:** Ask when bleeding begins, whether it is spotting or heavy, how long bleeding lasts, whether it is daily spotting, and how heavy the heavy days **(Note**: Daily spotting is suggestive of a polyp or infectious cause; heavy flow tapering to spotting, with no bleeding for several days, then returning to heavy flow again is characteristic of anovulatory bleeding)
3. **Determine if menstrual cycles are associated with premenstrual molimina that accompanies ovulatory cycles**: Ask about symptoms of breast fullness/tenderness, abdominal bloating, mood changes, edema, weight gain, and menstrual cramps
4. **Associated signs and symptoms**: Ask about presence of abdominal/pelvic pain, vaginal discharge, pain on intercourse, pain with urination or defecation, or pelvic heaviness **(Note**: Pelvic pain/heaviness may indicate an ovarian cyst [functional, dermoid, corpus luteum], endometriosis, or myoma)
5. **Contraceptive use and sexual practices/history**: Obtain this essential information
6. **Drugs and medications**: Ask about medications, including oral contraceptives and long-acting contraceptives such as Depo-Provera and Norplant
7. **Past medical history**: Inquire about past/present problems including endocrine, hematological, and gynecological problems **(Note**: Ask: "Are you seeing or have you recently seen a healthcare provider for any other problem?") Ask about family history of bleeding disorders
8. **Reproductive history**: Obtain complete history in these areas

> Obstetric history includes number of pregnancies (gravidity) and outcome of each (parity); by convention, this information is recorded as follows:
>
> **Gravida (G) a, Para (P) b, c, d, e**
>
> a = number of pregnancies
> b = number of term pregnancies (≥37 weeks)
> c = number of preterm pregnancies (viability through 36 weeks)
> d = number of abortions (spontaneous and induced) and ectopic pregnancies
> e = number of living children

9. **Behavior/lifestyle**: Ask about recent changes in weight, life, activity, exercise patterns

B. Physical Examination
   1. First, perform rapid assessment of hemodynamic stability (determine if patient is hypotensive or has orthostatic hypotension)
   2. Inspect skin for bruising, petechia, or purpura
   3. Always do pelvic and speculum examinations
      a. Insure that bleeding is uterine and not from urethra, rectum, or superficial surface of cervix
      b. Assess for foreign body in vault, examine cervical os for erosion, polyps, and mucopurulent discharge and obtain specimens for testing (see IV. D. below)
      c. Evaluate the uterus for tenderness, size, and shape
      d. Carefully assess the adnexa
   4. Assess thyroid and check for abdominal masses and tenderness

C. Differential Diagnosis: Rule out all conditions noted under Clinical Presentation (see III. above)

D. Diagnostic Tests
   1. If ectopic pregnancy is suspected, obtain an immediate pelvic ultrasound; refer to emergency OB/GYN care if confirmed
   2. Always obtain pregnancy test (βhCG) to determine if bleeding is due to a complication of pregnancy [may be the most important test!]. A positive pregnancy test should be followed up with a pelvic ultrasound; refer to a specialist as in IV.D.1. above
   3. Obtain a coagulation profile (adolescents are at significant risk for coagulopathy and are at very low risk for an endometrial lesion or atypia)
   4. Obtain complete blood count and platelet count
   5. Papanicolaou (Pap) smear if not done within past year
   6. Test for sexually transmitted diseases (gonorrhea and chlamydia)
   7. If symptoms suggest, TSH to evaluate for thyroid dysfunction
   8. Clinical findings of androgen excess suggest polycystic ovarian syndrome (PCOS) and appropriate studies should be obtained

V. Plan/Management

A. Patients with complications of pregnancy should be referred to the ED for emergent management

B. Adolescents with excessive uterine bleeding who are found to have an abnormal coagulation profile require further testing and should be referred to a hematologist for further evaluation and management

C. Treat obvious benign causes of vaginal bleeding such as the following
   1. Removal of foreign body from the vagina (most often impacted tampon)
      a. Under good visualization, and with the patient in the lithotomy position, grasp the tampon with a pair of sponge holding forceps (may also perform bimanual exam and sweep tampon out)
      b. Place a basin of water as close to the introitus as possible (to minimize malodor)
      c. Quickly immerse the tampon under water without releasing the forceps
      d. Flush the tampon and water down toilet
      e. **Note**: The unpleasant odor that envelopes the room is the most problematic; immersing the removed tampon into water the instant it is removed from the vagina reduces the malodor and the embarrassment to the patient
      f. May provide antibiotics 7-10 days if tampon in place for several days or has caused cervical erosion (doxycycline 100 mg BID x 7-10 days)

2.   For breakthrough bleeding from oral contraceptives
  a.   Counsel that breakthrough bleeding decreases dramatically after first 3 months of pills
  b.   Instruct to take pills at same time each day
  c.   Last, change oral contraceptive to one with a higher progestational activity (usually effective regardless of when bleeding occurs in the cycle) such as Desogen, Loestrin 1.5/30, or Yasmin

D.   Management of the adolescent with DUB can be divided into three categories based on CBC and degree of hemodynamic stability

---

TREATMENT OF DUB

Category 1: Patients with mild DUB, **defined as a hemoglobin >11 g/dL, a hematocrit of >33%, and stable vital signs can be managed as follows:**
Counseling and reassurance:
✓   The young woman and her parents should be educated about alterations in menstruation patterns associated with immaturity in HPG functioning and anovulation with a focus on the common occurrence and benign course of these alterations
✓   Patients should be advised to keep a menstrual calendar to document the duration of bleeding and to accurately determine cycle intervals
Pharmacologic management:
✓   For sexually active adolescents, a low dose combination oral contraceptive should be prescribed when there are no contraindications to OC use
✓   In addition, nonsteroidal anti-inflammatory drugs (NSAIDS) should be prescribed to decrease the amount of bleeding (see E. below)

Category 2: Patients with **moderate DUB**, defined as a hemoglobin value of 9 to 11 g/dL, a hematocrit of 27% to 33%, and stable vital signs can be managed as follows:
Counseling and reassurance: As above
Pharmacologic Management:
✓   If the adolescent is **not bleeding** at the time of the evaluation, a 21-day regimen of a monophasic oral contraceptive should be started (Sunday start) now
✓   Continue the therapy for 3-4 months to regulate the cycles and prevent recurrences
✓   Prescribe iron supplementation for 4-6 weeks (see section on IRON DEFICIENCY ANEMIA for products and dosing) to correct the mild anemia
✓   Patients who are **acutely bleeding** at the time of the evaluation should be placed on a tapering regimen using a monophasic OC with an estrogen content of 35 µg—the approach utilizes the healing effect of estrogen on the endometrium with the stabilizing effect of progesterone
✓   Use the 4-3-2 method—instruct the patient as follows
   •   For 4 **days**, take one pill 4 x/day
   •   For 3 **days**, take one pill 3 x/day
   •   For 2 **weeks**, take one pill 2 x/day
   •   After 21 days of pill taking (4 days, then 3 days, then 2 weeks), advise the patient that no pills should be taken for 7 days to allow for a withdrawal bleed
✓   **Note:** The high dose of estrogen may cause nausea; an antiemetic such as promethazine 25 mg BID should be prescribed (taking OCs with food does not appear to help)
✓   The patient is then cycled with a monophasic pill for 3-4 months and iron supplementation (see above) should be prescribed to correct the mild anemia

Category 3: Patients with severe DUB, **defined as a hemoglobin lower that 7 or 8 g/dL, or a value <10 g/dL with signs of hypovolemia should be referred to an expert for emergent management**

E.   Nonsteroidal anti-inflammatory drugs (NSAIDs) are prostaglandin synthetase inhibitors that have been shown to decrease bleeding in women with menorrhagia
  1.   Prescribe mefenamic acid (Ponstel) 250 orally TID for 5 days starting with menses to correct relative prostaglandin overproduction
  2.   Other NSAIDS that may be helpful include:
    a.   Naproxen 250-500 mg BID for 5 days beginning with onset of menses
    b.   Ibuprofen 600-1200 mg per day (in divided doses) for 5 days beginning with onset of menses

F.   Follow Up
  1.   Adolescents with mild DUB should be followed up in 6 months and those with moderate DUB should be followed up in 2-3 months to evaluate treatment efficacy

  2.   Follow up for adolescents with severe DUB should be by the expert to whom they were referred

AMENORRHEA

I. Definition: Absence of menses for at least 3 months duration at any age when menstrual function should be present

II. Pathogenesis

   A. An intact hypothalamic-pituitary-ovarian-axis, a hormonally responsive uterus, and an intact outflow tract need to function in a coordinated manner for menstruation to occur

   B. If any part of the system functions incorrectly, withdrawal menses do not occur and amenorrhea is the symptom

III. Clinical Presentation

   A. Diagnostic Criteria: Primary Amenorrhea
      1. No bleeding by age 14 in the absence of growth and development of secondary sexual characteristics
      2. Failure to have menses by age 16, regardless of presence of normal growth and development with the appearance of secondary sexual characteristics

   B. Diagnostic Criteria: Secondary Amenorrhea
      1. Adolescents must have had at least one spontaneous menstrual period
      2. Six months of amenorrhea (some say 3)

   C. Common causes of primary amenorrhea along with usual presenting signs are the following
      1. Gonadal dysgenesis—there is a lack of mature (stages 4 or 5) breast/pubic hair development, but small amounts of development (stages 2 or 3) may be present secondary to only adrenal hormone secretion
      2. Müllerion (uterovaginal) anomalies—normal breast/pubic hair development occurs
      3. Hypothalamic/pituitary disorders—normal breast/pubic hair development does not occur
      4. Constitutional delay secondary to an immature hypothalamic-pituitary axis—short stature (under 5 feet at age 14) is found

   D. Common causes of secondary amenorrhea in adolescent girls
      1. Pregnancy (most common cause)
      2. Hypothalamic hypofunction secondary to excessive stress, significant weight loss, and/or strenuous exercise (as many as half of all competitive female athletes may experience some menstrual abnormality, with luteal phase deficiency, anovulation, and amenorrhea the three most common)
      3. Hyperandrogenism and polycystic ovary syndrome
      4. Prolactin-secreting pituitary tumors
      5. Premature ovarian failure; endocrine disorders such as thyroid disease and diabetes mellitus
      6. Medications such as oral and injectable contraceptive steroids

   E. Hypothalamic induced amenorrhea is a universal feature of anorexia nervosa

IV. Diagnosis/Evaluation

   A. History: Primary Amenorrhea
      1. Question about growth and development; occurrence of growth spurt (ask: "Was there a period of 6 months - 1 year when you grew out of all your clothes, shoes?")
      2. Ask questions about puberty (breasts and pubic hair—when development began and how far it has advanced)
      3. Ask about diet, exercise patterns, stress

   B. Physical Examination: Primary Amenorrhea
      1. Height, weight
      2. Observe for common anomalies associated with gonadal dysgenesis
         a. Neck folds, low setting of ears
         b. Chest configuration, whether 4th metacarpal is short, cubitus, valgus

3. Assess breast and pubic hair development using Tanner stages
4. Inspect external genitalia for abnormalities
5. Speculum exam for imperforate hymen, presence of vagina and uterus, and bimanual exam for adnexal masses
   a. Estrogen exposed vaginal mucosa is thick, with rugae
   b. Presence of cervix at end of canal is sufficient evidence that uterus is present
   c. Clear cervical mucus in os is good indication that estrogen is present
   d. Bimanual exam to confirm presence, size of uterus, and any masses

C. Differential Diagnosis: Primary amenorrhea is a symptom. There are numerous etiologies for this symptom

D. Diagnostic Tests: Primary Amenorrhea (should be ordered by the specialist to whom patient was referred)

E. History: Secondary Amenorrhea
   1. Question patient regarding the following
      a. Age at menarche, cycle regularity, duration of menstrual flow (was it fairly constant month to month?) (**Note**: The presence of cycle regularity leads to a strong presumption of ovulation)
      b. Presence of symptoms suggesting ovulation--mittelschmerz, bloating, breast tenderness
      c. When and how deviation from prior menstrual cyclicity occurred
      d. Number and outcomes of pregnancies, postpartal course
      e. Type of contraception and possibility of pregnancy
   2. Obtain past medical history, medications currently taking (and recently discontinued such as oral contraceptives—" post-pill amenorrhea")
   3. Question regarding growth of excess hair on face, chest, abdomen, upper back; ask about presence of acne
   4. Ask about galactorrhea (breast milk). Persistent galactorrhea, even slight and unilateral, is significant
   5. Question regarding weight changes, skin texture, energy level, bowel habits, and temperature tolerance
   6. Take social history including exercise, eating habits and patterns, and stress at home, school, and work
   7. If woman is competitive athlete, obtain information about intensity and duration of training (**Note**: A triad of disordered eating, amenorrhea, and osteoporosis occurs in the elite athlete)

F. Physical Examination: Secondary Amenorrhea
   1. Vital signs, height and weight, and calculate BMI (see OBESITY section for how to calculate and interpret BMI) [a BMI <17 is associated with decreased GnRH production, which reduces LH and FSH production, causing amenorrhea]
   2. Examine skin for signs of androgen excess—acne and hirsutism
   3. Examine thyroid for size, presence of nodularity
   4. Assess breast development for Tanner staging and presence of galactorrhea
   5. Speculum exam for degree of vaginal rugation, type of cervical mucus (amount, stretchability, ferning pattern when dried on glass slide)
   6. Bimanual exam for masses; for example, a unilateral ovarian enlargement can mean a steroid-producing tumor. Assess deep tendon reflexes as index of thyroid status

G. Differential Diagnosis: Secondary amenorrhea is a symptom. There are numerous etiologies for this symptom

H. Diagnostic Tests: Secondary Amenorrhea
   1. Focused diagnostic tests based on history and physical examination findings are useful to isolate the underlying cause to the hypothalamic/pituitary, ovarian, or uterine/vaginal compartments, or to other organ systems
   2. First, measure βhCG to rule out the most common cause (pregnancy); also order serum prolactin, TSH, FSH, LH, and estradiol level (refer to V. Plan/Management for test interpretation)
   3. CBC, serum chemistries, and urinalysis should also be ordered to rule out systemic disease

V.   Plan/Management

      A.   Primary Amenorrhea: Refer all patients with primary amenorrhea to specialist for further work-up

      B.   Secondary Amenorrhea: Consult the table below

INTERPRETATION OF DIAGNOSTIC TESTING

➤ If sensitive thyroid-stimulating hormone (TSH) is abnormal, an asymptomatic thyroid disorder is present; refer for evaluation

➤ If prolactin is elevated, refer for a diagnostic evaluation of the etiology of the hyperprolactinemia

➤ If prolactin and FSH levels are normal, and history and physical exam suggest androgen excess, order a free testosterone level and refer patient for sonography to evaluate for evidence of polycystic ovary syndrome (PCOS); [women with this disorder do not always display clinical evidence of androgen excess]; refer for evaluation

➤ If estradiol level is subnormal, FSH and LH levels are normal or decreased, and patient has history of severe dietary weight loss or anorexia nervosa, a BMI <17, engages in highly strenuous exercise, or has severe stress, hypothalamic dysfunction is the likely cause; decreased gonadotropin levels are failing to stimulate sufficient estradiol production to produce endometrial proliferation

    • Screen for eating disorders and refer appropriately; consider referral for bone mineral density testing

    • Refer for dietary counseling for prudent diet, high in calcium rich foods

    • Counsel regarding risks of estrogen deficiency

    • Prescribe calcium and vitamin D supplements (amenorrhea of even a few months may be associated with osteopenia)

    • Prescribe low-dose oral contraceptives (if no contraindications)

      C.   Follow-up: Variable depending on the diagnosis

CONTRACEPTION

I.   Definition: Prevention of pregnancy by reversible or irreversible methods used by either or both sexual partners

II.   Pathogenesis: Not applicable

III.   Clinical Presentation

      A.   Requests for contraceptives and contraceptive counseling are among the most frequent reasons women visit a healthcare clinician

      B.   The proportion of never-married women currently in a sexual relationship has increased for all age categories over the past decade

      C.   Pregnancy rates among teens are greater in the US than in any other developed country in spite of a very small declining trend in teen pregnancy

      D.   Almost one half of pregnancies in the US are unintended in spite of the fact that there are many safe contraceptive methods available

      E.   Female sterilization, oral contraceptives, male condoms, and male sterilization are the dominant contraceptive methods in the US today

IV.   Diagnosis/Evaluation

      A.   History
          1.   **Obtain a menstrual history** including age at menarche, duration of, frequency of, and interval between menstrual periods, the last menstrual period (LMP, which is dated from the first day of last normal menses), any intermenstrual bleeding, pain with menses, and perimenstrual symptoms
          2.   **Obtain an obstetric history**, including number of pregnancies and outcome of each (see section on ABNORMAL UTERINE BLEEDING [IV.A.] for information on taking an obstetric history)

3. **Obtain a gynecologic history** including breast history, previous gynecologic surgery, infectious diseases involving the reproductive tract, any history of infertility, and use of douching/feminine hygiene products
4. **Obtain a sexual history** eliciting age at first intercourse; present sexual partner(s) and their gender; number of lifetime partners; types of sexual practices; level of satisfaction with sex life
5. **Obtain a contraceptive history** including contraceptive method currently used and reason for its choice; when begun, any problems, and satisfaction with method; inquire about previous methods used and why discontinued
6. **Inquire about** past or present **sexual abuse** or assault; screen for intimate-partner violence
7. **Obtain a complete medical and surgical history**, including information about cardiovascular disease, thromboembolic disease, liver problems, diabetes mellitus, blood transfusions, and migraine headaches
8. **Inquire about substance use** including tobacco, alcohol, and drug use; ask what medications are currently being taken
9. **Question about allergies** and any history of adverse drug reactions
10. **Determine childhood diseases** and immunization status
11. **Obtain family history**, asking about stroke, CVD, cancer, DM in first degree relative

B. Physical Examination
  1. **General Principles**: Hormonal contraception can safely be provided based on careful review of medical history and blood pressure measurement; for most women, no further evaluation is necessary
  2. Measure blood pressure
  3. If pelvic examination is performed (e.g., woman requests to be fitted for a diaphragm, or Pap smear screening or chlamydia screening are required [based on US Preventive Services Task Force (USPSTF) recommendations]), the following components should be considered
     a. Inspection and examination of external genitalia
     b. Speculum examination of the internal structures
     c. Pap smear and specimens as appropriate
     d. Bimanual examination of the pelvic organs
     e. Rectovaginal exam of posterior aspect of pelvic organs (if indicated)
  4. Consider clinical breast examination (the USPSTF does not recommend clinical breast examination for women under age 40). Consider instruction in breast self-exam (BSE); patient should be advised that benefits of breast self-examination have not been established and that the USPSTF has no recommendations for or against teaching or performing routine BSE

C. Differential Diagnosis: Not applicable

D. Diagnostic Tests
  1. Variable depending on findings from history and physical examination/blood pressure evaluation
  2. Type of contraceptive method selected by patient also influences which diagnostic testing is required (e.g., pregnancy test may be required, depending on the method selected by the patient)

V. Plan/Management

> Throughout the last 3 decades in the US, a legal framework developed that supports the provision of confidential healthcare to minors in many circumstances. Recently, however, there have been increasing attempts to limit minors' access to confidential services for sensitive healthcare issues such as reproductive health through proposals to mandate either parental consent or parental notification. As legislatures, courts, and administrative agencies consider these initiatives, defining the risks of limiting adolescents' access to confidential health services is important
>
> Healthcare professionals should support the availability of confidential adolescent health services within existing legal frameworks and be aware that the risks of limiting adolescents' access to confidential healthcare through mandatory parental notification, or any other mechanism, are high. For more information see English, A., Morreale, M., Stinnett, A., Boburg, E., Hirsch, C., & Kenney, K. (2002). *State consent statutes: A summary.* Chapel Hill, NC: Center for Adolescent Health & Law

A. All patients should be counseled regarding the following and counseling must be documented in the chart
  1. Anatomy and physiology of reproduction
  2. Contraceptive methods, including how they work, effectiveness, advantages, and disadvantages
  3. The need to use condoms to prevent STDs, regardless of contraceptive method selected
  4. Risks and benefits of all methods, as well as informed consent that is signed by patient and placed in chart when IUD, implants, injections, or other hormonal contraceptives are chosen by patient

B.   Assist patient to select one of the methods contained in the following overview of commonly used contraceptive methods, and provide counseling appropriate to the method selected

VI.   Brief Overview of Commonly Used Contraceptive Methods

A.   **Spermicides** contain nonoxynol-9 (N-9), which disrupt integrity of sperm membrane; available as creams, gels, foams, film, tablets, and suppositories and should be placed deep in vagina near cervix prior to intercourse
   1.   **Effectiveness:** About 5-50% of women experience an unintended pregnancy during a year of typical use; there is no significant difference among various forms
   2.   **Advantages:** Inexpensive, easily available, convenient with infrequent intercourse, few side effects or user risk; provides some protection against some STDs
   3.   **Disadvantages:** May cause local irritation (**Note**: Use of N-9 has become controversial recently after studies of prostitutes in Africa using large amounts of spermicide vaginally with the aim of reducing transmission of HIV were actually found to have a greater risk of seroconversion than the control group who was not using spermicide. The relevance of these studies to patient groups in the US remains unclear, but it may be wise for women at extremely high risk [prostitutes; partners of HIV+ individuals] to avoid any substance, including large amounts of N-9, that can irritate and disrupt vaginal mucosal integrity)

B.   **Male condoms** are more commonly used today to prevent transmission of STDs than for pregnancy prevention. They are thin sheaths made from latex or polyurethane which serve as a physical barrier (patients should be advised to avoid "skin" condoms). The Centers for Disease Control and Prevention (CDC) no longer recommends condoms lubricated with the spermicide N-9
   1.   **Effectiveness:** There is a 3% probability of pregnancy during a year of perfect use; causes of failure include slippage and breakage during intercourse and improper application
   2.   **Advantages:** Inexpensive, easy to use, easily available, reduce risk of STDs
   3.   **Disadvantages:** May decrease tactile sensation; condoms made of polyurethane are compatible with oil-based lubricants, but those made from latex are not

C.   **Female condoms (Reality)** have been in use since 1992 and are the first barrier contraceptive for women offering some protection against STDs. Composed of a thin polyurethane sheath that is 7.8 cm in diameter and 17 cm in length, the sheath has two polyurethane rings. The inner ring is at the closed end of the sheath that is placed inside the vagina and a larger ring remains outside the vagina providing some protection to the labia and the base of the penis. The inner ring provides stability for the condom, which is prelubricated with a dry silicone-based lubricant. The condom can be inserted up to 8 hours prior to intercourse and is intended for one-time use
   1.   **Effectiveness:** About 5% of women have an unintended pregnancy during a year of perfect use
   2.   **Advantages:** Controlled by woman and provides some STD protection
   3.   **Disadvantages:** Anatomy of woman may make stable placement difficult

---

Patient Education Relating to Use of Spermicides and Condoms

The correct way to use spermicides and condoms (appropriate lubricants to use with condoms, and how to put on and remove both male and female condoms) should be discussed
➢   Follow Up: In 1 year for annual exam
➢   Discuss emergency contraception and offer prescription

D.   **Diaphragms** are dome-shaped rubber caps with flexible rims that fit over the cervix and block the passage of sperm; spermicides are applied to the inner aspect of the dome, which is placed against the cervix
   1.   **Effectiveness:** About 6% of women have an unintended pregnancy during a year of perfect use
   2.   **Types**: Three types are commonly used
      a.   Flat spring rim: A thin rim with gentle spring strength, appropriate for use in women with normal vaginal size, contour, a shallow arch behind the symphysis pubis and normal vulvar tone
      b.   Arching spring rim: A sturdy rim with considerable strength, used in women with less than optimal vaginal support (indicated for women who have had a vaginal delivery which usually causes some amount of first degree cystocele) [**Note:** This type is the most commonly used]
      c.   Coil spring rim: A thin but sturdy rim useful in women with normal vaginal size, contour, and with an average or deep arch behind the symphysis pubis

3. **Goal** for fitting is to find the largest size that remains comfortable for the patient; most common problem in diaphragm fitting is selecting a size that is **too small**
   a. Generally, a nulliparous woman will be fitted with sizes 65, 70, or 75
   b. A multiparous woman, with sizes 75, 80, or 85
4. **Procedure** for fitting with diaphragm
   a. May use fitting rings or sets of various sizes of diaphragms (for the purpose of this explanation, a diaphragm will be used)
   b. Begin with a size in the middle of the probable range or estimate diaphragm size by using technique described below

---

DIAPHRAGM FITTING

- Insert your index and middle fingers into vagina until middle finger reaches vaginal posterior wall
- With tip of your thumb, mark the place where your index finger touches the pubic bone
- Remove your fingers
- Diaphragm is sized appropriately if it fits between mark on index finger and tip of middle finger

---

   c. After selecting the size believed to be appropriate, introduce the diaphragm into the vagina (first, lubricate the rim of the diaphragm; then compress the sides with fingers and thumbs of one hand, and place in vagina, inserting downward and inward)
   d. Check placement to make certain that the lower rim is in the posterior fornix, the circumference is against the lateral vaginal walls, and the upper rim is secured behind the symphysis pubis
   e. Determine if the size is right by referring to the box below

---

It's Too Small if
- it moves around in the vagina
- it can't be stabilized behind the symphysis pubis
- it comes out when woman coughs/bears down
- there is more than enough space to place your fingertips between rim and symphysis pubis

It's Too Large if
- rim buckles forward against the vaginal walls
- woman feels discomfort when the diaphragm is in place
- there is not enough space to place your fingertips between rim and symphysis pubis

It's Just Right if
- it fits snugly in the vagina without buckling forward and covers the cervix
- it fits both into posterior fornix and up behind symphysis pubis
- woman cannot feel the diaphragm and it does not cause discomfort
- there is just enough space to place your fingertips between rim and symphysis pubis

---

   f. Teach the woman how to insert, place, check, and remove the diaphragm; give woman detailed instructions on how to use and care for diaphragm
   g. Should be refitted after childbirth or a significant weight loss/gain.
5. **Advantages:** May be inserted up to 6 hours prior to intercourse; reduced risk of STDs and a reduced risk of cervical cancer; works well with infrequent intercourse
6. **Disadvantages:** UTIs are more common; some women are sensitive to contraceptive jelly; use has been associated with toxic shock syndrome (TSS), so should be avoided during menses and left in place no longer than 24 hours; requires fitting by a healthcare clinician and yearly replacement

E. **Cervical caps** are soft rubber cups with a firm, round rim (Prentif Cavity Rim Cervical Cap) that fit snugly around the base of the cervix. Spermicide is placed inside the cap prior to insertion
   1. **Effectiveness:** About 9-26% of women experience an unintended pregnancy during a year of perfect use (nulliparous women are less likely than parous women to become pregnant)
   2. **Advantages:** Provides continuous contraception protection for 48 hours with no need to remove for additional spermicide
   3. **Disadvantages:** Must be removed after 48 hours because of possible risk of TSS; some women experience odor problems with use for more than a few hours. Device must be fitted by a health care clinician and thus requires a visit and replacement every year at annual exam

F. **Intrauterine devices (IUDs)** are inserted into the uterus and their mechanisms of action are believed to prevent sperm from fertilizing ova

1. **Effectiveness:** About 0.6 to 1.5% of women experience unintended pregnancy in first year of use with perfect use

2. **Types:** Presently there are two intrauterine contraceptive devices marketed in the US: the Copper T-380A (ParaGard) and the intrauterine levonorgestrel-releasing system (Mirena) [Production of Progestasert has been suspended]

    a. The ParaGard is a T-shaped polyethylene device whose stem is wrapped with copper wire, and whose cross-arms are partly covered by copper tubing; fertilization is prevented primarily through creation of an intrauterine environment that is spermicidal; it is approved for 10 years of use

    b. Mirena is a plastic T-shaped device that releases 20 mcg of levonorgestrel daily; it is approved for 5 years of use. The levonorgestrel produces a contraceptive effect in a number of ways—by thickening cervical mucus and by inhibiting sperm mobility and endometrial growth; there is minimal systemic absorption of the progestin

    c. IUDs are not abortifacients

3. **Precautions** to IUD use are outlined in following table

---

PRECAUTIONS TO IUD USE

Refrain from providing an IUD for women with the following diagnoses (World Health Organization [WHO] category #4)

- Known or suspected pregnancy
- Active, recent (within past 3 months), or recurrent pelvic infection
- Severely distorted uterine cavity caused by anatomical abnormalities of the uterus including:
  - Leiomyomata
  - Endometrial polyps
  - Cervical stenosis
  - Bicornuate uterus
  - Small uterus

Exercise caution if an IUD is used or considered in the following situations and carefully monitor for adverse effects (WHO category #3)

- Risk factors for pelvic inflammatory disease
  - Purulent cervicitis, until treated
  - Any history of gonorrhea or chlamydia (especially recent infections)
- Risk factors for sexually transmitted diseases, including multiple sexual partners or a partner who has multiple partners
- Impaired response to infection
- Risk factors for infection with HIV and AIDS
- Undiagnosed, irregular, heavy or abnormal uterine bleeding, cervical or uterine malignancy, unresolved Pap smear
- Previous problems with IUD (any and all)
- Past history of severe vasovagal reactivity or fainting
- Difficulty in obtaining emergency follow-up care and treatment for PID

Adapted from Hatcher, R.A., Trussel, J., Stewart, F., Cates, W., Stewart, G., Guest, F., & Kowal, D. (1998). *Contraceptive technology*, 17th edition, New York: Ardent Media, Inc., pp 517-518.

---

4. **Timing of insertion:** Usually recommended during menses to avoid pregnancy

5. Provide a copy of the FDA-approved and manufacturer-supplied leaflet or pamphlet to each IUD user; consent forms can be written to include a statement such as "I have been given a copy of (title) and have been encouraged to read it carefully"

6. **Follow up** after patient's next menses (3-6 weeks after insertion) to make certain IUD is in place and that there are no signs of infection; further routine visits are not required

7. **Advantages:** High efficacy, which is sustained over 10 years for the ParaGard and 5 years for the Mirena; absence of systemic metabolic effects; not related to coitus; immediately reversible

8. **Disadvantages:** Risk of uterine perforation, increase in spontaneous abortion, ectopic pregnancy, uterine bleeding and pain, pelvic infection; need for clinician to insert and remove

Adapted from Nelson, A,, Hatcher, R.A., Zieman, M., Watt, A., Darney, P.D., & Creinin, M.D., et al. (2000) *Managing contraception*, Tiger, GA: Bridging the Gap Foundation

G.   **Combination oral contraceptives** prevent pregnancy by a number of effects of estrogen and progestin: they inhibit ovulation, presumably as a result of gonadotropin suppression induced by the estrogen and progestin effects on the hypothalamic/pituitary axis; they act directly on the cervical mucus, making it thicker which inhibits sperm penetration; they act directly on the endometrium, inhibiting its development into a state favorable for implantation

   1.   **Effectiveness:** About 0.1% of women experience an unintended pregnancy within the first year of use with perfect use (combined pills); the figure is 0.5% with progestin-only pills

   2.   **Advantages:** Easy to use, convenient, rapidly reversible, use controlled by woman, many noncontraceptive benefits such as prevention of gynecologic malignancies (endometrial and ovarian), prevention of benign conditions such as fibrocystic breast changes

   3.   **Disadvantages:** Dependent on user adherence to daily use, provides no protection against STDs, expensive, prescription needed, many possible side effects

   4.   World Health Organization (WHO) precautions to the use of oral contraceptives are contained in the following table

---

REFRAIN FROM PROVIDING COMBINED OCs

Refrain from providing combined oral contraceptives for women with the following diagnoses (World Health Organization [WHO] category #4)

- Deep vein thrombosis or pulmonary embolism, or history thereof
- CVA, coronary artery or ischemic heart disease, or history thereof
- Structural heart disease, complicated by pulmonary hypertension, atrial fibrillation, or history of subacute bacterial endocarditis
- Diabetes with vascular disease of >20 years duration
- Breast cancer
- Pregnancy
- Lactation (<6 weeks postpartum)
- Liver problems (all types)
- Headaches, including migraine with focal neurologic symptoms
- Major surgery with prolonged immobilization or any leg surgery
- Over 35 years of age and currently a heavy smoker (15 or more cigarettes a day)
- Hypertension, 160+/100+ or with vascular disease

Exercise caution if combined oral contraceptives are used or considered in the following situations and carefully monitor for adverse effects (WHO category #3)

- Postpartum <21 days
- Lactation (6 weeks to 6 months)
- Undiagnosed abnormal vaginal/uterine bleeding
- Over 35 years of age and light smoker (fewer than 15 cigarettes/day)
- Past history of breast cancer but no evidence of recurrence for 5 years
- Use of drugs that affect liver enzymes (Consult PDR)
- Gallbladder disease

Adapted from Hatcher, R.A., Trussel, J., Stewart, F., Cates, W., Stewart, G., Guest, F., & Kowal, D. (1998). *Contraceptive Technology*, 17th edition, New York: Ardent Media, Inc., pp 517-518.

   5.   Whereas some experts (see Hatcher et al., 1998) believe that no single OC in the sub-50 mcg (estrogen content) is clearly superior to another, other experts (see Vandenbroucke et al., 2001) recommend that third-generation progestins in combination preparations **not** be the first choice for new users because of the increase in the extent of adverse hemostatic changes and the associated risk of thrombosis associated with this class of progestins

   a.   One approach is to start with low-dose (estrogen content) combination OCs without regard to the progestin used in the preparation (see table that follows for product examples)

   b.   Another approach is to **avoid** third-generation progestins in combination preparations as the **first choice for new users** (third generation progestins used in combination OCs are desogestrel and, outside the US, gestodene) [see table that follows for product examples]

6. The newest progestin, drospirenone, is an analogue of spironolactone, an aldosterone antagonist with antimineralocorticoid and antiandrogenic activities (see table that follows for product example)
7. Women who are not candidates for estrogen-containing OCs should be considered for progestin-only pills such as Micronor or others listed in table of oral contraceptives categorized according to composition, or may consider other highly effective non-estrogen contraceptives
8. The following table lists oral contraceptives categorized according to composition:

Type	Drug	Estrogen (mcg)	Progestin (mg)	Color of active tablets
COMBINATION ESTROPHASIC				
Ethinyl estradiol/norethindrone acetate	Estrostep Fe	(5 tabs) 20	1	white (triangle)
		(7 tabs) 30	1	white (square)
		(9 tabs) 35	1	white (round)
COMBINATION TRIPHASIC				
Ethinyl estradiol/norethindrone	Ortho-Novum 7/7/7	(7 tabs) 35	0.5	white
		(7 tabs) 35	0.75	light peach
		(7 tabs) 35	1	peach
	Tri-Norinyl	(7 tabs) 35	0.5	blue
		(9 tabs) 35	1	yellow-green
		(5 tabs) 35	0.5	blue
Ethinyl estradiol/norgestimate	Ortho Tri-Cyclen	(7 tabs) 35	0.18	white
		(7 tabs) 35	0.215	light blue
		(7 tabs) 35	0.25	blue
Ethinyl estradiol/levonorgestrel	Tri-Levlen	(6 tabs) 30	0.05	brown
		(5 tabs) 40	0.075	white
		(10 tabs) 30	0.125	light yellow
	Triphasil	(6 tabs) 30	0.05	brown
		(5 tabs) 40	0.075	white
		(10 tabs) 30	0.125	light yellow
Ethinyl estradiol/desogestrel	Cyclessa	(7 tabs) 25	0.1	yellow
		(7 tabs) 25	0.125	orange
		(7 tabs) 25	0.15	red
COMBINATION BIPHASIC				
Ethinyl estradiol/norethindrone	Ortho-Novum 10/11	(10 tabs) 35	0.5	white
		(11 tabs) 35	1	peach
	Jenest-28	(7 tabs) 35	0.5	white
		(14 tabs) 35	1	peach
Ethinyl estradiol/desogestrel	Mircette	(21 tabs) 20	0.15	white
		(5 tabs) 10	0	yellow
COMBINATION MONOPHASIC				
Ethinyl estradiol/norethindrone combination	Loestrin 1/20*	20	1	white
	Loestrin (Fe) 1/20*	20	1	white
	Loestrin 1.5/30*	30	1.5	green
	Loestrin (Fe) 1.5/30*	30	1.5	green
	Brevicon	35	0.5	blue
	Modicon	35	0.5	white
	Norinyl 1+35	35	1	yellow-green
	Ortho-Novum 1/35	35	1	peach
	Ovcon-35	35	0.4	peach
	Ovcon-50	50	1	yellow
*As norethindrone acetate				
Ethinyl estradiol/levonorgestrel	Alesse	20	0.1	pink
	Levlite	20	0.1	pink
	Levlen	30	0.15	light orange
	Nordette	30	0.15	light orange
Ethinyl estradiol/norgestrel	Lo/Ovral	30	0.3	white
	Ovral	50	0.5	white

(Continued)

ORAL CONTRACEPTIVES CATEGORIZED BY COMPOSITION *(CONTINUED)*

Type	Drug	Estrogen (mcg)	Progestin (mg)	Color of active tablets
COMBINATION MONOPHASIC *(Continued)*				
Ethinyl estradiol/	Demulen 1/35	35	1	white
Ethynodiol diacetate	Demulen 1/50	50	1	white
Mestranol/norethindrone	Norinyl 1/50	50	1	white
	Ortho-Novum 1/50	50	1	yellow
Ethinyl estradiol/desogestrel	Desogen	30	0.15	white
	Ortho-Cept	30	0.15	orange
Ethinyl estradiol/norgestimate	Ortho-Cyclen	35	0.25	blue
Ethinyl estradiol/drospirenone	Yasmin	30	3	yellow
PROGESTIN-ONLY				
Norethindrone	Micronor	---	0.35	lime
	Nor-QD		0.35	yellow
Norgestrel	Ovrette	---	0.075	yellow

Adapted from Murphy, J.L. (2002, January). Tables: Oral contraceptives. *Monthly prescribing reference*. New York: Prescribing References, Inc.

Patient Education Relating to Use of Oral Contraceptives

➢ Instruct to use a backup method of birth control during first pack of pills

➢ Provide instructions on when to start the pills based on information in the table that follows

➢ Instruct patient to contact you if she does not have a menstrual period when expected while taking OCs

➢ Teach the patient the OC danger signs and symptoms that signal that the OC should be discontinued immediately. Use the acronym ACHES (*A*bdominal pain, *C*hest pain, *H*eadaches, *E*ye problems, *S*evere leg pain) and also include teaching on unilateral numbness, weakness, or tingling, slurring of speech (possible stroke), hemoptysis (possible pulmonary embolism)

➢ Provide a copy of the FDA-approved and manufacturer-supplied leaflet or pamphlet to each oral contraceptive user; consent forms can be written to include a statement such as "I have been given a copy of (title) and have been encouraged to read it carefully"

➢ When starting a woman on OCs for the first time, give her a 3 month supply and have her return for a BP check and for evaluation on how she is doing on the OCs; then give her enough OCs to last for the remainder of the year

➢ Follow Up: In 1 year for annual exam

RETIMING MENSES FOR CONVENIENCE

➢ Many patients are interested in skipping placebo pills to retime or skip menses

➢ Users of monophasic 30 mcg EE OCs may take as many as 3 packs of pills without using the placebo pills, which establishes a menstrual cycle with bleeding every 10th week rather than every 4th week

➢ This practice works less effectively with triphasic OCs

➢ Patients should be cautioned to never take active OCs for less than 21 days when they retime menses for convenience

---

DRUG INTERACTIONS

➢ Drug interactions involving oral contraceptives are of two types
  - Effects of other drugs on OC efficacy
  - Effects of OCs on efficacy of other drugs

➢ **Selected interactions only are listed here!**

➢ **Consult PDR** for possible interactions when prescribing medications for patients taking oral contraceptives; advise patients to remind other health care providers to whom they present for care to do the same

➢ As a general rule, patients should use condoms throughout any cycle during which they receive antibiotic therapy (especially rifampin) and some antiseizure medications as these medications interfere with OC efficacy (may need pill with higher estrogen component to prevent BTB and pregnancy)

➢ Fluconazole, a medication frequently taken by women of childbearing age, does not interfere with OC effectiveness

INSTRUCTIONS FOR STARTING ORAL CONTRACEPTIVES

> Advise woman to start OCs on the first day of her menstrual cycle or on the first Sunday after her period begins (if period begins Sunday, she should take the first pill on that day)
> Instruct patient to take 1 pill a day until pack is finished, then
> If on 28-day pack, begin a new pack immediately; skip no days
> If using 21-day pack, stop for 7 days, and then restart (**Note**: Caution patient not to wait until period starts, but to wait 7 days after completing pack, and then start next pack)
> Instruct to take at the same time each day and to associate with something that is done regularly at same time of day (going to bed, brushing teeth, etc.)
> Explain that a backup method such as condoms or foam should be used for first seven days during the first few cycles

Adapted from Dickey, R.P. (2002). *Managing contraceptive pill patients.* 11th Edition, Durant, OK: EMIS, Inc.

INSTRUCTIONS ABOUT EARLY SIDE EFFECTS

> Advise that some side effects are common during the first few cycles of use, but that they should disappear after that time
> Side effects to expect include the following
>   • Breakthrough bleeding (BTB) and spotting
>   • Symptoms associated with early pregnancy, especially nausea
> Encourage patient to delay making a decision about discontinuing the pill until after 3rd cycle to give side effects a chance to resolve

Adapted from Dickey, R.P. (2002). *Managing contraceptive pill patients.* 11th Edition, Durant, OK: EMIS, Inc.

INSTRUCTIONS FOR DEALING WITH MISSED PILLS

First, explain to patients the difference between the 21-pill pack and the 28-pill pack (first 21 pills in 28-pill pack contain hormones and the last 7 contain no hormones)

Patients who are taking the 28-pill pack and miss any of the last 7 (reminder pills) pills can discard the missed pill(s), and take the remaining "reminder" pills as scheduled to finish the pack
They should then start the next pack on usual schedule

Patients who miss any of the 21 hormonal pills must do the following

Use back-up contraception even if one pill was missed, or even if a pill was taken as much as 12 hours late (if only 1 pill was missed or taken late, back-up contraception such as condoms should be used for 7 days or patient should abstain from sex for 7 days)

Advise Patient to Get Back on Schedule by Following These Guidelines

If patient is <24 hours late in taking a pill	Take the missed pill immediately and return to the daily pill-taking routine making sure to take the next pill at the regular time
If patient is 24 hours late in taking a pill	Take both the missed pill and today's pill at the same time
If patient is >24 hours late in taking one pill, and is late for or completely missed a second pill as well	Take the last pill that was missed immediately; take the next pill on time; throw out the other missed pills, and take the rest of the pills in pack right on schedule. Use condoms for 7 days or abstain from sex for 7 days

If a pill was completely missed during the third week of pills (pills 15-21), advise the patient to do the following
  • Finish the remainder of the hormonal pills in pack (take through pill 21 if using a 28-pill pack)
  • Do not take a week off pills if using a 21-day pill pack OR do not take the last 7 pills (the nonhormonal pills) in the 28-pill pack
  • Begin taking a new pack of pills as soon as the hormonal pills in the current pack have been taken
  • Advise patient that she might not have a period until the end of the second pack of pills, but missing a period is not harmful
  • In all cases, back-up contraception for at least 7 days must be used

Adapted from Hatcher, R.A., Trussel, J., Stewart, F., Cates, W., Stewart, G., Guest, F., & Kowal, D. (1998). *Contraceptive technology,* 17th edition, New York: Ardent Media, Inc., pp 517-518.

H. **Norplant** is a long-acting subdermal contraceptive implant that is currently not available in the United States. Look for Norplant to return as Norplant II, a 2-rod levonorgestrel-releasing system providing highly effective contraception for up to 3 years. Other products that are currently in controlled clinical trials include Implanon, a 1-rod 3-ketodesogestrol-releasing system, and Annuelle, norethindrone-releasing pellets. Some of these products will be biodegradable within the subcutaneous tissue, requiring no removal after completion of the effective period of contraception

I.   **Depo-Provera** is an injectable form of long-acting progesterone with a mechanism of action similar to that of other progestin-only contraceptives; a good choice for women in whom estrogen-containing OCs are contraindicated, barrier methods are inadvisable because of compliance problems, and in women older than age 35 who smoke

    1.   **Effectiveness**: About 0.3% of women experience an unintended pregnancy within the first year with perfect use

    2.   **Advantages**: Easy to use, decreased menstrual flow and avoidance of the rare but serious complications attributable to estrogen use

    3.   **Disadvantages**: Unpredictable vaginal bleeding, adverse changes in lipids, patients are more likely to experience weight gain than patients using combined hormonal methods

    4.   How Administered: Usual dose is 150 mg, given IM every 12 weeks

        a.   Initial dose should be administered by the 5th day of menses in nonpostpartum women

        b.   In non-nursing postpartum women, initial dose should be given within first 5 days postpartum and at 6 weeks postpartum for breastfeeding mothers (breastfeeding must be well established)

        c.   Approximately half of women using this method experience amenorrhea after a year of injections (a harmless side effect that may be desired by the patient)

Patient Education Relating to Use of Depo-Provera

➢ Advise to use a backup form of contraception for the first seven days after the initial injection (may not be necessary if first injection given during first 5 days after the beginning of a normal menstrual period)

➢ Remind to return every 12 weeks for a repeat injection

➢ Explain that unpredictable menstrual bleeding, most often decreased blood flow, is common

➢ Review "red flags" with patient--repeated, very painful headaches, heavy bleeding, depression, severe pain in the lower abdomen, prolonged pain or bleeding at injection site

➢ Remind patients that this method provides no protection against sexually transmitted diseases

➢ Back-up methods of contraception must always be used when >one week late for injection

➢ For patients who are late for their injection and have unprotected intercourse, advise them to contact healthcare clinician regarding options; one option is emergency contraception; by calling (1-888-NOT-2-LATE) patients can be provided with phone numbers of 5 providers of emergency contraception in the area

---

J.   **Lunelle** is an injectable contraceptive administered every 28 days (may be given up to 33 days after the previous injection). Each 0.5 cc dose contains 25 mg medproxyprogesterone acetate and 5 mg estradiol cypionate. The injection is given intramuscularly into the deltoid or gluteus maximus; the initial dose is given within the first 5 days of the menstrual cycle. Suitable candidates for the use of Lunelle include women who prefer regular cycles to amenorrhea and who find monthly injection acceptable and accessible (not currently available in the US)

    1.   **Effectiveness:** Failure rate within the first year is 0.1-0.4/100 women

    2.   **Advantages:** Menstrual regularity, decreased ovulatory and menstrual pain, convenient, a good method for women who are forgetful with daily pills; does not disrupt spontaneity of intercourse; rapidly reversible; may have less adverse effects on lipid profile than combined OCs.

    3.   **Disadvantages:** Possible increased spotting in the first month of use, side effects such as depression, anxiety, irritability, fatigue and other mood changes. Not suitable for women who fear injections

    4.   **Precautions**: See precautions for combined OCs

    5.   **Patient teaching**: Advise patients to be alert for "ACHES," as with Combined OCs

    6.   **Lunelle (in the pre-filled syringe delivery system) has been voluntarily recalled** by the manufacturer, Pharmacia, because of a production error that may have resulted in insufficient dosing. Lunelle packaged in vials is not affected by this recall. For more information, healthcare clinicians may call 800-323-4204 and patients may call 800-691-6813

K.   **Ortho Evra** is a new transdermal contraceptive patch that is changed weekly for three weeks, then reapplied after a 7-day patch-free interval during which a withdrawal bleed will occur (i.e., a new patch is applied weekly for 3 weeks; week 4 is patch-free). The thin matrix-type transdermal patch contains three layers; the middle layer holds and releases the active hormones norelgestromin (150 mcg/day) and ethinyl estradiol (20 mcg/day). Evra is similar to combined OCs in contraceptive effectiveness and cycle control, and may be considered as a contraceptive option for women who are eligible to take combined OCs and other estrogen-containing contraceptives

1. **Advantages:** Ortho Evra may be a good method for women who are forgetful with daily pill-taking or fearful of injections; highly effective; rapidly reversible
2. **Disadvantages:** Visibility of the patch decreases user privacy; site reactions; may come off with exercise or swimming (detachment is uncommon); shares similar side effects with combined OCs; may be less effective in women weighing greater than 198 pounds
3. **Precautions:** See precautions for Combined OCs.
4. **Patient teaching** should include:
   a. Apply the patch to the abdomen, upper chest (not the breasts), upper outer arm, or buttocks at the beginning of the menstrual cycle
   b. A new patch is applied weekly for three weeks; week four is patch-free
   c. No decals, stickers, or other decorations should be applied to the patch
   d. Patients should be instructed to rotate the application site (may use the same anatomical area but rotate the site)
   e. Dispensed in packages of 3 patches for use in 1 cycle; single replacement patches are also available
   f. Patients should be alert for "ACHES" as with combined OCs

L. **NuvaRing** is a combined contraceptive vaginal ring containing the progestin etonogestrel and ethinyl estradiol (EE). It is inserted by the patient and worn within the vagina for a three-week period, then discarded. After 7 days, during which a withdrawal bleed occurs, a new ring is inserted. Contraceptive efficacy is similar to combination OCs. This is another good method for women who are candidates to use combined OCs but worry about forgetting daily pills
   1. **Advantages:** No fitting by healthcare clinician is needed; good for patients who dislike taking pills; may be removed for short intervals (i.e. during sexual intercourse); highly effective
   2. **Disadvantages:** May not be a suitable method for women with uterine prolapse; may forget to re-insert ring if taken out for intercourse; may forget to take ring out and insert a new one after menses
   3. **Precautions:** See precautions for Combined OCs
   4. **Patient teaching** should include:
      a. The ring may be removed for short periods of time but should be inserted again without undue delay (no longer than 3 hours)
      b. Patients should mark their calendars when a ring should be removed and when the next one should be inserted
      c. Patients should be alert for "ACHES", as with combined OCs

---

Patient Education Relating to Use of All Contraceptive Methods

➤ **Always** remind patients that condoms must be used with each sexual encounter to provide protection against STDs regardless of the method used for contraception

---

M. **Postcoital emergency contraception** (EC) for patients who have unintended unprotected intercourse can be provided via two hormonal regimens—combined estrogen-progestin (Preven and Yuzpe) and progestin only (Plan B). Both Preven and Plan B are **dedicated** products specifically marketed for emergency contraception; however, the products listed in the following table have been declared safe and effective by the FDA for use as emergency contraception (Yuzpe method)
   1. The Preven kit utilizes a combined estrogen-progestin regimen
      a. Contains 4 tabs containing both ethinyl estradiol 50 mcg and levonorgestrel 250 mcg as well as a home pregnancy test and a patient education booklet
      b. Dosing: 2 tabs PO within 72 hours of unprotected intercourse or a contraceptive failure and 2 tabs 12 hours later **(see M.8.b. below for comments on the 72-hour time limit)**
   2. The Plan B kit utilizes a progestin-only regimen
      a. Contains 2 doses of 0.75 mg levonorgestrel and patient education booklet; no pregnancy test is included
      b. Dosing: 1 tab PO as soon as possible or within 72 hours of unprotected intercourse followed by the second tab 12 hours later **(see M.8.b. below for comments on the 72-hour time limit)**
   3. The Yuzpe regimen, standard therapy for EC for many decades utilizes large doses of ethinyl estradiol plus levonorgestrel or norgestrel per dose
      a. These hormones are found in many brands of combined oral contraceptives available in the US
      b. The following table presents selected regimens for administering these drugs for emergency contraception

    c.   No laboratory testing including a pregnancy test is necessary before prescribing EC

    d.   Assessment can be done entirely by history; examination and laboratory tests are not necessary

    e.   A strong medical and legal case exists for prescribing EC over-the-counter as is done in many other countries

    f.   Patient will report whether she had unprotected/inadequately protected intercourse; the determination of whether the act was not adequately protected should be left to her judgment

4.   Clinicians should use encounters for emergency contraception as an opportunity to counsel patients about contraceptive options and avoidance of unintended pregnancies

5.   **Effectiveness**: Reduces the risk of pregnancy by about 75% (**Note**: Risk of becoming pregnant during unprotected intercourse during 2nd or 3rd week of cycle is about 8 of every 100 women; with ECs, this is reduced to about 2 out of every 100 women, which represents a 75% reduction)

6.   **Side effects**: About 42% of women who take ECs have nausea and about 16% have vomiting; patients can minimize nausea and vomiting by using the levonorgestrel regimen (Plan B); in addition, pretreatment with the antiemetic drug meclizine can significantly reduce the chance of these side effects. Once nausea occurs, antiemetics are unlikely to be effective (Note: Advising patient to take with food to reduce nausea and vomiting lacks merit with these particular drugs)

    a.   Preferred patient management when vomiting occurs shortly after taking EC is unknown

    b.   Some experts believe that vomiting indicates that sufficient quantities of steroid have been absorbed and the dose need not be repeated

    c.   Others recommend repeating the dose, particularly if vomiting occurs shortly after the dose is taken (within 1 hour)

7.   **Safety**: Almost all women can safely use ECs

    a.   Not indicated for women with a suspected or confirmed pregnancy because the treatment will not work if the woman is already pregnant (however, evidence suggests that no harm would occur to her, the course of her pregnancy, or the fetus if emergency contraception were used in error)

    b.   Treatment may not be appropriate in women with active migraine or marked neurologic symptoms

    c.   In women with a history of stroke or blood clots in the lungs or legs, treatment with progestin-only pills may be preferable (Plan B)

8.   Some data indicate that emergency contraceptive hormones are more effective the sooner after intercourse they are taken

    a.   In a large WHO clinical trial, pregnancy was prevented in 77% of cases if the Yuzpe regimen was used on the first day after intercourse, but only 31% of cases if it was used on the third day—other studies have found no decrease in effectiveness with delay of treatment

    b.   The 72-hour time limit should be considered a guideline only; women should be advised to use the treatment as soon as possible after unprotected intercourse, but treatment should **not be withheld** from those women who present past the 72-hour time limit

    c.   To avoid delays in treatment, consideration should be given to prescribing over the telephone, having after-hours systems in place, and providing prescriptions for EC to patients at their annual examination

9.   The Copper-T IUD has also been approved for emergency contraception and can be inserted up to five days after unprotected intercourse; reduces the risk of pregnancy following unprotected intercourse by more than 99%

DYSMENORRHEA

I.   Definition: Pain that occurs in lower abdomen/pelvis around the time of menses that has no anatomic cause

II.   Pathogenesis

A.   Primary dysmenorrhea results from a cascade of events precipitated by increased levels of prostaglandin $F_2\alpha$ ($PGF_2\alpha$), leukotrienes, and vasopressin
1.   These hormones lead to alterations in uterine basal tone, and increases in uterine contraction strength and frequency, resulting in vasospasm and reductions in uterine blood flow
2.   Pain occurs as a result of tissue hypoxia and ischemia

B.   Secondary dysmenorrhea is painful uterine contractions due to a clinically identifiable cause, and may be classified as follows:
1.   External to the uterus (examples are endometriosis, tumors, adhesions, and nongynecologic causes)
2.   Within the wall of the uterus (examples are adenomyosis, leiomyomas)
3.   Within the cavity of the uterus (examples are polyps and infection)

III. Clinical Presentation

A.   Painful menses is a common complaint in young women and one of the most common causes of missed school days and interference with social and recreational activities

B.   Many teens do not seek healthcare, but instead rely on over-the-counter products which often provide suboptimal pain relief

C.   Pain of primary dysmenorrhea is characterized by the following
1.   Onset is within 6-12 months after menarche and occurs only during ovulatory cycles
2.   Occurs within a few hours before or at the onset of menstruation (lasts 24-72 hours each month)
3.   Located in suprapubic area and radiates to back, upper thighs
4.   Associated with diarrhea, nausea, and vomiting in some women

D.   Secondary dysmenorrhea increases in incidence as women grow older due to the increased prevalence of processes that cause the condition among older women

E. Secondary dysmenorrhea is uncommon in adolescence usually occurring at a later gynecologic age. Adolescents with secondary dysmenorrhea usually experience pain consistent with the underlying pathology such as the following
   1. GI symptoms, UTI symptoms, and so on suggest nongynecologic causes
   2. Dyspareunia and pelvic pain unrelated to menses (but also occurring with menses) suggest causes such as endometriosis, infection (PID), adenomyosis, and leiomyomas

IV. Diagnosis/Evaluation

   A. History
      1. Obtain a complete menstrual history and contraceptive history
      2. Question patient about location of pain, when it begins, if it radiates, if there are associated symptoms of nausea, vomiting, or diarrhea
      3. Inquire if pain occurs independently of menses in addition to occurring with menses. Ask if there is dyspareunia
      4. Ask if there are urinary tract symptoms, if there is any vaginal discharge
      5. Question patient about treatments tried and results, and level of incapacitation (missed school days, interference with normal daily activities)

   B. Physical Examination
      1. Measure blood pressure, pulse rate, temperature
      2. Evaluate heart and lungs
      3. Perform abdominal exam, evaluating for bowel sounds, tenderness, masses, rigidity, guarding, rebound tenderness
      4. Perform pelvic exam; inspect cervix for mucopurulent discharge from the endocervix; gently scrape cervix to test for friability
      5. Perform bimanual exam to check for adnexal tenderness, uterine tenderness, and cervical motion tenderness
      6. Sexually active adolescents should be screened for sexually transmitted diseases

   C. Differential Diagnosis
      1. For primary dysmenorrhea, the most important differential diagnosis to consider is that of secondary dysmenorrhea
      2. For secondary dysmenorrhea, must consider the following
         a. Intrauterine causes such as adenomyosis, myomas, polyps, IUDs, infection
         b. Extrauterine causes such as endometriosis, tumors, inflammation, adhesions, and nongynecologic causes

   D. Diagnostic Tests
      1. For primary dysmenorrhea, none indicated
      2. For secondary dysmenorrhea, H & P should guide test selection; suspicious findings should be evaluated by ultrasound or MRI

V. Plan/Management

   A. For secondary dysmenorrhea, treatment of the underlying cause is indicated; if no obvious cause is uncovered, refer to expert for management

   B. For primary dysmenorrhea, drugs that suppress the production of prostaglandins (PGs) are indicated; best accomplished by using nonsteroidal anti-inflammatory drugs (NSAIDs) at scheduled intervals to prevent re-formation of prostaglandin metabolites and pain recurrence

   C. NSAIDs inhibit prostaglandin synthesis and exhibit antiinflammatory and analgesic activity
      1. The most commonly used NSAIDs for dysmenorrhea come from two classes: fenemates and propionic acids. Important to remind patient to take at scheduled intervals and not PRN
      2. Fenemates are considered the best choice of NSAIDs because they act as antiprostaglandins preventing both the production of PGs and binding of PG to its receptor
         a. Mefenamic acid (Ponstel) 500 mg initial dose, then 250 mg Q 6 H
         b. Has the advantage of more rapid onset and longer duration of activity (naproxen has the same advantage)

3. Propionic acids are also a good choice
   a. Naproxen (Naprosyn) 500 mg initial dose, then 250 mg Q 6-8 H, OR
   b. Ibuprofen (Motrin) 400-800 mg Q 4-8 H, OR
   c. Naproxen sodium (Anaprox) 550 mg initial dose, then 275 mg Q 8-12 H
4. Drug that is selected for treatment should be tried over the course of 2-4 cycles before success or failure is judged
5. If treatment failure occurs with one class, the second trial should utilize the other class
6. Patients almost always respond to this therapy; because this treatment is very successful, a failure to achieve pain relief in the patient should prompt a reevaluation of the diagnosis of primary dysmenorrhea

D. The newest class of NSAIDs, the cyclooxygenase-2 (COX-2) specific inhibitor, includes several drugs that have been approved for treatment of primary dysmenorrhea: one example is rofecoxib (Vioxx)
   1. Dosing is 25-50 mg once daily x 2-3 days each month for women 18 years of age and older; adolescents <18 years, not recommended
   2. May or may not be beneficial in treatment of women with history of GI bleeding or ulceration (but with short course of NSAID treatment needed each month, this is usually not an issue); use in healthy women may not be warranted because of the very high cost (about $3/tablet) and the reluctance of some insurance companies to pay for the medication unless need can be clearly demonstrated (patient must have failed treatment with other, much cheaper, NSAIDs)

E. Oral contraceptives are also highly effective and may be used in addition to or instead of NSAIDs if NSAIDs prove inadequate or if the patient also has contraceptive needs
   1. Oral contraceptives prevent fluctuations of endogenous progesterone levels and are first-line therapy for patients who also desire contraception
   2. Almost all patients with primary dysmenorrhea achieve good pain relief with use of OCs
   3. Low dose combination oral contraceptives should be prescribed if there are no contraindications

F. Nonpharmacologic management
   1. A regular aerobic exercise program may be helpful and should be recommended
   2. Use of acupuncture and acupressure on a weekly basis may also be helpful
   3. Use of a transcutaneous electrical nerve stimulation (TENS) unit is effective in some patients

G. Follow Up
   1. In 3-6 months to evaluate treatment efficacy
   2. If neither NSAIDs nor hormonal therapy provide relieve after 3-6 months of therapy, refer patient for workup for causes of secondary amenorrhea

LABIAL ADHESIONS IN YOUNG CHILDREN

I. Definition: Flap of skin formed by the adherence of the labia minora that completely or partially covers the vaginal opening

II. Pathogenesis: Condition is caused by a combination of inflammation and hypoestrogenization of the labia minora

III Clinical Presentation

A. Occurs primarily in girls younger than 5 years of age, with the peak incidence between 13 and 23 months; average age at diagnosis is 2.5 years

B. Parents are often concerned that the child does not have a vagina or that there is some type of anatomical abnormality

C. Adhesions present as a thin flat membrane of variable length in the midline when the labia majora are spread apart
   1. In most cases, the membrane extends from the clitoris to the posterior fourchette
   2. There is usually a small separation near the urethral meatus which allows for passage of urine
   3. The vaginal orifice is obscured

IV.   Diagnosis/Evaluation

    A.   History
        1.   In children who are able to respond (children 4-5), inquire about dysuria and difficulty voiding
        2.   Ask parent about amount, color, and odor of any vaginal discharge noted on child's underwear
        3.   In children who are able to respond, ask about discomfort and pain
        4.   Cautiously explore whether there is a history of trauma or injury (sexual abuse has been theorized to relate to labial adhesions)
        5.   Explore hygiene practices such as whether the child takes a shower or bath

    B.   Physician Examination

        1.   Visually inspect the vulva
        2.   Check for signs of physical and sexual abuse
        3.   Gently separate the labia majora to visualize the characteristic appearance and location of the adhesions

    C.   Differential Diagnosis: Imperforate hymen (hymen is apparent within the vaginal introitus and the labia are normal)

    D.   Diagnostic Tests: None are indicated

V.   Plan/Management

    A.   Adhesions completely resolve spontaneously in 6-12 months; therefore no treatment beyond explanation and reassurance is necessary in children in whom there is no evidence of obstruction to voiding, urinary tract infection, or discomfort

    B.   Should treatment be indicated or desired by the parent despite counseling, the topical application of estrogen cream (0.1% or 0.01% dienestrol) is effective
        1.   Instruct parent to apply cream BID for 2 weeks followed by once daily application at bedtime for another 2 weeks
        2.   Must show parent how to apply a thin layer of cream directly to the line of the labial adhesion rather than over the entire vulva and to apply gentle traction on the labia laterally at the time of application.

    C.   After separation, labia can be maintained apart by daily baths, good hygiene, and application of gland ointment at bedtime for 6-12 months

    D.   Forceful separation is contraindicated because it may cause adhesions to form again and is traumatic for the child

    E.   Occasionally a second course of treatment is needed

    F.   Follow Up: None indicated

VULVOVAGINAL CANDIDIASIS

I. Definition: Infection of the vulvar area and vagina by *Candida albicans* and other *Candida* sp. or yeasts

II. Pathogenesis

   A. Little is known about factors that contribute to the overgrowth of normal flora in the vagina

   B. When the complex balance of microorganisms changes, however, potentially pathogenic endogenous microorganisms that are part of the normal flora such as *Candida albicans* proliferate to numbers that cause symptoms

   C. Usually caused by *C. albicans* but occasionally caused by other *Candida* sp. or yeasts

III. Clinical Presentation

   A. Approximately 25% of all vaginal infections are due to vulvovaginal candidiasis (VVC); this condition is not transmitted sexually but is often diagnosed in women being evaluated for STDs

   B. An estimated 75% of women will have at least one episode of VVC, and 45% will have two or more episodes; approximately 10-20% of women will have complicated VVC (see box below for definition)

   C. Vulvar pruritus is the cardinal symptom and a white discharge may also be present; vulvar erythema is the most often observed sign, with edema and excoriation of the vulva also often observed; vaginal secretions have a normal pH (3.5-4.5)

   D. Primarily a disease of the childbearing years; pregnancy is the most common predisposing factor

   E. Depressed cell-mediated immunity (such as with HIV+ status, chemotherapy) also is risk factor

   F. Most healthy women with uncomplicated VVC have no precipitating factors; in a minority of women with asymptomatic *Candida* colonization, antibiotic use precipitates VVC

   G. On the basis of clinical presentation, microbiology, host factors, and response to therapy, VVC can be classified as either uncomplicated or complicated

Uncomplicated VVC	Complicated VVC

• Sporadic or infrequent vulvovaginal candidiasis
  OR
	• Recurrent vulvovaginal candidiasis
	  OR

• Mild-to-moderate vulvovaginal candidiasis
  OR
	• Severe vulvovaginal candidiasis
	  OR

• Likely to be *C. albicans*
  OR
	• Non-albicans candidiasis
	  OR

• Non-immunocompromised women	• Women with uncontrolled diabetes, debilitation, or immunosuppression or those who are pregnant

Source: Centers for Disease Control and Prevention (CDC). (2002) Sexually transmitted diseases treatment guidelines 2002. *MMWR 51* (No. RR-6) p. 45

IV. Diagnosis/Evaluation

   A. History
      1. Question about vulvar itching, discharge, odor, dysuria, dyspareunia
      2. Ask about previous occurrences of yeast infections
      3. Ask about predisposing factors such as pregnancy, recent antibiotic or estrogen therapy, history of diabetes, HIV+ status
      4. Ask about douching and use of feminine hygiene products (regular douching should always be discouraged; patients often try douching to relieve symptoms of vaginal infection that instead should be diagnosed and properly treated)

B.   Physical Examination
    1.   Examine vulva for erythema, edema, and excoriation
    2.   Perform pelvic exam and examine vagina for erythema, white patches/plaques; note odor of secretions (should not be malodorous)

C.   Diagnostic Tests
    1.   Obtain sample of vaginal secretions from anterior or lateral vaginal walls on a dry swab and apply to pH paper. In candidiasis, pH of vaginal secretions is ≤4.5 (normal pH of vagina is 3.5-4.5)
    2.   Microscopic examination of slide containing vaginal secretions mixed with 10% potassium hydroxide (KOH) shows typical hyphae and budding yeast

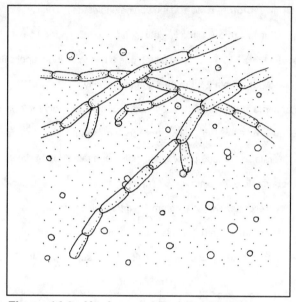

Figure 14.3. Hyphae and Budding Yeast

D.   Differential Diagnosis
    1.   Other common causes of vaginitis--bacterial vaginosis and trichomoniasis
    2.   Common causes of cervicitis--chlamydia and gonorrhea which can sometimes cause a vaginal discharge

V.   Plan/Management

A.   Short-course topical formulations (i.e., single dose and 1-3 day regimens) effectively treat uncomplicated VVC

RECOMMENDED REGIMENS FOR TREATMENT OF UNCOMPLICATED VULVOVAGINAL CANDIDIASIS

Intravaginal Agents:

Butoconazole 2% cream 5 g intravaginally for 3 days, ***

OR

Butoconazole 2% cream 5 g (Butoconazole 1-sustained release), single intravaginal application,

OR

Clotrimazole 1% cream 5 g intravaginally for 7-14 days, ***

OR

Clotrimazole 100 mg vaginal tablet for 7 days,

OR

Clotrimazole 100 mg vaginal tablet, two tablets for 3 days,

OR

Clotrimazole 500 mg vaginal tablet, one tablet in a single application,

OR

Miconazole 2% cream 5 g intravaginally for 7 days,***

OR

Miconazole 100 mg vaginal suppository, one suppository for 7 days,***

OR

Miconazole 200 mg vaginal suppository, one suppository for 3 days,***

OR

Nystatin 100,000-unit vaginal tablet, one tablet for 14 days,

OR

Tioconazole 6.5% ointment 5 g intravaginally in a single application.

OR

Terconazole 0.4% cream 5 g intravaginally for 7 days,

OR

Terconazole 0.8% cream 5 g intravaginally for 3 days,

OR

Terconazole 80 mg vaginal suppository, one suppository for 3 days.

Oral Agent:

Fluconazole 150 mg oral tablet, one tablet in single dose

*** Over-the-counter (OTC) preparations
NOTE: The creams and suppositories in this regimen are oil-based and may weaken latex condoms and diaphragms. Refer to condom product labeling for further information
Source: Centers for Disease Control and Prevention (CDC). (2002) Sexually transmitted diseases treatment guidelines 2002. *MMWR 51* (No. RR-6) p. 45

B. Self-medication with OTC products should be used only in women who have previously been diagnosed with VVC and who experience a recurrence of the same symptoms
1. Persistence of symptoms after self-treatment signals need to seek health care
2. Recurrence within 2 months of self-treatment also indicates need to seek health care

C. Treatment of sexual partners is not necessary unless candidal balanitis is present

D. Follow-up of patients with uncomplicated VVC: Return visits only for those patients in whom symptoms persist or who experience a recurrence within 2 months of onset of initial symptoms

E. **Complicated VVC includes the following categories**: Recurrent VVC (RVVC), severe VVC, non-*albicans* VVC, compromised host, pregnancy, and HIV infection; treatment considerations for each of these categories are considered below

F. **Recurrent VVC (RVVC)** [defined as *four* or more episodes of symptomatic VVC in a 12-month period] affects a small percentage of women (<5%)
1. Pathogenesis of RVVC is poorly understood and most women with RVVC have no apparent predisposing conditions
2. Vaginal cultures should be obtained to confirm the clinical diagnosis and to identify unusual species; *Candida glabrata* does not form pseudohyphae or hyphae and is not easily recognized on microscopy
3. Conventional antimycotic therapies are not as effective against these species as against *C. albicans*
4. Routine treatment of sex partners is controversial
5. Recommended regimens for both initial and maintenance therapy are contained in the table that follows

RECOMMENDED REGIMENS FOR RECURRENT VULVOVAGINAL CANDIDIASIS

Initial Therapy: A longer duration of initial therapy is recommended

7-14 days of topical therapy (see table RECOMMENDED REGIMENS FOR TREATMENT OF UNCOMPLICATED VULVOVAGINAL CANDIDIASIS for medications)

OR

150 mg oral dose of fluconazole repeated 3 days later

This regimen is designed to achieve mycologic remission before initiating a maintenance antifungal regimen

Maintenance Therapy: Long-term treatment with antifungals is recommended for RVVC
Ketoconazole, 100 mg dose once daily OR
Fluconazole, 100-150 mg dose once weekly OR
Itraconazole, 400 mg dose once monthly OR
Itraconazole, 100 mg dose once daily

All maintenance regimens should be continued for 6 months (30%-40% of women will have recurrent disease after maintenance therapy is stopped)

Note: Patients receiving long-term ketoconazole therapy should be monitored for liver toxicity

Source: Centers for Disease Control and Prevention. (2002). Sexually transmitted diseases treatment guidelines 2002. *MMWR, 51* (No. RR-6), p. 46

G. **Severe VVC** is defined as extensive vulvar erythema, edema, excoriation, and fissure formation
   1. Clinical response rates are lower in these patients when treatment is with short courses of topical or oral therapy
   2. Either 7-14 days of topical azole or 150 mg of fluconazole in two sequential doses (second dose 72 hours after initial dose) is recommended

H. Optimal treatment of patients with **non-*albicans* VVC** remains unknown
   1. Longer duration therapy (7-14 days) with a non-fluconazole azole drug is recommended as first-line therapy
   2. If recurrence occurs, 600 mg of boric acid in a gelatin capsule is recommended, administered vaginally once daily for 2 weeks; this regimen has clinical and mycologic eradication rates of about 70%
   3. Referral to a specialist is advised if recurrences continue

I. Treatment of patients with VVC and an underlying debilitating medical condition (**compromised host**)
   1. Efforts to correct modifiable conditions should be made
   2. More prolonged (i.e., 7-14 days) conventional antimycotic treatment is necessary as these patients usually have poor response to short-term therapies

J. Treatment of **pregnant women** with VVC: Only topical azole therapies, applied for 7 days, are recommended for use among pregnant women

K. Treatment of **HIV-infected women** with VVC should not differ from that for seronegative women
   1. Symptomatic VVC is more frequent in seropositive women and correlates with severity of immunodeficiency
   2. Although long-term prophylactic therapy with fluconazole at a dose of 200 mg weekly has been effective in reducing *C. albicans* colonization and symptomatic VVC, it is not recommended for routine primary prophylaxis in HIV-infected women in the absence of recurrent VVC

L. Follow-up of women with complicated VVC is variable, depending on patient diagnosis and recurrence rate

REFERENCES

Abramowicz, M. (2002). Ortho Evra: A contraceptive patch. *The Medical Letter, 44*, 5-8.

Abramowicz, M. (2002). Yasmin—an oral contraceptive with a new progestin. *The Medical Letter, 44*, 55-57.

Ballagh, S.A. (2001). Vaginal ring hormone delivery systems in contraception and menopause. *Clinical Obstetrics & Gynecology, 44*, 106-113.

Barbieri, R.L. (1999). Amenorrhea. In R.L. Barbieri, S.L. Berga, A.H. DeCherney, J. Hade, & E.F. Sheets (Eds.), *Gynecology in primary care: A step-by-step approach* (pp. 1-6). New York: Scientific American, Inc.

Beckman, C.R., Ling, F.W., Laube, D.W., Smith, R.P, Barzansky, B.M., & Herbert, W.N. (2002). *Obstetrics and gynecology* (4th ed.). Philadelphia: Lippincott Williams & Wilkins.

Berga, S.L. (1999). Premenstrual syndrome. In R.L. Barbieri, S.L. Berga, A.H. DeCherney, J. Hade, & E.F. Sheets (Eds.), *Gynecology in primary care: A step-by-step approach* (pp. 11-15). New York: Scientific American, Inc.

Burkman, R.T. (2001). Oral contraceptives: Current status. *Clinical Obstetrics & Gynecology, 44*, 62-72.

Centers for Disease Control and Prevention. (2002). Sexually transmitted diseases treatment guidelines 2002. *MMWR, 51*(No.RR-6), 1-78.

Chan, P.D., & Winkle, C.R. (2002). *Current clinical strategies: Gynecology and obstetrics.* Laguna Hills, CA: CCPS Publishing.

DeCheney, A.H., & Hade, J. (1999). Abnormal vaginal bleeding. In R.L. Barbieri, S.L. Berga, A.H. DeCherney, J. Hade, & E.F. Sheets (Eds.), *Gynecology in primary care: A step-by-step approach* (pp. 7-11). New York: Scientific American, Inc

Dickey, R.P. (2002). *Managing contraceptive pill patients* (11th ed.). Durant, OK: Emis Medical Publishers

Greydanus, D.E., Patel, D.R., & Rimsza, M.E. (2001). Contraception in the adolescent: An update. *Pediatrics, 107*, 562-573.

Grimes, D.A. (2002). Switching emergency contraception to over-the-counter status. *New England Journal of Medicine, 347*, 846-848.

Grimes, D.A., & Raymond, E.G. (2002). Emergency contraception. *Annals of Internal Medicine, 137*, 180-189.

Hatcher, R.A., Trussell, J., Stewart, F., Cates, W., Stewart, G., Guest, F., & Kowal, D. (1998). *Contraceptive technology.* New York: Adrent Media.

Henshaw, S.K. (1998). Unintended pregnancy in the United States. *Family Planning Perspectives, 30,* 329-336.

Kaunitz, A.M. (2001). Injectable long-acting contraception. *Clinical Obstetrics & Gynecology, 44*, 73-91.

Kovalevsky, G., & Barnhart, K.T. (2001). Norplant and other implantable contraceptives. *Clinical Obstetrics & Gynecology, 44*, 92-100.

Krattenmacher, R. (2000). Drospirenone: Pharmacology and pharmacokinetics of a unique progestogen. *Contraception, 62*, 29-38.

Mishell, D.R., Goodwin, T.M., & Brenner, P.F. (2002). *Management of common problems in obstetrics and gynecology.* United Kingdom: Blackwell Publications.

Mulders T.M. & Dieben, T.O. (2001). Use of the novel combined contraceptive vaginal ring NuvaRing for ovulation inhibition. *Fertility & Sterility, 75,* 865-70

Munro, M.G. (2000). Medical management of abnormal bleeding. *Obstetrics and Gynecology Clinics of North America, 27,* 287-301.

Nelson, A., Hatcher, R.A., Zieman, M., Watt, A., Darney, P.D., & Creinin, M.D. (2000). *Managing contraception.* Tiger, GA: Bridging the Gap Foundation.

Nuovo, J. (2002). Evaluation and management of abnormal pap smear. *Primary Care Reports, 8*, 29-36.

Nyirjesy, P. (2001). Chronic vulvovaginal candidiasis. *American Family Physician, 63,* 697-702.

Pena, K.S., & Rosenfeld, J.A. (2001). Evaluation and treatment of galactorrhea. *American Family Physician, 63,* 1763-1775.

Pennachio, D.L. (2001). New approaches to emergency contraception. *Patient Care*, (March 15), 19-27.

Petrozza, J.C., & Poley, K. (1999). Dysfunctional uterine bleeding. In M.G. Curtis & M.P. Hopkins (Eds.), *Glass's office gynecology,* (pp. 241-264). Baltimore: Williams & Wilkins.

Raab, S.S. (2001). Subcategorization of Papanicolaou tests diagnosed as atypical squamous cells of undetermined significance. *American Journal of Clinical Pathology, 116,* 631-634.

Sawaya, G.R., Brown, A.D., Washington, A.E., & Garber, A.M. (2001). Current approaches to cervical-cancer screening. *New England of Medicine, 344,* 1603-1610.

Schwetz, B.A. (2002). New contraceptive patch. *Journal of the American Medical Association, 287,* 1006-1007.

Smallwood, G.H., Meador, M.D., Lenihan, J.P., et al. (2001). Efficacy and safety of a transdermal contraceptive system. *Obstetrics & Gynecology, 96,* 799-805.

Solomon, D., Davey, D., Kuman, R., Moriarty, A., O'Connor, D., Prey, et al. (2002). The 2001 Bethesda system: Terminology for reporting results of cervical cytology. *Journal of the American Medical Association, 287,* 2114-2119.

Stennchever, M.A., Droegmueller, W., Herbst, A., & Mishell, D.R. (2001). *Comprehensive gynecology* (4th ed.). St. Louis: Mosby.

Stephenson, J. (2000). Widely used spermicide may increase, not decrease, risk of HIV transmission. *Journal of the American Medical Association. 284,* 949.

Stewart, F.H., Harper, C.C., Ellertson, C.E., Grimes, D.A., Sawaya, G.F., Trussell, J. (2001). Clinical breast and pelvic examination requirements for hormonal contraception: Current practice vs. evidence. *Journal of the American Medical Association. 285,* 2232-2239.

US Preventive Services Task Force. (1996). *Guide to clinical preventive services.* Baltimore: Williams & Wilkins.

US Preventive Services Task Force. (2002). Screening for breast cancer: Recommendations and rationale. *Annals of Internal Medicine, 137,* 344-346.

Vandenbroucke, J.P., Rosing, J., Bloemenkamp, K.W., Middeldorp, S., Helmerhorst, F.M., Bouma, B.N., et al. (2001). Oral contraceptives and the risk of venous thrombosis. *New England of Medicine, 344,* 1527-1535.

Varila, E., Wahlstrom, T., Rauramo, I. (2001). A 5-year follow-up study on the use of a levonorgestrel intrauterine system in women receiving hormone replacement therapy. *Fertility & Sterility, 76,* 969-973.

Wright, T.C., Cox, J.T., Massad, S., Twiggs, L.B., & Wilkinson, E.J. (2002). 2001 consensus guidelines for the management of women with cervical cytological abnormalities. *Journal of the American Medical Association, 287,* 2120-2129.

Sexually Transmitted Diseases

Mary Virginia Graham

Bacterial Vaginosis
Figure: Clue Cell, White Blood Cell (WBC), & Trichomonas Vaginalis
Table: Recommended & Alternative Regimens for Nonpregnant Women
Table: Recommended Regimens for Pregnant Women

Trichomoniasis

Chlamydial Infection
Table: Special Considerations: Management During Pregnancy

Gonorrhea
Table: Recommended Regimens: Uncomplicated Gonococcal Infections
Table: Recommended Regimens: Uncomplicated Gonococcal Infections of the Pharynx

Mucopurulent Cervicitis

Nongonococcal Urethritis
Table: Recommended & Alternative Regimens for Management of Patients with NGU
Table: Recommended Regimens for Management of Recurrent/Persistent Urethritis

Pelvic Inflammatory Disease
Table: Diagnostic Criteria for PID
Table: Situations When Hospitalization of Patients with Acute PID is Indicated
Table: Recommended Regimens for Ambulatory Treatment of Acute PID

Syphilis
Table: Recommended Treatment of Syphilis in Adults
Table: Management of Sex Partners
Table: Guidelines for Follow-Up of Patients with Syphilis

Genital Herpes Simplex Virus (HSV) Infection
Table: Recommended Regimens: First Clinical Episode
Table: Counseling for Management of Patients with Genital Herpes
Table: Episodic Therapy for Recurrent Genital Herpes
Table: Suppressive Therapy for Recurrent Genital Herpes
Table: Recommended Regimens for Episodic Infection in Persons Infected with HIV
Table: Recommended Regimens for Daily Suppressive Therapy in Persons Infected with HIV

Human Papillomavirus Infection (Genital Warts)
Table: Overview of Treatment
Table: External Genital Warts: Recommended Regimens
Table: Education and Counseling of Patients with Genital Warts

BACTERIAL VAGINOSIS

I. Definition: Clinical syndrome resulting from replacement of the normal H_2O_2-producing *Lactobacillus sp.* in the vagina with high concentrations of anaerobic bacteria (e.g., *Prevotella* sp. and *Mobiluncus* sp.), *Gardnerella vaginalis*, and *Mycoplasma hominis*

II. Pathogenesis

    A. Cause of the microbial alteration is not fully understood

    B. Bacterial vaginosis (BV) is associated with having multiple sex partners, douching, and lack of vaginal lactobacilli

    C. Remains unclear whether BV results from acquisition of a sexually transmitted pathogen

    D. Women who have never been sexually active are rarely affected

III. Clinical Presentation

    A. BV is the most prevalent cause of vaginal discharge and malodor in women

    B. Approximately half of the women with BV may not report symptoms of BV

    C. Clinical criteria require three of the following symptoms or signs
        1. Homogenous, white, noninflammatory discharge that smoothly coats the vaginal walls
        2. Presence of clue cells on microscopic examination
        3. Vaginal fluid pH >4.5
        4. Fishy odor of vaginal discharge before or after addition of 10% KOH (whiff test)

    D. Although it is unclear whether BV is transmitted sexually, this vaginal infection is included in this section because it is often diagnosed in women being evaluated for STDs

IV. Diagnosis/Evaluation

    A. History
        1. Question about onset of symptoms, description of discharge-whether malodorous, its appearance, and amount
        2. Ask if other signs and symptoms are present
        3. Ask if woman uses frequent douching, feminine hygiene products to control odor
        4. Obtain complete menstrual history and history of contraceptive use including condom use

    B. Physical Examination
        1. Examine introitus for homogenous, white discharge
        2. Perform speculum exam and look for homogenous discharge coating vaginal walls; vaginal walls should not appear inflamed; note odor for characteristic foul, fishy odor and obtain specimens for diagnostic testing (see IV.D. below)
        3. Inspect cervix (should be normal) and perform bimanual exam

    C. Differential Diagnosis
        1. Other common cause of vaginitis-trichomoniasis and vulvovaginal candidiasis
        2. Common causes of cervicitis-chlamydia and gonorrhea

    D. Diagnostic Tests
        1. Obtain sample of vaginal secretions from anterior or lateral wall on a dry swab and apply to pH paper. In bacterial vaginosis, pH of vaginal secretions is >4.5 (normal pH of vagina is 3.5-4.5)
        2. Microscopic examination of slide containing vaginal secretions mixed with saline shows clue cells. Secretions have an amine odor before or after being mixed with a drop of 10% KOH (positive whiff test)
        3. Figure 15.1 depicts a clue cell, which is an epithelial cell to which many bacteria are attached

4. When a Gram stain is used to diagnose BV, a determination of the relative concentration of the bacterial morphotypes characteristic of the altered flora of BV is an acceptable laboratory method
5. Culture of *G. vaginalis* is not recommended as a diagnostic tool because it is not specific
6. A DNA probe based test for high concentrations of *G. vaginalis* (Affirm VP III, manufactured by Becton Dickinson, Sparks, MD) may have clinical utility
7. Other commercially available tests that may be useful for diagnosing BV include a card test for the detection of elevated pH and trimethylamine (FemExam test card, manufactured by Cooper Surgical, Shelton, CT) and prolineaminopeptidase (Pip Activity Test Card, manufactured by Litmus Concepts, Inc., Santa Clara, CA)

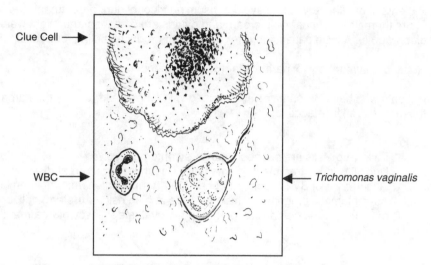

Figure 15.1. Clue Cell, WBC, & *Trichomonas vaginalis*

V. Plan/Management

A. The principal goals of therapy in non-pregnant women are to a) relieve vaginal symptoms and signs of infection and b) reduce the risk for infectious complications after abortion or hysterectomy

B. All women with symptomatic disease require treatment

C. All **symptomatic** pregnant women should be tested and treated: BV during pregnancy is associated with adverse outcomes, including premature rupture of the membranes, preterm labor, preterm birth, and postpartum endometritis

D. Because treatment of BV in **asymptomatic** pregnant women at high-risk for preterm delivery with a recommended regimen has reduced preterm delivery in several clinical trials, some specialists recommend the screening and treatment of these women
   1. Optimal treatment regimens have not been established
   2. Screening (if conducted) and treatment should be performed at the first prenatal visit

E. Data are conflicting regarding whether treatment of asymptomatic pregnant women at low risk for preterm delivery reduces adverse outcomes of pregnancy; therefore consultation/referral to a specialist is recommended

RECOMMENDED REGIMENS FOR NONPREGNANT WOMEN
Metronidazole 500 mg orally twice a day for 7 days, OR
Metronidazole gel 0.75%, one full applicator (5 g) intravaginally once a day for 5 days, OR
Clindamycin cream 2%, one full applicator (5 g) intravaginally at bedtime for 7 days
ALTERNATIVE REGIMENS FOR NONPREGNANT WOMEN
Metronidazole 2 g orally in a single dose, OR
Clindamycin 300 mg orally twice a day for 7 days, OR
Clindamycin ovules 100 mg intravaginally once at bedtime for 3 days

Source: Centers for Disease Control and Prevention. (2002). Sexually transmitted diseases treatment guidelines 2002. *MMWR, 51*(No.RR-6), pp. 43-44

F.   Patients should be advised to avoid consuming alcohol during treatment with metronidazole and for 24 hours thereafter. Clindamycin cream and ovules are oil-based and might weaken latex condoms and diaphragms. Advise patients to refer to condom product labeling for additional information

G.   Routine treatment of sex partners is **not** recommended

H.   Patients who have BV and also are infected with HIV should receive the same treatment regimen as those who are HIV-negative

I.   Follow Up
  1.   Follow-up visits are not necessary if symptoms resolve
  2.   Use alternative treatment regimens for treatment of recurrent disease
  3.   Recurrence of BV is common but no long-term maintenance regimen is recommended
  4.   Asymptomatic pregnant women who are at high risk for preterm delivery should receive follow-up one month after completion of therapy to evaluate efficacy of treatment

TRICHOMONIASIS

I.   Definition: Infection of the vagina by *Trichomonas vaginalis*. May also involve Skene's ducts and lower urinary tract in women, and the lower genitourinary tract in men

II.   Pathogenesis

A.   *Trichomonas vaginalis*, a unicellular flagellated protozoan, causes this primarily STD

B.   Incubation period is 4-28 days with the average being 1 week

III.   Clinical Presentation

A.   Trichomoniasis comprises about 10% of all vaginal infections and is observed primarily in women with normal estrogen levels

B.   Infection is frequently asymptomatic. If symptomatic, symptoms are usually worse immediately after menstruation and during pregnancy

C.   Cardinal symptoms are a diffuse, malodorous, yellow-green discharge and vulvar irritation

D.   Diffuse edema and redness is usually apparent in vulvar and vaginal tissue; the cervix may be inflamed and friable. Rarely, punctate lesions on the cervix give a "strawberry" appearance

E.   Flagellated protozoa are seen in wet prep of vaginal secretions. Vaginal secretions have a pH of >4.5 (normal pH of the vagina is 3.5-4.5)

F.   Most men who are infected with *T. vaginalis* do not have symptoms; others have nongonococcal urethritis (NGU)

IV.   Diagnosis/Evaluation

    A.   History
        1.   Question about presence of discharge, characteristics of discharge (odor, color, amount), and associated symptoms (vulvar irritation, dysuria, dyspareunia)
        2.   Obtain menstrual history and ask if menstruation makes symptoms worse
        3.   In males, question about dysuria
        4.   Obtain history of previous STDs; ask about condom use

    B.   Physical Examination
        1.   Examine external genitalia for signs of vulvar irritation, discharge pooling at introitus or posterior fourchette
        2.   Perform pelvic exam to determine if vagina has erythema, edema; note type, color, and amount of discharge; examine cervix for erythema, friability, discharge
        3.   Obtain specimens for diagnostic testing (see IV.D. below)

    C.   Differential Diagnosis
        1.   Other common causes of vaginitis—bacterial vaginosis and vulvovaginal candidiasis
        2.   Common causes of cervicitis—chlamydia and gonorrhea

    D.   Diagnostic Tests
        1.   Obtain sample of vaginal secretions from anterior or lateral wall on a dry swab and apply to pH paper. In trichomoniasis, pH of vaginal secretions is >4.5 (normal pH of the vagina is 3.5-4.5)
        2.   Microscopic examination of slide containing vaginal secretions mixed with saline solution shows organisms with whip-like flagellae that are motile and slightly larger than WBCs (see Figure 15.1 of trichomonad)
        3.   In men, collect the first 5-30 mL of an early morning specimen of urine. Examine under microscope for trichomonads (this test should be reserved for situations in which this infection is suspected [e.g., contact with trichomoniasis])
        4.   Culture is the most sensitive commercially available method of diagnosis
        5.   No FDA-approved PCR test for *T.vaginalis* is available in US

V.   Plan/Management

    A.   Recommended regimen is metronidazole 2 g orally in a single dose

    B.   Alternative regimen is metronidazole 500 mg twice daily for 7 days

    C.   Management of treatment failure
        1.   If treatment failure occurs with either regimen, retreat with metronidazole 500 mg twice daily for 7 days
        2.   If treatment failure occurs again, patient should be treated with a 2 g dose of metronidazole once daily for 3-5 days
        3.   Patients with laboratory-documented infection who do not respond to the 3-5 days treatment regimen and who have not been reinfected should be managed in consultation with a specialist; consultation is available from CDC (tel.770-488-4115; website: http://www.cdc.gov/std/)

    D.   Sex partners should be treated and patients should be instructed to avoid sex until they have been cured (after therapy has been completed and patient and partner are asymptomatic)

    E.   Patients should be advised to avoid consuming alcohol during treatment with metronidazole and for 24 hours thereafter

    F.   Pregnant women who are symptomatic with trichomoniasis should be treated to ameliorate symptoms with 2 g of metronidazole in a single dose

    G.   Data have not indicated that treating asymptomatic trichomoniasis during pregnancy lessens the association between vaginal trichomoniasis and adverse pregnancy outcomes

    H.   Patients who have trichomoniasis and also are infected with HIV should receive the same treatment regimen as those who are HIV-negative

I.   Follow Up: None indicated for men and women who become asymptomatic after treatment (or who are initially asymptomatic) [See V.C. above for management of treatment failures]

CHLAMYDIAL INFECTION

I.   Definition: A sexually transmitted disease caused by *Chlamydia trachomatis*

II.   Pathogenesis

   A.   *C. trachomatis,* a bacterial agent with at least 18 serologic variants (serovars) divided between the following two biologic variants: oculogenital (serovars A-K) and LGV (serovars L1-L3); genital infections are usually caused by serovars B and D through K

   B.   Infects the genital tract of women most commonly at the transition zone of the endocervix and infects the urethra in men

   C.   Incubation period is variable but is usually at least 1 week

III. Clinical Presentation

   A.   A frequent cause of cervicitis in women and urethritis in men, particularly among sexually active adolescents and young adults

   B.   Asymptomatic sexually active women aged 25 and under should be routinely screened for chlamydial infection; other asymptomatic women at risk for infection should also be screened

   C.   In women, chlamydial infection can cause mucopurulent cervicitis, urethritis, salpingitis, and proctitis; several important sequelae can result from infection including pelvic inflammatory disease (PID), ectopic pregnancy, and infertility

   D.   In men, chlamydial infection can cause nongonococcal urethritis (NGU) and acute epididymitis (see NGU and EPIDIDYMITIS)

   E.   Women may complain of abnormal vaginal discharge, dysuria, abnormal vaginal bleeding, and pelvic pain; commonly they are asymptomatic

   F.   Men may complain of discharge of mucopurulent or purulent material from the urethra and burning during urination; commonly they are asymptomatic

IV.   Diagnosis/Evaluation

   A.   History
         1.   In women, ask about presence of abnormal vaginal discharge, dysuria, abnormal bleeding, pelvic pain, and dyspareunia
         2.   In women, obtain menstrual history and contraceptive history
         3.   In men, ask about presence of mucopurulent/purulent discharge from urethra, presence of burning on urination
         4.   Inquire about sexual history including age at first intercourse, number of partners in past year, types of sexual practices, use of condoms
         5.   Ask about past history of STDs including types, frequency, and treatment

   B.   Physical Examination
         1.   In women, perform speculum exam to inspect cervix for mucopurulent discharge from the endocervix. Obtain specimens for diagnostic testing and gently scrape cervix to test for friability
         2.   Bimanual exam to check for adnexal tenderness, uterine tenderness, and cervical motion tenderness
         3.   In men, examine the urethra for mucopurulent/purulent discharge and obtain specimens for diagnostic testing

C. Differential Diagnosis
   1. PID in women
   2. Gonorrhea

D. Diagnostic Tests
   1. Nucleic acid amplification tests (NAATs) enable detection of *N. gonorrhoeae* and *C. trachomatis* on all specimens; these tests are more sensitive than traditional culture techniques and are the preferred method of detection of *C. trachomatis*
   2. Perform microscopic analysis of vaginal secretions in women (wet-prep and/or Gram stain) to detect coexisting vaginal infections

V. Plan/Management

A. Chlamydia is a reportable disease in every state; such reports are kept strictly confidential, and in most jurisdictions, such reports are protected by statute from subpoena
   1. Reporting can be provider-and/or laboratory-based
   2. Clinicians who are unsure of local reporting requirements should seek advice from local health departments or state STD programs

B. Recommended regimens for treatment of chlamydial infection are azithromycin 1 g orally in a single dose OR doxycycline 100 mg orally twice a day for 7 days

C. Alternative regimens: Erythromycin base 500 mg orally four times a day for 7 day, OR erythromycin ethylsuccinate 800 mg orally four times a day for 7 days, OR ofloxacin 300 mg orally twice a day for 7 days, OR levofloxacin 500 mg orally for 7 days

D. Selecting a treatment
   1. Doxycycline has the advantage of low cost and a long history of safety and efficacy
   2. Azithromycin has the advantage of single-dose administration and may be more cost effective in patients in whom compliance is an issue (single-dose, directly observed therapy [DOT] in the clinical setting is possible)
   3. Ofloxacin is similar in efficacy to doxycycline and azithromycin, but it is more expensive to use and offers no advantage with regard to the dosage regimen
   4. Erythromycin is less efficacious than either azithromycin or doxycycline; in addition, gastrointestinal side effects frequently discourage patients from complying with this regimen
   5. Levofloxacin has not been evaluated for treatment of *C. trachomatis* infection in clinical trials, but its pharmacology and in vitro microbiologic activity are similar to that of ofloxacin

E. To maximize compliance with recommended therapies, medications for chlamydial infections should be dispensed on site, and the first dose should be directly observed

F. To minimize further transmission of infection, patients treated for chlamydia should be instructed to abstain from sexual intercourse for 7 days after single-dose therapy or until completion of a 7-day regimen

G. To minimize the risk for reinfection, patients also should be instructed to abstain from sexual intercourse until all of their sex partners are treated

H. Treatment of sex partners: Patients should be instructed to refer their sex partners for evaluation, testing, and treatment, based on the following guidelines
   1. Sex partners should be evaluated, tested, and treated if they had sexual contact with the patient during the 60 days preceding onset of symptoms in the patient or diagnosis of chlamydia
   2. The most recent sex partner should be evaluated and treated even if the time of the last sexual contact was >60 days before symptom onset or diagnosis

Adapted from: Centers for Disease Control and Prevention. (2002). Sexually transmitted diseases treatment guidelines 2002. *MMWR, 51*(No.RR-6), p. 34.

I. Patients who have chlamydia and also are infected with HIV should receive the same treatment regimen as those who are HIV-negative

J. Follow Up
1. Patients do not need to be retested for chlamydia after completing treatment with doxycycline or azithromycin unless symptoms persist or reinfection is suspected
2. A test-of-cure (TOC) may be considered 3 weeks after completion of treatment with erythromycin; the CDC makes no recommendations relating to retesting for chlamydia after completing treatment with either ofloxacin or levofloxacin
3. Most post-treatment infections result from reinfection, often occurring because sex partners were not treated or because the patient resumed sex among a network of persons with a high prevalence of infection
4. Consider advising all women with chlamydial infection to be rescreened 3-4 months after treatment; rescreening is especially a high priority for adolescents (Note: Rescreening is different from early retesting to detect therapeutic failure [TOC])
5. Rescreen all women treated for chlamydia whenever they next present for care within the following 12 months; regardless of whether patient believes her sex partners were treated
6. See above table, SPECIAL CONSIDERATIONS: MANAGEMENT DURING PREGNANCY for follow-up recommendations for pregnant women

GONORRHEA

I. Definition: A sexually transmitted disease caused by *Neisseria gonorrhoeae,* a Gram-negative diplococcus that prefers columnar and pseudo-stratified epithelium

II. Pathogenesis

A. *N. gonorrhoeae* organisms are Gram-negative diplococci present in exudate and secretions of infected mucous surfaces

B. Transmission results from intimate contact, such as sexual acts and parturition; incubation period is usually 2-7 days

III. Clinical Presentation

A. In the US, an estimated 600,000 new *N. gonorrhoeae* infections occur each year, with the highest rate of infection in sexually active young adults

B. Transmission risk from an infected male to a woman is 70% after one exposure; from infected woman to male is as low as 20% with one exposure but rises to 60-90% with four exposures

C. At least 20% of neonates of infected women delivered vaginally acquire the disease

D. Most infections among men produce symptoms that cause them to seek treatment before serious sequelae develop; however, this may not be soon enough to prevent transmission to others

E. Many infections among women, on the other hand, do not produce symptoms until complications (e.g., PID) have occurred

F. In women, common sites of infection are the urethra, endocervix, upper genital tract, pharynx, and rectum
1. Presenting symptoms include increased vaginal discharge, abnormal uterine bleeding, and dysuria
2. Up to 40% of pelvic inflammatory disease (PID) is caused by gonorrhea
3. Disseminated disease occurs most often when gonorrhea is acquired during menses or pregnancy; common features of disseminated disease include tenosynovitis, petechial or pustular acral skin lesions, fever, and asymmetrical arthralgias
4. A primary measure for controlling gonorrhea is the screening of high-risk women

G. In men, common sites of infection are the urethra, epididymis, prostate, rectum, and pharynx; disseminated disease may also occur

IV. Diagnosis/Evaluation

A. History
1. Inquire about onset and duration of symptoms
2. In women, ask about presence of vaginal discharge, dysuria, abnormal bleeding, abdominal/pelvic pain, and dyspareunia; obtain menstrual history and contraceptive history
3. In men, ask about dysuria, urethral discharge, rectal pain or discharge
4. Inquire about sexual history including age at first intercourse, number of partners in past year, types of sexual practices, and use of condoms
5. Ask about past history of STDs, including types, frequency, treatments

B. Physical Examination
1. Take temperature to determine if febrile
2. In women, perform pelvic exam; inspect Bartholin's and Skene's glands for tenderness and enlargement and the urethra for discharge; inspect cervix for mucopurulent discharge and obtain specimens for diagnostic testing (see IV. D. below); gently scrape cervix to test for friability
3. In women, perform a bimanual exam to check for adnexal tenderness and masses, for uterine tenderness, and cervical motion tenderness
4. In men, examine for urethral discharge and obtain specimens for diagnostic testing (see IV. D. below); if anal sex practiced, perform rectal exam for tenderness and discharge

C. Differential Diagnosis: Chlamydia and pelvic inflammatory disease in women

D. Diagnostic Tests
1. Microscopic examination of Gram-stained smears (for Gram-negative intracellular diplococci) of exudate from the endocervix in females and the urethra in males is helpful in the initial evaluation
2. A number of nonculture gonococcal tests are available which enable detection of both *N. gonorrhoeae* and *C. trachomatis* on specimens—direct fluorescent antibody (DFA) tests, enzyme immunoassays (EIA), and nucleic acid amplification tests (NAATs)

V. Plan/Treatment

A. Gonorrhea is a reportable disease in every state; such reports are kept strictly confidential, and in most jurisdictions, such reports are protected by statute from subpoena
1. Reporting can be provider-and/or laboratory-based
2. Clinicians who are unsure of local reporting requirements should seek advice from local health departments or state STD programs

B. Recommended regimens for treatment of adults and adolescents with uncomplicated gonococcal infections of the cervix, urethra, and rectum are contained in the following table

<table>
<tr><td colspan="1" align="center">**RECOMMENDED REGIMENS: UNCOMPLICATED GONOCOCCAL INFECTIONS
OF THE CERVIX, URETHRA, AND RECTUM**</td></tr>
</table>

Cefixime 400 mg orally in a single dose*
OR
Ceftriaxone 125 mg IM in a single dose
OR
Ciprofloxacin 500 mg orally in a single dose[1]
OR
Ofloxacin 400 mg orally in a single dose[1]
OR
Levofloxacin 250 mg orally in a single dose[1]
PLUS
IF CHLAMYDIAL INFECTION IS NOT RULED OUT
Azithromycin 1 g orally in a single dose
OR
Doxycycline 100 mg orally twice a day for 7 days

* In July 2002, WYETH PHARMACEUTICALS discontinued manufacturing cefixime (Suprax) in the US—no other pharmaceutical company manufactures or sells cefixime tablets or suspension in the US. Cefixime is the only CDC-recommended oral antimicrobial agent to which *N. gonorrhoeae* has not developed significant resistance. In the absence of cefixime, the primary recommended treatment option for gonorrhea if the infection was acquired in Asia, the Pacific Islands (including Hawaii), or California is ceftriaxone

[1]Quinolones should not be used for infections acquired in Asia, the Pacific Islands, (including Hawaii) or California.

Source: Centers for Disease Control and Prevention. (2002). Sexually transmitted diseases treatment guidelines 2002. *MMWR, 51* (No.RR-6), p. 37

C. Alternative Regimens: Spectinomycin 2 g in a single IM dose, OR ceftizoxime 500 mg in a single IM dose, OR cefotaxime 500 mg in a single IM dose

D. Many other antimicrobials are active against *N. gonorrhoeae*, but none have substantial advantages over the recommended regimens

E. **Dual therapy** for gonococcal and chlamydial infections
   1. Routine dual therapy without testing for chlamydia can be cost-effective for populations in which chlamydial infection accompanies 10%-30% of gonococcal infections (cost of therapy is less than cost of testing)
   2. However, in geographic areas in which the rates of coinfection are low, some clinicians might prefer a highly sensitive test for chlamydia rather than treating presumptively
   3. Presumptive treatment is indicated for patients who may not return for test results

F. Gonococcal infections of the pharynx are more difficult to eradicate than infections at urogenital and anorectal sites. Recommended regimens for treatment of adults with uncomplicated gonococcal infections of the pharynx are contained in the table below

RECOMMENDED REGIMENS: UNCOMPLICATED GONOCOCCAL INFECTIONS OF THE PHARYNX
Ceftriaxone 125 mg IM in a single dose
OR
Ciprofloxacin 500 mg orally in a single dose
PLUS
IF CHLAMYDIAL INFECTION IS NOT RULED OUT
Azithromycin 1 g orally in a single dose
OR
Doxycycline 100 mg orally twice daily for 7 days

Source: Centers for Disease Control and Prevention. (2002). Sexually transmitted diseases treatment guidelines 2002. *MMWR, 51* (No.RR-6), pp. 37-38

G. Pregnant women should be treated with a recommended or alternate cephalosporin as listed above. Pregnant women who cannot tolerate a cephalosporin should be administered a single, 2-g dose of spectinomycin IM . Either erythromycin or amoxicillin is recommended for treatment of presumptive or diagnosed *C. trachomatis* infection (see CHLAMYDIAL INFECTIONS section above for treatment of pregnant women) [**Note: Pregnant women should not be treated with quinolones or tetracyclines**]

H.   Treatment of sex partners: Patients should be instructed to refer their sex partners for evaluation, testing, and treatment, based on the following guidelines
      1.   All sex partners of patients who have *N. gonorrhoeae* infection should be evaluated and treated for *N. gonorrhoeae* and *C. trachomatis* infections if their last sexual contact with the patient was within 60 days before onset of symptoms or diagnosis of infection in the patient
      2.   If the patient's most recent sexual encounter was >60 days before onset of symptoms or diagnosis, the patient's most recent sex partner should be treated

I.   Patients should be instructed to avoid sexual intercourse until therapy is completed and until they and their sex partners no longer have symptoms

J.   Persons with disseminated gonococcal infection (bacteremia) should be hospitalized for initial parenteral antibiotic therapy

K.   Patients who have gonorrhea and also are infected with HIV should receive the same treatment regimen as those who are HIV-negative

L.   Follow Up
      1.   Patients with uncomplicated gonorrhea and who are treated with any of the recommended regimens need not return for a test of cure
      2.   Patients with persistent symptoms after treatment need to be re-evaluated for antimicrobial susceptibility
      3.   Persistence of symptoms usually results from reinfection rather than treatment failure (indicates need to improve patient education and partner referral)

MUCOPURULENT CERVICITIS

I.   Definition: A sexually transmitted syndrome in which there is purulent or mucopurulent endocervical exudate visible in the endocervical canal or in an endocervical swab specimen

II.   Pathogenesis

      A.   Mucopurulent cervicitis (MPC) can be caused by *Chlamydia trachomatis* and *Neisseria gonorrhoeae*, but in **most cases** neither organism can be isolated

      B.   Other non-microbiologic determinants (e.g., inflammation in the zone of ectopy) may be involved

III. Clinical Presentation

      A.   MPC is often asymptomatic, but some women have an abnormal vaginal discharge and vaginal bleeding (e.g., after sexual intercourse)

      B.   Speculum examination of cervix reveals a purulent or mucopurulent endocervical exudate visible in the endocervical canal or in an endocervical specimen examined under the microscope

      C.   MPC can persist despite repeated courses of antimicrobial therapy

      D.   Some experts consider an increased number of polymorphonuclear leukocytes (PMNs) on Gram stain of endocervical secretions as being helpful in the diagnosis of MPC; however, this criterion has not been standardized and is not available in some settings

IV.   Diagnosis/Evaluation

      A.   History
            1.   Inquire about the onset and duration of symptoms, if present
            2.   Ask about presence of vaginal discharge, dysuria, abnormal bleeding particularly after sexual intercourse
            3.   Obtain menstrual history and contraceptive history

4. Inquire about sexual history including age at first intercourse, present partner(s), types of sexual practices, and use of condoms
5. Inquire about past history of STDs, including types, frequency, treatments

B. Physical Examination
1. Determine if febrile
2. Perform speculum exam to inspect cervix, to sample secretions for purulent or mucopurulent discharge, and to obtain specimens for diagnostic testing (see IV.D. below); assess for cervical motion tenderness and gently scrape cervix to determine friability
3. Perform bimanual exam, checking for adnexal tenderness, masses

C. Differential Diagnosis
1. Urinary tract infection
2. Chlamydia
3. Gonorrhea
4. Trichomonal vaginitis

D. Diagnostic Tests
1. Gram stain of endocervical secretions looking for PMNs and intracellular Gram-negative diplococci
2. Perform nucleic acid amplification tests (NAATs) or other nonculture tests which enable detection of both *C. trachomatis* and *N. gonhrrhoeae*
3. Wet mount exam for trichomonas
4. Urine for culture and sensitivity (if symptomatic)

V. Plan/Management

A. Results of sensitive tests for *C. trachomatis* and *N. gonorrhoeae* should determine the need for treatment

B. Empiric treatment should be considered for patients suspected of having ghonorrhea and/or chlamydia if a) the prevalences of these infections are high in the patient population, and b) the patient might be difficult to locate for treatment

C. Sex partners of women with MPC should be notified, examined, and treated for the STD identified or suspected in the index patient
1. A microbiologic test of cure is usually not recommended
2. Patients and their sex partners should be counseled to abstain from sexual intercourse until therapy is completed (i.e., 7 days after a single-dose regimen or after completion of a 7-day regimen)

D. Patients who have MPC and who also are infected with HIV should receive the same treatment regimen as those who are HIV-negative

E. Follow Up
1. Should be as recommended for the infections for which the woman is being treated
2. If symptoms persist, woman should be instructed to return for reevaluation and to abstain from sexual intercourse even if the course of prescribed therapy has been completed

NONGONOCOCCAL URETHRITIS (NGU)

I. Definition: Inflammation of the urethra not caused by gonococcal infection and characterized by a mucoid or purulent urethral discharge

II. Pathogenesis

A. *Chlamydia trachomatis* is a frequent cause of NGU (15%-55% of cases); however, the prevalence differs by age group with lower prevalence of this organism among older men

B. Etiology of most cases of nonchlaymdial NGU is unknown; *Ureaplasma urealyticum* and *Mycoplasma genitalium* have been implicated as causes in some studies

C. *Trichomonas vaginalis* and herpes simples virus (HSV) sometimes cause NGU

III. Clinical Presentation

A. Most common STD syndrome in males living in industrialized countries

B. NGU is substantially more common than gonococcal urethritis in most areas of US

C. Many men are entirely asymptomatic; primary complaints are urethral discharge (yellow, white, or cloudy), dysuria, or urethral itching

D. Urethritis can be documented by the presence of **any** of the following signs:
1. Mucopurulent or purulent discharge
2. Gram stain of urethral secretions demonstrating ≥5 WBCs per oil immersion field; Gram stain is the preferred rapid diagnostic test for evaluating urethritis
3. Positive leukocyte esterase test on first-void urine, or microscopic examination of first-void urine demonstrating ≥10 WBCs per high power field

IV. Diagnosis/Evaluation

A. History
1. Ask about onset, duration of symptoms
2. Inquire about presence and color of discharge, presence of dysuria, and urethral itching
3. Inquire about sexual history including age at first intercourse, number of partners in the past year, types of sexual practices, use of condoms
4. Inquire about past history of STDs, including types, frequency, and treatments

B. Physical Examination: Examine urethra for mucopurulent discharge and obtain specimens for diagnostic testing (see IV.D. below)

C. Differential Diagnosis: Gonorrhea

D. Diagnostic Tests
1. Gram-stain urethral smear (≥5 WBCs per oil immersion field PLUS no intracellular Gram-negative diplococci are expected findings)
2. Positive leukocyte esterase test on first void urine, or microscopic examination of first-void urine demonstrating ≥10 WBCs per high power field
3. Test for *N. gonorrhoeae* and *C. trachomatis* using nonculture tests such as nucleic acid amplification tests (NAATs), which enable detection of both organisms

V. Plan/Management

A. Treatment should be initiated as soon as possible after diagnosis; to improve compliance, medication should be provided in the clinic/office

B. Recommended regimens and alternative regimens are contained in the tables that follow

RECOMMENDED REGIMENS FOR MANAGEMENT OF PATIENTS WITH NGU
Azithromycin 1 g orally in a single dose   OR   Doxycycline 100 mg orally twice a day for 7 days

Source: Centers for Disease Control and Prevention. (2002). Sexually transmitted diseases treatment guidelines 2002. *MMWR, 51*(No.RR-6), p. 31.

ALTERNATIVE REGIMENS FOR MANAGEMENT OF PATIENTS WITH NGU
Erythromycin base 500 mg orally four times a day for 7 days
OR
Erythromycin ethylsuccinate 800 mg orally four times a day for 7 days
OR
Ofloxacin 300 mg twice a day for 7 days
OR
Levofloxacin 500 mg once daily for 7 days

Source: Centers for Disease Control and Prevention. (2002). Sexually transmitted diseases treatment guidelines 2002. *MMWR, 51*(No.RR-6), p. 31.

C. If none of the criteria for confirming urethritis are met (see III.D. above), treatment should be deferred until the diagnostic test results for *N. gonorrhoeae* and *C. trachomatis* are obtained
    1. If the results are positive for either infection, the appropriate treatment should be given and sex partners referred for evaluation and treatment
    2. Empiric treatment of symptoms without documentation of urethritis is recommended only for patients at high risk for infection who are unlikely to return for follow-up (such patients should be treated for both gonorrhea and chlamydia) [see GONORRHEA and CHLAMYDIA for treatment recommendations]
    3. Partners of patients empirically treated should be evaluated and treated

D. Management of sex partners: Patients should refer for evaluation and treatment all sex partners within the preceding 60 days. Because a specific diagnosis may facilitate partner referral, testing for gonorrhea and chlamydia is encouraged

E. Recurrent and persistent NGU may be due to a lack of compliance, or more often, reinfection by untreated sex partner
    1. Men with persistent or recurrent urethritis should be re-treated with the initial regimen if they failed to comply with the treatment regimen or if they were re-exposed to an untreated sex partner
    2. Otherwise, a culture of an intraurethral swab specimen and a first-void urine specimen for *T. vaginalis* should be performed
    3. If the patient was compliant with the initial regimen and re-exposure can be excluded, the following regimen is recommended

RECOMMENDED REGIMENS FOR MANAGEMENT OF PATIENTS WITH RECURRENT/PERSISTENT URETHRITIS **(FOR USE IN PATIENTS WHO WERE COMPLIANT WITH INITIAL THERAPY AND RE-EXPOSURE CAN BE EXCLUDED)**	
Metronidazole 2 g orally in a single dose **PLUS**	Erythromycin base 500 mg PO four times a day for 7 days **OR** Erythromycin ethylsuccinate 800 mg PO four times a day for 7 days

Source: Centers for Disease Control and Prevention. (2002). Sexually transmitted diseases treatment guidelines 2002. *MMWR, 51* (No.RR-6), p. 31

    4. Refer for evaluation by an expert if objective signs of urethritis continue after adequate treatment

F. Patients who have NGU and also are infected with HIV should receive the same treatment regimen as those who are HIV-negative

G. Follow Up
    1. Patients should be instructed to return for evaluation if symptoms persist or recur after completion of therapy
    2. Patients should be instructed to abstain from sexual intercourse until 7 days after therapy is initiated

PELVIC INFLAMMATORY DISEASE (PID)

I. Definition: A spectrum of inflammatory disorders of the upper female genital tract, including any combination of endometritis, salpingitis, tubo-ovarian abscess, and pelvic peritonitis

II. Pathogenesis

    A. Sexually transmitted organisms, especially *Neisseria gonorrhoeae* and *Chlamydia trachomatis*, are implicated in many cases

    B. Microorganisms that can be part of the vaginal flora (e.g., anaerobes, *G. vaginalis*, *H. influenzae*, enteric Gram-negative rods, and *S. agalactiae*) also have been associated with PID

    C. In addition, cytomegalovirus (CMV), *M. hominis* and *U. urealyticum* may be etiologic agents in some cases of PID

III. Clinical Presentation

    A. Incidence of PID is highest among sexually active adolescents

    B. Variables that **increase** risk of PID include adolescence, multiple sex partners, previous episode of STD, use of an intrauterine device, and douching

    C. Variables that **decrease** risk include use of oral contraceptives and barrier contraceptives

    D. Most typical presentation is continuous bilateral lower abdominal or pelvic pain that may be accompanied by fever, nausea, and vomiting

    E. In many patients the infection is asymptomatic (silent PID) or symptoms are vague and mild with abnormal vaginal bleeding, dyspareunia, or change in vaginal discharge as the only signs and symptoms (atypical PID); many episodes of PID go unrecognized

    F. PID symptoms most often begin within one week of onset of menses

    G. The diagnosis of PID usually is based on clinical findings; no single historical, physical, or laboratory finding is both sensitive and specific for the diagnosis

    H. The following recommendations for diagnosing PID are made by the CDC to help healthcare providers recognize when PID should be suspected and when there is a need to obtain additional information to increase diagnostic certainty

DIAGNOSTIC CRITERIA FOR PID

Minimum Criteria

Empiric treatment of PID should be instituted in sexually active young women and others at risk for STDs if all the following **minimum criteria** are present and no other cause(s) for the illness can be identified
- Uterine/adnexal tenderness or
- Cervical motion tenderness

Additional Criteria

More elaborate diagnostic evaluation often is needed because incorrect diagnosis and management may cause unnecessary morbidity. These additional criteria may be used to increase the specificity of the minimum criteria listed above
- Oral temperature >101F (>38.3C)
- Abnormal cervical or vaginal mucopurulent discharge
- Presence of white blood cells (WBCs) on saline microscopy of vaginal secretions
- Elevated erythrocyte sedimentation rate
- Elevated C-reactive protein
- Laboratory documentation of cervical infection with *N. gonorrhoeae* or *C. trachomatis*

Definitive Criteria

The **most specific criteria** for diagnosing PID include the following
- Endometrial biopsy with histopathologic evidence of endometritis
- Transvaginal sonography or magnetic resonance imaging techniques showing thickened fluid-filled tubes with or without free pelvic fluid or tubo-ovarian complex, and
- Laparoscopic abnormalities consistent with PID

Adapted from: Centers for Disease Control and Prevention. (2002). Sexually transmitted diseases treatment guidelines 2002. *MMWR, 51*(No.RR-6), pp. 48-49

IV. Diagnosis/Evaluation

    A. History
        1. Ask about presence of lower abdominal/pelvic pain, including onset, duration, location, and character or pain
        2. Ask the patient if she has had fever
        3. Inquire about presence of vaginal discharge, postcoital bleeding, spotting between menstrual periods, and gastrointestinal symptoms
        4. Obtain sexual history including age at first intercourse, number of partners in past year, types of sexual practices, and contraceptive history (ask if IUD is used)
        5. Inquire about past history of STDs, including type, frequency, treatments; ask about HIV+ status
        6. Obtain complete menstrual history including pattern of recent menstrual cycles and a description of the last menses (Ask: "Did onset of pain coincide with LMP?")

    B. Physical Examination
        1. Determine if febrile
        2. Examine abdomen for tenderness, masses, signs of peritonitis
        3. On speculum exam, inspect cervix for inflammation; insert swab(s) into cervix to sample mucus in order to obtain specimens for diagnostic testing, and to examine gross appearance of cervical secretions (a transparent discharge similar to clear hair styling gel is normal; secretions that appear yellow or green on swab are not normal)
        4. Perform bimanual exam to check for adnexal masses, uterine tenderness, and for cervical motion tenderness (pain that occurs when cervix is moved from side to side)

    C. Differential Diagnosis
        1. Appendicitis
        2. Ectopic pregnancy
        3. Tubo-ovarian abscess
        4. Ovarian cyst
        5. Pyelonephritis

D. Diagnostic Tests
1. Pregnancy Test
2. Nonculture tests such as nucleic acid amplification tests (NAATs) which enable detection of both *N. gonorrhoeae* and *C. trachomatis* should be obtained before treatment
3. CBC with differential and sedimentation rate
4. Wet prep or Gram stain of endocervical secretions
   a. If number of epithelial cells > than number of WBCs per high-powered field, then patient almost certainly does not have PID
   b. If WBCs outnumber epithelial cells per high powered field, patient may have PID
5. VDRL or RPR

V. Plan/Management

A. PID treatment regimens must provide empiric, broad-spectrum coverage of likely pathogens. Antimicrobial coverage should include *N. gonorrhoeae, C. trachomatis*, anaerobes, Gram-negative facultative bacteria, and streptococci

B. Inpatient therapy for every case of PID is unrealistic. The CDC has made recommendations for when to select inpatient therapy and these recommendations are contained in the following table

SITUATIONS WHEN HOSPITALIZATION OF PATIENTS WITH ACUTE PID IS INDICATED
• Surgical emergencies such as appendicitis and ectopic pregnancy cannot be excluded • Patient has a tubo-ovarian abscess • Patient is pregnant • Patient has severe illness, nausea and vomiting, or high fever • Patients is unable to follow or tolerate an outpatient oral regimen • Patient fails to respond clinically to oral antimicrobial therapy

Adapted from: Centers for Disease Control and Prevention. (2002). Sexually transmitted diseases treatment guidelines 2002. *MMWR, 51* (No.RR-6), p. 49

C. Outpatient therapy for PID is described in the table below

RECOMMENDED REGIMENS FOR AMBULATORY TREATMENT OF ACUTE PID
Regimen A
Ofloxacin 400 mg orally twice a day for 14 days **OR** Levofloxacin 500 mg orally once daily for 14 days ***WITH OR WITHOUT*** Metronidazole 500 mg orally BID for 14 days
Regimen B
Cefoxitin 2 g IM plus Probenecid 1 g orally in a single dose concurrently, **OR** ceftriaxone 250 mg IM in a single dose, **OR** other parenteral third-generation cephalosporin (e.g., ceftizoxime or cefotaxime) ***PLUS*** Doxycycline 100 mg orally twice a day for 14 days ***WITH or WITHOUT*** Metronidazole 500 mg orally twice a day for 14 days

Source: Centers for Disease Control and Prevention. (2002). Sexually transmitted diseases treatment guidelines 2002. *MMWR, 51*(No.RR-6), p. 51-52

D. Management of sex partners:
1. Male sex partners of women with PID should be examined and treated if they had sexual contact with patient during the 60 day period preceding onset of symptoms in patient
2. Evaluation and treatment are imperative because of the risk of reinfection of the patient and the strong likelihood of urethral gonococcal or chlamydial infection in the sex partner
3. Sex partners should be treated empirically with regimens effective against both *C. trachomatis* and *N. gonorrhoeae* regardless of the apparent etiology of PID

E. Pregnant women who have suspected PID should be hospitalized and treated with parenteral antibiotics

F. Whether the management of immunodeficient HIV-infected women with PID requires more aggressive interventions (e.g., hospitalization or parenteral antimicrobial regimens) has not been determined

G. Follow Up
1. Patients treated on an ambulatory basis need to be monitored closely and reevaluated within 72 hours for clinical improvement (**Note**: Clinical improvement is defined as defervescence; reduction in direct or rebound abdominal tenderness; reduction in uterine, adnexal, and cervical motion tenderness within 72 hours of initiation of therapy)
2. Patients who do not demonstrate improvement within 72 hours usually require hospitalization, additional diagnostic tests, and surgical intervention
3. Some experts recommend rescreening for *C. trachomatis* and *N. gonorrhoeae* 4-6 weeks after therapy is completed in women with documented infection with these pathogens

SYPHILIS

I. Definition: A systemic sexually transmitted disease involving multiple organ systems and caused by *Treponema pallidum*, a spirochete

II. Pathogenesis

A. *T. pallidum* is a thin, delicate organism with humans as the sole host

B. Organism penetrates intact skin or mucous membrane during sexual contact, multiplies, and rapidly spreads to regional lymph nodes

C. Spirochetes enter the blood stream within hours and are transported to other tissues

D. Congenital syphilis results from transplacental passage of the organism

E. Incubation period for acquired primary syphilis is about 3 weeks, but ranges from 10-90 days after exposure

III. Clinical Presentation

A. The pattern of syphilis infection in the US has changed during recent years; although the South continues to have the highest rate (56.2% in 2001) of primary and secondary (P&S) syphilis, rates actually decreased in the South over the two-year period (2000-2001) by 8.1%
1. In the West, rates increased 40% and in the Northeast rates increased 57.1% over that same time period
2. Racial/ethnic disparities in syphilis rates are decreasing because of declining rates among non-Hispanic blacks and increasing rates among non-Hispanic whites
3. The number of P&S cases increased among men during 2000-2001, ending the decade-long trend characterized by annual declines in syphilis cases among both men and women
4. This increase in syphilis cases among men is associated with reports in several cities of syphilis outbreaks among men having sex with men (MSM); these outbreaks were characterized by high rates of HIV co-infection and high-risk sexual behavior among subpopulations of MSM

B. To guide therapeutic decisions and disease intervention strategies, acquired syphilis has been divided into the following stages: primary, secondary, latent, and tertiary

C. Primary syphilis: Characterized by appearance of ulcer or chancre at site of inoculation, usually on genitals 3-4 weeks after exposure
1. Genital lesions are usually indurated and painless
2. Extragenital lesions (e.g., lips, breast) are often painful
3. Regional lymphadenopathy usually present
4. Chancre persists for 1-5 weeks and heals spontaneously

D. Secondary syphilis: Occurs about 6-8 weeks later and is characterized by flu-like symptoms—headache, generalized arthralgia, malaise, fever, and lymphadenopathy, followed by a generalized rash
1. Rash is macular, papular, annular, or follicular; often involves the palms and soles
2. Rash persists for 2-6 weeks then spontaneously heals
3. Mucous patches often occur in mouth, throat, on cervix; flat, papular lesions (condylomata lata) occur in intertriginous areas

4. About 25% of infected persons have at least one cutaneous relapse
5. Secondary syphilis is the most contagious state of the disease
6. Even without treatment, signs of first 2 stages resolve spontaneously, and infected persons enter the next state: the latent state

E. Latent syphilis: Defined as those infections characterized by seroactivity without other evidence of disease
1. Patients can be diagnosed as having early latent syphilis if, within the year preceding the evaluation, they had
    a. A documented seroconversion,
    b. Unequivocal symptoms of primary or secondary syphilis, or
    c. A sex partner documented to have primary, secondary, or early latent syphilis
2. All other cases of latent syphiilis are either late latent syphilis or latent syphilis of unknown duration
3. Difficult to make this distinction in practice, because exact date of infection is usually difficult to establish
4. Nontreponemal serologic titers usually are higher during early latent syphilis than late latent syphilis; this characteristic cannot be relied upon as the sole distinguishing factor
5. About 1/3 of persons with latent syphilis are little inconvenienced by the disease
6. After a variable period of latency, about 1/3 of untreated cases go on to develop tertiary syphilis, and about 28% of these will die because of the disease

F. Tertiary syphilis: Refers to gumma and cardiovascular syphilis, but not to all neurosyphilis (when there is evidence of central nervous system infection); since the advent of penicillin therapy, all forms of tertiary syphilis have become uncommon

G. Congenital syphilis involves multiple organ systems with the stage of syphilis in the mother determining the effects on the fetus
1. Early congenital syphilis occurs from birth to age 2 and is characterized by mucocutaneous lesions, rhinitis, and other symptoms
2. Congenital syphilis can be asymptomatic, especially in the first weeks of life
3. Late congenital syphilis is characterized by bone and joint disorders, cranial neuropathies, and interstitial keratitis which causes blindness if untreated

IV. Diagnosis/Evaluation

A. History
1. Question about onset, duration of symptoms
2. Ask about presence or history of chancre (when it appeared, where located, if symptomatic, when healed)
3. Inquire about presence (or history of) rash, mucous patches, condylomata lata
4. Ask about sexual behavior, use of condoms
5. Determine if sex partner has had similar symptoms
6. Obtain past history of STDs, including types, frequency, duration, treatment; establish HIV status
7. Obtain past medical history, medication history, drug and alcohol use, allergies

B. Physical Examination
1. Examine genital area and other skin surfaces (breast, buttocks) for characteristic chancre (primary syphilis)
2. Look for mucocutaneous lesions of secondary syphilis

C. Differential Diagnosis
1. Primary syphilis: Syphilis can mimic all lesions that appear to be genital ulcers: genital herpes, chancroid, lymphogranuloma venereum, scabies, balanitis should all be suspect
2. Secondary syphilis: Syphilis can mimic many skin disorders: all undiagnosed mucous or cutaneous eruptions should be suspect

D. Diagnostic Tests
1. Darkfield microscopy and direct fluorescent antibody tests of lesion exudate or tissue are the definitive methods for diagnosing early syphilis
2. A presumptive diagnosis is possible with the use of two types of serologic tests for syphilis
    a. Nontreponemal-specific tests: Rapid Plasma Reagin (RPR) test and Venereal Disease Research Laboratory (VDRL) test

b. Treponemal-specific tests: Fluorescent treponemal antibody absorbed (FTA-ABS) and *T. pallidum* particle agglutination (TP-PA)

c. Use of only one type of serologic test is insufficient for diagnosis, because false-positive nontreponemal test results may occur secondary to some medical conditions

3. VDRL and RPR are used for initial screening, to monitor disease activity, and to determine efficacy of treatment

   a. A fourfold change in titer, equivalent to a change of two dilutions (e.g., from 1:16 to 1:4 or from I:8 to 1:32) is considered necessary to demonstrate a clinically significant difference between two nontreponemal test results that were obtained using the same serologic test

   b. A decline in titers equivalent to a change of two dilutions indicates effective treatment, and a failure of test titers to decline fourfold by 6 to 12 months after therapy indicates treatment failure

   c. RPR is test most often used today, but the tests are comparable

4. For sequential serologic tests, the same test (VDRL or RPR) should be used

5. Treponemal tests are used to confirm diagnosis of syphilis in persons with reactive VDRL or RPR

   a. Usually remain reactive for life regardless of treatment or disease activity

   b. About 15%-25% of patients treated during primary stage revert to being serologically nonreactive after 2-3 years

6. Nontreponemal tests usually become nonreactive with time after treatment; in some patients, nontreponemal antibodies can persist at a low titer for a long period of time; response is referred to as the "serofast reaction"

V. Plan/Treatment

A. Report all cases of syphilis to appropriate public health authorities so that case finding can be performed

B. Treatment is based on clinical and serologic staging of the disease and is summarized in the following table

RECOMMENDED TREATMENT OF SYPHILIS IN ADULTS	
Stage	**Treatment***
Primary and Secondary Syphilis	Benzathine penicillin G 2.4 million units IM in a single dose *Other Management Considerations:* Always test for HIV infection. If symptoms or signs of neurologic or ophthalmic disease are present, refer for evaluation (invasion of CSF by *T. pallidum* is common among adults with primary or secondary syphilis; however, CSF analysis is not recommended for routine evaluation of patients unless clinical signs or symptoms are present)
Latent syphilis: Early latent syphilis and late latent syphilis (syphilis of unknown duration)	**Early Latent:** Benzathine penicillin G 2.4 million units IM in a single dose **Late Latent (or when duration is unknown):** Benzathine penicillin G 7.2 million units total, given as three doses of 2.4 million units IM each at 1-week intervals *Other Management Considerations:* Always test for HIV infection. All patients who have latent syphilis should be evaluated clinically for evidence of tertiary disease (e.g., aortitis, gumma, and iritis) and for evidence of neurologic involvement (e.g., cognitive dysfunction, motor or sensory deficits). Some experts recommend performing a CSF examination on all patients with latent syphilis and a nontreponemal serologic test of ≥1:32
Tertiary disease (no evidence of neurosyphilis)	As for **late latent** disease, with appropriate management of complications (refer to infectious diseases [ID] specialist)
Neurosyphilis	Aqueous crystalline penicillin G, 18-24 million units/day given as 3-4 million units IV every 4 hours for 10-14 days, or procaine penicillin 2-4 million units IM a day PLUS Probenecid 500 mg orally QID both for 10-14 days (refer to ID specialist)

*For patients allergic to penicillin, see alternatives under V.D. below

Adapted from Centers for Disease Control and Prevention. (2002). Sexually transmitted diseases treatment guidelines 2002. *MMWR,51* (No.RR-6), pp. 20-23

C. The Jarisch-Herxheimer reaction is an acute febrile reaction frequently accompanied by headache, myalgia, and other symptoms that usually occur within the first 24 hours after any therapy for syphilis

1. Patients should be informed about this possible adverse reaction

2. Occurs most often among patients who have early syphilis

3. Antipyretics may be used, but they have not been shown to prevent the reaction

D. Management of nonpregnant, penicillin-allergic patients who have primary and secondary syphilis

1. Data to support the use of alternatives to penicillin in the treatment of primary and secondary syphilis are limited

2. Doxycycline (100 mg twice daily for 14 days) and tetracycline (500 mg four times daily for 14 days) are regimens that have been used for many years; compliance is usually better with doxycycline as it causes fewer gastrointestinal side effects than tetracycline
3. Some experts recommend ceftriaxone 1 g daily either IM or IV for 8-10 days
4. Also, preliminary data suggest that azithromycin 2 g may be effective as a single oral dose
5. Patients with penicillin allergy whose compliance with alternative therapies or follow-up cannot be ensured should be desensitized and treated with benzathine penicillin (consult expert)

E. Management of nonpregnant, penicillin-allergic patients who have latent syphilis—early latent and late latent syphilis or syphilis of unknown duration
1. Effectiveness of alternatives to penicillin in the treatment of latent syphilis has not been well documented
2. **Early latent:** Should respond to therapies recommended as alternatives to penicillin for the treatment of primary and secondary syphilis (under V.D. above)
3. **Late latent syphilis or latent syphilis of unknown duration:** The only acceptable alternatives for treatment of this stage of the disease are doxycycline 100 mg orally twice daily for 28 days, **or** tetracycline 500 mg orally four times daily for 28 days
4. These therapies should be used only in conjunction with close serologic and clinical follow-up

F. Management of nonpregnant, penicillin-allergic patients who have tertiary syphilis: Treat according to alternative regimens for **late latent** syphilis (refer to ID specialist for management)

G. Patients with neurosyphilis require expert management (refer to ID specialist)

H. Management of sex partners should be guided by the following recommendations

---

MANAGEMENT OF SEX PARTNERS

Sexual transmission of *T. pallidum* occurs only when mucocutaneous syphilitic lesions are present; such manifestations are uncommon after the first year of infection. **However, patients exposed sexually to a patient who has syphilis in any stage should be evaluated both clinically and serologically as follows:**

Persons exposed within the 90 days preceding the diagnosis of primary, secondary, or early latent syphilis in a sex partner might be infected even if seronegative--**Treat presumptively**

Persons exposed >90 days before the diagnosis of primary, secondary, or early latent syphilis in a sex partner and in whom serologic test results are not available immediately and the opportunity for follow-up is uncertain--**Treat presumptively**

For purposes of **partner notification and presumptive treatment of exposed sex partners**, patients with syphilis of unknown duration with high nontreponemal serologic test titers (defined as ≥1:32) can be assumed to have early syphilis. However, serologic titers should not be used to differentiate early from late latent syphilis for the purpose of determining treatment for the index case

Long-term sex partners of patients who have latent syphilis should be evaluated clinically and serologicaly for syphilis and treated on basis of findings

---

Adapted from Centers for Disease Control and Prevention. (2002). Sexually transmitted diseases treatment guidelines. 2002. *MMWR,51* (No.RR-6), p. 20

I. Congenital syphilis
1. Infants born to mothers who have reactive nontrepnemal and treponemal test results should be evaluated with a quantitative nontreponemal serologic test (RPR or VDRL)
   a. Test should be performed on infant serum
   b. Umbilical cord blood may be contaminated with maternal blood and might yield a false-positive result
   c. A treponemal test of a newborn's serum is not necessary
2. Evaluation of infant includes the following
   a. Complete physical exam of neonate for evidence of congenital syphilis
   b. Pathologic examination of the placenta or umbilical cord using specific fluorescent antitreponemal antibody staining
   c. Darkfield microscopic examination or direct fluorescent antibody staining of any suspicious lesions or body fluids (example, nasal discharge)
3. Consult expert regarding therapy decisions and treatment guidelines for all infants born to seroreactive mothers

J.   Special Considerations: Management of Syphilis in Pregnancy
1.   All women should be screened serologically for syphilis at the first prenatal visit (with additional screening at 28 weeks and at delivery for high-risk patients)
2.   Seropositive pregnant women should be referred for expert care

K.   Syphilis in HIV infected persons
1.   Diagnostic considerations
a.   Both treponemal and non-treponemal serologic tests for syphilis can be interpreted in usual manner for most patients who are coinfected with *T. pallidum* and HIV (aberrant serologic responses do occur, but are uncommon)
b.   When clinical findings suggest syphilis, but serologic tests are nonreactive or unclear, alternate tests such as biopsy of lesion, darkfield examination or direct fluorescent antibody staining of lesion material may be helpful
2.   Treatment
a.   The recommended treatment is the same as that for HIV-negative patients
b.   HIV-infected patients who have either late latent syphilis or syphilis of unknown duration should have a CSF examination before treatment
c.   Refer these patients for expert care if available

3.   Follow Up
a.   HIV infected persons should have clinical follow-up and serologic testing at 3, 6, 9, 12, and 24 months after therapy
b.   If at any time clinical symptoms develop or nontreponemal titers rise fourfold, a repeat CSF examination should be performed (refer to expert for management)

L.   Treatment failure can occur with any regimen. Assessing response to treatment is often difficult, and definitive criteria for cure or treatment failure have not been established; follow-up guidelines for patients with primary, secondary, latent, and tertiary syphilis are contained in the following table

---

GUIDELINES FOR FOLLOW-UP OF PATIENTS WITH PRIMARY, SECONDARY, LATENT, AND TERTIARY SYPHILIS

Patients with Primary and Secondary Syphilis
- Patients in this category should be examined clinically and serologically at 6 months and 12 months; more frequent evaluation may be prudent if follow-up is uncertain
  - ✓ Patients who have a fourfold or greater decline in titers (e.g., A 1:32 titer that declines to 1:8 or lower) at 6 and 12 months has received effective treatment
  - ✓ Patients who have signs or symptoms that persist or recur or who have a sustained fourfold increase in nontreponemal test titer (i.e., compared with the maximum or baseline titer at the time of treatment) most probably either failed treatment or were reinfected
  - ✓ Such patients should be re-treated and also reevaluated for HIV infection; because treatment failure usually cannot be reliably distinguished from reinfection with *T. pallidum*, a CSF analysis also should be performed
  - ✓ Re-treatment (as recommended by most experts): 3 weekly injections of benzathine penicillin G 2.4 million units IM [unless CSF examination indicates neurosyphilis is present]

Patients with Latent Syphilis: Early Latent and Late Latent Syphilis or Latent Syphilis of Unknown Duration
- Quantitative nontreponemal serologic tests should be repeated at 6, 12, and 24, months
- Patients with a normal CSF examination should be retreated for latent syphilis if
  - ✓ Titers increase fourfold
  - ✓ An initially high titer (≥1:32) fails to decline at least fourfold; a fourfold change in titer is equivalent to a change of two dilutions (e.g. from 1:32 to 1:8) within 12-24 months of therapy, or
  - ✓ Signs or symptoms attributable to syphilis develop

Patients with Tertiary Syphilis
- Patients require CSF examinations to assess treatment response (refer to expert for management)

Adapted from Centers for Disease Control and Prevention. (2002). Sexually transmitted diseases treatment guidelines. 2002. *MMWR, 51* (No.RR-6), p. 20-25

GENITAL HERPES SIMPLEX VIRUS INFECTION

I. Definition: Infection with herpes simplex viruses (HSV). Two serotypes of HSV have been identified: HSV-1 and HSV-2. Most cases of recurrent genital herpes are caused by HSV-2. (see SKIN PROBLEMS IN CHILDREN AND ADULTS for herpes simplex infections of the skin and mucous membranes)

II. Pathogenesis

    A. HSV-1 and HSV-2 are epidermotropic viruses with infection occurring within keratinocytes

    B. Transmission is only by direct contact with active lesions, or by virus-containing fluid such as saliva or cervical secretions in persons with no evidence of active disease

    C. Inoculation of the virus into skin or mucosal surfaces produces infection, with an incubation period of 2-14 days

    D. About 48 hours after entering the host, the virus transverses afferent nerves to find host ganglion
        1. The trigeminal ganglia are the target of the oral virus--primarily HSV-1
        2. The sacral ganglia are the target of the genital virus--most often HSV-2

    E. Upon reactivation, the virus retraces its route, causing recurrence in the cutaneous area affected by the same nerve root, but not necessarily in the original site

    F. Generally HSV-1 is associated with infection of the lips, face, buccal mucosa, and throat; HSV-2, with the genitalia

    G. In spite of the distinctive sites of herpetic lesions with each serotype, there is overlap in site of infection in approximately 25% of individuals who are infected
        1. Type 1 strains can be recovered from the genital tract
        2. Type 2 strains probably can be recovered from the pharynx as a result of oral-genital activity
        3. Whereas type 1 HSV genital infections in children also can result from autoinoculation of virus from the mouth, sexual abuse must always be considered in prepubertal children with genital herpes

III. Clinical Presentation

    A. Genital herpes is a recurrent, life-long viral infection; at least 50 million persons in the U.S. have genital HSV infection

    B. Most HSV-2 infected persons have not been diagnosed
        1. Infections are either mild or unrecognized with the virus shed intermittently in the genital tract
        2. Most infections are transmitted by persons unaware that they are infected or asymptomatic when transmission occurs

    C. The usual sequence of disease in which signs/symptoms occur is painful papules followed by vesicles, ulceration, crusting, and healing

    D. First clinical episode of genital herpes
        1. Symptoms of primary infection that is symptomatic often consists of hyperesthesia, burning, itching, dysuria, pain, and tenderness in the genital area
        2. Fever and lymphadenopathy are frequently present
        3. More systemic manifestations are present than with recurrent episodes
        4. Viral shedding is prolonged (average 12 days) and healing of lesions takes 21 days on average
        5. Persons with genital infection with HSV-1 (about 30% of patients with first episode herpes) have a much lower risk of symptomatic recurrent outbreaks

    E. Recurrent episodes of HSV infection
        1. Most patients (about 50%) with symptomatic first episode HSV-2 infection will have recurrent episodes within 6 months after the first clinical episode
        2. Frequently have prodrome with recurrences

3. Lesions often localized in recurrent episodes
4. Length of viral shedding reduced compared to primary episode (average 7 days)
5. Healing of lesions is also faster (5 days on average)

IV. Diagnosis/Evaluation

A. History
1. Question regarding location, onset, duration, and appearance of lesions; ask if pain, burning, or paresthesia present prior to eruption
2. Ask about associated symptoms of fever, myalgia, malaise
3. Ask regarding previous occurrence of similar lesions, symptoms
4. Inquire about exposures to infected persons and use of condoms

B. Physical Examination
1. Examine genital area for characteristic location, distribution, appearance of lesions
2. Check for enlarged lymph nodes in inguinal area

C. Differential Diagnosis
1. Syphilis
2. Chancroid
3. Folliculitis
4. Molluscum contagiosum

D. Diagnostic Tests
1. Isolation of HSV in cell culture is the preferred virologic test in patients who present with genital ulcers or other mucocutaneous lesions (**Note:** Sensitivity of culture declines rapidly as lesions begin to heal, usually within a few days of onset)
   a. Unroof vesicle and scrape the material with Dacron-tipped swab
   b. Place swab in viral transport media
   c. Virus grows rapidly and cultures may be positive within 2-3 days (can take longer)
2. Because false-negative HSV cultures are common, particularly in patients with healing lesion or recurrent infections, type-specific serologic tests are useful in confirming a clinical diagnosis of genital herpes; additionally, such tests can be used to diagnose persons with unrecognized infection and to manage sex partners of persons with genital herpes
   a. Currently, the FDA-approved gG-based type-specific assays include POCkit HSV-2 (manufactured by Diagnology); HerpeSelect-1 ELISA IgG or HerpeSelect-2 ELISA IgG (manufactured by Focus Technology, Inc.); and HerpeSelect 1 and 2 Immunoblot IgG (manufactured by Focus Technology, Inc.)
   b. The POCkit HSV-2 assay is a point-of-care test that provides results for HSV-2 antibodies from capillary blood or serum during a clinic visit
   c. The Focus Technology assays are laboratory-based
   d. Sensitivities of these tests for detection of HSV-2 antibody vary from 80% to 90%
   e. Specificities of these assays are ≥96%
3. The Tzanck test is not recommended by the CDC for diagnosing HSV infection

V. Plan/Management

A. Healthcare providers often must treat patients before test results are available because early treatment decreases the possibility of transmission and because successful treatment of genital herpes depends upon prompt initiation of therapy
1. Treat for the diagnosis considered most likely on basis of clinical presentation and epidemiologic circumstances
2. Even after complete diagnostic evaluation, at least 25% of patients who have genital ulcers have no laboratory-confirmed diagnosis

B. Many patients with first-episode genital herpes present with mild clinical manifestations but later develop severe or prolonged symptoms. Most patients with initial genital herpes should receive antiviral therapy as outlined in the following table

RECOMMENDED REGIMENS: FIRST CLINICAL EPISODE

Select one of the following regimens

Acyclovir 400 mg orally 3 times a day for 7-10 days, OR
Acyclovir 200 mg orally 5 times a day for 7-10 days, OR

Famciclovir 250 mg orally 3 times a day for 7-10 days, OR
Valacyclovir 1 g orally twice a day for 7-10 days

Note: Treatment may be extended if healing is incomplete after 10 days of therapy

Adapted from Centers for Disease Control and Prevention. (2002). Sexually transmitted diseases treatment guidelines 2002. *MMWR, 51*(No.RR-6), p. 14

COUNSELING FOR MANAGEMENT OF PATIENTS WITH GENITAL HERPES

Two main goals of counseling are to help patient cope with infection and to prevent sexual and perinatal transmission

Information and Lifestyle Counseling
✓ Counsel patient regarding natural history of disease emphasizing recurrent episodes, asymptomatic viral shedding, and sexual transmission; partner notification should be encouraged
✓ Sexual and perinatal transmission can occur during asymptomatic periods; sex partners of infected persons should be advised that they might be infected even if they have no symptoms
✓ Type-specific serologic testing of asymptomatic partners of persons with genital herpes can determine whether risk for HSV acquisition exists
✓ Asymptomatic viral shedding occurs more frequently in persons with genital HSV-2 than HSV-1 and also occurs more frequently in those with infection <12 months
✓ Latex condoms when used consistently and correctly, can reduce risk for genital herpes when infected areas are covered by condom
✓ Need to abstain from all sexual activity when lesions or prodromal symptoms are present

Counseling Relating to Role of Antiviral Drugs
✓ Systemic antiviral drugs partially control the signs and symptoms when used to treat initial and recurrent episodes or when used as daily suppressive therapy
✓ Episodic and suppressive therapy is effective in preventing or shortening the duration of recurrent episodes

Resources Available for Patients
✓ Refer to educational resources: CDC National STD/HIV Hotline (800-227-8922); web site http://www.ashastd.org

Adapted from Centers for Disease Control and Prevention. (2002). Sexually transmitted diseases treatment guidelines 2002. MMWR, 51(No.RR-6), p. 15

C.   Patients with recurrent episodes of HSV infection can be managed in one of two ways--either episodically, to shorten the duration of lesions, or continuously with the use of suppressive therapy to reduce the frequency of recurrences
    1.   Options for treatment of recurrent episodes should be discussed with all patients
    2.   The following tables outline episodic therapy and suppressive therapy for recurrent HSV disease

EPISODIC THERAPY FOR RECURRENT GENITAL HERPES

Select <u>one</u> of the following regimens

- Acyclovir 400 mg orally three times a day for 5 days
- Acyclovir 200 mg orally 5 times a day for 5 days
- Acyclovir 800 mg orally twice a day for 5 days

- Famciclovir 125 mg orally twice a day for 5 days
- Valacyclovir 500 mg orally twice a day for 3- 5 days
- Valacyclovir 1.0 g orally once a day for 5 days

About Episodic Therapy
✓ Treatment is most efficacious when begun during the prodrome or within 1 day after onset of lesions

✓ If episodic therapy for recurrence is chosen, patient should be provided with antiviral therapy, or a prescription for the medication, so that treatment can be initiated at the first sign of prodrome or genital lesions

Adapted from Centers for Disease Control and Prevention. (2002). Sexually transmitted diseases treatment guidelines 2002. *MMWR, 51*(No.RR-6), p. 14

SUPPRESSIVE THERAPY FOR RECURRENT GENITAL HERPES

Select one of the following regimens

- Acyclovir 400 mg orally twice a day
- Famciclovir 250 mg orally twice a day

- Valacyclovir 500 mg orally once a day*
- Valacyclovir 1.0 gram orally once a day

About Suppressive Therapy
✓ Daily suppressive therapy reduces the frequency of genital herpes recurrences by ≥75% among patients who have frequent recurrences (defined as 6 or more recurrences per year)
✓ Suppressive therapy with acyclovir reduces but does not eliminate asymptomatic viral shedding
✓ Suppressive therapy has not been associated with emergence of acyclovir resistance among immunocompetent patients
✓ After 12 months of continuous suppressive therapy, discontinuation should be discussed with patient
✓ Famciclovir and valacyclovir should not be used for over 12 months
✓ Safety and efficacy have been documented among patients using daily acyclovir for as long as 6 years

---

*May be less effective than other valacyclovir or acyclovir dosing regimens in patients who have very frequent recurrences (≥10 outbreaks per year)

Adapted from Centers for Disease Control and Prevention. (2002). Sexually transmitted diseases treatment guidelines 2002. *MMWR, 51*(No.RR-6), p. 14

D. Management of sex partners
  1. Partners can usually benefit from evaluation and counseling
  2. Symptomatic partners should be evaluated and treated
  3. Asymptomatic partners should be questioned concerning history of genital lesions, educated to recognize symptoms of herpes, and offered type-specific serologic testing for HSV infection

E. Lesions caused by HSV are common among HIV-infected patients and may be severe, painful and atypical. Episodic or suppressive therapy with oral antiviral agents is often beneficial; see recommendations in the tables that follow

---

RECOMMENDED REGIMENS FOR EPISODIC INFECTION IN PERSONS INFECTED WITH HIV

Acyclovir 400 mg orally three times a day for 5-10 days
OR
Acyclovir 200 mg five times a day for 5-10 days
OR
Famciclovir 500 mg orally twice a day for 5-10 days
OR
Valacyclovir 1.0 g orally twice a day for 5-10 days

Source: Centers for Disease Control and Prevention. (2002). Sexually transmitted diseases treatment guidelines. *MMWR, 51*(No.RR-6), p. 16

RECOMMENDED REGIMENS FOR DAILY SUPPRESSIVE THERAPY IN PERSONS INFECTED WITH HIV

Acyclovir 400-800 mg orally two to three times a day
OR
Famciclovir 500 mg orally twice a day
OR
Valacyclovir 500 mg orally twice a day

Source: Centers for Disease Control and Prevention. (2002). Sexually transmitted diseases treatment guidelines 2002. *MMWR, 51*(No.RR-6), p. 16

F. If lesions persist or recur in patients receiving antiviral treatment, resistance should be suspected and patients should be referred to a specialist for management; patients should also be referred to a specialist if lesions are severe as hospitalization and IV therapy may be necessary

G. Pregnant women with genital herpes should be referred to a specialist for management (**Note**: The safety of acyclovir, valacyclovir, and famciclovir therapy in pregnant women has not been established)

H. Infants exposed to HSV during birth, as proven by virus isolation or presumed by observation of lesions should be followed by a specialist

I. Follow Up: Variable depending on clinical needs of patient

HUMAN PAPILLOMAVIRUS INFECTION (GENITAL WARTS)

I.   Definition: A sexually transmitted disease caused by certain types of the human papillomavirus (HPV) that produces epithelial tumors of the skin and mucous membranes

II.   Pathogenesis

    A.   More than 30 types of HPV can infect the genital tract

    B.   The virus enters the body via an epithelial defect and infects the stratified squamous epithelium of the lower genital tract

    C.   Visible genital warts usually are caused by HPV types 6 or 11

    D.   Other HPV types in the anogenital region--types 16, 18, 31, 33, and 35--have been strongly associated with cervical neoplasia

III. Clinical Presentation

    A.   Most HPV infections are asymptomatic, unrecognized, or subclinical

    B.   Clinical HPV infections develop following an incubation period of unknown length but it is estimated to range from 3 months to several years; depending on the size and anatomic location, genital warts can be painful, friable, and pruritic

    C.   In addition to the external genitalia, (i.e., the penis, vulva, scrotum, perineum, and perianal skin), genital warts can occur on the uterine cervix and in the vagina, urethra, anus, and mouth

    D.   Intra-anal warts are seen predominantly in patients who have had receptive anal intercourse; these warts are distinct from perianal warts, which can occur in men and women without a history of anal sex

    E.   In addition to the genital area, HPV types 6 and 11 have been associated with conjunctival, nasal, oral, and laryngeal warts

    F.   Individual warts may become confluent and appear as a single, large fleshy lesion

    G.   Growth of warts may be stimulated by pregnancy, oral contraceptive use, immunosuppression, and local trauma

IV.   Diagnosis/Evaluation

    A.   History
        1.   Question about location, onset, duration, and presence of any associated symptoms
        2.   Inquire about exposures to sexually transmitted diseases (unprotected intercourse)
        3.   Ask if partner has similar lesions
        4.   Inquire about past history of HPV
        5.   Question regarding pregnancy, use of oral contraceptives, and immune status

    B.   Physical Examination
        1.   Examine external genitalia and rectal areas for characteristic lesions
        2.   To assist in visualization of warts, apply 3-5% acetic acid to the vulva (women), penis (men) and perianal areas to reveal acetowhitening
        3.   Perform Pap smear to detect cervical dysplasia in women who have not had a Pap test within the past year

C.   Differential Diagnosis
1.   Herpes simplex
2.   Syphilis
3.   Molluscum contagiosum

D.   Diagnostic Tests: Visible anogenital warts are diagnosed by clinical inspection; no data support the use of type-specific HPV nucleic acid tests in the routine diagnosis or management of visible genital warts

V.   Plan/Management

A.   Primary goal of treating visible warts is the removal of symptomatic warts
1.   Treatment can induce wart-free periods in most patients; most patients have fewer than 10 warts with a total wart areas of 0.5-1.0 cm^2
2.   Currently available treatments do not affect the natural history of HPV infection
3.   Most genital warts are asymptomatic and, left untreated, often resolve on their own
4.   Existing data indicate that currently available therapies for genital warts may reduce, but probably do not eradicate, infectivity
5.   Patients should be advised that no available treatment is superior to the others; no single treatment is ideal for all patients or all warts
6.   A treatment protocol is important because many if not most patients require a course of therapy rather than a single treatment

---

OVERVIEW OF TREATMENT

Treatment of Genital Warts Should be Guided by
- Preference of the patients after they have been informed of the options
- Available resources
- Experience of healthcare provider

Factors that Influence Selection of Treatment
- Wart size, morphology, number, and anatomic site (in general, warts located on moist surfaces and/or intertriginous areas respond better to topical treatment than do warts on drier surfaces)
- Patient preference and provider experience
- Convenience, cost of treatment, and adverse treatment effects

Treatment Modality Should be Changed if
- Patient has not improved substantially after 3 provider-administered treatments, OR
- Warts have not cleared after 6 treatments

Avoid overtreatment: Risk/benefit ratio of treatment should be evaluated throughout course of therapy

To Increase Efficiency and Efficacy, Clinicians Should be Knowledgeable about
- At least one patient-applied treatment
- At least one provider-administered treatment that is available

Note: Opinion is divided regarding the practice of employing combination therapy (i.e., the simultaneous use of two or more modalities on the same wart at the same time). Because of the limitations of currently available treatments, some providers employ combination therapy; others believe that combining modalities may increase complications without improving efficacy

---

Adapted from Centers for Disease Control and Prevention. (2002). Sexually transmitted diseases treatment guidelines 2002. *MMWR, 51*(No.RR-6), p. 53-55

EXTERNAL GENITAL WARTS: RECOMMENDED REGIMENS

Patient-Applied
(**Note**: For patient-applied treatments, patient must be able to identify and reach warts)

Podofilox 0.5% solution or gel (relatively inexpensive, easy to use, safe, antimitotic drug) **Not for use in pregnancy**
- Dosing:
  - ✓ Apply BID x 3 days, followed by 4 days of no therapy
  - ✓ May repeat cycle as necessary for a total of 4 cycles
- Instruction to patient: Apply solution with cotton swab, gel with finger to visible genital warts
- Comments:
  - ✓ Most patients experience mild/moderate pain or local irritation after treatment
  - ✓ If possible, provider should apply initial treatment to demonstrate proper application technique and identify which warts should be treated
  - ✓ Total wart area treated should be ≤10 cm^2, and total volume of podofilox should be ≤0.5 mL per day

Imiquimod 5% cream (immune enhancer that stimulates production of interferon and other cytokines) **Not for use in pregnancy**
- Dosing: Apply QD at bedtime, 3 times/week for up to 16 weeks
- Instructions to patient: Apply cream with a finger at bedtime and wash off with mild soap/water after 6-10 hours
- Comment: Many patients may be clear of visible warts by 8-10 weeks

Follow up: Traditionally, follow-up visits are not required for patients using self-administered therapy; however, follow-up may be useful several weeks into therapy to determine appropriateness of medication use and response to treatment

Provider-Administered

Select **one** of the following

Cryotherapy with liquid nitrogen or cryoprobe (destroys warts by thermal-induced cytolysis)
- Repeat applications Q 1-2 weeks
- Pain after application, followed by necrosis and sometimes blistering, is common

  Note: Major limitation of this modality is that proper use requires substantial training; most warts are overtreated or undertreated by providers who have not been trained resulting in poor efficacy or increased complications

Podophyllin resin 10-25% in compound tincture of benzoin (contains several compounds including antimitotic podophyllin lignans)
- Apply small amount (thin layer) to each wart and allow to air dry
- Limit application to ~0.5 mL of podophyllin or an area of ≤10 cm^2 of warts per session
- Instruct patient to thoroughly wash preparation off 1-4 hours after application (to reduce local irrittion)
- Repeat weekly if necessary

  Note: Not for use in pregnancy

Trichloroacetic acid (TCA) or bichloracetic acid (BCA) 80%-90% (caustic agents that destroy warts by chemical coagulation of the proteins)
- Apply sparingly to warts only (TCA has low viscosity comparable with that of water and can spread rapidly)
- Allow to dry--a white "frosting" develops
- Powder with talc or sodium bicarbonate to neutralize acid (if acid is applied excessively, can damage adjacent tissues)
- Repeat weekly if necessary

Surgical removal either by tangential scissor excision, tangential shave excision, curettage, or electrosurgery

Adapted from Centers for Disease Control and Prevention. (2002). Sexually transmitted diseases treatment guidelines 2002. *MMWR, 51*(No.RR-6), p. 54-55

B.   Alternative regimens for treatment of external genital warts are intralesional interferon or laser surgery

C.   For treatment of cervical and vaginal warts, referral to an expert is recommended

D.   For treatment of urethral meatus warts, referral to an expert is recommended

E.   For treatment of external anal warts, use of cryotherapy with liquid nitrogen or TCA or BCA 80%-90%; apply as directed above under EXTERNAL GENITAL WARTS: RECOMMENDED REGIMENS

F.   Management of warts on rectal mucosa and on oral mucosa should be by an expert

G.   Management of pregnant women: Refer to expert for management

H.   Management of immunodeficient patients: Refer to expert for management (increased incidence of squamous cell carcinoma arising in or resembling genital warts may occur more frequently among immunosuppressed persons, thus requiring biopsy for confirmation of diagnosis)

EDUCATION AND COUNSELING OF PATIENTS WITH GENITAL WARTS

Patients can be educated through patient education materials including pamphlets, hotlines, and web sites (http://www.ashastd.org)

Emphasize the Following Key Messages
- Genital HPV infection is a viral infection that is common among sexually active persons
- Infection is almost always sexually transmitted, but because the incubation period is highly variable, it is often difficult to determine source of infection
- With ongoing relationships, sex partners usually are infected by the time of the patient's diagnosis, although they may have no symptoms or signs of infection
- Natural history of genital warts is usually benign; types of HPV that usually cause external genital warts are not associated with cancer
- Recurrence of genital warts within first several months after treatment is common; usually indicates recurrence rather than reinfection
- Likelihood of transmission to future partners and the duration of infectivity after treatment are unknown; condom use is associated with a lower rate of cervical cancer, an HPV-associated disease

Adapted from Centers for Disease Control and Prevention. (2002). Sexually transmitted diseases treatment guidelines 2002. *MMWR, 51*(No.RR-6), p. 56-57

I. Management of sexual partners of patients with visible warts
1. Examination of partners not necessary for the management of genital warts because no data indicate that reinfection plays a role in recurrences
2. The value to treatment in reducing infectivity is not known
3. Use of condoms reduces, but does not eliminate risk of transmission

J. Subclinical genital HPV infection (without exophytic warts)
1. Subclinical genital HPV infection is a term used to refer to manifestations of infection in the absence of visible genital warts, including situations where infection is detected on the cervix by Pap test, colposcopy, or biopsy; on the penis, vulva, or other genital skin by the appearance of white areas after application of acetic acid; or on any genital skin by a positive test for HPV
2. Subclinical genital HPV infection occurs more frequently than visible warts in both men and women
3. Screening for subclinical genital HPV infection using DNA or RNA tests is not recommended
4. In the absence of coexistent squamous intraepithelial lesion (SIL), treatment is not recommended for subclinical genital HPV infection diagnosed by colposcopy, biopsy, acetic acid soaking of genital skin/mucous membranes, or the detection of HPV by laboratory tests
5. The diagnosis of subclinical genital HPV infection is often not definitive, and no therapy has been identified that eradicates infection

K. Management of sexual partners of patients with subclinical genital HPV infection
1. Examination of sex partners is unnecessary
2. Most sex partners of infected patients probably are already infected subclinically with HPV
3. No screening tests for subclinical infection are available
4. Whether patients who have subclinical HPV infection are as infectious as patients who have exophytic warts is unknown

L. Recommendations relating to cervical cancer screening for women who attend STD clinics or have a history of STDs
1. Precursor lesions for cervical cancer occur about five times more frequently among women attending STD clinics than among women attending family planning clinics
2. If woman has not had a Pap smear during previous 12 months, a Pap smear should be obtained as part of the routine pelvic examination in the STD clinic
   a. The sequence of Pap testing in relation to collection of other cervicovaginal specimens does not appear to influence Pap test results/interpretation
   b. Thus, when other cultures or specimens are collected for STD diagnosis, the Pap test can be obtained last
3. Provide woman with printed information about Pap smears and a report containing a statement that a Pap smear was obtained during her clinic visit
4. A copy of the Pap smear result should be provided to the patient for her records
5. Counsel woman about need for an annual Pap smear, and provide her with names of local clinics/providers where Pap smears can be obtained on an annual basis and adequate follow-up is available

6.   Women who have external genital warts do not need to have Pap tests more frequently than women who do not have warts, unless otherwise indicated

7.   See ABNORMAL CERVICAL CYTOLOGY section for information on management of patients with cervical cytological abnormalities

M.   Follow Up

1.   After visible warts have cleared (which may require several visits for provider-administered treatments), a follow-up evaluation is not mandatory but may be helpful

2.   Patient should be advised to watch for recurrences, which occur most frequently during first 3 months after treatment; patients concerned about recurrences should be offered a follow-up evaluation 3 months after treatment

3.   Women should be counseled to undergo regular Pap screening as recommended for women without genital warts (see screening for cervical cancer in HEALTH MAINTENANCE chapter)

REFERENCES

Centers for Disease Control and Prevention. (2002). Discontinuation of cefixime tablets—United States. *Morbidity and Mortality and Weekly Report, 51*, 1052.

Centers for Disease Control and Prevention. (2002). Increases in fluoroquinolone-resistant *Neisseria gonorrhoeae*—Hawaii and California, 2001. *Morbidity and Mortality and Weekly Report, 51*, 1041-1044.

Centers for Disease Control and Prevention. (2002). Primary and secondary syphilis—United States. *Morbidity and Mortality and Weekly Report, 51*, 971-973.

Centers for Disease Control and Prevention. (2002). Sexually transmitted diseases treatment guidelines 2002. *Morbidity and Mortality Weekly Report, 51*(No. RR-6).

Hatcher, R.A., Trussell, J., Stewart, F., Cates, W., Stewart, G., Guest, F., & Kowal, D. (1998). *Contraceptive technology*. New York: Ardent Media.

Hill, Y.L., & Brio, F.M. (2001, March). Adolescents and sexually transmitted infections. *Medical Aspects of Human Sexuality*, 7-13.

Hook, E.W., & Marra, C.M. (1992). Acquired syphilis in adults. *New England Journal of Medicine, 326*, 1060-1067.

Obata-Yasuoka, M. (2002). Bacterial vaginosis: Making the diagnosis and reducing the incidence. *Obstetrics and Gynecology, 100*, 759-764.

Turner, C.F., Rogers, S.M., & Miller, H.G. (2002). Untreated gonococcal and chlamydial infection in a probability sample of adults. *Journal of the American Medical Association, 287*, 726-733.

Human Immunodeficiency Virus Infection and Acquired Immunodeficiency

CONSTANCE R. UPHOLD

Human Immunodeficiency Virus (HIV) Infection and Acquired Immunodeficiency Syndrome (AIDS) in Children

Human Immunodeficiency Virus (HIV) Infection and Acquired Immunodeficiency Syndrome (AIDS) in Adults and Adolescents

Occupational Exposure to Blood and Other Body Fluids That May Contain Human Immunodeficiency Virus (HIV)

HUMAN IMMUNODEFICIENCY VIRUS INFECTION AND ACQUIRED IMMUNODEFICIENCY SYNDROME IN CHILDREN

I.   Definition: Children under age 13 with Human Immunodeficiency Virus (HIV) infection and/or Acquired Immunodeficiency Syndrome (AIDS)

    A.   HIV Infection: Infection with human retrovirus, Human Immunodeficiency Virus

    B.   Acquired Immunodeficiency Syndrome: Definition of AIDS in children <13 years incorporates the age-dependent decline in CD4+ T-cells (see table on Immune Categories in IV.D.3.b.) and differentiates mild, moderate, and severe degrees of clinical symptoms (see table on Clinical Categories in IV.D.3.b.)

II.   Pathogenesis:

    A.   Human immunodeficiency virus enters and destroys cells, predominantly CD4+ T-lymphocyte cells (CD4+ T-cells) which are involved in cell-mediated immunity; the progressive destruction of CD4+ T-cells results in increased susceptibility of the patient to infections by opportunistic organisms

    B.   Transmission of HIV infection in children
        1.   Perinatal transmission is the most common mode of acquisition of HIV infection among US children
            a.   The estimated perinatal transmission rates in untreated women to their infants ranges from 13% to 30%, with the majority of children born to infected mothers being uninfected
            b.   Transmission from mother to infant can occur during the following times:
                (1)   Pregnancy or gestation (*in utero*); accounts for about 25-30% of perinatal HIV transmission
                (2)   Labor and delivery (intrapartum); accounts for about 70-75% of perinatal transmission
                    (a)   Possible mechanisms for neonatal HIV acquisition include direct exposure to maternal blood and genital tract secretions and transplacental microtransfusions
                    (b)   Cesarean delivery has a partially protective role against transmission
                (3)   Postpartum period through breastfeeding; accounts for a small percentage of transmission
            c.   The following factors increase the risk of vertical HIV transmission: Low maternal peripheral blood CD4+ T-cell counts, high maternal plasma HIV RNA levels, smoking, prolonged rupture of amniotic membranes, and invasive procedures such as amniocentesis, and possibly scalp electrodes, intrauterine pressure catheters, and fetal blood sampling
            d.   Zidovudine (AZT) therapy to mothers during the antepartum and intrapartum periods and to newborns for 6 weeks after birth reduced perinatal transmission by 70% in the Pediatric AIDS Clinical Trials Group Protocol (PACTG) 076
        2.   Other means of transmission in children include exposure to HIV-contaminated blood or blood products, sexual abuse, and sexual transmission during adolescence

III. Clinical Presentation

    A.   Epidemiology
        1.   The annual number of perinatally acquired AIDS cases in the U.S. has declined in recent years
        2.   The AIDS epidemic disproportionately affects African American and Hispanic children

    B.   Disease progression
        1.   Generally, HIV infection progresses to AIDS more rapidly in infants than in adults due to the immature immune systems of infants or exposures to increased viral loads relative to body masses
        2.   Approximately 20% of infants progress rapidly and are symptomatic during the first few months after birth; infants infected *in utero* are believed to be rapid progressors
        3.   Slower progression occurs in the majority of children who are probably infected during labor and delivery; these children typically become symptomatic within the first several years of life
        4.   A small percentage of children do not develop manifestations of disease progression until after 8-10 years of age

C.   Clinical manifestations
1.   At birth the majority of infants are asymptomatic
2.   A triad of symptoms often develop: Failure to thrive, chronic interstitial pneumonitis, and hepatosplenomegaly
3.   Other common manifestations include lymphadenopathy, recurrent diarrhea, chronic parotid swelling, hepatitis, malignancies, recurrent infections, recurrent febrile episodes, skin rashes, cardiomyopathy, and dysmorphic syndrome
4.   Features associated with lipodystrophy syndrome (fat redistribution, hyperlipidemia, peripheral insulin resistance) arise in some children taking highly active antiretroviral therapy (HAART), but the incidence is lower than that observed in adults on HAART

D.   When a significant quantity of CD4+ T-cells has been destroyed by the virus, immunosuppression occurs and children develop opportunistic infections (OI) and other complications (also see section on HIV/AIDS IN ADULTS AND ADOLESCENTS for further discussion of common clinical presentations of OIs)
1.   The lung is the most common site of infection with *Pneumocystis carinii* pneumonia (PCP), the most common OI
2.   The gastrointestinal tract is the next most common site for OIs with candida esophagitis the most common GI infection
3.   Central nervous system involvement is common in children; one of the earliest signs of CNS involvement is failure to achieve developmental milestones
4.   Chronic otitis media and sinusitis are common
5.   Endocrine and skeletal muscle manifestations are common and include short stature and delay of puberty

E.   The clinical presentation of HIV infection is different in children and adults
1.   The following AIDS-related problems are more common in children than adults: Hypergammaglobulinemia, lymphocytic interstitial pneumonia, bacterial sepsis, recurrent bacterial infections, failure to thrive, and parotitis
2.   Manifestations more common in adults than children: Kaposi's sarcoma, B-cell lymphoma, peripheral lymphopenia, acute mononucleosis-like presentations, opportunistic infections, and tumors of the central nervous system

IV.   Diagnosis/Evaluation

A.   History
1.   Determine if the child is at risk for HIV infection based on the HIV positive status of the mother
2.   Gather a complete pregnancy history of the mother including drug use and labor and delivery information
3.   Obtain a neonatal history including birth weight and complications
4.   Carefully explore feeding behaviors and developmental milestones
5.   Inquire about associated symptoms such as fevers, rashes, and diarrhea
6.   Carefully explore frequency and duration of infections

B.   Physical Examination
1.   Measure and plot height and weight on growth chart; compare with previous measurements
2.   Observe general appearance, noting alertness, responsiveness, and level of activity
3.   A complete physical examination is required with focus on the skin, lymph nodes, mouth, lungs, heart, abdomen, and neuromuscular systems
4.   Perform a neurodevelopment assessment every 6 months; order head CT if assessment is abnormal

C.   Differential Diagnosis
1.   Failure to thrive
2.   Recent therapy with an immunosuppressive agent
3.   Lymphoproliferative disease
4.   Congenital immunological states
5.   Congenital cytomegalovirus infection
6.   Congenital toxoplasmosis

D. Diagnostic Tests
1. Early identification of HIV-infected women is essential for the health of such women and for the care of HIV-exposed and HIV-infected children
   a. Universal counseling and voluntary testing with HIV tests are recommended as the standard of care for all pregnant females; in some states, offering HIV testing to pregnant women is mandated by law
   b. If women are not tested for HIV during pregnancy, counseling and HIV testing should be recommended during immediate postpartum period
   c. When maternal serostatus has not been determined during pregnancy or immediate postpartum period, newborn should be HIV antibody tested with counseling and consent of mother unless state law allows testing without consent (see IV.D.2.)
   d. Positive diagnosis of HIV infection requires both of the following tests which detect antibodies to HIV: A positive enzyme-linked immunosorbent assay (ELISA) as a screening test and a positive Western blot for confirmation
2. Diagnosis of HIV infection in infants
   a. Diagnosis of HIV infection in neonates is difficult because most children born to HIV-infected mothers are initially HIV positive because of placental transfer of maternal antibodies
   b. However, HIV infection can be definitively diagnosed in most infected infants by age 1 month and in virtually all infected infants by age 6 months by using viral diagnostic assays
      (1) HIV DNA polymerase chain reaction (PCR) is the preferred method; HIV cultures are not readily available and HIV RNA assays are investigational tests
      (2) Perform testing 48 hours after birth, at age 1-2 months, and at age 3-6 months (testing at age 14 days is also recommended by some experts)
      (3) Positive tests indicate possible HIV infection and should be confirmed by a repeat virologic test on a separate occasion; HIV infection is confirmed by 2 positive results of HIV DNA PCR
   c. Testing for HIV infection in children who are over 18 months of age is similar to testing of adults with a positive ELISA and positive Western blot tests for confirmation
3. Monitoring immunologic parameters in children with CD4+ T-cell counts is used in conjunction with other measurements to guide antiretroviral treatment decisions and primary prophylaxis of PCP after age 1 year
   a. Obtain CD4+ T-cell counts as soon as possible after child has a positive virologic test for HIV and every 3 months thereafter
   b. The following two tables on CD4+ T-cells and clinical categories present a pediatric clinical and immunologic staging system for HIV infection
   c. Change in CD4+ T-cell percentage, not number, may be better marker of identifying disease progression in children

1994 REVISED HIV PEDIATRIC CLASSIFICATION SYSTEM: IMMUNE CATEGORIES BASED ON AGE-SPECIFIC CD4+ T-LYMPHOCYTE COUNT AND PERCENTAGE

Immune category	<12 mos		1-5 yrs		6-12 yrs	
	No./µL	(%)	No./µL	(%)	No./µL	(%)
Category 1-- no suppression	≥1,500	(≥25%)	≥1,000	(≥25%)	≥500	(≥25%)
Category 2-- moderate suppression	750-1,499	(15%-24%)	500-999	(15%-24%)	200-499	(15%-24%)
Category 3-- severe suppression	<750	(<15%)	<500	(<15%)	<200	(<15%)

Source: Centers for Disease Control. (1998). Guidelines for the use of antiretroviral agents in pediatric HIV infection. *MMWR, 47* (RR-4), 1-47.

1994 REVISED HIV PEDIATRIC CLASSIFICATION SYSTEM: CLINICAL CATEGORIES

Category N: Not Symptomatic

Children who have no signs or symptoms considered to be the result of HIV infection or who have only **one** of the conditions listed in category A

Category A: Mildly Symptomatic

Children with **two** or more of the following conditions but none of the conditions listed in categories B and C:

- Lymphadenopathy (≥0.5 cm at more than two sites; bilateral = one site)
- Hepatomegaly
- Splenomegaly
- Dermatitis
- Parotitis
- Recurrent or persistent upper respiratory infection, sinusitis, or otitis media

Category B: Moderately Symptomatic

Children who have symptomatic conditions other than those listed for category A or category C that are attributed to HIV infection. Examples of conditions in clinical category B include but are not limited to the following:

- Anemia (<8 gm/dL), neutropenia (<1,000/mm^3), or thrombocytopenia (<100,000/mm^3) persisting ≥30 days
- Bacterial meningitis, pneumonia, or sepsis (single episode)
- Candidiasis, oropharyngeal (i.e., thrush) persisting (>2 mo) in children >6 mo of age
- Cardiomyopathy
- Cytomegalovirus infection with onset before age 1 month
- Diarrhea, recurrent or chronic
- Hepatitis
- Herpes simplex virus (HSV) stomatitis, recurrent (i.e., more than two episodes within 1 year)
- HSV bronchitis, pneumonitis, or esophagitis with onset before age 1 month
- Herpes zoster (i.e., shingles) involving at least two distinct episodes or more than one dermatome
- Leiomyosarcoma
- Lymphoid interstitial pneumonia (LIP) or pulmonary lymphoid hyperplasia complex
- Nephropathy
- Nocardiosis
- Fever lasting >1 month
- Toxoplasmosis with onset before age 1 month
- Varicella, disseminated (i.e., complicated chickenpox)

Category C: Severely Symptomatic

Children who have any condition listed in the 1987 surveillance case definition for acquired immunodeficiency syndrome (see AIDS Surveillance Case Definition in section on HIV INFECTION IN ADULTS AND ADOLESCENTS), with the exception of LIP (which is a category B condition)

Source: Centers for Disease Control. (1998). Guidelines for the use of antiretroviral agents in pediatric HIV infection. *MMWR, 47* (RR-4), 1-47.

4. The viral load (burden) can be determined by using quantitative HIV RNA assays
   a. Measure baseline viral load and within 4 weeks after initiation or change of therapy; after a maximal virologic response is achieved, measure every 3 months
   b. Perinatally, infected children typically have high HIV RNA levels and their initial virologic responses following therapy may take longer than that observed in adults
   c. Several methods can be used to quantify HIV RNA; use one method consistently
   d. Changes greater than fivefold (0.7 log$_{10}$) in infants <2 years and greater than threefold (0.5 log$_{10}$) in children aged ≥2 years after repeated testing should be considered biologically and clinically substantial changes
   e. Therapy should not be altered based on the result of a change in HIV copy number unless the change is confirmed by a second measurement
   f. Due to the complexities of HIV RNA testing and age-related changes in HIV RNA in children, clinical decision-making based on HIV RNA levels should be made in consultation with an expert in pediatric HIV infection
5. Antiretroviral drug resistance testing: No specific recommendations are available because there are no long-term data on the impact of this testing in children
   a. May prove useful in guiding initial therapy and in changing failing regimens; if testing is done, child should still be receiving antiretroviral therapy
   b. When antiretroviral drug resistance is known or suspected in the mother of a newly diagnosed infant, consider resistance testing of the infant's viral isolate to assist in selection of initial antiretroviral therapy

      c.   The presence of viral resistance to a particular drug(s) suggests that the specific drug(s) is unlikely to suppress viral replication

      d.   Absence of resistance to a drug does not insure that its use will suppress viral replication, particularly if the drug shares cross-resistance with drugs previously used

6.   Order additional tests at baseline and then every 3-4 months: CBC with differential, reticulocyte count, BUN, creatinine, liver function tests, urinalysis, electrolytes

7.   Order at baseline and then annually: Chest x-ray; ECHO and ECG in symptomatic children (stages B and C); tuberculin skin test, serologies for hepatitis, toxoplasmosis, EBV, and CMV

8.   If neurodevelopment evaluation is abnormal, perform head CT

V.   Plan/Management

A.   To reduce perinatal transmission the following guidelines are recommended:

1.   Care of HIV-infected pregnant females and newborn should be coordinated with an HIV-specialist, obstetrician, and primary healthcare clinician

2.   Assessment of the pregnant female should include evaluation of existing immunodeficiency (CD4+ T-cell count), risk of disease progression (level of plasma HIV RNA), history of prior or current antiretroviral therapy, gestational age of the baby, and supportive care needs

3.   Females currently taking antiretrovirals should continue their regimens; however, efavirenz should be avoided during the first 10-12 weeks gestation; consider temporarily discontinuing all antiretroviral agents during the first 10-12 weeks gestation

4.   For all pregnant females not current taking antiretroviral therapy, administer the three-part PACTG 076 zidovudine (ZDV) regimen: ZDV given orally antenatally starting after 14 weeks' gestation, intravenously during labor, and orally to the infant for the first 6 weeks after birth

      a.   In antepartum, prescribe ZDV 100 mg 5 times/day or 200 mg TID or ZDV 300 mg BID (starting after 14-34 weeks gestation)

      b.   During labor, order intravenous administration of ZDV in 1-hour-initial dose of 2 mg/kg followed by continuous infusion of 1 mg/kg/hour until delivery

      c.   Infants should be given ZDV syrup 2 mg/kg orally every 6 hours for 6 weeks beginning 8-12 hours after birth

5.   Additionally, females with HIV RNA levels ≥1000 copies/mL should be offered combination therapy that includes ZDV as one of the agents; consider prescribing one of the combination therapies recommended for nonpregnant adults

      a.   Two nucleoside reverse transcriptase inhibitors plus a protease inhibitor or a nonnucleoside reverse transcriptase inhibitor

      b.   Three nucleoside reverse transcriptase inhibitors

6.   Females with HIV RNA levels <1000 copies/mL can be treated with combination therapy or with zidovudine prophylaxis alone; when therapy is given principally to reduce perinatal transmission, consider discontinuing all antiretroviral agents simultaneously postnatally and reinstitute treatment on the basis of standard criteria for nonpregnant women

7.   For women who present in labor without prior antiretroviral therapy the following options are available:

      a.   A single oral dose of 200 mg of nevirapine at onset of labor and a single oral dose of 2 mg/kg to the newborn within 48-72 hours of life

      b.   Zidovudine 600 mg PO at onset of labor and then 300 mg every 3 hours plus 150 mg PO of lamivudine at labor onset and then 150 mg PO every 12 hours until delivery; for the infant, prescribe 4 mg/kg PO of zidovudine and 2 mg/kg PO of lamivudine every 12 hours for 7 days

      c.   Intravenous zidovudine for the mother and 2 mg/kg of zidovudine orally every 6 hours for 6 weeks for the infant

      d.   Intravenous zidovudine plus a single dose of 200 mg PO nevirapine for the mother; zidovudine 2 mg/kg orally every 6 hours for 6 weeks plus a single oral dose of 2 mg/kg nevirapine at age 48-72 hours for the infant

8.   Provide primary *Pneumocystis carinii* pneumonia prophylaxis to the pregnant female when CD4+ T-cells fall below 200/mm^3: Prescribe trimethoprim/sulfamethoxazole (Bactrim) one DS tablet QD three times weekly or aerosolized pentamidine once a month if unable to tolerate Bactrim

9.   General counseling should be provided about risk factors for transmission including the need to refrain from breastfeeding

B.   Additional recommendations for caring for the newborn of the HIV-infected mother

1.   Order CBC and differential at birth and at 6 weeks of age

2.   Monitor for adverse reactions from zidovudine such as anemia, neutropenia, myositis, elevated transaminases; mild, transient anemia is common and resolves when therapy is discontinued

3. More intensive monitoring of hematologic and serum chemistry measurements is needed for infants whose mothers received combination antiretroviral therapy
4. Follow-up care of child at risk for HIV infection from birth until HIV status is determined must be aggressive until it is assured that the child is not HIV infected
5. Prophylaxis for PCP is important (see V.C.12. for specific guidelines)

C. Care of the child with confirmed HIV infection
1. CD4+ T-cell counts and viral loads should be performed regularly (every 3 months)
2. CBC with differential, reticulocyte count, liver function tests, BUN, creatinine, and urinalysis should be performed every 3 months
3. Neurodevelopmental assessments should be completed every 6 months
4. Tuberculosis should be screened for annually with skin tests (PPDs)
5. Annually perform serologies for hepatitis, toxoplasmosis, EBV, and CMV
6. Order chest x-ray and ECHO and ECG in symptomatic children (stages B and C)
7. Pulmonary status should be evaluated regularly
8. Growth and development should be evaluated at least every 6 months
9. Nutritional assessments should be periodically performed
   a. Encourage a high calorie, high protein diet
   b. Recommend daily vitamin supplements
   c. Eliminate irritating foods such as lactose and caffeine
   d. Oral supplements such as PediaSure and Ensure may be helpful
   e. Cyproheptadine HCl (Periactin) 0.25 to 0.5 mg/kg/day divided into 2 or 3 doses may be used in children >2 years to increase appetite; other agents such as dronabinol (Marinol) and megestrol acetate (Megace) may also be used, but there is little data assessing their effects
10. Immunization guidelines
    a. The inactivated polio vaccine (IPV) should be given in place of the oral polio vaccine (OPV)
    b. Varicella vaccine is now recommended for children with CDC stage N or A and immune class 1 with an age-specific CD4+ T-cell% ≥25%
       (1) Eligible children should receive 2 doses of vaccine with a 3-month interval between doses
       (2) Susceptible household members who are not HIV-infected themselves should be given vaccine
    c. Do not administer MMR to children who have profound immunosuppression (immune Stage 3)
    d. Pneumococcal vaccine is now recommended for universal use in children <24 months; HIV-infected children <8 years should also receive vaccine
    e. Annual influenza vaccinations are recommended beginning at 6 months; influenza vaccine is also recommended for household contacts of symptomatic HIV-infected patients
    f. The routine immunization schedule is recommended for the other vaccines
11. Prophylaxis for herpes simplex, mycobacterium avium complex, and chronic candidiasis is controversial in children (consult specialist); see section on HIV/AIDS IN ADULTS AND ADOLESCENTS for further information on patient education to prevent opportunistic infections
12. PCP prophylaxis should be initiated based on the following guidelines:
    a. Children born to HIV-infected mothers should be given prophylaxis with TMP-SMZ beginning at age 4-6 weeks
    b. Discontinue prophylaxis for children who subsequently are determined to not be infected with HIV
    c. HIV-infected children and children whose infection status remains unknown should continue to receive prophylaxis for first year of life
    d. Children who have a history of PCP need lifelong chemoprophylaxis
    e. The following HIV-infected children >1 year of age need prophylaxis:
       (1) Children aged 1-5 years with CD4+ T-cell count of <500/μL or CD4+ percentages of <15%
       (2) Children aged 6-12 years with CD4+ T-cell count of <200/μL or CD4+ percentages of <15%
    f. Trimethoprim-sulfamethoxazole (TMP/SMX) 150/750 mg/m^2/day in two divided doses by mouth three times weekly on consecutive days is the most effective choice with dapsone, pentamidine aerosol, and intravenous pentamidine as alternatives

D. Antiretroviral therapy for children
  1. Adolescents in early puberty (Tanner Stages I and II) should be given pediatric dosing schedules; adolescents in late puberty (Tanner Stage V) should follow adult dosing schedules; closely monitor adolescents who are in their growth spurt (females in Tanner Stage III and males in Tanner Stage IV) when using pediatric or adult dosing guidelines
  2. An infectious disease specialist should be consulted for recommendations on initiating and changing antiretroviral therapy in children
  3. The following tables provide guidelines on when to initiate therapy and recommendations on antiretroviral regimens for initial therapy

---

INDICATIONS FOR INITIATION OF ANTIRETROVIRAL THERAPY

- Clinical symptoms associated with HIV infection (i.e., clinical categories A, B, or C [Table: Classification System: Clinical categories])
- Evidence of immune suppression, indicated by CD4+ T-lymphocyte absolute number or percentage (immune category 2 or 3 [Table: Classification System: Immune categories])
- Age <12 months–regardless of clinical, immunologic, or virologic status
- For asymptomatic children aged ≥1 year with normal immune status, two options can be considered:
  Preferred Approach
    Initiate therapy–regardless of age or symptom status
  Alternative Approach
    Defer treatment in situations in which the risk for clinical disease progression is low and other factors (e.g., concern for the durability of response, safety, and adherence) favor postponing treatment. In such cases, the clinician should regularly monitor virologic, immunologic, and clinical status. Factors to be considered in deciding to initiate therapy include the following:
    ✓ High (>100,000 copies/mL) or increasing HIV RNA copy number (more than a 0.7 $\log_{10}$ [five fold] increase for children <2 years and more than 0.5 $\log_{10}$ [three fold] for children ≥2 years) on repeat testing; these children should be offered therapy regardless of clinical or immunologic status or absolute level of viral load
    ✓ Rapidly declining CD4+ T-lymphocyte number or percentage to values approaching those indicative of moderate immune suppression (i.e., immune category 2)
    ✓ Development of clinical symptoms

Source: Working Group on Antiretroviral Therapy and Medical Management of HIV-Infected Children. (2003). *Guidelines for use of antiretroviral agents in pediatric HIV infections.* Bethesda (MD): Department of Health and Human Services Public Health Service (PHS), Centers for Disease Control and Prevention (CDC). 55 pages.

  4. Always use combination antiretroviral therapy; monotherapy is appropriate only when used in infants of indeterminate HIV status during the first 6 weeks of life to prevent perinatal HIV transmission
  5. Remember that antiretroviral therapy interacts with other medications and has many adverse effects (see drug manual and section HIV INFECTION IN ADULTS AND ADOLESCENTS)

RECOMMENDED ANTIRETROVIRAL REGIMENS FOR INITIAL THERAPY*

Strongly Recommended Regimens

Evidence of clinical benefit and sustained suppression of HIV RNA in clinical trials in HIV-infected adults; clinical trials in HIV-infected children are ongoing

- One highly active protease inhibitor plus two nucleoside reverse transcriptase inhibitors (NRTIs)
  - Preferred protease inhibitor for infants and children who cannot swallow pills or capsules: nelfinavir or ritonavir. Alternative for children who can swallow pills or capsules: indinavir
  - Recommended dual NRTI combinations: the most data on use in children are available for the combinations of zidovudine (ZDV) and dideoxyinosine (ddl) and for ZDV and lamivudine (3TC) and stavudine (d4T) and ddl. More limited data are available for the combinations of d4T and 3TC and ZDV and zalcitabine (ddC)**
- Alternative for children who can swallow capsules: Efavirenz[†] (Sustiva) plus 2 NRTIs or efavirenz plus nelfinavir and one or two NRTIs

Alternative Regimens

These treatment combinations are not strongly recommended because experience in infants and children is limited and evidence of efficacy may not outweigh potential adverse consequences (toxicity, drug interactions, or cost)

- Nevirapine and two NRTIs
- Lopinavir/ritonavir (Kaletra) with two NRTIs or with one NRTI and one NNRTI
- Indinavir or saquinavir soft get capsule with 2 NRTIs for children who can swallow capsules

Offer in Special Circumstances

Consider these combinations but they are not strongly recommended because virologic suppression is less durable and data are inconclusive concerning their efficacy

- Two NRTIs
- Amprenavir[§] in combination with 2 NRTIs or abacavir

Not Recommended

Evidence against use because of overlapping toxicity and/or because use may be virologically undesirable

- Any monotherapy
- d4T and ZDV
- ddC and ddl
- ddC and d4T
- ddC and 3TC
- Use with caution d4T and ddl (risk of pancreatitis)

*When antiretroviral drug resistance is known or suspected in the mother of a newly diagnosed infant, consider resistance testing of the infant's viral isolate to assist in selection of initial antiretroviral therapy

**ddC is not available in a liquid preparation commercially, although a liquid formulation is available through a compassionate use program of the manufacturer (Roche Pharmaceuticals). ZDV and ddC is a less preferred choice for use in combination with a protease inhibitor

[†]Efavirenz is currently only available in capsule form but a liquid preparation is being evaluated. There are no data available on appropriate dosage of efavirenz in children under 3 years of age

[§] Liquid formulation of amprenavir should not be used under age 3 due to high content of propylene glycol and vitamin E

Adapted from Working Group on Antiretroviral Therapy and Medical Management of HIV-Infected Children. (2003). *Guidelines for use of antiretroviral agents in pediatric HIV infections.* Bethesda (MD): Department of Health and Human Services Public Health Service (PHS), Centers for Disease Control and Prevention (CDC). 55 pages.

6. See following table for when to change antiretroviral therapy

---

CONSIDERATIONS FOR CHANGING ANTIRETROVIRAL THERAPY

Virologic Considerations*

- Less than a minimally acceptable virologic response after 8-12 weeks of therapy. For children receiving antiretroviral therapy with two nucleoside reverse transcriptase inhibitors (NRTIs) and a protease inhibitor, such a response is defined as a <10-fold (1.0 $\log_{10}$) decrease from baseline HIV RNA levels. For children who are receiving less potent antiretroviral therapy (i.e., dual NRTI combinations), an insufficient response is defined as a less than fivefold (0.7 $\log_{10}$) decrease in HIV RNA levels from baseline
- HIV RNA not suppressed to undetectable levels after 4-6 months of antiretroviral therapy[†]
- Repeated detection of HIV RNA in children who initially responded to antiretroviral therapy with undetectable levels
- A reproducible increase in HIV RNA copy number among children who have had a substantial HIV RNA response but still have low levels of detectable HIV RNA. Such an increase would warrant change in therapy if, after initiation of the therapeutic regimen, a greater than threefold (0.5 $\log_{10}$) increase in copy number for children aged ≥ 2 years and a greater than fivefold (0.7 $\log_{10}$) increase is observed for children aged <2 years

Immunologic Considerations*

- Change in immunologic classification
- For children with CD4+ T-lymphocyte percentages of <15% (i.e., those in immune category 3), a persistent decline of five percentiles or more in CD4+ cell percentage (e.g., from 15% to 10%)
- A rapid and substantial decrease in absolute CD4+ T-lymphocyte count (e.g., a >30% decline in <6 months)

Clinical Considerations

- Progressive neurodevelopmental deterioration[‡]
- Growth failure defined as persistent decline in weight-growth velocity despite adequate nutritional support and without other explanation
- Disease progression defined as advancement from one pediatric clinical category to another (e.g., from clinical category A to clinical category B); however, in patients whose disease progression is not associated with neurologic deterioration growth failure, virologic and immunologic parameters should be considered before changing therapy

---

*At least two measurements (taken 1 week apart) should be performed before considering a change in therapy
[†]The initial HIV RNA level of the child at the start of therapy and the level achieved with therapy should be considered when contemplating potential drug changes. For example, an immediate change in therapy may not be warranted if there is a sustained 1.5 to 2.0 $\log_{10}$ fall in HIV RNA copy number, even if RNA remains detectable at low levels
[‡]New treatment for children with neurodevelopmental deterioration should include one antiviral drug with substantial CNS penetration such as zidovudine or nevirapine

Adapted from Working Group on Antiretroviral Therapy and Medical Management of HIV-Infected Children. (2003). *Guidelines for use of antiretroviral agents in pediatric HIV infections*. Bethesda (MD): Department of Health and Human Services Public Health Service (PHS), Centers for Disease Control and Prevention (CDC). 55 pages.

7. Principles to follow when choosing of a new antiretroviral regimen in children who have had previous treatment
   a. If therapy is toxic or intolerable, choose agents with different toxicities and side-effect profiles; change of a single drug in a multidrug regimen and, in certain circumstances, dose reductions are permissible options
   b. If change is due to treatment failure always assess medication adherence
   c. If patient is adherent to prescribed drug regimen, assume the development of drug resistance and if possible, change at least two drugs to new antiretroviral agents; the new regimen should include at least three drugs, if possible; always consider cross-resistance between drugs when choosing new regimens
   d. Always review medications for possible drug interactions before making changes
   e. Always consider the patient's quality of life when making regimen changes, particularly in a patient with advanced disease

8. See following table for dosing of nucleoside reverse transcriptase inhibitors

DOSAGE SCHEDULE OF NUCLEOSIDE REVERSE TRANSCRIPTASE INHIBITORS

Drug	Preparation	Neonatal Dose	Pediatric Dose	Adolescent Dose
Abacavir (ABC)* ZIAGEN	Solution: 20mg/mL; Tabs: 300 mg	1-3 months (investigational) 8 mg/kg q 12 hours	8 mg/kg of body weight BID (maximum 300 mg q 12 hours)	Body weight >60 kg: 300 mg BID
Didanosine (dideoxyinosine) (ddI), VIDEX, VIDEX EC	10 mg/mL pediatric powder for oral solution; Chewable tabs 25, 50, 100, 150, 200 mg	Infants <90 days: 50 mg per m^2 of body surface area every 12 hours	90 mg per m^2 of body surface area every 12 hours	Body weight ≥60 kg: 200 mg BID; body weight <60 kg: 125 mg BID
Lamivudine (3TC)**, EPIVIR	Solution: 10 mg/mL; Tablets: 150 mg	Infants aged <30 days: 2 mg per kg of body weight BID	4 mg per kg of body weight BID	Body weight ≥50 kg: 150 mg BID. Body weight <50 kg: 2 mg per kg body weight BID
Stavudine (d4T), ZERIT	Solution: 1 mg/mL; Caps: 15, 20, 30, 40 mg	Under evaluation in Pediatric AIDS Clinical Trial Group protocol 332	1 mg per kg of body weight every 12 hours (up to weight of 30 kg)	Body weight ≥60 kg: 40 mg BID. Body weight <60 kg: 30 mg BID
Zalcitabine (ddC), HIVID	Syrup: 0.1 mg/mL (investigational); Tablets: 0.375 and 0.75 mg	Unknown	0.01 mg per kg of body weight every 8 hours	0.75 mg TID
Zidovudine (ZDV, AZT), RETROVIR	Syrup: 10 mg/mL; Caps: 100mg; Tabs: 300 mg; concentrate for injection or IV infusion: 10mg/mL	Premature infant: 1.5 mg/kg q 12 hours from birth to 2 weeks Neonate: 2 mg/kg q 6-8 hours PO; IV 1.5 mg/kg q 6-8 hours	160 mg m^2 of body surface every 8 hours PO; IV intermittent infusion: 120 mg per m^2 of body surface q 6 hours	200 mg TID or 300 mg BID

* Tablets in combination with zidovudine and lamivudine: Trizivir (300 mg zidovudine, 150 mg lamivudine, 300 mg abacavir)
** Tablets in combination with zidovudine: Combivir (300 mg zidovudine and 150 mg lamivudine)
Adapted from Working Group on Antiretroviral Therapy and Medical Management of HIV-Infected Children. (2003). *Guidelines for use of antiretroviral agents in pediatric HIV infections*. Bethesda (MD): Department of Health and Human Services Public Health Service (PHS), Centers for Disease Control and Prevention (CDC). 55 pages.

9. See table for doses of non-nucleoside reverse transcriptase inhibitors

DOSAGE SCHEDULE OF NONNUCLEOSIDE REVERSE TRANSCRIPTASE INHIBITORS

Drug	Preparation	Neonatal Dose	Pediatric Dose	Adolescent Dose
Delavirdine (DLV), RESCRIPTOR	Tablets: 100, 200 mg	Not recommended	Not recommended	400 mg TID (initiate at 200 mg QD x14 days, then 200 mg BID to full dose)
Efavirenz (EFV), SUSTIVA	Susp: 30 mg/mL (investigational); Caps: 50, 100, 200 mg	Not recommended	≥3 years: 10 to <15 kg: 200 mg 15 to <20 kg: 250 mg 20 to <25 kg: 300 mg 25 to <32.5 kg: 350 mg 32.5 to <40 kg: 400 mg ≥40 kg: 600 mg	600 mg q HS
Nevirapine (NVP), VIRAMUNE	Suspension: 10 mg/mL Tablets: 200 mg	120 mg/m^2 (or 5 mg/kg) QD for 14 days, then 120 mg per m^2 of body surface area q 12 hours for 14 days; then 200 mg of m^2 of body surface q 12 hours	120-200 mg per m^2 of body surface every 12 hours; initiate therapy with 120 mg per m^2 of body surface QD for 14 days, then increase to full dose	200 mg every 12 hours; initiate therapy at 200 mg QD for first 14 days, then increase to full dose

Adapted from Working Group on Antiretroviral Therapy and Medical Management of HIV-Infected Children. (2003). *Guidelines for use of antiretroviral agents in pediatric HIV infections*. Bethesda (MD): Department of Health and Human Services Public Health Service (PHS), Centers for Disease Control and Prevention (CDC). 55 pages.

10. See the following table for dosing protease inhibitors

DOSAGE SCHEDULE OF PROTEASE INHIBITORS

Drug	Preparation	Neonatal Dose	Pediatric Dose	Adolescent Dose
Amprenavir (APV), AGENERASE	Oral solution: 15 mg/mL Capsules: 50 and 150 mg	Not recommended	**4-16 years and <50 kg**: 20 mg/kg/dose BID (caps) **or** 15 mg/kg/dose TID (caps) **or** 22.5 mg/kg/dose BID (liquid) **or** 17 mg/kg/dose TID (liquid)	1200 mg BID (caps) 1400 mg BID (liquid)
Indinavir (IDV), CRIXIVAN	Capsules: 100, 200, 333, and 400 mg	Unknown. Due to side effect of hyperbilirubinemia, should not be given to neonates	500 mg per m^2 of body surface every 8 hrs	800 mg every 8 hrs
Lopinavir/ Ritonavir (KAL), KALETRA	Oral solution: 80 mg/mL lopinavir plus 20 mg/mL ritonavir Capsules: 133.3 mg lopinavir plus 33.3 mg ritonavir	Not recommended	**6 months to 12 years:** 7 to <15 kg: 12/3 mg/kg BID ≥15 to 40 kg: 10/2.5 mg/kg BID ≥40 kg: 400/100 mg BID **Dosing when used with nevirapine or efavirenz:** 7 to <15 kg: 13/3.25 mg/kg BID ≥15 to 45 kg: 11/2.75 mg/kg BID ≥45 kg: 533/133 mg BID	400/100 mg BID (3 capsules or 5 mL BID) **Dosing when used with nevirapine or efavirenz:** 533/133 mg BID (4 capsules or 6.5 mL BID)
Nelfinavir (NFV), VIRACEPT	Powder for oral suspension: 50 mg per 1 level gram scoopful; Tablets: 250 mg	(Investigational) 10 mg per kg of body weight TID	20 to 30 mg per kg of body weight TID	750 mg TID
Ritonavir (RTV), NORVIR	Oral solution: 80 mg/mL Capsules: 100 mg	Unknown	400 mg per m^2 per body surface area q 12 hours; start at 250 mg per m^2 BID; increase every 2-3 days by 50 mg/m^2 BID to full dose	600 mg BID; initiate at 300 mg BID and increase to full dose over 5 days
Saquinavir (SQV-SGC), FORTOVASE (soft gel capsule)	200 mg soft gel capsule	Unknown	Investigational: 50 mg/kg every 8 hours **or** 33 mg/kg every 8 hours with nelfinavir	1200 mg TID

Adapted from Working Group on Antiretroviral Therapy and Medical Management of HIV-Infected Children. (2003). *Guidelines for use of antiretroviral agents in pediatric HIV infections.* Bethesda (MD): Department of Health and Human Services Public Health Service (PHS), Centers for Disease Control and Prevention (CDC). 55 pages.

11. New antiretroviral agents are available or will soon be available

NEW ANTIRETROVIRAL DRUGS WITH CLINICAL DATA	
Drug	**Comment**
Enfuvirtide (Fuzeon)	• Interferes with entry of HIV-1 into cells by inhibiting fusion of viral and cellular membranes; blocks HIV's ability to infect healthy CD4+ T-cells • Indicated for therapy in treatment-experienced patients with evidence of HIV-1 replication despite ongoing antiretroviral therapy • Adverse events include local injection site reactions (occur commonly), increased rate of bacterial pneumonia, and potential hypersensitivity reactions • Dose is 2 mg/kg twice daily injected subcutaneously into upper arm, anterior thigh, or abdomen • Does not interact with other antiretroviral agents or rifampin
Atazanavir (Reyataz)	• Protease inhibitor • Once-a-day dosing • Less lipid problems than other PIs • Most common laboratory abnormality is hyperbilirubinemia that results in jaundice or scleral icterus • Adult dose is 400 mg (two 200 mg capsules) QD with food
Emtricitabine (ETC)	• Drug similar to, but more potent than lamivudine
Amdoxovir (DAPD)	• Nucleoside active against NRTI resistant strains

12. CD4+ T-cell counts and HIV viral loads should be monitored regularly to determine the effectiveness of therapy
13. In children, clinical parameters such as growth failure, abnormal neurodevelopmental function, and frequency and severity of infections are also helpful in evaluating drug efficacy

E. Adherence is a major issue
    1. Frequent evaluations (nursing, social, and behavioral) of adherence are needed
    2. Multidisciplinary team effort is recommended to enhance adherence
    3. Patient education, cues or reminders to administer drugs, and individualized plans are helpful
    4. Teach strategies to make drugs more palatable to increase adherence such as mixing liquid formulations with chocolate milk, pudding or ice cream; dulling senses prior to drug administration with popsicles, iced drinks, ice cream, or ice; coating mouth with peanut butter before drug administration; ingesting strong-tasting foods after drugs

F. Treatment of opportunistic infections in children: Typically a specialist in infectious disease will manage the care of children who develop opportunistic infections (see section on HIV/AIDS IN ADULTS AND ADOLESCENTS for additional information)

G. Nutritional, psychiatric, behavioral and neuropsychological problems are important clinical issues and should be evaluated and addressed at each visit

H. Patient education and counseling are extremely important and best managed with an interdisciplinary team of professionals who are specialists in the care of children

I. Follow up is individualized based on immune status and clinical parameters

HUMAN IMMUNODEFICIENCY VIRUS (HIV) INFECTION AND ACQUIRED IMMUNODEFICIENCY SYNDROME (AIDS) IN ADULTS AND ADOLESCENTS

I. Definitions:

A. HIV infection: Infection with human retrovirus, Human Immunodeficiency Virus (HIV)

B. AIDS: Disease characterized by opportunistic infections (see following table for case definition)

CONDITIONS INCLUDED IN THE 1993 AIDS SURVEILLANCE CASE DEFINITION

- HIV+ persons with CD4 cell counts <200/µL or a CD4 percent <14%*
- Candidiasis of bronchi, trachea, or lungs
- Candidiasis, esophageal
- Cervical cancer, invasive*
- Coccidioidomycosis, disseminated or extrapulmonary
- Cryptococcosis, extrapulmonary
- Cryptosporidiosis, chronic intestinal (>1 mo duration)
- Cytomegalovirus disease (other than liver, spleen, or nodes)
- Encephalopathy, HIV-related
- Herpes simplex: Chronic ulcer(s) (>1 mo duration); or bronchitis, pneumonitis, or esophagitis
- Histoplasmosis, disseminated or extrapulmonary
- Isosporiasis, chronic intestinal (>1 mo duration)
- Kaposi's sarcoma
- Lymphoma, Burkitt's (or equivalent term)
- Lymphoma, immunoblastic (or equivalent term)
- Lymphoma, primary, of brain
- *Mycobacterium avium* complex or *M. kansasii*, disseminated or extrapulmonary
- *Mycobacterium tuberculosis*, any site (pulmonary* or extrapulmonary)
- *Mycobacterium*, other species or unidentified species, disseminated or extrapulmonary
- *Pneumocystis carinii* pneumonia
- Pneumonia, recurrent*
- Progressive multifocal leukoencephalopathy
- *Salmonella* septicemia, recurrent
- Toxoplasmosis of brain
- Wasting syndrome due to HIV

---

*Added January 1993

Source: Center for Communicable Diseases. 1992. 1993 revised classification system for HIV infection and expanded surveillance case definition of AIDS among adolescents and adults. *MMWR, 41* (RR-17)

II. Pathogenesis

    A.   HIV invades the body and may enter any cell, but it has a propensity to infect and kill cells of the immune system, particularly the CD4+ T-cells (T-lymphocytes)

    B.   HIV actively replicates which leads to immune system damage and results in susceptibility to opportunistic infections (OIs), cancer, neurologic diseases, wasting, and death

    C.   Transmission occurs by direct contact of a person's blood or body secretions with the blood or body secretions of a person infected with HIV virus
        1.   Body fluids considered to be infectious include blood, tissues, cerebrospinal fluid, synovial fluid, peritoneal fluid, pleural fluid, pericardial fluid, amniotic fluid, semen, and vaginal secretions
        2.   Body fluids that are **not** considered infectious include feces, nasal secretions, sputum, sweat, tears, urine, vomitus, and saliva (unless contaminated with blood)
        3.   Certain activities are associated with high risk of infection such as unprotected anal, oral, or vaginal sex with multiple partners; unprotected sex with an HIV positive person; IV drug abuse; blood transfusions outside the US or during 1977-1985; unprotected sex with a person who has recent or past history of sexually transmitted diseases
        4.   Highest percentage of HIV transmissions occurs during sex acts where body fluids are exchanged
        5.   IV drug use is the second most frequent route of transmission

III. Clinical Presentation

    A.   Epidemiology
        1.   The first AIDS cases were reported in 1981
        2.   Seroprevalence of HIV in US is 0.3%
        3.   Highly active antiretroviral therapy (HAART), defined as a combination of three or more antiretroviral drug therapy (ART) agents, has revolutionized HIV/AIDS care with substantial decreases in AIDS-defining complications, hospitalizations, and deaths
        4.   The largest decline in cases of HIV/AIDS occurred among persons aged 25-44 years
        5.   Increasing proportions of individuals living with AIDS are black or Hispanic, female, residents of the South, and individuals exposed to HIV through heterosexual contact
        6.   Approximately one fourth of individuals living with HIV infection are unaware of their infection
        7.   Rising drug resistance to all three classes of ART has been found in new HIV infections

    B.   Viral load and CD4+ T-cell counts help to assess the prognosis of HIV-infected patients
        1.   Viral load measures the level of circulating plasma HIV-RNA; the greater the number of virus, the more active the infection, and the worse the prognosis
        2.   CD4+ T-cell counts assess the general level of immunity or the extent of HIV-induced immune damage already suffered; the lower the CD4+ T-cell count the greater the risk for OIs
        3.   A decrease in viral load of one log is associated with an average increase in CD4+ T-cells of about 85/mm^3

    C.   The natural history of HIV infection encompasses a wide spectrum of disease but infection is always harmful and true long-term survival free of major immune damage is uncommon

    D.   The acute retroviral syndrome develops after HIV exposure and a 1-3 week incubation period
        1.   Symptoms resemble those of infectious mononucleosis and are self-limited, lasting 1-3 weeks
            a.   Fever, fatigue, lymphadenopathy, pharyngitis, and arthralgias are typical
            b.   Rash, diarrhea, nausea, vomiting, hepatosplenomegaly, thrush, weight loss, and neurological disorders (aseptic meningitis, Guillain-Barré) are less common problems
        2.   Best diagnostic tests to detect disease are p24 antigen or plasma HIV RNA (viral load)
        3.   Syndrome is associated with rapid HIV replication or high viral load
        4.   Seroconversion occurs 3-5 weeks after transmission and is accompanied by sharp drop in viral load

    E.   Early HIV disease: Period between seroconversion to 4 months following HIV transmission
        1.   At approximately 4 months, the plasma levels of HIV RNA reach a set point that shows a very gradual increase, averaging 7% a year over several years in the absence of antigenic stimuli such as intercurrent illness or immunizations or antiretroviral therapy; this set point predicts the subsequent rate of progression
            a.   High concentrations (>100,000 copies/mL) are associated with median survival of 4.4 years
            b.   Low concentrations (<5,000 copies/mL) are associated with median survival >10 years

2. Patients in early course of disease are usually asymptomatic, but may have the following:
   a. Lymphadenopathy and dermatologic abnormalities (seborrheic dermatitis, psoriasis, eosinophilic folliculitis)
   b. Oral lesions such as aphthous ulcers, herpes simplex labialis, and oral hairy leukoplakia usually occur later but may present
3. As the disease progresses, patients have more frequent skin disorders, oral lesions, and infections as well as diarrhea, intermittent fevers, night sweats, chills, unexplained weight loss, myalgias, arthralgia, headache, and fatigue

F. Symptomatic HIV disease: Complications are due to direct effects of the virus or to immunosuppression which occurs after a significant quantity of CD4+ T-cells has been destroyed
   1. Direct effect of HIV: Persistent generalized lymphadenopathy, HIV-associated dementia, lymphocytic interstitial pneumonia, HIV-associated nephropathy, and progressive immunosuppression; other possible consequences are anemia, neutropenia, thrombocytopenia, cardiomyopathy, myopathy, peripheral neuropathy, chronic meningitis, polymyositis, and Guillain-Barré syndrome
   2. Immunosuppression results in opportunistic infections and tumors, primarily from compromised cell-mediated immunity; see tables in V.F., V.G., V.H., V.I. for further clinical presentation of OIs
   3. Only about 2% or less of HIV-infected patients can maintain CD4+ T-cell counts in the normal range for lengthy periods of time (>12 years) without antiretroviral therapy
   4. In untreated patients, CD4+ T-cells average a 40-60/mm^3 decrease per year
   5. OIs, particularly pneumocystic pneumonia, occur when CD4+ T-cell counts fall below 200/mm^3
   6. Risk for opportunistic infections increases dramatically as CD4+ T-cell counts drop below 50/mm^3

G. HAART has extended patients' life expectancies but has potential adverse effects
   1. Lactic acidosis and hepatic steatosis occur from treatment with NRTIs (nucleoside reverse transcriptase inhibitor); syndrome is associated with high mortality rate
      a. Patients are considered to have lactic acidemia if they are asymptomatic with lactate >10 mmol/L or if they are symptomatic with lactate 5-10 mmol/L
      b. Clinical manifestations include unexplained onset and persistence of nausea, abdominal pain and distention, vomiting, diarrhea, anorexia, dyspnea, weakness, ascending neuromuscular weakness, myalgias, paresthesias, weight loss, and hepatomegaly
      c. Laboratory evaluation reveals increased serum lactate and may include increased anion gap, decreased serum bicarbonate, elevated aminotransferases, creatine phosphokinase, lactic dehydrogenase, lipase, and amylase
      d. Echotomography and computed tomography scans may detect enlarged fatty liver, and histologic examination may detect microvesicular steatosis
      e. If NRTI treatment continues, patients may have mitochondrial toxicity with severe lactic acidosis resulting in tachypnea, dyspnea, and ultimately respiratory failure
   2. Hepatotoxicity
      a. Defined as 3-5 times increase in serum transaminases with or without clinical hepatitis
      b. Typically, patients are asymptomatic
      c. Nevirapine has the greatest potential for causing clinical hepatitis and fatal hepatotoxicity
      d. Fatal hepatotoxicity was reported in 3 pregnant women using didanosine/stavudine
      e. Other risk factors include protease inhibitor (PI) use (major), hepatitis C infection (major), hepatitis B infection, alcohol abuse, baseline elevated liver enzymes, stavudine use, and use of other hepatotoxic agents
   3. Hyperglycemia, glucose intolerance, insulin resistance, new-onset diabetes mellitus, diabetic ketoacidosis, and exacerbation of pre-existing diabetes mellitus are strongly associated with PI use; conditions may also occur with PI-sparing regimens
   4. Fat maldistribution syndrome; often referred to as lipodystrophy or as lipodystrophy syndrome when combined with metabolic abnormalities including insulin resistance and hyperlipidemia
      a. Occurs primarily in association with PIs, but may occur in non-PI regimens
      b. The abdomen, dorsocervical fat pad, and breasts are sites for fat accumulation
      c. The face and extremities are most often affected by fat atrophy
   5. Hyperlipidemia with elevation of total serum cholesterol, low-density lipoprotein, and fasting triglycerides
      a. Occurs primarily with use of PIs; strongest association with ritonavir
      b. Association with NNRTIs (nonnucleoside reverse transcriptase inhibitor) is unclear and contradictory
      c. Very high triglycerides may be associated with pancreatitis
   6. Increased spontaneous bleeding episodes may occur with patients with hemophilia A and B

7. Osteonecrosis, osteopenia, and osteoporosis are other metabolic complications that have a definitive association with HIV itself; association with ART and PIs is unclear
   a. Factors associated with decreases in bone mineral density include alcohol abuse, hemoglobinopathies, corticosteroid treatment, hyperlipidemia, and hypercoagulability states
   b. Patients typically complain of pain in affected site of bone loss, but about 5% of those affected are asymptomatic
8. Skin rash
   a. Occurs most commonly with NNRTI class of drugs (predominantly with nevirapine); abacavir is the NRTI and amprenavir is the PI most often associated with rashes
   b. Most cases are mild to moderate and occur within first weeks of initiating therapy
   c. Serious manifestations include Stevens-Johnson syndrome, toxic epidermal necrosis (TEN), and a life-threatening syndrome with drug rash, eosinophilia, and systemic symptoms (DRESS)
   d. Abacavir may cause fatal hypersensitivity reaction that occurs with or without rash plus fever, fatigue, myalgia, nausea/vomiting, diarrhea, abdominal pain, pharyngitis, cough, dyspnea

IV. Diagnosis/Evaluation

A. History
   1. Determine risk factors for HIV (see following table); many primary care clinicians miss opportunities to identify and test persons at high risk for HIV infection

---

SCREENING STRATEGIES TO IDENTIFY PATIENTS AT RISK FOR HIV INFECTION

- Did you ever receive a transfusion of blood products outside the US or between 1977 and 1985?

- Open-ended question by provider, "What are you doing now or what have you done in the past that you think may put you at risk for HIV infection?"

- Screening questions* -- "Since your last HIV test (if ever), have you
  ✓ injected drugs and shared equipment (e.g., needles, syringes, cotton, water) with others?"
  ✓ had unprotected intercourse with someone that you think might be infected (e.g., a partner who injected drugs, has been diagnosed or treated for a sexually transmitted disease [STD] or hepatitis, has had multiple or anonymous sex partners, or has exchanged sex for drugs or money)?"
  ✓ had unprotected vaginal or anal intercourse with more than one sex partner?"
  ✓ been diagnosed or treated for an STD, hepatitis, or tuberculosis?"
  ✓ had a fever or illness of unknown cause?"
  ✓ been told you have an infection related to a 'weak immune system'?"

---

* Clients who respond affirmatively to ≥1 of these questions should be considered at increased risk for HIV
Adapted from Centers for Disease Control and Prevention. (2001). Revised guidelines for HIV counseling, testing, and referral. Technical Expert Panel Review of CDC Counseling, Testing and Referral Guidelines. *MMWR 50* (RR-9), 1-58.

   2. History at initial visit after the diagnosis is confirmed; patient's health status may range from asymptomatic to advanced immunodeficiency; this first encounter sets the stage for a partnership with the patient that may last for years
      a. Explore the duration of HIV positivity as well as when and how the patient was infected
      b. Document when the patient was first diagnosed with HIV infection
      c. Inquire about testing (when and where was it done?; what led to testing?)
      d. Ask about results of prior diagnostic tests
      e. Inquire about medications, treatments (including complementary therapies), responses to treatments, and history of adherence to medications
      f. Obtain past risk history (see preceding table)
      g. Inquire about sexual history such as number of partners within last year, use of condoms, history of other sexually transmitted diseases
      h. Ask about previous medical care including immunization status (pneumococcal, influenza, tetanus, hepatitis A and B, varicella) and prior TB skin tests
      i. Document significant past medical history (opportunistic infections, hospitalizations, surgeries, chickenpox, and chronic diseases, particularly tuberculosis, hepatitis, shingles, anemia, heart disease, neuromuscular conditions, alcoholism, and psychiatric disorders)
      j. Explore risk for cardiovascular disease such as obesity, smoking, hypertension, diabetes, family history, blood lipids
      k. In females, obtain a gynecological history including use and type of contraception, pregnancy history, current menstrual pattern, date of last pelvic exam and pap smear, history of abnormal pap smear, and history of vaginal bleeding; ask about desire for pregnancy

l.   Inquire about travel to Ohio and Mississippi River valleys (risk of histoplasmosis) and to Southwestern desert (risk of coccidioidomycosis)

m.   Assess patient's and family's knowledge about HIV

n.   Obtain a detailed social and mental health history to determine psychosocial assets/needs

o.   Screen for domestic violence (see section on DOMESTIC VIOLENCE for questions)

p.   Perform an HIV-related review of systems (ROS) directed toward uncovering symptoms of infection (fevers, night sweats, weight change, lymphadenopathy, visual changes, skin changes, new headaches, memory problems, mouth lesions, difficulty swallowing, cough/chest pain, diarrhea, nausea, vomiting, vaginitis, peripheral neuropathy, weakness, insomnia, depression)

3.   History on subsequent visits

    a.   Document most recent CD4+ T-cell count and HIV viral load

    b.   Document medications used for treating HIV infection

        (1)   Inquire about adverse effects from medications

        (2)   Always ask about adherence; a simple, direct question such as "How many doses have you missed in the past 24 hours?" may be nonthreatening

    c.   Inquire about new or worsening symptoms

    d.   Perform an HIV-related ROS (see IV.A.2.p.)

B.   Physical Examination

1.   Vital signs (fever is a sign of opportunistic infections and neoplasms)

2.   Measure weight (important in detecting "wasting syndrome" and determining the type of dietary intervention that is needed)

3.   Observe general appearance, noting signs of distress and depression

4.   Inspect for signs of weight maldistribution syndrome and measure waist/hip (or waist alone); measure breasts in females

5.   Examine skin for color, lesions, ecchymosis, and signs of dehydration

6.   Inspect nails for discoloration (e.g. due to zidovudine use or fungal infection)

7.   Carefully assess the eyes, including ophthalmoscopy for retinopathy

8.   Examine oropharynx, noting thrush, hairy oral leukoplakia, herpes simplex, periodontal problems, ulcerations

9.   Palpate for lymphadenopathy as generalized lymphadenopathy is frequently present; localized lymphadenopathy may indicate carcinoma

10.   Perform pulmonary and cardiac exams for pneumonia and cardiomyopathy

11.   Perform a complete breast examination; protease inhibitors and ketoconazole can cause gynecomastia in males

12.   Perform examination of abdomen, noting organomegaly

13.   Examine anal area for detection of sexually transmitted diseases, ulcerations, and fissures

14.   Perform pelvic and speculum exams on females for cervical dysplasia, vaginal candidiasis, and sexually transmitted diseases; perform a complete genitourinary examination on men

15.   Perform a musculoskeletal exam, noting muscle mass, strength, and tenderness (to detect myositis that may be associated with antiretroviral therapy [ART])

16.   Perform complete neurologic exam, including testing of cranial nerves, cerebellar function, reflexes, sensory function, and mental status for dementia and neuropathy

17.   Perform a psychiatric examination

C.   Differential diagnosis

1.   Mononucleosis

2.   Chronic fatigue syndrome

3.   Cancer

4.   Anemia

5.   Infections

6.   Autoimmune diseases

7.   Adrenal insufficiency

D.   Diagnostic tests

1.   **Testing to determine the diagnosis of HIV**

    a.   **Antibody testing** uses enzyme-linked immunoabsorbent assay (ELISA) and a Western blot to make the diagnosis (both tests must be positive to confirm the diagnosis)

        (1)   ELISA, the initial test, is sensitive but not highly specific (may have false positives)

        (2)   Either a Western blot (WB) or an immunofluorescence assay (IFA) is used for confirmation of positive ELISA tests; WB and IFA are specific but labor intensive

b. Other tests for detection of antibodies
    (1) Calypte HIV-1 Urine EIA uses urine for screening; positive results require confirmation by standard serology
    (2) OraSure can detect antibodies from a sample of oral saliva
    (3) Home Access Express Test is an anonymous, finger-stick blood test for antibodies which can be done by an individual at home and purchased over-the-counter

c. SUDS and OraQuick are FDA-approved rapid tests
    (1) Tests are definitive if negative; positive results need confirmation with standard serology
    (2) Advantageous in settings in which there are occupational exposures and where reliable follow-up is unlikely such as in emergency rooms and STD clinics

d. Persons with positive antibody tests are considered HIV seropositive; however, a negative antibody test does not guarantee that an individual is seronegative
    (1) A window period exists; it may take 1-3 months after HIV exposure for seroconversion or for antibodies to form in sufficient amounts to be detectable by antibody tests
    (2) Because of this window period, persons with initial negative antibody tests and low risks should be retested at 6 months and high risk persons should be retested at 6 months and 1 year

e. **Antigen tests** can determine diagnosis by direct detection of virus, but they are expensive; useful in diagnosing persons with acute retroviral syndrome which occurs before antibody tests become positive
    (1) Viral load testing (RNA polymerase chain reaction [RT-PCR], branched DNA [bDNA] assays), and in vitro nucleic amplification test for HIV-RNA (Nucli-Sens HIF-1 QT) can measure the amount of HIV RNA in the plasma
    (2) p24 antigen can identify the presence of the HIV protein, but cannot quantify the amount of HIV; useful for diagnosing acute retroviral syndrome if RNA testing is unavailable
    (3) Diagnosis of HIV infection based on HIV RNA testing should be confirmed by standard methods (Western blot serology performed 2-4 months after the initial indeterminate or negative test)

2. **Tests to monitor disease progress: CD4+ T-cells and HIV RNA** (viral load)
a. Recommended schedule for ordering CD4+ T-cell and viral load tests:
    (1) At time of diagnosis and after initiation of therapy at 4, 8-12, and 16-24 weeks to assess response to therapy
    (2) Once viral suppression (2 sequential viral load measurements below the limit of detection of the most sensitive assay available) has been attained, monitor every 8-12 weeks
    (3) Consider more frequent monitoring in cases of intercurrent illness, change of antiretroviral therapy (ART), if adherence is questionable, or for patients with discordant responses (CD4+ T-cells that do not increase with successful viral suppression)

b. Measurement of CD4+ T-cell counts
    (1) Determine effectiveness of antiretroviral therapy, prognosis of disease, and need for prophylaxis of opportunistic infections
    (2) Typically, counts increase by more than 50 cells/mm^3 at 4-8 weeks after ART has been started or changed; additional increase of 50-100 cells/mm^3 per year thereafter
    (3) A substantial decrease in CD4+ T-cells is a decrease of >30% from baseline for absolute cell numbers

c. Measurement of HIV RNA levels or viral loads
    (1) RNA polymerase chain reaction (RT-PCR) and branched DNA (bDNA) and in vitro nucleic amplification assays can measure the amount of HIV RNA in the plasma; results with RT-PCR test are twice the levels with bDNA
    (2) Effective therapy reduces viral load by more than 90% (a 1-$\log_{10}$, or 10-fold, reduction) within 8 weeks of treatment; consider poor adherence, viral resistance, or inadequate drug exposure (e.g., malabsorption) if viral load fails to decrease to these levels
    (3) After 16-24 weeks of ART, plasma viral levels should be undetectable
    (4) Rates of viral load decline are affected by baseline CD4+ T-cells, the initial viral load, potency of drug regimen, medication adherence, previous exposure to ART, and presence of any opportunistic infections

        (5)   A threefold or 0.5-$\log_{10}$ increase or decrease in viral levels is considered a minimal change

        (6)   Viral load results may be inaccurate during or within 4 weeks after successful treatment of any intercurrent infection, resolution of symptomatic illness, or immunization because of the immune activation of virus associated with these events

3. **Tests to screen for concomitant diseases, immunity status, and as a base-line before drugs are administered;** ordered at first visit after diagnosis is confirmed and thereafter as recommended

   a.   Mantoux method using the purified protein derivative (PPD) to screen for tuberculosis and annually for high-risk patients (anergy testing is no longer recommended)

        (1)   Do not order if patient has history of positive PPD or history of TB treatment

        (2)   Positive PPD for person with HIV is >5 mm of induration

   b.   Rapid plasma reagin (RPR) or the Venereal Disease Laboratories (VDRL) to screen for syphilis which occurs in approximately 20% of patients with HIV infection; for patients with high-risk of developing STDs, order annually

   c.   Pap smear for women to screen for cervical dysplasia at baseline and at 6 months; then, annually if negative

   d.   Chemistry panel including liver function tests and renal profile; useful as baseline measures since patient may be receiving drugs with potential hepatic or renal toxicities

   e.   Hepatitis screen

        (1)   Anti-HBc to determine hepatitis immunity and need for HBV vaccine

        (2)   HBsAg and anti-HCV to detect active hepatitis if patient has unexplained elevated transaminase levels; obtain anti–HCV in all injection drug users

        (3)   Positive anti-HCV should be verified with recombinant immunoblot assay (RIBA) or reverse transcriptase-polymerase chain reaction (RT-PCR)

   f.   Toxoplasmosis serology (anti-toxoplasma antibody or IgG titer)

        (1)   Patient is at risk for reactivation toxoplasmosis when CD4+ T-cells drop below 100/mm^3

        (2)   Consider repeating in seronegative patients when their CD4+ T-cell counts are <100/mm^3

   g.   CBC with differential and platelet count; anemia, leukopenia, or thrombocytopenia are common in HIV infection and can also result from drug therapy; order every 3-6 months

   h.   Order lipid profile and glucose at baseline before antiretroviral therapy and at switch of therapy, 3-6 months after starting or switching therapy, and at least annually thereafter

   i.   The following are optional tests:

        (1)   Chest x-ray to screen for latent TB and as a baseline test

        (2)   Cytomegalovirus (CMV) IgG; CMV retinitis is a common complication and develops in seropositive patients when CD4+ T-cell drops below 50-75/mm^3

        (3)   Glucose-6-phosphate dehydrogenase deficiency (G-6-PD), particularly for high risk patients (African Americans and men of Mediterranean heritage): If test is positive, patient has a deficiency and should not use dapsone and possibly should not use a sulfonamide

        (4)   Varicella IgG to determine need for post-exposure prophylaxis with varicella zoster immune globulin

        (5)   Gonorrhea and chlamydia screens for women

        (6)   CD4+ cell subset determinations to enumerate memory and naive cells are used primarily in clinical trials to help define the degree of immune reconstitution

4. **Therapeutic drug monitoring**

   a.   In patients on zidovudine, order CBC at least every 3 months

   b.   Closely monitor liver enzymes after ART initiation; after nevirapine initiation monitor every 2 weeks for first month, then monthly for first 12 weeks, then every 1-3 months

   c.   Order routine fasting blood glucose tests at baseline and then every 3-6 months when PIs are used, particularly in patients with preexisting diabetes

   d.   Closely monitor lipid levels in patients with risk for atherosclerotic disease; in all patients assess at baseline, 3-6 months after ART is started or changed, and annually thereafter

   e.   Routine measurements of lactate levels and bone density (dual energy X-ray absorptiometry or quantitative ultrasound) among asymptomatic patients are not currently recommended; patients with symptoms of avascular necrosis should have CT ordered

   f.   There are no clear recommendations for monitoring body fat composition abnormalities; serial waist/hip (or waist alone) and breast measurement in women may be helpful

5. **Drug-resistance testing**
   a. Considered standard of care in management of treatment failure
      (1) Provides guidance on which drugs to exclude or include in new regimens
      (2) Perform testing when patient is on ART
   b. Strongly consider testing in patients who may have been infected with a resistant viral strain, particularly patients with a recent infection, or when the initial response to ART is suboptimal, despite excellent drug adherence, or when there is virologic failure during combination therapy
   c. Resistance testing is **not** recommended in following circumstances
      (1) Chronic infection in treatment naïve patients
      (2) After patient has discontinued ART for >2 weeks
      (3) When viral load is <1000 copies/mL
   d. Order either genotypic or phenotypic assays; for patients with complex treatment history, both assays may provide important and complementary information
      (1) Both assays measure only the dominant HIV species and thus some resistant strains may not be detected; assays are best at identifying drugs that will be ineffective rather than drugs that will work
      (2) Genotypic assays measure mutations on the reverse transcriptase or protease gene; results are available in 1-2 weeks
      (3) Phenotypic assays are more analogous to conventional antibacterial sensitivity tests; these assays are more costly and take 2-3 weeks to run
6. **Drug concentration monitoring**
   a. Not universally recommended
   b. May be beneficial in cases of treatment failure or when salvage therapy with a ritonavir-enhanced PI-based regimen has been started (particularly if other drugs have known pharmacological interactions such as efavirenz)

V. Plan/Management (care should be supervised by infectious disease specialist); because treatment of HIV infection changes rapidly consult following websites for updated information: CDC Clearinghouse (http://www.cdc.org) and the HIV Information Network (http://www.hivatis.org)

   A. Considerations for therapy among **HIV-infected adolescents**; medication dosages used to treat HIV and OIs should be based on Tanner staging of puberty and not specific age
      1. For patient in early puberty (Tanner stages I and II) prescribe dosages based on pediatric guidelines
      2. For patients in late puberty (Tanner stage V) prescribe dosages based on adult guidelines
      3. For patients in the midst of growth spurt (Tanner stage III females and Tanner stage IV males) choose either adult or pediatric dosing guidelines and closely monitor for medication efficacy and toxicity

   B. Provide **patient education and counseling** at each visit; adjust amount and complexity of teaching and counseling based on patient's degree of stress, prior knowledge, readiness to learn, and cognitive abilities
      1. Provide information about transmission and how to prevent spread of infection such as not sharing razors or toothbrushes, carefully cleaning up blood spills, disposing of used feminine sanitary products
      2. Discuss lifestyle choices and safe sex practices such as latex barriers including condoms, female vaginal pouches, and dental dams
         a. Even patients with undetectable viral loads should be considered infectious and should practice safe sex
         b. HIV-infected males should wear condoms even when engaging in sexual activity with other HIV-infected individuals to prevent transmission of drug-resistant strains of HIV and other sexually transmitted diseases
         c. Spermicides containing *nonoxynol-9* are not effective means of HIV prevention
      3. Provide education and support to stop injecting drugs; for patients that continue to inject discuss safety issues such as never sharing needles, disposing of syringes after use, and using sterile injection equipment
      4. Discuss ways to avoid exposure to infection from opportunistic infections
         a. Recommend that patient wash hands after changing diapers, handling pets, and gardening or having other contact with soil
         b. Avoid changing cat liter box due to risk of toxoplasmosis; avoid rough play with kittens due to risk of cat scratch disease
         c. Avoid animals aged <6 months when obtaining a pet
         d. Discuss susceptibility to contagious disease and how to protect self

  e. Travel, specifically to developing countries, may be hazardous due to high risk for food-borne and waterborne infections

    (1) Antimicrobial prophylaxis is not routinely recommended, but may be warranted in patients with high risk (consider ciprofloxacin 500 mg daily for high risk persons)

    (2) All travelers to developing countries should have a supply of antibiotics (e.g. ciprofloxacin 500 mg BID for 3-7 days) to take empirically if diarrhea occurs

    (3) Consult specialist in travel medicine for advice concerning immunizations, chemoprophylaxis against malaria, and protection against arthropod vectors

  f. Teach about food safety

    (1) Foods should be well done and thoroughly cooked; avoid raw/rare meat, fish and poultry, raw eggs, or unpasteurized dairy products

    (2) Wash hands after contact with raw meat

    (3) Wash fruits and vegetables before eating

    (4) Avoid foods from delicatessen counters or heat/reheat these foods until steaming

    (5) Consider using filtered or bottled water

5. Discuss ways to handle notification of partners and others; the local health department can assist with anonymous partner notification/elicitation

6. Discuss healthy diet; referral to nutritionist is beneficial

  a. Recommend eating a variety of foods from different food groups

  b. Encourage nutrient density or making every bite of food count; avoid foods with little protein, vitamins, and minerals

  c. Choose foods that are as close to their natural states as possible; use whole wheat instead of white bread or brown rice instead of white

  d. Use olive and canola oils instead of margarine and vegetable oils which are rich in polyunsaturated fatty acids and may suppress the immune system

  e. Recommend low-fat diets to reduce risk of developing hyperlipidemia

  f. To prevent decreased bone density, suggest an adequate intake of calcium and vitamin D

  g. One or two daily multivitamin/mineral supplement(s) is(are) recommended

7. Encourage smoking cessation and decreasing or eliminating other types of substance abuse (alcohol, recreational drugs)

8. Reinforce the importance of healthy lifestyles such as good oral hygiene, good sleep habits, and ways to reduce stress such as exercise, relaxation techniques, and guided imagery; massage therapy and referral to a psychologist may be beneficial

9. Exercise, including weight-bearing exercise, helps prevent adverse effects of HAART such as hyperlipidemia and bone density problems

10. Provide information on prognosis and future therapy plans; emphasize that advances in HIV therapy have dramatically improved outcomes and that patients who adhere to therapy can usually lead fairly normal lives and have a long life (however, remind that cure of HIV is unlikely)

11. Discuss what to do if an emergency arises and which symptoms require immediate attention

12. Help empower patients to become actively involved in their care through support groups, learning about the disease and treatments, and developing a partnership with the clinician

13. For patients in the late stage of disease offer information on advance directives; discuss living wills, health care surrogates; consider referral for home care or hospice care

14. Provide information on community resources and website resources (see following table)

WEB SITE RESOURCES	
HIV Prevention	http://hivinsite.ucsf.edu
Medical information	www.hopkins-aids.edu
Medical information	www.medscape.com

C. Medication adherence is crucial; nonadherence is the strongest predictor of virologic failure

  1. Determine patient's readiness before initiating ART

  2. Effective communication and trust between patient and clinician is essential

  3. Negotiate a treatment plan that the patient understands and to which he/she can commit

  4. Reinforce the need to adhere at every visit; emphasize that 90-95% of doses must be taken for optimal viral suppression

  5. Inform patient of potential side effects, ways to manage side effects, and possible adverse drug interactions

  6. Enlist support of friends/family, provide written drug schedules, pill boxes, or alarm clocks

  7. Factors to consider in improving adherence are pill volume, pill size, dietary restrictions, and toxic adverse effects

D. **Immunization** recommendations
   1. Influenza vaccine should be administered annually; pneumococcal, Hepatitis A and B vaccines should be administered to susceptible patients according to recommended guidelines (see table PROPHYLAXIS TO PREVENT FIRST EPISODE OF OPPORTUNISTIC DISEASE)
   2. *Haemophilus influenzae* type B vaccine is no longer recommended as most infections in HIV-infected persons involve nontypeable strains
   3. Administer tetanus-diphtheria, mumps, rubella, measles vaccines identical to patients without HIV
   4. If polio vaccine is needed, use enhanced inactivated polio vaccine (eIPV)
   5. Do **not** use any of the following vaccines: Live polio, varicella zoster, BCG, or any live or attenuated vaccine except measles, mumps, and rubella

E. **Health maintenance referrals** are optional
   1. Twice-yearly dental examinations
   2. Periodic ophthalmology examinations: screening for CMV retinitis by a trained ophthalmologist or optometrist should be considered every 4-6 months once the patient's CD4+ T-cell count falls below 75-100/mm^3

F. Medications should be given to **prevent opportunistic infections** when a person's CD4+ T-cell counts fall to certain levels or after exposure to certain pathogens (see following table)

PROPHYLAXIS TO PREVENT FIRST EPISODE OF OPPORTUNISTIC DISEASE

Pathogen	Indication Discontinuing/Restarting Primary Prophylaxis	Preventive regimens	
		First Choice	Alternative
I. Strongly recommended as standard of care			
Pneumocystis carinii pneumonia (PCP)*	CD4+ count <200 cells/μL or oropharyngeal candidiasis; also consider prophylaxis for persons with a CD4+ percentage of <14% or for persons with a history of AIDS-defining illness and possibly for those with CD4+ counts of >200 cells/μL but <250 cells/μL Discontinue in patients who have responded to HAART with an increase in CD4+ count >200 cells/μL for ≥3 mos; restart if CD4+ count decreases to <200 cells/μL or if PCP recurs	Trimethoprim-sulfamethoxazole (TMP-SMZ), 1 DS PO QD or TMP-SMZ, 1 SS PO QD*	TMP-SMZ, 1 DS PO three times a week; dapsone, 50 mg PO BID or 100 mg PO QD; dapsone, 50 mg PO QD plus pyrimethamine, 50 mg PO weekly plus leucovorin, 25 mg PO weekly; dapsone, 200 mg PO plus pyrimethamine, 75 mg PO plus leucovorin, 25 mg PO weekly; or aerosolized pentamidine, 300 mg every month via Respirgard II nebulizer
Mycobacterium tuberculosis Isoniazid-sensitive†	Tuberculin skin test (TST) reaction ≥5 mm or prior positive TST result without treatment or contact with case of active tuberculosis, regardless of TST result	Isoniazid, 300 mg PO plus pyridoxine, 50 mg PO QD x 9 mos or isoniazid, 900 mg PO plus pyridoxine, 100 mg PO twice a week x 9 mos	Rifampin, 600 mg PO QD x 4 mos or rifabutin, 300 mg PO QD X 4 mos; pyrazinamide, 15-20 mg/kg PO QD X 2 mos plus either rifampin, 600 mg PO QD X 2 mos or rifabutin, 300 mg PO QD X 2 mos
Isoniazid-resistant	Same as above	Rifampin, 600 mg PO QD or rifabutin, 300 mg PO QD X 4 mos	Pyrazinamide, 15-20 mg/kg PO QD X 2 mos plus either rifampin, 600 mg PO QD X 2 mos or rifabutin, 300 mg PO QD X 2 mos
Multidrug-resistant	Same as above	Consult Public Health authorities	----
Toxoplasma gondii	IgG antibody to *Toxoplasma* and CD4+ count <100/μL Discontinue when CD4+ count increases to >200 cells/μL for ≥3 mos; restart prophylaxis when CD4+ count decreases to <100-200 cells/μL	TMP-SMZ, 1 DS PO QD	TMP-SMZ, 1 SS PO QD; dapsone, 50 mg PO QD plus pyrimethamine, 50 mg PO weekly plus leucovorin, 25 mg PO weekly; atovaquone, 1,500 mg PO QD with or without pyrimethamine, 25 mg PO QD plus leucovorin, 10 mg PO QD *(Continued)*

PROPHYLAXIS TO PREVENT FIRST EPISODE OF OPPORTUNISTIC DISEASE (CONTINUED)

Pathogen	Indication Discontinuing/Restarting Primary Prophylaxis	Preventive regimens First Choice	Alternative
Mycobacterium avium complex	CD4+ count <50 cells/μL Discontinue when CD4+ count increases to >100 cells/μL for ≥3 mos; restart when CD4+ count <50-100 cells/μL	Clarithromycin, 500 mg PO BID or azithromycin, 1,200 mg PO weekly	Rifabutin, 300 mg PO QD; azithromycin, 1,200 mg PO QD plus rifabutin, 300 mg PO QD
Varicella-zoster virus (VZV)	Significant exposure to chickenpox or shingles for patients who have no history of either condition or, if available, negative antibody to VZV	Varicella-zoster immune globulin (VZIG), 5 vials (1.25 mL each) IM administered ≤96 h after exposure, ideally within 48 hours	None

II. Usually recommended

Pathogen	Indication	First Choice	Alternative
Streptococcus pneumoniae	CD4+ count of ≥200 cells/μL; also consider prophylaxis for persons with CD4+ counts of <200 cells/μL	23-valent polysaccharide vaccine, 0.5 mL IM (Revaccination ≥5 years after the first dose is optional; consider revaccinating sooner if the initial vaccination was administered when the CD4+ count was <200 cells/μL and the CD4+ count has increased to >200 cells/μL while on HAART)	None
Hepatitis B virus[§]	All susceptible patients (i.e., antihepatitis B core antigen-negative)	Hepatitis B vaccine: 3 doses	None
Influenza virus	All patients (annually, before influenza season)	Inactivated trivalent influenza virus vaccine: one annual dose (0.5 mL) IM	Oseltamivir, 75 mg PO QD (influenza A and B); rimantadine, 100 mg PO BID, or amantadine, 100 mg PO BID (influenza A); reduce doses in patients with decreased renal or hepatic function or who have seizure disorders
Hepatitis A virus[§]	All susceptible patients at increased risk for hepatitis A infection (i.e., antihepatitis A virus-negative) (e.g., illegal drug users, men who have sex with men, hemophiliacs) or patients with chronic liver disease, including chronic hepatitis B or C	Hepatitis A vaccine: two doses	None

III. Evidence for efficacy but not routinely indicated

Pathogen	Indication	First Choice	Alternative
Bacteria	Neutropenia	Granulocyte-colony-stimulating factor (G-CSF), 5-10 μg/kg SQ QD X 2-4 weeks or granulocyte-macrophage colony-stimulating factor (GM-CSF), 250 μg/m^2 SQ QD X 2-4 weeks	None
Cryptococcus neoformans	CD4+ count <50 cells/μL	Fluconazole, 100-200 mg PO QD	Itraconazole, 200 mg PO QD
Cytomegalovirus (CMV)	CD4+ count <50 cells/μL and CMV antibody positivity	Oral ganciclovir, 1 g PO TID	None
Histoplasma capsulatum	CD4+ count <100 cells/μL, endemic geographic area	Itraconazole, 200 mg PO QD	None

* TMP-SMZ reduces the frequency of toxoplasmosis and some bacterial infections. Patients receiving dapsone should be tested for glucose-6 phosphate dehydrogenase deficiency.

[†]Directly observed therapy (DOT) is recommended for isoniazid (e.g. 900 mg twice weekly); isoniazid regimens should include pyridoxine to prevent peripheral neuropathy. If rifampin or rifabutin is administered concurrently with protease inhibitors or nonnucleoside reverse transcriptase inhibitors, potential pharmacokinetic interactions may occur. Fatal and severe liver injury associated with treatment of latent tuberculosis infection among HIV patients treated with 2 month regimen of daily rifampin and pyrazinamide has occurred.

[§]For persons requiring vaccination against both hepatitis A and B, a combination vaccine is available.

Adapted from Centers for Disease Control and Prevention. (2002). Guidelines for preventing opportunistic infections among HIV-infected persons – 2002: Recommendations of the U.S. Public Health Service and the Infectious Diseases Society of America. *MMWR, 51*(RR-8), 1-52.

G.   It is important to recognize the signs and symptoms of **opportunistic diseases**, diagnose and treat appropriately, and then provide prophylaxis to prevent recurrences (**see V.K . for prevention of recurrences**) (see following table for diagnosis and treatment of bacterial infections)

ASSESSMENT, DIAGNOSIS, AND TREATMENT OF COMMON BACTERIAL OPPORTUNISTIC INFECTIONS

Transmission	Clinical Characteristics	Diagnosis	Treatment
Mycobacterium Avium Intracellulare (MAI) or M. Avium Complex Infections			
Widely dispersed in environment and found in most water supplies	Diarrhea, abdominal pain, organomegaly, high fevers, weight loss, fatigue, enlarged nodes, elevated alkaline phosphatase	Cultures of blood, stool, or bone marrow; lymph node and liver biopsy	Clarithromycin 500 mg BID **plus** ethambutol (EMB)15-25 mg/kg/day ± rifabutin (RFB) 300 mg QD; alternatively, azithromycin 600 mg QD plus EMB ± RFB; duration is indefinite in absence of immune reconstitution; with HAART may discontinue when MAC treatment is >1 year and CD4+ T-cell count is >100/mm^3 for 3-6 months, and patient is asymptomatic
Mycobacterium Tuberculosis			
Spread through droplet nuclei coughed up by persons with untreated TB	Productive, prolonged cough; fever, chills, night sweats, fatigue, weight loss, hemoptysis, lymphadenopathy	PPD skin test, chest x-ray, sputum smear and culture	**+ PPD but no active disease:** If patient is not receiving HAART: rifampin (RIF) 600 mg QD plus pyrazinamide (PZA) 20 mg/kg/day x 2 months; if patient is on HAART: Isoniazid (INH) 300 mg QD plus pyridoxine 50 mg QD x 9 months
			Active disease: 12 months treatment; If patient is not taking PI or NNRTI: INH/RIF/PZA/EMB (or streptomycin [SM]) daily x 2 months then INH/RIF daily or 2-3 times/week x 18 weeks (other regimens are available)
			If patient is receiving PI or NNRTI: INH/RFB/PZA/EMB daily x 8 weeks, then INH/RFB daily or 2 times per week x 18 weeks (other regimens are available)
Syphilis			
Caused by *Treponema pallidum*; Sexually transmitted disease	Primary: chancre Secondary: Rash on palms and soles Tertiary: No outward signs Neurosyphilis: CNS problems	RPR or VDRL and then FTA-ABS; lumbar puncture recommended with neurologic symptoms, treatment failure, and late latent syphilis	**Primary, secondary and early latent (<1 year):** benzathine penicillin G 2.4 mil units IM x 1 with follow-up 2, 3, 6, 9 & 12 months, if titer fails to decrease 4-fold at 6-12 months or patient is symptomatic, retreat with benzathine penicillin G 2.4 mil units IM once a week x 3 weeks **Latent and tertiary, not neurosyphilis:** benzathine penicillin G 2.4 mil units IM weekly x 3 weeks **Neurosyphilis:** aqueous penicillin G 18-24 mil units/day IV x 10-14 days (3-4 mil units q 4 hours); retreat if CSF WBC fails to decrease at 6 mos or CSF still abnormal at 2 years

H.   See following table for diagnosis and treatment of fungal infections

ASSESSMENT, DIAGNOSIS, AND TREATMENT OF COMMON FUNGAL OPPORTUNISTIC INFECTIONS

Transmission	Clinical Characteristics	Diagnosis	Treatment
Candidiasis			
Caused by *candida albicans* when CD4+ T-cells drop below 500/mm^3	Oral: White plaques anywhere in oral cavity, burning sensation, absence of taste, pain when swallowing	Swab lesion: KOH prep	Clotrimazole 10 mg troches; dissolve in saliva, 1 troche 5 times daily for 14 days; or - fluconazole 100 mg PO QD for 7-14 days
	Vaginal: Thick white vaginal discharge; itching, burning, redness in vaginal area	Swab vagina: KOH prep	Miconazole vaginal suppository 200 mg: 1 suppository HS X 3 nights; or - fluconazole 150 mg tab PO single dose
	Esophageal: Dysphagia, odynophagia	Diagnosed empirically or with endoscopy	Fluconazole 200 mg tab PO QD; up to 400 mg/day x 2-3 weeks
Cryptococcal Meningitis			
Yeast-like fungus found widely in environment, especially in soil contaminated with bird excrement	Fever, headache, fatigue, nausea, memory loss, confusion, problems with coordination	Cryptococcal serum antigen; lumbar puncture: India ink, cryptococcal antigen, culture	Amphotericin B 0.7 mg/kg/day IV plus flucytosine 100 mg/kg/day PO x 14 days, then fluconazole 400 mg/day for 8-10 weeks; lifelong suppressive therapy with fluconazole 200 mg/day

I.   See following table for diagnosis and treatment of protozoal infections:

ASSESSMENT, DIAGNOSIS, AND TREATMENT OF COMMON PROTOZOAL OPPORTUNISTIC INFECTIONS

Transmission	Clinical Characteristics	Diagnosis	Treatment
Pneumocystis Carinii Pneumonia (PCP) (Has characteristics of both protozoa & fungi)			
Believed to infect most humans during childhood, and then remains dormant	Dry, non-productive cough; shortness of breath, fever, fatigue, weight loss	Chest X-ray; Induced sputum; Broncho-alveolar lavage	Mild-Moderate Disease: TMP/SMX* PO 15 mg/kg/day, TMP equivalent in 3-4 divided doses x 21 days (usually 2 DS tabs TID or IV x 21 days); or - TMP 15 mg/kg/day PO plus dapsone 100 mg/day times 21 days for sulfa allergy Severe Disease: TMP/SMX PO 15 mg/kg TMP equivalent/day in 4 divided doses for 21 days with prednisone 40 mg PO BID x 5 days, then 40 mg QD x 5 days, then 20 mg QD to completion
Toxoplasmic Encephalitis			
30% U.S. adults infected with parasite which remains dormant until immune system is damaged	Fever, headache, neurological problems such as seizures, changes in mental status, coma	CT scan or MRI of brain for ring enhancing lesions; Positive toxoplasma IgG in serum	Pyrimethamine 100-200 mg PO loading dose, then 50-100 mg QD with sulfadiazine or trisulfapyrimidine 4-8 g PO QD plus folinic acid 10 mg PO QD for at least 6 weeks
Cryptosporidiosis			
Transmitted to humans via contact with feces, contaminated water or food	Chronic watery diarrhea, abdominal cramps, nausea, fever, weight loss, headache	Modified acid fast stain of stool; endoscopy with biopsy or bowel biopsy	Treatment is difficult – consider referral to specialist; sometimes paromomycin 500 mg PO TID or 1000 mg PO BID with food x 14-28 days then 500 mg BID may be effective

*Trimethoprim/sulfamethoxazole

J.   See following table for diagnosis and treatment of viral infections:

ASSESSMENT, DIAGNOSIS, AND TREATMENT OF COMMON VIRAL OPPORTUNISTIC INFECTIONS

Transmission	Clinical Characteristics	Diagnosis	Treatment
Cytomegalovirus Retinitis			
High percentage of US adults are infected with virus which remains dormant until immune system is damaged	Cytomegalovirus may infect GI tract, brain, and other organs but common site is the eye with blurred vision, floaters, flashing lights, loss of peripheral vision	Diagnosis of CMV retinitis made with indirect funduscopy by a trained ophthalmologist	Consult ophthalmologist; ganciclovir (IV, oral, implant), valganciclovir (oral), foscarnet (IV, intraocular injection), cidofovir (IV), fomivirsen (injection into vitreous) are effective therapies
Oral Hairy Leukoplakia			
Caused by Epstein-Barr virus	White, non-removable lesion with a corrugated surface on lateral margins of tongue	Clinical presentation	None usually needed; may treat with acyclovir 800 mg PO 5 times a day x 2-3 weeks
Progressive Multifocal Leukoencephalopathy (PML)			
Caused by J.C. virus; most people are infected by 2 years of age, but virus remains latent in brain until immune system is sufficiently damaged	Insidious onset with rapid progression; confusion, lack of energy, loss of balance, memory and speech problems, blurred or double vision, hallucinations, seizures, paralysis and eventual death	CT scan or MRI which may reveal focal brain lesions which do not enhance or cause surrounding edema	HAART may be effective; treatment with cidofovir is questionable; consult with specialist
Herpes Simplex, Herpes Zoster, and Molluscum Contagiosum (see chapter on SKIN PROBLEMS)			

K.   See following table for diagnosis and treatment of cancers:

ASSESSMENT, DIAGNOSIS, AND TREATMENT OF CANCERS ASSOCIATED WITH HIV INFECTION

Transmission	Clinical Characteristics	Diagnosis	Treatment
Kaposi's Sarcoma			
May be sexually transmitted and is caused by herpes virus, HHV-8	Red, brown or pink blotches on skin which change to hard, raised purplish-red lesions; can be on internal organs as well as common places of arms, legs, and chest	Visual examination or skin biopsy	Referral to specialist; generally responds to HAART; often left untreated or can treat with topical liquid nitrogen, alpha interferon, radiation, laser therapy, chemotherapy
Lymphomas			
Cancers of lymphoid cells; B-cell non-Hodgkin's lymphoma is most common	Spreads quickly, occurs in brain and outside of the lymph nodes	Depending on site; biopsy, CT/MRI, bone marrow biopsy, lumbar puncture	Refer to specialist

L. Patients who have a history of opportunistic diseases should be administered chemoprophylaxis to prevent recurrence (see following table)

PROPHYLAXIS TO PREVENT RECURRENCE OF OPPORTUNISTIC DISEASE AFTER CHEMOTHERAPY FOR ACUTE DISEASE

Pathogen	Indication Discontinue/Restart Prophylaxis	Preventive Regimens	
		First choice	Alternatives
I. Recommended as standard of care			
Pneumocystis carinii	Prior *P. carinii* pneumonia Discontinue when CD4+ count has increased to >200 cells/μL for ≥3 mos; Restart if CD4+ count decreases to <200 cells/μL or if PCP recurred at a CD4+ count of >200 cells/μL	Trimethoprim-sulfamethoxazole (TMP-SMZ), 1 DS PO QD or TMP-SMZ, 1 SS PO QD	Dapsone, 50 mg PO BID or 100 mg PO QD; dapsone 50 mg PO QD plus pyrimethamine, 50 mg PO weekly plus leucovorin, 25 mg PO weekly; aerosolized pentamidine, 300 mg every mo via Respirgard II nebulizer; atovaquone, 1,500 mg PO QD; TMP-SMZ, 1 DS PO three times a week
*Toxoplasma gondii**	Prior toxoplasmic encephalitis Discontinue with patients who complete initial therapy, remain asymptomatic, and have sustained (e.g., ≥6 mos) increase in CD4+ count >200 cells/μL; restart if CD4+ count decreases to <200 cells/μL	Sulfadiazine 500-1000 mg PO QID plus pyrimethamine 25-50 mg PO QD plus leucovorin 10-25 mg PO QD	Clindamycin, 300-450 mg PO Q 6-8 h plus pyrimethamine, 25-50 mg PO QD plus leucovorin, 10-25 mg PO QD; atovaquone, 750 mg PO Q 6-12 hours with or without pyrimethamine, 25 mg PO QD plus leucovorin, 10 mg PO QD
Mycobacterium avium complex**	Documented disseminated disease Discontinue when patient has completed a course of ≥12 months of treatment, remains asymptomatic, and has a sustained (≥6 mos) increase in CD4+ counts to >100 cells/μL; restart if CD4+ count decreases to <100 cells/μL	Clarithromycin,** 500 mg PO BID plus ethambutol, 15 mg/kg PO QD with or without rifabutin, 300 mg PO QD	Azithromycin, 500 mg PO QD plus ethambutol, 15 mg/kg PO QD with or without rifabutin, 300 mg PO QD
Cytomegalovirus	Prior end-organ disease Consult ophthalmologist; discontinue when CD4+ count has sustained (≥6 mos) increases to >100-150 cells/μL, and no evidence of active disease; restart if CD4+ count decreases to 100-150 cells/μL	Valganciclovir, 900 mg PO QD; ganciclovir, 5-6 mg/kg IV 5-7 days/wk or 1,000 mg PO TID; or foscarnet, 90-120 mg/kg IV QD; or (for retinitis) ganciclovir sustained-release implant every 6-9 mos plus ganciclovir, 1.0-1.5 g PO TID	Cidofovir, 5 mg/kg IV every other week with probenecid 2 g PO 3 hours before the dose followed by 1 g PO 2 hours after the dose, and 1 g PO 8 hours after the dose (total of 4 g); fomivirsen 1 vial (330 μg) injected into vitreous, then repeated every 2-4 weeks; valganciclovir 900 mg PO QD
Cryptococcus neoformans	Documented disease Discontinue when patient has completed a course of initial therapy, remains asymptomatic, and has a sustained increase (≥6 mos) in CD4+ count to >100-200 cells/μL; restart if CD4+ count decreases to 100-200 cells/μL	Fluconazole, 200 mg PO QD	Amphotericin B, 0.6-1.0 mg/kg IV weekly--three times weekly; itraconazole, 200 mg PO QD
Histoplasma capsulatum	Documented disease; no recommendation to discontinue prophylaxis	Itraconazole, 200 mg PO BID	Amphotericin B, 1.0 mg/kg IV weekly
Coccidioides immitis	Documented disease; no recommendation to discontinue prophylaxis	Fluconazole 400 mg PO QD	Amphotericin B, 1.0 mg/kg IV weekly; itraconazole, 200 mg PO BID
Salmonella species	Bacteremia	Ciprofloxacin, 500 mg PO BID for ≥2 mos	Antibiotic chemoprophylaxis with another active agent

(Continued)

PROPHYLAXIS TO PREVENT RECURRENCE OF OPPORTUNISTIC DISEASE AFTER CHEMOTHERAPY FOR ACUTE DISEASE (CONTINUED)

Pathogen	Indication Discontinue/Restart Prophylaxis	Preventive Regimens	
		First choice	Alternatives
II. Recommended only if subsequent episodes are frequent or severe			
Herpes simplex virus	Frequent/severe recurrences	Acyclovir, 200 mg PO TID or 400 mg PO BID; famciclovir, 250 mg PO BID	Valacyclovir, 500 mg PO BID
Candida (oral, vaginal, or esophageal)	Frequent/severe recurrences	Fluconazole, 100-200 mg PO QD	Itraconazole solution, 200 mg PO QD

*Pyrimethamine-sulfadiazine confers protection against PCP as well as toxoplasmosis; clindamycin-pyrimethamine does not offer protection against PCP

**Drug interactions can be problematic (e.g. those observed with clarithromycin and rifabutin); rifabutin has been associated with uveitis, chiefly when administered at daily doses of >300 mg or concurrently with fluconazole or clarithromycin

Adapted from Centers for Disease Control and Prevention. (2002). Guidelines for preventing opportunistic infections among HIV-infected persons – 2002: Recommendations of the U.S. Public Health Service and the Infectious Diseases Society of America. *MMWR, 51(*RR-8), 1-52.

M. **Antiretroviral drug therapy (ART)** or **highly active antiretroviral therapy (HAART)** should be individualized; see the following table for principals of therapy; also see V.P. through V. R. for discussion of specific drug classes, drug interactions, etc.; remember adolescents in Tanner stages I and II should follow pediatric guidelines; patients in late puberty (Tanner stages V) should follow adult guidelines and those in Tanner stage III females and Tanner stage IV males should follow either adult or pediatric guidelines

PRINCIPLES OF THERAPY

1. Treatment decisions must be individualized using a number of criteria: Efficacy and durability of antiretroviral activity, tolerability and adverse effects, convenience of regimen, drug-drug interactions, and potential salvageability of the initial regimen

2. Because currently available antiretroviral regimens do not eradicate HIV, the goal of therapy is to durably inhibit viral replication, to enable patient to attain and maintain an effective immune response to most potential microbial pathogens, and to improve quality of life

3. Simultaneous initiation of combinations of effective anti-HIV drugs that the patient has not previously received and that are not cross-resistant with antiretroviral agents that the patient has previously received is the most effective method to achieve durable suppression of HIV replication

4. Drug monotherapy is **NOT** a recommended option as it presents risk for development of drug resistance and potential development of cross-resistance to related drugs

5. Each antiretroviral drug should be used according to optimum schedules and dosages

6. Any change in antiretroviral therapy increases future therapeutic constraints

7. Women need optimal antiretroviral therapy regardless of pregnancy status

8. Structured, supervised, or strategic treatment interruptions are not currently recommended

9. If ART needs to be discontinued, stop all antiretroviral agents simultaneously

10. Patient adherence is extremely important as intermittent use leads to resistance; emphasize that patient should not stop any medications without consulting clinician

N. Recommendations for **initiating antiretroviral therapy in treatment-naïve individuals** (see following table)
1. CD4+ T-cell count is the major determinant of when to initiate therapy
2. Viral loads offer additional information to help make timing decisions; CD4+ T-cell counts decrease more rapidly in untreated patients with high viral loads
3. Be aware of risk of immune reconstitution that may occur concomitantly with increase in CD4+ T-cell counts in patients starting ART when there is confirmed or suspected opportunistic infection
4. In collaboration with the patient, consider both the benefits and risks of early initiation of ART when the CD4+ count is in the >200 cells/mm^3 – 350 cell/mm^3 range (see table BENEFITS AND RISKS)
5. When initiating ART, start all drugs simultaneously and at full dose with the following exceptions: Dose escalation regimens are recommended for ritonavir, nevirapine, and for certain patients, ritonavir plus saquinavir

6. Dosages of ART must be altered when used with certain medications (see tables under V.Q. and V.R.)
7. Always consider overlapping toxicities when prescribing ART with other medications (consult drug manual) (see table HIV-RELATED DRUGS WITH OVERLAPPING TOXICITIES)

RECOMMENDATIONS FOR INITIATING THERAPY IN TREATMENT-NAÏVE INDIVIDUALS

Disease Type	Recommendation
Symptomatic HIV disease	Treatment recommended
Asymptomatic HIV disease ≤200 CD4+ cells/µL	Treatment recommended
Asymptomatic HIV disease, >200 CD4+ cells/µL but ≤350	Treatment decision should be offered although controversial
Asymptomatic HIV disease, >350 CD4+ cells/µL	Treatment is usually not recommended; individualize therapy based on: • CD4+ cell count and rate of decline* • HIV RNA level in the plasma** • Patient interest in and potential to adhere to therapy • Individual risks of toxicity and drug-drug pharmacokinetic interaction

* Some clinicians and guidelines use a CD4+ count threshold of 350 cells/µL to initiate therapy, a high rate of CD4+ cell count decline is >100 cells/µL per annum
** A high viral load is >50,000-100,000 copies/mL. The frequency of CD4+ cell measurements before therapy is initiated may be guided by the plasma HIV RNA level

Adapted from Panel on Clinical Practices for Treatment of HIV Infection (Convened by Department of Health and Human Services [DHHS]). (2003). Guidelines for use of antiretroviral agents in HIV-infected adults and adolescents. Available at http://AIDSinfo.nih.gov.

BENEFITS AND RISKS OF EARLY INITIATION OF ANTIRETROVIRAL THERAPY

Potential Benefits:
- ✓ Easier control of viral replication and mutation
- ✓ Preservation of immune function
- ✓ Delayed progression to AIDS
- ✓ Decreased risk of increased HIV genetic complexity
- ✓ Decreased risk for selection of resistant virus
- ✓ Decreased risk for drug toxicity
- ✓ Decreased risk for immune reconstitution syndrome
- ✓ Decrease in risk of viral transmission

Potential Risks:
- ✓ Reduction in quality of life from adverse drug effects
- ✓ Limitation of future choices of ART agents
- ✓ Unknown long-term toxicity of drugs
- ✓ Inconvenience of drug administration
- ✓ Earlier development of drug resistance if viral suppression is suboptimal
- ✓ Unknown duration of effectiveness of current antiretroviral agents

HIV-RELATED DRUGS WITH OVERLAPPING TOXICITIES

Bone Marrow Suppression	Peripheral Neuropathy	Pancreatitis	Nephrotoxicity	Hepatotoxicity	Rash	Diarrhea	Ocular Effects
Cidofovir	Didanosine	Cotrimoxazole	Adefovir	Azithromycin	Abacavir	Atovaquone	Didanosine
Cotrimoxazole	Isoniazid	Didanosine	Aminoglycosides	Clarithromycin	Amprenavir	Didanosine	Ethambutol
Cytotoxic chemo-therapy	Stavudine	Lamivudine (children)	Amphotericin B	Fluconazole	Atovaquone	Clindamycin	Rifabutin
Dapsone	Zalcitabine	Pentamidine	Cidofovir	Isoniazid	Cotrimoxazole	Nelfinavir	Cidofovir
Flucytosine		Ritonavir	Foscarnet	Itraconazole	Dapsone	Ritonavir	
Ganciclovir		Stavudine	Indinavir	Ketoconazole	Delavirdine	Lopinavir/ritonavir	
Hydroxyurea		Zalcitabine	Pentamidine	Nucleoside reverse transcriptase inhibitors	Efavirenz	Tenofovir	
Interferon-α				Nonnucleoside reverse transcriptase inhibitors	Nevirapine		
Pegylated interferon-α				Protease inhibitors	Sulfadiazine		
Primaquine				Rifabutin			
Pyrimethamine				Rifampin			
Ribavirin							
Rifabutin							
Sulfadiazine							
Trimetrexate							
Valganciclovir							
Zidovudine							

Adapted from Centers for Disease Control and Prevention. (2002) Guidelines for the use of antiretroviral agents among HIV-infected adults and adolescents: Recommendations of the Panel on Clinical Practices for Treatment of HIV. *MMWR, 51*(RR-7), 1-55.

8. Choose one of the following preferred combination regimens when initiating therapy; discuss advantages and disadvantages of each regimen with the patient (see table that follows)

PREFERRED INITIAL COMBINATION REGIMENS FOR TREATMENT-NAÏVE PATIENTS*

Regimen	Possible Advantages	Possible Disadvantages	Drug-interaction Complications	Impact on Future Options
NNRTI-sparing regimen PI (with or without low-dose ritonavir** with 2 NRTIs)	• Clinical, virologic, and immunologic efficacy well-documented • Continued benefits despite viral breakthrough • Resistance requires multiple mutations • Targets HIV at 2 steps of viral replication (reverse transcriptase and PI)	• Might be difficult to use and adhere to • Long-term side effects might include lipodystrophy,§ hyperlipidemia, and insulin resistance	• Mild to severe inhibition of cytochrome P450 pathway; ritonavir is most potent inhibitor, but this effect can be exploited to boost levels of other PIs	• Preserves NNRTIs for use in treatment failure • Resistance primes for cross-resistance with other PIs
PI-sparing regimen NNRTI with 2 NRTIs	• Spares PI-related side effects • Easier to use and adhere to, compared with PIs	• Comparability to PI-containing regimens regarding clinical results unknown • Resistance conferred by a single or limited number of mutations	• Fewer drug interactions compared with PIs	• Preserves PIs for later use • Resistance can lead to cross-resistance throughout entire NNRTI class
NNRTI- and PI-sparing Triple NRTI	• Easy to use and adhere to • Spares PI and NNRTI side effects • Cross-resistance to all drugs in the NRTI class is unlikely with initial regimen failure	• Virologic efficacy inferior to efavirenz-based regimen	• No cytochrome P450 interaction	• Preserves both PI and NNRTI classes for use in treatment failure

* PI = Protease inhibitor; NNRTI = nonnucleoside reverse transcriptase inhibitor; NRTI = nucleoside reverse transcriptase inhibitor
** Low-dose ritonavir can boost saquinavir, indinavir, amprenavir, or lopinavir; nelfinavir is not sufficiently enhanced by low-dose ritonavir to justify this combination
§ Certain side effects being attributed to PI therapy (e.g., lipodystrophy) have not been reported to be associated strictly with using PI-containing regimens. Lipodystrophy has also been described among patients on NRTIs alone and among patients not on antiretroviral therapy
Adapted from Panel on Clinical Practices for Treatment of HIV Infection (Convened by Department of Health and Human Services [DHHS]). (2003). Guidelines for use of antiretroviral agents in HIV-infected adults and adolescents. Available at http://AIDSinfo.nih.gov.

9. Other combination regimens when initiating therapy may be selected (see following table)

OTHER COMBINATION REGIMENS WHEN INITIATING THERAPY

Regimen	Comment
PI-sparing/NNRTI-sparing regimens 3 NRTIs	• National Institutes of Allergy and Infectious Diseases (NIAID) (2003) study found that in treatment-naïve patients, a combination of three NRTIs, Trizivir, was inferior to two other efavirenz-containing treatment regimens • Not routinely recommended as initial therapy for patients with high viral loads (>100,000 copies/mL) or with low CD4+ T-cells • Preserves both PI and NNRTI classes for later use • Limited cross-resistance within the NRTI class
PI (with or without low-dose ritonavir) with an NNRTI plus 1 or 2 NRTIs	• Not routinely recommended due to risks of multiclass drug resistance and high toxicity, but may be beneficial for patients with advanced disease for which no effective therapy exists, and for cases in which *in vitro* resistance testing suggests regimen may be effective
NRTI-sparing regimen PI (with low-dose ritonavir) plus NNRTI	• Limited information available on this regimen

10. Carefully select specific ART agents for combination regimens (see following table for acceptable antiretroviral combinations); monotherapy and dual therapy regimens should **not** be selected

ANTIRETROVIRAL REGIMENS RECOMMENDED FOR TREATMENT OF HIV-1 INFECTION IN ANTIRETROVIRAL NAÏVE PATIENTS		
NNRTI-Based Regimens		# of pills per day
Preferred Regimens	**Efavirenz + lamivudine + (zidovudine or tenofovir DF or stavudine*) – except for pregnant women or women with pregnancy potential**	**3-5 pills/day**
Alternative Regimens	Efavirenz + lamivudine + didanosine – except for pregnant women or women with pregnancy potential	3-5 pills/day
	Nevirapine + lamivudine + (zidovudine or stavudine or didanosine)	4-6 pills/day
PI-Based Regimens		
Preferred Regimens	**Kaletra (lopinavir + ritonavir) + lamivudine + (zidovudine or stavudine)**	**8-10 pills/day**
Alternative Regimens	Amprenavir + ritonavir ** + lamivudine + (zidovudine or stavudine)	12-14 pills/day
	Indinavir + lamivudine + (zidovudine or stavudine)	8-10 pills/day
	Indinavir + ritonavir** + lamivudine + (zidovudine or stavudine)	8-12 pills/day
	Nelfinavir† + lamivudine + (zidovudine or stavudine)	6-14 pills/day
	Saquinavir (sgc or hcg)‡ + ritonavir ** + lamivudine + (zidovudine or stavudine)	14-16 pills/day
Triple NRTI Regimen – As Alternative to PI- or NNRTI-Based Regimens		
Alternative Regimens	Abacavir + lamivudine + zidovudine	2 pills/day
	Abacavir + lamivudine + stavudine	4-6 pills/day

Preferred regimens are in bold type; these regimens were selected by experts based on totality of virologic, immunologic, and toxicity data
Individualize therapy based on advantages and disadvantages of each combination
* Preliminary 96-week data comparing stavudine + lamivudine vs tenofovir + lamivudine revealed higher incidence of lipodystrophy and lipid abnormalities in the stavudine group
** Low-dose (100-400 mg) ritonavir
† Nelfinavir 625 mg tablet – available as of July 2003
‡ sgc = soft gel capsule; hgc = hard gel capsule

Adapted from Panel on Clinical Practices for Treatment of HIV Infection (Convened by Department of Health and Human Services [DHHS]). (2003). Guidelines for use of antiretroviral agents in HIV-infected adults and adolescents. Available at http://AIDSinfo.nih.gov.

O. Consider discontinuing ART for patient who began ART at CD4+ T-cell $>350/mm^3$; closely monitor patients who discontinue ART as they may have rebound in viral replication and renewed immunologic decline

P. Considerations for **changing an antiretroviral regimen** (see following table)
  1. If change is due to drug toxicity or inability to comply with regimen, substitute one or more alternative drugs of same potency from the same class of agents as causing suspected toxicity
  2. If change is due to failure to achieve acceptable viral suppression or immune response, use ≥2 or ≥3 new drugs

---

GUIDELINES FOR CHANGING AN ANTIRETROVIRAL REGIMEN BECAUSE OF SUSPECTED DRUG FAILURE

➡ Criteria for changing therapy include 1) a suboptimal reduction in plasma viremia after initiation of therapy, 2) reappearance of viremia after suppression to undetectable levels, 3) substantial increases in plasma viremia from the nadir of suppression, and 4) declining CD4+ T-cell numbers

➡ Before deciding to change therapy on the basis of viral load, a second test should be used to confirm viral load determination

➡ Clinicians should distinguish between the need to change a regimen because of drug intolerance or inability to comply with the regimen versus failure to achieve sustained viral suppression; single agents can be changed for patients with drug intolerance

➡ Usually a single drug should not be changed or added to a failing regimen; using ≥2 new drugs or using a new regimen with ≥3 new drugs is preferable. If susceptibility testing indicates resistance to one agent only in a combination regimen, replacing only that drug is possible; however, this approach requires clinical validation

➡ In some cases treatment failure is not associated with viral resistance, particularly if virus remains detectable at lower levels after several months of ART; if there is no evidence of resistance or nonadherence, regimen intensification is acceptable; addition of ritonavir, abacavir, or tenofovir disoproxil fumarate may be used; do not use NNRTIs and lamivudine alone as intensification agents

➡ Certain patients have limited options for new regimens of desired potency; in selected cases, continuing the previous regimen if partial viral suppression was achieved is a rational option

➡ In certain situations, regimens identified as suboptimal for initial therapy because of limitations imposed by toxicity, intolerance, or nonadherence are rational options, including in late-stage disease. For patients with no rational options who have virologic failure with return of viral load to baseline (i.e., pretreatment levels) and declining CD4+ T-cell counts, discontinuing antiretroviral therapy should be considered, but continuing regimens that maintain selective pressure on virus is preferred

➡ Experience is limited regarding regimens that use combinations of two protease inhibitors or combinations of protease inhibitors with NNRTIs; for patients with limited options because of drug intolerance or suspected resistance, these regimens provide alternative options

➡ Tenofovir may have a role in management of treatment-experienced patients

➡ Information is limited regarding the value of restarting a drug that the patient has previously received. Susceptibility testing might be useful if clinical evidence indicating emergence of resistance is observed; however, testing for phenotypic or genotypic resistance in peripheral blood virus might fail to detect minor resistant variants. Thus, the presence of resistance is more useful information in altering treatment strategies than the absence of detectable resistance

➡ Clinicians should avoid changing from ritonavir to indinavir or vice versa for drug failure because high-level cross-resistance is probable

➡ Clinicians should avoid changing among NNRTIs for drug failure because high-level cross-resistance is probable

➡ Decisions to change therapy and choices of new regimens require the clinician to have substantial experience and knowledge regarding the care of persons living with HIV infection. Clinicians who are less experienced are strongly encouraged to obtain assistance through consultation with or referral to a knowledgeable clinician

Adapted from Centers for Disease Control and Prevention. (2002). Guidelines for using antiretroviral agents among HIV-infected adults and adolescents: Recommendations of the Panel on Clinical Practices for Treatment of HIV. *MMWR, 51*(RR-7). 1-55.

3. Possible regimens following initial antiretroviral regimen failure (see following table)

TREATMENT OPTIONS WHEN CHANGING ANTIRETROVIRAL REGIMENS		
Initial Regimen	Predicted Early Resistance Pattern*	Possible Interventions
Generally Recommended		
NNRTI-sparing regimen PI (with/without low-dose ritonavir) plus 2 NRTIs	M184V** if regimen includes lamivudine	Revise/strengthen NRTI/NtRTI component Ritonavir boost PI component, if not part of initial regimen Change to NNRTI-based regimen
PI-sparing regimen NNRTI plus 2 NRTIs	M184V** with/without NNRTI-associated mutation, if regimen includes lamivudine	Revise/strengthen NRTI/NtRTI component Change to PI-based regimen if NNRTI resistance present
PI-sparing/NNRTI-sparing regimen 3 NRTIs (including abacavir)	M184V** if regimen includes lamivudine	Change to PI- or NNRTI-based regimen with revision or strengthening of NRTI component or consider adding NtRTI
Special Circumstances		
PI (with/without low-dose ritonavir) plus NNRTI plus 1 or 2 NRTIs	M184V** with/without NNRTI-associated mutation, if regimen includes lamivudine	Revise/strengthen NRTI component Ritonavir boosts PI component if not part of initial regimen Eliminate NNRTI if associated mutation present
Under Investigation		
NRTI-sparing regimen PI (with low-dose ritonavir) plus NNRTI	NNRTI-associated mutation	Eliminate NNRTI and add 2 NRTIs or consider adding NtRTI

* The likely drug resistance patterns are listed for illustrative purposes assuming virological failure is detected early. Drug-resistance testing is recommended to determine the actual genotype or phenotype profile of the patient's viral strain
** The M184V mutation confers high-level resistance (500- to 1000-fold decrease in susceptibility) to lamivudine and low-level resistance (2- to 4-fold decrease in susceptibility) to abacavir

Adapted from Yeni, P.G., Hammer, S.M., Carpenter, C.C.J., Cooper, D.A., Fischl, M.A., Gatell, J.M., et al. (2002). Antiretroviral treatment for adult HIV infection in 2002: Updated recommendations of the International AIDS Society—USA Panel. *JAMA, 288,* 222-235.

Q. Nucleoside or nucleotide reverse transcriptase inhibitors (NRTIs): Block the conversion of virus RNA into viral DNA through inhibition of reverse transcriptase; inhibit viral spread to uninfected cells rather than eradicating the virus (see following table of factors to consider when selecting a NRTI)

NUCLEOSIDE OR NUCLEOTIDE REVERSE TRANSCRIPTASE INHIBITORS

Generic Name/ Trade Name	Form	Dosing Recommendations	Adverse Effects	Contraindications/ Precautions	Comments
Zidovudine/ Retrovir	100 mg capsules, 300 mg tablets, 10 mg/mL intravenous solution, or 10 mg/mL oral solution Each Combivir tab contains 300 mg zidovudine and 150 mg lamivudine Each Trizivir tab contains 300 mg zidovudine, 150 mg lamivudine, and 300 mg abacavir	200 mg TID or 300 mg BID or with lamivudine as Combivir, 1 dose BID or with abacavir and lamivudine as Trizivir, 1 dose BID	✓ Major: bone marrow suppression with anemia and/or neutropenia ✓ Common subjective: nausea, headaches, insomnia, fatigue, malaise, vomiting, GI pain ✓ Less common: myopathy and muscle pain ✓ Long-term: nail pigmentation ✓ Rare but life-threatening: lactic acidosis with hepatic stenosis	Consider dose adjustment in patients with liver dysfunction	✓ Take without regard to food ✓ Cautiously use with ganciclovir or other marrow-suppressing drugs ✓ Do **not** use with stavudine, doxorubicin, ribavirin ✓ Consider discontinuing if hemoglobin falls below 7.5 g/dL ✓ Monitor CBC 2-4 weeks after initiating and then periodically ✓ Superior CNS effects compared to other NRTIs
Didanosine/ Videx or Videx EC	25, 50, 100, 150, 200 mg chewable/ dispersible buffered tablets; 100, 167, 250 mg buffered powder for oral solution; 125, 200, 250, or 400 mg enteric coated capsules	Body weight >60 kg: 200 mg BID (buffered tablets), 250 mg BID (buffered powder) or 400 mg QD (buffered tablets or enteric coated capsules) Preferred dosing is BID; once-daily dosing reserved for patients who need simplified regimen	✓ Pancreatitis (potentially fatal) ✓ Peripheral neuropathy ✓ Diarrhea and GI problems ✓ Rare but life-threatening: lactic acidosis with hepatic stenosis	Consider dose adjustment in patients with renal and liver dysfunction; do not prescribe to alcoholics, patients with history of pancreatitis, and possibly those with poor seizure control	✓ Take ½ hour before or 2 hours after meals ✓ Do not give within two hours following drugs requiring an acid environment (ketoconazole, dapsone, tetracyclines, quinolones, cimetidine) ✓ Monitor amylase levels and assess for abdominal pain, nausea, and vomiting ✓ Separate dosing of delavirdine, indinavir, tenofovir by 1-2 hours ✓ Use cautiously with alcohol, stavudine, pentamidine, hydroxyurea, allopurinol, ganciclovir
Zalcitabine/ HIVID	0.375, 0.75 mg tablets	0.75 mg TID	✓ Peripheral neuropathy ✓ Aphthous ulcers ✓ Pancreatitis (less frequently than with didanosine) ✓ Rare but life-threatening: lactic acidosis with hepatic stenosis	Extreme caution when given to patients with hepatitis B; consider dose adjustment in patients with renal and liver disease Avoid in patients with peripheral neuropathy or history of pancreatitis	✓ Take without regard to food ✓ Less efficacious than other NRTIs ✓ Numerous drug interactions *(continued)*

NUCLEOSIDE OR NUCLEOTIDE REVERSE TRANSCRIPTASE INHIBITORS *(CONTINUED)*

Generic Name/ Trade Name	Form	Dosing Recommendations	Adverse Effects	Contraindications/ Precautions	Comments
Lamivudine/ Epivir	150 mg tablets or 10 mg/mL oral solution	150 mg BID; or with zidovudine as Combivir, 1 dose BID or with zidovudine and abacavir as Trizivir, 1 dose BID	✓ Minimal toxicity but may have headache, nausea, diarrhea, abdominal pain, insomnia ✓ Rare but life-threatening: lactic acidosis with hepatic stenosis	Consider dose adjustment in patients with renal dysfunction	✓ Take without regard to food ✓ Increased drug absorption when given with trimethoprim/ sulfamethoxazole ✓ Delays or reverses resistance of zidovudine ✓ Resistance develops rapidly if not given with another antiretroviral ✓ Not recommended with ddC and ddI ✓ Do not add as single agent to a failing regimen ✓ Has activity against Hepatitis B
Stavudine/Zerit	15, 20, 30, 40 mg capsules or 1 mg/mL oral solution	Body weight >60 kg: 40 mg BID; body weight <60 kg: 30 mg BID	✓ Pancreatitis (possibly fatal) ✓ Peripheral neuropathy ✓ Neuromuscular weakness (possibly fatal) ✓ Rare but life-threatening: lactic acidosis with hepatic stenosis	Consider dose adjustment in patients with renal and liver dysfunction	✓ Take without regard to food ✓ Do not take with zidovudine ✓ Use cautiously with other drugs that cause peripheral neuropathy
Abacavir/ Ziagen	300 mg tablets or 10 mg/mL oral solution	300 mg BID or with zidovudine and lamivudine as Trizivir, 1 dose BID	✓ Hypersensitivity reaction that can be fatal: fever, rash, nausea, vomiting, malaise, fatigue, anorexia, or possibly respiratory symptoms (sore throat, cough, SOB) ✓ Rare but life-threatening: lactic acidosis with hepatic stenosis	Use cautiously in patients with liver disease	✓ Take without regard to meals ✓ <u>Discontinue</u> if hypersensitivity reaction occurs and do <u>not</u> restart ✓ Do not add as a single agent to a failing regimen ✓ Alcohol increases abacavir levels ✓ May antagonize methadone
Tenofovir disoproxil fumarate/Viread	300 mg tablets	300 mg daily for patients with creatinine clearance ≥60 mL/min; not recommended for patients with creatinine clearance <60 mL/min	✓ Asthenia, headache, diarrhea, nausea, vomiting, and flatulence ✓ Rare but life-threatening: lactic acidosis with hepatic stenosis	Contraindicated in patients with renal insufficiency	✓ Take with food to increase bioavailability ✓ Separate 1-2 hours from didanosine ✓ Limited information about efficacy

Adapted from Centers for Disease Control and Prevention. (2002) Guidelines for the use of antiretroviral agents among HIV-infected adults and adolescents: Recommendations of the Panel on Clinical Practices for Treatment of HIV. *MMWR, 51*(RR-7), 1-55.

    R.   Protease inhibitors (PI) (see following table)
          1.   Mechanisms of action: Inhibit HIV replication in cells that are chronically infected with HIV; competitively inhibit the HIV protease enzyme, a necessary enzyme for formation of the protein capsule surrounding the viral RNA in mature virions
          2.   Toxicities of PIs sometimes limit their use; elevated glucose, serum triglycerides, and cholesterol are often reported along with changes in body habitus
          3.   Always check drug manual and drug insert before prescribing PI
          4.   Certain drugs should not be used with PIs (see table DRUGS THAT SHOULD NOT BE USED WITH PIs)
          5.   When PIs are used with other PIs or NNRTIs, dosage modifications must be made (See tables DOSAGE CHANGES WITH OTHER PIS AND DOSAGE CHANGES WITH NNRTIS)
          6.   PIs interact with numerous medications and require dose modifications or cautious use (See table DOSAGE ADJUSTMENTS WHEN PRESCRIBING PIs)

PROTEASE INHIBITORS (PIs)

Name/Form	Dosing Recommendations	Food Effect	Adverse Events	Comments
Indinavir/Crixivan 200, 333, 400 mg capsules	800 mg every 8 hours; separate dosing with didanosine buffered preparation by 1 hour, Videx EC and indinavir can be administered together	Take 1 hour before or 2 hours after meals; may take with skim milk or low-fat meal	Nephrolithiasis; gastrointestinal intolerance and nausea; increased indirect bilirubinemia (inconsequential); transaminase elevation; headache, asthenia, blurred vision, dizziness, rash, metallic taste, thrombocytopenia, alopecia, hyperglycemia, hemolytic anemia; fat redistribution and lipid abnormalities, possible increased bleeding episodes among patients with hemophilia	✓ Drink >48 ounces of fluid to reduce risk of nephrolithiasis ✓ Can use oral contraceptives ✓ Separate dosing of didanosine by 1-2 hours
Ritonavir/Norvir 100 mg capsules 600 mg/7.5 mL solution by mouth	600 mg every 12 hours; separate dosing with didanosine by 2 hours Dose escalation: Days 1&2: 300 mg BID Days 3-5: 400 mg BID Days 6-13: 500 mg BID Day 14: 600 mg BID	Take with food, if possible; this might improve tolerability	Gastrointestinal intolerance, nausea, vomiting, diarrhea; paresthesias (circumoral and extremities); hepatitis; pancreatitis, asthenia; taste perversion; triglycerides increase >200%; elevated creatinine phosphokinase and uric acid; hyperglycemia, fat redistribution and lipid abnormalities, possible increased bleeding episodes among patients with hemophilia	✓ Refrigerate capsules; capsules can be left at room temperature for ≤30 days ✓ Capsule and liquid contain alcohol ✓ Coadministration with certain other drugs can be fatal ✓ Combination regimen with saquinavir is 400 mg BID plus ritonavir 400 mg BID ✓ Antagonizes oral contraceptives
Nelfinavir/Viracept 250, 625 mg tablets 50 mg/g oral powder	750 mg TID or 1,250 mg BID	Take with meal or snack	Diarrhea; hyperglycemia, fat redistribution and lipid abnormalities, possible increased bleeding episodes among patients with hemophilia; transaminase elevation	✓ May crush or dissolve tabs and mix in small amount water ✓ Powder may be mixed with non-acidic food or beverage ✓ Antagonizes oral contraceptives
Saquinavir/ Invirase 200 mg hard-gel capsules	400 mg BID with ritonavir; **otherwise Invirase is not recommended**	No food effect when taken with ritonavir	Gastrointestinal intolerance, nausea, and diarrhea; headache; elevated transaminase; hyperglycemia, fat redistribution and lipid abnormalities; possible increased bleeding episodes among patients with hemophilia	✓ Use only in combination with ritonavir
Saquinavir/ Fortovase 200 mg soft-get capsules	1200 mg TID (1600 mg BID is **not** recommended)	Take with large meal	Gastrointestinal intolerance, nausea, diarrhea, abdominal pain, and dyspepsia; headache; elevated transaminase; hyperglycemia; fat redistribution and lipid abnormalities; possible increased bleeding episodes among patients with hemophilia	✓ Refrigerate or store at room temperature (≤3 months)
Amprenavir/ Agenerase 50 mg, 150 mg capsules or 15 mg/mL oral solution (Capsules and solution are not interchangeable on mg/mg basis)	Body weight >50 kg: 1200 mg BID (capsules) or 1400 mg BID (oral solution) Body weight <50 kg: 20 mg/kg BID (capsules) maximum 2400 mg daily total; 1.5 mL/kg BID (oral solution) maximum 2800 mg daily total; With ritonavir: amprenavir 600 mg BID plus ritonavir 100 mg BID or amprenavir 1200 mg QD plus ritonavir 200 mg QD	Can be taken with or without food, but high-fat meal should be avoided	Gastrointestinal intolerance, nausea, vomiting, diarrhea; rash; oral paresthesias; transaminase elevation; hyperglycemia; fat redistribution and lipid abnormalities; possible increased bleeding episodes among patients with hemophilia; oral solution contains propylene glycol; therefore, contraindicated among pregnant women, children aged <4 years, patients with hepatic or renal failure, and patients treated with disulfiram or metronidazole	✓ Do not take with vitamin E supplements ✓ Separate dosing of didanosine, antacids by 1-2 hours ✓ Reduces effectiveness of oral contraceptives ✓ Contraindicated in patients with renal or hepatic failure, pregnant patients treated with disulfiram or metronidazole

(Continued)

PROTEASE INHIBITORS (PIs) *(CONTINUED)*

Name/Form	Dosing Recommendations	Food Effect	Adverse Events	Comments
Lopinavir plus ritonavir/Kaletra 133.3 mg lopinavir plus 33.3 mg ritonavir capsules, 80 mg lopinavir plus 20 mg ritonavir per mL oral solution	400 mg lopinavir plus 100 mg ritonavir BID	Take with food	Gastrointestinal intolerance, nausea, vomiting, diarrhea; asthenia; elevated transaminase enzymes; hyperglycemia; fat redistribution and lipid abnormalities; possible increased bleeding episodes among patients with hemophilia	✓ Separate dosing of didanosine by 1-2 hours ✓ May antagonize oral contraceptive ✓ Refrigerated capsules are stable until expiration date on label; if stored at room temperature, stable for 2 months ✓ Oral solution contains alcohol

DRUGS THAT SHOULD NOT BE USED WITH PIs

Drug Category	Calcium Channel Blocker	Cardiac	Lipid-lowering Agents	Antimyco-bacterial	Anti-histamine	GI Drugs	Neuroleptic	Psychotropic	Ergot Alkaloids (Vasoconstrictor)	Herbs
Protease Inhibitors										
Indinavir	None	None	Simvastatin Lovastatin	Rifampin	Astemizole Terfenadine	Cisapride	None	Midazolam Triazolam	Dihydroergotamine (D.H.E.45) Ergotamine (various forms)	St. John's wort
Ritonavir	Bepridil	Amiodarone Flecainide Propafenone Quinidine	Simvastatin Lovastatin	None	Astemizole Terfenadine	Cisapride	Pimozide	Midazolam Triazolam	Dihydroergotamine (D.H.E.45) Ergotamine (various forms)	St. John's wort
Saquinavir	None	None	Simvastatin Lovastatin	Rifampin	Astemizole Terfenadine	Cisapride	None	Midazolam Triazolam	Dihydroergotamine (D.H.E.45) Ergotamine (various forms)	St. John's wort
Nelfinavir	None	None	Simvastatin Lovastatin	Rifampin	Astemizole Terfenadine	Cisapride	None	Midazolam Triazolam	Dihydroergotamine (D.H.E.45) Ergotamine (various forms)	St. John's wort
Amprenavir	Bepridil	None	Simvastatin Lovastatin	Rifampin	Astemizole Terfenadine	Cisapride	None	Midazolam Triazolam	Dihydroergotamine (D.H.E.45) Ergotamine (various forms)	St. John's wort
Lopinavir plus Ritonavir	None	Flecainide Propafenone	Simvastatin Lovastatin	Rifampin	Astemizole Terfenadine	Cisapride	Pimozide	Midazolam Triazolam	Dihydroergotamine (D.H.E.45) Ergotamine (various forms)	St. John's wort

Suggested Alternatives
Simvastatin, lovastatin: Atorvastatin, pravastatin, fluvastatin, cerivastatin (alternatives should be used with caution)
Rifabutin: Clarithromycin, azithromycin (*Mycobacterium avium-intracellulare* prophylaxis); clarithromycin, ethambutol (*Mycobacterium avium-intracellulare* treatment)
Rifampin: Rifabutin (*Mycobacterium tuberculosis*)
Astemizole, terfenadine: Loratadine, fexofenadine, cetirizine
Midazolam, triazolam: Temazepam, lorazepam

Adapted from Centers for Disease Control and Prevention. (2002) Guidelines for the use of antiretroviral agents among HIV-infected adults and adolescents: Recommendations of the Panel on Clinical Practices for Treatment of HIV. *MMWR, 51*(RR-7), 1-55.

DOSAGE CHANGES WHEN PIs ARE PRESCRIBED WITH OTHER PIs

Drug affected	Ritonavir	Saquinavir	Nelfinavir	Amprenavir	Lopinavir/ritonavir
Protease inhibitors					
Indinavir	Indinavir 400 mg BID plus ritonavir 400 mg BID; or indinavir 800 mg BID plus ritonavir 100 or 200 mg BID	No changes	Indinavir 1200 mg BID plus nelfinavir 1250 mg BID	No change	Indinavir 600 mg BID; lopinavir, standard dose
Ritonavir	---	Invirase or Fortovase 400 mg BID plus ritonavir 400 mg BID; or Invirase or Fortovase 800 mg BID plus ritonavir 200 mg BID	Ritonavir 400 mg BID plus nelfinavir 500-750 mg BID	Amprenavir 600 mg BID plus ritonavir 100 mg BID or amprenavir 1200 mg QD plus ritonavir 200 mg QD	Lopinavir is coformulated with ritonavir as Kaletra
Saquinavir	---	---	Standard nelfinavir; Fortovase 800 mg TID or 1200 mg BID	No change	Saquinavir 800 mg BID; lopinavir, standard dose
Nelfinavir	---	---	---	No change	---
Amprenavir	---	---	---	---	Amprenavir 600-750 mg BID; lopinavir, increase to 500 mg BID

Adapted from Centers for Disease Control and Prevention. (2002) Guidelines for the use of antiretroviral agents among HIV-infected adults and adolescents: Recommendations of the Panel on Clinical Practices for Treatment of HIV. *MMWR, 51*(RR-7), 1-55.

DOSAGE CHANGES WHEN PIs AND NNRTIs ARE PRESCRIBED TOGETHER

Drug affected	Nevirapine	Delavirdine	Efavirenz
Protease inhibitors and nonnucleoside reverse transcriptase inhibitors			
Indinavir	Indinavir 1000 mg every 8 hours; nevirapine, standard dose	Indinavir 600 mg every 8 hours; delavirdine, standard dose	Indinavir 1000 mg every 8 hours; efavirenz, standard dose
Ritonavir	Standard dose	Delavirdine, standard dose; ritonavir, data unavailable	Ritonavir 600 mg BID (500 mg BID for intolerance); efavirenz, standard dose
Saquinavir	Data unavailable	Fortovase 800 mg TID; delavirdine, standard but monitor transaminase levels	Coadministration not recommended when saquinavir is used as a single PI
Nelfinavir	Standard dose	Data unavailable but monitor for neutropenic complications	Standard dose
Amprenavir	Data unavailable	---	Amprenavir 1200 mg TID as single protease inhibitor or 1200 mg BID plus ritonavir 200 mg BID; efavirenz, standard dose
Lopinavir/ritonavir	Consider lopinavir 533/133 mg BID for protease inhibitor-experienced patients; nevirapine, standard dose	Insufficient data	Consider lopinavir 533/133 mg BID for protease inhibitor-experienced patients; efavirenz, standard dose
Nevirapine	---	---	Standard dose
Delavirdine	---	---	---

Adapted from Centers for Disease Control and Prevention. (2002) Guidelines for the use of antiretroviral agents among HIV-infected adults and adolescents: Recommendations of the Panel on Clinical Practices for Treatment of HIV. *MMWR, 51*(RR-7), 1-55.

DOSAGE ADJUSTMENTS WHEN PRESCRIBING PIs AND OTHER DRUGS*

Drugs affected	Antifungals Ketoconazole	Antimycobacterials			
		Rifampin	Rifabutin	Clarithromycin	Miscellaneous
Protease Inhibitors					
Indinavir	Indinavir 600 mg TID	Contraindicated	Decrease rifabutin to 150 mg daily or 300 mg 2-3 times/week; indinavir, 1,000 mg TID	No dose adjustment	Grapefruit juice decreases levels Do not exceed 25 mg of sildenafil in 48-hour period
Ritonavir	Use with caution: do not exceed 200 mg/day of ketoconazole	No data; increased liver toxicity possible	Decrease rifabutin to 150 mg every other day or dose three times/week; ritonavir: standard dose	Adjustment for renal insufficiency	Multiple interactions (always check drug manual)
Saquinavir	Standard dose of saquinavir	Contraindicated, unless using ritonavir plus saquinavir, then use rifampin 600 mg daily or 2-3 times/week	No dose adjustment unless using ritonavir plus saquinavir; then use rifabutin 150 mg 3 times/week	No dose adjustment	Grapefruit juice increases levels; Dexamethasone decreases levels; Use sildenafil 25 mg starting dose
Nelfinavir	No dose adjustment	Contraindicated	Decrease rifabutin to 150 mg QD or 300 mg 2-3 times/week; increase nelfinavir dose to 1000 mg TID	---	Do not exceed 25 mg of sildenafil in 48-hour period
Amprenavir	No data available	Avoid concomitant use	Decrease rifabutin to 150 mg QD or 300 mg 3 times/week	No dose adjustment	Do not exceed 25 mg of sildenafil in 48-hour period
Lopinavir	Do not exceed 200 mg/day of ketoconazole	Avoid concomitant use	Decrease rifabutin dose to 150 mg every other day; lopinavir: standard dose	---	Do not exceed 25 mg of sildenafil in 48-hour period

* Lipid lowering agents and anticonvulsants frequently interact with PIs; check package insert and drug manual before prescribing drugs from these classes

Adapted from Centers for Disease Control and Prevention. (2002) Guidelines for the use of antiretroviral agents among HIV-infected adults and adolescents: Recommendations of the Panel on Clinical Practices for Treatment of HIV. *MMWR, 51*(RR-7), 1-55.

    S.   Nonnucleoside reverse transcriptase inhibitors (NNRTI) (see following table)
           1.   Act on a nonsubstrate binding site of the enzyme which alters the shape of the active site (see following table)
           2.   Always check drug manual or drug insert before prescribing NNRTI
                a.   Certain drugs should not be used with NNRTIs (see table DRUGS THAT SHOULD NOT BE USED WITH NNRTIs)
                b.   NNRTIs often interact with other medications and require dose modifications or cautious use (see table DOSAGE ADJUSTMENTS WHEN PRESCRIBING NNRTIs)
                c.   Some NNRTI dosages should be modified when used with PIs (see table DOSAGE CHANGES WHEN PIS AND NNRTIs ARE PRESCRIBED TOGETHER in V.Q.)

NONNUCLEOSIDE REVERSE TRANSCRIPTASE INHIBITORS (NNRTIs)

Generic/Trade Name	Form	Dosing Recommendations	Food effect	Adverse Events
Nevirapine/Viramune	200 mg tablets or 50 mg/5mL oral suspension	200 mg by mouth daily for 14 days; thereafter, 200 mg by mouth BID	Take without regard to meals	✓ Rash* ✓ Severe, life-threatening hepatotoxicity including hepatic necrosis (monitor patients intensively during first 12 weeks of therapy)
Delavirdine/Rescriptor	100 mg tablets or 200 mg tablets	400 mg by mouth TID; 4, 100 mg tablets can be dispersed in ≥3 oz water to produce slurry; 100 mg tablets should be taken as intact tablets; separate buffered preparations dosing with didanosine or antacids by 1 hour	Take without regard to meals	✓ Rash* ✓ Increased transaminase levels ✓ Headaches
Efavirenz/Sustiva	50, 100, 200 mg capsules or 600 mg tablets	600 mg by mouth daily on an empty stomach, preferably at bedtime	Take on empty stomach	✓ Rash* ✓ Central nervous system symptoms** ✓ Increased transaminase levels ✓ False-positive cannabinoid test

* During clinical trials, NNRTI was discontinued because of rash among 7% of patients taking nevirapine, 4.3% of patients taking delavirdine, and 1.7% of patients taking efavirenz. Rare cases of Stevens-Johnson syndrome have been reported with the use of all three NNRTIs
** Adverse events can include dizziness, somnolence, insomnia, abnormal dreams, confusion, abnormal thinking, impaired concentration, amnesia, agitation, depersonalization, hallucinations, and euphoria

DRUGS THAT SHOULD NOT BE USED WITH NNRTIs

Drug Category	Calcium Channel Blocker	Cardiac	Lipid-lowering Agent	Anti-mycobacterial	Antihistamine	GI Drugs	Neuroleptic	Psychotropic	Ergot Alkaloids (Vasoconstrictor)
Nevirapine	None	None	None	Insufficient data	None	None	None	None	None
Delavirdine	None	None	Simvastatin Lovastatin	Rifampin Rifabutin	Astemizole Terfenadine	Cisapride Hydrogen-2 blockers Proton pump inhibitors	None	Midazolam Triazolam	Dihydroergotamine (D.H.E.45) Ergotamine (various forms)
Efavirenz	None	None	None	None	Astemizole Terfenadine	Cisapride	None	Midazolam Triazolam	Dihydroergotamine (D.H.E.45) Ergotamine (various forms)

Suggested Alternatives

Simvastatin, lovastatin: Atorvastatin, pravastatin, fluvastatin, cerivastatin (alternatives should be used with caution)
Rifabutin: Clarithromycin, azithromycin (*Mycobacterium avium-intracellulare* prophylaxis); clarithromycin, ethambutol (*Mycobacterium avium-intracellulare* treatment)
Rifampin: Rifabutin (*Mycobacterium tuberculosis*)
Astemizole, terfenadine: Loratadine, fexofenadine, cetirizine
Midazolam, triazolam: Temazepam, lorazepam

DOSAGE ADJUSTMENTS WHEN PRESCRIBING NNRTIs*

| Drugs affected | Antifungals | Antimycobacterials | | | Miscellaneous |
	Ketoconazole	Rifampin	Rifabutin	Clarithromycin	
Nonnucleoside reverse transcriptase inhibitors					
Nevirapine	Not recommended	Use only if clearly indicated	No dose adjustment	No dose adjustment	Methadone levels decreased
Delavirdine	No data available	Contraindicated	Not recommended	Adjust dose for renal failure	May increase levels of dapsone, warfarin, quinidine; do not exceed 25 mg of sildenafil in 48-hour period
Efavirenz	No data available	Unknown	Increase rifabutin dose to 450-600 mg QD or 600 mg 3 times/week; efavirenz: standard dose	Alternative recommended	Methadone levels decreased. Monitor warfarin when used concomitantly

* Lipid-lowering agents and anticonvulsants may interact with NNRTIs; check package insert and drug manual before prescribing drugs from these classes

Above tables adapted from Centers for Disease Control and Prevention. (2002) Guidelines for the use of antiretroviral agents among HIV-infected adults and adolescents: Recommendations of the Panel on Clinical Practices for Treatment of HIV. *MMWR, 51*(RR-7), 1-55.

T. New antiretroviral agents are available or will be available soon (see following table)

NEW ANTIRETROVIRAL DRUGS WITH CLINICAL DATA

Drug	Comment
Enfuvirtide (Fuzeon)	• Interferes with entry of HIV-1 into cells by inhibiting fusion of viral and cellular membranes; blocks HIV's ability to infect healthy CD4+ T-cells • Indicated for therapy in treatment-experienced patients with evidence of HIV-1 replication despite ongoing antiretroviral therapy • Adverse events include local injection site reactions (occur commonly), increased rate of bacterial pneumonia, and potential hypersensitivity reactions • Dose is 2 mg/kg twice daily injected subcutaneously into upper arm, anterior thigh, or abdomen • Does not interact with other antiretroviral agents or rifampin
Atazanavir (Reyataz)	• Protease inhibitor • Once-a-day dosing • Less lipid problems than other PIs • Most common laboratory abnormality is hyperbilirubinemia that results in jaundice or scleral icterus • Adult dose is 400 mg (two 200 mg capsules) QD with food
Emtricitabine (ETC)	• Drug similar to, but more potent than lamivudine
Amdoxovir (DAPD)	• Nucleoside active against NRTI resistant strains

U. Adjuvant therapy to antiretroviral drugs
    1. Approaches that augment (interleukin 2) or dampen (cyclosporin A, corticosteroids, hydroxyurea, and mycophenolic acid) immune response may prove beneficial, but at present there is insufficient clinical data to recommend their use
    2. Hydroxyurea has significant toxicities which also limit its use

V. Treatment regimen for **primary HIV infection** (acute retroviral syndrome)
    1. When suspicion of acute infection is high, a test for HIV RNA should be performed; positive results should have confirmatory testing performed (Western blot serology)
    2. Aggressive treatment of primary HIV infection may be best time to alter disease course, however some experts believe the risks of ART are too great to recommend drug therapy to all patients
    3. If patient and clinician agree, prescribe a combination antiretroviral regimen (see table, INITIAL COMBINATION REGIMENS FOR TREATMENT-NAÏVE PATIENTS [V.M.8.])
    4. Testing for plasma HIV RNA levels and CD4+ T-cell counts should be performed on initiation of therapy, and then after 4, 8-12, 16-24 weeks on ART
    5. The optimal duration and composition of therapy is unknown but because of latently infected CD4+ T-cells, several years of treatment may be needed (some experts recommend that treatment should be indefinite whereas others treat for 1 year and then provide close monitoring)

W. Treatment of **patients with HIV- and HCV-coinfection**
1. Advise to avoid (best) or limit alcohol intake
2. Vaccinate against hepatitis A and possibly hepatitis B if susceptible
3. Regularly evaluate for liver disease and treat as these patients experience liver disease in a shorter time course than patients infected with only HCV

X. **Treatment of HAART-associated adverse clinical events**
1. Lactic acidosis
   a. Immediately discontinue ART: Lactate >5 mmol/L with symptoms or lactate >10 mmol/L
   b. Consider discontinuing ART: Lactate >5 mmol/L with or without symptoms
   c. Carefully monitor lactate levels if asymptomatic and lactate is 2-5 mmol/L
   d. Although there is limited empirical data, thiamine and riboflavin may be helpful
2. Hepatotoxicity
   a. Closely monitor liver enzymes after ART is initiated; for example, after nevirapine initiation monitor every 2 weeks for first month, then monthly for first 12 weeks; then every 1-3 months
   b. Discontinue the drug causing the adverse event
3. Hyperglycemia (see section on DIABETES MELLITUS)
   a. Closely monitor patients when PIs are used; some clinicians recommend routine fasting blood glucose tests every 3-6 months
   b. Avoid use of PI as initial therapy in patients with pre-existing glucose intolerance or diabetes
   c. Teach patients the warning signs of hyperglycemia (polydipsia, polyphagia, polyuria)
   d. Most clinicians recommend continuation of ART in absence of severe diabetes
   e. Emphasize diet, exercise, weight loss; antidiabetic drug therapy should follow guidelines for non-HIV infected population (preference should be given to insulin sensitizing agents such as metformin [except those with history of renal disease or lactic acidemia] or thiazolidinediones [except those with liver disease])
4. Fat accumulation
   a. No effective therapy is available but some clinicians switch antiretrovirals or switch to another class of drugs
   b. Carefully evaluate for cardiovascular events and pancreatitis
5. Hyperlipidemia (also see section on HYPERLIPIDEMIA)
   a. Recommend low-fat diets, regular exercise, control of blood pressure, and smoking cessation
   b. Avoid use of PI, if possible, in patients with preexisting cardiovascular risk factors, family history of hyperlipidemia
   c. Hypercholesterolemia may respond to statins; with continuing high cholesterol levels, fibrates may be added to statin therapy after 3-4 months of treatment
      (1) Remember that certain statins interact with PIs
      (2) Atorvastatin is probably the best statin to use with PIs, but should be used cautiously and in reduced doses
   d. Isolated triglyceride elevations respond best to low-fat diets and fibrates
   e. If lipid elevations are severe and unresponsive to above therapies, consider modifying antiretroviral therapy; switching PI component to nevirapine or abacavir may be effective
6. Osteonecrosis, osteopenia, and osteoporosis
   a. No recommendations are made for routine measurement of bone density or for prophylaxis or treatment to prevent decreases in bone density
   b. Teach patients to have an adequate intake of calcium and vitamin D and to engage in appropriate weight-bearing exercises
   c. If osteoporotic fractures occur, more aggressive therapies with bisphosphonates, raloxifene, or calcitonin may be prescribed
   d. Surgical resection of involved bone is only effective therapy for symptomatic osteonecrosis
7. Skin rashes
   a. Discontinue nevirapine and do not use another NNRTI if patient has severe skin reaction
   b. Discontinue abacavir if skin rash occurs as this may be a symptom of abacavir-associated systemic hypersensitivity
   c. For mild skin rashes from NNRTI, some clinicians manage with antihistamines and do not discontinue drug, but this practice has been questioned

Y. **Symptom management**
1. Wasting syndrome was previously defined as otherwise unexplained loss of 10% of body weight; proposed new definition is presented in following table

PROPOSED NEW DEFINITION OF HIV-ASSOCIATED WASTING

Patient must meet one of following criteria:

- 10% unintentional weight loss over 12 months
- 7.5% unintentional weight loss over 6 months
- 5% body cell mass (BCM) loss within 6 months
- In men: BCM <35% of total body weight and body mass index (BMI) <27 kg/m^3
- In women: BCM <23% of total body weight and BMI <27 kg/m^3
- Body mass index (BMI) <20 kg/m^3

Adapted from Polsky, B., Kotler, D., & Steinhart, C. (2001). HIV-associated wasting in the HAART era: Guidelines for assessment, diagnosis, and treatment. *AIDS Patient Care, 15,* 411-423.

    a.   Causative factors include
        (1)   Decreased food intake due to mouth or esophageal ulcers, anorexia (often related to depression), early satiety, nausea, or financial problems
        (2)   Decreased absorption from loss of enzymes causing lactose intolerance; to avoid this problem teach patient to avoid all milk products by reading labels
        (3)   Increased metabolic demand from infection, fever, and malignancies
        (4)   Malabsorption due to infections and bacterial overgrowth
        (5)   In rare cases may be due to lactic acidosis; with this condition, wasting is accompanied by abdominal pain, fatigue, and exercise-induced dyspnea
    b.   Order following diagnostic tests to rule-out infection and treat as needed: Stool culture, blood culture, cryptococcal serum antigen, and other tests based on patient's clinical presentation; consider lactic acid levels and liver enzymes if lactic acidosis is suspected
    c.   Treat cause (i.e., infection), but if etiology is unclear, consider the following:
        (1)   Daily multivitamin
        (2)   If patient has anorexia, consider prescribing one of the following appetite stimulants:
            (a)   Megestrol acetate (Megace) 40 mg/mL susp.; 800 mg/day; adverse effects include impotence, decreased libido, hypertension
            (b)   Dronabinol (Marinol): 2.5 mg BID before lunch and supper, may gradually increase to maximum of 20 mg/day; adverse effects include abuse potential, euphoria, psychomimetic reactions, altered mental status
        (3)   Recommend nutritional supplements (10 cans per day are needed for total daily caloric needs)
            (a)   If patient needs to gain weight and can tolerate milk use Carnation Instant Breakfast
            (b)   If the patient needs to gain weight but cannot tolerate milk give Ensure or Sustacal
            (c)   If patient has severe malabsorption state use an elemental diet (with easily absorbed nutrients) such as Vivonex TEN
    d.   Consider other beneficial therapies such as growth hormone (Serostim) 6 mg subcutaneous injection QD X 12 weeks, thalidomide 50-300 mg/day PO x 2-12 weeks with starting dose of 100 mg/day, or anabolic steroids such as oxandrolone (men: 20-40 mg/day PO and women: 5-20 mg/day PO)

2.   Testosterone failure may cause wasting as well as a decrease in energy levels and muscle mass
    a.   To diagnose, order serum testosterone level
    b.   Treatment is testosterone enanthate or testosterone cypionate IM injections 200-400 mg every 2 weeks or 100-200 mg every week or testosterone patch (Testoderm TTS), apply 5 mg patch every 22-24 hours to arm, back or upper buttocks (application site rotation is not necessary)

3.   Diarrhea
    a.   Acute diarrhea is often due to medications, anxiety, irritable bowel syndrome, or untreatable viral agents such a Norwalk agent; presence of severe diarrhea, fever, and fecal leukocytes and/or blood increase the likelihood of a treatable pathogen
    b.   Chronic diarrhea is often due to infections; about 20-30% of chronic diarrhea cases are idiopathic
    c.   Initially, order following diagnostic tests to rule-out parasites or infection: Stool for ova and parasites, bacterial stool culture, *C-difficile* toxin, acid-fast bacterial smear of stool can sometimes detect *Mycobacterium avium* and cryptosporidiosis; consult specialist for further tests such as CT, colonoscopy, endoscopy

      d.   If infection is ruled-out, prescribe one of following

          (1)   Loperamide (Imodium) 2 mg caps, two in AM and one after each BM up to maximum of 8 caps

          (2)   Alternative: Diphenoxylate (Lomotil) 2.5 mg; 2 tabs or 10 mL QID

      e.   Patient education

          (1)   Increase fluids

          (2)   Follow a low lactose, low fat, high fiber diet

          (3)   Use LactAid instead of milk

          (4)   Avoid caffeine, fried foods, carbonated beverages, cabbage, broccoli

4.   Nausea and vomiting

      a.   Rule out infections

      b.   Symptomatically treat with prochlorperazine (Compazine) 5-10 mg QID, or ondansetron (Zofran) 4-10 mg QID

5.   Pain is a common symptom (see section on PAIN)

6.   Fever without focal symptoms

      a.   Common causes are *Mycobacterium avium complex*, tuberculosis, lymphoma, cytomegalovirus infection, secondary syphilis

      b.   Following diagnostic tests should be obtained: Blood culture for conventional bacteria and for acid-fast bacteria, cryptococcal serum antigen, CBC; consider PPD, RPR, chest x-ray, liver enzymes, LDH, urinalysis, blood gases for PCP, urine culture

      c.   Symptomatic treatment (see section on FEVERS)

7.   Anemia may be caused by numerous factors

      a.   Order the following diagnostic tests to identify cause of anemia:

          (1)   CBC: if patient has normal WBCs but decreased RBCs consider infection with parvovirus

          (2)   Bleeding (stool guaiac), hemolysis (smear), iron deficiency (serum iron, transferrin, % saturation, ferritin, reticulocyte count), B_{12} and folate deficiencies (serum $B_{12,}$ serum folate)

      b.   If patient is on zidovudine, consider switching to another NRTI

      c.   If cause of anemia cannot be corrected and if hemoglobin is <9 g/dL, prescribe erythropoietin (Epogen, Procrit); some experts recommend erythropoietin should be given when patients have mild symptomatic anemia (13 g/dL in men & 11 g/dL in women) or moderate anemia (12 g/dL in men and 10 g/dL in women)

          (1)   Measure ferritin levels; patient must have adequate iron stores to respond to drug

          (2)   Initially administer 100 units/kg SQ 3 times per week to maximum of 300 units/kg 3 times per week or 40,000 units subcutaneous injection every week (investigational dosing schedule, but increasingly used in practice)

              (a)   If hemoglobin increases by >1 g/dL at 4 weeks, continue same dose and continue to monitor response; when hemoglobin is >11-13 g/dL, hold erythropoietin or decrease by 10,000 units per week

              (b)   If hemoglobin increase is <1 g/dL at 4 weeks, increase to 60,000 units a week; if hemoglobin increase is <1 g/dL at week 12, discontinue

8.   Neutropenia

      a.   May be due to drugs such as zidovudine or ganciclovir or to HIV infection

      b.   Prescribe G-CSF (Neupogen) or GM-CSF (Leukine) 1-10 μg/kg/day; usual initial dose of G-CSF is 1μg/kg/day SQ with increases of 1μg/kg/day at 5-7 day intervals to maintain absolute neutrophil count (ANC) at 1000-2000 cells/mm^3; usual maintenance dose is 300 μg given 3-7 times per week

9.   Mouth ulcers are common, particularly if patient is on zalcitabine (See sections on APHTHOUS ULCERS, HERPES SIMPLEX, CANDIDIASIS)

10.   Dermatological problems: Common causes are infection, neoplastic diseases, and reaction to medications

      a.   Eosinophilic folliculitis or red, itchy bumps is a common manifestation

          (1)   Generally disappears when CD4+ T-cells rise above 200/mm^3 and viral load is undetectable

          (2)   For symptomatic treatment, prescribe cetirizine (Zyrtec) 5-10 mg QD or loratadine (Claritin) 10 mg QD and one of following:

              (a)   Camphor 0.5/Menthol 0.5 lotion (Sarna)

              (b)   Topical steroids

              (c)   Ultraviolet light

      b.   See treatment of other dermatological conditions in SKIN chapter

11. Peripheral neuropathy: discontinue implicated NRTIs and treat with one of following:
    a. Nortriptyline (Pamelor) 10 mg HS; increase dose by 10 mg q 5 days to maximum of 75 mg HS or 10-20 mg TID
    b. Ibuprofen 600-800 mg TID
    c. Capsaicin-containing ointments (Zostrix) for topical application
12. Mental health problems are common (see sections on DEPRESSION, INSOMNIA, and ANXIETY)

Z. Follow Up: Adjust follow-up to clinical condition of patient
    1. Patients who are asymptomatic and not on antiretroviral therapy should be seen every 3-6 months
    2. Patients who begin antiretroviral therapy or begin a new antiretroviral regimen should be re-evaluated in one month
    3. Patients who are stable and on antiretroviral therapy should be seen every 1-3 months depending on their clinical situations

HUMAN IMMUNODEFICIENCY VIRUS (HIV) OCCUPATIONAL EXPOSURE

I. Definitions:

A. Health care personnel (HCP) are persons (employees, students, contractors, attending clinicians, public-safety workers, or volunteers) whose activities involve contact with patients or with blood or other body fluids from patients in a health care, laboratory setting, or public-safety setting

B. An exposure that may place the HCP at risk for HIV infection includes incidents involving blood, tissue or other body fluids contaminated with visible blood; semen, vaginal, cerebrospinal, synovial, pleural, peritoneal, pericardial, and amniotic fluids have an undetermined risk; examples include the following:
    1. Percutaneous injury such as a needlestick or cut with a sharp object
    2. Contact of mucous membrane or nonintact skin (e.g., exposed skin that is chapped, abraded or has dermatitis) with blood, tissues, or other potentially infectious body fluids
    3. Any direct contact with concentrated HIV in a research laboratory or production facility
    4. Human bites; possibility of infection for both the person bitten and the person who inflicted bite

II. Pathogenesis: (see section on HIV/AIDS in Adults and Adolescents)

III. Clinical Presentation

A. As of June 2000, 56 US HCP have reported documented occupationally acquired HIV infection (negative HIV-antibody tests at the time of exposure and subsequent seroconversion); another 138 HCP have possible occupationally acquired HIV infection (lack of documented seroconversion as result of exposure)

B. Nurses are the most commonly exposed professional group

C. Risk after a needlestick when the source patient is HIV positive is approximately 0.3%; risk of mucocutaneous transmission is less than 0.1%

IV. Diagnosis/Evaluation

A. History
    1. Evaluate exposure (determine type of incident, amount of fluid involved, and duration of exposure)
    2. Evaluate exposure source person
        a. Explore prior HIV testing results and CD4+ T-cell levels
        b. History of possible HIV exposures such as IV drug use, sexual contact with a known HIV infected partner, unprotected sexual contact with multiple partners, etc.
        c. Ask exposure source about clinical symptoms that may suggest acute syndrome or undiagnosed HIV infection

          d.   If exposure source is HIV positive, determine current HIV RNA levels, CD4+ T-cells, and current and previous antiretroviral therapies; resistance to antiretroviral agents should be suspected in source persons with clinical progression of disease or persistently increasing viral loads or decreasing CD4+ T-cell counts

     3.   For purposes of considering postexposure prophylaxis (PEP), ask HCP about current use of medications and underlying medical conditions

B.   Physical Examination
     1.   Thoroughly assess site of wound
     2.   Explore mental status and anxiety level of HCP

C.   Differential Diagnosis: None

D.   Diagnostic Test
     1.   Evaluation of occupational exposure source
          a.   Test for HIV antibody; consider rapid HIV-antibody test
          b.   For exposure sources whose infection remains unknown (exposure source refuses testing), consider medical diagnoses, clinical symptoms, and history of risk behaviors when making management decisions
     2.   Evaluation of HCP
          a.   Perform HIV antibody testing to establish serostatus at time of exposure if the source person is HIV infected or has recently engaged in high risk behaviors; routine use of direct virus assays (HIV p24 antigen EIA or tests for HIV RNA) are not recommended
          b.   Consider using a rapid HIV-antibody test
          c.   Perform follow-up HIV antibody testing at 6 weeks, 12 weeks, and 6 months if the exposure source person is HIV infected or has high risk for HIV infection; extended follow-up (12 months) is needed for HCP who become infected with HCV following exposure to an exposure source coinfected with HIV and HCV; extended follow-up should be individually considered for all HCP depending on type of exposure, etc.
          d.   Pregnancy testing should be offered to all nonpregnant women of childbearing age if pregnancy status is unknown
          e.   See section "Follow-Up" (V.D.2.) for monitoring of drug toxicity if PEP is used

V.   Plan/Management

A.   Wound and skin sites should be washed with soap and water; flush mucous membranes with water

B.   Postexposure prophylaxis (PEP)
     1.   Discuss risks and benefits of PEP
     2.   Selection of type of PEP regimen should involve consideration of the comparative risk of the exposure (see table POSTEXPOSURE PROPHYLAXIS)
     3.   Selection of drug regimens (see table POSTEXPOSURE PROPHYLAXIS DRUG REGIMENS)
          a.   Two-drug regimens are used for most exposures but three-drug regimens should be used for exposures that have increased risk
          b.   Drug selection should also be based on whether the exposure source person's virus is known or suspected to be resistant to one of more the potential drugs for PEP
     4.   If indicated, PEP should be started as soon as possible
     5.   Re-evaluation of exposed person should be considered within 72 hours postexposure, especially as additional information about exposure source person or exposure becomes available
     6.   PEP should be administered for 4 weeks, if tolerated
     7.   If PEP is taken and the source is later determined to be HIV negative, discontinue PEP

POSTEXPOSURE PROPHYLAXIS FOR PERCUTANEOUS INJURIES, MUCOUS MEMBRANE EXPOSURES, AND NONINTACT SKIN EXPOSURES

| Exposure Type | Infection Status of Source | | | |
	HIV-Positive Class 1*	HIV-Positive Class 2*	Source of Unknown HIV Status**	Unknown Source†
Percutaneous (less severe: solid needle and superficial injury) -or- Mucous membrane or skin (small volume: few drops)	Recommend basic 2-drug PEP	Recommend expanded 3-drug PEP	Generally, no PEP warranted; however, consider basic 2-drug PEP for source with HIV risk factors	Generally, no PEP warranted; however, consider basic 2-drug PEP in settings where exposure to HIV-infected persons is likely
Percutaneous (more severe: large-bore needle, deep puncture, visible blood on device, needle used in artery or vein) -or- Mucous membrane or skin (large volume: major blood splash)	Recommend expanded 3-drug PEP	Recommend expanded 3-drug PEP	Generally, no PEP warranted; however, consider basic 2-drug PEP for source with HIV risk factors	Generally, no PEP warranted; however, consider basic 2-drug PEP in settings where exposure to HIV-infected persons is likely

* HIV-Positive, Class 1 – asymptomatic HIV infection or known low viral load (e.g., <1,500 RNA copies/mL). HIV-Positive, Class 2 – symptomatic HIV infection, AIDS, acute seroconversion, or known high viral load. If drug resistance is a concern, obtain expert consultation. Initiation of postexposure prophylaxis (PEP) should not be delayed pending expert consultation, and, because expert consultation alone cannot substitute for face-to-face counseling, resources should be available to provide immediate evaluation and follow-up care for all exposures
** Source of unknown HIV status (e.g., deceased source person with no samples available for HIV testing)
† Unknown source (e.g., a needle from a sharps disposal container)

Adapted from Center for Disease Control. (2001). Updated U.S. Public Health Service guidelines for the management of occupational exposures to HBV, HCV, and HIV and recommendations for postexposure prophylaxis. *MMWR, 50*(RR11), 1-42

POSTEXPOSURE PROPHYLAXIS DRUG REGIMENS*

Regimen Category	Drug Regimen
Basic Regimen	Zidovudine, 600 mg per day in two or three divided doses plus lamivudine 150 mg BID; available as Combivir (one tab BID)
Alternate Basic Regimen	Lamivudine 150 mg BID plus stavudine 40 mg BID (if body weight is <60 kg, 30 mg BID)
Alternate Basic Regimen	Didanosine 400 mg QD on empty stomach (if body weight is <60 kg, 125 mg BID) plus stavudine 40 mg BID (if body weight is <60 kg, 30 mg BID)
Expanded Regimen	Basic regimen plus one of the following: indinavir 800 mg every 8 hours, nelfinavir 750 mg TID, nelfinavir 1250 mg BID, efavirenz 600 mg QD HS, abacavir 300 mg BID (available as Trizivir, a combination of zidovudine, lamivudine, and abacavir [1 tab BID])

*Ritonavir, saquinavir, amprenavir, delavirdine, lopinavir/ritonavir are agents that can used as PEP with expert consultation; nevirapine is generally not recommended for use as PEP

Adapted from Center for Disease Control. (2001). Updated U.S. Public Health Service guidelines for the management of occupational exposures to HBV, HCV, and HIV and recommendations for postexposure prophylaxis. *MMWR, 50*(RR11), 1-42

C. Counseling and education
    1. The emotional effect of exposure is great; HCP need social support and accurate information
    2. Advise HCP to use the following measures to prevent secondary transmission: Practice sexual abstinence or use condoms, refrain from donating blood, plasma, organs, tissue, or semen; refrain from breastfeeding, if applicable
    3. Counsel on importance of completing the prescribed drug regimen
    4. Inform of possible drug toxicities and the need for monitoring, and possible drug interactions
    5. Advise to seek medical evaluation for any acute illness that occurs during follow-up period as this may indicate acute HIV infection, a drug reaction, or another medical problem needing attention
    6. Resources for guidance on management of occupation exposures (see table)

RESOURCES FOR OCCUPATION EXPOSURES

National Clinician's Postexposure Prophylaxis Hotline	http://www.ucsf.edu/hivcntr
Needlestick (management of blood exposures)	http://www.needlestick.mednet.ucla.edu

D. Follow Up
1. HCP need counseling, postexposure testing and medical evaluation regardless of whether they receive PEP; HIV antibody testing should be performed at 6 weeks, 12 weeks, and 6 months
2. If PEP is used, monitor for drug toxicity at baseline and again 2 weeks after starting PEP
   a. Select tests based on medical conditions of exposed person and toxicity of drugs
   b. Minimally order CBC and renal and hepatic function tests
   c. Order serum glucose if regimens include a protease inhibitor
   d. If indinavir is used, monitor for crystalluria, hematuria, hemolytic anemia, and hepatitis

REFERENCES

Amaya, R.A., Kozinetz, C.A., McMeans, A., Schwarzwald, H., & Kline, M.W. (2002). Lipodystrophy syndrome in human immunodeficiency virus-infected children. *Pediatric Infectious Disease Journal, 21,* 405-410.

American Academy of Pediatrics Committee on Pediatric AIDS. (1997). Evaluation and medical treatment of the HIV-exposed infant. *Pediatrics, 99,* 909-917.

American Academy of Pediatrics Committee on Pediatric AIDS. (1998). Surveillance of pediatric HIV infection. *Pediatrics, 101,* 315-319.

American Academy of Pediatrics, Committee on Pediatric AIDS and Committee on Infectious Diseases. (1999). Issues related to human immunodeficiency virus transmission in schools, child care, medical settings, the home, and community. *Pediatrics, 104,* 318-324.

American Academy of Pediatrics, Committee on Pediatric AIDS. (2000). Identification and care of HIV-exposed and HIV-infected infants, children, and adolescents in foster care. *Pediatrics, 106,* 149-153.

American Psychiatric Association. (2000). Practice guideline for the treatment of patients with HIV/AIDS. *American Journal of Psychiatry, 156,* 1-62.

Barnhart, H.X., Caldwell, M.B., Thomas, P., Mascola, L., Ortiz, I., Hsu, H., Schulte, J., Parrott, R., Maldonado, Y., Byers, R. & the Pediatric Spectrum of Disease Clinical Consortium. (1996). Natural history of human immunodeficiency virus disease in perinatally infected children: An analysis from the Pediatric Spectrum of Disease Project. *Pediatrics, 97,* 710-716.

Barrett, D.J. & Sleasman, J.W. (1997). Pediatric AIDS: So now what do we do? *Contemporary Pediatrics, 14,* 111-124.

Bartlett, J.G. (2001). *The John's Hopkins Hospital 2002 guide to medical care of patients with HIV infection* (10th ed.). Philadelphia: Lippincott Williams & Wilkins.

Center for Communicable Diseases. (1992). 1993 revised classification system for HIV infection and expanded surveillance case definition of AIDS among adolescents and adults. *MMWR, 41* (RR-17).

Centers for Disease Control and Prevention. (2001). Updated U.S. Public Health Service guidelines for the management of occupational exposures to HBV, HCV, and HIV and recommendations for postexposure prophylaxis. *MMWR, 50*(RR11), 1-42

Centers for Disease Control and Prevention. (2002). Approval of a new rapid test for HIV antibody. *MMWR, 51,* 1051-1052.

Centers for Disease Control and Prevention. (2002). Guidelines for using antiretroviral agents among HIV-infected adults and adolescents: Recommendations of the Panel on Clinical Practices for Treatment of HIV. *MMWR, 51*(RR-7). 1-55.

Centers for Disease Control and Prevention. (2002). Guidelines for preventing opportunistic infections among HIV-infected persons – 2002: Recommendations of the U.S. Public Health Service and the Infectious Diseases Society of America. *MMWR, 51*(RR-8), 1-52.

Centers for Disease Control and Prevention. (2002). Update: AIDS—United States, 2000. *MMWR, 51,* 592-595.

Cheseaux, J.J., Jotterand, V., Aebi, C., Gnehm, H., Kind, C., Nadal, D., et al. (2002). Hyperlipidemia in HIV-infected children treated with protease inhibitors: Relevance for cardiovascular diseases. *Journal of Acquired Immune Deficiency Syndrome, 30,* 288-293.

Ferri, R.S., Adinolfi, A., Orsi, A.J, Sterken, D.J., Keruly, J.C., Davis, S. et al. (2001). Treatment of anemia in patients with HIV infection, Part 1: The need for adequate guidelines. *Journal of the Association of Nurses in AIDS Care, 12,* 39-51.

Ferri, R.S., Adinolfi, A., Orsi, A.J, Sterken, D.J., Keruly, J.C., Davis, S. et al. (2002). Treatment of anemia in patients with HIV infection, Part 2: Guidelines for management of anemia. *Journal of the Association of Nurses in AIDS Care, 13,* 50-59.

Gerberding, J.L. (2003). Occupational exposure to HIV in health care settings. *New England Journal of Medicine, 348,* 826-833.

Green, M.L. (2002). Evaluation and management of dyslipidemia in patients with HIV infection. *Journal of General Internal Medicine, 17,* 797-810.

Joffe, B.I., Panz, V.R., & Raal, F.J. (2001). From lipodystrophy syndromes to diabetes mellitus. *Lancet, 351,* 1379-1381.

Keithley, J.K. (2001). Management of antiretroviral-related nutritional problems: State of the science. *Journal of the Association of Nurses in AIDS Care, 12*(Suppl), 67-74.

Kirton, C. (Ed.). (2003). *ANAC's core curriculum for HIV/AIDS nursing* (2nd ed.). Thousand Oaks: Sage.

Laufer, M., & Scott, G. B. (2000). Medical management of HIV disease in children. *Pediatric Clinics of North America, 47,* 127-152.

Little, S.J., Holte, S., Routy, J.P., Daar, E.S., Markowitz, M., Collier, A.C., et al. (2002). Antiretroviral-drug resistance among patients recently infected with HIV. *New England Journal of Medicine, 347,* 385-394.

Luzuriaga, K., & Sullivan, J.L. (1998). Prevention and treatment of pediatric HIV infection. *JAMA, 280,* 17-18.

Moyle, G.J., Datta, D., Mandalia, S., Asbol, D., & Gazzard, B.G. (2001). Hyperlactataemia and lactic acidosis during antiretroviral therapy. *Antiretroviral Therapy, 6*(Suppl), 66.

National Institute of Allergy and Infectious Diseases. (2003). Important interaction results from a phase III, randomized, double-blind comparison of three protease inhibitor-sparing regimens for initial treatment of HIV infection (AACTG Protocol A5095). Available at http:www.nlm.nih.gov/databases/alerts/hiv.html.

Panel on Clinical Practices for Treatment of HIV Infection (Convened by Department of Health and Human Services [DHHS]). (2003). Guildelines for use of antiretroviral agents in HIV-infected adults and adolescents. Available at http://AIDSinfo.nih.gov.

Piscitelli, S.C., & Gallicano, K.D. (2001). Interactions among drugs for HIV and opportunistic infections. *New England Journal of Medicine, 344,* 984-996.

Pollock, B.H., Jenson, H.B., Leach, C.T., McClain, K.L., Hutchison, R.E, Garzarella, L., Joshi, V.V., Parmley, R.T., & Murphy, S.B. (2003). Risk factors for pediatric human immunodeficiency virus-related malignancy. *JAMA, 289,* 2393-2399.

Polsky, B., Kotler, D., & Steinhart, C. (2001). HIV-associated wasting in the HAART era: Guidelines for assessment, diagnosis, and treatment. *AIDS Patient Care, 15,* 411-423.

Schambelan, M., Benson, C.A., Carr, A., Currier, J.S., Dubé, M.P., Gerber, J.G., et al. (2002). Management of metabolic complications associated with antiretroviral therapy for HIV-1 infection: Recommendations of an International AIDS Society – USA Panel. *Journal of Acquired Immune Deficiency Syndrome, 31,* 257-275.

Shearer, W.T., & Hanson, I.C. (2003). *Medical management of AIDS in children.* Philadelphia: Saunders.

Smith, K. Y. (2002). Selected metabolic and morphologic complications associated with highly active antiretroviral therapy. *Journal of Infectious Disease, 185*(Suppl 2), S123-S127.

Steinhart, C., Orrick, J.J., & Simpson, K. (2002). *HIV/AIDS primary care guide.* Gainesville, FL: University of Florida.

US Food and Drug Administration. (2003). FDA approves first drug in new class of HIV treatments for HIV infected adults and children with advanced disease. Available at: http://www.fda.gov/bbs/topics/NEWS/2003/NEW00879.html

US Public Health Service Task Force. (2002). US Public Health Task force recommendations for use of antiretroviral drugs in pregnant HIV-1 infected women for maternal health and interventions to reduce perinatal HIV-1 transmission in the United States. *MMWR, 51*(RR18), 1-38.

Working Group on Antiretroviral Therapy and Medical Management of HIV-Infected Children. (2003). *Guidelines for use of antiretroviral agents in pediatric HIV infection.* Bethesda (MD): Department of Health and Human Services Public Health Service (PHS), Centers for Disease Control and Prevention (CDC). 55 pages.

Yeni, P.G., Hammer, S.M., Carpenter, C.C.J., Cooper, D.A., Fischl, M.A., Gatell, J.M., et al. (2002). Antiretroviral treatment for adult HIV infection in 2002: Updated recommendations of the International AIDS Society—USA Panel. *JAMA, 288,* 222-235.

Musculoskeletal Problems

CONSTANCE R. UPHOLD

ANKLE SPRAIN

I. Definition: Injury to the ligaments of the ankle

II. Pathogenesis

   A. Due to sudden stress on one or more of the supporting ligaments of the ankle

   B. Often occurs from stepping off a curb or into a hole

   C. If injury is sports-related, it is often due to jumping or falling on outstretched ankle; basketball, football, and cross-country running are the sports in which sprains occur most frequently

   D. Inversion injuries which involve the anterior talofibular or the calcaneofibular ligaments occur most often
      1. Occurs when the foot is plantarflexed and inverted
      2. Physical findings include anterolateral swelling, tenderness over anterior talofibular ligament, and, with severe sprains, a positive anterior drawer sign

   E. Eversion injuries which usually involve the deltoid ligament are the second most common type
      1. Occurs when foot is dorsiflexed and everted
      2. Location of maximal pain, swelling, and tenderness is medial rather than lateral

III. Clinical Presentation

   A. Most common musculoskeletal injury; approximately 85% of all ankle injuries in adults are due to sprains

   B. Classification of sprains (see table the follows)

CLASSIFICATION OF ANKLE SPRAINS	
Grade	**Clinical Manifestations**
I. First degree: Partial tear of ligament	Joint is stable with minimal pain, swelling, and ecchymosis Slight or no functional loss (able to bear weight with minimal pain)
II. Second degree: Incomplete tear of ligament, with moderate functional loss	Ligament appreciably torn but the joint remains stable Severe swelling (>4 cm about the fibula) and severe ecchymosis
III. Third degree: Complete tear and loss of integrity of ligament	Loss of function and motion (unable to bear weight); unstable joint

   C. Immediate pain is noticed and swelling over the injured ligament often occurs within 1 hour of the injury

   D. Persons with previous ankle injuries have increased risk of reinjuring the same ankle

   E. Characteristics of severe ankle injuries
      1. Eversion injury
      2. Syndesmosis sprain: Mechanism of injury is excessive dorsiflexion and eversion of the ankle joint with internal rotation of the tibia (suspect this injury if swelling or ecchymosis occurs above the malleolus)
      3. Immediate diffuse swelling which may indicate bleeding
      4. Inability to bear weight immediately
      5. Sensation of a "pop", "snap", locking of joint, or kick into the heel
      6. On physical exam, patient often has a positive drawer sign and a positive squeeze test

IV. Diagnosis/Evaluation

   A. History
      1. Ask patient to precisely describe how the injury occurred
      2. Ask patient to describe the foot position at the time of injury
      3. Ask patient to point to the location of the maximum pain
      4. Determine whether the patient was able to bear weight after injury

5. Determine whether the patient had a sensation of a "pop," a "snap," or had any locking of the joint which may indicate a partial- or full-tendon rupture
6. Question when and where the swelling and ecchymosis were first noticed
7. Ascertain whether there is any associated pain in the leg, knee, or foot
8. Inquire about previous musculoskeletal injuries
9. Inquire about self-treatment

B. Physical Examination
1. Always compare injured side with unaffected side; examine most painful area last
2. Observe ankle, concentrating on the lateral and medial aspects of the foot and ankle, for swelling, ecchymosis, and deformity
3. Assess neurovascular status of foot; evaluate distal pulses (tibialis posterior and/or dorsalis pedis) and dermatomes for sensation
4. Palpation should be systematic (see Figure 17.1 of anatomical structures)
   a. Start with bony structures: Shaft of fibula, distal fibula over lateral malleolus, medial malleolus, base of the fifth metatarsal, all the tarsals, metatarsals, and phalanges
   b. In children, it is important to carefully palpate the growth plates to detect tenderness
   c. Next palpate the ligamentous structures:
      (1) Anterior tibiofibular ligament
      (2) Anterior talofibular ligament
      (3) Calcaneofibular ligament
   d. Palpate tendons including the Achilles, the peroneal tendons, and the anterior tibial tendon

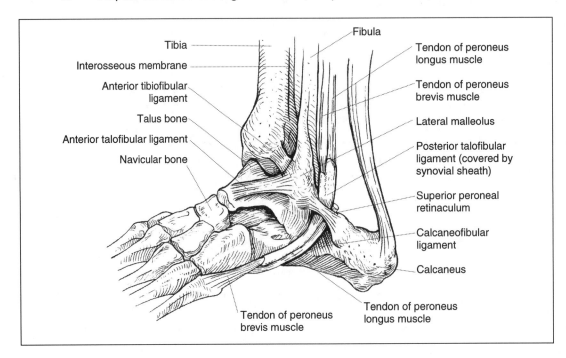

Figure 17.1. Anatomical Structures of the Ankle.

5. Perform active range of motion and assess the limits of unassisted movement
6. Perform passive range of motion and assess the limits of manipulation by the examiner without effort of the patient
7. Perform resisted range of motion to determine muscular strength by measuring the patient's active movement against resistance
8. Perform three special tests:
   a. Anterior drawer test is used to assess the anterior talofibular and other ligaments of the lateral side of the ankle (see Figure 17.2)

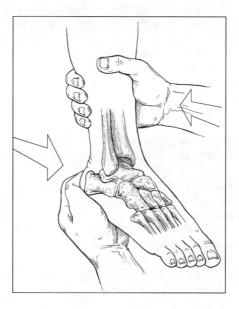

Figure 17.2. Anterior Drawer Sign.

Examiner grasps distal tibia with one hand and heel with other hand; patient's foot is held firmly while backward force is applied to tibia; Positive test is graded 1+ for slight movement, 2+ for moderate movement, and 3+ for marked movement

      b.   Talar tilt test is used to assess stability of the calcaneofibular ligament (see Figure 17.3)

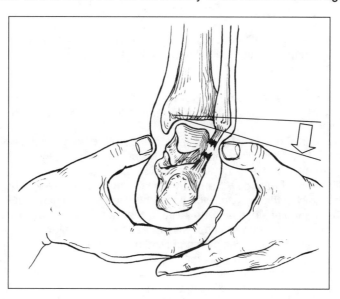

Figure 17.3. Talar Tilt Test.

Grasping the distal tibia and heel with other hand, apply gentle inversion force to affected ankle; ligaments are probably damaged if the talar tilt around the ankle is 5-10° greater around injured than around uninjured ankle

      c.   Squeeze test should be done if medial or severe lateral injury has taken place
          (1)   Examiner's hands are placed 6 inches inferior to the knee with thumbs on the fibula and fingers on the medial tibia
          (2)   Leg is squeezed as if to bring fibula and tibia together
          (3)   Pain with this test denotes syndesmotic injury which is a severe injury
    9.   Assess joints above and below injury

C.   Differential Diagnosis
    1.   Strains: Injuries to the tendons and muscles; usually have gradual onset of pain due to overuse rather than trauma
    2.   Tendonitis presents with pain with active stretching and plantar flexion against resistance; pain is worse with hill running (see section LOWER EXTREMITY PAIN)

3. Tendon ruptures such as Achilles have a sudden onset of shooting pain in calf, followed by weakness in leg and inability to walk on toes (see section LOWER EXTREMITY PAIN)
4. Fractures often occur in persons who engage in high velocity, high impact sports
   a. Four basic injury mechanisms for fractures: Lateral displacement of talus (most common), medial displacement of talus, axial compression of talus, and repetitive microtrauma
   b. Refer to orthopedist
5. Gout, arthritis, or infection may present with a painful ankle, but examination findings and history are inconsistent with trauma

D. Diagnostic Tests
   1. When to order x-rays is controversial; some authorities suggest x-rays should be routinely ordered to rule out bony involvement whereas the recently-developed Ottawa rules recommend the following:
      a. Order ankle series if there is pain near the malleoli and either inability to bear weight both immediately and in the emergency department, or bone tenderness at the posterior edge or tip of either malleolus
      b. Order foot x-ray series if there is pain in the midfoot and either inability to bear weight both immediately and in emergency department, or bone tenderness at the navicular or the base of the fifth metatarsal
   2. Consider ordering stress films when the ankle cannot be easily manipulated to test for stability or when the patient has chronically unstable ankles
   3. Consider computed tomography (CT) scan or magnetic resonance imaging (MRI) for the following: Ankle sprains that remain symptomatic for >6 weeks, injuries that involve crepitus or catching and locking, and suspected syndesmosis sprains (see III.E.2.)
   4. For children or adolescents with open growth plates, the chances of a growth plate fracture are higher and x-rays should be considered to rule out a Salter-Harris fracture

V. Plan/Management

A. Refer to orthopedist patient with Grade III sprains, injuries with neurovascular compromise, tendon rupture or subluxation, a wound that penetrates the joint, and injuries with mechanical "locking" of the joint, and injuries to the syndesmosis; consider orthopedist referral for all eversion injuries

B. In children, any tenderness or swelling over the growth plate should be treated as a Salter I fracture with splinting (or casting), elevation, crutches, and referral to an orthopedist

C. Early treatment (approximately first 48 hours) of less severe sprains focuses on regaining range of motion, early mobilization of joints, limiting soft-tissue effusion while protecting ankle against reinjury; follow the **PRICE** therapy (**P**rotection, **R**est, **I**ce, **C**ompression, **E**levation)
   1. Protected weight-bearing with an orthosis is permitted with weight bearing to tolerance as soon as possible following the injury; crutches can be used until painless-weight bearing is achieved
      a. Taping the ankle, a lace-up splint, a thermoplastic ankle stirrup splint, a functional walking orthosis, or a short-leg cast will protect ankle and allow mobility
      b. For severe injuries initial immobilization is required and a simple plaster posterior splint or plastic ankle-foot orthosis may facilitate early rehabilitation and prevent the ankle from stiffening in a plantar flexed, slightly inverted position; air-filled or gel-filled ankle braces that restrict flexion-dorsiflexion may also help
      c. Generally, protected range of motion is superior to rigid immobilization with a cast
   2. Apply ice to injury as many times as possible a day for 20 minutes for the first 48 hours or until edema and inflammation have stabilized
   3. Compression can be accomplished by using an Ace wrap to hold ice in place and after ice application to prevent swelling (when wrapping ankle, make sure to include heel)
   4. Elevate ankle above the level of heart
   5. For pain, prescribe a nonsteroidal anti-inflammatory agent (NSAID) such as ibuprofen (Motrin) 400 mg every 4-6 hours prn or a COX-2 selective nonsteroidal anti-inflammatory drug (NSAID) such as celecoxib (Celebrex) 100 mg BID or rofecoxib (Vioxx) 25 mg QD if the patient has a history of gastrointestinal, liver, or kidney problems; in children, use ibuprofen (Motrin) caplets, chewables, or drops; ≥6 months prescribe 10 mg/kg every 6-8 hours; maximum 40 mg/kg/day

D. Functional rehabilitation is critical regardless of grade of injury (consider referral to physical therapist)
1. The exact time to begin exercising varies with the severity of the sprain; generally the following exercises can be started after first 48 hours if the patient's pain and swelling are resolving normally
    a. Toe alphabet in which entire foot and ankle trace letters of alphabet in air
    b. Isometrics in which side of injured foot/ankle is placed against an immovable object and pressed
    c. Toe raising in which patient raises up and down on toes while holding onto object to maintain balance
2. Approximately 2 weeks post-injury begin the following:
    a. Resistive exercises with surgical or bicycle tubing (see Figure 17.4)
    b. Remind patient that once an injury has occurred, the joint will never be as strong which will increase likelihood of reinjury unless strengthening exercises are continued

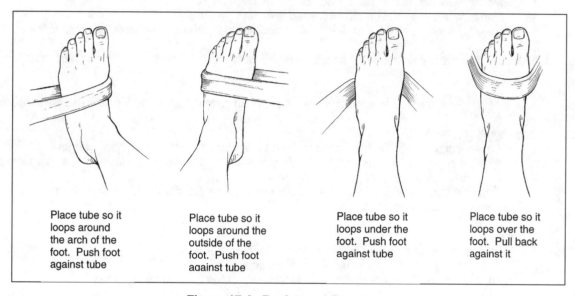

Place tube so it loops around the arch of the foot. Push foot against tube

Place tube so it loops around the outside of the foot. Push foot against tube

Place tube so it loops under the foot. Push foot against tube

Place tube so it loops over the foot. Pull back against it

Figure 17.4. Resistance Exercises

3. Last phase of functional rehabilitation
    a. When the patient achieves full weight-bearing without pain, proprioceptive training should be started for the recovery of balance and postural control (i.e., walk on normal or in heel-to-toe fashion over various surfaces and progress from hard, flat floor to uneven surfaces)
    b. There should be full resolution of swelling, normal joint motion, strength, and proprioception before the patient begins running; start with 50% walking and 50% jogging and gradually increase percentage of jogging until pain is no longer present

E. In children, a general rule for return to sports is 1 month for grade I sprains, 2 months for grade II sprains, and up to 3 months for grade III sprains

F. In all phases of recovery and rehabilitation, protect the ankle from further injuries by taping ankle or using high-top lace-up shoes or a combination of proper shoes with a lace-up brace underneath

G. Follow Up
1. Examine ankle in 7-10 days or sooner if pain and swelling do not decrease
2. If there is little improvement or the condition has worsened in 2-3 weeks, consider referral to orthopedist or the ordering of additional films or bone scans

COMMON ORTHOPEDIC DEFORMITIES IN CHILDHOOD

I.   Definition: Orthopedic problems usually not related to trauma or other musculoskeletal disease

II.   Pathogenesis

    A.   Developmental dysplasia of hip (DDH) (formerly known as congenital dislocation of the hip)
        1.   Condition in which the femoral head has an abnormal relationship to the acetabulum; includes hips that are unstable, subluxated, dislocated and/or have malformed acetabula
        2.   Mechanical factors such as breech birth may have a role
        3.   Hormonal factors may create increased laxity of ligaments
        4.   Heredity seems to be a factor as 20% of affected children have positive family histories

    B.   Increased femoral anteversion results when the femur is medially rotated on its long axis at birth and is usually idiopathic

    C.   Internal tibial torsion is due to a medially rotated tibia on its long axis at birth and is usually idiopathic

    D.   Pes planus (flat feet)
        1.   Longitudinal arch of the foot appears flat on the floor when child is bearing weight
        2.   Flexible or pseudo flat feet are familial in origin and due to increased laxity of the ligaments and joint capsules of the plantar aspect of the foot
        3.   Rigid flat feet are uncommon and considered a congenital deformity caused by a fibrous or bony connection between various bones

    E.   Metatarsus adductus
        1.   Results when the forefoot is turned in or adducted
        2.   Hypothesized to be caused by *in utero* molding
        3.   Rigidity and tightness of muscles and ligaments of forefoot cause in-toeing

    F.   Talipes equinovarus (type of club foot) is characteristic of cerebral palsy, spina bifida, or muscular disease, but the majority of children with this condition are healthy and the etiology may have a genetic basis or be idiopathic

    G.   Genu varum (bowlegs)
        1.   Angular variation which involves symmetrical bowing of the tibia and femur
        2.   Physiologic genu varum is often familial and a normal developmental variation
        3.   Pathologic genu varum is rare and due to rickets, dwarfing conditions, epiphyseal injury, dyschondroplasia, osteogenesis imperfecta, or Blount's disease

    H.   Genu valgum (knock-knees)
        1.   Angular variation in which there is deviation of the axis of the thighs and calves
        2.   Frequently has a positive family history
        3.   Often a normal developmental variation
        4.   Extreme or unilateral genu valgum may be associated with underlying, generalized bone disease

III. Clinical Presentation

    A.   Developmental dysplasia of the hip (DDH) (see table below for signs by ages)
        1.   May occur *in utero*, perinatally, or during infancy
        2.   Hip is at greatest risk for dislocation during 4 time periods: The 12th gestational week, the 18th gestational week, the final 4 weeks of gestation, and the postnatal period
        3.   Higher incidence in breech deliveries, infants with oligohydramnios, first born children, and females; left side is affected in 60% of cases (right 20%, bilateral 20%); less prevalent in African Americans
        4.   In newborns, there is ligamentous laxity resulting in hip instability without fixed deformity
        5.   About 60% of unstable hips in newborns spontaneously become normal within the first 2-4 weeks
        6.   In some children as they age, dislocation becomes more fixed and pathologic changes occur such as flattening of femoral head, excessive femoral anteversion, and valgus neck-shaft angle; these changes result in limitation of movements

7. In the ambulating child, the pelvis may tilt with weight-bearing and gait may be asymmetrical
8. The earlier the dislocated hip is detected, the more effective the treatment
9. Long-term complications include flexion contractures, osteoarthritis, pain, abnormal gait, and decreased agility; most serious complication is vascular necrosis of the hip

SIGNS OF DEVELOPMENTAL DYSPLASIA OF HIP BY AGES		
Birth to 8-12 weeks	**Older Infant**	**Walking Child**
Barlow's maneuver causes hip to dislocate (see Figure 17.5. in physical examination)	Limited abduction of hip	Curvature of spine (scoliosis)
	Unequal leg lengths	Leg length discrepancy
Ortolani's maneuver reduces the joint and a clunk is felt (see Figure 17.5.)	Unequal knee heights when supine and knees are flexed (Galeazzi sign)	Occasional asymmetric intoeing or outtoeing
	Asymmetry of thigh folds	

B. Increased femoral anteversion
   1. Often familial and occurs more frequently in females
   2. Typically presents between 3-10 years of age
   3. "Kissing knees," toeing in, and a clumsy gait are characteristic; child often sits in "W" position
   4. Patella and feet are rotated inwardly; internal rotation of hip is increased; usually external rotation of the hip in flexion is normal
   5. Usually is bilateral and symmetrical
   6. In most children, the condition significantly improves or resolves by age 7-8 years
   7. In late childhood and early adolescence, this condition can lead to abnormalities above the knee

C. Internal tibial torsion (ITT)
   1. Is the most common cause of in-toeing between the ages of 1 and 3 years
   2. Often has a familial tendency
   3. More common in precocious walkers and dark-skinned races
   4. Often is accompanied by metatarsus adductus
   5. May be associated with increased running speed; study found that sprinters were more internally rotated than a control group
   6. Typically, the majority of affected children have spontaneous improvement by age 7

D. Pes planus
   1. Feet have depression of the longitudinal arch; rigid flat foot may be associated with pathological conditions whereas flexible flat foot is common and not associated with problems
   2. Plantar fat pad is normal until ages of 4-6; therefore, diagnosis is difficult before age 6
   3. With flexible flat feet, the heel cord is flexible and the longitudinal arch is depressed during weight-bearing but reconstituted when non-weight-bearing
   4. Patients may have pain, particularly in the calcaneus, on the plantar surface, or on the lateral subtalar joint or the sinus tarsi
   5. A history of difficulties during birth, delay in motor development, or recent onset of flat feet may suggest a neuromuscular problem
   6. Fractures and tendon ruptures can result in flat foot

E. Metatarsus adductus
   1. Occurs at birth to 6 months
   2. Feet turn inward when child is both weight-bearing and non-weight-bearing
   3. Approximately 85% of the cases of metatarsus adductus spontaneously correct
   4. Usually the more flexible the foot, the more rapidly resolution takes place
   5. Differential diagnosis
      a. Talipes equinovarus; (see III.F.)
      b. Congenital metatarsus varus involves uncorrectable turning in of forefoot; heel is positioned outward and there is limitation of dorsiflexion of the ankle
   6. Often associated with torticollis and developmental dysplasia of hip

F. Talipes equinovarus: Forefoot is rigidly fixed and ankle cannot be dorsiflexed
  1. Strong family history is usually present
  2. Child may have unilateral or bilateral involvement
  3. If unilateral, foot is usually smaller and shorter than uninvolved foot
  4. Three cardinal findings:
     a. Toes point inward (metatarsal adduction and stiffness)
     b. Hindfoot and ankle are plantar flexed
     c. Heels roll inward (varus)
  5. Ranges from mild and easily correctable to a severe and difficult-to-treat form
  6. Children with talipes equinovarus have a higher incidence of DDH and neck anomalies such as torticollis as well as other system abnormalities

G. Genu varum (bowlegs)
  1. Genu varum up to 20° is normal in children until age of 18 months
  2. By 24-35 months of age there should be spontaneous resolution and the knees should touch when the child is positioned supine; as growth occurs genu varum changes to genu valgum until age 7-9 years when there is normal straightening as child ages
  3. If bowing is unilateral or extreme consider pathologic genu varum (see II.G.)

H. Genu valgum (knock-knees)
  1. Considered normal from ages 2-6 years; spontaneous resolution with growth is expected
  2. Occurs with pronation of feet and ligamentous relaxation; more marked in overweight children
  3. If genu valgum is present before age 2 years, developmental disorders such as metaphyseal dysplasia may be present

IV. Diagnosis/Evaluation

A. History
  1. Specifically ask parents to discuss their concerns and to describe their child's musculoskeletal problem
  2. If child is walking, inquire about gait and falling
  3. Determine when child reached developmental milestones
  4. Inquire about birth history, family history, nutritional problems, and incidents of trauma

B. Physical Examination
  1. Measure height; short stature may indicate metabolic growth disturbance which is sometimes present with genu varum
  2. Inspect skin; café-au-lait spots may indicate neurofibromatosis
  3. Observe for alignment of bones, deformities, and muscle development in supine, prone, and standing positions
  4. Observe gait if child is walking; scissor gait is suggestive of cerebral palsy; waddling with a wide stance suggests bilateral hip dysplasia
  5. Observe for unequal leg length
  6. Observe the shape of the bones such as lateral bowing of tibia in genu varum
  7. Perform passive and active range of motion, noting limitations in movement
  8. Assess motor strength
  9. Perform special tests for each suspected problem
     a. Developmental hip dysplasia: Perform Barlow's and Ortolani's tests (see Figure 17.5)
        (1) Newborn examination
           (a) Do not perform forceful and repeated examinations as they can break the seal between the labrum and the femoral head
           (b) A clunk must be felt to have positive signs; high-pitched clicks are common and inconsequential
           (c) If a positive Ortolani's or Barlow's sign is found, refer the infant to an orthopedist
           (d) If the physical examination at birth has equivocal findings (soft click, mild asymmetry, but neither a positive Ortolani's nor a positive Barlow's sign), - OR - there are risk factors (female gender, positive family history, breech birth) then a follow-up hip examination at 2 weeks by the primary care clinician is recommended; most clicks resolve by 2 weeks and do not lead to later hip dysplasia

(2) Examination at 2 weeks
    (a) If Ortolani's or Barlow's signs are positive, refer to orthopedist
    (b) If Ortolani's or Barlow's signs are absent, but physical findings are suspicious - **OR** - risk factors are present, consider referral to orthopedist or request ultrasonography at age 3-4 weeks (also see diagnostic testing)
    (c) If results of physical examination are negative at 2 weeks, follow-up is recommended at scheduled well-child periodic examinations

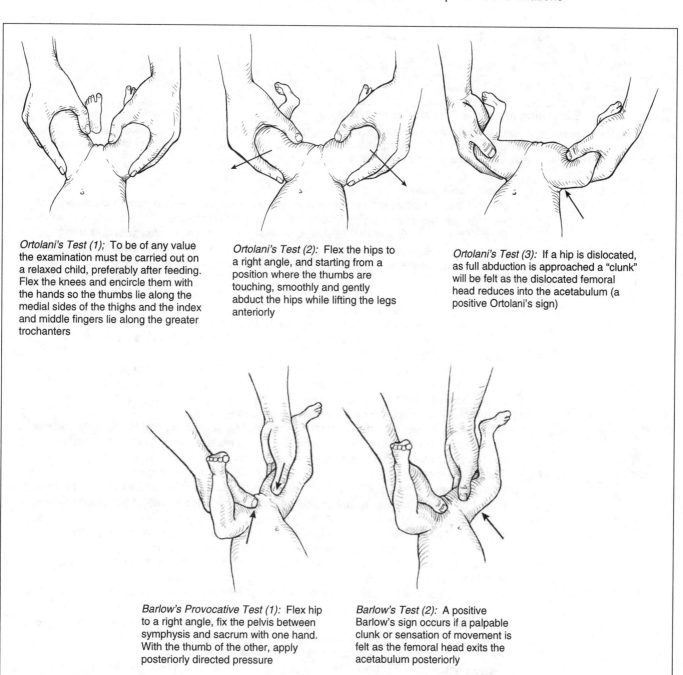

Ortolani's Test (1); To be of any value the examination must be carried out on a relaxed child, preferably after feeding. Flex the knees and encircle them with the hands so the thumbs lie along the medial sides of the thighs and the index and middle fingers lie along the greater trochanters

Ortolani's Test (2): Flex the hips to a right angle, and starting from a position where the thumbs are touching, smoothly and gently abduct the hips while lifting the legs anteriorly

Ortolani's Test (3): If a hip is dislocated, as full abduction is approached a "clunk" will be felt as the dislocated femoral head reduces into the acetabulum (a positive Ortolani's sign)

Barlow's Provocative Test (1): Flex hip to a right angle, fix the pelvis between symphysis and sacrum with one hand. With the thumb of the other, apply posteriorly directed pressure

Barlow's Test (2): A positive Barlow's sign occurs if a palpable clunk or sensation of movement is felt as the femoral head exits the acetabulum posteriorly

Figure 17.5. Ortolani's Test and Barlow's Test.

b.   Increased femoral anteversion (see Figure 17.6)

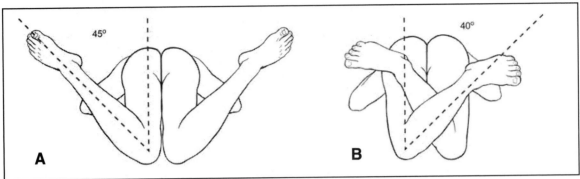

Figure 17.6. Evaluating Increased Femoral Anteversion.

With child lying prone and knees flexed to 90° measure ability to internally (A) and externally (B) rotate femur (make sure pelvis is level); in children with no problem, the external and internal measurements are similar; with increased femoral anteversion, internal rotation is increased (up to 90°) and external rotation is decreased (to as little as 20-30°)

c.   Internal tibial torsion
(1)   Observe legs and feet while child walks; knee-caps will be positioned straight ahead or slightly outward with one or both feet pointing inward
(2)   Observe legs and feet with patient sitting on examining table with thighs together and both knees bent over edge of table; feet will point inward toward each other and medial malleolus will be posterior to the lateral malleolus
d.   Pes planus
(1)   Assess heel cord flexibility by passively dorsiflexing the ankle with the knee in extension and the foot inverted
(2)   Assess eversion and inversion of foot and abduction and adduction of the forefoot
(3)   Heel cord and foot should be flexible; inflexibility suggests rigid flat feet
e.   Metatarsus adductus
(1)   Examiner should grasp heel with nondominant hand and gently push the inward-turning forefoot outward with the dominant hand, attempting to realign the foot in normal position; degree to which forefoot is passively correctable will allow classification as flexible, partially correctable, or rigid
(2)   Another way to determine foot flexibility is by scratching first the outside and then the inside of the lower border of the foot. With metatarsus adductus the foot will flex, but with metatarsus varus or talipes equinovarus the foot will straighten
f.   Talipes equinovarus
(1)   Grasp the foot by the heel with sole lying in examiner's hand and dorsiflex (inflexible cords are present if dorsiflexion cannot be carried to about 20-30° beyond a right angle)
(2)   Carefully ascertain that the child with clubfoot does not have a generalized neuromuscular disorder such as spina bifida or cerebral palsy
g.   Genu varum (see Figure 17.7): Bowing may also occur with internal tibia torsion; be certain that foot is pointing forward during the following measurements:
(1)   Position child supine with medial malleoli together and measure the distance between the knees (intercondylar distance)
(2)   Normally, by 24-36 months the knees should be touching or have a only a small space between the medial surfaces of the knees
(3)   Assess the child with genu varum every 4 months
h.   Genu valgum (see Figure 17.7)
(1)   Position child supine with knees touching and measure distance between the medial malleoli
(2)   Genu valgum in children over age 6 should be assessed every 6 months

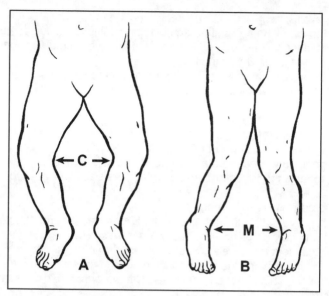

Figure 17.7. Measurement of Genu Varum and Genu Valgum.

For genu varum (bowing) (A) the intercondylar distance (C) is measured with ankles touching. In genu valgum (knock-knees) (B) the intermalleolar distance (M) is measured with the knees together. A measurement of more than 5 to 6 inches suggests a severe condition requiring further evaluation

C. Differential Diagnosis: See disorders under Pathogenesis

D. Diagnostic Tests
1. **Developmental dysplasia of hip**
   a. Ultrasonography is most effective if the infant is younger than 4-6 months
   b. Radiography is most effective if the infant is older than 4-6 months
   c. Between 4-6 months of age, ultrasonography and radiography are equally effective
   d. Specific guidelines for ordering tests:
      (1) Order ultrasonography at 3-4 weeks if Ortolani's or Barlow's signs are absent, but physical findings are suspicious; consider ultrasonography if risk factors are present
      (2) In girls with a positive family history of DDH, order ultrasonography at 6 weeks of age or a radiograph of the pelvis and hips at 4 months
      (3) In girls with breech presentation, order ultrasonography at 6 weeks of age or a radiograph of the pelvis and hips at 4 months
      (4) Consider ultrasonography at 6 weeks of age or a radiograph of the pelvis and hips at 4 months for ALL children born breech, not just girls
      (5) Consider ultrasonography or radiograph if parental concerns suggest DDH
2. Computed tomogram is best for quantifying **femoral anteversion**, but is usually not needed
3. X-rays can be ordered to measure the degree of **tibial torsion**, but usually are not needed
4. For children with **talipes equinovarus**, clinical findings are more reliable than any imaging; foot radiographs can be used at baseline and then to monitor improvement, but radiographs may not be interpretable until 2-3 months of age
5. Order x-rays if **genu varum** or **genu valgum** is extreme or unilateral to rule out bone disease and other systemic conditions; also order x-rays if genu valgum is present in any child less than 2 years of age to rule out a developmental disorder

V. Plan/Management

A. Early detection of developmental dysplasia of hip results in more effective treatment
1. Refer to orthopedist all children with positive physical examinations or imaging findings; consider referral if risk factors are present, if physical findings raise suspicion, or if parental concerns suggest DDH
2. Infants <6 months are treated with a Pavlik harness
3. Infants 6-18 months usually need traction and closed reduction with cast immobilization
4. Older children usually need surgical reduction; beyond 4 years of age in bilateral cases and 8 years in unilateral cases, reduction is usually not attempted

B. Increased femoral anteversion
1. Teach child to avoid the prone, in-toed sleeping position and the "reverse tailor" sitting position; instruct to sit in the tailor, modified lotus, or Indian-style sitting position
2. Re-evaluate child every 6-12 months
3. Refer to orthopedist if there is no improvement in in-toeing on subsequent visits, if in-toeing causes child problems, or if in-toeing persists beyond 7 years of age (surgery is rarely indicated)

C. Internal tibial torsion
1. Teach child to avoid the prone, intoed sleeping position and the "reverse tailor" sitting position (limited research data to support this practice)
2. If parents are unduly concerned or child trips and falls frequently, passive stretching exercises (externally rotating the foot at the ankle), corrective shoes, or application of torque heels may be beneficial
3. Re-evaluate child every 4-12 months
4. Children who have a 20° internal rotation that persists past age 15 months should be referred to orthopedist and may be given braces or corrective shoes
5. Usually no treatment is needed until child is older than 36 months; although controversial, a Denis-Brown bar which positions the feet and lower legs in outward-turning position during night and nap time may be used; this bar should not used without orthopedic consultation because it may cause abnormal stress on the hip joint
6. Surgical intervention is sometimes recommended by age 7 if condition has not resolved

D. Pes planus
1. Refer to orthopedist if no arch is visible when the child is non-weight-bearing, if there is heel cord tightness or foot rigidity, or if the child has marked foot or ankle pain
2. No treatment is needed for children who are asymptomatic; shoe modifications may be beneficial for children who experience rapid shoe wear because of excessive pronation or who experience discomfort
3. Child and parents should be told that shoe modifications will not change the foot structure and are used for comfort

E. Metatarsus adductus
1. For flexible metatarsus adductus, teach parents to do passive exercises several times a day to bring forefoot into a straight position
   a. Heel should be held firmly in palm while opposite hand pushes forefoot toward its outer side
   b. Stretch should be held for count of 3 seconds and repeated ten times
   c. Perform exercises 4 times a day
   d. Care should be taken to not twist forefoot on the heel as this may result in stretching of the longitudinal arch
2. If condition persists beyond 6 weeks with stretching, refer to orthopedist
3. Fixed metatarsus adductus should be referred to orthopedist
4. Ineffective strategies: Reverse shoes, bars, or shoe wedges

F. Talipes equinovarus: Refer immediately to orthopedist; often treated with abductor shoes, serial casting, and surgery

G. Genu varum: Refer to orthopedist if condition persists past 2 years of age, if bowing is increasing rather than decreasing, if bowing is severe (>5-6 inches between knees or intercondylar distance), or if there is bowing of only one leg

H. Genu valgum: Refer to orthopedist if condition presents before 2 years, persists beyond 8 years of age, or if condition is severe or unilateral

I. Follow up is variable depending on condition

ELBOW PAIN

I.   Definition: Chronic or recurrent pain or discomfort of the elbow caused by selected common problems

II. Pathogenesis (see Figure 17.8. of anatomical structures of the elbow)

   A.   Lateral epicondylitis or "tennis elbow"
      1.   Inflammation of the common tendinous origin of the extensor muscles of the forearm on the humeral lateral epicondyle
      2.   Exact mechanism of injury is uncertain but activities that combine excessive pronation and supination of the forearm with an extended wrist are probably responsible

   B.   Medial epicondylitis or "golfer's elbow"
      1.   Inflammation of the common forearm flexor origin at the humeral medial epicondyle
      2.   Occurs in persons performing repetitive pronation activities

   C.   Subluxation of the proximal radial head or "nursemaid's elbow"
      1.   Sudden traction on the outstretched arm pulls the radius distally causing it to slip partially through the annular ligament and tearing it in the process
      2.   When traction is released, the radial head recoils, trapping the proximal portion of the ligament between it and the capitellum

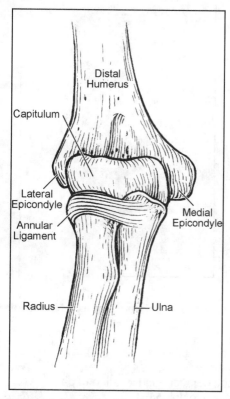

Figure 17.8. Anatomical Structures of the Elbow

III. Clinical Presentation

   A.   Lateral epicondylitis is one of the most common syndromes affecting the upper extremities
      1.   Commonly occurs in patients who frequently play tennis, badminton, or bowl
      2.   Also occurs in persons who engage in occupations that require using a wrench or screwdriver repetitively
      3.   The commonality among these activities is use of a strong grasp during wrist extension
      4.   Onset of symptoms is usually gradual with the patient complaining of tenderness on the lateral aspect of the elbow; swelling may occasionally be present

B. Medial epicondylitis is similar in presentation to "tennis elbow" described above but occurs less commonly
    1. Occurs in golfers, but more commonly associated with certain manual activities such as the frequent carrying of objects with elbows flexed; in children, condition occurs in baseball and softball pitchers
    2. Clinical presentation is similar to that of lateral epicondylitis except that the pain is located in the area of the medial, rather than the lateral epicondyle
    3. Inflammation can involve the ulnar nerve and compression of the nerve may cause numbness in the little and ring fingers on the affected side
    4. In children, medial epicondylitis may cause the growth plate that attaches the medial epicondyle to the body of the humerus to break down (i.e., olecranon apophysitis)

C. Nursemaid's elbow is the most common elbow injury in childhood, occurring most commonly in children between the ages of 1 and 4 years
    1. Typical history involves an adult suddenly and vigorously pulling the child by the arm or of the child being swung by the arms (see Figure 17.9. for mechanism of injury)
    2. Pain in the involved arm may be immediately present causing the child to cry; the pain quickly subsides, but the child is unable to use the arm, which is held close to the body with the elbow flexed and the forearm pronated
    3. The child resists attempts to supinate or rotate the forearm and mild limitation of elbow flexion and extension may also be present
    4. Usually, there is no bony tenderness or evidence of swelling of the affected elbow

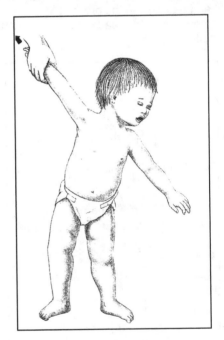

Figure 17.9. Mechanism of Injury: Nursemaid's Elbow.

IV. Diagnosis/Evaluation

A. History
    1. Inquire about onset, duration, and location of pain
    2. Determine mechanism of injury
    3. Determine what activities exacerbate the pain
    4. Determine if associated symptoms of swelling, numbness and tingling of hand/fingers, or loss of strength in arm or hand are present
    5. Inquire about participation in activities, either occupational or recreational, that require the following:
        a. Strong grasp during wrist extension (if lateral epicondylitis is suspected)
        b. Repetitive pronation of the arm or the carrying of heavy objects with elbows flexed (if medial epicondylitis is suspected)

6. If nursemaid's elbow is suspected (and to rule out an infectious disease), ask if there is a history of fever, recent illness, or prior joint pain
7. Inquire about what makes the pain better or worse
8. Determine what treatments (either by the patient or another clinician) have been tried and their results
9. Ask about past medical history and medication history

B. Physical Examination
   1. If lateral epicondylitis is suspected, examine the elbow to determine the following
      a. Assess for tenderness over the lateral epicondyle or over the radiohumeral joint
      b. Assess range of motion (flexion and extension should be normal although extension may cause minimal pain)
      c. Evaluate motor function of the hand by asking patient to abduct the thumb, index, and little fingers against resistance
      d. Evaluate sensation at the dorsal web space between thumb and index finger (radial nerve), the tip of the long finger (median nerve), and the tip of the little finger (ulnar nerve)
      e. Have the patient perform supination (palms up) and pronation (palms down) against resistance
      f. To reproduce the patient's symptoms, perform the maneuver in Figure 17.10.; sharp, localized tenderness in area of palpation or just distal is diagnostic of tennis elbow

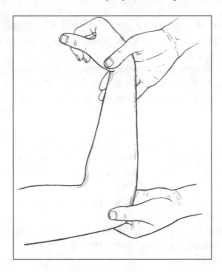

Figure 17.10. Palpation of the Lateral Epicondyle with the Thumb

   2. If medial epicondylitis is suspected, examine the elbow to determine the following:
      a. Assess for point tenderness over the medial epicondyle
      b. Assess range of motion (flexion and extension should be normal although extension may cause minimal pain)
      c. Evaluate motor function of the hand by asking patient to abduct the thumb, index, and little fingers against resistance
      d. Evaluate sensation at the dorsal web space between thumb and index finger (radial nerve), the tip of the long finger (median nerve), and the tip of the little finger (ulnar nerve)
      e. Palpate the medial epicondyle (see Figure 17.11) to determine degree of tenderness
      f. Valgus stress applied to the elbow may reproduce pain

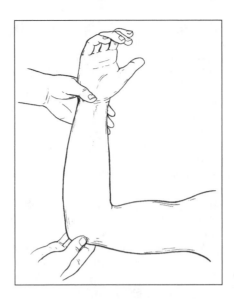

Figure 17.11. Palpation of the Medial Epicondyle with the Thumb

      3.   If nursemaid's elbow is suspected, examine the elbow to determine the following:
          a.   Look for swelling, deformity, or point tenderness of the affected elbow (none of these features should be present)
          b.   Examine the elbow joint for warmth and/or erythema (should be absent)
          c.   Evaluate the fingers for neurovascular compromise (rare)
          d.   Compare the affected and uninjured arms

  C.   Differential Diagnosis
      1.   Differential diagnosis for lateral and medial epicondylitis in children and adolescents:
          a.   Panner's disease (lateral compression injury of the throwing elbow in young baseball pitchers, often resulting in osteochondrosis of the capitellum)
          b.   Osteochondritis dissecans (results from chronic repetitive compression forces that may lead to avascular necrosis and osteochondral fragments that can displace and cause a locked elbow and pain)
      2.   Differential diagnosis for nursemaid's elbow includes fracture, infection, congenital radial head dislocation, arthritis (rare), or neoplasm (rare)

  D.   Diagnostic Tests
      1.   If lateral epicondylitis is suspected, no tests are indicated when the history and physical examination are consistent with the suspected diagnosis; order x-rays if atypical findings are noted on history or physical examination
      2.   If medial epicondylitis is suspected in children, order plain x-rays with oblique views of both the injured and uninjured elbow to rule out Panner's disease, osteochondritis dissecans, and olecranon apophysitis
      3.   If nursemaid's elbow is suspected, diagnosis can usually be made on the basis of clinical findings; reserve x-rays for unusual cases or those with uncertain histories

V.   Plan/Management

  A.   Lateral epicondylitis
      1.   Focus is on reduction of the inflammation, strengthening the involved muscle, and avoidance of further injury
      2.   Rest (immobilization in a sling for several days), ice, and use of rapidly acting NSAIDs (such as naproxen 375 mg BID or ibuprofen 600 mg TID or in children ≥6 months, ibuprofen [Motrin] 10 mg/kg every 6-8 hours) are helpful in reducing the inflammation
      3.   Referral to physical therapy can reduce symptoms and strengthen the involved muscle groups in the forearm and wrist through an appropriate exercise program, possibly preventing recurrences
      4.   Avoidance of the activity that caused the problem for several weeks or months is necessary
      5.   Use of an elbow strap (available at sporting goods stores) in the area of the muscle mass of the proximal portion of the forearm can be helpful, but is usually of limited value
      6.   Physiotherapy that includes massage, ultrasound therapy, and exercises may be helpful
      7.   Patients who fail to respond to conservative therapy should be referred to a specialist for management; local steroid injections may eventually be needed

B. Medial epicondylitis
1. Treatment is the same as described under V.A.
2. If ulnar nerve involvement is suspected based on history and physical examination, prompt orthopedic referral is indicated

C. Nursemaid's elbow
1. Apply pressure over the proximal radial head, and at the same time, rapidly supinate the child's forearm with the elbow in a flexed position (see Figure 17.12 for reduction maneuver); some experts suggest that the elbow should be extended maximally and then fully flexed while maintaining supination
2. Often, a click can be felt as the annular ligament is freed from the joint
3. Symptoms resolve within 30 minutes, and immobilization after reduction is usually not required
4. Acetaminophen may be prescribed for the aching discomfort in the arm that may persist for several hours after the reduction
5. Parents should be cautioned to avoid pulling on the child's arms as there is a significant risk of recurrence
6. Refer to orthopedist cases that do not reduce within 2-3 attempts, cases with abnormal findings, or cases that involve recurrent dislocations (>2-3 recurrences)

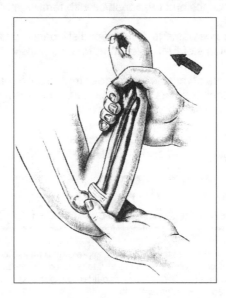

Figure 17.12. Nursemaid's Elbow: Reduction Maneuver Technique.

D. Follow Up
1. For lateral and medial epicondylitis, schedule return visit within one month to determine treatment effectiveness and to assess whether referral to a specialist is warranted
2. In nursemaid's elbow, no follow up is necessary unless the child fails to resume normal activities involving use of the arm in 1-2 days

FIBROMYALGIA

I. Definition: Complex syndrome involving fatigue and widespread, nonarticular musculoskeletal pain

II. Pathogenesis

A. Etiology is unknown

B. The following mechanisms have been hypothesized to trigger fibromyalgia (FMS): Dysregulation of the autonomic and neuroendocrine system, metabolic processes, immunological abnormalities, sleep disturbances, stress and trauma from accidents or surgery, and infection due to Epstein Barr virus, cytomegalovirus, human herpesvirus 6, enteroviruses, or *B. burgdorferi*

III.   Clinical presentation

    A.   Age of onset is typically between 20-40 years; prevalence increases with age but can occur in childhood

    B.   Females are affected 8-10 times more than men

    C.   Most common symptoms are diffuse musculoskeletal pain, sleep disturbance, and persistent fatigue

    D.   Other symptoms include swelling of hands and feet, morning stiffness, headaches, paresthesias, sensitivity to cold and/or hot, dyspnea, chest pain, night sweats, visual problems, dizziness, painful menses, gastrointestinal complaints, memory impairment, anxiety, and depression

    E.   Patients may have associated conditions or comorbidities such as mitral valve prolapse, episodic hypoglycemia, Raynaud's disease, irritable bowel syndrome, myofascial pain syndrome, migraine headaches, depression, and chronic fatigue

    F.   Symptoms can be severe and patients may become functionally disabled

    G.   Because patients have chronic, multiple, vague complaints and no outward signs, they are often misdiagnosed as hypochondriacs and relationships with family and friends may deteriorate

    H.   Patients often have disturbance of stage 4 of sleep; disturbance of this stage for 2-3 consecutive nights can produce physical symptoms of FMS even in normal controls

    I.   Tender points (localized areas of muscle tenderness that result in pain when pressure is applied) are essential to the diagnosis; trigger points (pain is elicited at initial site of palpation as well as in a linear or circumferential pattern surrounding the site or at a distant site) are also common

    J.   The American College of Rheumatology (ACR) established clinical criteria for diagnosing FMS (see table on ACR CRITERIA and Figure 17.13. on TENDER POINT SITES)

THE AMERICAN COLLEGE OF RHEUMATOLOGY
1990 CRITERIA FOR CLASSIFICATION OF FIBROMYALGIA

*1.   History of widespread pain

Definition. Pain is considered widespread when all of the following are present: pain in the left side of the body, pain in the right side of the body, pain above the waist, and pain below the waist. In addition, axial skeletal pain (cervical spine or anterior chest or thoracic spine or low back) must be present. In this definition, shoulder and buttocks pain are considered as pain for each involved side. "Low back" pain is considered lower segment pain.

2.   *Definition.* Pain, on digital palpation, must be present in at least 11 of the following 18 tender point sites:
- Occiput: Bilateral, at the suboccipital muscle insertions
- Low cervical: Bilateral, at the anterior aspects of the intertransverse spaces at C5-C7
- Trapezius: Bilateral, at the midpoint of the upper border
- Supraspinatus: Bilateral, at origins, above the scapula spine near the medial border
- Second rib: Bilateral, at the second costochondral junctions, just lateral to the junctions on upper surfaces
- Lateral epicondyle: Bilateral, 2 cm distal to the epicondyles
- Gluteal: Bilateral, in upper outer quadrants of buttocks in anterior fold of muscle
- Greater trochanter: Bilateral, posterior to the trochanteric prominence
- Knee: Bilateral, at the medial fat pad proximal to the joint line

Note: For a tender point to be considered "positive" the subject must state that the palpation was painful

*For classification purposes, patients must satisfy both criteria. Widespread pain must have been present for at least 3 months

Source: Wolfe, F., Smythe, H.A., Yunus, M.B., Bennett, R.M., Bombadier, C., Goldenberg, D.L., et al. (1990). The American College of Rheumatology 1990 criteria for the classification of fibromyalgia. *Arthritis and Rheumatism, 33*, 160-173.

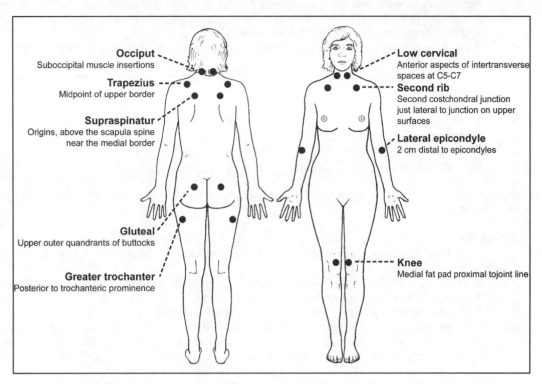

Figure 17.13. Tender Points Identified by American College of Rheumatology

In the figure:

Occiput - Suboccipital muscle insertions

Trapezius - Midpoint of upper border

Supraspinatur - Origins, above the scapula spine near the medial border

Gluteal - Upper outer quandrants of buttocks

Greater trochanter - Posterior to trochanteric prominence

Low cervical - Anterior aspects of intertransverse spaces at C5-C7

Second rib - Second costchondral junction just lateral to junction on upper surfaces

Lateral epicondyle - 2 cm distal to epicondyles

Knee - Medial fat pad proximal tojoint line

IV.   Diagnosis/Evaluation

A.   History: Obtain a thorough history and carefully listen to the patients describe their symptoms
   1.   Question about associated symptoms such as headaches, diarrhea, lack of concentration
   2.   Ask about factors that precipitate symptoms
   3.   Explore how the disease has impacted on the patient's family, interpersonal relationships, work, school, and activities of daily living

B.   Physical Examination
   1.   Measure vital signs
   2.   Observe general appearance
   3.   Assess neck for thyromegaly
   4.   Perform bilateral digital palpation using a force of about 4 kg/cm$_2$ which is approximately equal to pressing finger on bathroom scale until it registers 10 pounds, or until the nail bed just begins to blanch; to meet criteria of a positive tender point, patient must label the palpation as "painful," not just tender
   5.   Perform a complete musculoskeletal examination, particularly assess each joint
   6.   Assess mental status and perform a mental health assessment

C.   Differential Diagnosis
   1.   Chronic fatigue syndrome: These patients have vague, systemic symptoms but do not usually complain of pain as is characteristic of FMS (see section on FATIGUE)
   2.   Rheumatoid arthritis, in contrast to FMS, presents with warm, erythematous joints in addition to pain
   3.   Systemic lupus erythematosus (SLE): Patients with FMS may present with mildly elevated ANA but other criteria of SLE are absent (see section on RHEUMATOID ARTHRITIS for SLE criteria)
   4.   Somatization and depression often accompany FMS but are not the primary diagnoses; patients with psychological problems do not have characteristic tender points
   5.   Myofascial pain syndrome presents with referred trigger points and occurs more frequently in men than women, which is not characteristic of FMS
      a.   Trigger points, in contrast to tender points found in FMS, are usually nodular-type areas and cause radiating pain and muscle twitching
      b.   To complicate the situation, myofascial pain syndrome may occur in patients with FMS
   6.   Drug-induced myopathies: Particularly consider this problem in patients taking statins to lower lipids

7. Polymyalgia rheumatica can be diagnosed by an elevated erythrocyte sedimentation rate (ESR)
8. Severe hypothyroidism mimics FMS but usually these patients have signs such as lid lag, dry skin, and an elevated thyroid stimulating hormone
9. Sleep apnea often goes undiagnosed; this disorder presents with loud snoring and thrashing in bed

D. Diagnostic Tests: No tests are available to detect FMS, consider the following tests to exclude other possible diagnoses
1. Complete blood count
2. Erythrocyte sedimentation rate (order in all persons >50 years who present with symptoms)
3. Measurement of muscle enzymes
4. Thyroid stimulating hormone
5. Rheumatoid factor

V. Plan/Management: A multifaceted approach with an interdisciplinary team is ideal; clinical trials of FMS therapies are limited

A. Patient Education
1. Provide reassurance that patient has a distinct, recognizable disease and that symptoms are real and can be managed
2. Explain to patient that complete resolution of pain and associated symptoms is unlikely, but that therapies can reduce pain and improve quality of life
3. Discuss ways to improve sleep (see section on INSOMNIA)
4. Help patient shift from a sense of helplessness and frustration to a sense of self-efficacy and hope
   a. Self-management courses to control symptoms and promote health are effective
   b. Cognitive behavioral therapy such as helping patients to prioritize their time and activities to include meaningful work and enjoyable leisure is beneficial
   c. Social support interventions may be beneficial; support groups may be located through a local chapter of the Arthritis Foundation (AF); find support groups on the AF website (see table for helpful FMS websites)

WEBSITES FOR FIBROMYALGIA SYNDROME ORGANIZATIONS

Arthritis Foundation	http://www.arthritis.org
Fibromyalgia Network	http://www.fmnetnews.com
National Fibromyalgia Awareness Campaign	http://www.fmaware.com
National Fibromyalgia Partnership, Inc.	http://www.fmpartnership.org
American Chronic Pain Association	http://www.theacpa.org

B. Exercise: A program which includes pain reduction techniques of stretching, proper posture, and body mechanics with careful and gentle exercise such as walking, bicycling, and swimming is helpful
1. Strenuous or excessive exercise should be avoided
2. Referral to a physical therapist can be beneficial

C. Pharmacological treatment: In adults, medications are used to help patients receive a restful sleep, to treat muscle spasms, and to reduce pain; in children, nonpharmacological approaches should be used

D. Massage therapy, acupuncture, hypnosis, local infiltration of trigger points with 1% solution of lidocaine, stress management, relaxation techniques, transcutaneous electrical nerve stimulation, visualization, and meditation are additional effective therapies

E. Follow-up is variable and depends on the severity of symptoms as well as coping abilities and resources of the patients and their support systems

JOINT PAIN

I. Definition: Discomfort or tenderness in one or more joints

II. Pathogenesis: See clinical presentation for common causes

III. Clinical presentation of common forms of joint pain

    A. Pain involving multiple joints
- 1. Juvenile rheumatoid arthritis (JRA): Chronic inflammatory polyarthritis with symmetric joint involvement and rheumatoid factor positivity (see section on RHEUMATOID ARTHRITIS)
- 2. Systemic lupus erythematosus (SLE): American Rheumatism Association Classification (1982) (see following table)

CLASSIFICATION OF SYSTEMIC LUPUS ERYTHEMATOSUS

- Malar rash: Fixed, erythematous, flat, or raised rash over malar eminences
- Discoid rash: Erythematous raised patches with scaling
- Photosensitivity
- Oral ulcers
- Arthritis involving 2 or more peripheral joints
- Serositis involving either pleuritis or pericarditis
- Renal disorder involving persistent proteinuria or cellular casts
- Neurologic disorder involving seizures or psychosis
- Hematologic disorders of hemolytic anemia, leukopenia, lymphopenia, or thrombocytopenia
- Immunologic disorder such as positive lupus erythematosus cell preparation or anti-DNA antibody to native DNA in abnormal titer or anti-Sm or false positive serologic test for syphilis for at least 6 months
- Abnormal titer of antinuclear antibody

---

* A person is said to have SLE if 4 or more of 11 criteria are present

Adapted from Tan, E.M., Cohen, A.S., Fries, J.F., Masi, A.T., McShane, D.J., Rothfield, W.F., et al. (1982). The 1982 revised criteria for the classification of systemic lupus erythematosus. *Arthritis and Rheumatology, 25*, 1275-1277.

- 3. Systemic sclerosis or scleroderma initially involves arthralgia and inflammation of the hands; skin thickening, a hallmark of the disease, develops several months later
- 4. Fibromyalgia is a poorly understood syndrome involving widespread musculoskeletal pain and accompanied by fatigue, nonrestorative sleep, reduced functional ability, and sometimes accompanied by headaches, irritable bowel syndrome, paresthesias, restless leg syndrome, and cold sensitivity (see section on FIBROMYALGIA)
- 5. Reiter's syndrome, primarily a disease of young men, involves classic triad of arthritis, urethritis, and conjunctivitis
- 6. Psoriatic arthritis often presents with asymmetric joint involvement and characteristic nail and skin lesions
- 7. Gonococcal arthritis presents as migratory polyarthritis, tendinitis, and often has vesicular-pustular skin lesions
- 8. Lyme arthritis usually has classic history of tick bite and rash with arthritis in the knees (see section on LYME DISEASE)
- 9. Rheumatic heart disease presents in a migratory pattern of joint involvement with evidence of antecedent streptococcal infection
- 10. Inflammatory bowel disease, ulcerative colitis, and Crohn's disease are associated with gastrointestinal complaints
- 11. Ankylosing spondylitis or spondyloarthropathy involves large joints of lower extremities during childhood and early adolescence; in late adolescence presents with back pain and stiffness
- 12. Sickle cell disease causes pain, swelling, tenderness, and effusion in large joints
- 13. Growing pains occur in about 18% of school-aged children and peak at age 11 (see section on LOWER EXTREMITY PAIN)
- 14. Congenital syphilis may be seen in infants who have painful bony lesions and refuse to move the involved limb
- 15. Hypermobility syndrome is found in children and adolescents who have increased joint laxity; with vigorous activities involving extreme joint flexion and extension, these children experience pain

16. Vasculitic syndromes such as Henoch-Schönlein, Kawasaki disease in children, and polyarteritis nodosa usually have associated physical findings such as a purpuric rash
17. Malignancies such as leukemia and lymphoma sometimes affect the joints; bone pain, fever, and weight loss are typically present
18. Infections such as subacute bacterial endocarditis, influenza, rubella, mumps, chickenpox, infectious mononucleosis, hepatitis, Rocky Mountain-spotted fever, tularemia, and rat-bite fever can also involve joints
19. Physical abuse presents with signs of trauma and there is a suspicious history

B. Pain involving single joint
1. Infection
   a. Septic arthritis due to disseminated gonorrhea or gram positive bacteria, especially *Staphylococcus aureus,* is a serious condition, presenting with fever, chills, necrotic skin lesions, joint pain, and swelling
   b. Gram-negative bacterial infections and infections due to anaerobes are becoming frequent causes of monoarthritis due to the rising number of persons who are parenteral drug users and immunosuppressed persons
   c. Tuberculous arthritis with subsequent periarticular bone lesions and synovial involvement may occur even if pulmonary tuberculosis is not present
   d. Monoarthritis can herald the onset of HIV infection
2. Primary gout is rare in children but hyperuricemia and subsequent joint disease may occur with leukemia, hemolytic anemia, and glycogen storage disease
3. Pseudogout resembles gout but primarily affects a knee or wrist joint; results from crystals of calcium pyrophosphate inducing joint inflammation and is often associated with hyperparathyroidism and hemochromatosis in the older patient
4. Trauma and foreign-body reactions may present with sudden pain and swelling in one joint
5. Osteomyelitis involves localized swelling, limitation of joint mobility, erythema, and tenderness over the involved area, fever, and and/or an associated ulcer or skin lesion with possibly a sinus tract draining infected fluid; risk factors include history of bacteremia, peripheral vascular disease, diabetes mellitus, trauma, or surgery in the affected area
6. Toxic synovitis is found in children <10 years of age who have unilateral hip pain; typically occurs after an upper respiratory infection
7. Diskitis presents with low-grade fever, back pain, and tenderness over spinous process closest to involved disk space
8. Chondromalacia or patellofemoral pain syndrome causes knee pain (see section on LOWER EXTREMITY PAIN)
9. Localized tumors (e.g., osteogenic sarcoma) and metastatic processes (e.g., neuroblastoma) may cause solitary joint pain; typically accompanied by fever and weight loss

C. Rheumatoid arthritis, systemic lupus erythematosus, arthritis of inflammatory bowel disease, Lyme disease, psoriatic arthritis, Behçet's disease, Reiter's syndrome, and hemarthrosis (bleeding into a joint commonly due to a clotting abnormality) can result in pain in single or multiple joints

IV. Diagnosis/Evaluation

A. History
1. Ascertain pain characteristics, onset, location at onset, what aggravates pain, and what functional loss has occurred
2. Ask about distribution of involved joints (symmetric involvement of metacarpophalangeal joints [MCP] and wrists suggests rheumatoid arthritis [RA])
3. Determine severity of pain by asking if it awakens patient at night or hinders activities of daily living
4. Explore history of previous attacks; past episodes lend support for a crystalline or other noninfectious cause
5. Inquire about previous trauma to joint or surrounding tissues
6. Question about tick bites, fever, sexual risk factors, intravenous drug use, alcohol abuse, immunosuppression, and travel in foreign countries -- all of which suggest an infectious cause
7. Inquire about rash, diarrhea, urethritis, or uveitis which supports a diagnosis of arthritides
8. Explore systemic symptoms such as fatigue, fever, sleep problems which suggest rheumatoid arthritis, SLE, fibromyalgia
9. Ask about history of gastrointestinal problems and determine whether there is a history of an ulcer, because this will affect choice of analgesic medication
10. A complete family history is important
11. Often a complete review of systems is needed to determine other involved organs

B. Physical Examination
1. Measure temperature and other vital signs (fever suggests infection such as septic arthritis)
2. Observe gait and general appearance
3. Examine joints for presence of tenderness, erythema, warmth, effusion, bony enlargement, and mechanical abnormalities
   a. Assessment must distinguish an arthritis, which involves the articular space, from conditions involving the periarticular area, such as bursitis, cellulitis, or tendinitis; painful limitation of motion probably indicates joint involvement
   b. Helpful to compare paired joints
   c. Remember to inspect, palpate, perform range of motion activities, and perform special tests as needed
4. Assess for muscle atrophy
5. Detailed physical examination is often needed to detect extra-articular manifestations
   a. Observe skin for malar and discoid lesions of SLE, exanthem of gonococcal arthritis, tophi of gout, and nodules of rheumatoid arthritis
   b. Observe nails for pitting (psoriatic arthritis)
   c. Examine eyes for conjunctivitis of Reiter's syndrome and also observe eyes, nose, and mouth for dryness as occurs with sicca syndrome which suggests Sjögren's syndrome that often accompanies rheumatoid arthritis
   d. Inspect mouth for ulcers in Behçet's syndrome, Reiter's syndrome, and SLE
   e. Auscultate heart and lungs noting pleural rubs and heart murmurs from RA , SLE, and rheumatic diseases
   f. Palpate elbows, Achilles tendons, and pinnae for nodules and tophi (rheumatoid arthritis and gout, respectively)
   g. Examine spine for restriction of motion and tenderness that indicates spondylitis
   h. Urethral or cervical discharge suggests gonococcal arthritis

C. Differential Diagnosis: Rule out all conditions listed in section III.

D. Diagnostic tests: No standard battery of tests exists; base selection of tests on history and physical examination
1. Order x-rays if trauma or focal bone pain is present
2. Joint aspiration with fluid cell count is done if signs of inflammation are present to differentiate inflammatory from non-inflammatory joint disease and to determine whether a joint is infected
3. Complete cell count (CBC) and erythrocyte sedimentation rate (ESR) are useful as screens for inflammatory disease
4. Rheumatoid factor may be helpful in confirming the diagnosis of RA, but is also often positive when the patient has other conditions
5. Antinuclear antibody (ANA) is sensitive but not specific in diagnosing SLE
6. Uric acids levels are often elevated in gout
7. Magnetic resonance imaging can sometimes localize an infectious or inflammatory process in a joint, tissue, or bone; best utilized in soft tissue evaluation
8. Tests for HIV antibodies should be ordered when risk factors for this disease are present
9. Blood cultures are needed when sepsis is suspected
10. Bone biopsy or culture is needed when osteomyelitis is suspected

V. Plan/Management

A. Determine severity of disease and the need for hospitalization; rapid onset of pain, heat, swelling, and erythema of joint should be evaluated immediately for septic arthritis or osteomyelitis which can lead to rapid joint destruction and sepsis

B. Treat known causes. For example, ceftriaxone (Rocephin) should be used to treat gonococcal arthritis

C. Immobilization and rest of the involved joint, and hot and/or cold therapy are often helpful

D. Pharmacological therapy for pain
1. Anti-inflammatory pain agents should be postponed for at least 12-24 hours so that cultures can grow and joint aspiration can be repeated if needed; If pain is unbearable use acetaminophen or codeine which do not have anti-inflammatory effects
2. Later NSAIDs can be used (see section on PAIN)

E. Follow up is variable

KNEE INJURY, ACUTE

I.   Definition: Injury to the knee from acute trauma (also see sections LOWER EXTREMITY PAIN, OVERUSE INJURIES, and JOINT PAIN)

II.   Pathogenesis: Injuries are due to trauma but excessive pronation of the foot or misalignment of an extremity can cause inappropriate stress on structures of the knee and predispose the knee to injury

    A.   Strains and sprains of the collateral and cruciate ligaments are caused by forces that create abduction of the leg at the knee, hyperextension of the knee, or a direct blow to the knee
        1.   Grade I sprains involve stretching fibers without significant structural damage
        2.   Grade II sprains involve partial disruption of fibers with increased laxity
        3.   Grade III sprains involve complete tearing of ligamentous tissues
            a.   Anterior cruciate ligament (ACL) tear typically occurs when the foot is planted, the knee is flexed, and the individual suddenly changes direction, applying a rotational force to the knee
            b.   Posterior cruciate ligament tear (PCL) usually occurs from a blow to the anterior proximal tibia with the knee flexed
            c.   Medial collateral ligament (MCL) injuries result from valgus stress or external rotational force with the legs firmly planted; occurs frequently in sports such as football or basketball; often associated with an ACL injury
            d.   Lateral collateral ligament (LCL) injuries are caused by varus stress or rotational force sustained when the feet are planted or hyperextended

    B.   Tears of the medial and lateral meniscus are common and typically involve a simple twisting motion or a rotary force applied to a flexed knee joint; often caused by a noncontact injury

    C.   Patellar subluxation or dislocation usually occurs with knee near extension and the tibia externally rotated or may result from a direct blow to knee; may accompany an anterior cruciate ligament (ACL) injury

    D.   Fractures are found in about 6% of patients with acute knee trauma
        1.   Patella: Result from falls, direct blows to the knee, or a powerful contraction of the quadriceps muscle
        2.   Femoral condyles: Common causes are falls and motor vehicle accidents
        3.   Tibial plateau: Due to compression forces, twisting forces, or a combination of both

III. Clinical Presentation

    A.   Ligament injuries
        1.   Most frequently injured ligament is the medial collateral ligament, followed by the anterior cruciate ligament
        2.   Patients have variable amounts of pain, stiffness, tenderness, and swelling depending on severity of ligament damage
        3.   Anterior cruciate ligament injury is serious and the diagnosis is often missed
            a.   Patient typically falls to the ground and is unable to arise without assistance
            b.   An audible pop and "giving way" sensation may occur
            c.   A large, hemorrhagic effusion develops within first few hours
            d.   A positive Lachman test or anterior drawer test indicates instability of the ACL
        4.   Posterior cruciate ligament injuries are relatively uncommon
            a.   Patient usually has a positive posterior drawer test and observation of knee may reveal hyperflexion
            b.   Patients typically present with less instability and swelling than patients with ACL injuries
        5.   Collateral ligament injury (medial and lateral ligaments) involves local swelling, ecchymosis, laxity, localized medial or lateral tenderness; effusion is usually minimal

    B.   Meniscus injury
        1.   Uncommon in prepubescent patients, but frequently found in the adolescent athlete
        2.   Often occurs in combination with injuries of the ACL or MCL
        3.   Medial meniscus injuries are more common than lateral meniscus injuries
        4.   Patient often recalls a twisting flexion injury of the knee followed by a popping sound, pain with rotational movements and difficulty flexing the knee and bearing weight
        5.   May have clicking, locking, catching, or giving way of knee

6. Knee joint effusion and tenderness over the joint line are often noted
7. Inability to squat or hop because of pain is characteristic
8. Often associated with ligamentous injury

C. Patellar subluxation or dislocation occurs more frequently in females than males and is a common childhood injury
   1. Involves severe pain, medial tenderness, effusion, and inability to move knee
   2. On pivoting and running, patients often complain of "locking" or "popping" of knees
   3. About 20% of patients have recurrent dislocations

D. Fractures are difficult to differentiate from other injuries; may result in severe pain, inability to bear weight, swelling, limited range of motion, and unequal leg length
   1. Crepitus is palpable with patellar fractures; pain increases with active knee extension
   2. Neurovascular compromise may occur with femoral condylar fractures
   3. Pain with compression of the side of joint may occur with tibial plateau fractures

E. Musculoskeletal system of children differs from adults
   1. Children's bones are more porous and plastic than adults which creates a greater risk for fractures and unicortical or "greenstick" fractures
      a. Injuries, particularly fractures, to growth plates can lead to deformity and growth irregularities
      b. The Salter-Harris classification system groups fractures into 5 categories ranging from Type I which is a separation of the growth plate which does not affect future bone growth to Type V which is a crush injury and has the worst prognosis for normal growth
   2. Avulsion injuries in which a piece of bone is torn off at the point where a tendon or ligament attaches are common
   3. Meniscal injuries occur less frequently in children than adults

IV. Diagnosis/Evaluation

A. History
   1. Ask patient to precisely describe circumstances surrounding injury and mechanism of the injury; particularly ask if injury involved hyperextension of the knee, a direct blow to knee, or a twisting injury
   2. Inquire about location of pain, tenderness, and swelling in knee as well as hip, thigh, shin, ankle and foot
   3. Inquire about sensations of locking, clicking, catching, giving way or buckling of the knee
   4. Ask if there was an audible "pop"
   5. Ask patient to point to site of greatest pain
   6. Ask how quickly after the injury the swelling developed; swelling in the joint within 24 hours suggests hemarthrosis
   7. Ask about previous musculoskeletal injuries; important to determine if this is an acute problem or a pre-existing condition which has been aggravated
   8. Inquire about systemic symptoms such as fever, chills, night sweats
   9. Determine patient's occupation and job requirements
   10. Determine whether patient is involved in leisure or competitive athletics which will affect decisions about management
   11. Inquire about self treatments

B. Physical Examination
   1. Always compare injured side with unaffected side during observation, palpation, range of motion, and special tests
   2. Observe gait and stance, noting lower extremity alignment
   3. Examination of the entire lower extremity is required
   4. Observe knee while standing for deformity, discoloration, swelling, and abrasions
   5. With patient seated and knee flexed at 90°, look for bulge of fluid on either side of patellar ligament
   6. Palpate in a proximal to distal direction with patient sitting and supine (see Figure 17.14. for anatomical structures)
      a. Begin with thigh, palpating quadriceps, hamstrings, and articular surfaces of the femoral condyles; consider measuring thigh girth to detect disuse atrophy
      b. Palpate patella and all around the joint line (tenderness at joint line suggests meniscal tear, whereas tenderness slightly above or below joint line suggests ligament damage)
      c. Palpate muscles around patella and collateral ligaments
      d. Palpate around each growth plate
      e. Palpate tibial plateau and tibial tuberosity

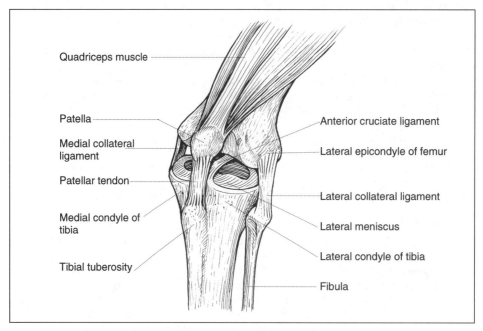

Figure 17.14. Anatomical Structures of the Knee.

Quadriceps muscle

Patella

Medial collateral ligament

Patellar tendon

Medial condyle of tibia

Tibial tuberosity

Anterior cruciate ligament

Lateral epicondyle of femur

Lateral collateral ligament

Lateral meniscus

Lateral condyle of tibia

Fibula

7.   Assess for effusion or fluid in knee joint (see Figure 17.15.)

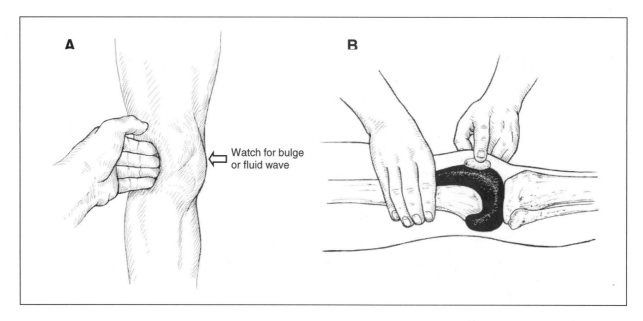

A

B

Watch for bulge or fluid wave

Figure 17.15. Testing for Fluid in the Knee Joint
A. The bulge sign. B. The patellar tap will suggest fluid in the knee as the patella clicks against the femur. With greater amounts of knee fluid, the patella will be ballottable.

8.   Perform range of motion of knee
9.   Assess mobility of patella by flexing knee 30° and applying medial and lateral pressure to determine amount of subluxation that is possible
10.   Determine the quadriceps or Q angle (see Figure 17.20. in section on LOWER EXTREMITY PAIN)
      a.   This angle is formed by lines drawn from center of patella to the tibial tubercle and from the center of patella to anterior superior spine
      b.   When angle exceeds 15° it is abnormal and may be associated with patellar subluxation and dislocation

11. Determine ligament stability (see Figure 17.16.)
   a. Apply valgus (medial) or varus (lateral) stress when knee is at full extension and then at 30° flexion to assess stability of medial and lateral collateral ligaments
      (1) In first-degree sprains, end point is solid
      (2) In second-degree sprains, laxity is evident at 30° flexion but not at full extension
      (3) In third-degree sprains, there are no solid end points at either 30° flexion or full extension

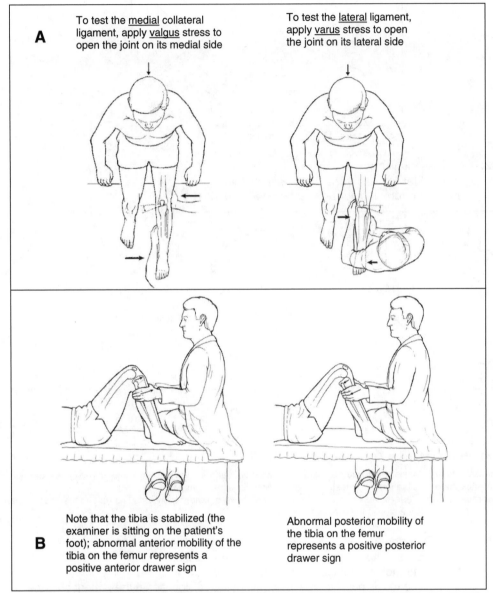

A

To test the medial collateral ligament, apply valgus stress to open the joint on its medial side

To test the lateral ligament, apply varus stress to open the joint on its lateral side

B

Note that the tibia is stabilized (the examiner is sitting on the patient's foot); abnormal anterior mobility of the tibia on the femur represents a positive anterior drawer sign

Abnormal posterior mobility of the tibia on the femur represents a positive posterior drawer sign

Figure 17.16. Collateral Ligament Testing
A: Collateral ligament testing. B: The "drawer" sign for cruciate ligament testing

   b. Assess stability of cruciate ligaments with the drawer test by applying anterior (see aforementioned illustration) and posterior forces to the proximal tibia when the knee is flexed and the foot is stabilized
   c. Lachman's test can also test cruciate ligaments and is performed with knee flexed to 30°; anterior drawer force is applied to the proximal tibia with one hand while the other hand stabilizes the femur (see Figure 17.17.)

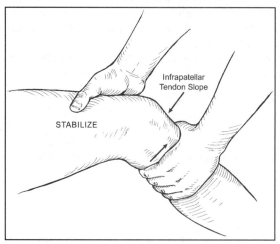

Figure 17.17. Lachman's Test

12. Assess meniscus
    a. Flex knee to 90° and palpate joint line
    b. Perform McMurray's test (see Figure 17.18.)

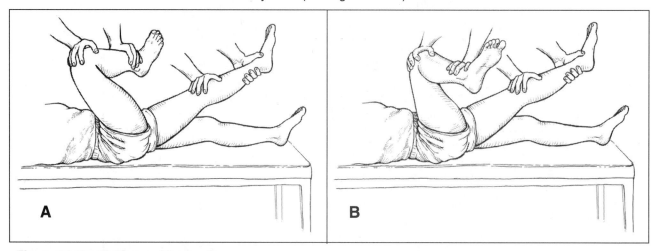

Figure 17.18. McMurray Maneuver.

A. Extension in internal rotation: Maximally flex knee, externally rotate tibia and apply varus stress as the knee is extended to test for lateral meniscus injury. A palpable or audible snap suggests a lesion in the lateral meniscus

B. Extension in external rotation: Perform flexion, external rotation as above but then apply valgus stress to test medial meniscus injury. A palpable or audible snap suggests a lesion in the medial meniscus

13. The apprehensive test is performed to detect patella dislocation
    a. Extend the knee but in a slightly flexed position
    b. Attempt to displace the patella laterally
    c. The test is positive and indicates patella dislocation if the patient becomes apprehensive about the procedure
14. Assess neurovascular status of extremity
15. Assess hip and back whenever a history of knee pain is combined with normal findings on the knee exam

C. Differential Diagnosis: Important to differentiate acute injuries from overuse injuries, inflammatory processes, infection, and neoplasms (see sections, LOWER EXTREMITY PAIN and JOINT PAIN)
    1. Overuse injuries have insidious onset and usually result from repetitive stress
        a. Chondromalacia patellae
        b. Osgood-Schlatter disease
        c. Patellar tendinitis
        d. Stress fractures
    2. Consider osteochondritis dissecans (see section LOWER EXTREMITY PAIN) for patients who have clinical findings of torn meniscus without a history of meniscal injury

3. Hemarthrosis or blood collecting in joint is a serious injury and results from extensive trauma and is often associated with ACL injuries
4. Inflammatory processes, infections, autoimmune diseases, and neoplasms are typically associated with systemic symptoms
5. Hip problems should be considered; referred pain from the hip occurs, especially in children

D. Diagnostic Tests
1. To rule out knee fractures, consider ordering x-rays of the knee including anteroposterior, lateral and sunrise patella views; the Ottawa Knee and Pittsburgh Decision Rules are helpful in deciding when to use radiography (see following tables)

OTTAWA KNEE RULE

Order knee x-ray series for patients with the following findings:

1) Age 55 years or older
   Or
2) Isolated tenderness of patella*
   Or
3) Tenderness at head of fibula
   Or
4) Inability to flex to 90°
   Or
5) Inability to bear weight immediately or walk more than four steps immediately after injury

---

*No bone tenderness of knee other than patella

Adapted from Stiell, I.G., Wells, G.A., Hoag, R.H., Sivilotti, M.L., Cacciotti, T.F., Verbeek, P.R., et al. (1997). Implementation of the Ottawa Knee Rule for the use of radiography in acute knee injuries. *JAMA, 278,* 2075-2079.

PITTSBURGH DECISION RULES

Blunt trauma or a fall as mechanism of injury plus either of the following:

- Age younger than 12 years or older than 50 years
- Inability to walk four weight-bearing steps in the emergency department

---

Adapted from Bauer, S.J., Hollander, J.E., Fuchs, S.H., & Thode, H.C., Jr. (1995). A clinical decision rule in the evaluation of acute knee injuries. *Journal of Emergency Medicine, 13,* 611-615.

2. Although ligament injuries can usually be detected based on history and physical examination, joint laxity and rupture may be missed; magnetic resonance imaging (MRI) is accurate in diagnosing ligamentous injuries; ultrasound examination is inexpensive and may be useful; arthroscopy of the knee is the gold standard test for detection of ruptured anterior cruciate ligaments
3. MRI is accurate in diagnosing meniscal injuries
4. Patellar subluxation: Order knee x-rays (AP, lateral, obliques, and sunrise views); consider an arteriogram
5. Perform arthrocentesis for patients with knee effusion who do not have history of trauma or in whom infection is a possible diagnosis; order cell count, Gram's stain, and culture
6. Injuries that do not heal after 2 weeks of conservative treatment may require magnetic resonance imaging or in the case of a meniscus injury, an arthrogram which is less accurate

V. Plan/Management

A. With all types of injuries, the initial treatment is immobilization of the knee in a splint or rigid knee immobilizer, ice, compression, and elevation

B. Refer patients with the following conditions to an orthopedist; surgery or special therapeutic procedures and/or braces are often needed
1. Neurovascular compromise
2. Suspected fractures
3. Dislocation and subluxation of the patella
4. Suspected growth plate injury
5. Torn ligaments (Grade II and III sprains)
6. Suspected ACL injuries
7. Locked knee which is unable to be manipulated into place

8. Torn meniscus
9. Hemarthrosis
10. Suspected infection or tumor
11. Patellar dislocation

C. Treatment for grade I sprains and minor injuries of the meniscus; management depends on the patient's age, athletic participation, occupation, and lifestyles
1. Rest depending on extent of injury; minor injuries may need only 1-2 days of rest
2. Apply ice (never directly to skin) 20 to 30 minutes with at least 10 minute breaks in application as often as possible during first 48 hours after injury
3. Elevate extremity
4. Consider prescribing NSAIDs such as ibuprofen (Motrin) 200-800 mg TID every 6 to 8 hours or in children ≥6 months 10 mg/kg every 6-8 hours with maximum of 40 mg/kg/day; some clinicians believe that NSAIDs hamper early healing and should be used conservatively
5. Teach crutch walking and the need to avoid weight-bearing until acute inflammation subsides
6. For injuries with pronounced symptoms, immobilize knee in brace for a minimal period of time
7. Exercise is important
   a. For minor injuries, exercise can be permitted within 1-2 days, but patient should be cautioned to gradually increase activity
   b. For more extensive injuries, activity should initially consist of isometric quadriceps tensing exercises
   c. Begin isotonic quadriceps exercises and range of motion exercises after acute inflammation subsides
8. Incision and drainage of large and fluctuant hematomas may be needed

D. Follow Up
1. For extensive injuries, schedule return visit in 24 hours
2. For less extensive injuries, return visits should be scheduled in two weeks or sooner if problems occur
3. Consult specialist for patients with ligament and meniscus injuries that improved only minimally after 2 weeks of conservative treatment
4. At the return visit, all patients should be taught ways to prevent further injuries to their knees particularly by proper exercising and conditioning and possibly the use of prophylactic braces

LOW BACK PAIN, ACUTE

I. Definition: Activity intolerance due to lower back or back-related leg symptoms of less than 3 months duration

II. Pathogenesis: In preadolescents isolated back pain is uncommon and often indicates an underlying pathology that needs increased attention; from early adolescence into adulthood, back pain is frequent and usually is a benign problem due to mechanical stress or trauma

A. Acute low back pain may be caused by mechanical factors, systemic diseases, or visceral diseases (see following table)

CAUSES OF ACUTE LOW BACK PAIN		
Mechanical Low Back Pain or Leg Pain	**Nonmechanical Spinal Disorders**	**Visceral Disease**
Lumbosacral strain	Neoplasia such as multiple myeloma, metastatic cancer, tumors	Diseases of pelvic organs such as pelvic inflammatory disease, prostatitis
Herniated disk	Infections	Renal diseases such as pyelonephritis, nephrolithiasis
Discitis	Inflammatory arthritis such as ankylosing spondylitis, Reiter's syndrome	Aortic aneurysm
Traumatic fractures	Paget's disease of bone	Gastrointestinal diseases such as penetrating ulcer, pancreatitis, cholecystitis
Spondylolisthesis		
Spondylolysis		
Congenital diseases such as kyphosis & scoliosis		

Adapted from Deyo, R.A., & Weinstein, J.N. (2001). Low back pain. *New England Journal of Medicine, 344*, 363-370.

B. Spondylolysis and spondylolisthesis are the most common causes of low back pain in children
1. Spondylolysis is a break of the pars interarticularis; usual site is L4 or L5
2. Spondylolisthesis is a slip of the vertebrae (after spondylolysis) which allows one vertebral body to slide forward on its neighbor; usual site is L5 or S1

C. Discitis occurs primarily in preschool-age children; most likely due to bacterial infection
1. Probably due to vascular disruption in hyaline epiphyseal endplates of vertebrae distal to T12 which results in vascular necrotic changes to disc
2. Disc becomes permanently deformed and narrowed

D. Lumbosacral strain
1. Etiology is often unclear but results from stretching or tearing of muscles, tendons, ligaments, or fascia of back secondary to trauma or chronic mechanical stress
2. Predisposing factors include chronic occupational strain, obesity, exaggerated lumbar lordosis, abnormal forward-tipped pelvis, weak paraspinal and/or abdominal muscles, leg length discrepancy, chronic poor posture, inadequate/inappropriate conditioning and suboptimal lifting habits

E. Herniated intervertebral discs are uncommon in children
1. Intervertebral discs are composed of collagenous annulus fibrosis and gelatinous nucleus pulposus
2. Herniation occurs with tears in annulus fibrosis which allows contents of nucleus pulposus to protrude
3. When nerve roots are compressed by these contents, pain and other neurological signs and symptoms develop

F. Scoliosis is rarely painful but in some children may cause back discomfort

G. Tumors most commonly occur in adolescents after their peak of growth
1. The most common benign tumors are osteoblastoma, hemangiomas, and aneurysmal bone cysts
2. Malignant tumors (leukemias, chondrosarcomas, Ewing's tumor, histiocytic lymphoma) primarily involve the pelvis in the early stages and may cause low back pain

H. Juvenile ankylosing spondylitis, infections such as spinal tuberculosis, and nontuberculosis vertebral osteomyelitis are less common causes of back pain

III. Clinical presentation of common syndromes of acute low back problems; 90% of patients with acute low back problems will recover spontaneously in 4 weeks

A. Spondylolysis
1. Often occurs from a stress fracture of the posterior vertebral elements or from hyperextension sports such as gymnastics, diving, or weight lifting
2. Family history for spondylolysis is often positive
3. Usually has gradual onset of pain that may be unilateral or bilateral
4. Pain is worse in sitting position
5. Typically patient does not experience night pain, but may have pain on awakening
6. Neurologic examination is usually normal, but patients may have tight hamstrings and hyperextension (back bending) that often reproduces pain at L5 or just below the iliac crests

B. Spondylolisthesis
1. Symptoms are similar to those found with spondylolysis
2. On physical examination, excess lumbar lordosis is often found; spine appears to have a shelf at the base of the lordotic curvature

C. Discitis: Patients' mains complaints are related to their ages:
1. Children <3 years refuse to walk or crawl
2. Children >3 years complain of abdominal pain and tenderness of hamstrings
3. Children may or may not have a fever
4. Most children have irritability which is relieved by lying in a prone, lumbar lordotic position

D. Lumbosacral strain
1. Most patients recover spontaneously within 4 weeks
2. Typically, patient experiences minimal discomfort during or immediately after injury or activity with stiffness and pain occurring 12-36 hours later as soft tissue swells

3. Pain is located in back, buttocks, or in one or both thighs
4. Pain is aggravated by standing or flexion, and is relieved with rest and reclining

E. Herniated intervertebral disc
1. Characterized by radicular pain which is described as shooting, sharp, electric-type pain, associated with foot and leg pain and worsened with Valsalva maneuvers
2. Paresthesia or numbness may occur in sensory distribution of nerve root
3. Deep tendon reflexes are absent or depressed in distribution of nerve root
4. Muscular weakness and atrophy may result
5. Most common disc ruptures affect L-5 or S-1 nerve roots
6. Most patients begin to improve within 6 weeks; with time, the herniated portion of disc regresses and about 2/3s of the patients have either partial or complete recovery after 6 months
7. Cauda equina involvement (compression of the lower portion of the nerve roots inferior to spinal cord proper) may occur secondary to central disc herniation and presents as insidiously worsening rectal and/or perineal pain with decreased perineal sensation, loss of sphincter control, and disturbances in bowel and bladder functions
8. Signs and symptoms depend on level of herniation (see Figure 17.19 on COMMON DISC SYNDROMES)

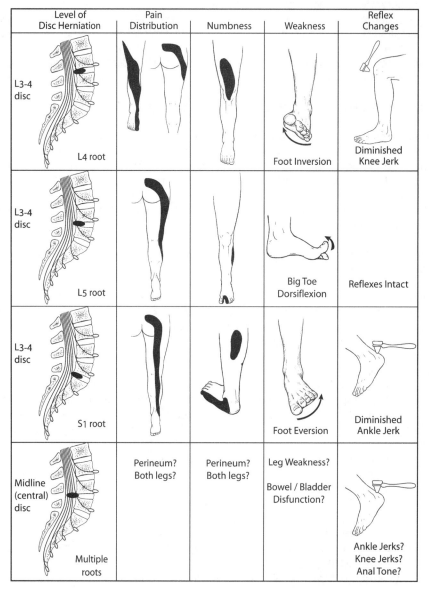

Figure 17.19. Common Disc Syndromes: Neurologic Findings

F. Scoliosis (see section on SCOLIOSIS)

G. Worrisome findings include constant pain in child <11 years that lasts for several weeks or occurs spontaneously at night, interferes with school or play, or is associated with marked stiffness, limitation of motion, fever, or neurologic abnormalities

IV. Diagnosis/Evaluation

A. History should uncover whether there is systemic disease, neurologic involvement that may require surgery, and social or psychological disease that can intensify and prolong the pain
   1. Ask patient to point with one finger where he/she feels pain and then to describe pain and/or radiation of pain
   2. Determine mechanism of onset; acute onset without trauma may signal serious conditions such as dissecting aortic aneurysm
   3. Specifically ask about duration of pain; pain is considered chronic if it persists >6-9 weeks
   4. Differentiate whether pain is mechanical and worsens after bending or lifting or is nonmechanical, occurring at rest, and related to extraspinal disorders such as pelvic or intra-abdominal conditions
   5. Determine whether pain and paresthesia occur after walking which typically indicate neurologic involvement
   6. Ask if sneezing, coughing, or performance of Valsalva maneuver intensifies pain (suggests disk herniation)
   7. Inquire about pattern of symptoms; ask whether symptoms are constant or intermittent
   8. Ask if patient has night-time pain which could suggest cancer or infection
   9. Explore occurrence of systemic symptoms, such as weight loss and fever which could signal malignant disease or a serious infection
   10. Ask about possible associated symptoms such as dysuria, bowel or bladder incontinence, muscle weakness, paresthesia, and loss of sensations
   11. Obtain careful past medical history, noting previous trauma, TB, cancer, immunosuppression, urinary infection, osteoporosis, previous back problems, back surgery, and mental health problems
   12. Inquire about steroid and other drug use
   13. Determine patient's limitations and the effects of pain on occupational, social, recreational, and family activities
   14. Use of pain drawings or visual analog scales may augment history

B. Physical Examination
   1. Observe gait and general appearance
      a. Patients with herniated disks usually are uncomfortable sitting and gait is cautious and awkward
      b. Limping or coordination problems suggest a possible neurological problem
      c. Severe guarding of lumbar motion may indicate spinal infection, tumor, or fracture
   2. Determine temperature; fever is an ominous sign
   3. Observe spine for alignment and abnormalities; observe skin overlying spine for signs of trauma or infection
   4. Perform range of motion
      a. Increased pain with extension often indicates osteoarthritis
      b. Increased pain with flexion most often indicates strain or injured or herniated disk
   5. Palpate spine and paraspinal structures noting point tenderness and paravertebral muscle spasm
   6. If patient fell on tailbone, perform a rectal exam checking for stability of coccyx
   7. Palpate ischial tuberosity and greater trochanter to rule out bursitis
   8. Perform traction maneuvers
      a. Straight leg raise (SLR): Elevate each leg passively with flexion at hip and extension of knee (see Figure 17.20)
         (1) Positive SLR is radicular symptoms (involving the leg and/or foot) when leg is raised to 45° (A)
         (2) Dorsiflexion of foot sometimes exaggerates SLR responses (B)
         (3) Crossed leg raise is very diagnostic for disk injury; positive when patient complains of pain in leg that is not raised (C)

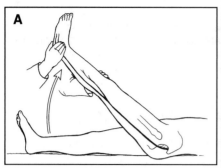
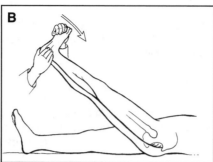
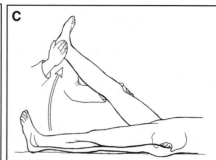

Figure 17.20. Straight Leg Raise

b.   Patrick's test: Heel is placed on opposite knee and lateral force is exerted on knee and pressure is exerted on anterior superior iliac spine of the opposite side; increased pain indicates hip or sacroiliac disease (see Figure 17.21)

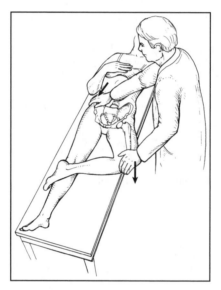

Figure 17.21. Patrick's Test

c.   Gaenslen's sign: Ask patient to lie supine on the table and draw both legs onto chest; then shift patient to side of table and allow unsupported leg to drop over edge while opposite leg is flexed; pain upon execution of this maneuver indicates pathology of the sacroiliac joint (see Figure 17.22)

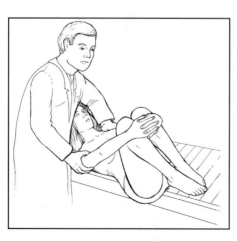
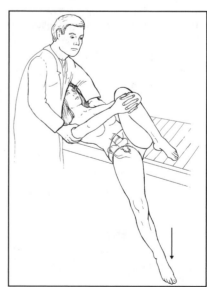

Figure 17.22. Gaenslen's Sign

9. Check for malingering
   a. Observe for overreaction
   b. Perform axial loading (apply slight pressure to top of head); this test should not produce pain unless malingering is present
   c. Perform pelvic rotation which should not elicit pain except with malingering
   d. Perform distracted straight leg raise; inconsistent responses suggest malingering
   e. Observe for nonanatomical motor or sensory regional disturbances
10. Perform complete neurological examination
    a. Determine pain and sensation distribution; pain and diminished or absent sensation should follow nerve root distribution
    b. Do complete motor strength assessment, including dorsiflexion of great toe (only abnormality of the common L4-5 disk protrusion may be great toe weakness)
       (1) Ask patient to toe walk which tests calf muscles and mostly S1 nerve root
       (2) Ask patient to heel walk which tests ankle and toe dorsiflexor muscles, L5, and some L4 nerve roots
       (3) Ask patient to perform a single squat and rise which tests quadriceps muscles, mostly L4 nerve root
    c. Circumferential measurements of calf and thigh bilaterally can detect muscle atrophy; differences of greater than 2 cm in measurements of the two limbs often indicate an abnormality
    d. Deep tendon reflex testing
       (1) Ankle jerk tests mostly the S1 nerve root
       (2) Knee jerk tests mostly the L4 nerve root
       (3) Up-going toes in response to stroking the plantar footpad (Babinski or plantar response) may indicate motor-neuron abnormalities such a myelopathy or demyelinating disease
11. Check sensation of perineum to rule out cauda equina syndrome (compression of the lower portion of the nerve roots inferior to the spinal cord proper)
12. Examine abdomen, noting masses or bruits
13. Assessment of the legs and feet is necessary to differentiate spinal stenosis from vascular insufficiency
    a. Inspect legs and feet for loss of hair and color changes that may accompany vascular insufficiency
    b. Palpate legs and feet for temperature and tenderness
    c. Palpate femoral, popliteal, and pedal pulses
14. Consider pelvic and rectal examinations
15. Consider measuring chest expansion (measurement of <2.5 cm may indicate ankylosing spondylitis)

C. Differential diagnosis (also see table under PATHOGENESIS II.A.-H.)
   1. Important to rule out red flags for potentially serious conditions (see following table)

RED FLAGS FOR POTENTIALLY SERIOUS CONDITIONS		
Possible Fracture	*Possible Tumor or Infection*	*Possible Cauda Equina Syndrome*
Major trauma such as vehicle accident or fall from a high place	Age <20 years	Saddle anesthesia
Use of corticosteroids	History of cancer	Recent onset of bladder dysfunction such as urinary retention, increased frequency, or overflow incontinence
	Constitutional symptoms such as fever, chills, or unexplained weight loss	
		Severe or progressive neurologic deficit in legs
	Risk factors for infection: Recent bacterial infection, IV drug abuse, or immunosuppression	Unexpected laxity of anal sphincter
		Perianal/perineal sensory loss
	Pain that worsens when supine; severe nighttime pain; rest pain; pain that fails to improve with therapy	Major motor weakness such as knee extension weakness or foot drop

Adapted from Bigos, S., Bowyer, O., Braen, G., Brown, K., Deyo, R.A., Haldeman, S., et al. (1994). *Acute low back problems in adults. Clinical practice guideline No. 14.* AHCPR Publication No. 95-0642. Rockville, MD: Agency for Health Care Policy and Research, Public Health Service, U.S. Department of Health and Human Services.

2. Differential diagnosis is extensive; always consider nonspinal pathology that occurs with systemic diseases and referred back pain that occurs with visceral diseases
3. Psychosocial pathology may complicate the diagnosis and management of low back pain; consider malingering (see IV.B.9.)
4. Pseudosciatica with a normal neurologic exam includes simple mechanical back pain, disorders of hip, thigh, pelvis, rectum, and vascular claudication
5. True radicular pain (sciatica or shooting, sharp pain down to the lower leg and foot) includes herniated intervertebral disk, spondylolisthesis, compression fracture, degenerative spondylosis, herpes zoster, and neoplasm
6. Fever or meningeal symptoms suggest vertebral osteomyelitis

D. Diagnostic Tests: In children diagnostic testing is more comprehensive than in adults
  1. If trauma occurred, order plain radiograph; if x-ray is normal, computed tomography (CT) or magnetic resonance imaging (MRI) may be needed unless strain or sprain is most likely; if fracture is still suspected after 10 days or there are multiple sites of pain, consider bone scan or consultation
  2. In preadolescent children when there is no history of trauma, order tests to rule out infections such as discitis:
    a. Order CBC, erythrocyte sedimentation rate (ESR), and blood culture
    b. Also order one of the following radiologic studies
      (1) MRI is sensitive in detecting disc space involvement
      (2) Technetium Tc99 bone scan can detect early discitis
      (3) By 4 weeks, discitis can usually be detected on plain x-ray by disc space narrowing
    c. Aspiration or biopsy of the disc space should be performed if child does not respond to therapy, when involvement of the vertebral body is extensive, or when clinical presentation is atypical for discitis
  3. For patients over 13 years of age consider the following:
    a. X-rays are useful in only a minority of cases
      (1) If spondylolysis or spondylolisthesis is suspected, order x-rays; if x-rays are negative and suspicion is high, order bone scan
      (2) If spinal fracture is a possibility, order plain x-ray of lumbosacral spine; if x-ray is negative and fracture is still suspected after 10 days, or there are multiple sites of pain, consider bone scan or consultation
      (3) For patients with low back pain less than 4-6 weeks and in the absence of signs and symptoms of dangerous conditions (see preceding table on RED FLAGS FOR POTENTIALLY SERIOUS CONDITIONS), no tests are needed
    b. If cancer and/or infection are/is suspected, order CBC, erythrocyte sedimentation rate, urinalysis; if after these tests, there is still suspicion consider consultation or order bone scan, MRI, or CT
      (1) MRI is best at imaging soft tissue (herniated disks, tumors; infections); poor choice of test to visualize fractures
      (2) CT is better at imaging cortical bone (osteoarthritis)
      (3) Bone scans with radioactive compounds are useful when radiographs of spine are normal, but patient has suspicious clinical findings for osteomyelitis, spondylolysis, neoplasm, metastatic disease, or occult fracture
    c. For patients whose back pain does not improve over 4 weeks:
      (1) If symptoms are primarily in the low back consider ordering CBC, ESR, x-rays, CT, MRI, or bone scan depending on symptomatology and risk factors
      (2) If spinal stenosis is suspected, spinal x-ray (not diagnostic, but may demonstrate degenerative changes), MRI, or CT should be considered

V. Plan/Management of common mechanical low back pain disorders

A. Immediately arrange for emergency care for patients with cauda equina

B. Consult specialist for patients with suspected discitis, tumors, infections, juvenile ankylosing spondylitis, and rapidly progressing neurologic deficits

C. Management of spondylolysis
  1. Begin with rest, analgesics, and hamstring stretching exercises
  2. Back muscle strengthening exercises are recommended when the pain has subsided
  3. Immobilization with back braces may be needed to achieve healing of fractures or to relieve irritation if patient is not responding to analgesics and exercises
  4. Surgical fusion is rarely required

D.   Management of spondylolisthesis
     1.   Begin with an adequate trial of conservative, symptomatic therapy
     2.   Progressive or severe neurologic deficit with severe functional impairments that persist for a year or longer are indications for surgery

E.   Management of discitis; usually hospitalization for initial treatment is recommended
     1.   Prescribe oral antibiotics based on results of blood culture for 3-4 weeks
     2.   If blood culture is negative or not performed, prescribe an antistaphylococcal drug such as cephalexin 100 mg/kg/day divided every 6 hours for 3-4 weeks
     3.   Also, prescribe an NSAID if the patient can tolerate one; acute acting NSAIDs such as ketorolac (30-60 mg IM or IV every 6 hours for 48 hours) may be needed initially
     4.   Initially, child should be on bedrest; some authorities recommend rigid bracing after child responds to antibiotics
     5.   Surgical debridement may be needed if there is no clinical response in 48 hours after treatment or if ESR shows no improvement

F.   Management of lumbosacral strain and probable herniated intervertebral disk; remember that back pain in preadolescents is uncommon and a diagnosis of exclusion
     1.   **Pharmacological therapy**
          a.   Generally, drugs should be prescribed on a regular rather than on as-needed basis
          b.   Safest effective medication is acetaminophen which may be used safely in combination with non-steroidal anti-inflammatory drugs (NSAIDs) or physical therapeutics
          c.   NSAIDs including aspirin are also effective but can cause gastrointestinal, renal, or allergic problems; COX-2 selective nonsteroidal anti-inflammatory drugs (NSAIDs) such as celecoxib (Celebrex) and rofecoxib (Vioxx) have better safety profiles than nonselective NSAIDs and are becoming the drugs of choice (see section on PAIN)
          d.   Muscle relaxants are no more effective than NSAIDs in relieving low back symptoms and have adverse effects; they are seldom indicated for children and adolescents
          e.   Opioids should be avoided if possible, and if selected, used only for a short time
          f.   For some patients with herniated intervertebral disks, epidural corticosteroids injections provide relief
          g.   The following therapies are not recommended: Long-term oral steroids and colchicine
     2.   **Physical methods**
          a.   Referral for manipulation (manual loading of the spine using short or long leverage methods) may be beneficial
               (1)   Often reserved for patients who have pain for >3 weeks, because half of all patients improve spontaneously without any treatment within this time period
               (2)   Safe and effective for patients if they do NOT have radiculopathy
               (3)   Stop manipulation if there is no symptomatic or functional improvement after 4 weeks
          b.   Self application of heat and cold therapy may provide temporary symptom relief
               (1)   Cold therapy for 20-30 minutes several times a day for first 24 hours
               (2)   Topical heat 20-30 minutes several times a day after first day
          c.   Massage therapy has not been well studied; preliminary results have been promising
          d.   The following are ineffective: Traction, diathermy, ultrasound, biofeedback, shoe lifts, transcutaneous electrical nerve stimulation, acupuncture, back corsets, back belts
     3.   **Activity**
          a.   For most patients, bed rest is not needed; prolonged bed rest may have debilitating consequences
          b.   For patients with severe limitations, 2-4 days of bed rest may be beneficial
          c.   Low-stress, aerobic exercise (walking, riding bike, swimming, and eventually jogging) can be gradually and incrementally started within the first 2 weeks of symptoms; conditioning exercises for trunk muscles are not recommended during the first few weeks of symptoms
          d.   For patients with chronic back pain, intensive exercise reduces pain and improves functioning
     4.   **Surgery** should not be performed for patients with lumbosacral strain and most patients with probable herniated disks within the first 4 months; consider surgery if the patient has any of the following:
          a.   Cauda equina syndrome
          b.   Progressive or severe neurologic deficit
          c.   Persistent neuromotor deficit after 4-6 weeks of nonoperative treatment
          d.   Radicular pain for 4-6 weeks (surgery is elective); even patients with clinical findings of nerve root dysfunction due to disk herniation may recover activity tolerance within one month; no research has found that delaying surgery for one month worsens outcomes

5. **Patient education**
    a. Discuss the natural history of the disorder; typically patients make a slow but complete recovery with conservative therapy, but problems often recur
    b. Explain that diagnostic tests and special therapies are not needed unless red flags are present or symptoms markedly worsen or persist
    c. Teach patient to minimize stress to the back (see table that follows)

STRATEGIES TO MINIMIZE STRESS TO THE BACK

- Avoid jerky, hurried movements when lifting
- Lift with legs by straddling the load; bend knees to pick up load; keep back straight (do not bend back)
- Keep objects close to the body at navel level when lifting
- Avoid twisting, bending, reaching while lifting
- Avoid prolonged sitting
- Change positions often while sitting
- A soft support at small of back, armrests to support some body weight, a slight recline in chair back may make sitting more comfortable
- Firm mattress/bed board, lying supine with hips and knees flexed on pillows is beneficial when sleeping

---

G. Prevention of further back problems
    1. Discuss that low back pain, like other chronic conditions, will get worse unless preventive measures are taken
    2. Exercises to condition specific trunk muscles can be added a few weeks after acute symptoms; encourage patient to do exercises such as partial sit-ups or extension exercises such as lying prone and lifting legs off floor or upper torso off floor for at least 5 minutes a day
    3. Instruct patient in proper lifting, sleeping position, and body mechanics (see table in V.B.5.)
    4. Weight loss and smoking cessation may be beneficial

H. Follow Up
    1. Re-evaluate patients with severe pain which does not improve in 24 hours
    2. If patient is in moderate pain, re-evaluate in 7-10 days
    3. For patients with mild pain, re-evaluate in 4-6 weeks; instruct patient to return sooner if neurological symptoms worsen or bowel/bladder dysfunction occurs
    4. Children with spondylolysis should be followed at least yearly to rule out spondylolisthesis

LOWER EXTREMITY PAIN, OVERUSE INJURIES

I. Definition: Acute or chronic discomfort or pain in the foot, leg, or hip due to overuse and repetitive stress (also see sections ANKLE SPRAIN and KNEE INJURY, ACUTE)

II. Pathogenesis: Overuse injuries are a result of extrinsic factors such as improper footwear and poor athletic training and intrinsic factors such a structural abnormalities, malalignment, or poor flexibility

    A. Growing pains: Etiology is unknown; possibly involves edema of muscle bodies within tight fascial sheaths during periods of activity or overuse

    B. Shin splints: Microtears and inflammation of the sites of origin of the muscles originating from the shaft of the tibia; often due to overactivity

    C. Stress fractures are due to repetitive forces being applied to the lower leg during strenuous activity that causes the bony architecture to exceed a given threshold; a malaligned lower leg may be a predisposing factor

    D. Osgood-Schlatter disease
        1. Degeneration of the tibial tubercle at the insertion site of the quadriceps ligament
        2. Associated with overuse and rapid growth, particularly during adolescence
        3. Result of repetitive, microstress fractures

E. Patellofemoral pain syndrome (PFPS) is due to one or both of the following:
   1. Mild malalignment of the extensor mechanism of the knee
   2. Repetitive microtrauma from overuse

F. Chondromalacia patellae is due to degeneration of the cartilage on the articular surface of the patella; overuse and malalignment of the lower leg predispose individuals to this condition

G. Iliotibial band syndrome is caused by overuse and excessive friction between the iliotibial band and the lateral femoral condyle, resulting in inflammation; related to change in footwear, increase in running schedule, or prolonged downhill running

H. Osteochondrosis includes a group of conditions in which degeneration or aseptic necrosis of bone and overlying cartilage occurs at the ossification center and is followed by recalcification; conditions include the following:
   1. Legg-Calvé-Perthes disease results from compromise of the vascular supply to the femoral capital epiphysis; disorder may be idiopathic or due to one of following: Slipped capital femoral epiphysis, trauma, steroid use, sickle cell crisis, congenital dislocation of the hip
   2. Osteochondritis dissecans involves degeneration of bone and cartilage at the articular surface of the knee as a result of fatigue injury or a disruption of blood supply to the bone

I. Slipped capital femoral epiphysis is a disorder of the growth and development of the upper femur due to a sudden or gradual dislocation of the head of the femur from its neck and shaft at the upper epiphyseal plate level; may be associated with endocrinopathies and heredity

J. Tendonitis occurs from a direct blow or overuse with repetitive overloads or faulty technique; tendon ruptures may occur while exercising or with trauma

K. Bursitis may be caused by acute trauma, contusion over bursae, overuse, or acute or chronic intra-articular inflammation (Baker's cyst)

L. Plantar fasciitis results from small tears near the origin of the plantar fascia and causes foot pain, particularly on dorsiflexion of toes or when taking first steps in the morning (see section on PLANTAR FASCIITIS)

M. Injuries from acute trauma such as sprains, fractures, tenosynovitis, subluxations, dislocations, ligament injuries, etc. occur (see sections on ANKLE SPRAINS and KNEE INJURY, ACUTE)

N. Other important causes of lower extremity pain include rheumatoid arthritis, osteomyelitis, neoplasms, fractures, sprains, fibromyalgia, sickle cell anemia, septic arthritis, thyroid disorders, and conditions with psychosocial origins

III. Clinical Presentation

A. Growing pains
   1. Most common in children 3-5 years old or 8-12 years old
   2. Usually bilateral and intermittent with deep, aching pain or restlessness that spares the joints; pain typically resolves in 12-24 months
   3. Commonly occurs at night with resolution by morning

B. Shin splints
   1. Usually do not occur before age 10
   2. Most often develop in persons who undergo exercise and are not properly conditioned, do not warm up properly, run on hard or uneven surfaces, wear improper shoes, and/or have anatomical abnormalities
   3. Achy pain over the medial tibia that increases with exercise and improves with rest
   4. Tenderness over the medial tibia; may also have warmth

C. Stress fractures of the lower extremities (metatarsal, tibial, fibular, femoral, and pelvic); most fractures heal in approximately 4-12 weeks
   1. Metatarsal stress fractures typically involve the second and third metatarsals and are common in athletes who are frequently on their feet
   2. Tibial stress fractures occur primarily in athletes
      a. Fractures most often occur in distal third of bone; fractures in the middle third of the tibia are of more concern because they are prone to nonunion

        b.   Initially the pain occurs at the start of running activity and resolves with rest; eventually the pain lasts longer after running and finally persists even at rest

        c.   Diffuse tenderness over medial aspect of tibia is typical

3.   Fibular stress fractures are found primarily in runners; symptoms are similar to those found in tibial stress fractures

4.   Femoral neck stress fractures occur primarily in long-distance runners and dancers

        a.   Pain occurs in the groin, initially with activity and ultimately also at rest

        b.   May result in long-term disability; complications include avascular necrosis, non-union, varus deformity, and bone displacement

5.   Pelvic stress fractures are most common in long-distance runners

        a.   Pain occurs in the inguinal, perineal, or adductor region after an increase in training activity

        b.   Patient may be unable to stand unsupported on the affected side

        c.   Healing may take longer than other stress fractures (i.e., 3-5 months)

D.   Osgood-Schlatter disease

1.   Most common in late childhood and adolescence; boys are more commonly affected than girls, although female gymnasts are particularly prone to this disorder

2.   Painful swelling and point tenderness that is localized to the tibial tubercle; resisting knee extension worsens pain

3.   Bilateral involvement occurs in 30% of cases

4.   Occurs with strenuous activity, particularly involving the quadriceps muscles

5.   May have a permanent prominence of the tibial tubercle

6.   Symptoms are usually self-limited and resolve by end of adolescence, but can last for 1-4 years with recurrences

E.   Patellofemoral pain syndrome (PFPS)

1.   Most common complaint in sports medicine clinics, particularly for the running athlete

2.   Females are affected more than males, probably due to females having increased width of the gynecoid pelvis which results in an exaggerated Q angle (see IV.B.7.); also associated with femoral anteversion, external tibial torsion, ankle valgus, and excessive foot pronation

3.   Insidious onset of dull, achy knee pain sometimes associated with clicking or popping of knee on movement; pain is often poorly localized and bilateral

4.   Pain is exacerbated with extended sitting and activity involving knee flexion such as running and climbing and descending stairs

5.   A positive patellar apprehension test (patient experiences pain when trying to contract the patella by tightening the quadriceps) is often present

6.   Knee is stable without swelling and erythema

7.   May lead to chondromalacia patellae and patellofemoral degenerative arthritis in adulthood

F.   Chondromalacia patellae

1.   Occurs mainly in adults, infrequent incidence in adolescents

2.   Diffuse pain especially with climbing stairs or getting up from a squatting position

3.   Usually has a greater degree of malalignment than occurs with PFPS

G.   Iliotibial band syndrome: Typically involves mild pain over lateral side of knee

H.   Osteochondrosis of the femoral head

1.   Legg-Calvé-Perthes disease is a serious disorder that is most common in males aged 4-8 years

        a.   Limp may be presenting complaint

        b.   Pain often is minimal, intermittent, and referred to medial aspect of knee

        c.   Limitation of internal rotation and abduction of the femur is often present

2.   Osteochondritis dissecans presents predominantly in boys 14-16 years

        a.   Knee pain and tenderness over the distal femur are common complaints

        b.   Snapping, giving way of the knee, and crepitus are typical

I.   Slipped capital femoral epiphysis

1.   Condition is a surgical emergency and requires immediate nonweight-bearing status to prevent further slippage

2.   Commonly affects sedentary, obese male adolescents

3.   Limp and varying degrees of achy pain in the groin or referred pain in the knee are typical

4.   May have sudden dislocation of the head of the femur resulting in severe pain with associated inability to bear weight or gradual dislocation resulting in increasing dull pain

5.   Abduction, internal rotation, and flexion of the hip are the movements most limited

6. Most cases are stable with a good prognosis if diagnosed early
7. Unstable cases have a poorer prognosis because of high risk of avascular necrosis

J. Tendonitis and tendon ruptures
1. Common sites: Achilles tendon (above its insertion into the calcaneus), tibialis posterior (behind medial malleolus), tibialis anterior (dorsum of foot, under the extensor retinaculum), peroneal tendon (behind lateral malleolus, at the insertion into the base of the fifth metatarsal), patella
2. Signs and symptoms include pain with active movement (aggravated in weight bearing) and passive stretching; localized swelling; morning stiffness; and possibly swelling or thickening in the tendon
3. Achilles tendonitis is a common example and presents with pain on palpation of tendon and pain which is worse with active stretching and plantar flexion against resistance; tenderness is worse with hill running
4. Patients with tendon ruptures such as Achilles have a sudden onset of shooting pain in calf
   a. Pain is followed by weakness in leg and inability to stand or walk on toes
   b. Signs include swelling, ecchymosis over the posterior aspect of the leg and heel, gap in tendon (approximately 5 cm proximal to its insertion), absence of normal plantar reflex, absence of active plantar flexion with good strength, and a positive Thompson test (with patient prone, flex the affected leg 90° at knee and squeeze calf; if foot doesn't move, the tendon is ruptured)

K. Bursitis
1. Typically has swelling and pain over respective bursae (prepatellar, infrapatellar, and anserine bursae)
2. May be associated with a Baker's cyst
3. Because there usually is no joint involvement, range of motion is not limited

IV. Diagnosis/Evaluation

A. History
1. Inquire about mode of onset, duration, frequency, location, and characteristics of pain; night pain or pain that wakes the patient from sleep is a possible indicator of a malignant process
2. Question about discomfort in areas above and below the stated location of pain
3. Ask about joint pain, especially without a history of trauma, as joint pain is often related to rheumatologic diseases and needs to be ruled out
4. Query patient about recent trauma involving the lower leg
   a. Determine how injury occurred
   b. Ask patient to specifically describe the position and movement of his/her leg during the trauma
5. Inquire about a history of a fever, limp, joint stiffness, joint redness, grinding, or any audible popping or snapping sound
6. Inquire about exercise without pretraining, change in intensity or duration of exercise, recent viral infections, previous musculoskeletal problems, or repetitive activity
7. Ask about medication use, particularly steroid use, and recent immunizations such as rubella
8. Inquire about recent infections and family history of musculoskeletal problems, autoimmune diseases, and sickle cell disease
9. Inquire about self-treatments and what aggravates and relieves pain
10. Perform a review of systems to rule-out systemic disease

B. Physical Examination
1. Assess vital signs, as increased temperature may point to a systemic disease
2. Observe gait
3. Observe for misalignment of bones such as femoral anteversion and external tibial torsion
4. Observe for signs of trauma, development of muscles, deformities, swelling, and erythema
5. May need to measure limb length
6. Compare opposite limb for swelling, muscle wasting, color, mobility, strength, pulses, and sensation
7. Determine quadriceps angle (Q angle) if PFPS and chondromalacia patellae are suspected (see Figure 17.23) QA

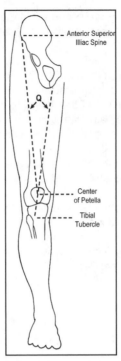

Figure 17.23: Measurement of Q-Angle or the Patellofemoral Angle

Q angle is measured as the angle between a line drawn from the center of the patella to the anterior superior iliac spine and a line drawn from the center of the patella to the tibial tubercle. Average Q angle is 10-13° in males and 15-18° in females. Any angle less than or greater than average angles may be associated with PFPS.

8. Palpate limb and joints for tenderness, swelling, and warmth
9. Perform range of motion of affected joints, noting any limitation in movement, crepitus, and tenderness
10. Assess muscle strength (distal weakness is often due to a neurological problem and proximal weakness is often due to a muscular problem)
11. Evaluate joint stability
12. Assess hamstring flexibility by having patient lie on back with hips flexed to 90° and then extend leg; failure to extend knee completely indicates hamstring tightness and may be a contributing factor in the extremity pain
13. If tendon rupture is suspected, perform the Thompson test (see III.J.4.b.)
14. Assess peripheral vascular status by palpating pulses and determining capillary refill time distal to site of pain
15. Perform a focused neurological examination of the affected extremity, assessing for sensation and deep tendon reflexes; observe patient walking on toes, heels, and hopping on one foot
16. A complete physical examination is often needed to rule out rheumatologic diseases

C. Differential Diagnosis (see conditions listed under Pathogenesis, II.A.-N.); other conditions include the following:
1. Toxic synovitis is an acute inflammatory reaction of the hip joint with unknown etiology
   a. Signs and symptoms resemble those found in patients with Legg-Calvé-Perthes, juvenile rheumatoid arthritis, or slipped capital femoral epiphysis; may need to order CBC, sedimentation rate, and x-rays to rule-out these more serious conditions
   b. Most common cause of limping and hip pain in children <10 years
   c. Often follows a viral upper respiratory infection
   d. Self-limited, unilateral hip or groin pain of insidious or acute onset; child may refuse to walk because of pain
   e. Hip is often held in flexion, abduction, and external rotation positions
   f. Symptoms usually persist no longer than one week with bed rest and analgesics; in rare cases, avascular necrosis of the femoral head may be a complication
2. Septic arthritis often involves abrupt onset of fever, malaise, pain, and a tense, hot joint effusion
3. Inflammatory arthritis presents with warm, swollen, tender joints
4. Osteomyelitis commonly has extremity pain along with systemic signs of infectious disease such as fever and a septic appearance

5. Neoplasms are rare causes of limb pain; usually the pain is deep and "boring" and patient has systemic complaints such as weight loss and fever
6. Acute injuries due to trauma (see sections on ANKLE SPRAIN and KNEE INJURY)

D. Diagnostic Tests
   1. If there is suspicion of systemic or infectious disease, or if pain has a longer duration than expected, is not relieved by common therapies, or is more intense than usually expected, the following tests may be helpful
      a. CBC
      b. Erythrocyte sedimentation rate
      c. Sickle cell preparation or hemoglobin electrophoresis
   2. Consider rheumatologic studies for chronic pain
   3. X-rays are usually ordered for the following:
      a. Pain due to trauma
      b. Suspected pathologic fractures, tumors, or metabolic defects
      c. Pain lasting longer than 4-6 weeks
      d. Any history of swelling
   4. Bone scan is often ordered if stress fractures or osteomyelitis is suspected
   5. Diagnostic tests are usually ordered for suspected common causes of extremity pain:
      a. Growing pains: None usually needed
      b. Shin splints: Order x-ray or bone scan if uncertain about diagnosis
      c. For suspected tibial and fibular stress fractures, x-rays (AP, lateral, and both oblique views of leg) are usually ordered; x-rays may be negative in early stages; technetium-99m bone scans and MRI are most helpful
      d. Osgood-Schlatter disease: None usually needed; may order x-ray to rule out other conditions or if diagnosis is uncertain; x-rays will reveal changes in the tibial tuberosity
      e. PFPS: Order x-rays if pain lasts longer than 4-6 weeks
      f. Chondromalacia patellae: Order knee x-rays which include a tangential or sunrise view to look for lateral subluxation of the patella
      g. Iliotibial band syndrome: None usually needed
      h. Legg-Calvé-Perthes disease and osteochondritis dissecans: Order x-rays (anteroposterior and frog-leg lateral pelvis), bone scan, or magnetic resonance imaging
      i. Slipped capital femoral epiphysis: Order x-rays
      j. Tendonitis: none usually needed
      k. Bursitis
         (1) Arthrography is ordered to definitively diagnose a Baker's cyst; otherwise no tests are needed
         (2) If there is swelling, warmth, erythema, and tenderness in the bursa, aspirate fluid from bursa and examine with a Gram's stain and send sample for leukocyte count and culture

V. Plan/Management

A. Growing pains: Symptomatic treatment with heat, massage, and acetaminophen (Tylenol) 5-10 mg/kg/dose every 4-6 hours

B. Shin splints
   1. Rest: Unless the pain is severe, the athlete does not need to completely stop exercising but needs to reduce intensity and duration of exercise
   2. Ice should be applied to reduce swelling and inflammation
   3. Anti-inflammatory medication such as naproxen (Naprosyn) 250-500 mg every 6-8 hours
   4. May need to treat concomitant hyperpronation of foot with flexible orthotics or sturdy, well-fitting footwear
   5. Instruct patient to run on soft, flat surfaces; begin a program of pre-activity conditioning exercises

C. Stress fractures
   1. Consider referral to orthopedic surgeon for patients who have fractures that have a potential to result in delayed union or nonunion and bone displacement (i.e., tibial stress fractures in middle third anterior cortex, femoral neck stress fractures, pelvic stress fractures)
   2. Initial treatment is rest until there is no longer point tenderness on palpation or pain with activity (usually takes 6-8 weeks for tibial and fibular fractures to resolve; whereas femoral neck fractures and pelvic stress fractures take much longer)
   3. Ice is helpful in tibial and fibular fractures

4. Anti-inflammatory medication may relieve pain
5. Usually fractures heal without casting or surgery
6. Activities such as biking and swimming typically produce less pain and help to maintain conditioning
7. In female athletes, obtain a menstrual history, looking for amenorrhea which is associated with osteopenia and a higher incidence of stress fractures

D. Osgood-Schlatter disease: Rest, ice, quadriceps strengthening exercises, hamstring stretching exercises, and limited use of anti-inflammatory medication

E. PFPS
1. Modify activities to avoid full flexion of the knee and stress on the patellofemoral joint
2. After a brief period of rest, ice, and NSAIDs, begin stretching and strengthening program for quadriceps muscles (perform three sets of 10 repetitions each day during the acute phase)
   a. Quadriceps setting: Patient lies supine with affected knee fully extended, dorsiflexes foot, then tightens the thigh muscles or pushes the thigh into the floor
   b. Straight leg raise: Patient sits on floor, leans back on elbows with one leg fully extended and the other leg flexed to 90°; the extended leg is raised until it is parallel with the thigh of the flexed leg and held in this position for 5 seconds
   c. Terminal-arc extension: Patient lies on floor with knees in about 20° of flexion over a rolled towel of about 6 inches in diameter; patient then extends knee fully and holds for 5 seconds
   d. After the acute phase, progressive resistance with ankle weights should be initiated
   e. Encourage flexibility exercises as well
3. Consider flexible orthotics for malalignment of lower extremities
4. For exacerbations, use ice and anti-inflammatory medication
5. Teach that pain tends to be chronic with exacerbations and remissions, but pain can be controlled; swimming or walking are better sports to participate in than running, basketball, and volleyball

F. Chondromalacia patellae: Plan is similar to treatment for PFPS (see above)

G. Iliotibial band syndrome: Rest for approximately 1-2 weeks (may take as long as 6 weeks), ice, limited use of NSAIDs, and gradual resumption of full activities with rehabilitation (quadriceps strengthening exercises); consider one-eighth-inch lateral heel wedge

H. Legg-Calvé-Perthes disease and osteochondritis dissecans: Refer to orthopedic surgeon

I. Slipped capital femoral epiphysis: Refer to orthopedic surgeon

J. Tendonitis and tendon ruptures
1. Initial treatment includes rest, ice, NSAIDs, and gentle stretching exercises
2. Early referral to a physical therapy program to improve flexibility, resolve strength deficits, and correct foot biomechanical problems is recommended
3. Heel lifts or orthotics may be helpful for tendonitis about the ankle
4. Refer patients with tendon ruptures to an orthopedist

K. Bursitis
1. Rest (couple days to weeks), ice for 24 hours, and limited use of NSAIDs
2. Aspirate tense, inflamed bursa or Baker's cyst to relieve pressure and pain
3. Consider injecting corticosteroid solution if infection has been ruled-out or injecting a local anesthetic such as lidocaine
4. Apply a bulky, compressive dressing for protection and comfort
5. If a bacterial infection is present, prescribe antibiotics; infections tend to be gram-positive cocci and respond well to cephalexin (Keflex) or dicloxacillin (Dynapen)

L. Follow up for extremity pain is variable depending on patient's problem

PLANTAR FASCIITIS

I.   Definition: Overuse injury of the plantar fascia (the thickened fibrous aponeurosis that originates from the medial tubercle of the calcaneus and runs forward to form the longitudinal foot arch; this structure maintains integrity of foot function and serves as a major shock absorber)

II.   Pathogenesis: Caused by collagen degeneration that results from repetitive microtears of the plantar fascia

III. Clinical presentation

      A.   Risk factors
           1.   Overuse (most common) from running or other weight-bearing activities
           2.   Anatomic conditions: Pes planus (flat feet), pes cavus (high arches), overpronation, discrepancy in leg length, excessive lateral tibial torsion, and excessive femoral anteversion
           3.   Functional factors: Tightness and weakness in the gastrocnemius, soleus, Achilles tendons, and intrinsic foot muscles
           4.   Obesity may be a predisposing factor

      B.   Classic sign is heel pain that occurs with first steps in the morning and resolves or lessens with activities but then returns over the course of the day

      C.   Point tenderness at the anteromedial region of the calcaneus that worsens with passive dorsiflexion of the toes or when patient stands on tips of toes is characteristic

      D.   Heel spurs may or may not be present

      E.   Condition is usually self-limited, but resolution of symptoms may take 6-18 months

IV.   Diagnosis/Evaluation

      A.   History
           1.   Determine onset, severity, and characteristics of pain
           2.   Question about possible risk factors such as athletic activity, frequent and prolonged standing on feet, history of anatomic problems of the structures and muscles of the feet
           3.   Inquire about success of current and previous treatments
           4.   Determine degree to which pain is interfering in activities of daily living

      B.   Physical Examination
           1.   Inspect feet and legs for anatomic abnormalities
           2.   Palpate foot; tenderness is typically along the medial plantar aspect of foot, about 3 finger breadths distal to posterior heel
           3.   Passively dorsiflex toes; this technique typically elicits pain
           4.   Ask patient to stand on toes which usually produces pain

      C.   Differential Diagnosis
           1.   Entrapment syndromes such as tarsal tunnel syndrome; results in radiating, burning pain and paresthesia
           2.   Calcaneal fractures and calcaneal stress fractures; history includes trauma or overuse; pain may be similar or more intense than pain related to plantar fasciitis; x-rays are abnormal
           3.   Paget's disease; anatomic deformities such as bowed tibia or kyphosis are usually observable
           4.   Calcaneal apophysitis; typically occurs in adolescents and causes posterior heel pain
           5.   Soft tissue causes
                a.   Fat pad syndrome; atrophy of the heel pad may be visible
                b.   Heel bruise; patient has a history of trauma
                c.   Bursitis; swelling and erythema of the heel usually occur
                d.   Tendonitis; pain occurs with resisted motion
                e.   Plantar fascia rupture; pain is acute and knifelike; ecchymosis may be present
           6.   Neuropathy secondary to diabetes; paresthesia is usually present
           7.   Arthritides; systemic signs of joint pain and swelling
           8.   Tumors present with deep bone pain and other constitutional symptoms

D. Diagnostic Tests: X-rays and additional tests are rarely needed unless there is suspicion of tumors or other serious conditions

V. Plan/Management

A. Rest and correction of the problems that place the patient at risk for plantar fasciitis are recommended initially

B. A stretching, flexibility, and strengthening exercise program should be started after the initial resting phase (see figure 17.24)

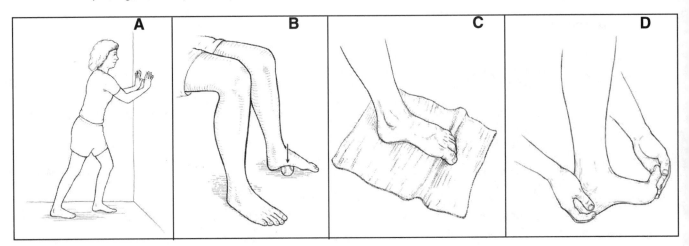

Figure 17.24: Stretching, Flexibility, and Strengthening Exercises
(A) Stretch calf muscles by performing wall exercises; (B) stretch foot muscles by rolling foot arch over a tennis ball; (C) strengthen intrinsic muscles of foot with towel curls; (D) strengthen intrinsic muscles of foot by dorsiflexing toes

C. Footwear
1. In some patients, simply changing shoes is all that is needed; shoes that are too small or worn often aggravate symptoms
2. Over-the-counter arch supports may be beneficial but simply taping the arch may be less expensive, but equally effective
3. Custom orthotics and heel cups are useful for some patients

D. Night splints may be tried to maintain the patient's ankle in a neutral position overnight

E. Nonsteroidal anti-inflammatory drugs may or may not be helpful (see section on PAIN for dosing)

F. Ice applied as a ice massage, ice bath, or an ice pack often relieves pain

G. Iontophoresis which uses electric impulses to drive topical corticosteroids into the soft tissue structures may be used as adjunct therapy

H. Cortisone injections may be prescribed in intractable cases

I. Surgical debridement of affected tissue is indicated for the most recalcitrant cases

J. Patient education: Suggest that patient avoid flat shoes, barefoot walking, and lose weight if obesity is a problem

K. Follow Up
1. Return evaluation is not needed if symptoms abate
2. Consider follow-up in 2-4 weeks for patients who continue to have pain or sooner if symptoms worsen
3. If no improvement occurs after six weeks, refer to podiatric foot and ankle surgeon

RHEUMATOID ARTHRITIS, JUVENILE

I. Definition: A chronic, systemic, inflammatory disease which primarily affects joints but often has generalized manifestations

II. Pathogenesis

    A. Autoimmune disorder of unknown etiology, associated with various factors: Inflammatory response mechanisms, immune system responses, bone resorption mechanism, endogenous hormonal response, neuronal response mechanics, and genetic predisposition (many patients have genetic marker HLA-DR4)

    B. Inflammation of synovial membranes results in panus or thickened synovium which adheres to articular cartilage and later erodes cartilage and underlying bone; adhesions develop between opposing joint surfaces and/or cysts grow

III. Clinical Presentation

    A. Juvenile rheumatoid arthritis (JRA)
        1. Criteria for diagnosing juvenile rheumatoid arthritis (JRA) (see following table)

DIAGNOSTIC CRITERIA FOR CLASSIFICATION OF JUVENILE RHEUMATOID ARTHRITIS (JRA)

- Age of onset less than 16 years
- Arthritis of one or more joints, defined as swelling or effusion or the presence of 2 or more of following signs: Limitation of range of motion, tenderness or pain in motion, increased heat
- Duration of disease is 6 weeks to 3 months
- Type of onset of disease during first 4-6 months classified as:
    ✓ Oligoarthritis or Pauciarthritis: 4 joints or fewer
    ✓ Polyarthritis: 5 or more joints
    ✓ Systemic disease: Arthritis with intermittent fever, light salmon-colored rash, extra-articular manifestations
- Exclusion of other forms of juvenile arthritis

Adapted from Cassidy, J.T., Levinson, J.E., Bass, J.C., Baum, J., Brewer, E.J. Jr., Fink, C.W., et al. (1986). A study of classification criteria for diagnosing juvenile rheumatoid arthritis. *Arthritis and Rheumatology, 29*, 274.

        2. In children, the mean age of onset is 1-3 years old
        3. Approximately 30% of children have severe long-term functional limitations
        4. Chief complaints are gait disturbance, joint swelling, and morning stiffness
        5. Chronic uveitis which can lead to blindness and delays in growth and development is a complication

    B. Systemic JRA (approximately 10% of cases)
        1. Occurs equally in both sexes; no age predilection
        2. Associated symptoms may include fever, joint pain, macular rash, and polyarthritis
        3. Some children have pericarditis, pleuritis, hepatomegaly, splenomegaly, or lymphadenopathy
        4. Often remission occurs within one year

    C. Pauciarticular JRA (approximately 40% of cases)
        1. Onset approximately 2 years; affects females more than males
        2. Involves four or fewer joints; typically affects large joints such as knees, wrists, ankles, elbows
        3. Most children limp or have a gait disturbance
        4. At risk for asymptomatic chronic iridocyclitis which can lead to visual loss if not treated
        5. Prognosis is excellent

    D. Polyarticular JRA (approximately 50% of cases)
        1. Typically presents with multiple symmetric involvement of joints or hands, feet, cervical spine, temporomandibular joint, and sternoclavicular joint
        2. May have short duration of systemic symptoms
        3. Many children (approximately 50-60%) do **not** have permanent joint disability

IV.	Diagnosis/Evaluation

    A.	History
1.	Exactly determine duration, location, and characteristics of pain, tenderness, inflammation, and morning stiffness
2.	Question about systemic symptoms such as weight loss, fever, and fatigue
3.	Inquire about associated symptoms such as nodules, eye pain, or conjunctivitis
4.	Ask about past medical history and medication use; comorbid conditions may be exacerbated by RA or by its treatment (infection, renal insufficiency, cardiovascular disease, chronic pulmonary disease, peptic ulcer disease, lymphoproliferative disease, and mental illness)
5.	Inquire about family medical history
6.	Specifically determine degree of limitation in patient's activities of daily living

    B.	Physical Examination
1.	Measure vital signs
2.	In children, assess growth and development; plot height and weight
3.	Count number of swollen joints, noting bilateral symmetry of joint involvement
4.	Check for various deformities of the hand such as swan-neck deformity, mallet finger, Boutonnière deformity
5.	Carefully palpate joints noting tenderness, temperature, and swelling
6.	Apply traction maneuvers to determine joint stability
7.	Assess muscular strength, particularly grip strength
8.	A complete physical examination is often needed because of systemic problems such as pleurisy, pericarditis, splenomegaly

    C.	Differential Diagnosis (see section on JOINT PAIN)
1.	Reiter's syndrome
2.	Systemic lupus erythematosus
3.	Gouty arthritis, gonococcal arthritis, psoriatic arthritis
4.	Lyme disease
5.	Acute rheumatic fever
6.	Ulcerative colitis and Crohn's disease
7.	Leukemia
8.	Serum sickness
9.	Hypothyroidism
10.	Sleep disturbance or depression

    D.	Diagnostic Tests
1.	Baseline laboratory information in patients suspected of RA includes CBC with differential, erythrocyte sedimentation rate, urinalysis, rheumatoid factor titer, and C-reactive protein
2.	Before initiating any drugs it is important to get the following: CBC, electrolytes, serum creatinine, liver function tests, hepatic panel, urinalysis, stool guaiac, and radiographs of affected joints
3.	In selected patients, consider ordering the following:
    a.	Synovial fluid analysis to rule out other diseases; may need repeated during disease flares to rule-out septic arthritis
    b.	X-rays of selected joints; limited diagnostic value early in disease, but helpful in establishing a baseline to periodically monitor progression and response to therapy
    c.	Additional serological studies such as antinuclear antibodies (ANAs) and serum hemolytic complement (CH50) may be needed to rule-out other diseases

V.	Plan/Management: Goals are to reduce inflammation, relieve pain, preserve joint function, prevent further disease progression, and preserve ability to perform daily activities

    A.	Initially, all children are treated by specialists; consultation is also needed when patients have exacerbations or flares of their symptoms

    B.	In children, a referral to an ophthalmologist should be made at the time of diagnosis of JRA and then periodically

    C.	Patient education includes discussion of chronicity of disease and ways to decrease exacerbations and prevent deformities; early referrals to a physical therapist and occupational therapist are recommended
1.	Maintain ideal body weight
2.	Exercise with emphasis on joint extension (physical therapy is always helpful)

3. Receive adequate rest with naps; balance rest therapy with an exercise plan that includes stretching, strengthening, and endurance
4. Perform correct body mechanics
5. Always use large joints, such as shoulders or hands, rather than fingers to carry pail of water, etc.
6. In children, management of behavior is important; parents should avoid overprotection
7. Tell patients about the Arthritis Foundation's educational resources and Web site (www.arthritis.org)

D. General management program
1. Prescribe splints and protheses to protect joints, to keep in functional position, and to reduce pain
2. Hot and cold therapy, ultrasound, electrical stimulation with transcutaneous nerve stimulator are often beneficial
3. Visual imagery, massage, acupuncture, and hypnosis may be helpful
4. Treat pain effectively because it limits joint use, interferes with ability to exercise, and is associated with depression and insomnia (see V.E.1., V.E.2.)
5. Screen and, if necessary, provide early treatment for depression and insomnia

E. Drug therapy
1. Nonsteroidal anti-inflammatory drugs (NSAIDs) are recommended for mild cases of JRA. NSAIDs provide symptomatic relief, but do not prevent joint damage; prescribe one of the following:
   a. Naproxen (Naprosyn) 10 mg/kg/day in 2 divided doses. Available in suspension 125 mg/5 mL
   b. Ibuprofen (Children's Motrin): 30-40 mg/kg/day in 3-4 divided doses; available 100 mg/5 mL suspension
   c. Tolmetin and choline magnesium trisalicylate are other FDA-approved drugs for JRA
   d. COX-2 inhibitors may be beneficial in children who experience gastrointestinal problems or who have adverse effects from NSAIDs such as pseudoporphyria
2. Disease-modifying drugs are used to prevent joint damage; If disease is rapidly progressing or symptoms are moderate or severe, a DMARDs is recommended (specialist consultation is recommended for initial treatment)
   a. Methotrexate (Rheumatrex) is first-line drug (consult specialist for dosage)
      (1) Adolescents should be counseled about teratogenic effects of drug
      (2) Do not administer live vaccines to patients taking this drug
   b. Sulfasalazine (Azulfidine) is sometimes effective, but toxicity may be a problem (hepatotoxicity, leukopenia, hypoimmunoglobulinemia, and gastrointestinal disorders); consult specialist for dosing
   c. Etanercept (Enbrel) is approved by FDA for reducing symptoms and delaying structural damage in patients with moderately to severely active polyarticular-course JRA that is refractory to one or more DMARDs
      (1) Not recommended for children <4 years; patients 4-17 years: 0.4 mg/kg subcutaneous (SC) injection, twice weekly, 72-96 hours apart (maximum 25 mg/dose); patients >17 years: 25 mg SC injection twice weekly, 72-96 hours apart
      (2) Assure that children receive all their immunizations before initiating this drug
      (3) Immunize with varicella in susceptible children and administer varicella zoster immune globulin in exposed children; do not give live vaccine concurrently with this drug
      (4) Patients exposed to varicella should temporarily discontinue the drug
      (5) Infections, neoplastic complications, hematologic complications, and multiple sclerosis-like neurologic diseases have occurred in small numbers of patients
   d. Other agents may be beneficial, particularly for etanercept nonresponders:
      (1) Hydroxychloroquine (Plaquenil), 5 mg/kg/day in divided doses
      (2) Gold sodium thiomalate (consult specialist for dosing)
      (3) Azathioprine (consult specialist for dosing)
      (4) Cyclosporine (consult specialist for dosing)
      (5) Intravenous cyclophosphamide is sometimes effective for patients with severe systemic JRA who have failed all other therapies
3. Oral corticosteroids are used only for severe systemic manifestations; topical corticosteroids may be beneficial in controlling eye problems; intra-articular corticosteroids can relieve pain
4. Disease modifying drugs have adverse effects and need frequent monitoring (see following table, RECOMMENDED MONITORING STRATEGIES)

RECOMMENDED MONITORING STRATEGIES FOR DISEASE MODIFYING AGENTS

Drugs	Toxicities Requiring Monitoring	Baseline Evaluation, Vaccines, & Screening Tests	Monitoring and Screening Tests
Hydroxychloroquine	Macular damage	None unless patient is >40 years or has previous eye disease	Funduscopic and visual fields every 6-12 months
Sulfasalazine	Myelosuppression	CBC, AST or ALT in patients at risk, G6PD	CBC every 2-4 weeks for first 3 months, then every 3 months
Methotrexate	Myelosuppression, hepatic fibrosis, cirrhosis, pulmonary infiltrates or fibrosis	CBC, chest radiography, hepatitis B and C serology in high-risk patients, AST or ALT, albumin, alkaline phosphatase, and creatinine	CBC, platelet count, AST, albumin, creatinine every 4-8 weeks
Gold, intramuscular	Myelosuppression, proteinuria	CBC, platelet count, creatinine, urine dipstick for protein	CBC, platelet count, urine dipstick every 1-2 weeks for first 20 weeks, then at the time of each injection
Gold, oral	Myelosuppression, proteinuria	CBC, platelet count, urine dipstick for protein	CBC, platelet count, urine dipstick for protein every 4-12 weeks
D-penicillamine	Myelosuppression, proteinuria	CBC, platelet count, creatinine, urine dipstick for protein	CBC, urine dipstick for protein every 2 weeks until dosage stable, then every 1-3 months
Azathioprine	Myelosuppression, hepatotoxicity, lympho-proliferative disorders	CBC, platelet count, creatinine, AST or ALT	CBC and platelet count every 1-2 weeks with changes in dosage, and every 1-3 months thereafter
Cyclophosphamide	Myelosuppression, myeloproliferative disorders, malignancy, hemorrhagic cystitis	CBC, platelet count, urinalysis, creatinine, AST or ALT	CBC and platelet count every 1-2 weeks with changes in dosage, then every 1-3 months, urinalysis and urine cytology every 6-12 months
Cyclosporine	Renal insufficiency	CBC, AST or ALT, creatinine, urinalysis, potassium	Creatinine every 2 weeks until dose is stable, CBC, AST or ALT every 3-6 months, potassium periodically
Minocycline	Hepatotoxicity	CBC, urinalysis, creatinine, AST or ALT	CBC, urinalysis, creatinine, AST or ALT every 3-6 months
Leflunomide	Hepatotoxicity, renal insufficiency, immunosuppression	CBC, AST or ALT, urinalysis, creatinine; screen for hepatitis B and C; perform pregnancy test	CBC, AST or ALT every 4-8 weeks
Etanercept	Immunosuppression, hematological abnormalities	CBC; update vaccines before initiating; screen for ANA and DNA antibodies, screen for TB with skin test	CBC every 3-6 months
Infliximab	Lymphoproliferative disorders, immunosuppression	CBC; TB skin test before initiating, screen for ANA and DNA antibodies	CBC every 3-6 months
Anakinra	Immunosuppression, hematological abnormalities	CBC, urinalysis, creatinine, AST or ALT	CBC monthly for first 3 months; then every 3 months up to 1 year; creatinine, AST or ALT periodically

5.   New biologic therapies, in addition to etanercept, are used in adults; their efficacy and safety are being researched in children (see table that follows)

NEW BIOLOGIC THERAPIES	
Drug	**Mechanism of Action**
Leflunomide (Arava)*	DMARD; pyrimidine synthesis inhibition
Etanercept (Enbrel)†	BRM; tumor necrosis factor-α (TNF-α) antagonist
Infliximab (Remicade)‡	BRM; tumor necrosis factor-α (TNF-α) antagonist
Anakinra (Kineret)†	BRM; interleukin-1 (IL-1) receptor antagonist
Adalimumab† (Humira)	BRM; tumor necrosis factor-α (TNF-α) antagonist

* Leflunomide (Arava) is contraindicated in pregnant females and premenopausal females should use birth control
† Etanercept, anakinra, and adalimumab package inserts carry a strong caution on the use of this drug in patients with a history of recurring infections or underlying conditions that may predispose to infection such as poorly controlled diabetes
‡ Infliximab must be administered with methotrexate

F.   Surgery is needed if there is marked structural damage on x-ray, lack of response to medical therapy, or significant pain and loss of function

G.   Follow Up
1.   When initiating new drug therapies, patient should be seen every 1-2 weeks
2.   Interval between follow up visits depends upon patient's condition and monitoring recommendations of medications (see table on RECOMMENDED MONITORING STRATEGIES V.E.4.)
3.   Patients in remission may be seen every 6 months (see table for the American College of Rheumatology criteria)

SCOLIOSIS

I.   Definition: Lateral curvature of the spine; usually thoracic or lumbar spine but may involve cervical spine

II.   Pathogenesis

A.   Etiology is usually unknown or idiopathic; genetic factors are probably involved

B.   Scoliosis can be congenital and caused by anomalous bony development

C.   Scoliosis can be associated with neuromuscular diseases (cerebral palsy), genetic diseases (neurofibromatosis), metabolic diseases (juvenile osteoporosis), infections, trauma, or tumors

III.   Clinical presentation

A.   Present in approximately 3% of children; 10% of these children have scoliosis that requires treatment

B.   Idiopathic scoliosis (65-75% of all cases) can be divided into three types according to age when scoliosis was first noticed
1.   Infantile type occurs in children <3 years, predilection for males, and resolves without treatment
2.   Juvenile type occurs in ages 3-10 years; affects both genders equally, and tends to progress during growth spurts
3.   Adolescent type affects mainly girls and tends to rapidly progress during growth spurts; accounts for the majority of cases of idiopathic scoliosis

C.   Condition is usually painless and discovered on routine physical examination

D.   Scoliotic curves progress less rapidly after skeletal growth is completed

E. Complications:
    1. If untreated, can result in severe deformity of the spinal column
    2. Spinal deformity can impair respiratory and cardiovascular functions as well as limit physical activity and cause pain

IV. Diagnosis/Evaluation

    A. History
        1. Determine onset and duration of any symptoms such as back pain
        2. Ask questions to rule out possible neurologic causes of scoliosis such as muscle weakness, lack of coordination, skin lesions
        3. Explore etiological factors such as family history and medical history of infection, trauma, congenital abnormalities
        4. Inquire about sexual development; onset of menses (end of puberty signals limited growth potential and less likelihood of curve progression)

    B. Physical Examination
        1. Observe gait
        2. Observe posture; evaluate shoulder, scapular, rib, iliac crest, and breast symmetry
        3. Inspect skin for hairy patches, nevi, café au lait spots, dimples, and lipomata
        4. Inspect back
            a. Curve may have one turn ("C curve") or two compensating curves ("S curve")
           b. Closely inspect spinal column as well as ribs to look for deviation and rotation of individual vertebra; increased or decreased thoracic kyphosis or lumbar lordosis may be associated with scoliosis
           c. Perform forward bend test (see Figure 17.25.)

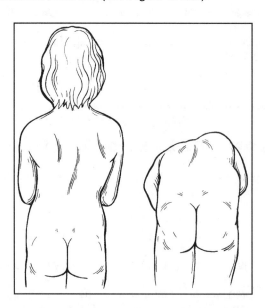

Figure 17.25. Bend Test

Ask patient to bend forward at hips with both palms held at midline; a simple, level-like instrument, the scoliometer, can document the degree of symmetry of the trunk; Prominence of one scapula or one side of rib cage or of the lumbar paraspinous muscles indicates scoliosis

        5. Observe thorax, noting unequal rib prominences and chest asymmetry
        6. Measure leg lengths
        7. Evaluate for secondary sex characteristics; determine Tanner stage (see section in PRECOCIOUS PUBERTY)
        8. Perform complete neurological and musculoskeletal examinations

    C. Differential diagnosis
        1. Important to differentiate functional scoliosis from structural or true scoliosis
           a. Functional or nonstructural scoliosis refers to the appearance of a lateral curve when there is no structural change in the vertebral column and may be due to unequal leg lengths, poor posture, muscle spasm, or herniated discs
           b. Functional scoliosis may eventually become structural if means to prevent progression are overlooked

2. Important to rule-out systemic problems such as neurofibromatosis, cerebral palsy, multiple sclerosis, rickets, tuberculosis, and tumor
3. The following are red flags that suggest the diagnosis of idiopathic scoliosis is unlikely and that a more extensive search is needed
   a. Pain
   b. Left thoracic curve
   c. Marked stiffness
   d. Sudden, rapid progression in a previously stable curve
   e. Extensive progression after patient has attained skeletal maturity
   f. Abnormal neurologic findings
   g. Onset of scoliosis before eight years of age

D. Diagnostic Tests
   1. Limit spinal x-rays to children in whom clinical findings are suggestive of scoliosis of at least 10°; a single, standing posteroanterior radiograph to allow measurement of the curve using the Cobb method or the Risser grading of the iliac apophysis is recommended
   2. X-rays determine degree of curvature and structure of vertebrae
   3. For children who present with red flags (see IV.C.3.), bone scans and/or MRIs may be needed

V. Plan/Management

A. Refer the following children to an specialist: Those with congenital scoliosis or who have curvature on initial examination that is greater than 15°; those with progressive scoliosis as indicated by a change of at least 5°; those with associated diseases such as neuromuscular, metabolic, infectious conditions; or any child if red flags are present

B. Typically, children with mild curves of <25° require no active intervention, but frequent re-evaluations are important; exercises, physical therapy, and chiropractic manipulation are ineffective

C. Children with curves >25° or 30° to 45° are usually given ambulatory brace treatments with rigid spinal instrumentation and an exercise program
   1. Braces prevent progression of curve in about 85% to 90% of cases
   2. Modern braces can usually be worn under the clothing
   3. Counsel patients that braces do not correct scoliosis but rather prevent progression of the curvature
   4. Braces are not recommended for patients who are skeletally mature

D. Surgery is indicated for children who have progressive curves despite brace treatment or for children with curves >40°-45°

E. Follow Up: Serial evaluations should be performed every 4-6 months, and are especially important during rapid growth spurts when progression is most likely

SHOULDER PAIN

I. Definition: Pain in the shoulder that is either acute or chronic

II. Pathogenesis (see figure 17.26 for anatomy of shoulder)

A. Acute shoulder pain
   1. Fractures, dislocations, sprains, separations, and strains are the most common causes
   2. Trauma is usually responsible

B. Chronic shoulder pain
   1. Subacromial impingement (SI) syndrome or rotator cuff disorders are common
      a. The rotator cuff, the dynamic stabilizer of the glenohumeral joint, is composed of four muscles--the subscapularis, the supraspinatus, the infraspinatus, and the teres minor, along with their musculotendinous attachments

b. Rotator cuff injury or dysfunction occurs when the space between the undersurface of the acromion and the superior aspect of the humeral head becomes so narrowed that there is impingement of the acromion onto the rotator cuff tendons

c. In the younger patient, SI causes inflammation with subsequent tendinitis and bursitis that occurs during forward shoulder elevation and with repetitive overhead activities

2. Adhesive capsulitis or frozen shoulder, is due to thickening and contraction of the capsule around the glenohumeral joint; typically results from immobility following a shoulder injury or due to a painful stimulus that causes the patient to limit movement

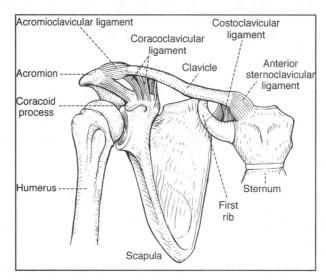

Figure 17.26. Anatomical Structures of the Shoulder Bones and Joints

III. Clinical Presentation: Shoulder pain is one of the most common orthopedic complaints in primary care

A. Fractures
1. Fractures of the clavicle
   a. Most common fracture that occurs in childhood
   b. Mechanisms of injury are usually either a fall on outstretched hand or a direct blow to the shoulder
   c. Considerable force is needed to crack the clavicle in an adult; therefore, if trauma is minor, look for an underlying cause (neoplastic disease, infection)
   d. Patients may have concomitant dislocation of the sternoclavicular joint and disruption of the ligaments of the acromioclavicular joint
   e. Patient usually presents with pain at the fracture site
   f. Patient may avoid moving the arm or may angle head toward the injured side to relax the pull of the trapezius to limit pain
   g. On examination, there is a visible and palpable deformity
2. Fractures of the proximal humerus
   a. Mechanism of injury is usually a fall on an outstretched hand or a direct blow to shoulder
   b. Incidence increases with age and women are twice as likely as men to sustain this injury
   c. Patient typically presents with complaints of pain, tenderness, and swelling in the area of the greater tuberosity
   d. Crepitus may or may not be present
3. Fractures of the scapula
   a. Uncommon fracture that results from a direct blow to the scapular area or from extremely high-force impact elsewhere to the thorax; may be associated with multiple fractures relating to severe trauma
   b. Patient complains of tenderness at fracture site and arm abduction is painful
   c. Fractures are easy to diagnose because the scapula is directly beneath the skin; palpation will detect point tenderness or an obvious deformity

B.	Dislocations make up about 25% of all shoulder injuries, with about 95% being anterior glenohumeral dislocations (following presentation pertains to anterior glenohumeral dislocations)
1.	Occurs when the arm is forcefully elevated and pulled backwards
2.	First-time dislocations are always the result of significant trauma; once glenohumeral instability is present, however, dislocations tend to recur
3.	Patient usually presents with the affected arm in external rotation and abduction; a dimple in the skin beneath the acromion may be present
4.	Shoulder is extremely painful, especially with passive range of motion
5.	Generalized weakness of entire arm may be present; active range of motion may be very difficult due to muscle spasm
6.	Shoulder is grossly deformed; shoulder appears as if deltoid muscle has disappeared; a protrusion inferior to the acromion and lateral to the coracoid (result of the head of the humerus being displaced) is usually apparent

C.	Acromioclavicular (AC) joint sprain and separation
1.	Common among athletes and results from direct blow to the superior aspect of the shoulder or a lateral blow to the deltoid area; infrequently may result from falling onto outstretched hands
2.	Classification of AC joint injuries
a.	Grade I sprain: Complete congruity, or overlap, of the distal clavicle and acromion
b.	Grade II sprain: Incomplete overlap of the clavicle and acromion
c.	Grade III sprain: Clavicle and acromion are completely separated, a result of a complete tear of the AC and coracoclavicular ligaments
d.	Grades IV, V, VI are variations of the completely disrupted AC joint, with the clavicle being displaced posteriorly, superiorly, or inferiorly, respectively
3.	Patients experience point tenderness and swelling directly over the joint
4.	Localized pain with elevation of arm usually occurs
5.	Patients with tears usually have a noticeable bump at the AC joint or what is referred to as a step-off between the acromion and the distal end of the clavicle

D.	Sternoclavicular joint sprain and separation
1.	Anterior sternoclavicular joint separation typically results from motor vehicle accident
a.	Medial end of clavicle is displaced anteriorly or anterosuperiorly with respect to the anterior border of the sternum
b.	Pain occurs primarily with adduction and is often exacerbated when patient is supine
c.	Localized tenderness and deformity are typically present and head may be tilted toward side of injury
2.	Posterior joint separation may be life-threatening due to compression of the trachea and great vessels of the neck

E.	Shoulder strain is a diagnosis of exclusion and is reserved for muscle injury, usually involving the large deltoid muscles

F.	Rotator cuff problems involve subacromial impingement syndrome; impingement syndrome is a general term that includes bursitis, tendinitis, and associated tears of the rotator cuff
1.	The most frequent cause of chronic shoulder pain is injury to the rotator cuff with pain, weakness, and loss of motion usually reported
2.	Patients typically complain of pain over the anterolateral aspect of the shoulder that does not radiate below the elbows
3.	May have a clicking or popping sensation in the affected shoulder
4.	Biceps tendonitis often accompanies syndrome; patient has discrete pain and tenderness in the area of the bicipital groove
5.	Disorder may be primary or secondary impingement
a.	Primary impingement occurs from chronic overuse and degeneration of the tendon; patient complains of anterior shoulder pain
b.	Secondary impingement is due to an underlying problem of instability; patient is typically young and complains of arm heaviness and numbness
6.	Rotator cuff impingement syndrome (and associated tears of the rotator cuff) is usually classified into three stages (see following table); stages II and III do not usually occur in childhood or adolescence

STAGES OF ROTATOR CUFF IMPINGEMENT SYNDROME	
Stage I	• Usually involves patients <25 years of age • Usually results from overuse and most often occurs in athletes, with pain developing after exercise • Pain is dull, aching, and diffuse • Rotator cuff edema and hemorrhage may by present • Process is reversible at this point
Stage II	• Typically occurs in laborers aged 25-40 • Work requires repeated and constant overhead reach for many hours during the day • Occurs both during and after activity • Pain frequently occurs at night, interfering with sleep • Pathologic changes become evident and include fibrosis and irreversible tendon changes
Stage III	• Final stage usually occurs in patients >40 years of age, but may occur to younger patients as a result of trauma • Usually, person has been a laborer or involved in repetitive overhead activities for many years • In addition to the pain described under Stage II, above, additional complaints of stiffness and weakness may be present • Patients present with a long history of shoulder problems • May also present with sudden, severe episode of pain with resultant shoulder disability from an apparently minor recent trauma • Rotator cuff is either partially or completely torn • Damage is irreversible at this stage

G.   Adhesive capsulitis or frozen shoulder occurs more commonly in adults than children
    1.   Pain is often slow in onset and localized near the deltoid insertion
    2.   Patient may have restricted glenohumeral elevation and external rotation; patient may be unable to sleep on affected side

IV.   Diagnosis/Evaluation

A.   History
    1.   Determine patient's age, dominant hand, and work or sports activities
    2.   Ask about the onset (sudden or gradual), duration, location, radiation, and intensity of pain (have patient rate on a scale of 1 to 10 with 1 being no pain at all and 10 being the worst pain the patient has ever experienced) [**Note**: Gradual onset of pain is the hallmark of impingement syndrome]
    3.   Ask what reduces the pain and what makes it worse
    4.   Ask if the shoulder feels loose or unstable; if there is muscle weakness, catching, stiffness, or paresthesias; inquire about swelling or deformity
    5.   Ask about problems with other joints, especially the neck and elbow
    6.   Ask about previous treatments (including diagnostic testing, hospitalizations, surgeries, and pain management)
    7.   Obtain past medical history including medication use and allergies
        a.   Ask about previous surgeries and orthopedic problems
        b.   Obtain complete neurologic history for the upper extremity
        c.   Obtain a complete ROS to detect referred, remote, or nonshoulder sources of symptoms (with a focus on respiratory, cardiovascular, gastrointestinal systems); ask about systemic symptoms including fevers, night sweats, and weight loss
    8.   Determine if the pain hampers normal work and recreational activities
    9.   Important to distinguish if problem is acute or chronic; for acute pain, determine the following:
        a.   Determine whether the onset of pain was related to a single event (macrotrauma) or to a reinjury of a chronically symptomatic joint
        b.   If macrotrauma was involved, ask about the activity or sport being performed at the time of the injury, the position of the arm when injured, and the exact mechanism of the injury. Ask if there was a direct blow to the shoulder or an indirect injury such as falling on the elbow or arm

      c.   If macrotrauma was involved, was there immediate pain, swelling, or deformity?

      d.   If reinjury of a chronically symptomatic joint is suspected, ask what activities were being engaged in when pain started (was the patient lifting overhead, pulling, throwing, or was there no apparent cause for the reinjury?) [**Note**: If no apparent cause, consider systemic arthritis, neoplasm, infection, or cardiac disease]

10.   For chronic pain, determine the following:

      a.   Determine if pain awakens patient from sleep and if lying on the affected shoulder is avoided because of discomfort

      b.   Ask appropriate questions to grade the patient's overuse pain in terms of impact on function (from less to most impact)

            (1)   Grade 1: Pain occurs only after activity (implies early inflammatory activity)

            (2)   Grade 2: Pain during activity but not restricting performance

            (3)   Grade 3: Pain during activity and restricting performance

            (4)   Grade 4: Pain chronic and unremitting, even at rest

B.   Physical Examination (see Figures 17.27 and 17.28 for specific assessment maneuvers); **Note**: Examination of the unaffected shoulder should be performed at each step of the exam for comparison with the involved shoulder

1.   Inspection; patient should be properly disrobed to permit inspection of both shoulders

      a.   Observe how the patient moves and carries shoulders

      b.   Inspect front and back of shoulders for swelling, discoloration, asymmetry, muscle atrophy, scars, abrasions, lacerations, and any venous distention

      c.   Observe the height of the shoulders and scapulae (common for the dominant shoulder to be slightly lower) and observe for deformities

            (1)   Squaring of shoulders occurs with anterior dislocations

            (2)   Scapular winging is associated with shoulder instability and muscle dysfunction

2.   Palpation should be done with patient at rest and with shoulder movement; palpate the following: acromioclavicular and sternoclavicular joints, the cervical spine, the biceps tendon, the anterior glenohumeral joint, coracoid process, acromion, and scapula

      a.   Palpate for point tenderness, snapping, grinding, and bony crepitus

      b.   Palpate the area distal and proximal to the pain location

3.   Assess passive and active (with and without resistance) range of motion: Forward elevation, abduction, external rotation, internal rotation

4.   Perform muscle strength testing as weakness is often both the underlying cause and the result of injury (on a standard scale of 0 to 5, results of muscle testing should be in 4 to 5 range)

5.   Assess for nerve injury

      a.   Sensation in the arm and hand on the affected side should be evaluated

      b.   Muscles that are innervated by the major nerves of the extremity should be examined for motor function

6.   Assess for arterial blood flow

      a.   Assess for circulatory compromise on the affected side

      b.   Color, warmth, and nail bed capillary refill time should be assessed in each finger

      c.   Radial, ulnar, and brachial pulses should be evaluated

7.   In the absence of trauma (i.e., patient denies a precipitating event for the acute onset of shoulder pain), it is important to carefully check the neck, chest, heart, and abdomen for sources of referred pain

8. Perform specific maneuvers (see figures that follow)

MANEUVERS TO ASSESS SHOULDER PAIN

Test	Description	Interpretation
Maneuvers to Test for Rotator Cuff Problems		
Empty Can Test (Drawing A)	• Patient attempts to elevate the arms against resistance while the elbows are extended and the thumbs are pointing downward	• Pain accompanied by weakness in the affected shoulder suggests rotator cuff problems
Neer's Test (Drawing B)	• Place the patient's arm in forced flexion with arm fully pronated; scapula should be stabilized during maneuver to prevent scapulothoracic motion	• Pain with this maneuver suggests subacromial impingement syndrome
Maneuver to Test for Acromioclavicular Joint Disease		
Cross-arm Test (Drawing C)	• Patient raises arm to 90 degrees then actively adducts arm (patient's arm crosses body so that hand grasps contralateral shoulder)	• Pain in the area of acromioclavicular joint suggests a disorder in this area
Maneuver to Test for Glenohumeral Joint Stability		
Apprehension Test (Drawing D)	• Shoulder should be in a neutral position at 90° of abduction. Examiner applies slight anterior pressure to the humerus and externally rotates the arm	• Pain or apprehension about the feeling of impending subluxation or dislocation suggests anterior glenohumeral instability

Figure 17.27

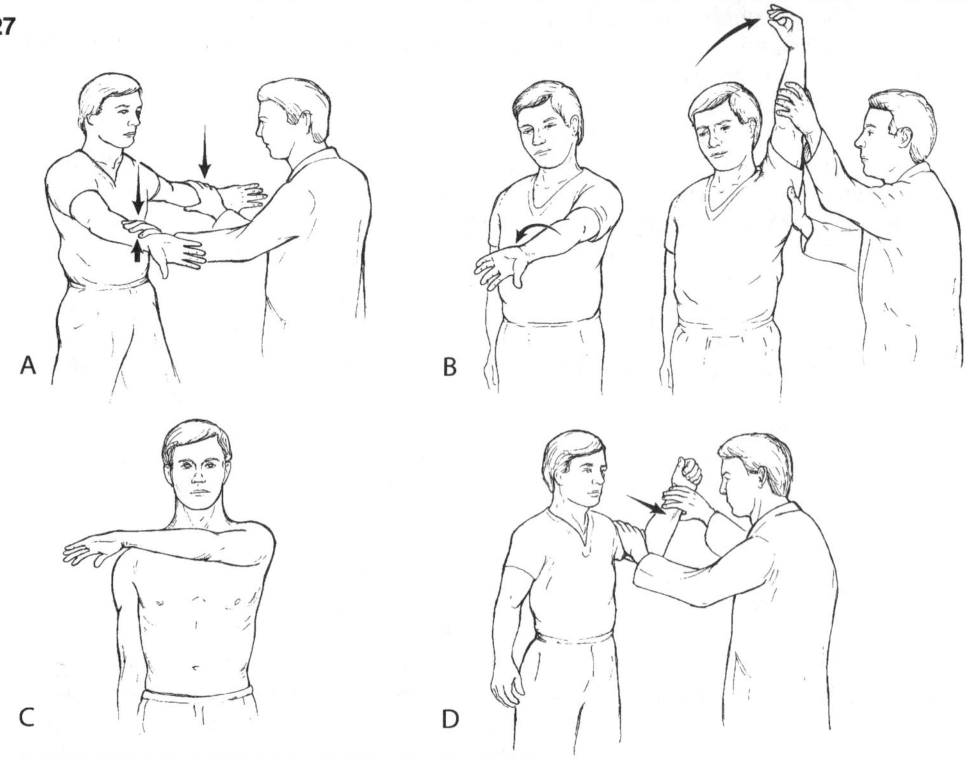

A

B

C

D

MANEUVERS TO ASSESS FOR CERVICAL SPINE PATHOLOGY AND TO TEST ROM

Maneuver to Screen for Cervical Spine Pathology

Head Compression Test (Drawing A)	• With patient sitting on low stool, stand behind patient, lock hands together, and then apply gentle but firm downward pressure on head, using both hands locked together	• Pain localized to neck suggests disk degeneration or facet joint arthritis • Burning pain or pain radiating to involved shoulder suggests nerve root involvement • If test is negative (shoulder pain is not reproduced), continue with exam

Maneuvers to Test Range of Motion

Scratch Test (Drawings B & C)	• Evaluate adduction and internal rotation by having patient place arm and hand behind back and reach toward the opposite scapula with the thumb pointed up • Evaluate abduction and external rotation by having patient place the hand behind the neck and touch the border of the scapula on the opposite side	• Repeat with the unaffected side and compare differences • Adhesive capsulitis reduces range of motion on the affected side
Painful Arc Test (Drawing D)	• Patient begins test with arm held at side, and then lifts arm to position over head. At 45° of abduction, pain is felt when inflamed tissue is forced under the acromion; pain continues until the 120° point on the arc is reached; then, pain subsides as the inflamed tissue passes from beneath the acromion as the arm moves into full abduction	• This pattern of pain strongly supports impingement

Figure 17.28

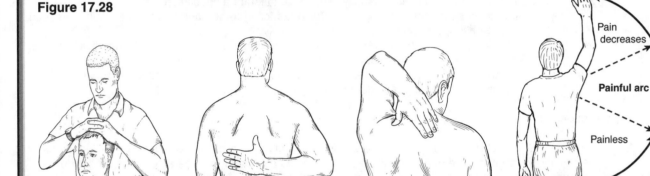

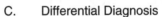

C. Differential Diagnosis
   1. Acute shoulder pain
      a. Necessary to differentiate among intrinsic causes (fracture, dislocation, strains, and sprains) and to determine if pain is being referred from areas such as the chest (myocardial infarction, thoracic outlet syndrome, diaphragmatic irritation), abdomen (gallbladder disease), or cervical spine (cervical spondylosis)
      b. Infection from osteomyelitis or septic arthritis may have an acute or more gradual onset; signs are severe pain, fever, and possibly swelling
   2. Chronic shoulder pain
      a. Septic arthritis, gout, rheumatoid arthritis, cervical radiculopathy, avascular necrosis may mimic impingement syndrome
      b. Malignant (i.e., osteosarcoma in young persons) and benign tumors may have gradual onset of pain

D. Diagnostic Tests
    1. X-rays should be ordered to evaluate acute shoulder injuries
        a. Clavicle fractures: Anteroposterior (AP) view of shoulder; in patients with substantial trauma, also order x-ray of chest
        b. Humerus fractures: AP and lateral views of the humerus
        c. Scapular fractures: AP and axillary or lateral views of the shoulder; order chest film in patient with substantial trauma (rule out co-existing pneumothorax, rib fractures)
        d. Glenohumeral dislocations: AP and axillary views of the shoulder; CT scan may detect subtle dislocations
        e. Acromioclavicular joint sprain and separation: AP view of shoulder; order axillary view if Grade 4 to Grade 6 injuries are suspected
        f. Sternoclavicular joint sprain and separation: This injury is difficult to visualize on plain films; a modified radiographic view, such as a 40° cephalic tilt view, may be needed; a CT scan is often recommended
    2. For patients with chronic shoulder problems, the following diagnostic testing is recommended:
        a. The routine radiograph or x-ray film should be used first before consideration of more sophisticated and expensive studies
        b. The standard views include the AP and lateral views (can reveal basic bony structures but are not helpful in viewing the coracoacromial arch or the glenohumeral joint)
        c. Scapular Y (outlet) view discloses the coracoacromial arch as well as the supraspinatus outlet
        d. West Point axillary view can be used to rule out dislocation and assess for avulsion fractures of the glenoid caused by dislocation
    3. Consider other imaging studies (usually with consultation of a specialist)
        a. Magnetic resonance imaging is helpful in detecting rotator cuff tears, partial cuff tears, cuff degeneration, and chronic tendonitis
        b. Ultrasonography detects complete rotator cuff tears but is less helpful in identifying partial tears; a disadvantage is that the interpretation of this test is operator-dependent
        c. Arthrography is helpful in detecting complete rotator cuff tears or adhesive capsulitis, but is invasive and less useful in detecting partial tears

V. Plan/Management

A. Simple clavicle fractures can be treated by a trained primary care clinician; fractures with evidence of neurovascular compromise or if acromioclavicular joint is displaced more than 1 cm require orthopedic consultation
    1. Patients are often in severe pain and require analgesics
    2. For children <12 years, place the arm in a sling that should be worn during the waking hours for at least the first two weeks or until the child can carry arm without discomfort
    3. For older patients, use a figure 8 strap in addition to a sling for 2-4 weeks
    4. Teach patients to be aware of possible signs and symptoms of neurovascular compromise; advise to avoid contact sports for 3 months
    5. Order a follow-up x-ray in a week to ensure adequate positioning and healing

B. Refer patients with humeral fractures; stable fractures can usually be treated with a shoulder immobilizer to prevent external rotation and abduction; surgical treatment is indicated for complex fractures

C. Simple scapular fractures can be treated by a trained primary care clinician; patients with acromial, neck, and glenoid fractures should be referred to orthopedist; for simple fractures:
    1. Apply ice, order analgesics, and use a sling for comfort
    2. Begin range-of-motion exercises as soon as acute pain resolves (usually within 2 weeks) to avoid a frozen shoulder
    3. Refer patients to a specialist if fractures are unstable or involve the articular site

D. Glenohumeral dislocations can be treated by a trained primary care clinician provided the axillary nerve has not been damaged (perform sensory test over shoulder and deltoid to rule-out)
    1. Treatment involves relocation of the humerus; several techniques are available, but should only be performed by an experienced clinician; Stimson's maneuver is one technique that can be performed
        a. Patient is placed prone on examining table with affected arm hanging over the side with a 5- to 10-pound weight strapped to affected arm
        b. If reduction does not occur within 15 minutes (light analgesia or a muscle relaxant may be helpful), place arm in sling and refer to a specialist

2. Following reduction, immobilize shoulder and elbow, and reassess neurovascular status of arm
3. Obtain postreduction x-rays; if pain persists for more than one week, repeat x-rays and refer to orthopedist
4. Apply ice every 3-4 hours during the first 2-3 days after the injury and order analgesics
5. Range-of-motion exercises should begin as soon as possible (usually within 7-10 days) to prevent frozen shoulder
6. Surgery is often needed for recurrent shoulder dislocations

E. Grade 1 and possibly Grade 2 acromioclavicular joint injuries can be treated by a trained primary care clinician; do not confuse AC joint injuries with shoulder dislocations (with shoulder dislocations the deltoid muscle looks like it has disappeared)
    1. Immobilize arm in sling for 2 days to 2 weeks depending on degree of injury
    2. Apply ice to painful area and give analgesics
    3. As soon as possible, begin pendulum exercises (patient swings arm back and forth, side-to-side, and around); typically, refer to physical therapist
    4. Gradually advance to exercises to strengthen trapezius and deltoid muscles

F. Patients with Grade 3 to Grade 6 acromioclavicular joint injuries need referral to a specialist; because a Grade 2 injury is difficult to differentiate from a Grade 3 injury, also consider referral of these patients

G. Simple sternoclavicular joint sprains can be treated with a sling or figure-eight appliance, ice, analgesics, and early, progressive range-of-motion exercises; refer more serious sprains and separations

H. Rotator cuff problems
    1. Patients with Stage I impingement (pain is Grade 1 or 2 which suggests mild to moderate inflammation) can be managed conservatively with the goal of decreasing the inflammation that is compressing the subacromial space before irreversible damage occurs

---

CONSERVATIVE TREATMENT FOR STAGE I SHOULDER IMPINGEMENT
ADVICE THAT SHOULD BE GIVEN TO PATIENT

- **Rest without** immobilization
- **Use** arm and shoulder in activities that do not require overhead motion
- **Refrain** from activities that precipitated the injury
- **Apply ice** as often as desired and as long as inflammation is present (**Note**: Ice is a potent anti-inflammatory agent that can reduce both pain and muscle spasm)
- **Use** nonsteroidal anti-inflammatory drugs (NSAIDs) for 2-4 weeks
- **Visit** physical therapist for therapeutic modalities such as high-voltage electrical stimulation and ultrasound, and training in stretching and strengthening exercises
- **Exercise programs** (see Figure 17.29)

---

    2. Patients with Stage I impingements that do not respond to conservative therapy in 4 weeks should be referred for further evaluation and possible corticosteroid injections
    3. Patients with Stages II and III impingement syndrome require referral to an orthopedist

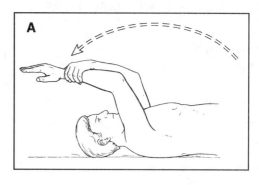
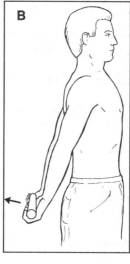
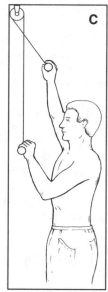
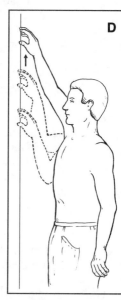
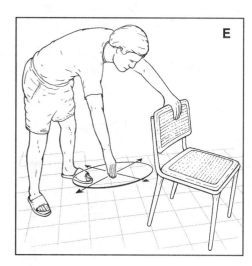
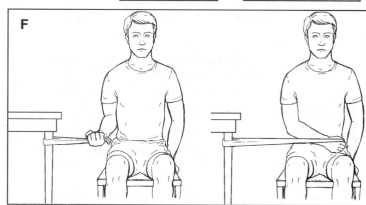

Figure 17.29. Exercise Programs

A. Forward evaluation: Grasp wrist of affected arm with unaffected hand and pull/stretch in an arc to head; repeat 5-10 times every day
B. Extension: Grasp stick with both hands behind back and push backwards; repeat 5-10 times every day
C. Pulley: Pull affected arm near pulleys and stretch; unaffected arm supplies the power; repeat 5-10 times every day
D. Wall climbing: Stand 1-2 feet from wall and slowly "walk" fingers up the wall so that stretch can be felt; increase distance walked up wall as motion improves
E. Pendulum: Lean forward, dangle affected arm, and swing arm back and forth, side-to-side, and around; increase length of swing as motion improves; repeat 5-10 times every day
F. Internal rotation: Anchor rubber tubing to solid object (table leg or doorknob); sit or stand with arm at side and elbow bent; slowly rotate arm inward toward body; hold 5-10 seconds, relax, and repeat; initially do 10 times in 1 set; try to increase number of sets per day as pain decreases

    I.   Adhesive capsulitis (frozen shoulder)
         1.   Conservative treatment with early, extensive physical therapy, analgesics, and occasionally intra-articular corticosteroid injections may be effective
         2.   Surgical referral is needed if conservative treatment fails

    J.   Follow Up
         1.   Patients with simple acute injuries (simple fractures, sprains, separations, dislocations) should be re-evaluated within 2 weeks
            a.   Repeat x-rays are needed for clavicle fractures a week after injury
            b.   Post-reduction x-rays are needed for shoulder dislocations
            c.   For patients with acute injuries who have persistent pain, consider repeat x-rays and refer to specialist
         2.   For patients with Stage I impingement syndrome (chronic pain) follow-up should be in 4 weeks to assess the efficacy of conservative management
         3.   For patients with Stages II and III impingement syndrome, follow-up should be with specialist to whom patient was referred
         4.   For patients with adhesive capsulitis and osteoarthritis follow-up is variable and depends on the patient's progress; typically re-evaluate patient within 2-4 weeks

REFERENCES

American Academy of Pediatrics Committee on Quality Improvement, Subcommittee on Developmental Dysplasia of the Hip. (2000). Clinical practice guideline: Early detection of developmental dysplasia of the hip. *Pediatrics, 105,* 896-905.

American College of Rheumatology Ad Hoc Committee on Clinical Guidelines. (1996). Guidelines for the management of rheumatoid arthritis. *Arthritis and Rheumatology, 39,* 713-722.

American Pain Society. (2002). *Guideline for the management of pain in osteoarthritis, rheumatoid arthritis, and juvenile chronic arthritis.* Glenview, IL: American Pain Society.

Anderson, S.J. (2002). Lower extremity injuries in youth sports. *Pediatric Clinics of North America, 49,* 627-641.

Arcuni, S.E. (2000). Rotator cuff pathology and subacromial impingement. *The Nurse Practitioner, 25,* 58-78.

Athreya, B.H., & Szer, I.S. (2002). Juvenile rheumatoid arthritis and spondyloarthropathy syndromes. In. F.D. Burg, J.R. Ingelfinger, R.A. Polin, & A.A. Gershon (Eds.), *Gellis and Kagan's current pediatric therapy.* Philadelphia: Saunders.

Austermuehle, P.D. (2001). Common knee injuries in primary care. *The Nurse Practitioner, 26,* 26-45.

Bachur, R. (2001). Minor trauma. In C. Green-Hernandez, J.K. Singleton, & D.Z. Aronzon, (Eds.). *Primary care pediatrics.* Philadelphia: Lippincott.

Bauer, S.J., Hollander, J.E., Fuchs, S.H., & Thode, H.C., Jr. (1995). A clinical decision rule in the evaluation of acute knee injuries. *Journal of Emergency Medicine, 13,* 611-615.

Bigos, S., Bowyer, O., Braen, G., Brown, K., Deyo, R.A., Haldeman, S., et al. (1994). *Acute low back problems in adults. Clinical practice guideline No. 14.* AHCPR Publication No. 95-0642. Rockville, MD: Agency for Health Care Policy and Research, Public Health Service, U.S. Department of Health and Human Services.

Brady, M.T. (2002). Bone and joint infections. In. F.D. Burg, J.R. Ingelfinger, R.A. Polin, & A.A. Gershon (Eds.), *Gellis and Kagan's current pediatric therapy.* Philadelphia: Saunders.

Bratton, R.L. (1999). Assessment and management of acute low back pain. *American Family Physician, 60,* 2299-2308.

Burke, M.G. (2001). Extremity pain. In R.A. Hoekelman (Ed.). *Primary pediatric care.* (4th ed.). St. Louis: Mosby.

Busch, M.T., & Hall, D.E. (2001). Sports injuries. In R.A. Hoekelman (Ed.). *Primary pediatric care.* (4th ed.). St. Louis: Mosby.

Cassidy, J.T., Levinson, J.E., Bass, J.C., Baum, J., Brewer, E.J. Jr., Fink, C.W., et al. (1986). A study of classification criteria for diagnosing juvenile rheumatoid arthritis. *Arthritis and Rheumatology, 29,* 274.

Della-Guistina, D., & Kilcline, B.A. (2002). Acute low back pain in children: A guide to diagnosis and treatment. *Consultant, December,* 1737-1743.

Deyo, R.A., & Weinstein, J.N. (2001). Low back pain. *New England Journal of Medicine, 344,* 363-370.

Gates, S.J., & Mooar, P.A. (1999). *Musculoskeletal primary care.* Philadelphia: Lippincott.

Gómez, J.E. (2002). Upper extremity injuries in youth sports. *Pediatric Clinics of North America, 49,* 593-626.

Goroll, A.H., & Mulley, Jr., A.G. (2000). Evaluation of acute monoarticular arthritis. In A.H. Goroll, & A.G. Mulley, Jr., (Eds.). *Primary care medicine,* (4th ed.). Lippincott: Philadelphia.

Goroll, A.H., & Mulley, Jr., A.G. (2000). Evaluation of polyarticular complaints. In A.H. Goroll, & A.G. Mulley, Jr., (Eds.). *Primary care medicine,* (4th ed.). Lippincott: Philadelphia.

Greiner, K. A. (2002). Adolescent idiopathic scoliosis: Radiologic decision-making. *American Family Physician, 65,* 1817-1822.

Halin, J. (2000). Treatment of rheumatoid arthritis: Etanercept, a recent advance. *Journal of American Nurse Practitioner, 12,* 433-441.

Hockenbury, R.T., & Sammarco, G.J. (2001). Evaluation and treatment of ankle sprains. *The Physician and Sportsmedicine, 29,* 57-64.

Hoekelman, R.A. (2001). Foot and leg problems. In R.A. Hoekelman (Ed.). *Primary pediatric care.* (4th ed.). St. Louis: Mosby

Ilowite, N.T. (2002). Current treatment of juvenile rheumatoid arthritis. *Pediatrics, 109,* 109-115.

Jarvik, J.G., & Deyo, R.A. (2002). Diagnostic evaluation of low back pain with emphasis on imaging. *Annals of Internal Medicine, 137,* 586-597.

Jarvis, J.N. (2002) Juvenile rheumatoid arthritis: A guide for pediatricians. *Pediatric Annals, 31,* 437-445.

Johnson, M.W. (2000). Acute knee effusions: A systematic approach to diagnosis. *American Family Physician, 61*, 2391-2400.

Jupiter, J.B., & Ring, D. (2000). Approach to minor orthopedic problems of the elbow, wrist, and hand. In A.H. Goroll, & A.G. Mulley, Jr., (Eds.). *Primary care medicine,* (4th ed.). Lippincott: Philadelphia.

Karol, L.A. (1997). Rotational deformities in the lower extremities. *Current Opinion in Pediatrics, 9,* 77-80.

Kremer, J.M. (2001). Rational use of new and existing disease-modifying agents in rheumatoid arthritis. *Annals of Internal Medicine, 134,* 695-706.

Kupecz, D., & Berardinelli, C. (2002). Using anakinra for adult rheumatoid arthritis. *The Nurse Practitioner, 27,* 62-65.

Leet, A.I., & Skaggs, D.L. (2000). Evaluation of the acutely limping child. *American Family Physician, 61,* 1011-1018.

Loder, R. (1998). Slipped capital femoral epiphysis. *American Family Physician, 57,* 2135-2142.

Mankin, K.P. (2001). Chronic orthopedic problems. In C. Green-Hernandez, J.K. Singleton, & D.Z. Aronzon, (Eds.). *Primary care pediatrics.* Philadelphia: Lippincott.

Mazzone, M.F., & McCue, T. (2002). Common conditions of the Achilles tendon. *American Family Physician, 65,* 1805-1810.

Millea, P.J., & Holloway, R.L. (2000). Treating fibromyalgia. *American Family Physician, 62,* 1575-1582, 1587.

Mortensen, S.E. (2002). Bursitis, tendonitis, myofascial pain, and fibromyalgia. In R.E. Rakel & E.T. Bope, (Eds.). *2002 Conn's current therapy.* Philadelphia: Saunders.

Owens, S., & Itamura, J.M. (2001). Differential diagnosis of shoulder injuries in sports. *Orthopedic Clinics of North America, 32,* 393-398.

Patel, A.T., & Ogle, A.A. (2000). Diagnosis and management of acute low back pain. *American Family Physician, 61,* 1779-1786, 1789-1790.

Pendergrast, R.A. (2001). Back pain. In R.A. Hoekelman (Ed.). *Primary pediatric care.* (4th ed.). St. Louis: Mosby.

Perron, A.D., Brady, W.J., & Keats, T.A. (2002). Management of common stress fractures. *Postgraduate Medicine, 111,* 95-106.

Reamy, B.V., & Slakey, J.B. (2001). Adolescent idiopathic scoliosis: Review and current concepts. *American Family Physician, 64,* 111-116.

Schroeder, B.M. (2002). American College of Foot and Ankle Surgeons: Diagnosis and treatment of heel pain. *American Family Physician, 65,* 1687-1688.

Siegel, D.M., & Baum, J. (2001). Joint pain. In R.A. Hoekelman (Ed.). *Primary pediatric care.* (4th ed.). St. Louis: Mosby.

Sills, E.M. (2001). Spinal deformities. In R.A. Hoekelman (Ed.). *Primary pediatric care.* (4th ed.). St. Louis: Mosby.

Smidt, N. (2002). Corticosteroid injections, physiotherapy, or a wait-and-see policy for lateral epicondylitis: A randomized controlled trial. *Lancet, 259,* 657-662.

Solomon, D.H., Simel, D.L., Bates, D.W., Katz, J.N., & Schaffer, J.L. (2001). Does this patient have a torn meniscus or ligament of the knee? *JAMA, 286,* 1610-1620.

Stiell, I.G., Wells, G.A., Hoag, R.H., Sivilotti, M.L., Cacciotti, T.F., Verbeek, P.R., et al. (1997). Implementation of the Ottawa Knee Rule for the use of radiography in acute knee injuries. *JAMA, 278,* 2075-2079.

Sussman, M., & Turker, R.J. (2002). Skeletal system. In. F.D. Burg, J.R. Ingelfinger, R.A. Polin, & A.A. Gershon (Eds.), *Gellis and Kagan's current pediatric therapy.* Philadelphia: Saunders.

Tan, E.M., Cohen, AS., Fries, J.F., Masi, A.T., McShane, D.J., Rothfield, W.F., et al. (1982). The 1982 revised criteria for the classification of systemic lupus erythematosus. *Arthritis and Rheumatism, 25,* 1275-1277.

Tandeter, H.B., Shvartzman, P., & Stevens, M.A. (1999). Acute knee injuries: Use of decision rules for selective radiograph ordering. *American Family Physician, 60,* 2599-2608.

Von Korff, M., & Moore, J.C. (2001). Stepped care for back pain: Activating approaches for primary care. *Annals of Internal Medicine, 134,* 911-917.

Wolfe, F., Smythe, H.A., Yunus, M.B., Bennett, R.M., Bombadier, C., Goldenberg, D.L., et al. (1990). The American College of Rheumatology 1990 criteria for the classification of fibromyalgia. *Arthritis and Rheumatism, 33,* 160-172.

Wolfe, M.W., Uhl, T.L., & McCluskey, L.C. (2001). Management of ankle sprains. *American Family Physician, 63,* 93-104.

Woodward, T.W., & Best, T.M. (2000). The painful shoulder: Part I. Clinical evaluation. *American Family Physician, 61,* 3079-3088.

Woodward, T.W., & Best, T.M. (2000). The painful shoulder: Part II. Acute and chronic disorders. *American Family Physician, 61,* 3291-3300.

Young, C.C., Rutherford, D.S., & Niedfeldt, M.W. (2001). Treatment of plantar fasciitis. *American Family Physician, 63,* 467-474, 477-478.

Neurologic Problems

MARY VIRGINIA GRAHAM

Acute Facial Paresis (Bell's Palsy)

Dizziness

Febrile Seizures

Headache

Seizures and Epilepsy

ACUTE FACIAL PARESIS (BELL'S PALSY)

I.   Definition: Acute, unilateral paresis of facial muscles due to inflammation and subsequent mechanical compression of the 7th (the facial) cranial nerve

II.   Pathogenesis

    A.   Believed to be a viral neuropathy caused by herpes simplex virus (HSV) type 1

    B.   Most likely the herpes virus spreads from the oral cavity along the chorda tympani nerve to the geniculate ganglion where it remains dormant until reactivated by various physiologic stressors

III.   Clinical Presentation

    A.   Disease is common, with an incidence each year of 20 per 100,000; affects all age groups but occurs most often in young and middle-age adults

    B.   Typical presentation is rapid onset of facial weakness with little or no progression beyond 48 to 72 hours
        1.   There is loss of facial expression, loss of voluntary movement of facial and scalp muscles on affected side, altered ability to close one eye, and numbness of the face
        2.   In addition, patient may experience loss of taste, be hypersensitive to sound, and have excessive tearing
        3.   Usually, the diagnosis is established without difficulty in patients presenting with unexplained, unilateral, isolated facial weakness

    C.   May have ear or facial pain (which is usually transient and may have resolved by time of presentation) on affected side for about 24 hours prior to onset of weakness

    D.   Most patients recover completely without treatment within weeks to a few months, but some have residual effects
        1.   Three months after initial onset of symptoms seems to be an important landmark in terms of recovery
        2.   Patients whose recovery is delayed beyond this time period often experience significant sequelae

    E.   Recurrent facial nerve palsy is unusual; if patient has more than two episodes of the condition, the possibility of tumor should be suspected

IV.   Diagnosis/Evaluation

    A.   History
        1.   Question about onset of symptoms as paresis in Bell's palsy is abrupt and does not occur gradually over days or weeks (waxing and waning of symptoms suggest another cause)
        2.   Ask about facial pain, particularly in area of mastoid process (not atypical to have pain in this area)
        3.   Include careful questioning about neurological symptoms in other areas of face and body
        4.   Ask about prior history of facial weakness (if positive, raises concern for another cause)
        5.   Inquire about cerebrovascular and cardiac risk factors
        6.   Ask about predisposing factors such as infection, trauma, recent outdoor activities in area endemic for Lyme disease

    B.   Physical Examination
        1.   Measure vital signs, noting elevations in blood pressure and temperature
        2.   Observe general appearance including gait, evidence of trauma or distress
        3.   Inspect skin for herpetic lesions or characteristic lesions of Lyme disease
        4.   Carefully examine the head, ears, eyes, nose, and throat
        5.   Special attention should be given to assessment of the cranial nerves and the neurological examination, looking for evidence of other cranial neuropathies or neurologic deficits
            a.   To differentiate between Bell's palsy and a central lesion (an ominous cause of facial weakness), have patient raise eyebrows and wrinkle forehead
            b.   With peripheral lesions, both the upper and lower face are affected (cannot wrinkle forehead)
            c.   With central lesions, mainly the lower face is affected (can wrinkle forehead)

C. Differential Diagnosis: Simultaneous bilateral facial palsies, unilateral facial weakness that slowly progresses over 3 weeks with or without facial hyperkinesis, and failure of facial function to return within 6 months after acute onset suggest a diagnosis other than Bell's palsy; possible alternative diagnoses are the following
1. Benign and malignant tumors
2. Infectious processes, viral, bacterial, or spirochete (acute or chronic otitis media; Lyme disease, herpes zoster, herpes simplex type 1)
3. Trauma (temporal bone fracture)
4. Guillain-Barré syndrome (typically has symmetric bilateral weakness)

D. Diagnostic Tests
1. In patients with a classic history for Bell's palsy and a physical examination that is otherwise normal, order an audiogram in the acute phase to help rule out a lesion in cerebellopontine angle and temporal bone (this is usually the only test needed during the acute phase)
2. Obtain Lyme titer if there is a history of exposure to ticks and patient resides in or has recently visited a geographic location where disease is prevalent
3. If there is uncertainty about the diagnosis, or if the patient has gradual progression of symptoms over the follow-up period (see below for follow-up), then refer the patient to a neurologist for further diagnostic testing
4. Additional diagnostic testing in patients with Bell's palsy usually involves tests to estimate the patient's prognosis
    a. Electrical testing during the first week or two involves use of the Hilger nerve stimulation test and electroneurography–these tests are used to determine prognosis and have little utility beyond the first 2-3 weeks after onset of symptoms
    b. Electromyography testing can be performed many weeks later (not in the early phases) to also provide information on recovery potential

V. Plan/Management

A. Explain that symptoms usually resolve in 3-4 weeks without any treatment and with no sequelae

B. Good eye care is paramount as corneal abrasion can easily occur in patients with facial paralysis; inability to close eye completely and blink, as well as decreased tearing and corneal hyperesthesia, predispose the eye to injury
1. Advise patient to use lubricant eye drops 1-2 drops every 2 hours when awake and ophthalmic ointment at night
2. Available products include Hypo Tears PF (preservative free), Gen Teal, Refresh Plus, and Tears Naturale Forte, all available over the counter
3. Glasses should be worn when outdoors to protect eye from drying effects of wind
4. Affected eye may need to be patched, especially at night, to reduce eye damage; care must be taken that the lid does not open and expose the cornea to material covering the eye

C. A physical therapy referral may be beneficial; usually involves heat therapy, electrical stimulation, or massage

D. Even though the benefit of corticosteroid use in Bell's palsy has not been definitively established, steroids are safe for short-term use and are probably effective in improving facial functional outcomes in affected patients
1. Whereas some have suggested that patients with complete paralysis (not paresis) benefit most from steroids, there is little evidence that severity of facial weakness at the onset of treatment influences effectiveness of oral prednisone therapy
2. If there are no contraindications, initiate short-term treatment with oral prednisone (1.0 mg/kg/day for 3 days, 0.75 mg/kg/day for 3 days, 0.50 mg/kg/day for 3 days, and then a rapid taper over the next 4-5 days)
3. Corticosteroids should be started as soon as possible after the onset of facial paralysis/paresis
4. Initiation of therapy within 3 days is considered optimal

E. The benefit of antiviral agents in the treatment of Bell's palsy has not been established; however, antivirals (combined with prednisone) are possibly effective in improving facial functional outcomes in affected persons; consider treatment with either famciclovir or valacyclovir for one week

F.   Follow Up
1.   Patients who present with facial weakness or paralysis believed to be due to Bell's palsy should be seen several times a week for the first week to make sure that symptoms are not progressing and that the eye on the affected side is receiving proper care
2.   If symptoms are resolving at that point, and proper eye care is being performed by the patient, then visits can be less often (every 1-2 weeks)
3.   Patients who have delayed or incomplete recovery should be referred to a neurologist for management
4.   Patient should be referred without delay to an ophthalmologist if any eye symptoms or signs develop

DIZZINESS

I.   Definition: Various abnormal sensations relating to perceptions of the body's position or motion in relation to the environment

II.   Pathogenesis

A.   There are four subtypes of dizziness–vertigo, presyncopal lightheadedness, disequilibrium, and other dizziness (does not fit into the first three categories)

B.   **Vertigo:** Sensation that the body or environment is moving, usually spinning
1.   Suggests disorder of the vestibular system
2.   Systemic causes of vertigo and dizziness include certain drugs, infectious disease, endocrine disease, and vasculitis

C.   **Presyncope:** Feeling of lightheadedness that produces the sensation of an impending faint; occurs episodically, and is usually caused by inadequate cerebral perfusion

D.   **Disequilibrium:** Sense of imbalance or postural instability generally described as involving legs/trunk without a sensation in the head
1.   Isolated symptoms of disequilibrium are usually due to some type of neurologic disorder–multiple sensory deficits are the most common cause
2.   Imbalance that accompanies other types of dizziness is most often a secondary rather than a primary symptom
3.   A rare cause of dizziness in children

E.   **Other dizziness:** A vague feeling of floating (patients often have difficulty describing this sensation)
1.   Often caused by psychological disorders and often accompanied by other somatic symptoms such as headache or abdominal pain
2.   Also, a distinct though rare form of dizziness is in this category–ocular dizziness due to rapid vision change (e.g., cataract surgery) or to a change in corrective lenses; an uncommon cause in children and adolescents

III. Clinical Presentation

A.   Dizziness occurs in all age groups and is a relatively common symptom in childhood and adolescence with girls reporting the symptom more often than boys

B.   Of the four dizziness subtypes, presyncope is the most common type that occurs in children and adolescents

C.   Other dizziness (i.e., dizziness that does not fit the first 3 sub-types) also commonly occurs in children, with migraine headache being a common cause of "other dizziness"

D. **Vertigo**: True vertigo is due to either vestibular or nonvestibular causes
1. Vestibular problems may be **peripheral** or **central**
2. Peripheral vestibular causes of vertigo are problems or conditions affecting labyrinthine structures or the vestibular nerve
3. Central vestibular causes of vertigo are a manifestation of progressive disease of the central nervous system

E. **Vertigo: Peripheral vestibular causes of vertigo** are characterized by isolated vertigo (i.e., without associated signs and symptoms, with the exception of tinnitus or hearing loss that occurs in Ménière's syndrome). Peripheral vestibular problems are the following
1. Benign paroxysmal positional vertigo (BPPV) is the most common type of vertigo and is caused by free-floating particulate matter, usually in a posterior semicircular canal, that moves within the canal with certain head movements by the patient, thereby disturbing the vestibular sensory receptors and producing vertigo
2. Ménière's syndrome is believed to be caused by endolymphatic hydrops manifested by excess fluid in the cochlea and vestibular labyrinth (rare in children)
3. Acute labyrinthitis (or vestibular neuronitis which is believed to be the same disorder without any cochlear involvement) is caused by a viral infection involving the cochlea and labyrinth

F. **Vertigo: Central vestibular causes of vertigo** are rare in children and include brainstem ischemia and infarction, intrinsic brainstem lesions, cerebellopontine angle tumor such as acoustic neurinoma, and demyelinating disease such as multiple sclerosis
1. Patients with central vestibular disorders typically present with vertigo in association with other brainstem deficits
2. Commonly associated neurologic symptoms and signs include diplopia and focal sensory or motor deficits

G. **Presyncope**: Inadequate cerebral perfusion can cause dizziness; patients often report feeling "light-headed"
1. This subtype of dizziness commonly occurs in children who have fever, dehydration, orthostatic hypotension, and vasovagal syncope; also seen with anemia in adolescent females
2. Patients typically report a worsening of symptoms with standing and an improvement with lying down
3. Postural changes in blood pressure and pulse are characteristic
4. See section on PRESYNCOPE/SYNCOPE for a discussion of this topic

H. **Disequilibrium**: Multiple sensory deficits are the most common cause in this type of dizziness that patients describe as a feeling of "unsteadiness on the feet" (rare in children)
1. Disequilibrium in this age group may reflect acute cerebellar problems such as postviral acute cerebellar ataxia and posterior fossa tumors
2. Sense of imbalance may come on with standing and can be aggravated by walking or turning
3. Typically, symptoms worsen in the dark–because of elimination of visual positional input–and improve with holding onto a railing
4. The child often has a history of falling

I. **Other dizziness**: Most often caused by psychological disturbances such as anxiety states, depression, or panic attacks, or the medications used to treat these disorders. Migraine headaches are a common cause of this subtype in children
1. Dizziness is usually ill-defined and is unrelated to position change; there is no history of underlying heart disease or conditions that would cause multiple sensory deficits
2. Precise mechanism of the dizziness is unknown, but is believed to be related to the confusional state induced by the illnesses or by the medications used to treat them
3. Hyperventilation can produce metabolic alkalosis, causing patients to experience light-headedness, and paresthesias

IV. Diagnosis/Evaluation

A. History
1. Ask patient to describe in a few words the sensation he/she experiences; if patient's description is too vague, prompt with the following questions
    a. "Do you feel like you or the room is spinning around?" (a positive response favors vertigo)
    b. "Do you feel like you might black out?" (a positive response favors presyncope)
    c. "Do you feel unsteady on your feet, like you are about to lose your balance?" (a positive response favors disequilibrium)

2. Guided by the patient's response, determine which of the subtypes of dizziness the patient is experiencing; determine if the symptoms are severe, moderate, or mild and ask what makes the symptoms better or worse
3. Determine how often the dizziness occurs and what makes the dizziness better or worse
4. Ask about associated symptoms; specifically ask about nausea and vomiting, and about auditory symptoms such as hearing impairment, tinnitus (whether pulsatile or constant), history of ear infections, sensation of aural pressure
5. Ask patient if dizziness is accompanied by headache
6. Ask about associated neurologic symptoms that suggest a central cause of dizziness; specifically ask if there is diplopia, facial numbness, weakness/numbness in arms or legs, confusion, slurring of speech, difficulty swallowing
7. Ask about recent life stressors (school problems, parental discord, abuse problems)
8. Determine if patient has (or is recovering from) a viral or bacterial infection that can present with dizziness
9. Determine if patient has recently had a change in a corrective prescription
10. Obtain past medical history including past episodes of dizziness, ear or head trauma, recent weight loss, or dieting (severe restriction of caloric intake)
11. Obtain complete medication history including over-the-counter products (specifically, weight loss drugs, stimulants) and alternative therapies to determine if dizziness is drug-related
12. Ask about drug and alcohol use

B. Physical Examination
1. Evaluation of an undifferentiated symptom such as dizziness is difficult; the steps in the physical examination below are considered most important but are not all inconclusive; findings from the history should also guide the physical examination
2. Measure vital signs; assess for orthostatic hypotension (see section on PRESYNCOPE/SYNCOPE for measurement procedure)
3. Perform a complete ear examination
4. Perform a complete cardiovascular exam to rule out conditions that can be life threatening
5. Do a careful neurological examination to rule out multiple sensory deficits as well as conditions that can be life threatening
   a. Test sensory function, peripheral vision, and gait
   b. Test cranial nerves (**Note**: Any cranial nerve abnormality suggests a serious cause for dizziness)
   c. Test cerebellar function (tandem gait or heel-to-toe walking) and perform the Romberg test (patient stands upright with feet close together and arms folded across chest with eyes open and then closed–minimal movement or sway is normal finding)
6. Symptom reproduction with hyperventilation may be helpful if suggested by history

C. Differential Diagnosis
1. The major challenge is identifying critical diagnoses (those that are life threatening)
2. The second challenge is to determine the subtype of dizziness—vertigo, presyncope, disequilibrium, or other dizziness that is causing the symptoms

D. Diagnostic Tests
1. Most episodes of dizziness in pediatric patients can be diagnosed by history and physical exam
2. Abnormalities on history and physical exam should direct additional testing (e.g., if actual fainting has occurred, an electrocardiogram [ECG] may be necessary)
3. Hemoglobin (Hb) in adolescent girls to rule out iron deficiency as cause

V. Plan/Management

A. Patients with abnormal neurologic or cardiac findings on history and physical examination should be immediately referred for emergent care

B. Management of patients with acute onset of dizziness that interferes with ability to function (but is not life-threatening) and with a cause not immediately identifiable should be referred to a specialty setting for urgent management; short-term use of the antihistamine dimenhydrate (Dramamine) may be helpful. Available OTC; advise patient to follow dosing instructions on label. Causes drowsiness and sedation, and may cause paradoxical excitement in children

C. Patients with true vertigo should be referred to a pediatric neurologist or otolaryngologist

D. For patients with presyncopal dizziness in whom cardiac and neurological abnormalities have been ruled out, management consists of reassurance and instructions about adequate hydration, care when arising suddenly, and putting the head lower than the heart when symptoms occur

E. Patients with psychogenic lightheadedness should be treated for the appropriate underlying cause; however, these patients frequently have significant comorbidity and disability and require an interdisciplinary evaluation; therefore, they are best referred for expert evaluation and management

F. For motion sickness in patients ≥18 ears of age, prescribe scopolamine transdermal patch (Transderm Scop) 1 disc applied behind ear at least 4 hours prior to travel; patch should be removed and replaced after 72 hours. In younger children (≥2 years), Dramamine may be used. Advise parents to follow instructions on label for dosing

G. Follow Up: Variable depending on diagnosis and whether the patient was referred for evaluation and management

FEBRILE SEIZURES

I. Definition: Seizures that occur in neurologically healthy young children who have fever but no evidence of intracranial infection or acute neurological illness

II. Pathogenesis

A. There is no clear etiology but age is one of the most important factors governing seizure threshold
   1. The cortex becomes increasingly prone to seizures during the early months of life
   2. At about three to six years of age, the neuronal excitability diminishes and children outgrow the tendency toward febrile seizures

B. Febrile seizure may be the first sign child is ill; unclear whether seizure activity is triggered by rapid rise of fever or the actual height (degree) of temperature

C. High rate of febrile seizures associated with roseola, shigellosis, salmonellosis which may be due to direct effect of the causative organism on CNS, or to a neurotoxin that is produced

D. Genetic factors may be involved as there is increased incidence of febrile seizures in first-degree relatives of affected children

III. Clinical Presentation

A. Occur in 2-5% of all children and are the most common convulsive event in children younger than 5 years of age, with boys being more susceptible than girls
   1. Median age of occurrence is 18 to 22 months
   2. Risk of having recurrent febrile seizures varies with age of the child
   3. Children <12 months of age at time of first febrile seizure have about a 50% probability of a second such event; children >12 months of age at time of first febrile seizure have about a 30% probability of a second such event

B. Febrile seizures may be simple or complex; simple febrile seizures are **by far** the most common type

C. Simple febrile seizures are benign events with an excellent prognosis
   1. Seizures are generalized and last <15 minutes with most lasting only 1-2 minutes
   2. Seizures usually occur in first few hours of child's illness and they do not recur within 24 hours
   3. EEG obtained 2 weeks after seizure is normal
   4. Otherwise healthy child with no central nervous system infection or abnormality

D. Complex febrile seizures are much less common
   1. Seizures are focal rather than generalized
   2. Seizures last >15 minutes (prolonged) and/or occur more than once in a 24-hour period (repetitive)

E. Febrile seizures can be triggered by any illness that causes fever; most commonly associated with otitis media and upper respiratory tract infections

IV. Diagnosis/Evaluation

A. History (**Note:** Assumes child presents after seizure activity has stopped)
1. Inquire about onset, duration, degree of fever, and parent's management of child's fever (i.e., antipyretic use)
2. Carefully determine characteristics (i.e., focal or generalized), and duration of seizure
3. Review of systems should concentrate on uncovering source of fever
4. Question about family history of febrile seizures and epilepsy
5. Assess developmental milestones

B. Physical Examination
1. Assess alertness, color, and vital signs
2. Perform a careful neurological examination
3. Assess for meningeal signs and symptoms
4. Complete physical examination must be done to search for the source of fever

C. Differential Diagnosis
1. Epilepsy
2. Meningitis or encephalitis
3. Metabolic disorder

D. Diagnostic Tests
1. Order diagnostic tests such as CBC, urinalysis, blood cultures, chest x-ray if source of fever is unknown (**Note**: The purpose of these diagnostic tests is to diagnose and treat the cause of the fever, not to identify the cause of the seizure)
2. After the first seizure with fever in infants younger than 12 months of age, performance of a lumbar puncture should be **strongly** considered because clinical signs and symptoms of meningitis in this age group may be minimal or absent; LP should also be considered in children between 12 and 18 months of age
3. EEG is not indicated as part of the evaluation of a neurologically healthy child with a first simple febrile seizure

V. Plan/Management

A. Children between the ages of 6 months and 5 years of age with a simple febrile seizure lasting only a few minutes, with no focal neurologic deficits, and with no (or minimal) postictal period need no further therapy relating to the seizure
1. Counsel family regarding benign nature of a simple febrile seizure; advise parents that the risk of subsequent epilepsy in children who have febrile seizure is less than 5%
2. Family education should include use of antipyretics at onset of fever and first aid for seizures; warn the parents that dosing of antipyretics must be appropriate and that high doses of antipyretics do not reduce the seizure recurrence rate but do involve the risk of toxicity from over-medication

B. Children with complex febrile seizures (prolonged, i.e., >15 minutes, focal or recurrent in 24 hours), or neurologic deficits must be referred to a pediatric neurologist for immediate/emergent care

C. Infants younger than 6 months of age should be referred to a pediatric neurologist for immediate/emergent care

D. Children with new-onset seizure not associated with a fever should be referred to a pediatric neurologist for immediate/emergent care

E. Neither continuous nor intermittent anticonvulsant therapy is recommended for children with one or more simple febrile seizures

F. Follow Up
1. For children with simple febrile seizure, telephone follow up within first 24-48 hours to ascertain that child is alert, active, and has no additional symptoms
2. For infants <6 months of age, and for children with seizures that cannot be classified as a simple febrile seizure, follow up should be by the pediatric neurologist to whom the child was referred

HEADACHE

I. Definition: Diffuse pain in various parts of the head with the pain not confined to the area of distribution of a nerve

II. Pathogenesis

   A. Primary headaches are caused by traction on pain sensitive structures, inflammation of vessels and meninges, vascular dilation, excessive muscle contraction, and dysregulation of the ascending brain stem serotonergic system

   B. Secondary headaches are due to an underlying organic cause; fewer than 2-10% of headaches are secondary

III. Clinical Presentation of Primary Headache

   A. Headache is one of the most common pain-related problems presenting in primary care settings

   B. Headaches are common during childhood and become more common and frequent during adolescence; boys are more often affected before puberty, and girls are more often affected after the onset of puberty

   C. Primary headache disorders–migraine, tension-type, and cluster–are usually acute-recurrent and have no underlying disease process as their cause; descriptions of the three types of primary headache are contained in the box that follows

	Migraine	*Tension-type*	*Cluster*
Patient population	More common in females; episodes often begin in adolescence or early adulthood but are quite common in childhood beginning as early as age 5-6 years	Most common headache type, occurs in both genders and all age groups (in children, most commonly begins between 8-12 years of age)	More common in men (mean age of onset in late 20s); incidence diminishes with age; compared with migraine and tension-type headache, an uncommon form of primary headache
Family history	Positive	Negative	Negative
Typical time of onset	Any time of day	Later in the day	Frequently nocturnal, waking patient from sleep
Untreated duration	4 to 72 hours	30 minutes to 7 days	15 minutes to 3 hours
Characteristics	Often unilateral, throbbing head pain that is made worse by movement and physical activity	Bilateral, often slowly progressing, non-throbbing, mild to moderate pain; patient may complain of dull pressure or band-like sensation about head; physical activity does not worsen pain	Unilateral, severe, sharp, orbital, supraorbital, or temporal pain always on the same side
Associated symptoms	Nausea, vomiting, phonophobia, and photophobia	Usually none	At least one of the following is present on the headache side: lacrimation, conjunctival injection, nasal congestion, ptosis or eyelid swelling, and rhinorrhea
Comments	Females often report relationship between migraine and menses Two categories: *Migraine with aura* (only about 15% of patients have this type) such as visual prodromes [flashing lights, zigzags, illusions of distorted shapes], strange odors, or paresthesias; previously known as classic migraine *Migraine without aura*; (most patients have this type) previously known as common migraine	Account for more than one half of headache patients who present to primary care settings; compared with migraine headache, tension-type receives little attention in the medical literature	Attacks may occur once a day or as frequently as 8 times/day; duration may be as short as 15 minutes or last more than 3 hours; occur in bouts which may last days to weeks; most patients experience one bout per year

IV.   Diagnosis/Evaluation

A.   History (**Note:** This approach assumes the patient presents for evaluation of acute-recurrent headaches, but is not experiencing attack at time of presentation)
1.   Ask patient how often headaches occur and if onset is usually gradual or sudden; ask how long headaches usually last
2.   Ask where pain is usually located and if the pain seems to spread to any other area; if yes, determine where; ask patient to describe the pain (throbbing, stabbing, dull, other)
3.   Ask patient to rate usual pain on a scale from 1 to 10 (with 1 being no pain at all and 10 being the worst pain ever experienced); ask if headaches are getting worse
4.   If patient presents with an acute headache as the chief complaint, ask if this is first or worst headache (see Red Flags in table below)
5.   Question about associated symptoms that frequently occur: Ask, "What symptoms do you have before the headache starts? What symptoms do you have during the headache? Do you have to stop whatever you are doing (playing, studying, watching TV) when you get a headache?"
6.   Ask about precipitating factors such as stress, diet, caffeine intake, physical exertion, sleep problems, or menses
7.   Inquire about prescription and over-the-counter medication use (especially caffeine-containing analgesics)
8.   Obtain past medical history and determine if any concurrent medical conditions are present
9.   Ask about previous trauma to the head and any medical or dental procedures
10.   Document family medical history, especially history of migraine headaches
11.   Explore present and previous treatments and responses to treatments including prescription, over-the-counter medications, herbal remedies, and home remedies
12.   Determine impact of headaches on patient's quality of life and daily functioning (for migraineurs, get a quick but accurate estimate about impact of temporary disability via use of the *Migraine Disability Assessment Scale (MIDAS)*, a well-validated five-item scale that is easy to use in clinical practice (for source, see Stewart et al., 1999, in reference list or access more information on MIDAS at www.migraine-disability.net)

B.   Physical Examination
1.   Keep in mind that the main purpose of the examination is to identify causes of secondary headache
2.   Observe general appearance, noting signs of acute distress, anxiety, or depression
3.   Measure blood pressure, pulse, pulse pressure
4.   Palpate head, face, and temporomandibular joint (TMJ); examine mouth and teeth for signs of inflammation/trauma/infection
5.   Perform ophthalmoscopic assessment
6.   Perform cardiovascular assessment
7.   Perform complete neurological exam including mental status, level of consciousness, cranial nerve testing (with particular attention to detecting problems related to the optic, oculomotor, trochlear, and abducens nerves–cranial nerves II III, IV, and VI, respectively), pupillary responses, motor strength testing, deep tendon reflexes, sensation, reflexes (e.g., Babinski's sign), cerebellar function, gait testing, and signs of meningeal irritation

C.   Differential Diagnosis
1.   Whereas a minority of headaches are secondary, diagnoses in this category are the most life-threatening and **must not** be missed
2.   Consult table below (Red Flags in Acute Headache Evaluation in Children) for differential diagnosis of important causes of secondary headache

RED FLAGS IN ACUTE HEADACHE EVALUATION IN CHILDREN

Red Flag	Differential Diagnosis
Headache in a child younger than 3 years	Children <3 years of age most often have secondary rather than primary cause
Sudden onset of severe headache "worst headache in life"	Subarachnoid hemorrhage, mass lesion, hemorrhage into a mass lesion or vascular malformation
Headaches increasing in frequency and severity	Mass lesion, subdural hematoma, medication overuse (rebound headache)
New-onset headache in a patient with risk factors for HIV infection or cancer	Meningitis, brain abscess, metastasis
Headache with signs of systemic illness (fever, stiff neck, rash)	Meningitis, encephalitis, Lyme disease, systemic infection, collagen vascular disease
Focal neurologic signs or symptoms of disease (other than typical aura)	Mass lesion, vascular malformation, stroke, collagen vascular disease
Papilledema	Mass lesion, pseudotumor cerebri, meningitis
Headache subsequent to head trauma	Intracranial hemorrhage, subdural hematoma, epidural hematoma, post-traumatic headache

D. Diagnostic Tests
1. If there is a likelihood of intracranial pathology based on abnormal findings on neurologic examination that are unexplained, the patient should be referred to a neurologist for further evaluation and possible neuroimaging
2. Random use of laboratory testing in the evaluation of headache is not warranted; if there is diagnostic uncertainty (clinician is unable to classify patient's headache as primary or secondary, or is uncertain about type of primary), referral to a headache subspecialist is recommended

V. Plan/Management

A. Management of patients with primary headache—migraine, tension, or cluster—is outlined below, beginning with management of patients with migraine headache

B. Goals of long-term migraine treatment, both nonpharmacologic and pharmacologic, are to (1) reduce attack frequency, severity, and patient disability, (2) reduce patient reliance on poorly tolerated or ineffective medications, and (3) improve quality of life

C. The initial step, after establishing a diagnosis, is to educate the patient (and family if patient is child) about his/her condition and its treatment
1. Provide a brief overview of what the problem is and how it can best be managed
2. Refer patient (or family) to web sites that may be helpful

> ### Selected Web Sites for Headache Patients
> www.ama-assn.org/special/migraine/migraine.htm
>
> www.headache.org
>
> www.achenet.org

D. Create a formal management plan with the patient (and family if patient is child) in order to implement preventive and/or acute episodic therapy for migraine; treatment choice depends on several factors
1. Frequency/severity of attacks
2. Presence and degree of temporary disability
3. Associated symptoms such as nausea and vomiting

E. General proactive counseling for all patients with migraine headache includes the following
1. Encourage patient (or family if patient is <10 years) to keep a headache diary to assist in identifying precipitating events and risk factors and for tracking progress of treatment approaches
2. Encourage the patient to identify and avoid triggers (examples are provided in the box below)

Common Migraine Triggers

- ✓ Disrupted sleep (not enough sleep/sleeping later than usual)
- ✓ Skipped meals
- ✓ Consumption of certain foods: Common triggers are cheese, chocolate, citrus fruits, foods containing nitrates (contained in some processed meats) and monosodium glutamate
- ✓ Alcoholic beverages, especially red wine
- ✓ Stress
- ✓ Caffeine overuse (soft drinks and coffee) as well as caffeine withdrawal
---

F.   Determine if patient is a candidate for preventive therapy for migraine headaches

---
Candidates for Preventive Therapy

Institution of preventive therapy should be considered for patients who:
- ✓ Have recurrent headaches that interfere with daily functioning despite treatment for acute attacks
- ✓ Exhibit a trend toward an increasing frequency of attacks as documented by patient in migraine diary
- ✓ Have contraindications to or adverse effects from acute therapy
- ✓ Experience failure/overuse of acute therapy

Rule of Thumb
If headaches occur 1-2 days per month, preventive therapy is usually not needed
If occurrence is 3-4 days per month or more, preventive therapy should be seriously considered
---

G.   **Nonpharmacologic therapies for the prevention of migraine** are contained in the box below

---
Nonpharmacologic Preventive Therapy

These therapies may be best suited to patients who have a poor tolerance of, or poor response to drug therapy, who have contraindications to drug therapy, who have a past history or excessive use of analgesics, and for patents who are pregnant (planning to become pregnant), or nursing
- ✓ Relaxation training
- ✓ Thermal biofeedback combined with relaxation training
- ✓ Electromyographic (EMG) biofeedback
- ✓ Cognitive-behavioral therapy

H.   **Drugs for treatment of migraine** can be divided into **two classes**
  1.   Drugs that are taken daily whether or not headache is present to reduce the severity of attack (called preventive therapy [adolescents ≥18 years])
  2.   Drugs that are taken to treat attacks as they arise

I.   **Drugs used to prevent migraine (preventive therapy)** in adolescents ≥18 years are contained in the table that follows
  1.   Initiate therapy with the lowest effective dose of the drug and increase it slowly until clinical benefits are achieved
  2.   Take coexisting conditions into account; select a drug that will treat the coexisting condition and migraine, if possible
  3.   Counsel patient that the prescribed medication must be given an adequate trial and that it may take 2-3 months to achieve clinical benefit

---
SELECTED RECOMMENDED DRUGS FOR USE IN PREVENTION OF MIGRAINE IN ADOLESCENTS 18 AND OLDER

Select one of the following:

Class/Drug	Dose	Selected Side Effects
β-Blockers		
Propranolol	40-120 mg twice daily	Reduced energy, tiredness, postural symptoms,
Timolol	5 mg twice daily	contraindicated in patients with asthma
Anticonvulsants		
Divalproex sodium	400-600 mg twice daily	Drowsiness, weight gain, tremor, hair loss, hematologic/liver abnormalities
Antidepressants		
Amitriptyline	25-75 mg at bedtime	Drowsiness

Adapted from Silberstein, S.D. for the US Headache Consortium. Report of the Quality Standards Subcommittee of the American Academy of Neurology. (2000). Practice parameter: Evidenced-based guidelines for migraine headache (an evidence-based review). *Neurology, 55*, p. 758.

J. **Drugs used for the acute treatment of migraine** in adolescents ≥18 years are contained in the table that follows
  1. Efficacy of acute treatment is determined by correct drug choice and timing of intervention
  2. Early intervention at the outset of the headache (when pain is mild) can abort headache in most cases within 2 to 4 hours with lower headache recurrence
  3. During migraine attacks, the oral absorption of many drugs is delayed; thus, consideration should be given to use of nonoral routes with quicker onset of action

---

SELECTED RECOMMENDED DRUGS FOR ACUTE TREATMENT OF MIGRAINE IN ADOLESCENTS 18 AND OLDER

Patients with **mild to moderate headache** often respond well to **nonspecific** therapy
  ✓ Ibuprofen (Motrin, generic), 400-800 mg/dose PO Q 6 hours as needed; maximum 3200 mg/day
  ✓ Acetaminophen, aspirin, plus caffeine (Excedrin Migraine), 2 tabs PO Q 6 hours as needed; maximum 8 tabs a day for 2 days
Patients with **moderate to severe headache** often require **specific** therapy; select a nonoral route of administration for patients with associated nausea or vomiting

Class/Drug	Dosing
Serotonin receptor agonists (triptans)	
Rizatriptan (Maxalt)	5-10 mg PO initially; available in orally-disintegrating tabs; may repeat after 2 hours, max 30 mg/day; if taking a β-blocker, use 5 mg per maximal dose up to 15 mg/day
Sumatriptan (Imitrex), available as PO, SC, IN	Oral Dose: 25-100 mg PO initially; may repeat after 2 hours, max 200 mg/day SC Dose: 6 mg SC initially; may repeat in 1 hour, max 12 mg/day Nasal Spray Dose: 5-20 mg spray nasally; may repeat once after 2 hours, max 40 mg/day
Zolmitriptan (Zomig),	1.25-2.5 mg PO initially; may repeat after 2 hours, max 10 mg day
Ergot alkaloids and derivatives	
Dihydroergotamine [DHE] (Migranal) Nasal spray	1 spray in each nostril; may repeat in 15 minutes, max 4 sprays per 24 hours and 8/week

Use of antiemetics should not be restricted to patients who are vomiting or likely to vomit as nausea in and of itself is a very disabling symptom (consult section on NAUSEA AND VOMITING for drug selection and dosing recommendations)

Silberstein, S.D. for the US Headache Consortium. Report of the Quality Standards Subcommittee of the American Academy of Neurology. (2000). Practice parameter: Evidenced-based guidelines for migraine headache (an evidence-based review). *Neurology, 55*, p. 759.

K. Nonpharmacologic therapies should be used in children <18 years of age for prevention of migraine (refer to box under V.G. above)

L. Few drugs used to treat headaches in adults are approved for use in children <18 years of age; only drugs that are approved for use in children for pain management are recommended here

M. Mainstay of acute treatment of migraine in children is intermittent use of oral analgesics and environmental manipulation

---

ACUTE TREATMENT OF MIGRAINE IN CHILDREN

Analgesics
  Most children respond well to ibuprofen
    Children <12 years of age: Dose at 10 mg/kg/dose Q 6-8 hours (available as suspension, 100 mg per 5 mL; chewable tabs, 50 mg and 100 mg)
    Children >12 years of age: Dose 200-400 mg Q 6 hours PRN (available as 200 mg tabs, caplets)

  A second option is acetaminophen
    Children <12 years of age: Dose at 10-15mg/kg/dose Q 6 hours (available as suspension, 160 mg per 5 mL; chewable tabs, 80 mg and 160 mg)
    Children >12 years of age: Dose 2 regular strength tabs (325 mg/tab) Q 4-6 hours

Environmental Manipulation
  Best therapeutic approach is to allow the child to rest in a quiet, dark room with a cool, wet cloth across the forehead; sleep is often the most effective treatment

If an antiemetic is needed to control nausea, see section on NAUSEA AND VOMITING for drug selection and dosing recommendations

N. Follow up for adolescents and children with migraine headache
    1. Monitor trends in headache frequency, severity, and response to therapies (both preventive and acute pharmacologic therapy) via a headache diary kept by patient and reviewed on every follow up visit (every 2-4 weeks in first 3 months, then every 3-6 months)
    2. If after 3-6 months, headaches are well controlled with preventive therapy, consider tapering or discontinuing treatment

O. Referral considerations
    1. Patients who do not respond to (or fail) treatments outlined above for moderate to severe migraine should be referred to an expert for management
    2. Patients who prefer nonpharmacologic treatments (e.g., behavioral treatments [see V.G. above] or complementary therapies such as acupuncture and cervical manipulation) should be referred to experts in these modalities for management
    3. Patients with migraine headache and who are pregnant or who want to become pregnant should be referred to an expert for management

P. **Management of patients with episodic tension-type headache** is described in the table below

MANAGEMENT OF ADOLESCENT PATIENTS WITH EPISODIC TENSION-TYPE HEADACHE
Nonpharmacologic   Because of the chronic nature of these headaches, nonpharmacologic approaches such as biofeedback, stress management, relaxation therapy, and aerobic exercise should be given a trial; provide patient with specific referral for any of these approaches that seem appropriate and that patient is willing to try   *Pharmacologic*   The following OTC medications are usually effective in adolescents ≥18 years   ✓ Ibuprofen, 400-600 mg every 4-6 hours; maximum 3200 mg/day   ✓ Acetaminophen, 650 mg every 4 hours OR 1000 mg every 12 hours   ✓ Aspirin, 650 mg every 4 hours   ✓ Acetaminophen, 250 mg/aspirin, 250 mg/caffeine, 65 mg (Excedrin Extra Strength), 2 tabs PO at start of attack; up to 8 per day

Q. In **children**, use the same medications recommended under V.M above (Acute Treatment of Migraine in Children)

R. Educate patient and parents about overuse of analgesics which can lead to rebound headaches; patients who take analgesics at least three times a day for 5 or more days a week are prone to rebound headache

S. **Management of adolescent patients with cluster headache** (a rare disorder in children) includes both preventive therapy and acute therapy and is described in the table below

MANAGEMENT OF PATIENTS ≥18 YEARS WITH CLUSTER HEADACHE
The brevity of cluster headache attacks precludes most oral acute-relief therapies

Triptans are very efficacious using the subcutaneous or nasal spray routes of administration
     Sumatriptan (Imitrex), 6 mg SC initially; may repeat in 1 hour, max 12 mg/day; the nasal spray dose is 5-20 mg spray nasally; may repeat after 2 hours, max 40 mg/day
 Also effective is 100% oxygen for 10-15 minutes; repeat as needed
 	
 Preventive therapy for cluster headache is indicated when there is high attack frequency
     Verapamil (Calan), 80-120 mg PO TID is effective and usually well tolerated (Not FDA approved for this indication)
 If this medication proves to be ineffective or poorly tolerated, refer patient for expert care (surgical procedures are available for refractory cases)

T. Follow Up
    1. Patients with migraine headaches, as outlined above under V.N.
    2. Patients with tension or cluster headache, follow up is necessary within 2-4 weeks after patient is placed on therapy to determine efficacy

SEIZURES AND EPILEPSY

I. Definitions

    A.   Seizures: Behavioral changes resulting from abnormal paroxysmal neuronal discharge and are a symptom of an underlying brain problem

    B.   Epilepsy: Recurrent unprovoked seizures with few other systemic or neurologic symptoms

II. Pathogenesis

    A.   Initiated by electrochemical abnormalities in brain such as alterations in concentration of excitatory or inhibitory neurotransmitter

    B.   Abnormal electrical discharge from one site is rapidly transmitted to other parts of the brain, producing disturbances in perception, motor control, attention, and consciousness

    C.   Important causes of seizure by age group are as follows:

Infancy and childhood	✓ Birth trauma, congenital malformations ✓ Inborn errors of metabolism ✓ Idiopathic
Adolescents	✓ Idiopathic ✓ Trauma ✓ Infection ✓ Alcohol or drug related

III. Clinical Presentation

    A.   Children have a high incidence of seizures and epilepsy; population-based studies show the incidence to be 100 per 100,000 in infancy and 50 per 100,000 for most of childhood

    B.   Children and adolescents are most likely to have idiopathic seizures or seizure secondary to trauma, inborn errors of metabolism, or infection. Alcohol and drug related causes are less common
        1.   Idiopathic seizures, known as epilepsy, often begin in childhood and adolescence
            a.   Cause is unknown, but there may be a hereditary predisposition
            b.   In many patients with idiopathic epilepsy, the physical, neurologic, and laboratory evaluations are normal
        2.   Traumatic causes, most often from accidental injuries
            a.   Birth and perinatal injuries can cause seizures but these are usually diagnosed early in life
            b.   Head trauma from MVCs, falls, and sports injuries are common causes, with the more severe the head injury, the greater the likelihood of developing post-traumatic seizures
        3.   Infectious causes, including infection of the brain: Presence of an epidemic of encephalitis, or recent history of febrile illness with changes in mental status suggest an infectious cause
        4.   Alcohol and drug related seizures occur via a number of mechanisms
            a.   Alcohol can cause seizures due to malnutrition, increased risk of head trauma, and during withdrawal
            b.   Cocaine and other stimulants are associated with increased risk of seizure; withdrawal from barbiturates can also cause seizures

    C.   Children with idiopathic (or genetically determined) epilepsy have the best prognosis, whereas those with preceding neurologic abnormalities are likely to have less positive outcomes

D. Principal types of seizures and their clinical features are listed in the table that follows:

PRINCIPAL TYPES OF SEIZURES	
Type of Seizure	**Clinical Features**
Partial Seizures	
Simple partial seizures (focal)	**No alteration/impairment of consciousness occurs** ✓ Signs and symptoms may be motor, sensory, autonomic, or psychic ✓ With motor symptoms, movements often begin in single muscle group and spread to entire side of body ✓ With sensory symptoms, sensory changes may involve paresthesia, or visualization of flashing lights ✓ With autonomic symptoms, patient experiences symptoms such as tachycardia, loss of bowel/bladder control ✓ With psychic symptoms, patients may report hallucinatory experiences, déjà vu, or a dreamlike state
Complex partial seizures (Temporal lobe or psychomotor)	**Impairment of consciousness occurs** ✓ Seizure may begin without warning or with motor, sensory, autonomic, or with psychic signs or symptoms ✓ Automatisms (automatic acts about which patient has no recollection) may occur ✓ Seizure is often followed by period of confusion
Secondarily generalized partial seizures (tonic-clonic or grand mal)	**Impairment of consciousness occurs** ✓ Seizures may begin with motor, sensory, autonomic, or psychic signs/symptoms ✓ A tonic increase in muscle tone occurs with subsequent rhythmic (clonic) jerks that slowly subside ✓ Seizure duration is one minute or longer and there is increased muscle tone during the event ✓ After seizure, patient is comatose and slowly recovers ✓ Tongue biting and incontinence may occur
Generalized Seizures	
Absence seizures	**Impairment of consciousness occurs** ✓ Very brief, frequent periods of nondistractible staring (average ~10 seconds) occurring primarily in children (age at first seizure is 3-20 years); recovery is rapid ✓ Increased or decreased muscle tone may also occur as well as automatisms or mild clonic movements (atypical absence seizures) [petit mal]
Primarily generalized tonic-clonic seizures (grand mal)	**Loss of consciousness occurs** ✓ Patient loses consciousness (without warning or is preceded by myoclonic jerks) ✓ Clinical features are similar to those of secondarily generalized partial seizure

Adapted from Brown, T.R., & Holmes, G.L. (2001). Epilepsy. *New England Journal of Medicine, 344*, p. 1146.

IV. Diagnosis/Evaluation

    A.   History: Initial step is to determine whether patient does or does not have seizures; next step is to determine type of seizure (by classifying it as focal or generalized in onset) and etiology (if identifiable)

        1.   Important to question family members and witnesses as well as patient (for much of the history, witnesses are better sources than patients, but patients are the best source for presence and type of aura)

        2.   Explore precipitating factors

        3.   Describe the focal onset, duration, and seizure characteristics

        4.   Inquire about the setting in which episode occurred

            a.   Determine whether the patient completely lost consciousness and/or was incontinent

            b.   Determine if there was an aura, antegrade amnesia, or postictal period

        5.   Determine if this was a first seizure or if patient has history of minor types of seizures (e.g., myoclonic or absence seizures) [**Note**: History of minor types of seizures in a person presenting with a possible tonic-clonic seizure helps establish the diagnosis of a seizure disorder]

        6.   Obtain past medical history including history of head trauma, birth complications, febrile convulsions, middle ear or sinus infections, alcohol or drug use, or symptoms of cancer

        7.   Inquire about possible toxic exposures (related to recreational pursuits or residence in a geographic location that places the child at risk, e.g., high levels of air pollutants

        8.   Determine if there is a family history of epilepsy

        9.   Ask parents about birth history and attainment of developmental milestones

        10.   For patients with known epilepsy who present with seizures, determine the following:

            a.   Precipitating factors

            b.   Similarity and differences between these seizures and ones in the past

            c.   Medications currently taking and adherence with regimen

            d.   If the seizures are occurring more frequently

B. Physical Examination
1. Assess vital signs and evaluate for orthostatic hypotension
2. Perform a complete physical examination with a focus on signs of disorders associated with seizures
   a. HEENT—look for signs of head trauma, infections of ears/sinuses
   b. Cardiovascular system
   c. Neurologic—assess pupils, fundi, cranial nerves, sensory, motor and reflexes exam (examine fontanelles and responsivity in infants) [**Note**: A normal neurologic exam is often found in persons with idiopathic seizure disorder]

C. Differential Diagnosis
1. Most common causes of seizures are listed under II.C. above and must be considered
2. Syncope does not cause seizures but is often confused with this disorder
   a. Whereas patients with syncope may exhibit repetitive clonic, myoclonic, or dystonic movements, these movements rarely last beyond 5-10 seconds and do not exhibit the organized progression from tonic to clonic phase seen in convulsive seizures
   b. Incontinence does not occur with syncope but may occur with seizures
   c. Tongue biting does not occur with syncope but may occur with seizures
   d. A few minutes of confusion immediately following the event is not likely with syncope but is likely with seizures
3. Pseudoseizures must be differentiated from seizures; pseudoseizures are more likely to be long in duration, may involve bizarre or unusual movements, and may be precipitated by stressful events

D. Diagnostic Tests
1. Basic laboratory evaluation to determine cause of a newly diagnosed seizure disorder includes the following
   a. CBC with differential
   b. Chemistry profile
   c. Electroencephalography in waking and sleeping states
   d. Magnetic resonance imaging (MRI) or computed tomography (CT), with MRI being the preferred test because it is more likely to reveal small tumors
   e. Toxicology screening should be performed in children across the entire pediatric age range if there is any question of drug exposure or substance abuse
   f. Lumbar puncture if infection or cancer is suspected (in children with a first nonfebrile seizure, LP is of limited value and should be used primarily when there is concern about possible meningitis or encephalitis)
2. American Academy of Neurology practice guidelines for neuroimaging studies in patients who have had a first seizure are outlined in the box below

---

Emergent neuroimaging (MRI preferred) should be performed in children of any age (with a first nonfebrile seizure) with a postictal focal deficit or altered mental status that does not quickly resolve

Nonemergent imaging studies with MRI should be considered for children in the following categories
   ✓ No cause of seizure has been determined
   ✓ Child with seizure of focal onset
   ✓ Child under age of one year with nonfebrile seizure
   ✓ Child with unexplained cognitive or motor dysfunction
   ✓ Child with abnormalities on neurologic examination

V. Plan/Management

A. Data from the history, physical examination, and laboratory studies are usually sufficient to diagnose a seizure disorder
1. If presence of seizure disorder or type of disorder cannot be established, additional data should be collected (e.g., additional information about the event from other witnesses, repeated electroencephalogram)
2. Referral a pediatric neurologist for this additional evaluation is essential

B. Management of children with epilepsy is based on the establishment of good clinician-patient interaction, including education, counseling, and advocacy—interventions that have a significant impact on the long-term adaptation of the family and child to the diagnosis and treatment plan
1. **Education/counseling:** Family (and child if age-appropriate) should be given detailed information about epilepsy and its treatment, including long-term prognosis. The importance of carefully following the medication regimen and monitoring of side effects and idiosyncratic reactions that are potentially fatal (see V.E. below) should be emphasized
2. **Advocacy:** Refer the patient and family to the Epilepsy Foundation of American (EFA), an organization dedicated to countering societal misconceptions and prejudices about epilepsy as well as improving the quality of life for persons affected by seizures

> - The national office can be contacted by writing EFA, 4351 Garden City Drive, Landover, MD 20785-2267 or by calling 301-459-3700 or 800-EFA-1000; the website is http://www.efa.org
> - Most states have local affiliates which provide community outreach programs, support groups, information and referral, employment services, respite care for families, and help with living arrangements

C. Treatment with an antiepileptic drug (AED) should be contemplated but not always automatically begun in children who have recurrent unprovoked seizures
1. The anticipated benefit of AED therapy needs to be considered in light of the likelihood of harm from the seizures and from the medications
2. Decision to institute drug treatment is complex and is influenced by the frequency and type of seizures, the estimated risk from further episodes, and the underlying epilepsy syndrome
3. **Because of the complexity of the decision, treatment decisions should always be made by a pediatric neurologist, or if that is not possible, in consultation with a pediatric neurologist**
4. Children are **rarely** treated for a first-time seizure (nearly 60% of children with an uncomplicated single seizure do not experience a second one)

D. Goal of pharmacologic treatment of patients with epilepsy is to provide optimal control of seizures without producing unacceptable side effects; thus the selection and adjustment of medications are important therapeutic decisions
1. Begin treatment with an average dose of a first line antiepileptic drug that is effective for the child's seizure disorder
2. Select one that best fits the patient based on both patient and medication characteristics including presence of other medical conditions and side-effect profile
3. Gradually make incremental changes that will enhance effectiveness and tolerability
4. A general rule of thumb is to initiate therapy with one-fourth to one-third of the anticipated maintenance dose and increase the dose to maintenance level over a 3-4 week period
5. Most side effects are experienced at the initiation of therapy and can be minimized by starting with a low enough dose
    a. Sedation, dizziness, ataxia, headache, and nausea are common dose-related side effects
    b. These side effects can be managed by reducing the dose by 25 to 50% and then waiting 2 weeks for tolerance to develop before gradually increased doses can be resumed
6. In addition to dose-related side effects, idiosyncratic reactions to AEDs can also occur; these reactions, some of which are potentially fatal, do not correlate with the dose of medication and occur unpredictably, most often early in the course of treatment
    a. Many AEDs can cause a rash during the first weeks of therapy which in some cases progresses to Stevens-Johnson syndrome or other serious conditions; rashes are usually erythematous, maculopapular or morbilliform eruptions, often beginning on trunk, face, or upper arms
        (1) Patients should immediately be evaluated at the onset of any new rash, especially rashes that blister, peel, bleed, or involve the mucous membranes, palms, or soles
        (2) Fever, dry cough, symptoms common with viral syndromes can be the initial features of Stevens-Johnson syndrome
    b. Liver dysfunction and bone marrow suppression can also occur
        (1) Protracted vomiting, lethargy, easy bruisability, protracted bleeding from minor cuts, or persistent infection may indicate liver dysfunction or bone marrow suppression
        (2) Routine measurement of blood chemistry profile, liver function tests, and complete blood count every 3-6 months are standard practice but are not likely to identify potentially life threatening conditions until late in the course of the condition
    c. The child's parents must be educated to recognize the warning signs of idiosyncratic reactions so that early intervention can occur

E. First-line antiepileptic drugs according to seizure type are listed in the table that follows:

FIRST-LINE ANTIEPILEPTIC DRUGS ACCORDING TO SEIZURE TYPE		
Seizure Type	First-Line Drugs Adolescents ≥16	First-Line Drugs Children <16
Generalized Seizures		
Absence seizures (petit mal)	Ethosuximide, divalproex sodium,	Ethosuximide
Primarily generalized tonic-clonic seizures (grand mal)	Divalproex sodium, phenytoin	Divalproex sodium
Partial Seizures		
Simple (focal) and complex (temporal lobe or psychomotor) partial seizures	Carbamazepine, divalproex sodium, oxcarbazepine, phenytoin	Carbamazepine, oxcarbazepine
Secondarily generalized partial seizures	Carbamazepine, divalproex sodium, oxcarbazepine, phenytoin	Carbamazepine, oxcarbazepine

F. If adequate seizure control is attained with the average dose of a first-line drug and the side effects are tolerable, no adjustment in dosing is needed

G. If the seizures are not controlled with the average dose of a first-line drug, and if there is no evidence of serious toxicity, the dose of the drug should be systematically increased until the seizures are controlled or until side effects preclude further increases in the dose
   1. If the maximal tolerated dose of the first-line AED does not control the seizures, one option is to substitute another first-line AED for use as monotherapy
      a. Start a second drug and taper the first. As the dosage of the new medication is titrated, the first medication is gradually tapered until monotherapy with the new agent is achieved. If control is not obtained with monotherapy with a second drug, then refer to a neurologist
      b. Never abruptly withdraw any drug; gradually taper
   2. A second option when the first AED does not control the seizures is to add another first-line (or second-line) AED while continuing the first
      a. Until very recently, therapy with 2 or more AEDs was used only after two or more first-line drugs given as monotherapy had been ineffective
      b. Since most of the newer AEDs for partial seizures (the most common types of seizures) are approved by the FDA only as adjunctive therapy, there has been an increased use of two-drug regimens that consist of one first-line drug and one of the newer second-line drugs approved for adjunctive therapy
      c. Selected adjunctive medications for use in patients with partial seizures are listed in the box below

> *Selected adjunctive medications for partial seizures*
>
> Divalproex sodium (Depakote) [approved for monotherapy or adjunctive therapy]
> Gabapentin (Neurontin)
> Levetiracetam (Keppra)
> Oxcarbazepine (Trileptal) [approved for monotherapy or adjunctive therapy]
> Tiagabine (Gabitril)

H. If trials of two sensibly selected drugs fail, referral should be made to a pediatric neurologist (if not done previously)

I. The newer AEDs include tiagabine, gabapentin, lamotrigine, levetiracetam, oxcarbazepine, zonisamide, and topiramate; these drugs are used primarily as adjunctive therapy in refractory patients

J. For drugs with established therapeutic range of plasma concentrations, titrate dosage to achieve adequate concentrations, recognizing that this is only a rough guide for determining the appropriate dosage
   1. Treat the patient, not the plasma drug concentration
   2. Plasma drug concentrations within the therapeutic range may have toxic effects
   3. Seizures may be controlled in some patients with plasma drug concentrations below the therapeutic range
   4. Titration of dose of phenytoin must be done with great caution because of its nonlinear pharmacokinetics

K. Once AED therapy is initiated, withdrawal of AEDs should be considered when the child is free of seizures for 2 years
1. Disadvantages of continuing therapy include the risks of side effects, drug interactions, and teratogenicity (in women) as well as the costs of therapy
2. Withdrawal of therapy should be gradual (with dose tapering over the course of 6-12 weeks) and at a mutually agreed upon time with the patient
3. Risk of recurrent seizures is 25% among patients without risk factors and about 50% in patients with such factors (risk is highest for children with symptomatic epilepsy, persistently abnormal EEGs and abnormal neurologic examination
4. About 80% of recurrences occur within 4 months after a regimen of tapering of dosage has been begun and 90% occur within the first year
5. Caution patients about driving and operating machinery for at least the first 4 months after the start of drug withdrawal

L. Patient education is an ongoing process
1. Understanding the disorder and the prescribed medications by both the child (if old enough to comprehend) and family is of the utmost importance; non-adherence to the medication regime has been identified as the single most common reason for treatment failure
   a. Review with family/child dosing, actions, side effects, and drug interactions of the particular AED that is being prescribed
   b. For adolescent girls of childbearing age or who are taking oral contraceptives, emphasize that AEDs are teratogenic and that they also reduce the effectiveness of oral contraceptives
   c. Patient education must be continuous and must be addressed at every visit
2. Instruct families regarding the fundamentals of emergency management of seizures

M. Review the law in your state concerning operating a motor vehicle by persons with seizure disorders
1. In most states, drivers are required to self-report a seizure disorder to the Department of Motor Vehicles at the time of diagnosis; healthcare clinicians may not report a patient's condition without a written release of information from the patient (there are exceptions to this, however)
2. Six states (CA, DE, NV, NJ, OR, and PA) require mandatory provider reporting of patients with seizures to regulatory authorities
3. Recognize that whereas regulating driving privileges of epileptic patients may seen beneficial, it actually is unnecessary and may hinder medical management
   a. The relative risk for MVCs involving epileptic drivers is comparable to or lower than those of more prevalent conditions not subject to similar mandatory reporting requirements
   b. Only about 25% of epileptic drivers experiencing a seizure in the past 12 months report the seizure to their healthcare clinician for fear of being reported to the licensing authorities
4. A summary of requirements for each state is available from the Epilepsy Foundation at http://www.efa.org

N. Follow Up
1. Children with a newly diagnosed seizure disorder should be managed by a pediatric neurologist who will determine the appropriate follow-up schedule
   a. In general, children who are placed on AED therapy are followed closely during period of adjusting medication dose, then every 3 months for the next 6 months, and then every 6 months thereafter
   b. Monitoring of plasma drug concentrations for therapeutic range is indicated for many of the AEDs and should be done on a regular basis and with any medication adjustment
   c. Periodic monitoring of blood cell counts and hepatic enzyme levels—every 3-6 months is recommended with many of the medications (package inserts contain monitoring requirements for prescribed medications)
2. Once the child is stabilized, follow-up by the primary care clinician is appropriate

REFERENCES

American Academy of Pediatrics, Committee on Quality Improvement, Subcommittee on Febrile Seizures. (1999). Practice parameter: Long-term treatment of the child with simple febrile seizures. *Pediatrics, 103,* 1307-1309.

Bahra, A., May, A., & Goadsby, P.J. (2002). Cluster headache: A prospective clinical study with diagnostic implications. *Neurology, 58,* 354-361.

Benbadis, S.R., & Tatum, W.O. (2001). Advances in the treatment of epilepsy. *American Family Physician, 64,* 91-98.

Breslau, N., & Rasmussen, B.K. (2001). The impact of migraine. *Neurology, 56,* S4-S12.

Brown, T.R., & Holmes, G.L. (2001). Epilepsy. *New England Journal of Medicine, 344,* 1145-1151.

Cargan, A.L. (2002). Febrile seizures. In F.D. Burg, J.R. Ingelfinger, R.A. Polin, & A.A. Gershon (Eds.), *Gellis & Kagan's current pediatric therapy* (pp. 453-455). Philadelphia: Elsevier Science.

Chutorian, A.M. (2002). Headaches in children. In F.D. Burg, J.R. Ingelfinger, R.A. Polin, & A.A. Gershon (Eds.), *Gellis & Kagan's current pediatric therapy* (pp. 457-460). Philadelphia: Elsevier Science.

Diaz-Arrastia, R., Agnostini, M.A., & Van Ness, P.C. (2002). Evolving treatment strategies for epilepsy. *Journal of the American Medical Association, 287,* 2917-2922.

Fountain, N.B. (2002). Seizures and epilepsy in adolescents and adults. In R.E. Rakel, & E.T. Bope (Eds.), *Conn's current therapy* (pp. 884-893). Philadelphia: Saunders.

Furman, J.M., & Cass, S.P. (1999). Benign paroxysmal positional vertigo. *New England Journal of Medicine, 341,* 1590-1598.

Goadsby, P.J., Lipton, R.B., & Ferrari, M.D. (2002). Migraine—Current understanding and treatment. *New England Journal of Medicine, 346,* 257-269.

Hirtz, D., Ashwal, S., Berg, A., Bettis, D., Camfield, C., Camfield, P., et al. (2000). Practice parameter: Evaluating a first nonfebrile seizure in children. *Neurology, 55,* 616-623.

Holland, K., & Wyllie, E. (2002). Epilepsy in infants and children. In R.E. Rakel, & E.T. Bope (Eds.), *Conn's current therapy* (pp. 893-898). Philadelphia: Saunders.

Hotson, J.R., & Baloh, R.W. (1998). Acute vestibular syndrome. *New England Journal of Medicine, 339,* 680-685.

Kapoor, W. N. (2000). Syncope. *New England Journal of Medicine, 343,* 1856-1862.

Kraus, G.L., Ampaw, L., & Krumholz, A. (2001). Individual state driving restrictions for people with epilepsy in the US. *Neurology, 57,* 1780-1785.

Lambert, P.R. (2002). Acute facial paralysis (Bell's palsy). In R.E. Rakel, & E.T. Bope (Eds.), *Conn's current therapy* (pp. 948-950). Philadelphia: Saunders.

Lewis, D.W. (2002). Headaches in children and adolescents. *American Family Physician, 65,* 625-632.

Logemann, G.D., & Ranking, L.M. (2000). Newer intranasal migraine medications. *American Family Physician, 61,* 180-186.

Louis, E.D. (2001). Essential tremor. *New England Journal of Medicine, 345,* 887-891.

Martin, C.O. (2002). Neurology. In M.A. Graver & M.L. Lanternier (Eds.). *The family practice handbook* (pp. 337-390). St. Louis: Mosby.

Millea, P.J., Brodie, J.J. (2002). Tension-type headache. *American Family Physician, 66,* 797-804.

Morey, S.S. (2000). Guidelines on migraine: Part 2. General principles of drug therapy. *American Family Physician, 62,* 1915-1918.

Morey, S.S. (2000). Guidelines on migraine: Part 3. Recommendations for individual drugs. *American Family Physician, 62,* 2145-2152.

Morey, S.S. (2000). Guidelines on migraine: Part 4. General principles of preventive therapy. *American Family Physician, 62,* 2359-2364.

Morey, S.S. (2000). Guidelines on migraine: Part 5. Recommendations for specific prophylactic therapy. *American Family Physician, 62,* 2359-2364.

Morey, S.S. (2000). Headache consortium releases guidelines for use of CT or MRI in migraine. *American Family Physician, 62,* 1699-1702.

Nordli, D.R. (2002). Medical treatment of the child with epilepsy. In. F.D. Burg, J.R. Ingelfinger, R.A. Polin, & A.A. Gershon (Eds.), *Gellis & Kagan's current pediatric therapy* (pp. 446-453). Philadelphia: Elsevier Science.

Oas, J.G. (2002). Episodic vertigo. In R.E. Rakel, & E.T. Bope (Eds.), *Conn's current therapy* (pp. 912-917). Philadelphia: Saunders

Silberstein, S.D., for the US Headache Consortium. Report of the Quality Standards Subcommittee of the American Academy of Neurology. (2000). Practice parameter: Evidenced-based guidelines for migraine headache (an evidence-based review). *Neurology, 55*, 754-762.

Sloane, P.D., Coeytaux, R.R., Beck, R.S., & Dallara, J. (2001). Dizziness: State of the science. *Annals of Internal Medicine, 134*, 823-832.

Stafstrom, C.E., Rostasy, K., & Minster, A. (2002). Usefulness of children's drawings in the diagnosis of headache. *Pediatrics, 109*, 460-472.

Stewart, W.F., Lipton, R.B., Kolodner, K., Liberman, J., & Sawyer, J. (1999). Reliability of the migraine disability assessment score in a population-based sample of headache sufferers. *Cephalalgia, 19*, 107-114.

Tatum, W.O., Galvez, R., Benbadis, S., & Carrazana, E. (2000). New antiepileptic drugs. *Archives of Family Medicine, 9,* 1135-1141.

Hematologic Problems

MARY VIRGINIA GRAHAM

IRON DEFICIENCY ANEMIA

I. Definition: Anemia characterized by small (microcytic), pale (hypochromic) red blood cells (RBCs), and depletion of iron (Fe) stores

II. Pathogenesis

   A. Iron loss exceeds intake so that storage iron (as measured by serum ferritin concentration) is progressively depleted

   B. As storage iron is depleted, a compensatory increase in absorption of dietary Fe and in the concentration of transport iron (as measured by transferrin saturation) occurs

   C. Iron stores are no longer able to meet the needs of the erythroid marrow; the plasma-transferrin level increases, the serum Fe concentration declines, resulting in a decrease in Fe available for RBC formation

   D. The shortage of iron leads to underproduction of iron-containing functional compounds, including hemoglobin

   E. The RBCs of persons who have iron deficiency anemia (IDA) are microcytic and hypochromic

   F. In early childhood and adolescence, poor dietary intake and increased demand are the most common causes

III. Clinical Presentation

   A. Iron deficiency anemia is the most common nutritional deficiency of infancy and childhood worldwide
      1. Toddlers (especially those aged 9 to 18 months) and adolescent females are most at risk for iron deficiency and iron deficiency anemia because of poor iron intake and increased iron needs with rapid growth
      2. Adolescent girls also have ongoing iron losses from menstruation; pregnant teens are at especially high risk because of the combination of rapid growth and the increased iron needs of pregnancy

   B. Iron status and iron requirements for children and adolescents are briefly reviewed in the box below

   - Eighty percent of fetal iron is produced during the third trimester so that the elemental iron concentration in the body of healthy full-term infants at birth is approximately 75 mg/kg—most (75%) of this iron is in circulating hemoglobin, and the remainder is divided between storage and tissue protein
   - During the first 4 months after birth, infants use iron from the breakdown of red blood cells (RBCs) and from their dietary intake; thus, iron stores of full-term infants can meet iron requirements until 4-6 months of life without becoming iron deficient (Preterm infants have inadequate stores and increased postnatal iron requirements)
   - A rapid rate of growth together with dietary intake that is frequently inadequate in dietary iron places children less than 24 months (especially those between 9-18 months of age) at the highest risk of any age group during childhood for iron deficiency
   - After 24 months of age, with the slowing of growth and increased diversification of diet, the risk for iron deficiency declines
   - In children ≥36 months of age, dietary iron and iron status are usually adequate; risk factors for iron depletion in this age group include low family income, a low iron or other specialized diet, and medical conditions that affect iron status such as inflammatory or bleeding disorders
   - During adolescence (defined here as ages 12 to <18 years of age), iron requirements and thus the risk for iron deficiency increase because of rapid growth
      ✓ Among males, the risk essentially ends after the peak pubertal growth period and adolescent boys are not likely to be iron deficient
      ✓ Adolescent girls continue to be at risk for iron deficiency because of menstrual blood loss

   C. Iron deficiency is the result of long-term negative iron balance—inadequate body iron stores are manifest along a continuum beginning with iron depletion, continuing to iron deficiency, and finally culminating in iron deficiency anemia—a late manifestation of prolonged negative iron balance

D. Clinical presentation depends on severity, age of the child, and ability of the cardiovascular and pulmonary systems to compensate for decreasing oxygen carrying capacity of the blood; in the early stages of the process, when iron depletion is occurring and iron deficiency is developing, the child's symptoms may be minimal

E. Children with iron depletion, iron deficiency, or mild to moderate iron deficiency anemia (hemoglobin 8 to 11 g/dL) may have nonspecific complaints of irritability, anorexia, headache, poor concentration, palpitations, and fatigue

F. Children with severe iron deficiency anemia (hemoglobin less than 8 g/dL) may have pallor (best seen in conjunctiva), fatigue, irritability, tachycardia, and dyspnea with exercise

G. Iron deficiency and iron deficiency anemia in infants and children has been associated with numerous long-term consequences that may be irreversible
1. For example, cognitive deficits, delays in psychomotor development, and behavioral problems can occur; further, growth may be impaired and the immune system may be depressed, resulting in an increased susceptibility to infection and immune system disorders
2. Iron deficiency anemia also contributes to lead poisoning in children by increasing the gastrointestinal tract's ability to absorb heavy metals such as lead

H. The Centers for Disease Control and Prevention (CDC) criteria for defining anemia in a healthy reference population are contained in the table below
1. Keep in mind that high altitudes and cigarette smoking increase anemia cutpoints
2. Altitudes above 3,000 feet raise the cutpoint for anemia because of lower oxygen partial pressure, a reduction in oxygen saturation of the blood, and an increase in red cell production
3. Cigarette smoking raises the cutpoint for anemia because carboxyhemoglobin formed from carbon monoxide during smoking has no oxygen carrying capacity
4. To illustrate, the Hb cutpoint for children living at altitudes between 3,000 and 4,000 feet is increased by 0.2 g/dL. The Hb cutpoint for children who smoke at least 10 but fewer than 20 cigarettes per day is increased by 0.3 g/dL
5. **Note:** The Institute of Medicine recommends lowering the hemoglobin concentration and hematocrit cutoff values for African American children ≤5 years of age by 0.4 g/dL and 1% respectively to reflect the observation that the mean hemoglobin concentration and hematocrit for African Americans are lower than those for Caucasians (these lower levels do not reflect a difference in iron status), but the CDC opposes using cutoff values based on race

MAXIMUM HEMOGLOBIN CONCENTRATION AND HEMATOCRIT VALUES FOR ANEMIA[a]		
Sex/Age, Years	Hemoglobin, < g/dL	Hematocrit, < %
Males and Females		
1 to <2[b]	11.0	32.9
2 to <5	11.1	33.0
5 to <8	11.5	34.5
8 to <12	11.9	35.4
Males		
12 to <15	12.5	37.3
15 to <18	13.3	39.7
≥18	13.5	39.9
Females[c]		
12 to <15	11.8	35.7
15 to <18	12.0	35.9
≥18	12.0	35.7

[a] Age- and sex-specific cutoff values for anemia are based on the 5th percentile from the third National Health and Nutrition Examination Survey (NHANES III)
[b] Although no data are available from NHANES III to determine the maximum hemoglobin concentration and hematocrit values for anemia among infants, the values listed for children ages 1 to <2 years can be used for infants ages 6-12 months
[c] Nonpregnant and lactating adolescents

Adapted from Centers for Disease Control and Prevention (1998). Recommendations to prevent and control iron deficiency in the United States. *MMWR 47* (RR-3), 1-29.

IV. Diagnosis/Evaluation

    A.   History
        1.   Inquire about onset and duration of symptoms
        2.   In infants, determine if preterm, and obtain data related to feeding, including type (if formula fed, specifically ask if iron-fortified formula is being fed to infant), amount, and frequency; ask if whole cow's milk is being given to infant
        3.   In children and adolescents, obtain dietary history with focus on types and amounts of iron enriched food consumed
        4.   In adolescents, determine if caloric intake is being severely restricted to lose weight (see section on EATING DISORDERS)
        5.   In both children and adolescents obtain a careful history of gastrointestinal complaints that might suggest gastritis, peptic ulcer disease, or other conditions that might produce gastrointestinal bleeding; ask if there has been change in stool patterns or color
        6.   In menstruating females, ask about usual blood loss during menses
        7.   Obtain medication history, particularly use of aspirin and other NSAIDs; ask about past history of anemia or GI bleeding
        8.   In infants, obtain developmental history via parent report to determine if developmental milestones are being achieved

    B.   Physical Examination
        1.   In infants and children, obtain height and weight (calculate BMI in children ≥2 years), plot on growth chart, and compare with previous parameters
        2.   In adolescents, obtain weight and compare with previous weights; calculate BMI
        3.   Observe for pallor, particularly the conjunctiva
        4.   Examine tongue, corners of mouth, and nails for characteristic changes
        5.   Perform abdominal exam for tenderness on palpation and enlargement of the spleen
        6.   Auscultate heart for systolic flow murmurs
        7.   Obtain stool for occult blood only if history suggests that blood loss from the GI tract is a possibility

    C.   Differential Diagnosis:
        1.   Inadequate intake of iron
        2.   Any condition that causes acute or chronic blood loss
        3.   Other causes of microcytic anemias

    D.   Diagnostic Tests
        1.   Hemoglobin concentration and hematocrit, because of their low cost and ease of measurement, are the tests most commonly used to screen for iron deficiency in infants and children

> **Hemoglobin:** Concentration of iron-containing protein Hb in circulating red blood cells and a more direct and sensitive measure than Hct
>
> **Hematocrit:** Proportion of whole blood occupied by the red blood cells; it falls only after the Hb concentration

        2.   Changes in Hb concentration and Hct occur only at the late stages of iron deficiency; thus both tests are **late** indicators of iron deficiency
        3.   Although measures of Hb concentration and Hct cannot be used to determine the cause of anemia, a diagnosis of iron deficiency anemia can be made if Hb concentration or Hct increases after a course of therapeutic iron supplementation
        4.   Additional indicators of iron depletion, iron deficiency, and iron deficiency anemia are contained in the box below. The costs and feasibility of using additional indicators of iron deficiency may preclude their routine use, but such tests may be indicated in circumstances when detection of earlier changes in iron status is important; such tests can also be used to differentiate iron deficiency from microcytic anemias due to other causes (see *Laboratory Values for Most Common Microcytic Anemias* in the table below)

- ➡ **Mean cell volume (MCV)**: Average volume of red blood cells, measured in femtoliters using an electronic counter. MCV is highest at birth, decreases during the first 6 months of life, then gradually increases during childhood to adult levels; a low MCV indicates microcytic anemia (Lead poisoning, anemias of infection, chronic disease, and thalassemia minor can also cause a reduction in MCV)
- ➡ **Red blood cell distribution width (RDW)**: Indication of variation in cell size. IDA usually causes greater variation in red blood cell size than do conditions such as thalassemia minor
- ➡ **Serum ferritin concentration**: Nearly all ferritin in the body is intracellular, but a small amount circulates in the plasma. A direct relationship exists between serum ferritin concentration and the amount of iron stored in the body (1 µg/L of serum ferritin concentration is equivalent to approximately 10 mg of stored iron). Serum ferritin concentration is an early indicator of the status of iron stores and is the **most specific indicator** available of depleted iron stores, especially when used in conjunction with other tests to assess iron status. Values ≤15 µg/L in infants older than 6 months, children, and adolescents indicate depleted iron stores
- ➡ **Erythrocyte protoporphyrin concentration**: The concentration of erythrocyte protoporphyrin in blood increases when insufficient iron is available for hemoglobin production; infection, inflammation, and lead poisoning can also elevate erythrocyte protoporphyrin concentration
- ➡ **Transferrin saturation**: An indicator of the extent to which transferrin has vacant iron-binding sites (**low** transferrin saturation indicates a **high** proportion of vacant iron-binding sites)
  - ✓ Saturation is highest in neonates, declines by age 4 months, and then increases throughout childhood until adulthood
  - ✓ Transferrin saturation is based on two laboratory measures – serum iron concentration and total iron-binding capacity (TICB)
  - ✓ Transferrin saturation is calculated by dividing serum iron concentration by TIBC and multiplying by 100 to express the result as a percentage
  - ✓ Transferrin saturation (%) = [serum iron concentration (µg/dL)/TIBC (µg/dL)] x 100
- ➡ **Serum iron concentration**: Measures the total amount of iron in the serum (concentration increases after each meal, rises in the AM and falls at night, and decreases with infections and inflammations); more variation of this measure than with Hb and Hct
- ➡ **Total iron binding capacity (TIBC)**: Measures the iron-binding capacity within the serum and reflects the availability of iron-binding sites on transferrin; TIBC increases when serum iron concentration and stored iron is low and decreases when serum iron concentration and stored iron is high. **Note**: factors other than iron status that can affect this measure are inflammation and chronic infection (result in lower TIBC); oral contraceptives and pregnancy can elevate this measure; however, a more stable measure than serum iron concentration. Changes in TIBC occur after iron stores are depleted

LABORATORY VALUES FOR MOST COMMON MICROCYTIC ANEMIAS

Laboratory Test	Iron Deficiency Anemia	α- or β-Thalassemia Trait	Lead poisoning
Hemoglobin	Reduced	Reduced	Normal*
MCV	Reduced	Reduced	Normal*
RDW	Increased	Normal	Normal
Serum iron	Reduced	Normal	Normal*
Transferring	Reduced	Normal	Normal
TIBC	Increased	Normal	Normal*
Ferritin	Reduced	Normal	Normal*

*May be decreased if the blood lead concentration is very high

Adapted from Tender, J., & Cheng, T.L. (2002). Iron deficiency anemia. In F.D. Burg (Ed.), *Gellis & Kagan's current pediatric therapy* (pp. 633-637). Philadelphia: Saunders

V. Plan/Management

A. The initial step in management is to confirm a positive anemia screening result by performing a repeat Hb concentration or Hct test; if the tests agree and the child is not ill, a presumptive diagnosis of iron deficiency anemia can be made and treatment begun

B. Children with a presumptive diagnosis of severe iron deficiency anemia (Hb less than 8 g/dL) require further diagnostic testing including CBC (if not already obtained), smear, reticulocyte count, serum ferritin, serum iron, TIBC or transferrin, quantitative hemoglobin electrophoresis (including hemoglobin A_2 and F) and urgent referral to a pediatric hematologist

C. Children with a presumptive diagnosis of mild to moderate iron deficiency anemia (Hb 8 to 11 g/dL) are treated with oral iron therapy; the most widely recommended oral iron agent is ferrous sulfate, which is inexpensive, well absorbed, and well tolerated

- Infants and children younger than 5 years: 3 mg/kg/day of elemental iron (Feosol Elixir contains 44 mg of elemental iron per 5 mL and is divided into 3 doses/day)
- Children ages 5 to 12 years: One 60 mg elemental iron tablet per day (one 300 mg ferrous sulfate tablet [generic] = 60 mg elemental iron)
- Adolescent males ages 12 to 18 years: two 60 mg elemental iron tablets per day
- Adolescent females ages 12 to 18 years: one to two 60 mg elemental iron tablets per day
- Advise parent/patients regarding the following
  - ✓ Iron should be taken between meals for better absorption; in infants and small children, liquid medication should be placed in back of mouth to reduce staining of teeth
  - ✓ Iron taken with vitamin C containing juice boosts absorption
  - ✓ Iron preparations should not be taken within one hour of substances that may inhibit iron absorption (e.g., dairy products, antacids, calcium supplements, coffee, tea, bran, and whole grains)
  - ✓ To prevent accidental poisoning, iron preparations should be stored out of reach of infants and children

D. Counsel the parent (or patient in the case of adolescents) about adequate dietary intake of iron rich foods to correct the underlying problem of low iron intake

> ✓ Heme iron, found only in meat, poultry, and fish, is two to three times more absorbable than non-heme iron which is found in plant-based foods and iron-fortified foods (liver is not recommended because of its high cholesterol content and potentially high level of environmental toxins)
> ✓ The bioavailability of non-heme iron is strongly affected by the kind of other foods consumed at the same meal
> ✓ Enhancers of iron absorption are heme iron (in meat, poultry, and fish) and vitamin C
> ✓ Inhibitors of iron absorption include polyphenols (in certain vegetables), tannins (in tea), phytates (in bran), and calcium (in dairy products)
> ✓ Vegetarian diets, by definition, are low in heme iron; iron bioavailability in a vegetarian diet can be increased by careful planning of meals to include other sources of iron and enhancers of iron absorption
> ✓ Servings of the non-meat sources of iron in the box below contain approximately 2 mg of iron
>
>> 1 baked potato with skin
>> ½ cup dried bean, cooked
>> ½ cup soybeans, cooked
>> ½ cup tofu
>> 1 cup spinach
>> 1 tablespoon blackstrap molasses
>> 5 pieces dried fruit, especially plums or figs

E. Repeat hemoglobin/hematocrit in 4 weeks; an increase in hemoglobin of more than 1 g/dL or in hematocrit of more than 3% is consistent with iron deficiency anemia

F. Patients who have an appropriate response to therapy after 4 weeks should be managed as follows

> ✓ Continue therapy and repeat Hb in 2 months
> ✓ Continue treatment for 2-3 months after anemia resolves
> ✓ Repeat anemia screen 6 months after successful treatment
> ✓ Continue to provide dietary counseling

G. Patients who have been compliant with the treatment regimen and who have an inadequate response to therapy require additional diagnostic testing: Obtain a CBC (MCV, RDW), smear, ferritin, TIBC or transferrin, quantitative hemoglobin electrophoresis (including hemoglobin A_2 and F) and refer to a pediatric hematologist for further evaluation and management

H. **Primary prevention** of iron deficiency during infancy and childhood is most important for children <2 years, because, among all age groups, these children are at the greatest risk for inadequate intake of iron. The table below contains counseling recommendations

PRIMARY PREVENTION OF IRON DEFICIENCY AMONG INFANTS AND TODDLERS

- Encourage breastfeeding for all infants for the first 12 months of life; although breast milk contains low concentrations of iron—approximately 0.5 mg/L, 50% of the iron is absorbed
- Encourage exclusive breastfeeding (without supplementary liquid, formula, or food) for the first 6 months of life; nursing mothers should continue taking prenatal vitamins
- When exclusive breastfeeding is discontinued, encourage use of an additional source of iron (approximately 1 mg/kg/day of iron) from supplementary foods such as iron fortified infant cereal (Two or more servings per day of iron-fortified infant cereal can meet an infants' requirements for iron)
- For breastfed infants who were preterm or had a low birthweight, recommend 2-4 mg/kg/day of iron drops (to a maximum of 15 mg/day) starting at 1 month after birth and continuing until 12 months after birth
- Infants <1 year who are formula-fed should be fed only iron-fortified formula
- Early introduction (i.e., before age 1 year) of whole cow's milk and consumption of more than 24 ounces of whole cow's milk daily after age 1 are risk factors for iron deficiency because this milk has little iron, may replace foods with higher iron content, and may cause occult gastrointestinal bleeding

I.   Secondary prevention of iron deficiency is contained in the table below

SECONDARY PREVENTION: IRON DEFICIENCY

- ✓ In populations of infants and preschool children at high risk for iron deficiency anemia (i.e., children from low-income families, children eligible for the Special Supplemental Nutrition Program for Women, Infants, and Children (WIC), migrant children, or recently arrived refugee children), screen for anemia between ages 9 and 12 months, 6 months later, and annually from ages 2 to 5 years
- ✓ Among school-age children and adolescent boys, only those who have a history of iron deficiency anemia, special healthcare needs, or low iron intake should be screened for anemia
- ✓ Beginning in adolescence, screen all nonpregnant females for anemia every 5-10 years throughout their childbearing years during routine health examinations
- ✓ Annually screen for anemia females having risk factors for iron deficiency—extensive menstrual or other blood loss, low iron intake, or a previous diagnosis of iron deficiency anemia

J.   Follow-up: See V.E., F., and G. above

REFERENCES

Bergin, J.J. (2002). Anemia: A strategy for the workup. *Consultant, 63*, 869-882.

Blackwell, S., & Hendrix, P.C. (2001). Common anemias: What lies beneath. *Clinician Reviews, 11*, 53-62.

Centers for Disease Control and Prevention. (1998). Recommendations to prevent and control iron deficiency in the United States. *MMWR, 47*, RR-3, 1-36.

Centers for Disease Control and Prevention. (2002). Iron deficiency – United States, 1999-2000. MMWR, 51, 897-899.

Chen, K., & Graber, M.A. (2002). Anemia. In M.A. Graber & M.L. Lanternier (Eds.), *University of Iowa: The family practice handbook* (pp. 216-223). St. Louis: Mosby.

Goroll, A.H., & Mulley, A.G. (2002). *Primary care recommendations.* Philadelphia: Lippincott Williams & Wilkins.

Hamilton, C.W. (1998). Hematologic disorders. In B.G. Wells, J.T. DiPiro, T.L. Schwinghammer, & C.W. Hamilton (Eds.), *Pharmacotherapy handbook* (pp 367-375). Stamford, CT: Appleton & Lange.

Irwin, J.J., & Kirchner, J.T. (2002). Anemia in children. *American Family Physician, 64*, 1379-1386.

Kohli-Kumar, M. (2001). Screening for anemia in children: AAP recommendations—A critique. *Pediatrics, 108*, e56.

McLaren, G.D., & Gordeuk, V.R. (2002). Iron deficiency. In R.E. Rakel & E.T. Bope (Eds.), *Conn's current therapy* (pp. 366-369). Philadelphia: Saunders.

Oski, F.A. (1993). Iron deficiency in infancy and childhood. *The New England Journal of Medicine, 329*, 190-193.

Story, M., Holt, K., & Sofka, D. (Eds.) (2002). *Bright futures in practice: Nutrition* (2nd ed.). Arlington, VA: National Center for Education in Maternal and Child Health.

Tender, J., & Cheng, T.L. (2002). Iron deficiency anemia. In F.D. Burg, J.R. Ingelfinger, R.A. Polin, & A.A. Gershon (Eds.), *Gellis & Kagan's current pediatric therapy* (pp. 633-637). Philadelphia: Saunders.

US Department of Health and Human Services. (2000). *Healthy people 2010.* McLean, VA: International Publishing, Inc.

20

Minor Emergencies

MARY VIRGINIA GRAHAM & CONSTANCE R. UPHOLD

AVULSED TOOTH

I. Definition: A total displacement of a tooth out of its socket, usually due to trauma, resulting in severance of the apical blood supply and damage to the periodontal ligament

II. Pathogenesis: Teeth not fully erupted have loosely structured periodontal ligaments; thus these are the teeth most likely to be displaced when trauma to mouth occurs

III. Clinical Presentation

    A. An upper central incisor is the most frequently avulsed tooth

    B. Children aged 7-10 years are most likely to have avulsed teeth, but avulsion can also occur in adults

IV. Diagnosis/Evaluation

    A. Determine if the avulsed tooth is a primary or a secondary tooth; primary teeth should not be replanted because they often ankylose or fuse to the bone

    B. Immediate replanting of a secondary tooth is necessary to maintain vitality of the tooth (each minute the tooth remains out if its socket greatly reduces the likelihood that replantation will be successful); thus, assess for fractures of the teeth and alveolar ridge while simultaneously performing steps to preserve tooth

V. Plan/Treatment

    A. The avulsed tooth should be replanted immediately if possible
        1. If the tooth was displaced from the mouth and has collected debris from the ground or floor, rinse gently with sterile water holding the tooth by the crown. (DO NOT TOUCH ROOT SURFACE)
        2. Holding the tooth by the crown, gently tease it back onto the socket and cover with gauze; instruct patient to gently bite down on gauze during transport to dentist office
        3. If the avulsed tooth cannot be placed into socket for transport, store tooth in physiologic medium to preserve vitality of tooth
            a. Best medium is a commercially available kit containing Hank's Balanced Salt Solution (Save-A-Tooth)
            b. Cold milk is also a good storage medium
            c. Saline and saliva are acceptable as storage media, and are certainly preferable to allowing the tooth to become dry
            d. If milk, saline, or Hank's balanced salt solution is not available, and placement back into socket cannot be done, placement of the tooth under the patient's tongue or in the buccal vestibule between gums and teeth is better than allowing to air dry which is destructive to the tooth (irreversible damage to the periodontal cells occurs in 30 minutes of air drying)
        4. Transport to the dentist must be immediate

    B. Provide appropriate tetanus prophylaxis within 48 hours

    C. Antibiotic prophylaxis with penicillin is often prescribed

    D. Patient education: Advise use of mouthpiece when involved in sports or other activities that may result in dental injuries

    E. Follow Up: By dentist to whom the patient was referred for replantation

BITE WOUNDS

I.   Definition: Mechanical trauma to skin and/or underlying tissue from bite of an animal or human

II.   Pathogenesis

    A.   Transmission of bacteria from animal's or human's mouth into wound may produce infection
        1.   *Pasteurella multocida* is the causative agent in 20-50% of infections from dog bites and 80% of infections from cat bites
        2.   Dog and cat bites also become infected with *Staphylococcus aureus*, streptococci, anaerobes, *Capnocytophaga, Moraxella, Corynebacterium, Neisseria*
        3.   Enteric gram-negative bacteria and anaerobes are likely to cause infections from reptile bites
        4.   Rat and mice bites may become infected from *Streptobacillus moniliformis*
        5.   Streptococci, *Staphylococcus aureus, Eikenella corrodens,* or anaerobes are likely to cause infections from human bites
        6.   Hepatitis B and human immunodeficiency virus (HIV) can be transmitted by human bites; especially consider if the biter is within a high-risk group

    B.   Rabies, an acute viral illness, may be transmitted to human beings by infected saliva or other secretions after an animal bite or by licking mucosa of an open wound; airborne transmission has been reported in bat-infested caves

III. Clinical Presentation

    A.   Dog bites account for over 90% of mammal bites

    B.   Most bites are minor and may include scratches, abrasions, lacerations, and puncture wounds

    C.   Potential complications of bites include to the following:
        1.   Infection is the most common problem
            a.   Cat bites become infected more frequently than dog bites because they are often deep puncture wounds; approximately 50% of all cat bites and 15-20% of all dog bites become infected
            b.   Bites on the hand have the highest infection rates; bites on the face have the lowest rates
            c.   Cellulitis and abscesses are common; infections of tendons, periosteum, and joint spaces can be devastating infections
        2.   Rabies may occur after a bite; transmission is more likely if the bite was unprovoked
            a.   Rabies in small rodents is rare
            b.   Rabies in domestic animals has been decreasing, but rabies in wild animals is on the increase
            c.   Skunks, bats, raccoons, bobcats, coyotes, and foxes may harbor the virus and may also bite and infect domestic dogs, cats, horses, and cows
            d.   Incubation period in humans averages 4-6 weeks, but ranges from 5 days to more than one year
            e.   Infection with rabies produces an acute febrile illness with central nervous system problems (anxiety, dysphagia, seizures) and death if untreated
        3.   Bites of large dogs and other animals may produce crush injuries, avulsions, and fractures
        4.   Human bites are generally more severe than animal bites
            a.   "Clenched-fist" injuries that occur during fistfights can cause potential tendon or joint capsule injuries and often require hospitalization
            b.   Osteomyelitis and pyogenic arthritis are possible complications

IV.   Diagnosis/Evaluation

    A.   History
        1.   Inquire about type of animal that bit patient
        2.   Ask if attack was provoked or unprovoked
        3.   If animal is known to the patient, obtain name and telephone number(s) of owner
        4.   Ask about condition of animal: Was the animal acting strangely or did the animal appear ill?
        5.   Determine the amount of time that elapsed since the bite

6. If patient receives a human bite, determine whether the biter is HIV infected or has hepatitis B or if biter is from a high risk group
7. Inquire about all self-treatments of injury
8. Determine immune status of the animal or human biter
9. Inquire about tetanus immunization status and prior rabies immunizations
10. Inquire about patient's past medical history, especially diseases such as diabetes mellitus and immunodeficiencies which would place patient at risk for infection and other complications

B. Physical Examination
1. Check distal to the injured site for neurovascular status and motor function
2. Assess range of motion of affected joint
3. Determine extent and depth of wound; check for foreign body
4. In patients with old wounds, check for signs of infection and palpate adjacent nodes for lymphadenopathy
5. Diagrams and photographs are useful

C. Differential Diagnosis: See Pathogenesis

D. Diagnostic Tests
1. Order x-rays if bony injury or presence of a foreign body such as tooth is suspected
2. Obtain wound cultures in following cases:
   a. If wound is ≥8 hours and <24 hours from time of injury
   b. All cases in which there are signs of infections regardless of time from injury
3. To determine if an animal is rabid, brain tissue can be examined by fluorescent microscopy
4. Consider sedimentation rate and C-reactive protein in patients with infected wounds

V. Plan/Management

A. Wound care
1. Sponge away visible dirt
2. Irrigate wound with copious amounts of sterile saline; do not irrigate puncture wounds
   a. Irrigate under pressure with either an 18 gauge needle and a 35 mL syringe or a Water-Pik
   b. Use at least 500-1000 mL of solution for irrigation and direct stream at all surfaces of wound
   c. Do not use antibiotic or anti-infective solutions as they may increase tissue irritation
3. Scrub the surrounding area
4. Débride all wounds to reduce risk of infection unless they are small and superficial
5. Trim jagged edge of wound

B. Open-wound management versus sutures
1. Do not suture wounds that are likely to become infected such as the following:
   a. Hand bites
   b. Bites that are older than 8 hours
   c. Deep or puncture bites
   d. Bites with extensive injury
2. See section on WOUNDS for suturing procedure

C. Antibiotic prophylaxis of bite wounds to prevent infection
1. Following type of wounds need prophylaxis:
   a. All wounds with signs of infections
   b. Moderate or severe wounds, especially if edema or crush injury is present
   c. Puncture wounds, especially if bone, tendon sheath, or joint penetration occurred
   d. Facial bites
   e. Hand and foot bites
   f. Genital area bites
   g. Wounds in immunocompromised and asplenic persons
2. Selection of antimicrobial agent is based on organism likely to cause infection and should be modified after receiving culture results (see following table for antibiotics)

ANTIBIOTICS FOR ANIMAL OR HUMAN BITE WOUNDS

	Dog/Cat	Reptile	Human
Oral Route	Amoxicillin-clavulanate*	Amoxicillin-clavulanate*	Amoxicillin-clavulanate*
Oral Alternatives for Penicillin-Allergic Patients**	Extended spectrum cephalosporin or trimethoprim-sulfamethoxazole **PLUS** clindamycin	Extended spectrum cephalosporin or trimethoprim-sulfamethoxazole **PLUS** clindamycin	Trimethoprim-sulfamethoxazole **PLUS** clindamycin
Intravenous Route	Ampicillin-sulbactam†	Ampicillin-sulbactam† **PLUS** gentamicin	Ampicillin-sulbactam†
Intravenous Alternative for Penicillin-Allergic Patients**	Extended spectrum cephalosporin or trimethoprim-sulfamethoxazole **PLUS** clindamycin	Clindamycin **PLUS** gentamicin	Extended spectrum cephalosporin or trimethoprim-sulfamethoxazole **PLUS** clindamycin

*Prescribe amoxicillin/clavulanate (Augmentin) 250-500 mg every 8 hours for 3-7 days or 40 mg/kg/day in 3 divided doses
**In patients with history of allergy to penicillin or one its many congeners, a cephalosporin or other β-lactam class drug may be acceptable. However, these drugs should not be used in patients with an immediate hypersensitivity (anaphylaxis) to penicillin because approximately 5% to 15% of penicillin-allergic patients also will be allergic to the cephalosporins
†Ticarcillin-clavulanate may be used as an alternative

Adapted from American Academy of Pediatrics. (2000). Bite wounds. In L.K. Pickering (Ed.). *Red book: Report of the Committee on Infectious Diseases* (25th ed., pp. 156-157). Elk Grove Village, IL: American Academy of Pediatrics.

D.   Prescribe appropriate tetanus prophylaxis; see WOUND section for guidelines

E.   If there is a high risk or known exposure to hepatitis B after a human bite, provide passive prophylaxis with hepatitis B immune globulin (HBIG) 0.06 mL/kg intramuscularly and begin hepatitis B vaccination three-shot series

F.   Consult infectious disease specialist if there is a high risk or known exposure to HIV after a human bite

G.   Control measures related to rabies
   1.   Contact personnel in local health department who can provide information on the risk of rabies in a particular area for each species of animals (unprovoked attack is more suggestive of rabid animal than provoked attack; properly immunized domestic animals have only a minimal chance of developing rabies)
   2.   A suspected domestic animal should be caught, confined, and observed by a veterinarian for 10 days; if animal develops signs of rabies it should be killed and its head removed and shipped to laboratory for examination. No treatment is necessary if examination of brain is negative
   3.   A suspected wild animal should be killed and its brain examined for evidence of rabies. No treatment is necessary if examination of brain is negative
   4.   Patients with bites from bats and wild carnivores need rabies prophylaxis (see V.H.) if the offending animal cannot be caught; because the injury inflicted by a bat bite or scratch may be small and not visibly evident, prophylaxis is indicated for situations in which the bat was physically present unless prompt testing of bat excludes rabies infection

H.   Care of patients exposed to rabies (consult with local health department); after local wound care, use both passive and active immunoprophylaxis as soon as possible after exposure, ideally within 24 hours, but even patients who have been exposed >24 hours should still be given therapy
   1.   Active immunization: Human diploid cell vaccine (HDCV), rabies vaccine absorbed (RVA), or purified chick embryo cell (PCEC) 1.0 mL is given intramuscularly in the deltoid or anterolateral aspect of thigh on first day of treatment, and repeat doses are administered on days 3, 7, 14, and 28
   2.   Passive immunization: Rabies immune globulin (Human) (RIG) should be used simultaneously with first dose of HDCV or RVA; recommended dose is 20 IU/kg of body weight; approximately one half of RIG is infiltrated into wound and the remainder is given intramuscularly

I.   Patient Education
   1.   Teach patient to watch for signs of infection
   2.   Educate about bite prevention
      a.   Caution against approaching unknown dogs, cats, and wild animals and avoid contact when animals are eating

b.   Secure garbage containers so that raccoons and other animals will not be attracted to home

c.   Chimneys and other potential portals of entry for wild animals should be identified and covered

d.   Teach children to avoid running and screaming in the presence of a dog; best to remain calm and avoid eye contact when threatened by a dog

J.   Referral/consultation is needed in the following cases:
1.   Bites of ears, face, genitalia, hands, and feet
2.   Large, contaminated wounds

K.   Follow Up: Inspect wound for signs of infection within 48 hours

BURNS, MINOR

I.   Definition: Lesions caused by heat or other cauterizing agents; the following burns are considered minor if they do not involve the eyes, ears, face, hands, feet, genitalia

A.   Partial-thickness burns <15% total percentage of body surface area (TBSA) in individuals >10 years of age

B.   Partial thickness burns <10% TBSA in child <10 years of age

C.   Full-thickness burns ≤2% TBSA

II.   Pathogenesis

A.   Cellular protein coagulation and destruction of enzyme systems occur as a result of excessive heat energy which is transferred into the skin

B.   Burns impair the skin's ability to retain water and heat, thereby increasing the risk of infection

C.   Common agents causing burns include the following:
1.   Scalds or burns from wet heat
2.   Direct burns from flames; matches and cigarettes are common sources; irons and ovens are other sources
3.   Chemicals
4.   Electricity
5.   Radiation; burns caused by exposure to sunlight

III.   Clinical Presentation

A.   Approximately 95% of burns are minor and can be managed in the ambulatory care setting

B.   Depth of burn depends on the intensity of the burning agent and the amount of time the burning agent was in contact with skin; the traditional classification of first-, second-, and third-degree burns has been replaced (see below)
1.   Superficial (first degree) burns have minimal epithelial damage and cause no skin loss
a.   Skin has slight erythema, blanches with pressure, and sometimes has small, dry blisters
b.   Heals without scarring or contractures in about 7-14 days
c.   Burns are very painful
2.   Partial thickness (superficial second degree) burns involve the upper layers of the epidermis, but spare epidermal appendages such as hair follicles, nails, sweat and sebaceous glands, and sensory nerve cells
a.   Present with tender, erythematous, weeping skin and blisters
b.   Skin blanches with pressure
c.   Wounds are painful as sensory function is preserved
d.   Heal within 14-21 days with minimal scarring and no contractures; changes in pigmentation may last for months or throughout life

3. Deep dermal partial thickness (deep second degree) burns typically have patchy areas of injury varying from superficial partial thickness to full thickness; wounds may progress to full thickness
   a. Epidermal appendages are usually spared
   b. Appear pale and waxy with patchy red areas and may have large blisters
   c. No blanching with pressure
   d. Decreased pinprick sensation but pressure sensation is intact
   e. Healing may take more than 21 days
   f. May have contracture formation and hypertrophic scarring
4. Full thickness (third degree) burns involve the entire thickness of the skin; may involve subcutaneous fat, connective tissue, muscle, and even bone
   a. Skin is charred or whitish in appearance
   b. Sensation is absent
   c. Unless burn is very small, the dermal elements needed to regenerate new skin are destroyed and surgical management with excision and grafting is needed

C. Scalds are the most common type of burn injury and generally result in superficial skin loss

D. Burns from flames are the second most common cause of burns; burns in which clothing catches on fire are almost always third degree and serious

E. The severity of chemical burns depends on the type of chemical, its concentration, and the contact time; cement and phenol are common sources

F. Electricity burns often cause small, punctate, deep burns at the entry point; electrical burns across the chest can cause cardiac problems

G. Radiation burns due to sun exposure are always superficial but can be extensive, painful, and result in hospitalization

H. Minor burns do not result in systemic problems (shock, acute renal failure, hypothermia, and severe depression of the immune system) which may occur with severe burns

I. Other injuries may accompany minor burns and include trauma and smoke inhalation; singed facial or nasal hairs, facial burns, change in voice, or altered mental status suggest an inhalation injury

J. Carbon monoxide and cyanide poisoning do not usually occur with minor burns, but should be considered in more extensive burns

K. Bacterial infection is a complication of minor burns

IV. Diagnosis/Evaluation

A. History
1. Ask what caused the burn or how the burn was acquired
2. Query about length of time the skin was in contact with the burning agent
3. Determine how much time has elapsed from burn occurrence to seeking treatment
4. Question about occurrence of smoke inhalation
5. Ask about associated injuries
6. When chemicals are involved ask the name and concentration of the chemical
7. Ask patients with electrical injury about the amount of voltage involved and whether there was loss of consciousness at time of injury
8. Ask about tetanus status
9. Ask about past medical history, particularly cardiac valvular disease (pre-existing medical problems can adversely affect healing of burns)
10. Inquire about history of alcohol and narcotic abuse; this information is important in managing the patient's pain
11. Ask about recent streptococcal infection
12. Because of possibilities of abuse and neglect, ask about prior injuries and burns; documentation of quotes should be recorded

B. Physical Examination; important to remove all clothing, dressings, jewelry, dentures and prostheses to thoroughly assess burns and any associated injuries
    1. Remember that it may require 3-5 days of serial examinations and debridement to determine whether partial-thickness wound is superficial or deep or has progressed to a full-thickness injury
    2. Observe general appearance for distress
    3. Observe for any signs that suggest abuse such as scald burns consistent with "dipping" injuries of the buttocks or arms and legs, cigarette burns, and iron burns
    4. Measure vital signs
    5. Estimate the area of burn from Lund-Browder burn charts (see figure that follows); surface area of the patient's palm can be used to estimate the extent of small or patchy burns (palm represents 0.4 percent of TBSA and entire hand represents 0.8 percent of TBSA)

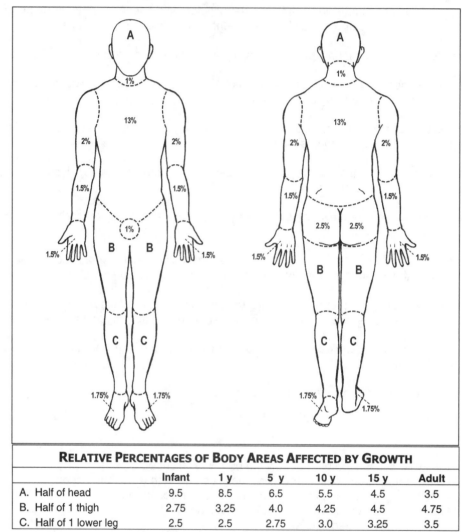

RELATIVE PERCENTAGES OF BODY AREAS AFFECTED BY GROWTH						
	Infant	1 y	5 y	10 y	15 y	Adult
A. Half of head	9.5	8.5	6.5	5.5	4.5	3.5
B. Half of 1 thigh	2.75	3.25	4.0	4.25	4.5	4.75
C. Half of 1 lower leg	2.5	2.5	2.75	3.0	3.25	3.5

Figure 20.1. Lund-Browder Burn Chart

    6. Determine depth of burn
    7. Assess sensation in the burn area by using a blunt sterile needle or pin
    8. Check distal to the burn site for neurovascular status and motor function
    9. Perform a complete exam of the lung and heart
    10. Other body systems should be examined depending on location and extent of burn and to determine any associated injuries such as fractures and dislocations from jumping from windows in house fires
    11. Assess for signs of infection

C. Differential Diagnosis:
    1. Always consider possibility of abuse or neglect, particularly if location of burn is inconsistent with the history
    2. Burn injuries may be the initial presentation of an alcohol or drug abuse problem

D.   Diagnostic Tests: None usually needed
1.   If inhalation injury is suggested, order chest radiograph and arterial blood gases
2.   Consider other studies based on coexisting trauma such as complete blood count, blood type and screen, x-rays

V.   Plan/Management

A.   Refer to a burn center patients who meet the following criteria:
1.   Age >10 years with partial-thickness burns ≥15-20% TBSA
2.   Age <10 years with partial-thickness burns ≥10% TBSA
3.   Any age with full-thickness burns ≥2-5% TBSA
4.   Partial- or full-thickness burns to hands, feet, face, eyes, ears, perineum, and/or major joints
5.   Circumferential burns to the chest or extremities
6.   Electrical injuries, including lightning injuries
7.   Significant burns from caustic chemicals
8.   Burns complicated by multiple trauma in which the burn poses the greatest risk of morbidity
9.   Significant inhalation injury
10.   Co-morbid conditions that could complicate the management
11.   Lack of social or emotional support and/or long-term rehabilitative support
12.   Suspected family violence

B.   Emergency treatment of severe burns while waiting transport of the patient to a burn center or an emergency department includes prompt IV fluid resuscitation with lactated Ringer's solution, elevating the burned areas, and administering 100% oxygen if inhalation injury is present

C.   First aid
1.   Remove the burning agent, maintain patent airway, and resuscitate if needed
2.   Remove all clothing, jewelry, and shoes before swelling develops
3.   Keep patients covered with blanket to prevent hypothermia
4.   Lavage burned area with cool water or normal saline; chemical burns require extensive lavaging (at least 15 minutes)

D.   Outpatient treatment of superficial burns from all causes except radiation
1.   Apply cool water- or saline-soaked gauze to burn (do not apply ice or immerse wound in fluid)
2.   Cleanse with water or saline with or without mild soap; do **not** use agents such as hydrogen peroxide or alcohol; even Hibiclens and Betadine are discouraged because they can delay healing
3.   May use topical anesthetic such as dibucaine (Nupercainal) cream or benzocaine (Americaine) spray 3-4 times a day as needed for pain
4.   Infection prophylaxis or dressings are not needed

E.   Outpatient treatment of partial-thickness burns from all causes except radiation
1.   Cool burn with water- or saline-soaked gauze; because of risk of hypothermia, exercise caution in cooling extensive burns
2.   Cleanse burned areas with saline or tap water and mild soap (may need to sedate patient before cleansing and debridement or use local or regional anesthesia [do not apply anesthesia topically to burn or inject directly into wound])
3.   Tar and asphalt residues should be removed with a mixture of cool water and mineral oil, but never débrided; application of polymyxin B-bacitracin zinc ointment over several days should emulsify and remove residual tar
4.   Manually débride or use whirlpool to remove necrotic tissue to minimize infection
5.   Leave intact all blisters that are clean with clear fluid unless they are large and thin-walled and likely to rupture (may use sharp debridement or use sterile aspiration with a 19-gauge hypodermic needle to remove fluid if likely to rupture)
6.   Remove blistered skin that is almost detached and other devitalized skin
7.   For small burns on face cover with bacitracin ointment and leave open; for other small burns cover with bacitracin and apply nonadherent dressing and a bulky dressing to absorb drainage from burn
8.   For larger burns:
       a.   Bacitracin is gaining favor as topical prophylactic antibiotic of first choice; this agent should always be used around mucous membranes and on the face
       b.   Silver sulfadiazine 1% cream (Silvadene) can be used; cover burned area with a thin layer; do not use if patient is allergic to sulfa drugs or is pregnant
       c.   Biologic dressings are expensive but effective; apply within first 6 hours after the burn; dressings gradually peel of as skin epithelializes

Bismuth-impregnated petroleum gauze and Biobrane dressings are other effective agents; both are applied as single layer over burn and covered with a bulky dressing that should be changed every other day

e. For burns not treated with biologic dressings, apply nonadherent gauze and bulky dressing to absorb drainage from burn; to reduce circulatory impairment apply nonadherent dressing in successive strips rather than wrapping around extremity
   (1) Dressings should be changed twice daily to once a week
   (2) Remove dressing whenever it becomes soaked with exudate
   (3) At each dressing change, completely clean wound with gentle washings

f. Splinting hands with burns is not usually recommended as it impedes patients in regaining range of motion

F. For mild sunburns use cool compresses and topical dexamethasone aerosol spray every 3 hours; most effective if treatment is started within 12 hours of injury

G. Pain management of all types of burns is important; recommend regular use of acetaminophen or a nonsteroidal anti-inflammatory drug
   1. During dressing changes or increased physical activity a narcotic may be needed
   2. Patient's worst pain score should be less than 5 on a scale from zero to 10

H. Tetanus prophylaxis is needed if the patient has not received either a course of immunizations or a booster within 10 years; see guidelines for tetanus prophylaxis in the WOUND section

I. Systemic antibiotics are given only if patient has a valvular disease or a concomitant streptococcal infection

J. Patient Education
   1. Teach patient to clean burned area completely with gentle soap and water, dry burn well, and reapply ointment or cream and dressing
   2. Keep dressing and/or burn clean and dry
   3. Increase fluid intake
   4. Elevate affected parts
   5. Maintain active range of motion of all joints with overlying burns
   6. Teach signs and symptoms of infection and need to return to clinician if they occur

K. Follow Up
   1. Patients should be re-evaluated in 24 hours to assess pain control, evidence of infection, and to change dressing
   2. At least once a week, partial-thickness burns should be assessed for signs of complications
   3. Wounds that have not healed in 3 weeks in adults or 2 weeks in children have a high incidence of hypertrophic scarring and these patients should be referred to surgeon

CORNEAL ABRASION

I. Definition: Partial or complete removal of a focal area of epithelium on the cornea

II. Pathogenesis

   A. The cornea is composed of three principal layers: epithelium (the outer layer), stroma, and endothelium

   B. Disruption of the epithelium on the cornea by mechanical or chemical factors results in corneal abrasion

   C. Because the epithelium is richly innervated with sensory nerve endings, even the tiniest injuries are painful

III. Clinical Presentation

   A. Corneal injuries are very painful, with the degree of pain generally related to the amount of epithelial disruption; motion of the eyeball and blinking increase the pain and foreign body sensation

B. Patients usually complain of a scratchy, gritty sensation (foreign body sensation) that develops suddenly and worsens with blinking

C. Redness of the eye follows corneal insult due to the reactive conjunctival vasodilation (injection)

D. Photophobia is often present and occurs because the disruption in the optical surface causes light to be scattered within the eye rather than focused so that bright light sources have a glaring appearance

IV. Diagnosis/Evaluation

A. History
   1. Ask which eye is injured
   2. Determine how, when, and where the eye was injured
   3. Ascertain if eye pain or vision loss is present
   4. Ask if any eye protection was being used at time of injury and if anyone witnessed the injury
   5. Ask if contact lenses are being worn (or were being worn at time of injury)
   6. Ask about tetanus immunization status

B. Physical Examination
   1. Measure visual acuity **(Note**: Even in the case of trauma, it is critically important to know visual ability is present; if patient is unable to read chart, acuity may be grossly evaluated by finger counting)
   2. Evert the eyelids and examine the conjunctival fornices for foreign body. The presence of a foreign body under the upper lid should **always** be looked for in the presence of a suspected corneal abrasion
   3. Using a bright hand-held light and oblique illumination, inspect the cornea; an abrasion may be apparent by noting that an obvious shadow is cast on the iris from a surface defect illuminated when the light strikes the cornea
   4. If trained and experienced in the technique of corneal staining with fluorescein, examine cornea using this technique which makes identification of abrasions much easier

---

CORNEAL STAINING WITH FLUORESCEIN TO ASSESS EPITHELIAL INTEGRITY

Technique

✓ Instill 1 or 2 drops of a rapid onset and short duration topical anesthetic (e.g., proparacaine HCl 0.5% [Ophthetic])

✓ Moisten the sterile fluorescein strip with sterile normal saline (can also touch strip to the tear film in the lower cul de sac of affected eye)

✓ Touch moistened fluorescein strip to lower conjunctiva of the eye being inspected (If tear film was used to moisten strip, this step is unnecessary as dye has already been placed in eye)

✓ Ask patient to blink eye

✓ Illuminate the eye with cobalt blue light and inspect for patterns of fluorescence

✓ Remove excess dye with sterile saline and remind patient not to rub eye

Interpretation

✓ If the corneal epithelium has been disturbed, fluorescein will pool within these areas and stain the hydrophilic stroma; the resultant brighter fluorescence of these pools will delineate the corneal abrasion from surrounding intact epithelium

✓ The size and pattern of the defect depends on nature and extent of injury

✓ A characteristic pattern that suggests the presence of a foreign body trapped underneath the upper lid is a faint vertically-oriented pattern on the cornea

---

C. Differential Diagnosis
   1. Corneal foreign body
   2. Viral keratitis
   3. Corneal laceration

D. Diagnostic Tests: None indicated beyond corneal staining with fluorescein described above (consider referral to an ophthalmologist for this test)

V.   Plan/Management

A.   Instill an antibiotic ointment such as erythromycin ophthalmic ointment (Ilotycin) OR gentamicin ophthalmic ointment (Garamycin) into the affected eye

B.   Instruct patient to close injured eye and then apply a two-pad pressure dressing over the closed lids of the affected eye
1.   The patch must be firm and tight such that the eye cannot be opened beneath it
2.   Leave pad in place for 24 hours
3.   Instruct patient to return after 24 hours for removal of dressing
4.   After removal of the dressing, a topical antibiotic ointment such as listed above, or drops such as sulfacetamide sodium solution (Sulamyd) should be continued for 5 days after the injury as protection against infection. Small amount of ointment or 2-3 drops of solution should be used 4 x/day
5.   Administer tetanus immunization if indicated

C.   If the type of injury sustained is chemical, thermal, or a mechanical injury that has qualities of both blunt and sharp trauma, immediate transport to an ophthalmologist is required because of threat to vision

D.   Follow Up: In 24 hours to remove patch and evaluate healing

HEAD TRAUMA, MINIMAL AND MILD

I.   Definition: Trauma to the head; simple linear skull fractures and concussions are the most common examples of minor head injuries

A.   Simple linear skull fractures: Small break in skull that is not associated with depressed bone fragments and underlying brain injury

B.   Concussion: Trauma-induced alteration in mental status that may or may not involve loss of consciousness (previously, to be diagnosed with a concussion, the patient had to have a loss of consciousness)

C.   Classification of head injuries
1.   American Academy of Pediatrics (1999) defines minor closed head injury in previously neurologically healthy children of either sex 2 through 20 years of age as the following:

MINOR CLOSED HEAD INJURY: DEFINITION OF THE AMERICAN ACADEMY OF PEDIATRICS
Children who have no abnormal or focal findings on neurologic (including funduscopic examination) examination, and who have no physical evidence of skull fracture (such as hemotympanum, Battle's sign, or palpable bone depression)

2.   The following table is a system for classifying head injuries

CLASSIFICATION OF HEAD INJURIES		
Minimal	**Mild**	**Moderately or Potentially Severe**
All of the following:	Any of the following:	Any of the following:
✓ No loss of consciousness or amnesia	✓ Brief (<5 min) loss of consciousness	✓ Prolonged (>5 min) loss of consciousness
✓ Glasgow Coma Scale score of 15	✓ Amnesia for the event	✓ Glasgow Coma Scale score of <14
✓ Normal alertness and memory	✓ Glasgow Coma Scale score of 14	✓ Focal neurologic deficit
✓ No focal neurologic deficit	✓ Impaired alertness and memory	✓ Post-traumatic seizure
✓ No palpable depressed skull fracture		✓ Intracranial lesion detected on CT scan

Adapted from Smith, E.E. (1993). Minor head injury: A proposed strategy for emergency management. *Annals of Emergency Medicine, 22,* 1193-1196.

II. Pathogenesis:

A. Common causes of traumatic head injuries; in all ages a fall is the most common cause
   1. In infants, head injuries are often associated with falls and abuse; "shaken baby syndrome" should always be considered
   2. In preschool and school-age children, auto accidents are common
   3. In adolescents, sports injuries and assault become more important etiologic factors
   4. In older adolescents and young adults, auto accidents, falls, and assaults are causative factors

B. Outcomes following head trauma:
   1. Seriousness of the head injury is related to the nature and extent of the cerebral injury rather than the damage to the overlying scalp or skull structures
   2. Clinical course is dependent on the degree of acute injury to brain at the time of the accident (primary brain injury) and to delayed neurochemical and metabolic changes that result during the initial hours and days after the injury (secondary brain injury)
   3. Even minimal head injuries can result in a secondary brain injury which involves tissue injury, swelling, and ischemia
      a. Delayed cerebral edema may occur within 8-12 hours
      b. Maximal cerebral edema occurs within 48-72 hours after the injury
   4. "Second impact syndrome" occurs when a person (particularly an athlete) has a second concussion without recovering from the first; may lead to massive acute-brain swelling and ultimately death; multiple head injuries can result in chronic impairment of brain function

III. Clinical Presentation

A. Epidemiology
   1. Head injury is the most common cause of traumatic mortality in the US
   2. Most patients with head injuries are between 15-24 years of age
   3. Males are 2-3 times more likely to have a head injury than females
   4. Positive blood alcohol is sometimes detected in head injuries involving adolescents

B. Head injuries in infants and children are different than those in adults
   1. "Shaken baby syndrome" is often fatal
      a. Typically, the baby is held by shoulders and shaken vigorously
      b. Diffuse cerebral swelling is often present
      c. Infants with minimal external signs of trauma with neurologic deficits should be suspected of this injury
   2. Children typically have a better prognosis than adults, especially elderly persons, with similar head injuries for the following reasons:
      a. The skull in younger children is thin and, in infants, the sutures are not fused which allows the skull to expand and decreases likelihood of increased intracranial pressure
      b. The base of children's skulls are smoother than in adults which reduces the incidence of basilar contusions and contré coup injuries

C. Simple or linear skull fractures
   1. Approximately 75% of skull fractures in children are linear
   2. Patients with linear fractures are usually asymptomatic, but any fracture requires close observation because the force required to fracture a skull, particularly a child's skull, is significant
   3. Skull fractures with underlying lacerations may predispose the patient to meningitis
   4. Infants can lose a significant amount of blood from skull fractures
   5. In children, a rare complication is a leptomeningeal cyst or "growing fracture" which presents as an enlarging bony defect due to a portion of leptomeninges squeezing between the edges of the fracture

D. Concussion
   1. Hallmarks are confusion and amnesia which occur immediately after injury or several minutes later
   2. Early symptoms (first few minutes or hours) include headache, dizziness or vertigo, lack of awareness of surroundings, and nausea and vomiting
   3. Postconcussive syndrome may occur and includes low-grade headaches, light-headedness, poor attention and concentration, memory dysfunction, reduced energy levels, intolerance of bright lights and noise, sleep disturbances, and irritability and depression; symptoms may last as long as 3 months post injury
   4. A grading scale based on severity of the injury follows:

SCALE FOR GRADING THE SEVERITY OF CONCUSSION

Grade 1	Grade 2	Grade 3
✓ Transient confusion ✓ No loss of consciousness ✓ Concussion symptoms or mental status abnormalities on examination **resolve in *less* than 15 minutes**. Grade 1 concussion is the most common yet the most difficult form to recognize	✓ Transient confusion ✓ No loss of consciousness ✓ Concussion symptoms or mental status abnormalities on examination **last *more* than 15 minutes**. Grade 2 symptoms (greater than 1 hour) warrant medical observation	✓ Any loss of consciousness either brief (seconds) or prolonged (minutes). Grade 3 concussion is usually easy to recognize--the patient is unconscious for any period of time

Adapted from American Academy of Neurology, Quality Standards Subcommittee: Practice parameter. (1997). The management of concussion in sports (summary statement). *Neurology, 48,* 581-585.

IV.   Diagnosis/Evaluation

    A.   History: Important to obtain information from the patient as well as a person at the scene of the injury as the patient may be amnestic or confused

        1.   Determine how the injury occurred and the incidents surrounding the injury; explore possibility of alcohol or illicit drug use

        2.   Ask whether the patient had a loss of consciousness and amnesia

        3.   Inquire about symptoms after the injury such as vomiting, headaches, confusion, drowsiness, or abnormal behaviors

        4.   Determine if there is any neck pain or pain in other areas of the body

        5.   Inquire about other injuries

        6.   Ask about self treatments

        7.   Always ask about previous head injuries, particularly in athletes, to determine "second impact syndrome"

    B.   Physical Examination

        1.   To quickly rule out a serious injury which needs immediate intervention, perform the following:

            a.   Assess airway patency, breathing, and circulation

            b.   Assess level of consciousness

            c.   Measure vital signs

            d.   Stabilize neck and check for signs of neck injury which often accompany head trauma

            e.   Assess the thorax for hemothorax and pneumothorax

            f.   Examine abdomen for signs of bleeding such as fullness and rigidity

            g.   Signs of increased intracranial pressure are listed in the following table

SIGNS OF INCREASED INTRACRANIAL PRESSURE[†]

Papilledema	Decreased pulse
Elevated systolic pressure	Slow respirations
Wide pulse pressure	

[†] In young children a full fontanelle (even when upright) and separation of cranial sutures are signs

        2.   A rapid system for evaluating athletes who suffer injuries during an event is presented in the following table

QUICK EVALUATION OF ATHLETES WITH HEAD INJURIES DURING THE SPORTS EVENT

Mental Status Testing

Orientation	Time, place, person, and situation (circumstances of injury)
Concentration	Digits backward (e.g., 3-1-7, 4-6-8-2, 5-3-0-7-4) Months of the year in reverse order
Memory	Names of teams in prior contest; recall of 3 words and 3 objects at 0 and 5 minutes Recent newsworthy events; details of the contest (plays, moves, strategies, etc)
External Provocative Testing	40-yard sprint; 5 push ups; 5 sit ups; 5 knee bends (any appearance of associated symptoms is abnormal, e.g., headaches, dizziness, nausea, unsteadiness, photophobia, blurred or double vision, emotional lability, or mental status changes)

Neurologic Tests

Pupils	Symmetry and reaction
Coordination	Finger-nose-finger, tandem gait
Sensation	Finger-nose (eyes closed) and Romberg

Adapted from McCrea, M., Kelly, J.P., Kluge, J., Ackley, B., & Randolph, C. (1997). Standardized assessment of concussion in football players. *Neurology, 48,* 586-588.

3.   After determining that the patient is not in acute distress, perform the following at frequent intervals:

    a.   Use the Glasgow coma scale to assess mental status which can be used later to evaluate the patient's progress (see following table)

GLASGOW COMA SCALE FOR EVALUATING CHILDREN AND ADULTS*

Eye-Opening Response

Score	Children <1 Year	Children >1 Year and Adolescents
4	Spontaneous	Spontaneous
3	To shout	To verbal command
2	To pain	To pain
1	None	None

Motor Response

Score	Children <1 Year	Children >1 Year and Adolescents
6	Spontaneous response	Obeys commands
5	Localizes pain	Localizes pain
4	Withdraws from pain	Withdraws from pain
3	Displays abnormal flexion to pain (decorticate rigidity)	Displays abnormal flexion to pain (decorticate rigidity)
2	Displays abnormal extension to pain (decerebrate rigidity)	Displays abnormal extension to pain (decerebrate rigidity)
1	None	None

Verbal Response

Score	Children <2 Years	Children 2-5 Years	Children >5 Years and Adolescents
5	Babbles, coos appropriately	Uses appropriate words and phrases	Is oriented and converses
4	Cries, but is consolable	Uses inappropriate words	Conversation is confused
3	Cries or screams persistently to pain	Cries or screams persistently to pain	Words are inappropriate
2	Grunts or moans to pain	Grunts or moans to pain	Sounds are incomprehensible
1	None	None	None

* Score of less than 8 denotes severe head injury

Adapted from Simon, J. (1992). Accidental injury and emergency medical services for children. In R.E. Behrman (Ed.). *Nelson textbook of pediatrics.* Philadelphia: WB Saunders.

    b.   Observe gait
    c.   Examine the eyes
        1)   Evaluate pupillary size, equality, and reaction to light
        2)   Perform funduscopy to detect retinal hemorrhage and papilledema
    d.   Carefully inspect and palpate head, noting wounds, indentations
    e.   Examine nasopharynx and ears for evidence of fresh blood

4. Palpate abdomen for signs of bleeding
5. Perform a complete neurologic examination including assessment of cranial nerves, reflexes, motor functioning, sensory functioning, and coordination
6. Assess mental status
7. Assess memory

C. Differential Diagnosis: Crucial to identify persons who are at risk for development of complications such as intracranial mass lesions, intracranial edema, and delayed neurological deterioration
   1. Age, co-morbidity, and mechanism of the injury are potential risk factors for severe head injuries (see following table)

RISK FACTORS FOR SEVERE HEAD INJURIES		
Mechanism	Age	Medical Condition
✓ High speed motor vehicle accident	✓ Greater than 65 years	✓ Long-term anticoagulant therapy
✓ Fall of more than 8 feet		✓ Presence of cerebrovascular malformation
✓ Injury with extensive damage to other areas of body		

Adapted from Marion, D.W. (1998). Acute head injuries in adults. In R.E. Rakel (Ed.), *1998 Conn's current therapy*. Philadelphia: WB Saunders.

   2. Common causes of serious head trauma include the following:
      a. Basilar skull fractures
         (1) Bruising around the eye (raccoon sign), blood in external auditory canal (Battle's sign), cerebrospinal fluid leakage in the ear or nose, and cranial nerve palsies often occur
         (2) Fractures may not be present on plain x-rays, but are apparent on computed tomography (CT)
      b. Cerebral contusion or laceration results from edema, hemorrhage, and possibly necrosis
         (1) Associated with trauma directly beneath the site of blunt or penetrating injury (coup) or may result from indirect trauma contralateral to the injury (contré coup)
         (2) Typically, the patient has loss of consciousness for >2 minutes
         (3) May result in death or severe residual neurologic deficits such as post-traumatic epilepsy
      c. Acute epidural hemorrhage results from a tear in the meningeal artery, vein, or dural sinus and is usually associated with a skull fracture
         (1) Several hours after injury the patient may have a headache, confusion, somnolence, seizures, or focal deficits
         (2) Without treatment, coma, respiratory arrest, and death follow
      d. Acute subdural hematoma is due to a tear in veins from cortex to superior sagittal sinus or from cerebral laceration
         (1) More common injury than acute epidural hemorrhage
         (2) The symptoms and complications are similar to an epidural hemorrhage but the interval before onset of symptoms is longer
      e. Cerebral hemorrhage develops immediately after the injury with symptoms of intracranial pressures and distress; a hematoma is usually visible on CT scan
   3. Typical characteristics of severe head injuries include the following:
      a. Loss of consciousness associated with one or more neurologic deficits
      b. Glasgow Coma Scale score of less than 8
      c. Alterations in mental status
      d. Prolonged memory deficit
      e. Persistent vomiting and severe headache
      f. Seizures
      g. Signs of primary brainstem injury include coma, irregular breathing, fixation of pupils to light, and diffuse motor flaccidity
   4. Child abuse or family violence should always be included in differential diagnosis

D. Diagnostic Tests:
    1. Diagnostic testing in children (recommendations of American Academy of Pediatrics, 1999)
        a. Evaluation and management of child with minor closed head injury and **no** loss of consciousness: Observation; no diagnostic tests are needed for initial evaluation
        b. Evaluation and management of child with minor closed head injury **with** brief loss of consciousness:
            (1) Patient observation alone is an acceptable option
            (2) CT scanning is the imaging modality of choice; CT scanning along with observation is another acceptable option
            (3) Skull radiography is an option and may be helpful if CT scanning is not readily available; remember that skull fractures may be detected on radiographs in the absence of intracranial injury and vice versa, intracranial injury may be present despite the absence of skull fracture on x-ray
            (4) MRI is an acceptable option but CT is more sensitive for hyperacute and acute intracranial hemorrhage (especially subarachnoid hemorrhage), and is quicker, less expensive, and more easily performed than MRI
    2. Diagnostic testing for older adolescents
        a. No tests are needed in patients with minimal head trauma (see classification system in I.C.) who have no abnormal neurological signs but monitoring for neurological abnormalities should extend for at least 48 hours after the injury
        b. Order CT scans in patients who are classified as having mild, moderate, or severe head injuries (see I.C.) and patients with minimal head trauma if they have evidence of a skull fracture on x-ray or if they later develop abnormal neurological symptoms and signs
    3. Always consider ordering cervical spine films or other radiographs for any patient depending on the mechanism and circumstances surrounding the injury
    4. Consider ordering a blood alcohol
    5. Consider serial CBCs in young children with skull fractures

V. Plan/Management

A. Hospitalization
    1. For patients with simple fractures and concussions without abnormal neurologic signs and symptoms, hospitalization is not required unless the patient is an infant who is predisposed to losing a significant amount of blood
    2. Hospitalization is recommended in the following situations:
        a. Suspicion of child abuse or family violence
        b. All head injuries categorized as mild, moderate, or severe
        c. Injuries accompanied by a neurologic deficit
        d. Any mechanism severe enough to cause concern of secondary brain injury

B. For patients who are not hospitalized, monitoring for delayed abnormal signs and symptoms is essential; careful assessment of the caregiver's anticipated compliance with instructions and abilities to care for patient (i.e., adequate transportation) is crucial; patient education includes the following:
    1. Provide printed information and teach family members that there is a need for thorough, frequent observation and precautions for at least 48 hours after the injury; recommend the following:
        a. Check whether pupils are equal and react to light
        b. Determine arousability and coherence by waking patient every 4 hours
        c. Time respiratory rate and check whether respiratory pattern is regular
    2. Call health care provider for any of the following:
        a. Headaches which worsen
        b. Vomiting becomes more frequent
        c. Pupils are unequal or do not react to light
        d. Symptoms such as seizures, neck pain, drowsiness, confusion, difficulty walking, talking, or visualizing occur
    3. Instruct family members that patient should be observed for the development of complications for at least 2 weeks after the injury; signs of complications include drowsiness, vomiting, gait disturbance, or severe headache
    4. Emphasize to family members of athletes that repeat head injuries can lead to permanent brain damage

C.   Guidelines for the management of sports-related concussions were developed by the American Academy of Neurology
   1.   Initial management following the head injury depends on the grade of the concussion (see III.D.4.)
      a.   Athletes with Grade 1 injuries may return to play the same day if the following are met: Normal on-site evaluation (see IV.B.2) while at rest and with exertion, including a normal, detailed mental status examination
      b.   Athletes with Grade 2 and Grade 3 injuries must have a complete neurologic examination and may not return to play the same day
   2.   Decisions on when to return to play after removal from the athletic event are based on grade of the concussion and whether previous head injuries have occurred (see table that follows)

RECOMMENDATIONS ON ATHLETE'S RETURN TO PLAY	
Grade of Concussion	**Time Until Return to Play***
Multiple Grade 1 concussion	1 week
Grade 2 concussion	1 week
Multiple Grade 2 concussions	2 weeks
Grade 3--brief loss of consciousness (seconds)	1 week
Grade 3--brief loss of consciousness (minutes)	2 weeks
Multiple Grade 3 concussions	1 month or longer, based on clinical decision of evaluating health care provider

*Only after being asymptomatic with normal neurologic assessment at rest and with exercise

Adapted from American Academy of Neurology, Quality Standards Subcommittee: Practice parameter. (1997). The management of concussion in sports (summary statement). *Neurology, 48*, 581-585.

D.   Prevention of head injuries
   1.   Remind patients to wear safety belts in motor vehicles and helmets when riding a bike or motorcycle
   2.   Proper safety equipment is needed for even recreational sports
   3.   Measures to prevent falls in the household such as removing loose carpets and maintaining uncluttered, well-lit walkways are important

E.   Follow Up
   1.   Frequent monitoring of all head injuries is important
   2.   Communicate with family members within first 4-12 hours after the injury and then periodically depending on the clinical condition of the patient

INSECT STING AND BROWN RECLUSE SPIDER BITE

I.   Definition: A sting or bite in which there is secretion of venom into skin by insect or spider

II.   Pathogenesis

A.   Insect Sting
   1.   Honeybees, wasps, hornets, and yellow-jackets of the order Hymenoptera embed a firm, sharp stinger in the skin; venom is secreted
   2.   Honeybees leave their stingers in the skin (with venom sac attached; other stinging insects of the order have a retractable stinger and thus may sting many times)
   3.   The injected venoms are proteins with enzyme activity that can cause local or general reactions, or both; reactions are classified as toxic or allergic

B.   Brown Recluse Spider Bite
   1.   Of the 50 or so species known to bite humans, the brown recluse spider (*Loxosceles reclusa*) is one of two species in the US (black widow is the other) capable of producing severe reactions
   2.   The brown recluse is the most widespread, well-studied, and clinically important of the *Loxosceles* species in North America

3. Brown recluse spider is small (1.5 cm or less) light brown, and lives in dark areas such as closets, under porches, or in basements; usually found in river country of mid-America, most commonly in the south-central US
   a. Endemic range of this spider is southeastern Nebraska through Texas, east to Georgia and southernmost Ohio
   b. Several additional species of this spider are native to the southwestern deserts, but are rarely found inside urban houses
4. Venom is composed of enzyme-spreading factor hyaluronidase, and a toxin distributed by the enzyme
5. Bite can cause local or general reactions, but does not cause allergic reactions

III. Clinical Presentation

A. Insect Sting
   1. A sharp, pinprick sensation is felt at the instant of stinging followed by burning pain at site
   2. A red papule or weal appears, enlarges, then subsides within hours
   3. Multiple stings can cause a toxic reaction producing symptoms such as syncope, dizziness, vomiting, diarrhea, and headache because of the large toxin load
   4. Allergic reactions may be localized or systemic
   5. Systemic reactions begin 2-60 minutes after sting and range from a few hives to anaphylaxis; 40% of persons with generalized allergic reactions have a previous history of similar reaction
   6. Anaphylaxis symptoms include generalized itching, hypotension, shortness of breath, throat tightness, dizziness, and wheezing which may subside spontaneously or progress to edema of upper airway, causing obstruction and death

B. Brown Recluse Spider Bite
   1. *Loxosceles* spiders are very shy creatures that are reticent to bite; bites typically occur when spider is accidentally trapped against human skin
   2. Bite may feel sharp, or, more often, remains unnoticed; within a few hours minor swelling and erythema with a surrounding pale halo from vasospasm at the site often occurs
   3. Severity of local reaction appears to depend on site of bite with fatty areas of body developing more severe reactions
   4. Tissue necrosis in bite area may develop as early as four hours after bite
   5. Cutaneous changes at the site include a blue-gray, macular halo around puncture site; emergence of pustule or vesicle/bulla at site; widening of macule and sinking of center of lesions producing a "sinking infarct"; sloughing of tissue leaves a deep ulcer which takes weeks or months to heal
   6. In rare cases, within 12 hours after bite, systemic symptoms of fever, chills, nausea, vomiting, and generalized weakness may appear; rarely, severe systemic reactions of generalized hemolysis, disseminated intravascular coagulation, and renal failure occur (usually only in children)
   7. There are no proven US fatalities involving brown recluse spider bites in which the spider bite was witnessed, and the spider was collected and identified by an expert
   8. Throughout the US, dermonecrotic wounds of uncertain etiology are often (incorrectly) attributed to the brown recluse spider

IV. Diagnosis/Evaluation

A. History
   1. Quickly question regarding type of bite or sting, time of occurrence, and location of bite/sting
   2. If sting, quickly determine if allergic reaction is present (generalized itching, shortness of breath, throat tightness, urticaria, or wheezing)
   3. If sting, question about history of previous allergic reactions

---

***** **ALERT** *****
**If allergic reaction is present or anticipated based on history,
go immediately for treatment**

---

   4. If bite is suspected, attempt to determine the following: Whether anyone witnessed the bite; whether spider was collected; and whether spider can be identified or described
   5. If bite is suspected, determine if dermonecrotic wound is present, and ask about the timing and progression of changes at the site of the suspected bite
   6. If bite is suspected, ask about presence of systemic symptoms such as fever, chills, nausea, vomiting, and weakness

B. Physical Examination
  1. If history suggests an anaphylactic reaction is imminent, do not complete exam or wait for symptoms to develop, institute treatment immediately (See V.B. below)
  2. If sting with no systemic allergic reaction evident or anticipated based on history, take pulse, respirations, and blood pressure
  3. Examine site of bite or sting for characteristic erythema and edema or localized allergic reactions
  4. Examine site of suspected spider bite for presence of characteristic dermonecrotic wound (not present until hours or days after event)

C. Differential Diagnosis
  1. Vasovagal attacks: May follow pain or upset and be accompanied by nausea, diaphoresis and hypotension; lasts only a few minutes and relieved by lying down
  2. Hyperventilation episodes: Accompanied by tachypnea, perioral tingling, but BP is maintained and other signs of anaphylaxis are absent
  3. Necrotic wounds may be caused by infectious (e.g., Lyme disease, cutaneous anthrax) or neoplastic processes; in general, brown recluse spider bite has been overdiagnosed as the cause of necrotic lesions and other, more likely causes of the wound should be considered
  4. Of recent interest, a 7 month-old child in New York who contracted cutaneous anthrax was initially diagnosed as having a brown recluse spider bite as the cause of the necrotic wound (the state of New York is outside the endemic range of the brown recluse and has no populations of the spider)
  5. The many causes of necrotic wounds should be considered before attributing such wounds to spider bites without any corroborating evidence

D. Diagnostic Tests: None indicated for bites or stings with no systemic symptoms

V. Plan/Treatment

  A. Treatment of anaphylactic reactions is based on type of reaction which can range from mild to life-threatening; in all cases, epinephrine is the drug of choice

  B. Treatment of mild anaphylaxis is outlined in the table that follows

TREATMENT OF MILD ANAPHYLAXIS
For mild symptoms of pruritus, erythema, urticaria, and wheezing, treat with epinephrine injected via the intramuscular route (now the recommended route rather than subcutaneous), followed by diphenhydramine, hydroxyzine, or other antihistamine given orally or parenterally
Epinephrine, 1:1000 (aqueous) 0.01 mL/kg per dose up to 0.5 mL. Usual dose:
Infants: 0.05-0.1 mL   **Children**: 0.1-0.3 mL   **Adolescents**: 0.3-0.5 mL
Repeat in 10-20 minutes up to 3 doses; monitor patient's condition constantly, and monitor BP every 5 minutes
Antihistamine: Give **one** of the following: Hydroxyzine, oral or IM: Give 0.5-1 mg/kg/dose (100 mg maximum single dose) Q 4-6 HRS PRN Diphenhydramine, oral or IM: Give 1-2 mg/kg/dose (100 mg maximum single dose) Q 4-6 HRS PRN
Ice: Immediately apply ice to the site of the sting
Also, give oral antihistamines for next 24 hours; see dosing above
Observe patient in office for several hours (a period of 4-6 hours is considered reasonable in patients who are responding well to initial therapy) before discharging to home. Instruct patient to continue to apply ice to site of insect sting and elevate the affected extremity to control local reaction
Advise patient to immediately seek emergency care if difficulty in breathing develops
Follow Up: By telephone in 12-24 hours.

  C. For severe and potentially life-threatening systemic anaphylaxis (bronchospasm, laryngeal edema, hypotension, shock, and cardiovascular collapse) institute the following and call 911 for immediate transport

TREATMENT OF SEVERE ANAPHYLAXIS

Promptly institute airway maintenance and oxygen therapy. Give Intravenous (IV) epinephrine
An initial bolus of intravenous epinephrine is given to patients not responding to intramuscular epinephrine using a dilution of 1:10 000 rather than a dilution of 1:1000. This dilution can be made using 1 mL of the 1:1000 dilution in 9 mL of physiologic saline solution. The dose is 0.01 mg/kg or 0.1 mL/kg of the 1: 10 000 dilution. A continuous infusion should be started if repeated doses are required. For a continuous infusion, add one milligram (1 mL) of 1:1000 dilution of epinephrine to 250 mL of 5% dextrose in water, resulting in a concentration of 4 µg/mL; initially infuse at a rate of 0.1 µg/kg/minute and increase gradually to 1.5 µg/kg/minute to maintain blood pressure

If bronchospasm is prominent, inhaled β_2 agonist: Albuterol (Ventolin) should be administered via nebulizer

Usual dose: Children: 0.1-0.15 mg/kg in 3 cc of saline   Adolescents: 2.5 mg (0.5 cc of 0.5% solution) in 3 cc
                                                                                                                  saline

Transport to emergency department

D.   Prevention of recurrence in patients with mild to severe anaphylactic reactions
    1.   Refer for allergy testing to identify the venom responsible for sensitization
    2.   Five Hymenoptera venoms are commercially available for this purpose: honeybee, yellow jacket, yellow hornet, white-faced hornet, and Polistes wasps
    3.   If skin tests produce ambiguous results, serologic methods (RAST) can be performed to detect IgE antibody to venoms
    4.   Immunization with insect venom can prevent future systemic reactions in patients with a previously documented reaction

E.   Emergency treatment kits (available by prescription) for self-treatment before reaching medical help should be obtained by all persons at risk for anaphylaxis from insect stings
    1.   Patients should be prescribed 3 kits: one for home, one for car, and one to carry; detailed information regarding when and how to use the kit should be given to patient
    2.   Ana-Kit (Hollister-Stier, Spokane, WA) contains a preloaded syringe
    3.   Epi-Pen or Epi-Pen Junior (Dey Laboratories, Napa, CA) are spring-loaded automatic injectors for individuals reluctant to perform self-injection

F.   Patients should also wear a medical alert tag and should be counseled to take special precautions such as the following:
    1.   Nesting areas should be avoided or eliminated
    2.   Avoid eating outdoors, going barefoot outdoors, and mowing the lawn
    3.   Insect repellents do not seem to prevent stings and thus should not be relied upon

G.   For insect stings which are localized with mild urticaria
    1.   Remove stinger if present using forceps, or by scraping out (do not attempt to squeeze out)
    2.   Wash the wound thoroughly and immediately apply ice packs
    3.   Prescribe oral antihistamines (see above for dosing of hydroxyzine and diphenhydramine) to relieve local reaction and discomfort
    4.   Recommend continued use of ice packs and elevation for the next 8-12 hours

H.   For moderate localized swelling, the interventions outlined above should be used. In addition, a burst of oral prednisone (40 mg on day 1, tapering over 4-7 days) is also recommended

I.   Diagnosis of brown recluse spider bite should be made only after corroborative evidence is sought; other, more likely causes of necrotic wounds should be sought in cases where no spider is recovered and identified by an expert

J.   Treatment of the brown recluse bite is controversial; there are no accepted, conclusively established guidelines
    1.   All experts recommend the following conservative treatment
        a.   Gently cleanse with soap and water
        b.   Apply ice and elevate
        c.   Avoid strenuous exercise
        d.   AVOID APPLICATION OF HEAT
        e.   Monitor the patient closely for the first 72 hours
        f.   Give tetanus toxoid if indicated

2. Controversy surrounds which drugs, if any, are indicated
   a. No drug treatments are indicated, according to most experts (excellent outcomes usually occur without any pharmacologic interventions)
   b. If systemic signs and symptoms are present, refer patient to an expert for management

K. Follow Up
   1. Stings: In 12-24 hours (may be by telephone) for patients with anaphylactic symptoms; none indicated for those with localized reactions only
   2. Brown recluse spider bite: No follow up is needed, but patients must be instructed to report any systemic problems such as headache, myalgia, fever, chills, gastrointestinal complaints, rash and darkening of urine (the presentation of hemolysis is within the first weeks); complications of wound healing may occur at any time until resolution and patients must be instructed in signs and symptoms of wound infection

OCULAR FOREIGN BODY

I. Definition: Presence of a foreign body in the cul-de-sacs and under the upper lid or on the cornea

II. Pathogenesis

   A. A foreign body of the conjunctiva occurs when particles become entrapped under the upper lid or in the cul-de-sacs

   B. Most often occurs with blowing dirt or sand; there is usually no trauma involved

   C. A foreign body of the cornea occurs when substances become embedded in the corneal epithelium, most often due to some traumatic event

   D. A sudden event such as an explosion, or an accident involving metal grinding may scatter small fragments onto the cornea

III. Clinical Presentation

   A. The most common conjunctival foreign bodies are dust, sand, and contact lenses

   B. The most common foreign bodies found on the cornea are metallic, often rusty particles

   C. Foreign bodies may be single or multiple, easily seen without magnification or barely detectable with slit-lamp examination

   D. Symptoms are photophobia, lacrimation, and foreign body sensation

IV. Diagnosis/Evaluation

   A. History
      1. Ask which eye is injured
      2. Determine how, when, and where the eye was injured
      3. Ascertain if eye pain or vision loss is present
      4. Ask if any eye protection was being used at time of injury and if anyone witnessed the injury (important for medicolegal reasons)
      5. Ask if contact lenses are in place (or were in place at time of injury)
      6. Ask about tetanus immunization status
      7. Note: Based on history, if foreign body is result of explosion, blunt or sharp trauma, (i.e., if **corneal** foreign body is suspected) eye should be protected from further damage by placing eye shield over eye (or if shield not available, a paper cup to prevent rubbing eye); at this point, arrangements should be made to transport the person for emergency care by a pediatric ophthalmologist

B. Physical Examination
1. Measure visual acuity (**Note**: Even in the case of trauma, it is critically important to know visual ability is present; if patient is unable to read chart, acuity may be grossly evaluated by finger counting)
2. Evert the eyelids and examine for foreign body
3. Technique for everting the eyelid is as follows:

EVERSION OF THE UPPER LID

✓ Instill 1 or 2 drops of a rapid onset, short duration topical ophthalmologic anesthetic such as proparacaine HCl (Ophthetic, 0.5%) into the affected eye

✓ Ask patient to look down

✓ Grasp the lashes with one hand and apply gentle pressure on the lid above the tarsal plate with a cotton-tip applicator with the other hand

✓ Foreign bodies such as soft contact lenses and grit are often found in superior temporal cul-de-sac of the orbit

---

4. Examine the inferior cul-de-sac by having the person look up while the lower lid is pulled down

V. Plan/Management

A. When foreign body is visualized, sweep sterile cotton-tipped swab moistened with topical anesthetic across conjunctival area to remove the object
1. If there is difficulty with removal or if patient complains of severe pain, attempts should be discontinued
2. Refer to ophthalmologist

B. After removal of conjunctival foreign body (or if conjunctival foreign body cannot be located), determine if corneal abrasion present (See CORNEAL ABRASION)
1. If no corneal abrasion present, prescribe topical antibiotic ointment or drops such as sulfacetamide sodium (Sulamyd); apply small amount of ointment or 2-3 drops to affected eye 4 x/day x 5 days
2. If corneal abrasion present, see CORNEAL ABRASION for treatment recommendations
3. Provide tetanus immunization if indicated

C. Follow Up: In 24 hours

SUBCONJUNCTIVAL HEMORRHAGE

I. Definition: A flat, bright-red hemorrhage under the conjunctiva

II. Pathogenesis

A. May occur spontaneously, with raised venous pressure from a forced Valsalva maneuver (as in coughing, sneezing)

B. May occur with major, minor, or no detectable trauma to the front of the eye

III. Clinical Presentation

A. Presents as a striking flat, deep-red hemorrhage under the conjunctiva and may become sufficiently severe to cause a "bag of blood" to protrude over lid margin

B. Subconjunctival hemorrhage is usually asymptomatic

IV. Diagnosis/Evaluation

    A.   History
        1.   Determine which eye affected and how, when, and where the injury occurred
        2.   Ascertain if eye pain, discharge of secretions, or vision loss is present
        3.   Ask if patient has had previous symptoms or complaints similar to the current complaint

    B.   Physical Examination
        1.   Measure visual acuity
        2.   Examine lids and the adnexa for symmetry, swelling, abnormal discharge, and erythema
        3.   Palpate the soft tissue of the orbit, lids, and zygoma
        4.   Inspect the conjunctiva and sclera for localized swelling, signs of hemorrhage
        5.   Examine pupils for size, shape, reaction to light, and perform funduscopic exam

    C.   Differential Diagnosis
        1.   Conjunctivitis
        2.   Conjunctival laceration

    D.   Diagnostic Tests: None indicated

V. Plan/Management

    A.   With no other signs and symptoms, no treatment is required; the patient should be reassured that the blood will clear over a 2-3 week period

    B.   If trauma with a sharp object is suspected, or if there is impaired vision, eye pain, foreign body sensation, discharge of secretions from the eye, change in the appearance of the globe, patient should be referred to a pediatric ophthalmologist for evaluation

    C.   Follow Up: None required; for patients with signs and symptoms described under V.B. above, follow-up should be by the ophthalmologist to whom the patient was referred

WOUNDS

I.   Definition: Breach in the external surface of the body

II.   Pathogenesis

    A.   Wounds such as lacerations and abrasions typically heal through a 3-stage process: Clotting, inflammatory, and proliferative stages

    B.   Devitalized tissue, oral secretions, toxic solutions, soil and dirt, and injurious forces can impede the healing process and possibly cause infection

    C.   *Staphylococcus aureus* and *β-hemolytic streptococcus* are the most common pathogens causing wound infection

    D.   Tetanus can also occur due to multiplication of *Clostridium tetani*, producing a toxin which can block motor neurons

III.   Clinical Presentation

    A.   Mechanism of injury is important in determining likelihood of infection and tissue damage
        1.   Sharp objects often make smooth cuts which can penetrate deep structures
        2.   Crushing injuries often damage underlying tissues and can result in fractures
        3.   Human bites have the greatest risk of bacterial infection and can also transmit hepatitis B and possibly human immunodeficiency virus (HIV)

    B.   Location or environment in which the wound occurred suggests potential problems; wounds which occur in dirty soil such as farmyards are at risk for contamination with spores of *Clostridium tetani*

C. The time interval between when the wound first occurred to when the patient received appropriate care affects the chances of infection; if 6 hours have elapsed, bacterial multiplication is likely

D. Site of the wound influences rate of healing and potential for complications:
   1. Due to rich vascular supply, wounds on face heal rapidly, but may create future cosmetic problems
   2. Hands are used extensively; wounds on hands have increased risk for reinjury and infection

E. Certain types of wounds may be problematic
   1. Dirty wounds are more at risk for infection
   2. Deep wounds can cause underlying tissue destruction and also have increased risk of contamination
   3. Wounds with untidy edges often heal slowly and may heal with disfigurement
   4. Wounds with tissue necrosis have potential for infection and delayed healing

F. Characteristics of the patient are also factors in wound healing; patients who are elderly, undernourished, who have underlying illness, and who are taking corticosteroids and chemotherapeutic agents are at greatest risk for adverse sequela from wounds

G. Tetanus is a rare but dangerous complication of a wound and is characterized by trismus and severe muscular spasms

IV. Diagnosis/Evaluation

A. History
   1. Ask patient to explicitly describe how the wound occurred
   2. Determine where the injury was sustained
   3. Question how much time has elapsed since the wound occurred
   4. Ascertain tetanus immunization status
   5. Ask about allergies to drugs, dressings, and local anesthetics
   6. Ask about current medication use, especially steroid and anticoagulant therapy
   7. Inquire about past medical history to determine if patient has underlying illness such as immunodeficiency which could affect healing process
   8. Ask whether the patient has a tendency to form keloids, because this could result in a poor scar

B. Physical Examination: Always use sterile technique when examining wounds; it may be necessary to apply local or regional anesthesia prior to the examination
   1. Measure wound
   2. Assess depth of wound
   3. Explore wound for foreign bodies
   4. Fully examine underlying structures
   5. Assess circulation, sensation, and movement distal to wound
   6. Palpate underlying bone
   7. Assess range of motion and strength against resistance of all body parts surrounding wound site
   8. Test tendon function against resistance; if function is intact but there is pain, suspect a partial tendon laceration
   9. Examination of the patient with an old wound includes the following:
      a. Carefully inspect wound and surrounding area
      b. Palpate for local lymphadenopathy
      c. Measure patient's temperature

C. Differential Diagnosis: Always consider the possibility of non-accidental injury (see following table)

INDICATORS OF POSSIBLE NON-ACCIDENTAL INJURY
✓ Delay between injury and seeking treatment
✓ The history of the accident does not match the observed injury
✓ The history changes
✓ Other injuries, especially if at different stages of healing
✓ Signs of general neglect or failure to thrive
✓ Signs of family tension or indications of alcohol or drug abuse

Adapted from Wardrope, J., & Smith, J.R.R. (1992). *The Management of wounds and burns.* New York: Oxford.

D. Diagnostic Tests
   1. Order x-rays for crushing and deep penetrating wounds
   2. Obtain wound swabs for culture on any wound which is slow to heal; fresh wounds do not require a culture

V. Plan/Management

A. The following wounds should be managed by a clinician with extensive experience in wound management
   1. Wounds involving nerve, tendon, or bone damage
   2. Wounds with full thickness skin loss
   3. Facial and hand wounds (small, superficial wounds, however, may be treated in outpatient setting)

B. Wound-cleansing is the first step of wound care (consider using anesthesia before cleansing)
   1. Irrigate wound with one of the following:
      a. Normal saline is an economical and effective irrigant
      b. Povidone-iodine, hydrogen peroxide, and other detergents can cause tissue toxicity and should not be used
      c. Use high-pressure irrigation which can be achieved with a 35- or 65-ml syringe and a 16- or 19- gauge needle; higher pressure may result in tissue trauma and should be reserved for highly contaminated wounds
      d. Alternatively, a plastic disposable splashguard (Zerowet) can be substituted for the needle to give high-pressure irrigation; less threatening to children and avoids inadvertent exposure to blood-contaminated fluid
   2. Apply mechanical force to clean wound: May use a fine-pore sponge such as an Optipore with a surfactant such as poloxamer 188 (Shur Clens)

C. Preparation of the wound site is next
   1. Debridement of devitalized tissue is important
   2. Clip, do not shave, surrounding hair as close to skin surface as possible; never shave an eyebrow

D. After appropriately preparing the wound, the next step is to decide whether to apply sutures; the following wounds require open-wound management:
   1. Abrasions and superficial lacerations
   2. Wounds with a great deal of tissue damage
   3. Wound which have a low risk for infection of >12-24 hours of age
   4. Wounds which have a high risk for infection of >6 hours of age
   5. Wounds contaminated by feces, human or animal saliva, or large amounts of soil or dirt
   6. Abrasions or wounds involving large superficial denudement of skin

E. Wound dressings: Best environment for wounds which are not sutured is a moist one; the following occlusive or semiocclusive dressings can promote a moist environment and all are effective
   1. Occlusive dressings such as DuoDERM, Telfa, and OpSite can be used
   2. Hydrocolloid dressing is another possible choice (good for leg ulcers and pressure sores)
   3. Hydrogel dressing such a Vigilon may be selected
   4. Foam dressings are another choice

F. Closure of the wound with tape (Steri-strip) is appropriate if the wound is superficial, has little tension, the edges are well approximated, and the injured area has full range of motion; strips can be left in place until they fall off on their own

G. Other wounds require sutures
   1. Anesthesia
      a. Topical anesthetics such a mixture of lidocaine 4% plus epinephrine 1:1000 plus tetracaine 0.5% (LET) are safe, effective, and inexpensive; put 3 mL on cotton ball and firmly place in wound for 15 minutes; before suturing assess effectiveness of anesthesia
      b. Alternatively inject plain lidocaine (Xylocaine) solution buffered by adding 1 mL of sodium bicarbonate solution to every 9-10 mL of lidocaine and allow to reach body temperature before use
      c. For crush injuries and lacerations with fractures, inject 0.25% bupivacaine (Marcaine) which has a slower onset, but longer duration of action; do not exceed dose of 3 mg/kg; some experts recommend avoiding use in children <12 years
      d. Do not use any anesthetic containing epinephrine in an area in which circulation is easily compromised such as fingers, toes, nose, penis, or ears

  e. Subdermally inject anesthesia slowly inside the cut margin of wound, avoiding piercing intact skin

  f. Use regional blocks to minimize distorting tissue or where there is no loose areolar tissue to infiltrate, such as the finger tip

 2. Wound edge approximation should be achieved with little or no tension to the surrounding area. Tension would be indicated by puckering of the skin

  a. In patients with a history of keloid formation, close skin with minimal tension and consider applying a pressure dressing for 3-6 months

  b. Many different suture techniques are available; suturing technique will depend on site and extent of injury

  c. Different suture materials are available

   (1) Skin is usually closed with nonabsorbable suture material such as nylon, Prolene, or silk

   (2) Subcutaneous tissue and mucosal surfaces are usually closed with absorbable material, such as Dexon, Vicryl, or plain or chromic gut

   (3) Rapidly dissolving suture forms may be used to close the skin in some patients to avoid the discomfort associated with follow up suture removal

 3. Delayed primary closures with sutures

  a. This technique is used for wounds that cannot be closed initially because of gross contamination, potential injury to joints or other deep structures, retained foreign bodies, host immune status, or an inability to adequately cleanse the wound

  b. Consider closing wound in 3-5 days when the risk of infection decreases

 4. Care of wound after suturing

  a. For simple lacerations, place gauze over suture line and cover with occlusive dressing for 24-48 hours. For more complex lacerations, immobilize injured body part for 5-7 days and apply bulky dressing; some advocate wound closure tape directly over the sutures

  b. Splint sutured wounds which are over or around a joint

  c. Instruct patient to keep wound clean and dry for at least 48 hours

H. Cyanoacrylate tissue adhesives can be used for skin closure of short (<6-8 cm), low tension (≤0.5 cm gap between wound edges), clean edged, straight or curved lacerations

 1. Dry wound edges are approximated with fingers or forceps; approximated edges are painted with adhesive using short brush strokes in a multilayering fashion, allowing 15 seconds to elapse between layers (usually about four layers are applied)

 2. At end of process, edges are held together for 30-60 seconds to dry

 3. Adhesives act as their own dressings and have antimicrobial effects against gram-positive organisms; a dry gauze dressing may or may not be applied

 4. Ointments and creams should not be used

 5. Suture removal is not necessary as adhesives slough off in 7-14 days

 6. Patients may shower and gently bathe wound, but should avoid prolonged wetness that occurs with swimming, scrubbing, or soaking

 7. Advantages: Less pain, decrease in time to perform procedure, reduction in risk of needlestick to health care workers, decrease in need for instruments and supplies, no need for follow-up suture removal, and good antibacterial effect

 8. Disadvantages: Adhesives have lower tensile strength than sutures and may break over high-tension areas such as joints; children may pick adhesive off; adhesive may drip into uninvolved areas; improperly applied adhesive may delay healing and have poor cosmetic results

I. Certain types of wounds require different therapy

 1. Puncture wounds should have very high-powered irrigation with saline; do not close puncture wounds with sutures

 2. Flap wounds which have edges which are not approximated should be cleaned, non-viable fat should be removed, and Steri-Strips should be applied to appose but not close the wound

 3. For small scalp lacerations, consider skin staples

J. Topical antibiotic ointments can be applied to open or sutured wounds; limit prophylactic ointments to high-risk wounds

 1. Polysporin, bacitracin, and mupirocin are appropriate choices

 2. Avoid Neosporin because it may cause allergies

K. Oral antibiotics are sometimes used for prophylactic purposes to prevent infection
1. Prophylactic antibiotics should be given in the following cases:
a. Most mammal bites (see section on BITE WOUNDS)
b. Puncture wounds in which cleansing was difficult
c. Patients with valvular disease or implants who are at risk for bacteremia
2. Also, consider prophylactic antibiotics in the following cases:
a. Heavily contaminated wounds
b. Wounds with delayed treatment
c. Wounds with tissue necrosis
3. Choose one of the following antibiotics for prophylaxis
a. Amoxicillin-clavulanate (Augmentin); prescribe 250-500 mg every 8 hours or 40 mg/kg/day in 3 divided doses
b. For patients with penicillin allergies, prescribe erythromycin (Ery-Tab) 250 mg QID for 7-10 days or 30-50 mg/kg/day in 4 divided doses

L. Prevention of tetanus is important (following table provides guidelines on tetanus prophylaxis)

GUIDE TO TETANUS PROPHYLAXIS IN WOUND MANAGEMENT				
History of Tetanus Immunization (doses)	Clean, Minor Wounds		All Other Wounds*	
	dT[†]	TIG	dT[†]	TIG
Uncertain or <3	Yes	No	Yes	Yes
3 or more[‡]	No[¶]	No	No[§]	No

*Such as, but not limited to, wounds contaminated with dirt, feces, soil, and saliva; puncture wounds; avulsions; wounds resulting from missiles, crushing, burns, and frostbite

[†] For children <7 years, diphtheria and tetanus toxoids and acellular pertussis vaccine (DTaP) are recommended; if pertussis vaccine is contraindicated, DT is given. For persons ≥7 years, dT is recommended. dT indicates adult-type diphtheria and tetanus toxoids; TIG, tetanus immune globulin (human)

[‡] If only 3 doses of fluid toxoid have been received, a fourth dose of toxoid, preferably an adsorbed toxoid, should be given

[¶] Yes, if >10 years since the last dose

[§] Yes, if >5 years since the last dose. More frequent boosters are not needed and can accentuate adverse effects

Adapted from American Academy of Pediatrics. (2000). Tetanus. In L.K. Pickering (Ed.), *2000 red book: Report of the Committee on Infectious Disease*. 25th ed. Elk Grove Village, IL: Author.

M. Patient Education
1. Teach patient to return if wound is increasingly painful, if there is significant discharge, or if there is spreading of redness around wound, or a red streak developing from the wound in the direction of the heart
2. Inform patient that appearance of the wound and subsequent scar will change substantially during the year after the injury; thus, decisions for scar revision should be made after one year
3. Advise patients to avoid sun exposure of their wounds to reduce the risk of developing hyperpigmentation

N. Follow Up
1. On return visits evaluate and consider hospitalization or aggressive antimicrobial therapy if signs and symptoms of pyogenic abscess, cellulitis, and ascending lymphangitis (red line spreading proximally on a limb) are present
2. Return for re-evaluation, dressing change, and/or suture removal in 2 days
3. Time to remove sutures depends on wound location; apply surgical adhesives or tape after sutures are removed
a. Facial wounds: 3-5 days
b. Scalp wounds: 7-10 days
c. Hand wounds: 10-14 days
d. Lower legs: 14 days
e. Other: 7-21 days

REFERENCES

American Academy of Neurology, Quality Standards Subcommittee: Practice parameter. (1997). The management of concussion in sports (summary statement). *Neurology, 48,* 581-585.

American Academy of Pediatrics (1999). The management of minor closed head injury in children. *Pediatrics, 104,* 1407-1415.

American Academy of Pediatrics. (2000). Bite wounds. In L.K. Pickering (Ed.), *2000 red book: Report of the Committee on Infectious Diseases* (25th ed., pp. 155-159). Elk Grove Village, IL: Author.

American Academy of Pediatrics. (2000). Rabies. In L.K. Pickering (Ed.), *2000 red book: Report of the Committee on Infectious Diseases* (25th ed., pp. 475-482). Elk Grove Village, IL: Author.

American Academy of Pediatrics. (2000). Tetanus. In L.K. Pickering (Ed.), *2000 red book: Report of the Committee on Infectious Diseases* (25th ed., pp. 563-568). Elk Grove Village, IL: Author.

American Academy of Pediatrics. (2000). Treatment of anaphylactic reaction. In L.K. Pickering (Ed.), *2000 red book: Report of the Committee on Infectious Diseases* (25th ed., pp. 51-53). Elk Grove Village, IL: Author.

American Burn Association. (1996). *Guidelines for transfer of patients in burn centers.* New York: Author.

Bachur, R. (2001). Minor trauma. In C. Green-Hernandez, J.K. Singleton, & D.Z. Aronzon (Eds.). *Primary care pediatrics* (pp. 513-531). Philadelphia: Lippincott.

Bower, M.G. (2001). Managing dog, cat, and human bite wounds. *The Nurse Practitioner, 26,* 36-45.

Brook, I. (2003). Microbiology and management of human and animal bite wound infections. *Primary Care Clinical Office Practice, 30,* 25-39.

Buttaravoli, P., & Stair, T. (2000). *Minor emergencies: Splinters to fractures.* Mosby: St. Louis.

Doody, D.P. (1999). Lacerations and abrasions. In R.A. Dershewitz (Ed.), *Ambulatory pediatric care.* Philadelphia: Lippincott.

Douglass, A.B. & Douglass, J.M. (2003). Common dental emergencies. *American Family Physician, 27,* 511-516.

Golden, D.B. (2002). Allergic reactions to insect stings. In R.E. Rakel & E.T. Bope (Eds.), 2002 *Conn's current therapy* (pp. 768-771). Philadelphia: Saunders.

Gound, P. (2003). Nurse practitioners' practice guidelines for avulsed tooth. *Clinical Excellence for Nurse Practitioners: The International Journal of NPACE, 7,* 14-18.

Hall, D.E., & Goldstein, E.M. (2001). Head injuries. In R.A. Hoekelman (Ed.), *Primary pediatric care* (4th ed., pp. 1970-1974). St. Louis: Mosby.

Knapp, J.F. (1999). Updates in wound management for the pediatrician. *Emergency Medicine, 46,* 1201-1212.

Kushner, D.S. (2001). Concussion in sports: Minimizing the risk for complications. *American Family Physician, 64,* 1007-1014.

Leclerc, S., Lassonde, M., & Delaney, J.S. (2001). Recommendations for grading of concussion in athletes. *Sports Medicine, 31,* 629-636.

Lewis, D.P. (2001). Burns: Initial management and outpatient follow-up. *Family Practice Recertification, 23,* 19-34.

Marion, D.W. (1998). Acute head injuries in adults. In R.E. Rakel (Ed.), *1998 Conn's current therapy.* Philadelphia: WB Saunders.

McCrea, M., Kelly, J.P., Kluge, J., Ackley, B., & Randolph, C. (1997). Standardized assessment of concussion in football players. *Neurology, 48,* 586-588.

Morgan, E.D., Beldsoe, S.C., & Barker, J. (2000). Ambulatory management of burns. *American Family Physician, 62,* 2015-2026.

Osterhoudt, K.C., Zaortis, T., & Zorc, J.J. (2002). Lyme disease masquerading as brown recluse spider bite. *Annals of Emergency Medicine, 39,* 558-561.

Pavan-Langston, D. (2002). Burns and trauma. In D. Pavan-Langston (Ed.), *Manual of ocular diagnosis and therapy* (5th ed., pp. 31-46). Philadelphia: Lippincott Williams & Wilkins.

Pavan-Langston, D. (2002). Cornea and external disease. In D. Pavan-Langston (Ed.), *Manual of ocular diagnosis and therapy* (5th ed., pp. 67-129) Philadelphia: Lippincott Williams & Wilkins.

Presutti, R.J. (2001). Prevention and treatment of dog bites. *American Family Physician, 63,* 1567-1572, 1573-1574.

Quayle, K.S. (1999). Minor head injury in the pediatric patient. *Pediatric Clinics of North America, 46,* 1189-1199.

Simon, J. (1992). Accidental injury and emergency medical services for children. In R.E. Behrman (Ed.). *Nelson textbook of pediatrics.* Philadelphia: WB Saunders.

Singer, A.J., Hollander, J.E., & Quinn, J.V. (1997). Evaluation and management of traumatic lacerations. *New England Journal of Medicine, 337,* 1142-1148.

Smith, E.E. (1993). Minor head injury: A proposed strategy for emergency management. *Annals of Emergency Medicine, 22,* 1193-1196.

Sorrentino, A., & Monroe, K. (2002). Insect stings In F.D. Burg, J.R. Ingelfinger, R.A. Polin, & A.A. Gershon (Eds.), Gellis and Kagan's current pediatric therapy (pp. 1052-1054). Philadelphia: Saunders.

Vetter, R.S., & Bush, S.P. (2002). The diagnosis of brown recluse spider bite is overused for dermonecrotic wounds of uncertain etiology. *Annals of Emergency Medicine, 39,* 544-546.

Wardrope, J., & Smith, J.R.R. (1992). *The management of wounds and burns.* New York: Oxford.

Index

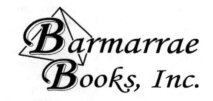

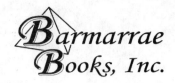

Barmarrae Books, Inc.

Ordering Information

Credit card orders (VISA or MasterCard) or institutional purchase orders may be placed toll free
8:00 AM to 5:00 PM EST weekdays at
888-276-7780

Credit card orders (VISA or MasterCard) or institutional purchase orders may be faxed to
352-378-1441

OR

Please photocopy or clip the order form below and mail with your check, money order, or purchase order to:
Barmarrae Books, Inc.
3017 NW 62nd Terrace
Gainesville, FL   32606

Visit our website at www.barmarrae.com

Note to Book Sellers:
All book returns require written permission and label from the publisher. Write to the address above or fax to the number above for permission.

Order Form
Barmarrae Books, Inc.
3017 NW 62nd Terrace
Gainesville, FL   32606

Order by mail, phone, or fax

Title	Unit Price	Qty	Total
Clinical Guidelines in Family Practice ISBN 0-9646151-6-9	$70.00		
Clinical Guidelines in Adult Health ISBN 0-9646151-8-5	$65.00		
Clinical Guidelines in Child Health ISBN 0-9646151-7-7	$65.00		

Subtotal		
Shipping and Handling (within the US)	$10.00	
Shipping outside US, Add $15.00		
Florida residents, add 6% sales tax		
TOTAL DUE (US funds **ONLY**)		

Name: _____

Address: _____

City: _____ **State/Zip** _____

Area Code/Phone No.: _____

Form of Payment: ☐ Check ☐ Money Order
☐ Purchase Order (Institutions Only) *Credit references may be required*
☐ MasterCard ☐ VISA
Credit Card # _____
Name as it appears on card _____
Expiration Date _____
Signature _____

Mail Order to:	**Barmarrae Books, Inc.** 3017 NW 62nd Terrace Gainesville, FL 32606	**Phone Order to:**	888-276-7780 or 352-378-5554
		Fax Order to:	352-378-1441

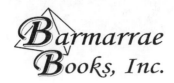

Barmarrae Books, Inc.

Ordering Information

Credit card orders (VISA or MasterCard) or institutional purchase orders may be placed toll free
8:00 AM to 5:00 PM EST weekdays at
888-276-7780

Credit card orders (VISA or MasterCard) or institutional purchase orders may be faxed to
352-378-1441

OR

Please photocopy or clip the order form below and mail with your check, money order, or purchase order to:
**Barmarrae Books, Inc.
3017 NW 62nd Terrace
Gainesville, FL   32606**

Visit our website at www.barmarrae.com

Note to Book Sellers:
All book returns require written permission and label from the publisher. Write to the address above or fax to the number above for permission.

Order Form
Barmarrae Books, Inc.
3017 NW 62nd Terrace
Gainesville, FL   32606

Order by mail, phone, or fax

Title	Unit Price	Qty	Total
Clinical Guidelines in Family Practice ISBN 0-9646151-6-9	$70.00		
Clinical Guidelines in Adult Health ISBN 0-9646151-8-5	$65.00		
Clinical Guidelines in Child Health ISBN 0-9646151-7-7	$65.00		
Subtotal			
Shipping and Handling (within the US)	$10.00		
Shipping outside US, Add $15.00			
Florida residents, add 6% sales tax			
TOTAL DUE (US funds **ONLY**)			

Name: _____

Address: _____

City: _____ State/Zip _____

Area Code/Phone No.: _____

Form of Payment: ☐ Check   ☐ Money Order
☐ Purchase Order (Institutions Only) *Credit references may be required*
☐ MasterCard   ☐ VISA
Credit Card # _____
Name as it appears on card _____
Expiration Date _____
Signature _____

Mail Order to: Barmarrae Books, Inc.
3017 NW 62nd Terrace
Gainesville, FL 32606

Phone Order to: 888-276-7780 or
352-378-5554

Fax Order to: 352-378-1441

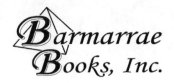

Barmarrae Books, Inc.

Ordering Information

Credit card orders (VISA or MasterCard) or institutional purchase orders may be placed toll free
8:00 AM to 5:00 PM EST weekdays at
888-276-7780

Credit card orders (VISA or MasterCard) or institutional purchase orders may be faxed to
352-378-1441

OR

Please photocopy or clip the order form below and mail with your check, money order, or purchase order to:
**Barmarrae Books, Inc.
3017 NW 62nd Terrace
Gainesville, FL   32606**

Visit our website at www.barmarrae.com

Note to Book Sellers:
All book returns require written permission and label from the publisher. Write to the address above or fax to the number above for permission.

Order Form
Barmarrae Books, Inc.
3017 NW 62nd Terrace
Gainesville, FL   32606

Order by mail, phone, or fax

Title	Unit Price	Qty	Total		
Clinical Guidelines in Family Practice ISBN 0-9646151-6-9	$70.00			**Name:** _____	
Clinical Guidelines in Adult Health ISBN 0-9646151-8-5	$65.00			**Address:** _____	
Clinical Guidelines in Child Health ISBN 0-9646151-7-7	$65.00			**City:** _____ **State/Zip** _____	
				Area Code/Phone No.: _____	
Subtotal				**Form of Payment:** ☐ Check ☐ Money Order	
Shipping and Handling (within the US)		$10.00		☐ Purchase Order (Institutions Only) *Credit references may be required* ☐ MasterCard ☐ VISA	
Shipping outside US, Add $15.00				Credit Card # _____	
Florida residents, add 6% sales tax				Name as it appears on card _____	
TOTAL DUE (US funds **ONLY**)				Expiration Date _____ Signature _____	

Mail Order to:	Barmarrae Books, Inc. 3017 NW 62nd Terrace Gainesville, FL 32606	**Phone Order to:** **Fax Order to:**	888-276-7780 or 352-378-5554 352-378-1441